# BASIC ANESTHESIA REVIEW

# BASIC ANESTHESIA REVIEW

EDITED BY

*Alaa Abd-Elsayed, MD, MBA, MPH, CPE, FASA*

MEDICAL DIRECTOR, UW HEALTH PAIN SERVICES

MEDICAL DIRECTOR, UW PAIN CLINIC; DIVISION CHIEF, CHRONIC PAIN MEDICINE,

DEPARTMENT OF ANESTHESIOLOGY

ASSOCIATE PROFESSOR OF ANESTHESIOLOGY, UNIVERSITY OF WISCONSIN-MADISON

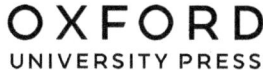

# OXFORD
## UNIVERSITY PRESS

Oxford University Press is a department of the University of Oxford. It furthers
the University's objective of excellence in research, scholarship, and education
by publishing worldwide. Oxford is a registered trade mark of Oxford University
Press in the UK and certain other countries.

Published in the United States of America by Oxford University Press
198 Madison Avenue, New York, NY 10016, United States of America.

© Oxford University Press 2024

CIP data is on file at the Library of Congress

ISBN 978–0–19–758456–9

DOI: 10.1093/med/9780197584569.001.0001

Printed by Sheridan Books, Inc., United States of America

*To my two beautiful children, Maro and George*

# CONTENTS

# PREFACE

The American Board of Anesthesiology (ABA) developed a new revised curriculum outline to address the relatively new Board exam structure (Basic and Advanced written exams). The majority of textbooks currently on the market were developed to address the previous curriculum and historical exam structure (only one written exam). This book represents a vital ally to all examinees as it provides a concise and complete outline of Basic exam content.

This book was developed with short chapters that address each item in the ABA outline and an emphasis on "high-yield" topics. While no review source can be entirely comprehensive, our intention was to provide a single source for general knowledge topics likely to occur on the Basic examination and "high-yield" points that can be mastered to provide a base of knowledge for patient care in the operating room.

This book highlights authors from a number of prestigious institutions who have poured considerable knowledge and experience into each page.

A complement to this book is another specifically tailored to the Advanced exam that utilizes the same information-presentation strategy. For many readers, consuming this Advanced exam review book will provide additional information breath that can be utilized throughout the course of residency.

This review book requires you to read everything; there are no wasted keystrokes. Every effort was made to supply large volumes of knowledge into short chapters. Also, some topics are mentioned more than once, as they may be related to different anesthesia topics. Do not think of this as unnecessary replication—the information was written by different authors with different perspectives, and there is significant benefit to be derived from approaching certain topics from multiple angles.

My advice to you is to read this book consistently and thoroughly during your residency training. Over time, expand your reading of topics that require mastery and utilize practice questions to consistently re-evaluate for areas of weakness. In this way, the knowledge gained from this book will be solidified and I am confident that, if you do this, you will pass your test. Always remember, reading is a process and habit that needs to be established throughout your training to solidify the practice for a lifetime of learning and expansion of clinical knowledge.

I would like to thank the publisher for supporting this large project and all my colleagues who contributed to this book.

Alaa Abd-Elsayed, MD, MBA, MPH, CPE, FASA
Anesthesiology, University of Wisconsin, School of Medicine and Public Health, Madison, Wisconsin

# CONTRIBUTORS

**Rany T. Abdallah, MD, PhD, MBA**
Center for Interventional Pain and Spine

**Alaa Abd-Elsayed, MD, MBA, MPH, CPE, FASA**
Medical Director, UW Health Pain Services
Medical Director, UW Pain Clinic
Division Chief, Chronic Pain Medicine, Department of
    Anesthesiology
Secretary, State Medical Board, Wisconsin
Editor in Chief of *Pain Medicine Case Reports*
Chronic Pain Physician and Associate Professor of
    Anesthesiology
University of Wisconsin School of Medicine and
    Public Health
Madison, WI, USA

**Ali Abdullah, MD**
Department of Anesthesiology
Allegheny General Hospital
Allegheny Health Network
Pittsburgh, PA, USA

**Furqan Ahmed, MBBS**
Department of Anesthesiology
Dow Medical College
Dow University of Health Sciences
Karachi, Pakistan

**Muhammad Fayyaz Ahmed, MBBS, MD**
Assistant Professor of Clinical Anesthesiology
Department of Anesthesiology
Temple University Hospital, Lewis Katz School of Medicine
Philadelphia, PA, USA

**Neal Al-Attar, MD**
Department of Anesthesiology
Beaumont Health
Royal Oak, MI, USA

**Mazin T. Albert, DO**
Department of Anesthesiology
Allegheny Health Network
Pittsburgh, PA, UAS

**Bozana Alexander, MD**
Department of Anesthesiology and Pain Management
John H. Stroger, Jr. Hospital of Cook County
Chicago, IL, USA

**Caroline Al-Haddadin, MBBS**
Anesthesiologist
Yale New Haven Children's Hospital
New Have, CT, USA

**Piotr Al Jindi, MD**
Cook County Health Systems
Chicago, IL, USA

**Kenan Alkhalili, MD**
Department of Anesthesia
Cook County Health and Hospital Systems
Chicago, IL, USA

**E. Saunders Alpaugh, MD**
Louisiana State University School of Medicine
New Orleans, LA, UAS

**Brannon Y. Altenhofen, MD**
UCLA Department of Anesthesiology and Perioperative
    Medicine
Los Angeles, CA, UAS

**Suwarna Anand, MD**
Associate Professor, Anesthesiology
Department of Anesthesiology
University of Mississippi Medical Center
Jackson, MS, USA

**Keith A. Andrews, DO**
Anesthesia and Perioperative Medicine
University Hospitals
Cleveland, OH, USA

**Santhalakshmi Angappan, MD**
Department of Anesthesiology, Pain Management, and
    Perioperative Medicine
Henry Ford Health System
Detroit, MI, USA

**Ben Aquino, MD**
Department of Anesthesiology
Illinois Masonic Medical Center
Chicago, IL, USA

**Lovkesh Arora, MD**
Clinical Associate Professor
Department of Anesthesia
University of Iowa Health Care
Iowa City, Iowa

**Jason Bang, MD**
Cook County Health Systems
Chicago, IL, USA

**Lauren Beck, MD**
UCLA Health
Los Angeles, CA, USA

**David S. Beebe, MD**
Professor, Department of Anesthesiology
University of Minnesota Medical School
Minneapolis, MN, USA

**Kumar G. Belani, MBBS, MS**
Professor, Department of Anesthesiology
University of Minnesota Medical School
Minneapolis, MN, USA

**Sean Beplate, MD**
Cook County Health Systems
Chicago, IL, USA

**Stefan Besada, MD**
David Geffen School of Medicine at UCLA
Los Angeles, CA, USA

**Leah Bess, MD**
Department of Pediatric Anesthesia
Anesthesiology Institute
Cleveland Clinic
Cleveland, OH, USA

**Prince Bonsu, MD**
Department of Anesthesiology
University at Buffalo
Buffalo, NY, USA

**Elaine A. Boydston, MD**
UCLA Department of Anesthesiology and
    Perioperative Medicine
David Geffen School of Medicine at UCLA
Los Angeles, CA, USA

**Meghan Brennan, MD**
Department of Anesthesiology
University of Florida College of Medicine
Gainesville, FL, USA

**J. Brown, MD**
Department of Anesthesiology and Perioperative Medicine
The University of Texas
MD Anderson Cancer Center
Houston, TX, USA

**Eileen Bui, MD**
Anesthesiology Specialist
Boston, MA, USA

**Brian J. Cacioppo, MD**
Department of Anesthesiology
University of Wisconsin-Madison
Madison, WI, USA

**Jeffrey W. Cannon, MD**
Department of Anesthesiology and Perioperative Medicine
University Hospitals, Cleveland Medical Center
Cleveland, OH, USA

**Jauhleene Chamu, MD**
Department of Anesthesiology and Perioperative Medicine
University Hospitals Cleveland Medical Center
Cleveland, OH, USA

**Michael Chang, MD**
Westchester Medical Center
Valhalla, NY, USA

**Pradeep R. Chawla, DO**
Cook County Health Systems
Chicago, IL, USA

**Pinxia Chen, MD**
Anesthesiologist and Intensivist
Anesthesia Specialists of Bethlehem
St. Luke's University Health Network
Bethlehem, PA, USA

**Paul K. Cheng, MD**
Volunteer Clinical Faculty/Assistant Clinical Professor
Department of Anesthesiology and Pain Medicine
UC Davis Medical Center
Sacramento, CA, USA

**Surendrasingh Chhabada, MD, FAAP**
Department of Pediatric and Congenital Cardiac Anesthesia
Anesthesiology Institute
Department of Outcome Research
Cleveland Clinic
Cleveland, OH, USA

**Adrian Ching, MD**
Department of Anesthesiology
University of Florida College of Medicine
Gainesville, FL, USA

**Katya H. Chiong, MD, FASA**
University Hospitals Cleveland Medical Center
Cleveland, OH, USA

**Emuejevoke Chuba, MBBS, MSCR**
Department of Anesthesia
Temple University Hospital
Philadelphia, PA, USA

**Lindsey Cieslinski, DO**
Tulane University School of Medicine
New Orleans, LA, USA

**Joseph Cody, DO**
The Ohio State University Wexner Medical Center
Columbus, OH, USA

**Till Conermann, MD**
Program Director, Pain Medicine Fellowship,
    Anesthesiologist
Allegheny Health Network/West Penn Pain Medicine
    Fellowship Program
Pittsburgh, PA, USA

**Jay I. Conhaim, MD**
University of Cincinnati Medical Center
Cincinnati, OH, USA

**Matthew T. Connolly, MD**
University of Wisconsin Hospitals and Clinics
Madison, WI, USA

**Rollin Cook, MD**
Department of Anesthesia
University of Iowa Hospitals Carver College of Medicine
Iowa City, IA, USA

**Daniel S. Cormican, MD, FCCP**
Anesthesiologist and Intensivist
Anesthesiology Institute
Allegheny Health Network
Pittsburgh, PA, UAS

**Elyse M. Cornett, PhD**
Assistant Professor
Department of Anesthesiology
LSU Health Shreveport
Shreveport, LA, USA

**Drew Cornwell, DO**
Department of Anesthesiology and Pain Medicine
Geisinger Medical Center
Danville, PA, UAS

**Adi Cosic, DO**
Department of Anesthesiology
University Hospitals Cleveland Medical Center
Cleveland, OH, USA

**Lucas Costa Santos, MD**
Department of Anesthesiology, Pain Management, and
    Perioperative Medicine
Henry Ford Hospital
Detroit, MI, USA

**Ettore Crimi, MD**
University of Central Florida/HCA GME Consortium,
    Orlando
Ocala Health Florida
Ocala, FL, USA

**Adam Cruz, MD**
Anesthesiology Specialist
Royal Oak, MI, USA

**Anthony D'Auria, DO**
Anesthesiology
University at Buffalo
Department of Anesthesiology
Buffalo, NY, USA

**Evan DaBreo, MD**
University of Virginia
Department of Anesthesiology
Charlottesville, VA, USA

**Talia H. Dagher, MD**
UCLA Health
Los Angeles, CA, USA

**Nadeen Dakhlallah, DO**
Department of Anesthesiology
Beaumont Health
Royal Oak, MI, USA

**Youssef Daklallah, MD**
Department of Anesthesiology
Beaumont Health
Royal Oak, MI, USA

**Charles deBoisblanc, MD**
Louisiana State University School of Medicine
Shreveport, LA, USA

**Aladino De Ranieri, MD, PhD**
Advocate Illinois Masonic Medical Center
Chicago, IL, USA

**F. Cole Dooley, MD**
Assistant Professor of Anesthesiology
Department of Pediatric Anesthesiology
University of Florida College of Medicine
Gainesville, FL, USA

**Zachary Drennen, DO**
Department of Anesthesiology
Allegheny Health Network
Pittsburgh, PA, USA

**Kirk Dressen, MD**
Department of Anesthesia
University of Iowa Hospitals
Iowa City, IA, USA

**Karthik Dwarki, MD**
Baystate Medical Center
Springfield, MA, USA

**Jeffery James Eapen, MD**
Cook County Health Systems
Chicago, IL, USA

**Maxim S. Eckmann, MD**
University of Texas Health Science Center at San Antonio
San Antonio, TX, USA

**Hila Elias, BA**
Maimonides Medical Center
Brooklyn, NY, USA

**Dalia Elmofty, MD**
Associate Professor of Anesthesia and Critical Care
Department of Anesthesia and Critical Care
University of Chicago Medical Center
Chicago, IL, USA

**Marwa El-Sabbahy, MD**
Staff Nephrologist
Lawrence General Hospital
Lawrence, MA, USA

**Lauren K. Eng, MD**
Tulane University School of Medicine
New Orleans, LA, USA

**Matthew Epelman, DO**
Department of Anesthesiology, Pain Management, and
    Perioperative Medicine
Henry Ford Health System
Detroit, MI, USA

**Christopher O. Fadumiye, MD**
Assistant Professor
Department of Anesthesiology
Medical College of Wisconsin
Milwaukee, WI, USA

**Evan Falgoust, MD**
Department of Anesthesiology
Louisiana State University School of Medicine
Shreveport, LA, USA

**Andrea Farela, MD**
Department of Anesthesiology
Yale New Haven Hospital
New Haven, CT, USA

**Mohamed Fayed, MD**
Department of Anesthesiology
Henry Ford Hospital
Detroit, MI, USA

**Kris Ferguson, MD**
Aspirus Health System
Antigo, WI, USA

**Kyle Ferguson, MD**
Department of Anesthesiology and Perioperative Medicine
University Hospitals
Cleveland Medical Center
Cleveland, OH, USA

**Karim Fikry, MD**
Staff Anesthesiologist and Intensivist
Assistant Professor, Tufts University School of Medicine
Lahey Hospital and Medical Center
Burlington, MA, USA

**Timothy F. Flanagan, MD**
Department of Anesthesia
Tufts University School of Medicine
Lahey Hospital and Medical Center
Burlington, MA, USA

**Amanda Frantz, MD**
University of Florida College of Medicine
Gainesville, FL, USA

**Eric D. Friedman, MD**
Department of Anesthesiology and Pain Management
John H. Stroger Hospital of Cook County
Chicago, IL, USA

**Ilana R. Fromer, MD**
University of Minnesota Medical School
Minneapolis, MN, USA

**Alina Genis, MD**
Department of Anesthesiology
New York Medical College
Westchester Medical Center
Valhalla, NY, USA

**Arun George, MD**
Department of Anesthesiology
Allegheny General Hospital
Allegheny Health Network
Pittsburgh, PA, USA

**Mark L. Germani, MD**
Department of Anesthesiology
Lahey Hospital & Medical Center
Burlington, MA, USA

**Laura Liss Gershon, MD**
Staff Anesthesiologist
West Penn Hospital; Allegheny Health Network

**Hussam Ghabra, MD**
Department of Anesthesiology and Perioperative Medicine
Ochsner Clinic Foundation
New Orleans, LA, USA

**Shirin Ghanavatian, MD**
University of Miami Hospital and Clinics-UHealth Tower
U.S. News Best Hospital
Durham, CA, USA

**Christina Gibson, DO**
Allegheny Health Network
Pittsburgh, PA, USA

**Chris Giordano, MD**
Department of Anesthesiology
University of Florida College of Medicine
Gainesville, FL, USA

**Brook Girma, MD**
Department of Anesthesiology
Louisiana State University School of Medicine
Shreveport, LA, USA

**Vicko Gluncic, MD, PhD**
Assistant Professor of Anesthesiology
Department of Anesthesiology
Advocate Illinois Masonic Medical Center, University of
    Illinois
Chicago, IL, USA

**Daniel Gotlib**
Department of Anesthesiology
University Hospitals Cleveland Medical Center
Cleveland, OH, USA

**Raymond Graber, MD**
Anesthesiology Specialist
State University of New York at Buffalo
Cleveland, OH, USA

**Ravi K. Grandhi, MD, MBA**
Anesthesiology
Maimonides Medical Center
Brooklyn, NY, USA

**Ellyn Gray, MD**
Department of Anesthesia
University of Iowa Hospitals
Iowa City, IA, USA

**Jayakar Guruswamy, MD**
Department of Anesthesiology, Pain Management, and
    Perioperative Medicine
Henry Ford Health System
Detroit, MI, USA

**David Guz, DO**
Department of Anesthesiology and Perioperative Medicine
University Hospitals
Cleveland, OH, USA

**Jacob Guzman, MD**
Faculty, Department of Anesthesiology
Allegheny General Hospital
Pittsburgh, PA, USA

**Chike Gwam, MD**
Cook County Health & Hospital Systems
Chicago, IL, USA

**Florian Hackl, MD**
Assistant Professor in Anesthesia
Department of Anesthesiology and Interventional Pain
    Management
Tufts University School of Medicine
Lahey Hospital and Medical Center
Burlington, MA, USA

**Jack Hagan, MD**
Department of Anesthesiology
University of Florida College of Medicine
Gainesville, FL, USA

**Matthew J. Hallman, MD**
University of North Carolina Health
Chapel Hill, NC, USA

**Joseph Salama Hanna, MD**
Henry Ford Health System
Detroit, MI, USA

**Rewais B. Hanna, MD**
University of Wisconsin School of Medical & Public Health
Madison, MI, USA

**Alain Harb, MD**
Department of Anesthesia and Perioperative Medicine
University Hospitals Cleveland Medical Center—Rainbow
	Babies and Children's Hospital
Cleveland, OH, USA

**Ronald Harter, MD, FASA**
Department of Anesthesiology
Wexner Medical Center
The Ohio State University
Columbus, OH, USA

**Muin Haswah, MD**
Cook County Hospital
Chicago, IL, USA

**Andrew Hayden, MD**
Department of Anesthesia
University of Iowa Hospitals
Iowa City, IA, USA

**Afshin Heidari, MD**
Department of Anesthesiology
Illinois Masonic Medical Center
Chicago, IL, USA

**Mada Helou, MD**
Program Director for Anesthesiology
Assistant Professor of Anesthesiology
Department of Anesthesiology and Perioperative Medicine
University Hospitals
Cleveland, OH, USA

**Jared Herman, DO**
Mount Sinai Medical Center
Miami Beach, FL, USA

**Candice C. Hithe, DO**
Kettering Health Network
Grandview Medical Center
Dayton, OH, USA

**Balazs Horvath, MD, FASA**
Associate Professor
Department of Anesthesiology
University of Minnesota
Minneapolis, MN, USA

**Nicholas Hozian**
John Carroll University

**Hao Hua, MD**
Anesthesiology Institute
Allegheny Health Network
Pittsburgh, PA, USA

**Maria Huarte, MD**
Anesthesiology Institute
Cleveland Clinic
Cleveland, OH, USA

**Jerome B. Huebsch, DO**
Kettering Health Network
Grandview Medical Center
Dayton, OH, USA

**Shahrose Hussain, MD**
Tufts University School of Medicine
Lahey Hospital and Medical Center
Burlington, MA, USA

**David Hutchinson, MD**
Department of Anesthesiology
University of Florida College of Medicine
Gainesville, FL, USA

**Fatima Iqbal, MD**
Intern at Raleigh Hospital
Raleigh, CA, USA

**Behdad Jahromi, MD**
Department of Anesthesia
Illinois Masonic Medical Center
Chicago, IL, USA

**Dominika Lipowska James, MD**
Associate Professor of Anesthesiology and Pain Medicine
University of North Carolina Health
Chapel Hill, NC, USA

**Tatiana Jamroz, MD**
Anesthesiology Residency Program Director
Department of Anesthesiology
Cleveland Clinic Florida
Weston, FL, USA

**Jai Jani, MD**
Attending
Advocate Aurora Health
Department of Anesthesia
Illinois Masonic Medical Center
Chicago, IL, USA

**Susan Jeffers, MD, MS**
Anesthesiology
Northern Colorado Anesthesia Professionals
Fort Collins, CO, USA

**Thomas Keith Jenkins, MD**
University of Florida College of Medicine
Gainesville, FL, USA

**Aparna Jindal, MD**
Department of Anesthesia
University of Iowa Hospitals
Iowa City, IA, USA

**Angela Johnson, MD**
Department of Anesthesiology and Perioperative Medicine
University Hospitals Cleveland Medical Center
Cleveland, OH, USA

**Savion D. Johnson, MD**
Department of Anesthesiology
Duke University Medical Center
Durham, NC, USA

**Courtney R. Jones, MD**
Assistant Professor of Anesthesiology
University of Cincinnati College of Medicine
Cincinnati, OH, USA

**Antony Joseph, MD**
Cook County Health Systems
Chicago, IL, USA

**Claire Joseph, DO**
Anesthesiology
Maimonides Medical Center
Brooklyn, NY, USA

**Maryam Jowza, MD**
Assistant Professor of Anesthesiology and Pain Medicine
University of North Carolina Health
Chapel Hill, NC, USA

**Charles Jun, DO**
Department of Anesthesiology and Pain Management
John H. Stroger Hospital of Cook County
Cook County Health
Chicago, IL, USA

**Daniel Gonzalez Kapp, PharmD, BCOP, BCPS**
UW Health
Madison, WI, USA

**Hisham Kassem, MD**
Department of Anesthesiology
Mount Sinai Medical Center
Miami Beach, FL, USA

**Alan D. Kaye, MD, PhD**
Vice Chancellor of Academic Affairs, Chief Academic Officer, and Provost
Professor, Department of Anesthesiology and Pharmacology, Toxicology, and Neurosciences
Louisiana State University School of Medicine
Shreveport, LA, USA

**Julia Kendrick, MD**
Cardiac Anesthesiology
Department of Anesthesiology
Medical University of South Carolina
Charleston, SC, USA

**Sahel Keshavarzi, MD**
Department of Anesthesiology
Advocate Illinois Masonic Medical Center
Chicago, IL, USA

**Jonathan I. Kim, MD**
UCLA Department of Anesthesiology and Perioperative Medicine
Los Angeles, CA, USA

**Lisa Klesius, MD**
Department of Anesthesiology
University of Wisconsin Hospital and Clinics
Madison, WI, USA

**Benjamin Kloesel, MD, MSBS**
Associate Professor
Department of Anesthesiology
University of Minnesota, Medical School
Minneapolis, MN, USA

**Nebojsa Nick Knezevic, MD, PhD**
Department of Anesthesiology
Advocate Illinois Masonic Medical Center
Chicago, IL, USA

**Nigel Knox, MD**
Assistant Professor
Department of Anesthesiology and Pain Management
Westchester Medical Center
Valhalla, NY, USA

**Lynn Kohan, MD**
Department of Anesthesiology, Division of Pain Medicine
University of Virginia
Charlottesville, VA, USA

**Igor Kolesnikov, MD**
Cook County Hospital
Chicago, IL, USA

**Elizabeth Kremen, MBBS**
Department of Anesthesiology
Advocate Illinois Masonic Medical Center
Chicago, IL, USA

**Donnie Laborde, DC, FACO**
Instructor
American Heart Association
Shreveport, LA, USA

**Kelsey E. Lacourrege, MD**
School of Medicine
Louisiana State University Health Sciences Center
New Orleans, LA, USA

**Jennifer Lamb, MD**
Anesthesiology
Department of Anesthesiology
University at Buffalo
Buffalo, NY, USA

**Vadzim Lapkouski, MD**
Department of Anesthesiology
Cleveland Clinic Florida
Weston, FL, USA

**Dustin Latimer, MD**
Department of Anesthesiology
Louisiana State University School of Medicine
Shreveport, LA, USA

**Sarah Lauve, MD**
School of Medicine
MSI
LSU Health Shreveport

**Melinda M. Lawrence, MD**
Associate Professor
Department of Anesthesiology
Division of Pain Medicine
University Hospitals Cleveland Medical Center
Cleveland, OH, USA

**Albert Lee, MD**
UCLA Department of Anesthesiology and Perioperative Medicine
Los Angeles, CA, USA

**Gretchen A. Lemmink, MD**
University of Cincinnati Medical Center
Cincinnati, OH, USA

**Richard Lennertz, MD, PhD**
Assistant Professor
Department of Anesthesiology
University of Wisconsin–Madison
Madison, WI, USA

**Ethan R. Leonard, MD**
Pediatric Infectious Diseases
UH Rainbow Babies and Children Hospital
Cleveland, OH, USA

**Lora B. Levin, MD**
Chief, Obstetric Anesthesia
Assistant Professor
Department of Anesthesiology and Perioperative Medicine
University Hospitals Cleveland Medical Center
Cleveland, OH, USA

**Hewenfei Li, MD**
UCLA Department of Anesthesiology and
    Perioperative Medicine
Los Angeles, CA, USA

**Austine Lin, MD**
University of Texas Harris County Psychiatric Center
McKinney, TX, USA

**Nathan Liu, MD**
Department of Anesthesia and Critical Care
University of Chicago
Chicago, IL, USA

**Tanya Lucas, MD**
UMass Memorial Healthcare
Worcester, MA, USA

**Santiago Luis, MD**
Cleveland Clinic Florida
Weston, FL, USA

**Samuel MacCormick, MBBCh**
Department of Anesthesiology
University of Virginia
Charlottesville, VA, USA

**Sohail K. Mahboobi, MD, FASA**
Department of Anesthesiology
Lahey Hospital & Medical Center
Burlington, MA, USA

**Neeraj Maheshwari, MD**
Department of Anesthesiology
Beaumont Health
Royal Oak, MI, USA

**Faraz Mahmood, MD**
Department of Anesthesiology and Interventional Pain
    Management
Tufts University School of Medicine
Lahey Hospital and Medical Center
Burlington, MA, USA

**Tariq M. Malik, MD**
Department of Anesthesia and Critical Care
University of Chicago Medical Center
Chicago, IL, USA

**Jillian A. Maloney, MD**
Department of Anesthesiology and Division of Pain
  Medicine
Mayo Clinic of Arizona
Phoenix, AZ, USA

**Larry Manders, MD, MBA**
Department of Anesthesiology
Beaumont Health
Royal Oak, MI, USA

**Sheridan Markatos, MD**
Department of Anesthesiology
Beaumont Health
Royal Oak, MI, USA

**Adriana Martin, MD**
Anesthesiology Institute
Cleveland Clinic, OH, USA

**David Matteson, MD, MS**
Allegheny Health Network
Pittsburgh, PA, USA

**Bryan Matusic, DO**
Acute Perioperative Pain Director
Department of Anesthesiology
Allegheny Health Network
Pittsburgh, PA, USA

**Hovik Mazmanyan, MD**
Department of Anesthesiology and Pain Management
John H. Stroger, Jr. Hospital of Cook County
Chicago, IL, USA

**Brendan McCafferty, DO**
University Hospitals Cleveland Medical Center
Cleveland, OH, USA

**Matthew McConnell, MD**
Allegheny Health Network
Pittsburgh, PA, USA

**Eric McDaniel, MD**
Harbor-UCLA Medical Center
Los Angeles, CA, USA

**Lauren McGinty, PharmD, BCOP**
Clinical Hematology/Oncology Pharmacist
Department of Pharmacy
UW Health—University Hospital
Madison, WI, USA

**Connor McNamara, MD**
Department of Anesthesiology and Perioperative Medicine
Cleveland, OH, USA

**Wilson Alfredo Medina II, MD**
Allegheny Health Network

**Steven Minear, MD**
Associate Professor, Department of Anesthesia
Anesthesia Research Department
Cleveland Clinic Florida
Weston, FL, USA

**Anna Moldysz, MD**
Department of Anesthesia
University of Iowa Hospitals
Iowa City, IA, USA

**Ruth E. Moncayo, MD**
Cook County Health Systems
Chicago, IL, USA

**Warner Moore, MD**
Department of Anesthesiology
Louisiana State University School of Medicine
Shreveport, LA, USA

**Monnica Morales, DO**
Department of Anesthesiology
Cleveland Clinic Florida
Weston, FL, USA

**Benjamin B. G. Mori, MD**
Cook County Health Systems
Chicago, IL, USA

**Gurpreet Mundi, MD**
Assistant Professor of Anesthesiology
Fox Chase Cancer Center (FCCC)
Temple University Health System
Philadelphia, PA, USA

**Ronny Munoz-Acuna, MD**
Universidad De Costa Rica
Framingham University Hospital
Framingham, MA, USA

**Ricardo Munoz-Acuna, MD**
Beth Israel Deaconess Medical Center
Harvard Medical School

**Ricardo Murguia-Fuentes, MD**
Department of Neurology
Louisiana State University Health Sciences Center-Shreveport
Shreveport, LA, USA

**Ned F. Nasr, MD**
Department of Anesthesia
Cook County Health and Hospital Systems
Chicago, IL, USA

**Harsh Nathani, MB, ChB**
Cook County Health Systems
Chicago, IL, USA

**Mallory Nebergall, MD**
Department of Anesthesiology
Allegheny Health Network
Pittsburgh, PA, USA

**Greta Nemergut, PharmD**
Clinical Pharmacist
UW Health Department of Pharmacy
University of Wisconsin Hospital and Clinics
Madison, WI, USA

**Christina T. Nguyen, MD**
Assistant Clinical Professor
UCLA Department of Anesthesiology and Perioperative Medicine
Los Angeles, CA, USA

**Tina Nowak, MD**
Allegheny General Hospital
Pittsburgh, PA, USA

**Alexandria Nickless, MD**
Department of Anesthesiology
Allegheny General Hospital
Allegheny Health Network
Pittsburgh, PA, USA

**Edward Noguera, MD**
Anesthesiologist/Intensivist
Medical Director SICU/CVICU
Cleveland Clinic
Weston, FL, USA

**Nazir Noor, MD**
Mount Sinai Medical Center
Miami Beach, FL, USA

**Brian A. Nordstrom, MD**
Anesthesiology Specialist
South Lake Tahoe, CA, USA

**Ryan Nowatzke, MD**
Department of Anesthesiology
Beaumont Health
Royal Oak, MI, USA

**Laurence Ohia, MD**
Department of Anesthesiology
Allegheny Health Network
Pittsburgh, PA, USA

**Asli Ozcan, DO**
Department of Anesthesiology
Allegheny Health Network
Pittsburgh, PA, USA

**John Ozinga, DO**
Department of Anesthesiology
Advocate Illinois Masonic Medical Center
Chicago, IL, USA

**David Padilla, MD**
Department of Anesthesia
University of Iowa Hospitals
Iowa City, IA, USA

**Nicole Palm, PharmD**
Surgical ICU Clinical Pharmacy Specialist
Department of Pharmacy
Cleveland Clinic Foundation
Cleveland, OH, USA

**Wenyu Pan, MD**
Department of Anesthesia and Critical Care
University of Chicago Medical Center
Chicago, IL, USA

**Peter Papapetrou, MD**
Aspirus Health System
Antigo, WI, USA

**Nicholas M. Parker, PharmD, RPh, CNSC**
Clinical Pharmacist—Surgery and Nutrition Support
Department of Pharmacy
UW Health
Madison, WI, USA

**Ahmad Reza Parniani, MD**
Department of Anesthesiology
University of Florida College of Medicine
Gainesville, FL, USA

**Nimesh Patel, MD**
Department of Anesthesiology
Henry Ford Hospital
Detroit, MI, USA
Priyanka H. Patel, DO
Allegheny Health Network
Pittsburgh, PA, USA

**Sheetal Patel, MD**
Anesthesiology and Pain Management
John H. Stroger, Jr. Hospital of Cook County
Chicago, IL, USA

**Robert Pellicer, DO**
Department of Anesthesiology
University of Wisconsin Hospitals & Clinics
Madison, WI, USA

**Huanhuan Peng, MD**
Anesthesiology
Allegheny Health Network Medication Education Consortium
Pittsburgh, PA, USA

**John Penner, MD, MS**
Assistant Professor, Clinical
Director of Anesthesia and Associate Medical Director
Madison Surgery Center
Department of Anesthesiology
School of Medicine and Public Health
University of Wisconsin
Madison, WI, USA

**Kayla Penny, MS (MD anticipated)**
LSU Health Shreveport
Shreveport, LA, USA

**Carlos M. Perez-Ruiz, MD, MSc**
Department of Anesthesiology
Allegheny General Hospital
Allegheny Health Network
Pittsburgh, PA, USA

**Nicholas Pesa, MD**
Assistant Professor of Anesthesiology
University Hospitals Cleveland Medical Center
Cleveland, OH, USA

**Elisha Peterson, MD, FAAP**
Department of Anesthesiology
Pain and Perioperative Medicine
Children's National Hospital
Washington, DC, USA

**Ba Hoang Nguyen Pham, MD**
Cook County Health Systems
Chicago, IL, USA

**Vincent Pinkert, MD**
Oregon Health & Science University
Portland, OR, USA

**Mariya Pogrebetskaya, MD**
Department of Anesthesiology and Perioperative Medicine
University Hospitals/Case Western Reserve University
    School of Medicine
Cleveland, OH, USA

**Harlee Possoit, MD**
Department of Anesthesiology
Louisiana State University School of Medicine
Shreveport, LA, USA

**Zack Powers, DO**
Department of Anesthesiology
University of Florida College of Medicine
Gainesville, FL, USA

**Rosemary Prejean, MD**
Louisiana State University School of Medicine–Shreveport
Shreveport, LA, USA

**Anand Prem, MD**
Associate Professor, Anesthesiology
Medical Director, University Pain Clinic
Department of Anesthesiology
University of Mississippi Medical Center
Jackson, MS, USA

**Nawal E. Ragheb-Mueller, DO, PhD, MPH, FASA**
Department of Anesthesiology & Pain Management
John H. Stroger, Jr. Hospital
Cook County Health
Chicago, IL, USA

**Abed Rahman, MD**
Cook County Health Systems
Chicago, IL, USA

**Shobana Rajan, MD**
Department of Anesthesiology
Allegheny General Hospital
Allegheny Health Network
Pittsburgh, PA, USA

**Maria F. Ramirez, MD**
Department of Anesthesiology and Perioperative Medicine
The University of Texas MD Anderson Cancer Center
Houston, TX, USA

**Akshatha Gururaja Rao, MD**
Department of Anesthesiology, Pain Management, and
    Perioperative Medicine
Henry Ford Health System
Detroit, MI, USA

**Douglas K. Rausch, DO, MS**
University of Miami/Jackson Memorial Health System

**Austin Reilly, MD**
Physician
Department of Anesthesia and Critical Care
University of Chicago Medical Center
Chicago, IL, USA

**Eric Reilly, DO**
Department of Anesthesiology
Beaumont Hospital
Royal Oak, MI, USA

**Rhett Reynolds**
LSU Health Shreveport
University of Alabama Birmingham
Al, USA

**Dmitry Roberman, DO**
Assistant Professor of Anesthesiology
Temple University School of Medicine
Philadelphia, PA, USA

**Shaun Roche, MD**
Cook County Health Systems
Chicago, IL, USA

**Gloria Rodriguez, MD**
Anesthesiology Institute
Cleveland Clinic Foundation
Cleveland, OH, USA

**Evgeny Romanov, MD**
Anesthesiology
Lahey Clinic

**John Rose, DO, Msc**
Department of Anesthesiology
Mount Sinai Morningside-West
New York, NY, USA

**Sydney E. Rose, MD**
Oregon Health & Science University
Portland, OR, USA

**David Rosenblum, MD**
Clinical Assistant Professor
Department of Anesthesiology
Director of Pain Management
Maimonides Medical Center
SUNY Downstate Medical Center
Brooklyn, NY, USA

**Raquel Montagner Rossi, MD**
Department of Anesthesiology, Pain Management, and
    Perioperative Medicine
Henry Ford Hospital
Detroit, MI, USA

**Timothy Rushmer, MD**
University of Wisconsin School of Medicine and Public
    Health
Madison, WI, USA

**Ramsey Saad, MD**
Henry Ford Health System
Detroit, MI, USA

**Samiya L. Saklayen, MD**
The Ohio State University Wexner Medical Center

**Sabrina S. Sam, MD**
Cook County Health Systems
Chicago, IL, USA

**Amit Samba, DO**
Specialist in Gainesville
FL, USA

**Syena Sarrafpour, MD**
Department of Anesthesia, Critical Care, and Pain Medicine
Beth Israel Deaconess Medical Center
Harvard Medical School
Boston, MA, USA

**Mariam Sarwary MD**
Department of Anesthesiology and Perioperative Medicine
University of California Los Angeles
Los Angeles, CA, USA

**Emily Young, MD**
Firelands Regional Medical Center

**Kathy D. Schlecht, DO**
William Beaumont Oakland University School of Medicine
Rochester, MI, USA

**Ben Schmitt, DO**
Advocate Aurora Health
Department of Anesthesia
Illinois Masonic Medical Center
Chicago, IL, USA

**Elizabeth Scholzen, MD, MHA**
Department of Anesthesiology
University of Wisconsin Hospital and Clinics
Madison, WI, USA

**Robert P. Schroell III, MD**
Department of Anesthesiology
The Ohio State University
Wexner Medical Center
Columbus, OH, USA

**Nathan Schulman, MD**
Assistant Clinical Professor
Department of Anesthesiology and Perioperative Medicine
University of California Los Angeles
Los Angeles, CA, USA

**Ruben Schwartz, DO**
Mount Sinai Medical Center
Miami, FL, USA

**Courtney L. Scott, MD**
UCLA Department of Anesthesiology and Perioperative Medicine
David Geffen School of Medicine at UCLA
Los Angeles, CA, USA

**Anish Sethi, DO**
Assistant Professor of Clinical Anesthesiology
Lewis Katz School of Medicine
Temple University
Philadelphia, PA, USA

**Nimit K. Shah, MBBS, FRCA, FCARCSI, DA, DNB, EDAIC, EDRA**

**Rutvij Shah, MD, MPH**
Ochsner LSU Health
Shreveport, LA, USA

**Ezra Shapiro, MD**
University of Central Florida/HCA GME Consortium, Orlando
Ocala Health
Ocala, FL, USA

**Archit Sharma, MD, MBA**
Clinical Assistant Professor
Department of Anesthesia
University of Iowa Hospitals Carver College of Medicine
Iowa City, IA, USA

**Sahil Sharma, MBBS**
Department of Anesthesia
University of Iowa Hospitals Carver College of Medicine
Iowa City, IA, USA

**Surangama Sharma, MD**
Clinical Assistant Professor
Department of Anesthesia
University of Iowa Health Care
Iowa City, IA, USA

**Derek Shirey, DO**
Allegheny Health Network Department of Anesthesiology
Pittsburgh, PA, USA

**Vasu Sidagam, MD**
Assistant Professor
Department of Anesthesiology and Perioperative Medicine
University Hospitals of Cleveland
Case Western Reserve University
Cleveland, OH, USA

**Simranjit Singh, MD**
Cook County Health Systems
Chicago, IL, USA

**Sarah C. Smith, MD**
Assistant Professor of Anesthesiology
Westchester Medical Center
New York Medical College
Valhalla, NY, USA

**Mahad Sohail (Illustrations)**
Department of Anesthesiology
Beth Israel Deaconess Medical Center
Boston, MA, USA

**Ramaiza Sohail**
Department of Anesthesiology
Beth Israel Deaconess Medical Center
Boston, MA, USA

**Jacqueline Sohn, DO**
Department of Anesthesiology and Perioperative Medicine
University Hospitals Cleveland Medical Center
Cleveland, OH, USA

**Amol Soin, MD**
Aspirus Health System
Antigo, WI, USA

**Allyson L. Spence, PhD**
Department of Pharmaceutical Sciences
Regis University School of Pharmacy
Rueckert-Hartman College for Health Professions
Denver, CO, USA

**Andrew Sprowell, MD**
Department of Anesthesia
University of Iowa Hospitals
Iowa City, IA, USA

**Brian M. Starr, MD**
Department of Anesthesiology
Duke University Medical Center
Durham, NC, USA

**R. Scott Stayner, MD, PhD**
Pain Medicine
Nura Pain Clinic
Edina, MN, USA

**Robin B. Stedman, MD, MPH, FASA**
Senior Staff Physician
Ochsner Health System
Assistant Professor of Anesthesiology
The University of Queensland School of Medicine,
    Ochsner Clinical School
Jefferson, LA, USA

**Natalie H. Strand, MD**
Mayo Clinic of Arizona
Department of Anesthesiology and Division of
    Pain Medicine
Phoenix, AZ, USA

**Charlotte Streetzel, MD**
University of Florida College of Medicine
Gainesville, FL, USA

**Ryan Stuckey, MD**
University of North Carolina Health
Chapel Hill, NC, USA

**Gunar G. Subieta-Benito, MD**
Attending Physician, Department of Anesthesiology and
    Pain Management
Assistant Professor, Rush Medical College
John H. Stroger, Jr. Hospital of Cook County
Chicago, IL, USA

**Felipe F. Suero, MD**
Assistant Professor of Anesthesiology
Fox Chase Cancer Center (FCCC)
Temple University Health System
Philadelphia, PA, USA

**David E. Swanson, MD**
University of Iowa
Iowa City, IA, USA

**Madiha Syed, MD**
Assistant Professor of Anesthesiology and Critical Care
Department of Intensive Care and Resuscitation
Anesthesiology Institute, Cleveland Clinic
Cleveland, OH, USA

**Camila Teixeira, MD**
Anesthesia Research Department
Cleveland Clinic Florida
Weston, FL, USA

**Ling Tian, MD, PhD**
UCLA Department of Anesthesiology and Perioperative Medicine
Los Angeles, CA, USA

**Samuel Tillmans, MD**
Department of Anesthesiology
University at Buffalo
Buffalo, NY, USA

**Daniel Tobes, DO**
Department of Anesthesiology
Beaumont Health
Royal Oak, MI, USA

**Jacob Topfer, DO**
University of Miami/Jackson Memorial Health System

**Felipe Vasconcelos Torres, MD, PhD**
Department of Anesthesiology, Pain Management, and
    Perioperative Medicine
Henry Ford Hospital
Detroit, MI, USA

**Maria Torres, MD**
Cook County Health Systems
Chicago, IL, USA

**Patrick Torres, MD**
Regional Anesthesiologist
Department of Anesthesiology and Perioperative Medicine
Ochsner Clinic Foundation
New Orleans, LA, USA

**Kenneth Toth, MD**
Cook County Health Systems
Chicago, IL, USA

**Gaurav Trehan, MD, MBA**
Associate Professor of Clinical Anesthesiology
Lewis Katz School of Medicine, Temple University
Philadelphia, PA, USA

**Michelle A. Carroll Turpin, PhD**
Assistant Professor of Pharmacology
Department of Biomedical Sciences
College of Medicine
University of Houston
Houston, TX, USA

**Ajay S. Unnithan, MD**
Physician of Anesthesiology
University of North Carolina Health
Chapel Hill, NC, USA

**Ivan Urits, MD**
Department of Anesthesiology, Critical Care, and Pain Medicine
Beth Israel Deaconess Medical Center
Harvard Medical School
Boston, MA, USA

**Shivani Varshney, MD**
Allegheny General Hospital
Pittsburgh, PA, USA

**Kris Vasant, MD**
Department of Anesthesiology
Temple University Hospital
Lewis Katz School of Medicine
Philadelphia, PA, USA

**Jasmin Villatoro-Lopez, DO**
Center for Interventional Pain and Spine

**Omar Viswanath, MD**
Department of Anesthesiology
Louisiana State University Health Sciences Center
Shreveport, LA, USA
Valley Anesthesiology and Pin Consultants
Envision Physician Services
Phoenix, AZ, USA

**Taruna Waghray-Penmetcha, MD**
Cook County Health Systems
Chicago, IL, USA

**Anureet Walia, MD**
Clinical Assistant Professor
Department of Anesthesia
University of Iowa Hospitals
Carver College of Medicine
Iowa City, IA, USA

**Syed Waqar, MD**
Anesthesiology
Henry Ford University
Detroit, MI, USA

**Stacey Watt, MD, MBA, FASA**
Clinical Professor of Anesthesiology
Program Director, Anesthesiology Residency Program
Jacobs School of Medicine & Biomedical Sciences
Chief of Service, Department of Anesthesiology, Kaleida Health
Department of Anesthesiology
University at Buffalo
Buffalo, NY, USA

**Peggy White, MD**
Department of Anesthesiology
University of Florida College of Medicine
Gainesville, FL, USA

**Alex Woodrow, DO**
Department of Anesthesia
University of Iowa Hospitals
Iowa City, IA, USA

**Caylynn Yao**
School of Medicine and Health Sciences
George Washington University
Washington, DC, USA

**Christopher Yates, DO, MBA**
Department of Anesthesia
University of Iowa Hospitals
Iowa City, IA, USA

**Joshua Younger, MD**
Henry Ford Health System
Detroit, MI, USA

**John Yousef, MD**
Department of Anesthesiology
Beaumont Health
Royal Oak, MI, USA

**Yasser M. A. Youssef, MD, MSc**
Department of Anesthesiology and Pain Management
John H. Stroger, Jr. Hospital Cook County Health
Chicago, IL, USA

**Raymond C. Yu, MD**
Department of Anesthesiology
AGH-WPH Medical Education Consortium
Allegheny Health Network
Pittsburgh, PA, USA

**Adam Yu Yuan, MD**
Allegheny General Hospital
Pittsburgh, PA, USA

**Sherif Zaky, Md, MSc, PhD**
Associate Professor of Anesthesiology
Ohio University, Heritage College of Medicine
Medical Director, Pain Management Services
Firelands Regional Medical Center

**Erica Zanath, MD**
Anesthesia and Perioperative Medicine
University Hospitals
Cleveland, OH, USA

**Muhammad Haseeb Zubair, MD**
Advocate Illinois Masonic Medical Center
Chicago, IL, USA

# Part I

# ANATOMY

# 1.

# TOPOGRAPHICAL ANATOMY AS LANDMARKS

*Derek Shirey and Bryan Matusic*

## NECK LANDMARKS

### CRICOTHYROID MEMBRANE

This is the landmark used for a cricothyrotomy procedure. Located between the cricoid and thyroid cartilage tissue, as shown in Figure 1.1, the membrane acts as a guide for establishing an airway for patients in emergency situations. Palpate superiorly to the sternal notch until the prominence of the cricoid cartilage is identified and a subtle step-off is felt just inferior to the thyroid cartilage.

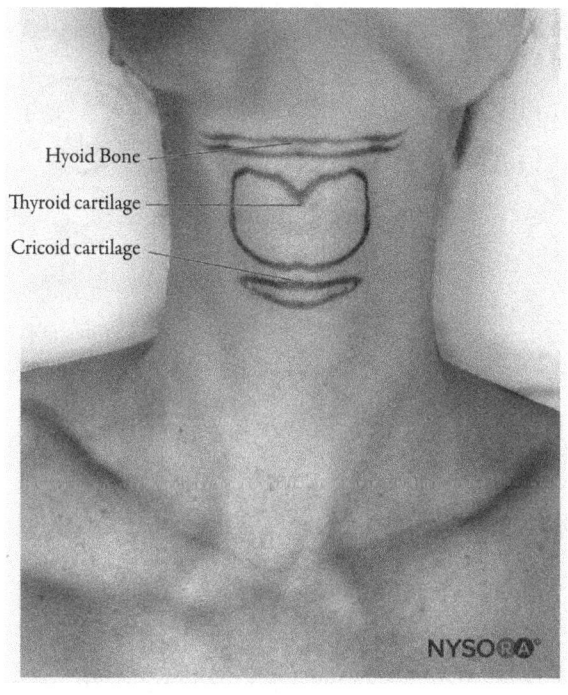

**Figure 1.1.** Surface anatomy of the neck.
Reproduced with permission from the New York School of Regional Anesthesia (NYSORA).
https://www.nysora.com/.

## INTERNAL AND EXTERNAL JUGULAR VEINS

Extending superiorly from the brachiocephalic veins, the internal jugular veins sit anterolateral to the carotid arteries. The anterior approach for cannulation for central venous access relies on identification of the area between the sternal and clavicular heads of the sternocleidomastoid muscle (SCM) by having the patient extend and rotate the head to the contralateral side. Alternatively, a posterior approach can be completed by identification of the point where the posterolateral border of the SCM for the entry point. The external jugular vein, more posterior and lateral in relation to the internal jugular vein, typically travels superficial to the SCM from the angle of the mandible to the middle third of the clavicle and is often visible in the neck. The common carotid artery splits into the external and internal carotid arteries at the level of C4 near the upper border of the thyroid cartilage. Located deep and medial to the internal jugular vein, as seen in Figure 1.2, the carotid artery can be visualized by ultrasound as the non-compressible, pulsating

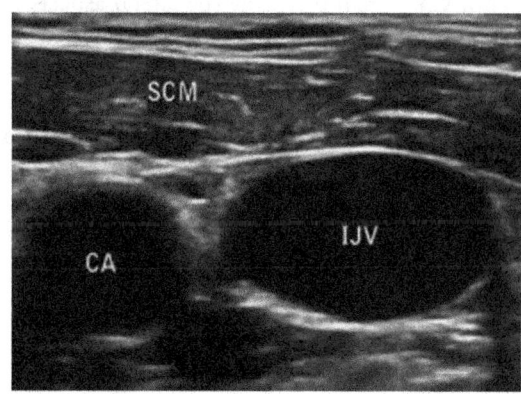

**Figure 1.2.** Ultrasound anatomy of the internal jugular vein and carotid artery.
Reproduced with permission from Ahmad H, Frderico P, Rosenthal R, *Mental Conditioning to Perform Common Operations in General Surgery Training*. Cham: Springer; 2020.

structure in the transverse plane. By utilizing ultrasound and a lateral approach, avoidance of the carotid artery during cannulation of the internal jugular vein can be achieved.

## SUBCLAVIAN VEIN

Cannulation for central venous access relies on identification of the middle third of the clavicle. Once deep to the clavicle, the needle should be directed cephalad to the sternal notch.

## STELLATE GANGLION

The stellate ganglion is the result of fusion of the inferior cervical ganglion and first thoracic ganglion. The sympathetic ganglion is located at the level C7, anterior to the C7 transverse process and the neck of the first rib, and sits just inferior to the subclavian artery.

## VERTEBRA PROMINENS

Another name for C7, this palpable landmark is the result of a prominent spinous process which becomes more distinct with flexion of the neck.

## CHASSAIGNAC'S TUBERCLE

Extending anteriorly from C6, this landmark separates the carotid artery from the vertebral artery. Also called the carotid tubercle, it is useful as a landmark for stellate ganglion, brachial plexus, and cervical plexus blocks which provide pain relief in the upper extremity and neck.

## HYOID BONE

Located in the anterior midline of the neck between the thyroid cartilage and chin, the hyoid bone can be found at the level of C3. When palpating the lateral aspects of the thyroid cartilage, as shown in Figure 1.1, move superiorly until the wings of the hyoid bone are felt. The wings serve as the landmark for the superior laryngeal nerve block, which is useful when attempting an awake intubation. In obese patients, the normally subtle hyoid bone can be extremely difficult to identify with palpation alone and requires ultrasound visualization.

## SUPERFICIAL CERVICAL PLEXUS

Arising from C1 to C4, the individual nerves travel lateral to the transverse processes between the paravertebral muscles. As the spinal nerves travel anteriorly, deep to the SCM, they create a plexus while forming an anastomosis with the accessory nerve, hypoglossal nerve, and sympathetic trunk. The branches emerge along the posterior border of the SCM, known as the nerve point or Erb's point.

## CHEST LANDMARKS

### CARDIAC AUSCULTATION LANDMARKS

Aortic valve: Second intercostal space to the right of the sternum

Pulmonic valve: Second intercostal space to the left of the sternum

Tricuspid valve: Fifth intercostal space to the left of the sternum

Mitral valve: Fifth intercostal space in the left midclavicular line

Subclavian vein: Cannulation for central venous access relies on identification of the middle third of the clavicle. Once deep to the clavicle, the needle should be directed toward the sternal notch.

## PELVIS AND BACK LANDMARKS

### VERTEBRAL LEVEL OF TOPOGRAPHICAL LANDMARKS

C6: Chassaignac's tubercle, cricoid cartilage, superior aspect of trachea

T4: Sternal angle

T7: Inferior angle of scapula

T9–L2: Artery of Adamkiewicz origin

T10: Umbilicus

T12–L4: Lumbar plexus

L1–2: Termination of spinal cord

L4: Iliac crest

L4–S3: Sacral plexus

S2: Termination of dural sac, posterior superior iliac spine (PSIS)[1,2]

## EXTREMITY LANDMARKS WITH ASSOCIATED NERVE BLOCKS

### UPPER EXTREMITY

#### Interscalene

Identify the posterior aspect of the SCM at the level of the cricoid cartilage. Palpate the groove between the anterior and middle scalene muscles and place the ultrasound probe in the transverse plane, as seen in Figure 1.3A. Direct the needle posterior to the clavicular head of the SCM. The brachial plexus is located between the anterior and middle scalene muscles, which is shown in Figure 1.3B.

## Supraclavicular

The needle insertion point of the lateral border of the SCM clavicular head while the patient faces away from you. Direct the needle perpendicular to the floor. If ultrasound-guided,

the brachial plexus can be seen as a collection of hypoechoic oval structures superficial and posterolateral to the subclavian artery, as shown in Figure 1.3C.

## Infraclavicular

Adduct the arm and mark a point 2 cm medial and inferior to the tip of the coracoid process. Insert the needle

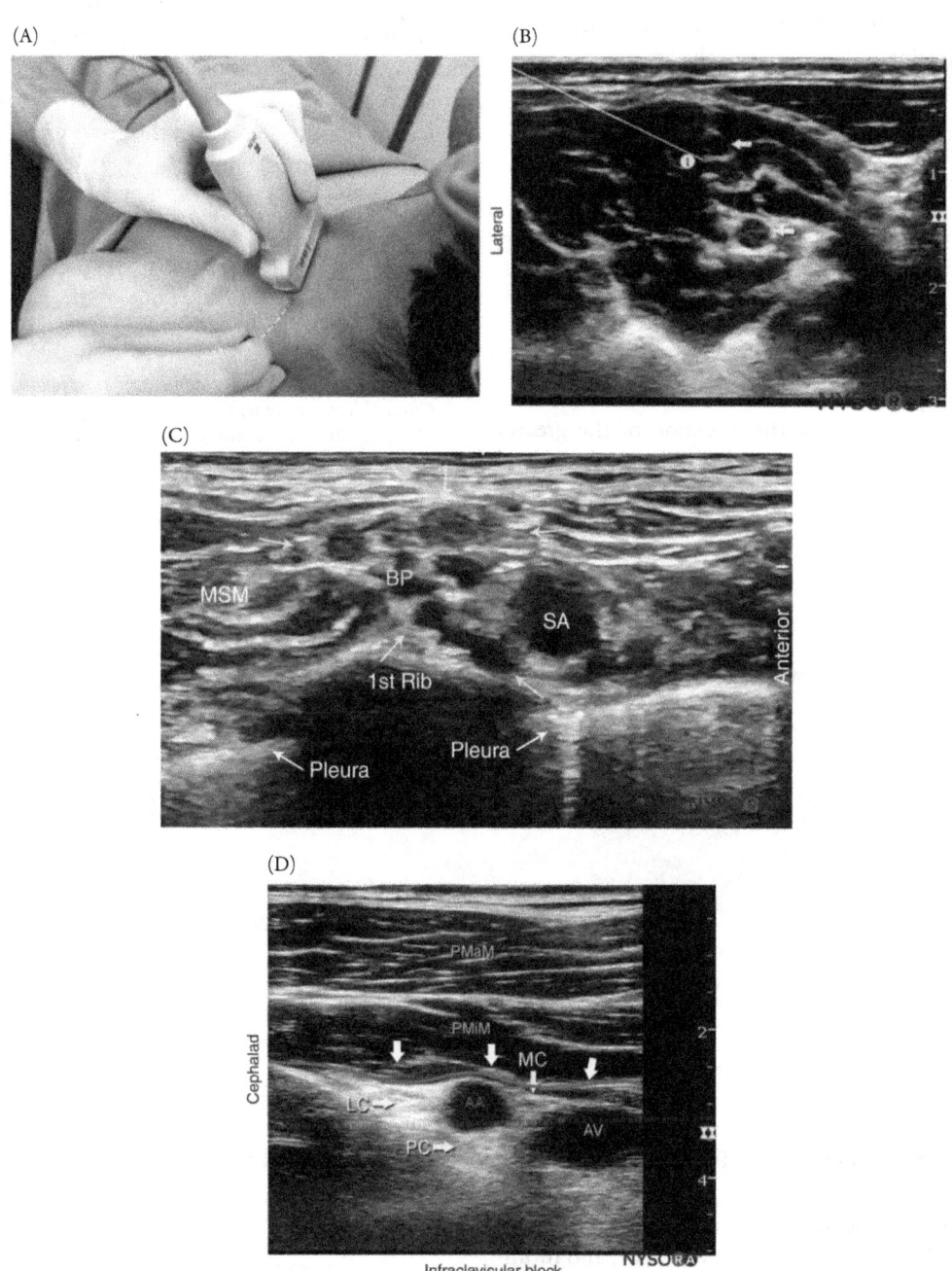

**Figure 1.3.** Ultrasound (US) anatomy of the interscalene (A and B), supraclavicular (C), and infraclavicular brachial plexus blocks. A: The US probe is oriented in the transverse plane with needle insertion posterior to the SCM. B: US image showing the needle tip lying lateral to the brachial plexus (yellow arrows). C: US image showing the brachial plexus (yellow arrows) lying superior and posterolateral to the subclavian artery and anterior to the middle scalene muscle (MSM). D: US imaging of the lateral (LC), posterior (PC), and medial cords (PC) surrounding the axillary artery (AA) and deep to the pectoralis major (PMaM) and minor (PMiM) muscles and fascia (red line). The axillary vein (AV) lies caudal to the AA.

perpendicular to the skin. With ultrasound guidance, the medial, lateral, and posterior cords of the brachial plexus can be seen surrounding the axillary artery, as seen in Figure 1.3D.

### Axillary

Abduct the arm, flex at the elbow, and palpate the axillary artery. Direct the needle superior to the artery to encounter the median nerve while the radial and ulnar nerves are encountered inferior and posterior to the artery.

### LOWER EXTREMITY

### Femoral Nerve

Palpate the femoral artery below the inguinal ligament. The femoral nerve sits lateral to the artery at the level of the femoral crease.

### Sciatic Nerve

Mark a point 4 cm distal to the bisection of the greater trochanter of the femur and the PSIS. Using ultrasound guidance, the femoral artery is identified deep to the sartorius muscle. Deep to the vastus intermedius muscle, the femur can be seen as a hyperechoic rim. Medial to the femur, the adductor magnus sits superiorly to a hyperechoic oval structure which is the sciatic nerve.

### Popliteal

Identify the biceps femoris and semitendinosus/semimembranous muscles in the posterior proximal leg. Mark a point midway between the muscles and 8 cm superior to the popliteal crease. Alternatively, a lateral approach inserts 8 cm above the popliteal crease in the grove created by the vastus lateralis and biceps femoris.[3]

### REFERENCES

1. Hansen JT, et al. *Netter's Clinical Anatomy.* Philadelphia, PA: Elsevier; 2019.
2. Valenta Jiří, Fiala P. *Topographical Anatomy with Autopsy Guide and Clinical Notes.* Prague: Karolinum; 2013.
3. Meier G, Büttner Johannes. *Atlas of Peripheral Regional Anesthesia: Anatomy and Techniques.* Stuttgart: Thieme; 2016.

# 2.

# GENERAL RADIOGRAPHIC ANATOMY

*Keith A. Andrews and Mada Helou*

## INTRODUCTION

Diagnostic imaging encompasses the use of various imaging technologies for diagnostic, surveillance, and monitoring purposes. Image interpretation combines subjective and objective information to assist in revealing a diagnosis, confirming line placement, monitoring response to treatment, and much more. The aim of this chapter is to provide a foundational reference for the anatomy visualized by plain radiographs (X-rays), computed tomography (CT), and magnetic resonance imaging (MRI), with brief mention of the utility of ultrasound to aid in central line placement.

## MODALITY OVERVIEW

### X-RAY IMAGING

X-ray photons traversing matter are either absorbed or scattered. Absorption—or attenuation—is directly proportional to the density of the medium through which the photons travel. High-density tissue like bone appears bright, compared to low-density mediums such as air, which appear dark.

## COMPUTED TOMOGRAPHY

CT uses an X-ray beam that moves in an arc around a patient, opposite from a detector, to reconstruct a three-dimensional anatomic image. Its advantages include better bone and soft tissue resolution compared to X-ray, with excellent imaging for the lungs, liver, and vasculature. Disadvantages include relatively high radiation exposure and potential intolerance to IV contrast agents.

## MAGNETIC RESONANCE IMAGING

In MRI, a pulsed radiofrequency beam excites protons in the patient's tissue into different energy levels. After the beam is turned off, the protons return to resting and emit energy, which is captured as light based on the excitation level of the proton, hydrogen density within a tissue, and time required for proton relaxation. Combined, these factors dictate whether an image is T1 or T2 weighted, a comparison of which is highlighted in Table 2.1.

## ULTRASOUND

Ultrasound utilizes high-frequency sound waves transmitted from a probe through tissues. Reflections are picked up by the probe and transformed into images, with less dense structures and mediums appearing dark, while denser tissues and structures appear bright. Bone is an exception; sound waves are strongly absorbed by bone, but rather than appearing bright, a shadow is cast on the image.

# IMAGING SPECIFICS BY BODY REGION

## BRAIN AND SKULL

CT scan is a preferred initial study for the evaluation of bony and intracranial abnormalities. Vascular structures appear opaque following IV contrast. It is indicated to rule out skull fracture, or with suspicion of epidural hematoma,

subdural hematoma, subarachnoid hemorrhage, space occupying lesions, hydrocephalus, and edema. MRI is more expensive and more time-consuming than CT. However, MRI will provide much greater detail when there is strong clinical suspicion for intracranial abnormality and CT imaging is equivocal.

## SPINE

MRI is considered the most sensitive for evaluating spinal disease and is most commonly utilized to assess conditions such as spinal stenosis, disc herniation, or radiculopathy of unknown etiology. *MRI is the imaging of choice for suspicion of epidural abscess and/or osteomyelitis following spinal procedures.*

## NECK ULTRASOUND

Ultrasound is the imaging of choice utilized for cannulation of major vessels, particularly the internal jugular vein, brachial artery, femoral artery, and femoral vein.

High-yield considerations include proximity of the median nerve to the brachial artery during cannulation.

## CHEST

Chest X-rays (CXR) can be performed with a posteroanterior (PA) view where the anterior chest is against a film plate to minimize heart size magnification, from a lateral view to see the retrocardiac space and thoracic spine, or as an anteroposterior (AP) view for bedridden patients. Chest radiographs are also valuable for verifying the position of tubes, lines, and catheters, as shown in Table 2.2.

CT scanning is often important to further define abnormalities seen on CXR, including pleural effusions and consolidations, or when significant vascular pathology is suspected, such as aortic dissection. Different modes of CT chest are shown in Table 2.3.

## ABDOMEN

Radiographs are typically performed as left lateral decubitus, supine, and erect upright. Indications include acute

*Table 2.1* COMPARISON OF T1 AND T2 MRI IMAGES

| IMAGING SEQUENCE | WHITE MATTER | GRAY MATTER | CSF | BLOOD | DETAILS |
|---|---|---|---|---|---|
| T1 | Bright | Dark gray | Black | Bright | Considered an "anatomic scan," since T1 provides excellent reference for landmarks in three-dimensional space |
| T2 | Dark | | Bright white | | Often considered a "pathologic scan," since edema and local tissue inflammation are well visualized |

*Table 2.2* CHEST X-RAY TO VISUALIZE TUBES, LINES, AND CATHETERS

| DEVICE | OPTIMAL LOCATION | POTENTIAL COMPLICATIONS |
|---|---|---|
| Central venous catheter | Tip should be proximal to right atrium, ideally between the first rib border superiorly and the RA inferiorly | Pneumothorax, mediastinal/pleural bleeding, air embolism |
| Endotracheal tube | <3 cm above carina | Right mainstem intubation, subcutaneous emphysema, or pneumomediastinum secondary to pharyngeal perforation |
| Nasogastric tube | Tip and sideport distal to esophagogastric junction | Pneumothorax |
| PA catheter (Swan-Ganz) | Within a large, lobar branch of either right or left main pulmonary artery | Pneumothorax, mediastinal bleed |

*Table 2.3* CT CHEST VARIATIONS

| MODALITY | ADVANTAGE | DISADVANTAGE | CONTRAST | INDICATION |
|---|---|---|---|---|
| Standard | Quick full thoracic imaging | Does not clearly demonstrate diffuse pathology | ± | CXR abnormality including pleural and mediastinal changes, empyema versus abscess |
| High resolution | Thinner slices providing high definition of lung parenchyma | | No | Hemoptysis, characterizing solitary nodules, diffuse lung disease, e.g., sarcoidosis |
| Low dose | 1/5 the radiation burden | Decreased detail | No | Screening imaging rather than diagnostic, follow-up infections, e.g., pneumonia |
| CTA | Clearly shows vasculature | Relatively high contrast load | Yes | PE, aortic pathology |

*Table 2.4* COMPARISON OF X-RAY, CT, AND MRI FOR VARIOUS EXTREMITY CIRCUMSTANCES

| MODALITY | DESCRIPTION | INDICATIONS | LIMITATIONS |
|---|---|---|---|
| X-ray | Useful initial study in acute and chronic bone and joint disorders | Acute trauma; review hardware after orthopedic placement; assess chronic disease, e.g., arthritis | Minimal soft tissue visualization |
| CT | Fine detail soft tissue imaging | Evaluate more complex acute pathology, e.g., acetabular | Higher radiation load |
| MRI | Most accurate for soft tissue illumination | Tendinous and muscular pathology; staging soft tissue malignancy; assess internal joint injuries, e.g., labral tears | Time-consuming, requires patient cooperation |

abdomen to evaluate for bowel perforation, toxic megacolon, and small/large bowel obstruction. Of note, radiographs are not helpful when there is suspicion of GI bleed.

Indications for plain abdominal CT include renal colic and suspected hemorrhage. Contrast images are indicated when there is concern for liver and/gallbladder obstructing tumors, or as oral contrast to evaluate the GI tract.

## EXTREMITIES

As outlined in Table 2.4, all three imaging modalities have utility in assessing a range of extremity pathologies. These modalaties can answer clinical questions preoperatively and intraoperatively. For instance, plain radiographs of the extremities are used to verify hardware placement during orthopedic surgeries. CT scanning and MRI are typically utilized as preoperative assessments, rather than intraoperative modalities to assess the extent of soft tissue pathology, for instance after acute trauma.[1,2]

## REFERENCES

1. Elsayes KM, Oldham SAA, eds. *Introduction to Diagnostic Radiology.* New York, NY: McGraw-Hill; 2014. Accessed June 8, 2020. http://accessmedicine.mhmedical.com/content.aspx?boo kid=1562&sectionid=95874473.
2. Kim, J. *Essential Med Notes 2017.* Toronto: Toronto Notes for Medical Students; 2017:MI1–MI31.

# 3.

# NECK ANATOMY

*Wenyu Pan and Tariq M. Malik*

## INTRODUCTION

Understanding the anatomy of the neck is essential for proper airway management, safe central venous catheter cannulation, and for an uncomplicated execution of cervical procedures. The side of the neck is divided by sternocleidomastoid muscle (SCM) into anterior and posterior part or triangles. The posterior triangle has most nerves of interest that are blocked for postoperative analgesia of shoulder and arm, while the anterior triangle has airway structure, thyroid, and major vessels of the neck. This chapter reviews the major landmarks of the neck and important learning points related to its anatomy.

## BASIC OVERVIEW

The neck structures are separated by four fascial layers; deep cervical fascia, prevertebral fascia, pretracheal fascia,

and carotid sheath. Of these four, the deep cervical and prevertebral are much more defined. The nerves of the superficial cervical plexus pierce the deep cervical fascia behind the midpoint of SCM to become superficial. The external jugular vein is superficial to this fascia. The cricoid cartilage is at the level of C6.

## ANTERIOR NECK TRIANGLE

The anterior neck triangle is bounded by midline in the middle, SCM laterally, and mandible superiorly. The key structures here are the trachea, thyroid cartilage, hyoid bone, and cricothyroid cartilage.

## CRICOTHYROID MEMBRANE

The cricothyroid membrane consists of the median and lateral cricothyroid ligaments. It attaches the thyroid cartilage to the cricoid cartilage. Accessibly located close to the skin, it can be palpated as a soft spot inferior to the thyroid cartilage and entered in emergency cricothyroidotomy and transtracheal jet ventilation.[1,2] This membrane is punctured to inject local anesthetic inside the trachea and to numb the inside wall of trachea and vocal cords when planning for awake fiberoptic intubation (FOI).

## THYROID CARTILAGE AND HYOID BONE

The vocal cords are present at the level of thyroid cartilage. The hyoid bone cornu is a landmark used to block superior laryngeal nerve for an awake FOI.

## AIRWAY INNERVATION

The vagus nerve (CN X) innervates the airway through two branches, the superior laryngeal nerves and the recurrent laryngeal nerves (RLNs). The superior laryngeal nerve descends along the lateral wall of pharynx behind and then medial to the internal carotid artery and splits into the internal and external branches at the level of thyroidhyoid membrane. The internal branch supplies sensory fibers to the upper airway from the back of the throat up to the vocal cords, including the epiglottis, piriformis sinus, and arytenoids. The external branch innervates the cricothyroid muscle that tenses the vocal cords. The RLN is the sensory supply of the airway from the vocal cord and below, and innervates all of the intrinsic muscles of the larynx (adductors and abductors) except for the cricothyroid muscle.[3]

## RLN INJURY AND VOCAL CORD POSITIONS

The RLN is the most commonly injured nerve in thyroidectomies and parathyroidectomies. Complete transection of bilateral RLNs affects both the abductors and adductors, and the vocal cords will be in the paramedian position (2–3 mm from the midline), leading to stridor and requiring intubation or tracheostomy in acute injury.[2] Partial paralysis of bilateral RLNs affects only the abductor muscle, resulting in unopposed adductor muscle action, closed vocal cords, and complete airway obstruction (Figure 3.1).

## COUGH REFLEX

The afferent component of the cough reflex is the internal branch of the superior laryngeal nerve. The RLN is primarily involved and can be blocked by transtracheal injection of local anesthetic (LA) after air is aspirated through the cricothyroid membrane or aerosolization of LA.[3]

## GAG REFLEX

The afferent component of the gag reflex is the glossopharyngeal nerve (CN IX), which provides innervation of the base of the tongue, vallecula, anterior epiglottis, and tonsils. It can be blocked by topicalization in the pharyngeal folds near the base of the tongue or injection of LA at the base of the fold in the floor of the mouth. If blood is aspirated, the needle should be directed medially to avoid the carotid artery.[3] The efferent component is the vagus nerve.

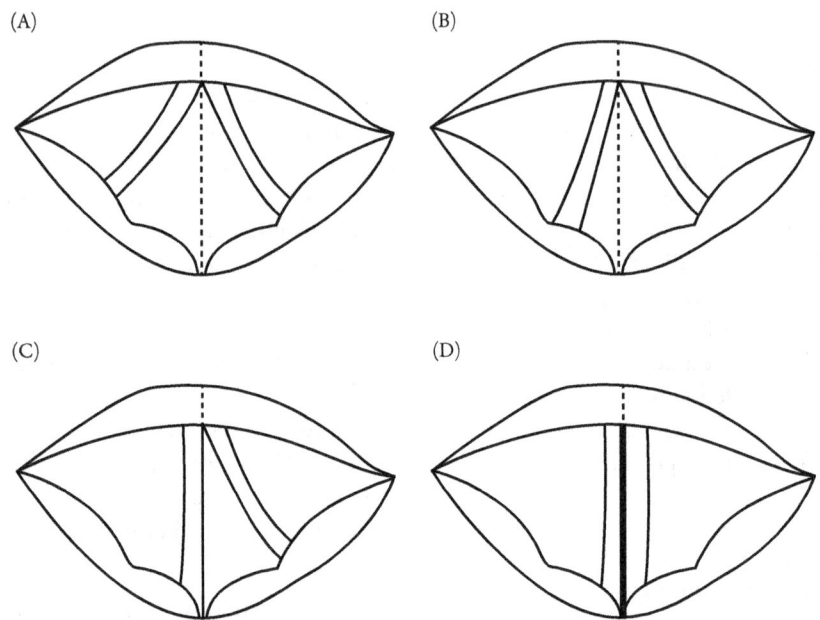

**Figure 3.1.** Vocal cord palsy during inspiration. A: normal vocal cord positions in abduction. B: complete unilateral palsy with the left vocal cord in the paramedian position. C: incomplete unilateral palsy with the left vocal cord in the closed position. D: incomplete bilateral palsy with both vocal cords in the closed position.

## INTERNAL AND EXTERNAL JUGULAR VEINS

The external jugular (EJ) vein begins near the angle of the mandible, crosses the sternocleidomastoid muscle, and terminates in the subclavian vein.[1] The EJ is superficial to deep cervical fascia; hence it is very mobile and hard to puncture. The subclavian vein joins the internal jugular vein (IJV) to form the brachiocephalic vein posterior to the medial clavicle. The IJV starts from the jugular foramen and runs in the carotid sheath lateral to the carotid artery.

## CENTRAL VENOUS ACCESS

The IJV is a common site for central venous catheter cannulation. Excessive head rotation can reposition the IJV anterior to the carotid artery under ultrasound view, increasing the risk for carotid artery cannulation (Figure 3.2). Cannulation of the IJV on the right side is preferred, due to its straight access to the superior vena cava on the right side, the presence of the thoracic duct on the left side, and the fact that performance of this procedure from the right side is easier for right-handed people.

With the patient's head turned to the opposite side, the course of the IJV is determined by drawing a line between the mastoid process and the medial insertion of the sternocleidomastoid muscle on the clavicle. The carotid artery should be palpated and identified before insertion of the needle. The needle is inserted through the skin and directed toward the ipsilateral nipple at about a 45-degree angle.

## CAROTID AND VERTEBRAL ARTERIES

### CAROTID ARTERIES

The left common carotid artery arises from the aorta arch, while the right common carotid artery arises from the brachiocephalic trunk.[1] The common carotid artery ascends within the carotid sheath and divides into the internal and external carotid arteries at the level of the superior thyroid cartilage. The internal carotid artery supplies the brain, while the external carotid artery supplies most structures outside of the cranium.

### CAROTID SINUS

Located at the bifurcation of the common carotid artery, the carotid sinus is a baroreceptor innervated by the vagus nerve.[1] During carotid endarterectomy, pressure on the carotid sinus may cause bradycardia and hypotension.

### CAROTID BODY

In close relation to the carotid sinus is the carotid body, a chemoreceptor supplied by the glossopharyngeal and vagus nerves that monitors the arterial partial pressure of oxygen.[1]

### VERTEBRAL ARTERY

The vertebral artery arises from the subclavian artery, passes the transverse foramina of C6–C1, and enters the cranial cavity through the foramen magnum, supplying the brain.[1]

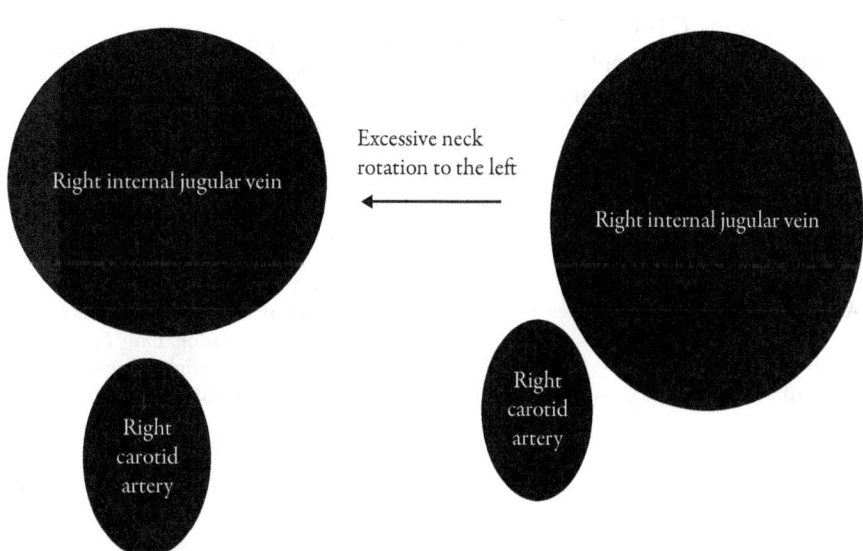

**Figure 3.2.** The internal jugular vein lies laterally to the carotid artery. With excessive head rotation, the internal jugular vein is repositioned anteriorly to the carotid artery, increasing the risk for carotid artery cannulation.

## THORACIC DUCT

The thoracic duct is the main lymphatic channel of the body, draining from the entire body, except the upper right quarter which drains through the right lymphatic duct.[1] The thoracic duct drains into the junction of the left subclavian and IJVs. Thus, left IJV cannulation may potentially damage the thoracic duct and cause chylothorax.[4]

## STELLATE GANGLION

The stellate ganglion is a sympathetic ganglion, the fusion of the inferior cervical and first thoracic ganglia. It receives preganglionic sympathetic fibers from T1–T6. The stellate ganglion block is often used to diagnose and treat complex regional pain syndrome of the upper extremities. Chassaignac's tubercle (anterior tubercle on the transverse process of C6) is the major landmark for stellate ganglion block, due to the ganglion's location anterior to the C7 vertebral body and directly inferior to the transverse process of C6. The vertebral artery lies anterior to the ganglion and is the closest vascular structure to the stellate ganglion.

## POSTERIOR NECK TRIANGLE

The posterior neck triangle is bounded by the SCM anteriorly, the trapezius muscle posteriorly, and the clavicle inferiorly. The accessory nerve and dorsal scapular nerve run through it in the upper half of the triangle deep to cervical fascia, while the brachial plexus and its branches run in the lower half.

## SUPERFICIAL CERVICAL PLEXUS

The cervical plexus arises from the C1–C4 spinal nerves and divides into a motor branch that supplies the deep neck muscles and a sensory branch that supplies the skin of the neck and the shoulder.[5] The superficial cervical plexus is blocked at the midpoint of the posterior border of the sternocleidomastoid muscle, resulting in cutaneous anesthesia.

## BRACHIAL PLEXUS

The brachial plexus emerges between the two scalene muscles just behind the subclavian artery and pierces the

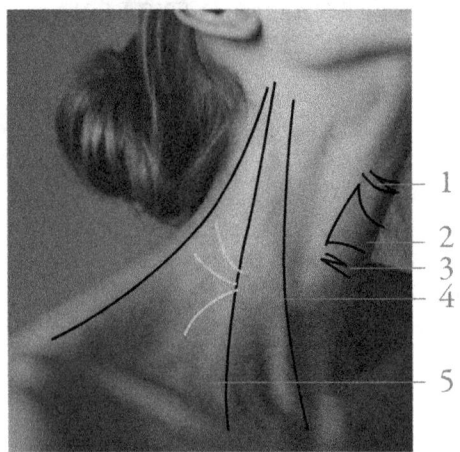

**Figure 3.3.** Neck topography. 1: hyoid bone; 2: thyroid cartilage; 3: cricoid cartilage; 4: superficial cervical plexus; 5: brachial plexus.

deep cervical fascia posterior to the SCM before running into the arm behind the midclavicular point (Figure 3.3).

## ANESTHETIC CONSIDERATIONS

- The cricoid cartilage is about the level of C6.
- The stellate ganglion is located superficial to pretracheal muscles but deep to the thyroid gland and carotid vessels.
- The superficial plexus nerves can be damaged during brachial plexus block as they lie just superficial to the brachial plexus (Figure 3.3).
- The thoracic duct is prone to damage on the left side during left-sided central line placement.

## REFERENCES

1. Moore KL, et al. Neck. In: Moore KL, Agur AMR, Dalley AF II, eds. *Essential Clinical Anatomy.* 5th ed. Philadelphia, PA: Lippincott Williams & Wilkins; 2015:581–626.
2. Doyle DJ. Anesthesia for ear, nose, and throat surgery. In: Miller RD, ed. *Miller's Anesthesia.* 8th ed. Philadelphia, PA: Elsevier; 2015:2523–2549.
3. Rosenblatt WH, Sukhupragarn W. Airway management. In: Barash PG, Cullen BF, Stoelting RK, Cahalan MK, Stock MC, Ortega R, eds. *Clinical Anesthesia.* 7th ed. Philadelphia, PA: Lippincott Williams & Wilkins; 2013:762–802.
4. Saxena P, et al. Bilateral chylothorax as a complication of internal jugular vein cannulation. *Lung India.* 2015;32(4):370–374.
5. Horlocker TT, et al. Peripheral nerve blocks. In: Miller RD, ed. *Miller's Anesthesia.* 8th ed. Philadelphia, PA: Elsevier; 2015:1721–1751.

# 4.

# CHEST

*Felipe F. Suero and Gurpreet Mundi*

## PULMONARY ANATOMY

The chest cavity contains the lungs, situated on both sides of the heart. Lungs have an apex with a rounded shape; the apex prolongs into the base of the neck, extending shortly above the level of the sternal end of the first rib. The base is concave and rests on the surface of the diaphragm. The pleura contains both lungs. Two different membranes form the pleura: the parietal pleura covers the inner wall of the chest, and the lungs are covert for the visceral pleura. The pleural cavity is a potential space between two layers of the pleura, filled with a small volume of pleural fluid.

The bronchial and pulmonary circulation provides blood to the lungs. This dual vascular system is unique in the body. The bronchial circulation forms for the bronchial arteries, branches of the aorta, delivering oxygen and nutrients to the tissues of the lungs. In the pulmonary circulation, the pulmonary arteries deliver deoxygenated blood to the lungs. The pulmonary veins return the oxygenated blood to the heart and the rest of the body.

The lungs are paired and separated into lobes; the left lung, smaller than the right, is divided into 2 lobes; the right lung is composed of 3 lobes. Each lung becomes divided into 9–10 segments: 3 segments form the upper lobes, 2 form the middle lobe/lingula, and 4–5 form the lower lobes. Two fissures, oblique and horizontal, divide the right lung; the upper and middle lobe are separated by the horizontal fissure, and the oblique fissure divides the middle and lower lobes. There is only an oblique fissure in the left lung, which separates the upper lobe from the lingula and lower lobe.[1]

## CARDIAC LANDMARKS

Cardiac landmarks are an integral part of comprehensive cardiac auscultation. Precordial auscultation of the valvular structure of the heart can be achieved using the following locations: at the right sternal border, at the second right intercostal space level (aortic valve), at the left sternal border, at the second left intercostal space (pulmonic valve), at the left sternal border fourth left intercostal space (tricuspid valve), and at the left mid-clavicular line at the level of the fifth intercostal space (mitral valve). Cardiac activity produces two primary sounds, S1 and S2. The close of the mitral and tricuspid valve generates the first sound—S1—after blood fills the ventricles. This sound marks the beginning of systole. The close of the aortic and pulmonary valves generates the second heart sound—S2—which occurs after the end of the ventricle contraction. This establishes the start of diastole.

### SYSTOLIC MURMURS

Systolic murmurs can be detected during the ventricular contraction. The main pathologies of systolic murmur are mitral regurgitation (MR), tricuspid regurgitation (TR), aortic stenosis (AS), and ventricular septal defect (VSD). Common causes of MR include degenerative, rheumatic, and myocardial infarction (acute MR). The most frequent cause of aortic stenosis is the congenital bicuspid aortic valve.

### DIASTOLIC MURMURS

Diastolic murmurs are audible during ventricular relaxation. The main pathologies of diastolic murmur include aortic regurgitation (AR), pulmonary regurgitation (PR), mitral stenosis (MS), and tricuspid stenosis (TS). Common causes of AR are congenital bicuspid valve and rheumatic fever. The most common cause of PR is pulmonary hypertension, while the most common cause of MS is rheumatic fever. TS is usually caused by rheumatic disease or Carcinoid syndrome.[2]

## VASCULAR ANATOMY

### ARTERIES

At the level of the trachea, the brachiocephalic artery arises from the aortic arch on the right. The right subclavian and right common carotid arteries emerge from the brachiocephalic artery. On the left side, the left common carotid artery and the left subclavian artery arise from the aortic arch.

## VEINS

The subclavian veins drain blood from the upper extremities and lay under the clavicle and anterior to the subclavian artery and first ribs. At the medial border of anterior scalene muscles, the subclavian veins converge with the internal jugular veins, to become the brachiocephalic veins (also known as the innominate veins). The left brachiocephalic vein passes through the superior mediastinum to the level of the aortic arch and joins with the right brachiocephalic vein to form the superior vena cava.[3]

## ANESTHETIC CONSIDERATIONS

- The lung and pleural cavity lay deep and inferior to the subclavian vein. This proximity means subclavian central line insertion and brachial plexus blocks have a high risk for pneumothorax.
- There is a lower risk for infection in subclavian access, but it is associated with a higher rate of insertion failure.

- The lower pleural apex and absence of the thoracic duct on the right result in a lower risk for right-sided subclavian line placement, with regard to pneumo and chylo thorax. Right subclavian access, however, is associated with higher rates of catheter malposition and vessel trauma.
- The brachiocephalic artery is vulnerable to compression during mediastinoscopy, leading to loss of the right radial pulse. Placement of right radial arterial catheter during mediastinoscopy is important to identify brachiocephalic compression.[4]

## REFERENCES

1. Standring S, et al. Thorax. In: *Pleura, Lung Trachea, and Bronchi*. Elsevier Health Sciences. *Gray's Anatomy* (41st ed.). E-book. 2016: 953–960.
2. Bonow RO. ACC/AHA 2006 Guidelines for the management of patients with valvular heart disease. *J Am Coll Cardiol*. 2006;48(3):e-8–e-13.
3. Standring S, et al. Thorax. In: *Great Vessels*. Elsevier Health Sciences. *Gray's Anatomy* (41st ed.). E-book. 2016: 1024–1028.
4. Apfelbaum JL, et al. Practice guidelines for central venous access 2020: An updated report by the American Society of Anesthesiologists Task Force on Central Venous Access. *Anesthesiology*. 1 2020;132:8–43.

# 5.

# BACK AND PELVIS

*Brian A. Nordstrom and Abed Rahman*

## SPINAL CORD AND NEURAXIAL ANALGESIA

The spine consists of cervical, 12 thoracic, 5 lumbar, and 5 sacral vertebrae encompassing the spinal cord. These vertebrae and their corresponding landmarks (see Box 5.1) can be used to provide precise neuraxial anesthesia to

specific regions, spanning from the thoracic cavity to the lower extremities. During a cesarean section the incision usually extends no further than the T10 dermatome (umbilicus), but epidural coverage is usually provided up to the T4 dermatome (nipple line), which helps provide analgesia to visceral plexus stimulated by peritoneal stretch during uterine manipulation. In contrast to spinal anesthesia,

**Box 5.1** VERTEBRAL LEVELS AND PERTINENT CORRESPONDING ANATOMY

IMPORTANT LANDMARKS

| | |
|---|---|
| C7 | Vertebra prominens, stellate ganglion level |
| T1–T4 | Cardioaccelerator fibers |
| T3 | Axilla level |
| T4 | Nipple line |
| T7 | Xiphoid process |
| T8 | Inferior border of scapula |
| T9–L2 | Origin of artery Adamkiewicz (in 85% of patients) |
| T10 | Umbilicus level |
| T12–L4 | Lumbar plexus |
| L1 | Celiac plexus |
| L2 | Caudal end of spinal cord (adults) |
| L3 | Caudal end of spinal cord (pediatrics) |
| L4 | Iliac crest |
| L4–S3 | Sacral plexus |
| S2 | Posterior superior iliac spine, caudal end of subarachnoid space in adults |
| S3 | Caudal end of subarachnoid space in pediatrics |
| S4 | Sacral hiatus |

thoracic epidurals can often be used to provide analgesia in surgeries where a large thoracic or upper abdominal incision is required.[1-5] The spinal epidural space and the ligamentum flavum extend from the foramen magnum to the sacral hiatus.[3] The anterior border of the epidural space is formed by the posterior longitudinal ligaments and the lateral border by the intervertebral foramina and pedicles. Its posterior border is the ligamentum flavum. *Spinal anesthesia* is most often administered below the L3–L4 level in an adult patient and at the L4–L5 level in a pediatric patient (over 1 year) to avoid trauma to the spinal cord during needle insertion.[1] In adults a circumferential line drawn from superior edge of both iliac crests will signify the L3–L4 interspace. In pediatrics the L4–L5 or L5–S1 interspace may be used by counting down the spinous processes from the L4 interspace. When using a midline approach through this space, one will pass through the following layers: skin, subcutaneous tissue, supraspinous ligament, interspinous ligament, ligamentum flavum, epidural space, dura matter, and arachnoid membrane.[1,3]

## LUMBAR REGION

The *lumbar plexus* originates from the anterior rami of L1–L4 but often can also contain branches from both T12 and L5. The lumbar plexus lies within the psoas compartment between the psoas major and quadratus lumborum and forms both the femoral and obturator nerves.

The *femoral* originates from the posterior divisions of L2–L4. Lateral femoral cutaneous is formed from L2–L3.

The *obturator* originates from anterior divisions of L2–L4.

## SACRUM

*Sacral plexus* nerve roots originate from L4–S3 level and later become two nerves that are relevant for lower extremity surgery: the sciatic nerve and posterior cutaneous nerve; the sciatic being a derivative from the L4–S3 level and the posterior cutaneous origin being S1–S3.[3]

### SCIATIC DIVISION

The sciatic is composed of two separate nerves within a shared sheath: the *tibial* and the *common peroneal*.

The *tibial* originates from the ventral branches of the anterior rami at the L4–S3 levels. The *common peroneal* originates from the dorsal branches of the anterior rami of L4–S3.

The sciatic nerve reaches the lower extremity initially by passing through the sacrosciatic foramen just inferior to the piriformis muscle.[3] It is then stationed between the greater trochanter of the femur and the ischial tuberosity.

Caudal epidural placement is a common practice used during pediatric anesthesia and anorectal surgery in adults. *Sacral hiatus* connects with the lumbar spinal cord and houses the terminal end of the cauda equina, epidural venous plexus, and meninges. The sacral hiatus lies just below the fourth sacral spinous tubercle and is created by the unfused S4–S5 laminae. This hiatus can be palpated as a step-off just above the coccyx and between the sacral cornua (two prominences that flank the hiatus). It can also be located by forming a triangle between the posterior superior iliac spines superiorly with the inferior apex being the sacral hiatus.[3] To enter this space, the physician gains passage through the sacrococcygeal ligament, which may be difficult in adult patients due to calcifications.[3]

## REFERENCES

1. Olawin AM, M Das J. Spinal anesthesia. [Updated July 3, 2020]. In: *StatPearls* [Internet]. Treasure Island, FL: StatPearls; 2020 Jan–. Available from: https://www.ncbi.nlm.nih.gov/books/NBK537299/.

2. Freeman BS, Berger JS. *Anesthesiology Core Review.* New York, NY: McGraw-Hill Education Medical; 2014.

3. Butterworth JF, et al. *Morgan and Mikhail's Clinical Anesthesiology.* New York, NY, McGraw-Hill Education Medical; 2018.

4. Ahmed A, Attia Mohamed Kassem M. Thoracic spinal anesthesia: To do or not to do! *Integr Anesthesiol.* 2018;1(1):001–003.

5. Manion SC, Brennan TJ. Thoracic epidural analgesia and acute pain management. *Anesthesiology.* 2011;115:181–188.

# 6.

# EXTREMITIES

*Jeffrey W. Cannon and Mada Helou*

## INTRODUCTION

Anatomy, particularly of the extremities, is very pertinent to the daily practice of anesthesiology. The anesthesiologist must have a good understanding of landmarks, i.e., comprehend how the observed surface anatomy correlates with underlying structures. In this chapter, the basics of the anatomy of the extremities will be explored to better understand the arteries, veins, and nerves and their usual course. Particular attention will be given to using physical exam skills to identify these landmarks and assess how to incorporate these data into a successful anesthetic plan.

## UPPER EXTREMITY

The shoulder is composed of the clavicle, scapula, and proximal humerus. These three bones articulate with a neurovascular bundle running nearby from the neck to the arm via the axilla. Also, the muscles of the neck, chest, and arm have various insertions and attachments in this region. The landmarks seen on physical exam of the shoulder in the standard anatomical position are as follows: the distal end of the acromion of the scapula along the posterior aspect of the shoulder, the distal end of the coracoid process of the scapula along the anterior aspect of the shoulder, and the greater tubercle of the humerus as the lateral prominence of the shoulder. It is important for the anesthesiologist to understand the topographical anatomy for injections in the glenohumeral joint and for performing a suprascapular peripheral nerve block.

The axilla is a conduit leading from the neck to the arm. The neurovascular bundles from the great vessels and the spinal cord run through the axilla as the axillary artery, axillary vein, and brachial plexus. The landmark structures of the axilla are the clavicle, under and along which the neurovascular bundle courses; and the deltohumeral groove, in which the cephalic vein lies, leading back to the axillary vein. The clavicle is a landmark important for various brachial plexus peripheral nerve blocks (supraclavicular, infraclavicular, etc).The deltohumeral groove can be palpated to approximate the point at which the cephalic vein joins the axillary vein on its way to the subclavian vein, thus marking a key point in the placement of a subclavian central venous catheter.[1]

The arm is the portion of the upper extremity from the shoulder to the elbow. The humerus is the bony framework of the arm. They key topographical anatomy is the point on the medial arm at which the biceps brachii and triceps brachii meet. In this groove, the brachial artery can be palpated.

The elbow and cubital fossa are made up of the humerus, radius, and ulna. The key topographical landmarks of this region are the antecubital fossa in which vascular access can often be achieved by means of the antecubital vein, and the brachial artery can be auscultated during the measuring of noninvasive blood pressure.[1]

The forearm is the portion of the upper extremity made up by the bony framework of the radius and the ulna. The key topographical landmarks of the forearm are the radial artery, which can be palpated for pulse monitoring or accessed with an arterial catheter for invasive monitoring of blood pressure. Typically, the artery is best palpated and accessed at the distal, anterior portion of the radius with the hand extended in order to bring the radial artery more superficial.[2]

The hand is the distal end of the upper extremity, made up of nearly 30 different bones. The key topographical features of the hand are the dorsal venous arch and the metacarpophalangeal (MCP) joints. On the dorsal surface of the hand is the dorsal venous arch, in which intravenous catheters can be placed for vascular access. The MCP joints can be identified by palpating the region where the individual phalanges meet the rest of the hand. This is the region around which local anesthetic can be injected to perform a digital peripheral nerve block.

## LOWER EXTREMITY

The gluteal region is contained inferior to the posterior iliac crest, posterior to the greater trochanter of the femur, and superior to the inferior gluteal fold. The key topographical landmarks of the gluteal region are the posterior superior iliac spine, ischial tuberosity, and greater trochanter. The posterior superior iliac spine can be palpated just lateral to the S2 spinous process. The ischial tuberosity can be palpated at the point where the gluteus meets a surface in the standard sitting position. The greater trochanter is the extrusion of the femur palpated at the extension of the midaxillary line. These are all important landmarks for performing subgluteal sciatic nerve blocks.[1,2]

The thigh is the region of the lower extremity that begins at the inguinal fold and continues to the knee. The femur makes up the bony framework. The key topographical anatomy of the thigh is the inguinal crease. Near the inguinal crease is the inguinal ligament, which can be identified by palpation along a line formed from the anterior superior iliac spine and the pubic symphysis. Just inferior and medial to the inguinal ligament is the femoral triangle, in which the femoral artery can be palpated. Situated from lateral to medial within the femoral triangle are the femoral nerve, femoral artery, femoral vein, and femoral lymphatics.

These vessels can be used for central venous access, arterial monitoring, and catheterization during procedures.

The knee is the region of the lower extremity where the femur articulates with the tibia and fibula. The key topographical landmarks are the patella, popliteal fossa, and patellar tendon. The patella can be seen and palpated as the irregularly round protrusion on the anterior surface of the knee. The popliteal fossa is palpated at the crease in the skin on the posterior surface of the knee. Within this fossa, the popliteal artery can be palpated, and a popliteal peripheral nerve block can be performed. The patellar tendon can be seen and palpated medially and inferior to the patella. The space felt immediately inferior and lateral to the patella is a site of potential injection into the synovial capsule of the knee joint.

The leg is made up of the region of the lower extremity from the knee to the ankle and includes the bony framework of the tibia and fibula. The important topographical anatomy of the leg are the tibial tuberosity and the tarsal tunnel. The tibial tuberosity can be seen and palpated inferior to the patellar ligament. Medial to this is a flat region of the tibia. This is a site which can be used for intraosseous catheter placement. The tarsal tunnel can be seen and palpated immediately posterior to the medial malleolus of the tibia. The tarsal tunnel is where the posterior tibial artery can be palpated.

The foot is made up of nearly 30 bones at the distal portion of the lower extremity. The key topographical landmarks of the foot are the metatarsophalangeal (MTP) joints. The MTP joints can be identified by palpating the region where the individual phalanges meet the rest of the foot. This is the region around which local anesthetic can be injected to perform a digital peripheral nerve block.

## REFERENCES

1. Drake R, et al. *Gray's Anatomy for Students.* 2nd edition. Churchill Livingstone (Elsevier); 2010:628–637, 777–785.
2. Bickley LS. *Bates' Guide to Physical Examination and History Taking.* 11th edition. Lippincott, Williams, & Wilkens; 2013:615–662.

# 7.

# DERMATOME ANATOMY

*Derek Shirey and Bryan Matusic*

## BASIC ANATOMY

Sensory information is relayed to the central nervous system by way of sensory neurons. The cell bodies of sensory neurons are located in the dorsal root ganglion (DRG) at each spinal level and convey sensory inputs from the corresponding skin distribution as shown in Figure 7.1. Dermatomal maps have defined local anesthetic injections at a single DRG and subsequent mapping of observed analgesic distribution. Myotomes are defined by neurons which travel through the ventral root at each spinal level and act on muscles to produce movement.

## DERMATOMAL MAPPING WITH ASSOCIATED ANATOMICAL LANDMARKS

### HEAD AND NECK

*Trigeminal nerve* (cranial nerve [CN] V1–V3): Skin of the face, including the forehead (V1), maxilla (V2), and mandible (V3)

*Cervical plexus* (C2–C4): Skin over the anterior and posterior portion of the ear, angle of the mandible, the neck, and posterior aspect of the head

*Greater occipital nerve* (C2), *third occipital nerve* (C3), and C4–C6: Posterior aspect of head (C2) and posterior aspect of neck (C3, C4–C6).

### TRUNK

T3: Third intercostal space

T4: Nipple line

T6: Level of the xiphoid process

T10: Level of the umbilicus

T12: Midpoint of inguinal ligament

L1: Groin area just inferior to inguinal ligament.

## UPPER EXTREMITIES

C5: Lateral aspect of arm extending just proximal to the elbow

C6: Lateral forearm and thumb

C7: Middle finger

C8: Little finger and medial forearm

T1: Medial arm extending proximally from the elbow to the axilla.

## LOWER EXTREMITIES AND GENITALIA

L2: Anterior and medial aspect of thigh

L3: Lateral thigh extending distally to the medial aspect of the knee

L4: Posterolateral thigh extending distally over the knee to the medial aspect of the leg involving the medial malleolus

L5: Posterolateral thigh extending distally over the lateral aspect of knee involving the anterior aspect of leg and dorsum of foot

S1: Heel, lateral malleolus, lateral foot, and lateral aspect of posterior thigh

S3: Medial aspect of buttock, penis, and scrotum

S5: Anus.

## MYOTOMES WITH ASSOCIATED MOTOR FUNCTION

C1–C2: Neck flexion and extension

C4: Shoulder elevation

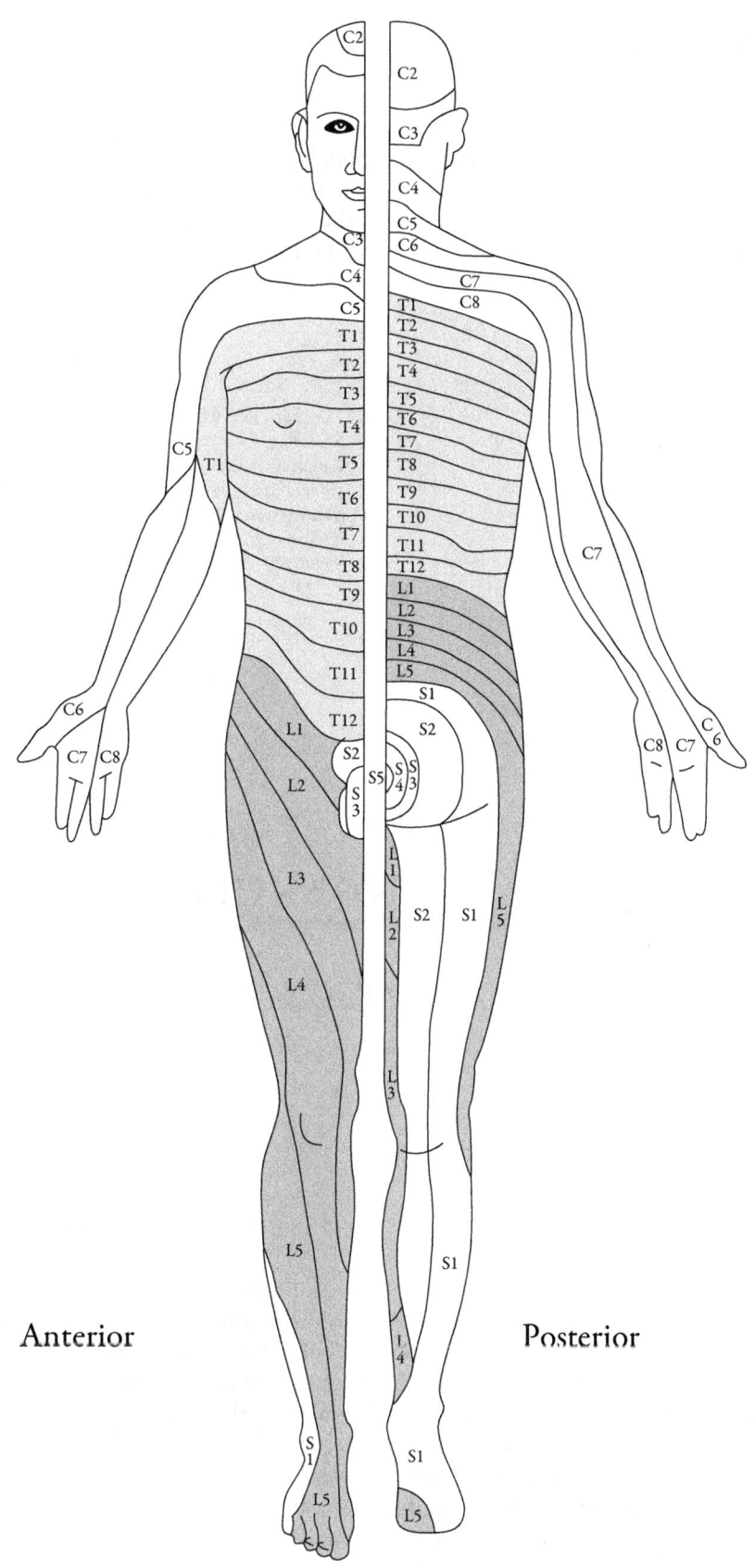

**Figure 7.1.** Sensory dermatome map.

Reproduced with permission from Mayer SA, Marshall RS, *On Call Neurology*, 3rd ed. Elsevier Books; 2007.

Anterior

Posterior

C5: Shoulder abduction and external rotation, elbow flexion

C6: Elbow flexion, wrist extension

C7: Elbow extension, wrist flexion, finger extension

C8: Finger flexion

T1: Finger abduction

L2: Hip flexion

L3: Knee extension

L4–L5: Inversion and dorsiflexion of the foot

S1: Eversion and plantarflexion of the foot, hip extension

S2: Knee flexion

S3–S4: Anal wink.[2,3]

## ANESTHETIC CONSIDERATIONS

Dermatomal anatomy has direct application in the preoperative setting, guiding the selection of appropriate regional nerve blocks, interventional pain procedures, and neuraxial anesthesia. The procedures provide focused anesthetic and analgesic effects directed at a specific area of the body to ensure proper analgesic effect in affected regions of the body.

## REFERENCES

1. Marshall RS, Mayer SA. *On Call Neurology*. Philadelphia, PA: Saunders/Elsevier; 2007.
2. Ladak A, et al. Mapping sensory nerve communications between peripheral nerve territories. *Clin Anat*. 2013;27(5):681–690.
3. Schwartzman R. Basic principles for the sensory examination. *Neurol Exam*. 2006 Jan;2:153–167. doi:10.1002/9780470753262.ch7.

# 8.

# BRAIN AND SKULL

*Nathan Liu and Tariq M. Malik*

## INTRODUCTION

A basic knowledge of skull and head anatomy, including familiarity with basic radiologic modalities of imaging, is helpful for anesthetic planning and considerations. The knowledge is useful when providing anesthetic care to a neurosurgical case. The detailed knowledge of anatomy is much more important for a chronic pain practioner who practices injection techniques for head and neck pain. The implications for airway management are most significantly impacted by abnormalities in the head and skull anatomy, and a working basic knowledge of this anatomy, as well as imaging, is important in a providing safe and effective anesthetic and post-procedural care to a critically ill patient.

## OSSEOUS ANATOMY OF THE SKULL

The skull consists of the cranium and the mandible. The cranium is a rounded structure with a top part made of flat bone. The skull is composed of 22 bones and is divided into two regions: the neurocranium (which protects the brain), and the viscero-cranium (which forms the face). The main bones are the frontal bone, a pair of parietal bones, a pair of temporal bones, sphenoid bones, zygomatic bones, and occipital bones. The cranial bones are joined by fibrous joints called sutures. The main sutures seen on the skull are coronal suture, sagittal suture, and lambda suture. The *pterion* is the meeting point/junction of the frontal, parietal, temporal, and sphenoid bones. The *asterion* is the articulation of the parietal, temporal, and occipital bones.[1] The midline meeting point of the frontal bone and the two parietal bones is called the *bregma*, the site of the anterior fontanelle. The parietal bones have holes through which emissary veins connect the sagittal sinus to scalp veins. The midline meeting point where the sagittal suture meet with the occipital bone is called the *lambda*. The lambda suture often contains small bones with the suture called *Wormian bones*. Further posteriorly, around 6 cm along the midline, the occipital bone has a small protuberance, called the external occipital protuberance. The superior nuchal line extends laterally from this protuberance toward the mastoid process. The line is the demarcation point where the scalp ends and the neck begins; the tentorium cerebelli is attached to the skull on the inside, and the transverse sinus is present along this line on the inside, while on the outside, the trapezius and sternocleidomastoid muscles are attached to the skull along this line on the outside (Figure 8.1).

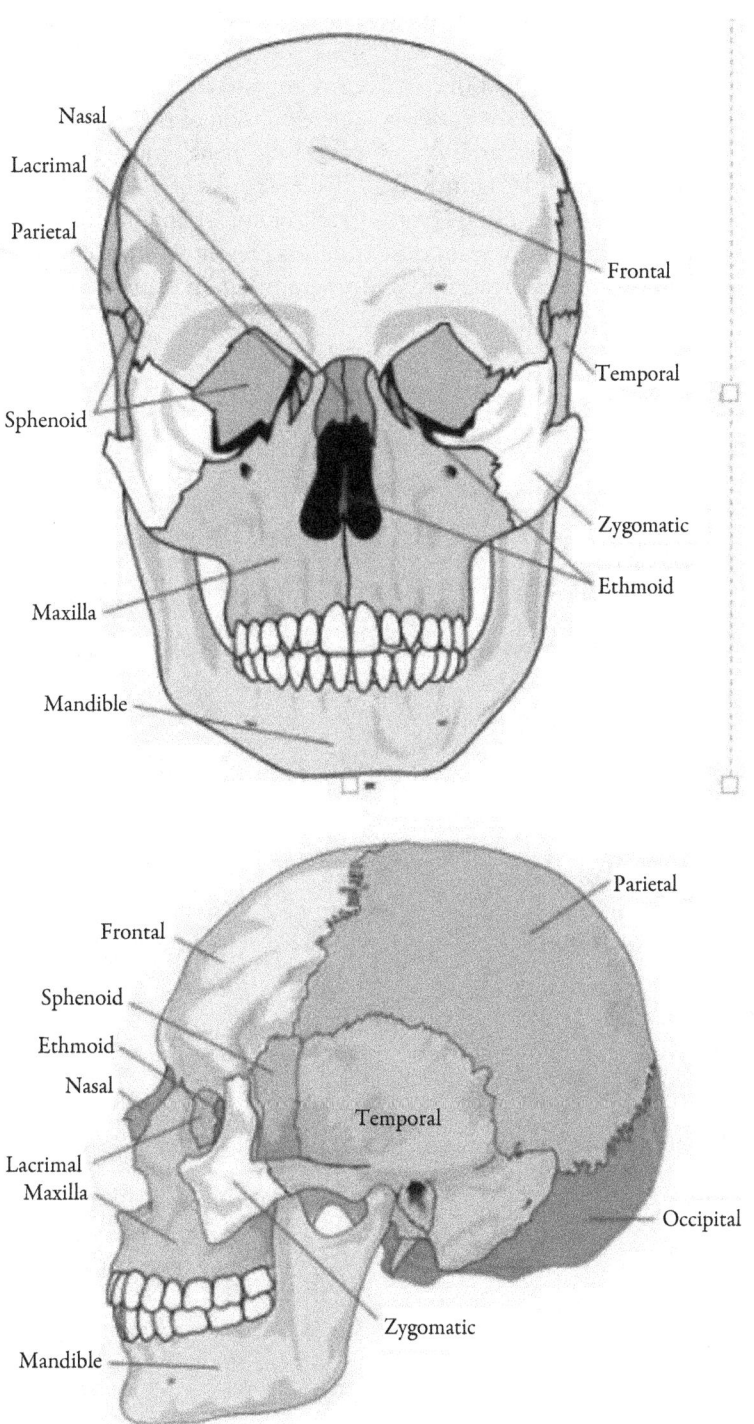

**Figure 8.1.** Bones of the skull.

Inferiorly, the foramen magnum is part of the occipital bone. Superior and inferior nuchal lines are visible on the undersurface and are concentric with the foramen magnum. The occipital condyles are kidney shaped on each side of the foramen, and are part of the ball-and-socket atlanto-occipital joints. The pharyngeal tubercle is present in front of the foramen magnum, to which fibers of pharyngeal fascia and superior constrictor muscles are attached. The prevertebral fascia and prevertebral muscles (longus capitus and rectus capitus anterior) are attached to the base of the skull behind the ridge. Important foramens in the base of skull are jugular foramen (internal jugular vein, 9th, 10th and 11th cranial nerves), carotid canal (internal carotid artery), foramen ovale (mandibular nerve, emissary veins, lesser petrosal nerve, accessory meningeal artery), and foramen spinosum (middle meningeal vessels) (Figure 8.2).[2]

The inside of the base of the skull has three fossae; the anterior fossa houses the frontal lobe, the middle fossa contains the temporal lobes, and the posterior fossa contains the cerebellum and brainstem. The roof of the posterior fossa is formed by tentorium cerebelli, a dural reflection. The 6th nerve often gets stretched at the free edge of the tentorium cerebelli and gets damaged.

The major osseous structures of the head and skull that primarily concern anesthetic management consist of the mandible, maxilla, and nasal bones. The maxilla is the bony structure that encompasses the nares and is the root of the upper incisors and molars. The mandible is the most inferior bony structure of the head, and anchors the lower teeth. The primary routes of airway management are generally orotracheal and nasotracheal, and thus, knowledge of the normal anatomy of these osseous structures is imperative for anesthesiologists. Care must be taken to avoid hyperextension of the temporomandibular joint (TMJ) with the "scissoring" maneuver during direct laryngoscopy to decrease risks of TMJ dislocation. Furthermore, when facial trauma or anomalous anatomy (pathologic or congenital) is present in a patient, careful examination of airway anatomy and possible imaging will be helpful in successful airway management.

**Outer surface**

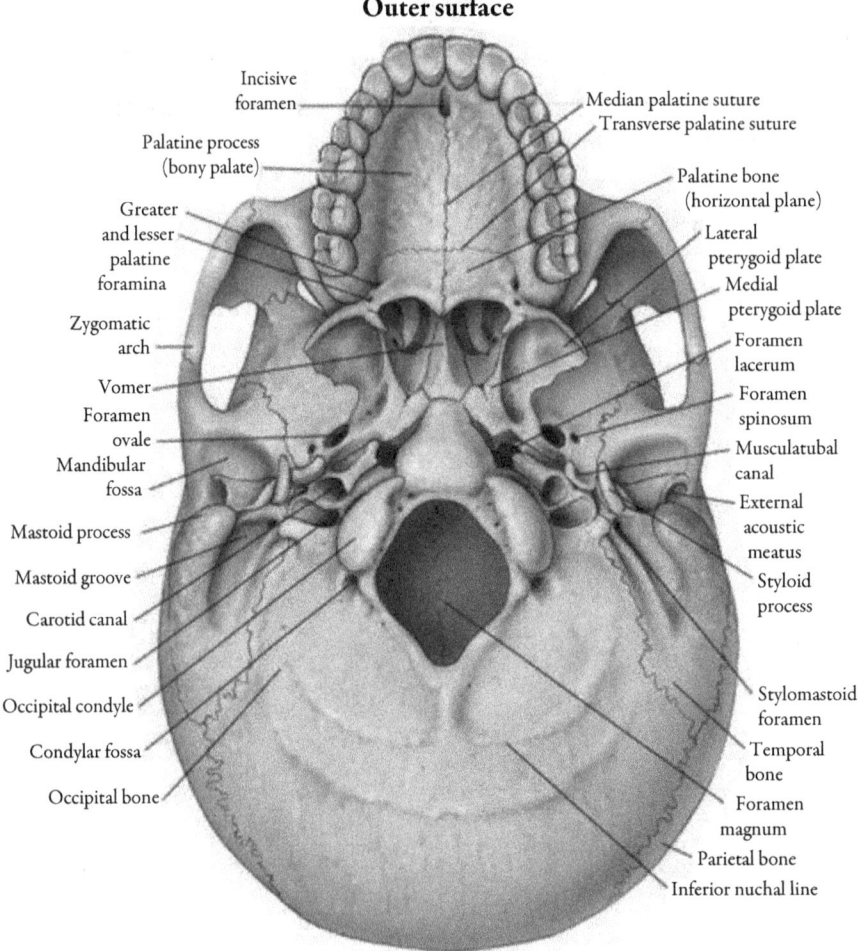

Incisive foramen — Median palatine suture — Transverse palatine suture — Palatine process (bony palate) — Palatine bone (horizontal plane) — Greater and lesser palatine foramina — Lateral pterygoid plate — Medial pterygoid plate — Foramen lacerum — Zygomatic arch — Foramen spinosum — Vomer — Foramen ovale — Musculatubal canal — Mandibular fossa — External acoustic meatus — Mastoid process — Styloid process — Mastoid groove — Carotid canal — Jugular foramen — Stylomastoid foramen — Occipital condyle — Temporal bone — Condylar fossa — Foramen magnum — Occipital bone — Parietal bone — Inferior nuchal line

Figure 8.2. Base of the skull.

## VASCULAR ANATOMY OF THE HEAD AND SKULL

Arterial blood supply to the head and skull is primarily provided by the common carotid arteries and its branches, as well as the vertebral arteries, posteriorly.[3,4] Venous drainage is predominantly carried by the internal jugular veins. These vessels have significant involvement primarily in the form of central venous cannulations. Knowledge of this anatomy and both landmark-based and ultrasound-guided cannulation techniques are valuable to anesthesiologists.

### CIRCLE OF WILLIS AND MAJOR BLOOD VESSELS OF THE BRAIN

1. ACA
2. MCA
3. PCA
4. Vertebral
5. Basilar
6. Superior cerebellar
7. Anterior inferior cerebellar
8. Anterior communicating
9. Posterior communicating (see Figure 8.3 for an illustration of the circle of Willis).

General knowledge of perfusion territories of major blood vessels is helpful for perioperative management of patients at risk for intracranial events. Motor deficits will localize to contralateral hemispheres. Speech deficits generally localize to L-hemisphere lesions. Coordination and balance deficits localize to the posterior circulation (Figure 8.4).

The circle of Willis plays a significant role in collateral circulation during situations where arterial flow is occluded (i.e., carotid endarterectomy).

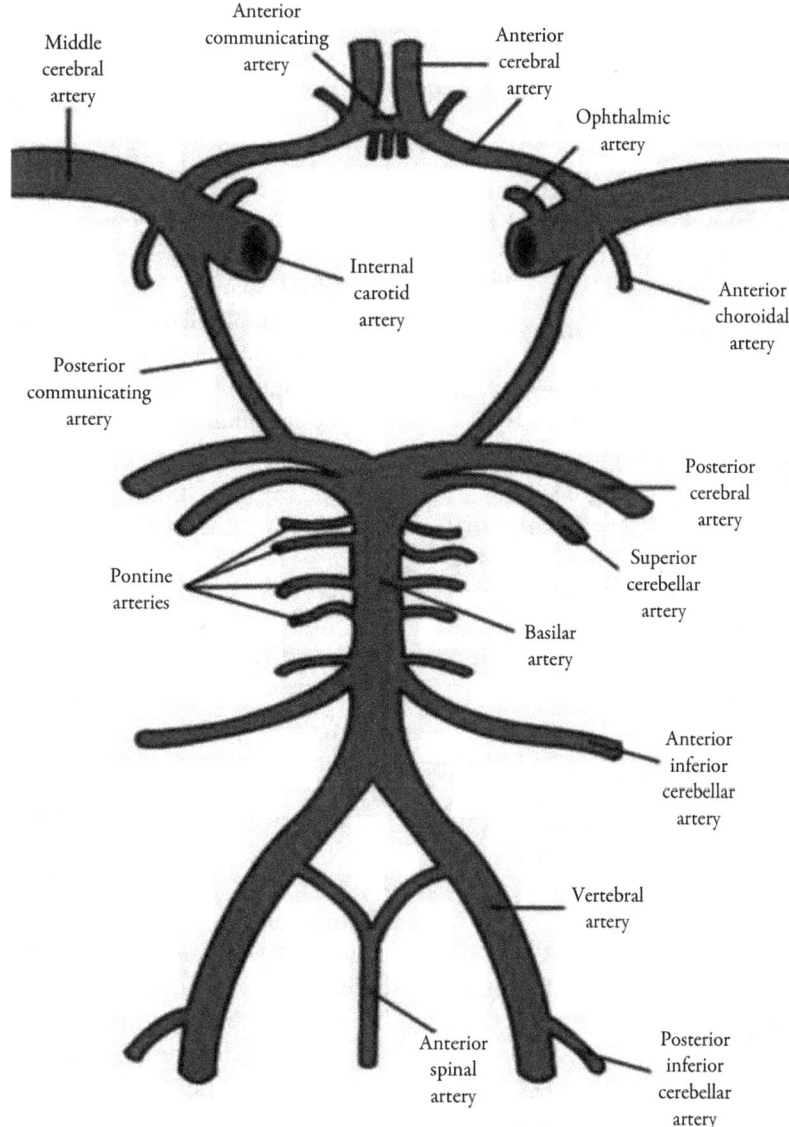

**Figure 8.3.** Circle of Willis.

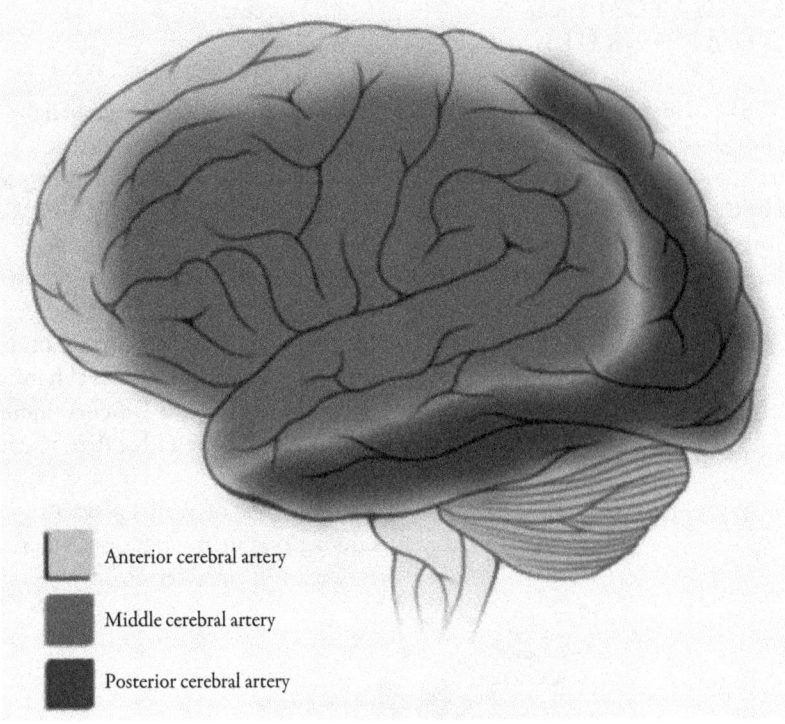

**Figure 8.4.** Cerebral vascular territories.

Anterior cerebral artery

Middle cerebral artery

Posterior cerebral artery

## NEUROLOGICAL ANATOMY OF THE HEAD AND SKULL

1. Triencephalon (cerebrum)[4]
   - Cerebral hemispheres
   - The center of higher-level thought, speech, abstract thinking, reasoning
   - Primary sensory cortex–postcentral gyrus
   - Primary motor cortex–precentral gyrus
   - Broca's area: prefrontal lobe (expressive dysphasia)
   - Wernicke's area: temporal lobe (receptive dysphasia)
   - Limbic system: set of structures involved with emotion, affective and behavioral aspect, also regulating endocrine and autonomic system
   - Components of limbic system: amygdala, hippocampus/parahippocampus, thalamus, hypothalamus, basal ganglia, and cingulate gyrus
   - Basal ganglia
   - Include the caudate, putamen, globus pallidus, and work in conjunction as a "relay station" between the cerebrum and thalamus to coordinate movement
2. Diencephalon
   - Thalamus
   - Involved in motor control and sleep-wake cycles
   - Major sensory relay station
   - Hypothalamus
   - Major autonomic and endocrine functions, regulating hunger, thirst, temperature, emotion (rage), as well as direct control of antidiuretic hormone (ADH) and oxytocin and indirect control of pituitary hormones
3. Brainstem
   - Comprised of midbrain, pons, medulla
   - Cranial nerve nuclei originate here (except I and II)
4. Cerebellum
   - Coordination of speech, motor, balance, posture.

## EMBRYOLOGY

The skull is derived from ectoderm (frontal bone, ethmoid bone, and sphenoid bone) and mesoderm (parietal bones and occipital bone). The temporal bones derive from both mesoderm and neural crest.

## PHYSIOLOGIC VARIANTS: FONTANELLES AND SUTURES

There are six fontanelles; the anterior and posterior are the largest. The anterior closes at age 1–2 years and hardens to become the *bregma*; the posterior closes at 6–8 weeks and becomes the *lambda*. There is a great deal of variation in the timing of the closure of individual sutures. The sagittal suture is first to close at around age 20, followed by the coronal suture, then the lambdoid at around the mid-20s; the squamous sutures close at about age 60.

## REFERENCES

1. Anderson BW, et al. Anatomy, head and neck, skull. [Updated July 27, 2020]. In: *StatPearls*. Treasure Island, FL: StatPearls; 2020 Jan–. Available from: https://www.ncbi.nlm.nih.gov/books/NBK499 834/?report=classic.

2. Sinnatamby SS. *Last's Anatomy: Regional and Applied*. 12th ed. Churchill Livingstone, 2011.
3. Ellis H, et al. *Clinical Anatomy: Applied Anatomy for Students and Junior Doctors*. 14th ed. New York, NY: Wiley and Sons; 2018.
4. Barash P. *Clinical Anesthesia Fundamentals*. 8th ed. Wolters Kluwer Health; 2017.

# 9.

# SPINE ANATOMY

*Wenyu Pan and Tariq M. Malik*

## INTRODUCTION

Knowledge of the spine anatomy is required for the safe and proficient administration of spinal and epidural anesthesia as well safe performance of regional anesthesia techniques around the spine. The spine consists of 7 cervical, 12 thoracic, 5 lumbar, 5 sacral, and 4 coccygeal vertebrae.[1] The sacral and coccygeal vertebrae are fused into the sacrum and the coccyx. These vertebrae form the body's basic structural support and enclose and protect the spinal cord which extends from the midbrain to approximately the second lumbar level in adults and continues caudally as the cauda equina.

## BASIC STRUCTURE

The vertebral column in its simplistic form consists of a series of vertebrae separated by discs and bound together by a network of ligaments. A typical vertebra has a body and a neural arch with three bony processes sticking out of the neural arch. The midline process is called spinous process (SP), and a side process on each side is called transverse process (TP). The neural arch between the transverse process and the spinous process is called the lamina, and the neural arch part between the transverse processes and the vertebral body is called the pedicle (Figure 9.1).

At the junction of lamina and pedicle on each side, two articular processes stick up and down, called superior and inferior articular processes, which articulate with the similar processes from the vertebrae above and below to form a synovial joint, the facet joint. The SP of adjacent vertebrae are connected by supraspinous ligament and interspinous ligament, and the interlaminar is bridged by the ligamentum flavum which runs between laminae of adjacent vertebrae.

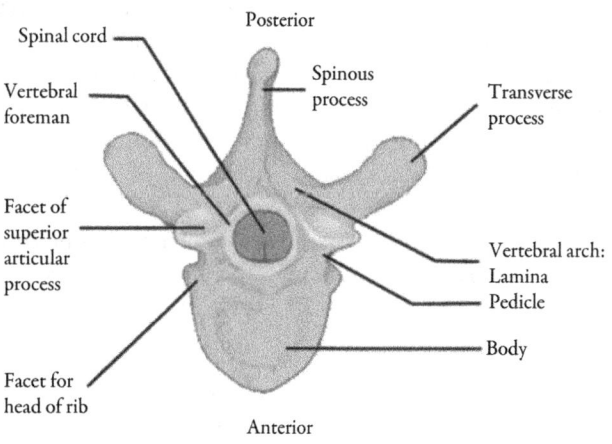

**Figure 9.1.** Anatomy of vertebra.

## VARIATIONS IN VERTEBRAL CONFIGURATION

From the cervical spine to the coccyx, there are regional variations in the shape and size of the vertebrae and in the orientation of the articular facets.

### CERVICAL SPINE

Cervical vertebrae (C1–C6) are characterized by the presence of foramina in their transverse processes, called the foramina transversaria, in which vertebral arteries and sympathetic and venous plexuses pass through.[2] The foramen is absent in the C1, has no spinous process or body, but has TP which extends laterally the most of all the cervical vertebrae transverse processes. Axis, C2, is the strongest cervical vertebra; its dens is a pivot around which the atlas turns and carries the cranium. The dens is kept in place by the transverse ligament of atlas, but if the ligament is damaged by trauma or disease processes (Down's syndrome/rheumatoid arthritis), the dens can damage the spinal cord during neck manipulation. The C2 SP tip is bifid, a useful ultrasound landmark. C6 TP has a very prominent anterior tubercle called the Chassaignac tubercle or carotid tubercle, an important landmark for stellate ganglion block. C7 has the most prominent SP, an important surface landmark, and the basis of C7 being named vertebral prominence. C7 and C2 TP have a rudimentary or absent anterior tubercle.

### THORACIC SPINE

The thoracic vertebral bodies are triangular in shape, with short pedicle. The TP of the thoracic vertebrae are long and extend posterolaterally.[2] Both the TP and the bodies have costal facets for articulation with the ribs. The TPs at thoracic level are long and slope posteroinferiorly, partially or even completely overlapping the vertebrae below, and often deviate from midline. The laminae and down sloping TP of T4–T9 thoracic vertebrae overlap, like roof shingles on a house, making access of the thoracic epidural space using midline approach technically challenging. The scapular spine is at the level of T3 spinous process and the tip of scapula around T7. Thoracic SPs below T9 project more dorsally than downward, opening up the interlaminar space for midline epidural space access.

### LUMBAR SPINE

The lumbar vertebrae have larger bodies than the cervical or thoracic vertebrae and shorter SPs than the thoracic vertebrae. The TP are thin and long, projecting directly laterally. The L4 tends to have the smallest TP and L5 the biggest TP. Lumbar rib is present in 8% of the population. The lumbar SPs are big, rectangular in shape, and project straight back in sagittal plane. L5 SP is the smallest of the lumbar SPs. L5–S1 is the largest interspace of the vertebral column—the Taylor approach to spinal anesthesia uses a paramedian approach to the L5–S1 interspace. L4 SP is located by drawing a line at the highest part of iliac crest when performing neuraxial anesthetic technique.

### SACRUM AND COCCYX

The sacrum is a wedge-shaped bone formed by the fusion of 5 vertebrae along with intervertebral discs. There is no TP. The SP of S1–S4 fuse to form a median sacral crest, while S5 SP often fails to fuse, creating an opening, sacral hiatus, which is covered by sacrococcygeal ligament and is pierced to access caudal epidural space. The TP fuse to create lateral sacral rest; fusion of articular processes creates an intermediate sacral crest which is least prominent and hardest to see. The neural foramina are located within bony sacral canal as a lateral opening. The posterior and anterior sacral foramina should not be misinterpreted as interneural foramina.[2] The beak-shaped coccyx consists of 4 fused vertebrae. Sacrum anatomy is highly variable due to variability in the extent of fusion among laminae, TP, and SP.

## EPIDURAL, SUBDURAL, AND SUBARACHNOID SPACES

### EXTENT OF DURAL SAC

In most adults, the spinal cord ends at L1–L2 and the dural sac ends at S2. In 30% of individuals the spinal cord may end at T12, and in 10% it may extend to L3.[3] In most infants, the spinal cord extends to L3, and the dural sac extends to S3–S4.

What tissue layers does the needle go through in the following procedures?

*Midline epidural*: skin, subcutaneous tissue, supraspinous ligament, interspinous ligament, ligamentum flavum, epidural space (Figure 9.2). The "snap" felt just before entering the epidural space is the dense ligamentum flavum.[3]

*Caudal epidural*: skin, subcutaneous tissue, sacrococcygeal ligament, epidural space.[1] The sacrococcygeal ligament covers the sacral hiatus and is related to the ligamentum flavum as it passes inferiorly.

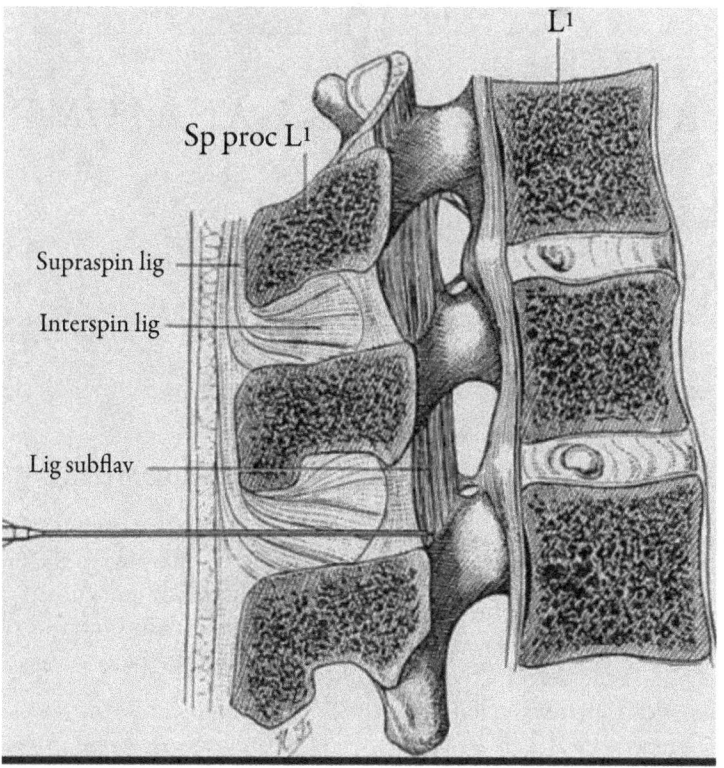

**Figure 9.2.** Anatomy of the spinal ligaments.

## ANESTHETIC CONSIDERATIONS

- In neck flexion, the most prominent midline projection is of C7 SP.
- With arm by the side, the medial end of scapular spine corresponds to T3 SP, while inferior scapular tip corresponds to T7 SP (Figure 9.3).
- The line that connects the lowest part of the rib cage on the back is usually at the level of L1.
- Intercristal line is usually at the level of L4 SP.
- SPs often deviate from midline. Therefore always review imaging if available before performing a neuraxial technique.
- Placing spinal needle at L3 or above can result in spinal cord damage.

## REFERENCES

1. Drasner K, Larson MD. Spinal and epidural anesthesia. In: Miller RD, Pardo MC, eds. *Basics of Anesthesia*. 6th ed. Philadelphia, PA: Elsevier; 2011:252–283.
2. Moore KL, et al. Back. In: Moore KL, Agur AMR, Dalley AF II, eds. *Essential Clinical Anatomy*. 5th ed. Philadelphia, PA: Lippincott Williams & Wilkins; 2015:265–307.
3. Bernards CM, Hostetter LS. Epidural and spinal anesthesia. In: Barash PG, Cullen BF, Stoelting RK, Cahalan MK, Stock MC, Ortega R, eds. *Clinical Anesthesia*. 7th ed. Philadelphia, PA: Lippincott Williams & Williams; 2013:905–933.
4. Jarvik JG, Deyo RA. Diagnostic evaluation of low back pain with emphasis on imaging. *Ann Intern Med*. 2002;137(7):586–597.

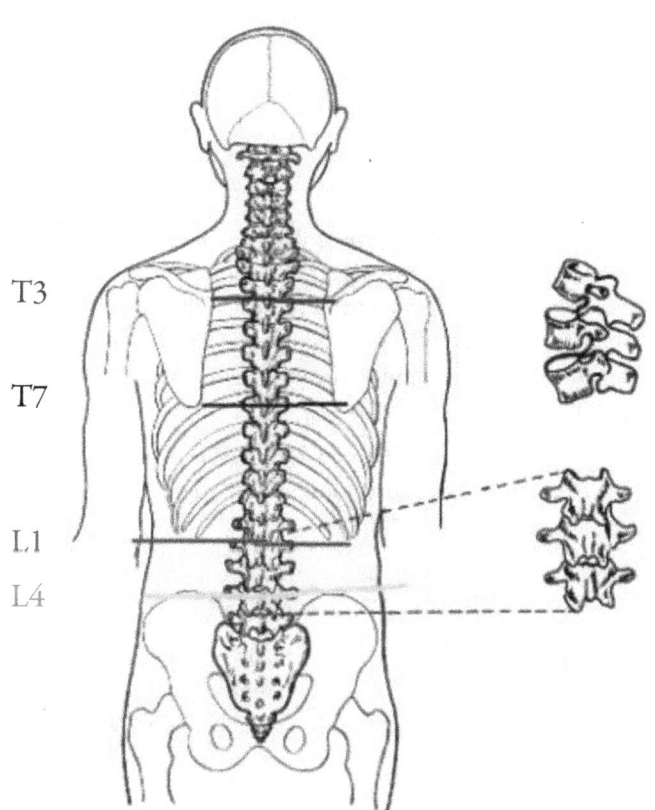

**Figure 9.3.** Anatomical landmarks.

# 10.

# ABDOMINAL WALL ANATOMY

*Wenyu Pan and Dalia Elmofty*

## INTRODUCTION

The abdominal wall is bounded by the costal margin and the xiphoid process superiorly, the inguinal ligament and pelvic bones inferiorly, and extends to the lumbar spine posteriorly.[1] The abdominal wall consists of multiple layers: skin, subcutaneous tissue, superficial fascia, external oblique muscle, internal oblique muscle, transversus abdominis muscle, transversalis fascia, preperitoneal adipose tissue, and peritoneum.[1] Vasculature, nerves, and lymphatics are present throughout these layers.

## ABDOMINAL WALL STRUCTURES

### ABDOMINAL WALL MUSCLES

The muscles of the abdominal wall support and protect the abdominal viscera, control the intra-abdominal pressure, maintain posture, and produce force for physiologic functions, such as defecation, micturition, and parturition.[1]

*Rectus abdominis*: a pair of strap-like muscles that form the anterior abdominal wall. It is mostly enclosed in the rectus sheath. It originates from the xiphoid process and costal cartilages and inserts into the linea alba medially and pubis and pubic crest inferiorly.

*External oblique*: the superficial layer that originates from the external surfaces of the ribs to linea alba, pubic tubercle, and anterior iliac crest.

*Internal oblique*: the middle layer that runs interior to the external oblique. Its fibers run upward and forward.

*Transverse abdominis*: the innermost muscle. Its fibers run horizontally and forward.

*Pyramidalis*: a small triangular muscle that arises from the pubic crest and attaches along the linea alba, anterior to the inferior part of the rectus abdominis.

## ABDOMINAL WALL FASCIA

*Rectus sheath*: a tough fascia spanning from the midclavicular line to the midline. It arises from the sheet-like aponeuroses of the three flat muscles: external oblique, internal oblique, and transversus abdominis.

*Linea alba*: a midline raphe arising from the interweaving aponeuroses of the rectus sheath between the left and right and between the superficial, intermediate, and deep layers. It spans from the xiphoid process to the pubic symphysis.

*Transversalis fascia*: it lies interior to the transversus abdominis and is separated from the peritoneum by a fat layer.

## ABDOMINAL WALL VASCULATURES

The *superior epigastric artery* (a branch of the internal thoracic artery) supplies the upper portion of the rectus abdominis and anastomoses with the inferior epigastric artery (a branch of the external iliac artery) which supplies the lower portion of the rectus muscle.[1]

The *subcostal* and 10th and 11th *posterior intercostals* (branches of the aorta) supply the lateral abdominal wall.

The *musculophrenic artery* supplies the hypochondriac region of the lateral abdominal wall.

The *deep circumflex*, *superficial circumflex*, and *superficial epigastric arteries* supply the inferior abdominal, inguinal, and inferior umbilical areas, respectively.[1]

## ABDOMINAL WALL NERVES

*Thoraco-abdominal nerves* (T7–T11): run between the internal oblique and transversus abdominis. They supply the muscles and overlying skin of the anterolateral abdominal wall from the lower costal area to the level just below the umbilicus.

*Subcostal nerve* (T12): runs inferiorly to the 12th rib and supplies the muscles and overlying skin between the umbilicus superiorly and the iliac crest, inguinal ligament, and pubic crest inferiorly.

*Ilio-hypogastric nerve* (L1): pierces the transversus abdominis muscle and supplies the inferior part of the internal oblique and transversus abdominis muscles along with skin overlying the iliac crest, inguinal, and hypogastric regions.

*Ilio-inguinal nerve* (L1): runs between the internal oblique and transversus abdominis muscles and transverses the inguinal canal. It supplies the skin of the genital area and medial aspect of the thigh, as well as the most inferior part of the internal oblique and transversus abdominis muscles.

## ABDOMINAL WALL NERVE BLOCKS

*Transverse abdominus plane* (TAP) blocks are suitable for lower abdominal surgery, such as appendectomy and abdominal hysterectomy.[2]

*Ilio-inguinal* and *ilio-hypogastric* blocks provide analgesia to the inguinal region and are suitable for inguinal herniorrhaphy and are alternatives to caudal blocks in pediatric patients.[3]

*Rectus sheath* blocks can be used for midline surgical incisions such as umbilical hernia repair and midline laparotomy.[3]

## ULTRASONOGRAPHY FOR ABDOMINAL WALL NERVE BLOCKS

The use of ultrasound can decrease the incidence of adverse events with nerve blocks including block failure, and puncture of surrounding structures including blood vessels and organs. Landmark anatomy can be identified with ultrasonography and can improve the efficacy of nerve blocks.

### ULTRASOUND TECHNIQUE

*TAP block*: Transducer is placed between the iliac crest and costal margin; local anesthetic is injected in the fascial plane between the internal oblique and transversus abdominis (Figure 10.1)

*Ilio-inguinal and ilio-hypogastric blocks*: Transducer is placed at the level of the iliac crest. The nerves can be seen between the internal oblique and transversus abdominis.[3]

*Rectus sheath block*: Transducer is placed above the umbilicus. The needle is advanced between the rectus abdominis muscle and the posterior rectus sheath.[3]

### ANESTHETIC CONSIDERATIONS

#### PREOPERATIVE

Regional anesthesia of the abdominal wall can provide perioperative analgesia and should be incorporated into the multimodal perioperative pain management plan. Various limitations may exist given underlying comorbidities.

#### INTRAOPERATIVE

The surgical team should be informed of the total amount of local anesthetic administered during the nerve block to

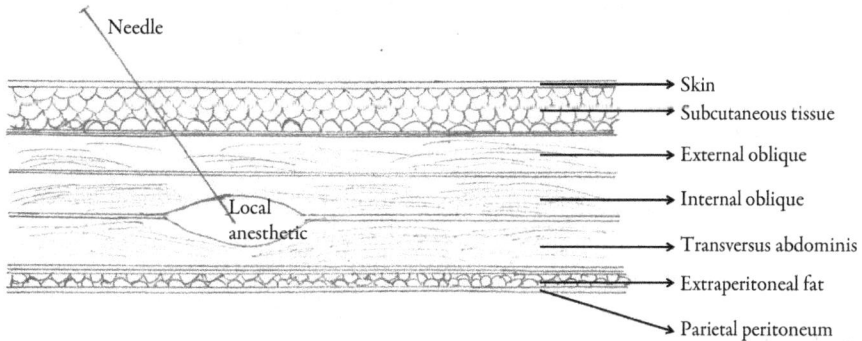

**Figure 10.1.** Illustration of the transversus abdominis plane block. The needle is seen in the fascial plane between the internal oblique and the transversus abdominis muscles, hydro-dissecting the fascial plane with local anesthetic deposition.

prevent inadvertent administration of supratherapeutic doses of local anesthetic.

## POSTOPERATIVE

Complications can occur with abdominal wall blocks. Peritoneal puncture, bowel perforation, vascular injury, and liver hematoma have been reported after TAP blocks.[2] Inadvertent block of the femoral nerve has been reported with ilio-inguinal and ilio-hypogastric blocks.[2] Incomplete analgesia can result due to anatomical variance, for example, of the anterior cutaneous nerves in 30% of the population.[3]

## REFERENCES

1. Moore KL, et al. *Essential Clinical Anatomy.* 5th ed. Philadelphia, PA: Lippincott Williams & Wilkins; 2015.
2. Horlocker TT, et al. Peripheral nerve blocks. In: Miller RD, ed. *Miller's Anesthesia.* 8th ed. Philadelphia, PA: Elsevier; 2015:1721–1751.
3. Yarwood J, Berrill A. Nerve blocks of the anterior abdominal wall. *Cont Educ Anaesth Crit Care Pain.* 2010;10(6):182–186.

# 11.

# UPPER EXTREMITY

*Amit Samba and Alexandria Nickless*

## INTRODUCTION

Upper extremity anatomy includes structures connecting to the shoulder girdle, arm, elbow, forearm, hand, and fingers. Compared to the lower extremity, the upper limb has a wider range of motion, denser sensory innervation, and finer control of movement. Formulating an anesthetic plan for surgery and nerve blockade of the upper extremity requires a deep understanding of the anatomy to prevent any postoperative complications.

## BONES

See Figure 11.1 for a depiction of the upper extremity skeleton.

## VASCULATURE

### BASILIC VEIN

- Medial to biceps brachii muscle tendon
- Courses from medial posterior forearm to anterior elbow.

### CEPHALIC VEIN

- Lateral to biceps tendon
- Begins at lateral wrist and courses lateral to biceps brachii muscle to anterior deltoid before joining with axillary vein inferior to clavicle.

### AXILLARY ARTERY

- Begins at first rib originating from subclavian artery
- Courses laterally to become brachial artery.

### BRACHIAL ARTERY

- Continuation of axillary artery that can be palpated medial to biceps brachii tendon in antecubital fossa
- Distally bifurcates into radial (lateral) and ulnar (medial) arteries.[1]

## INNERVATION

### BRACHIAL PLEXUS

- Originates from ventral rami of C5–T1 with occasional contribution from C4 and T2

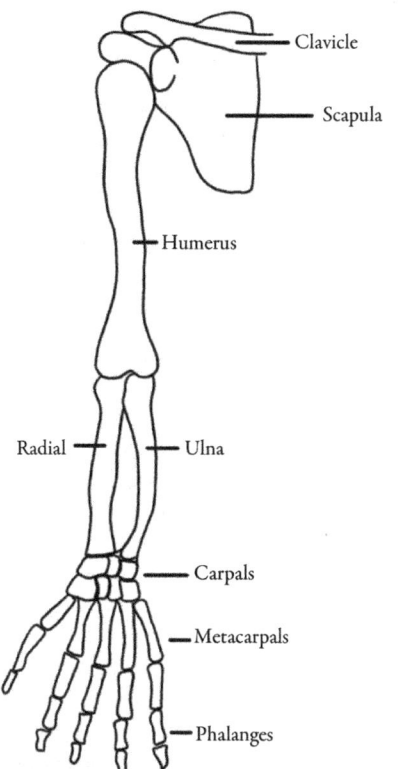

**Figure 11.1.** Anatomy of upper skeleton.
Reproduced with permission from Schünke M, Schulte E, Schumacher U, *Atlas of Anatomy*, 2nd ed. Thieme; 2015.

- After exiting the spinal column, C5–T1 *roots* form the superior (C5-6), middle (C7), and inferior *trunks* (C8–T1) which are located between the anterior and middle scalene muscles.
  - The superior trunk gives rise to the suprascapular nerve which innervates most of the shoulder.[1]
  - Interscalene nerve block is performed here; inferior trunk is usually spared. This can be overcome by increased volume.[2,3]
- The trunks are split into anterior and posterior *divisions*.
- The divisions are combined into lateral, medial, and posterior *cords* which are named after their orientation to subclavian artery.[1]
  - Infraclavicular nerve block usually covers all of the cords.[2]
- The cords further form the terminal *branches*: musculocutaneous, axillary, radial, median, and ulnar nerves.[1]
  - Axillary nerve block is performed here[2] (Figure 11.2) (Table 11.1).

## DERMATOMAL DISTRIBUTION

See Figure 11.3 and Table 11.2 for the dermatomal distribution.

C6: thumb

C7: middle finger

C8: 5th finger

T1: medial/lateral forearm[1]

## ANESTHETIC CONSIDERATIONS

### PREOPERATIVE

- Assessment of patient's preexisting neurovascular status and risk factors for intraoperative neuropathies should be documented.
  - Risk factors include: diabetes mellitus, obesity, male gender, alcohol abuse, peripheral vascular disease, preexisting peripheral neuropathy, and arthritis.
- Fall on outstretched hand can frequently cause:
  - Fracture to scaphoid leading to avascular necrosis
  - Dislocation to lunate leading to impingement on carpal tunnel and median nerve
- Reconstruction of ulnar collateral ligament has risk of injuring ulnar nerve due to proximity to medial epicondyle.
- During clavicular fracture, suprascapular nerve can be frequently injured, leading to weakness and/or atrophy of infraspinatus and supraspinatus muscles.
- When fracture to humeral neck, glenohumeral displacement, or poor crutch placement occurs, injury to the axillary nerve may occur, resulting in weakness and/or atrophy in deltoid muscle.
- Midshaft humeral fractures can lead to radial nerve injuries leading to wrist drop or flexion contractures.[1]
- Although the evidence is weak, consider the Allen's test prior to placing radial arterial line to assess collateral circulation in the hand.
- Ligation of brachial artery distal to axillary artery but proximal to bifurcation into radial and ulnar arteries can lead to significant decrease in perfusion to forearm and hand.
- If axillary vein is compromised, cephalic vein must be preserved for venous return from upper extremity.[1]
- The intercostobrachial nerve is formed by the lateral cutaneous branch of the T2 spinal nerve. It is responsible for sensation of the skin in the axilla and medial upper arm. If tourniquet will be applied to the upper arm during the procedure, consider an intercostobrachial nerve block to provide complete analgesia for skin over axilla and medial arm not innervated by brachial plexus.[3]
- Median nerve injury may occur with arterial or venous lines placed in the antecubital fossa.

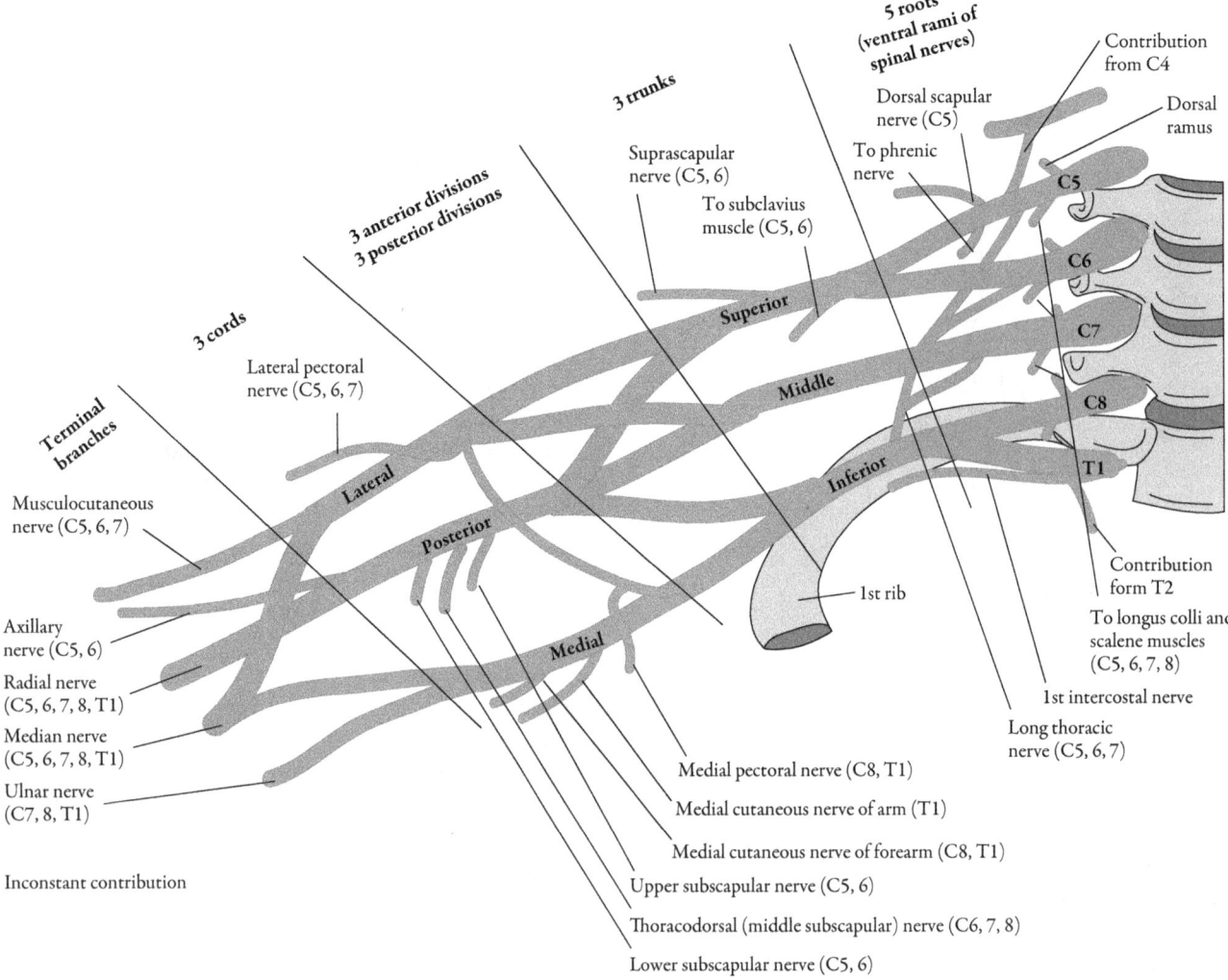

**Figure 11.2.** Anatomy of brachial plexus: roots, trunks, divisions, cords, and branches.
Reproduced with permission from Schünke M, Schulte E, Schumacher U, *Atlas of Anatomy*, 2nd ed. Thieme; 2015.

### *Table 11.1* NERVES OF THE UPPER EXTREMITY

| NERVE | VERTEBRAL LEVELS | MOTOR COMPONENT | SENSORY COMPONENT |
|---|---|---|---|
| Suprascapular nerve | C5–C6 | Lateral rotation of arm<br>Adduction of shoulder | Acromioclavicular and glenohumeral joint |
| Musculocutaneous nerve | C5–C7 | Flexion of arm at elbow | Lateral forearm |
| Axillary nerve | C5–C6 | Arm abduction at shoulder | Over deltoid muscle |
| Radial nerve | C5–C8, T1 | Wrist extension<br>Finger extension at MTP joints<br>Supination<br>Thumb extension and abduction | Posterior arm<br>Dorsal hand<br>Dorsal thumb |
| Median nerve | C6–8, T1 | Wrist flexion<br>Lateral finger flexion<br>Opposition of thumb | Palmar aspect of lateral 3½ fingers<br>Dorsal lateral 3½ fingers<br>Thenar eminence |
| Ulnar nerve | C8, T1 | Wrist flexion<br>Medial finger flexion<br>Abduction/adduction of fingers<br>Adduction of thumb<br>Extension of 4th and 5th fingers | Medial 1½ fingers<br>Hypothenar eminence |

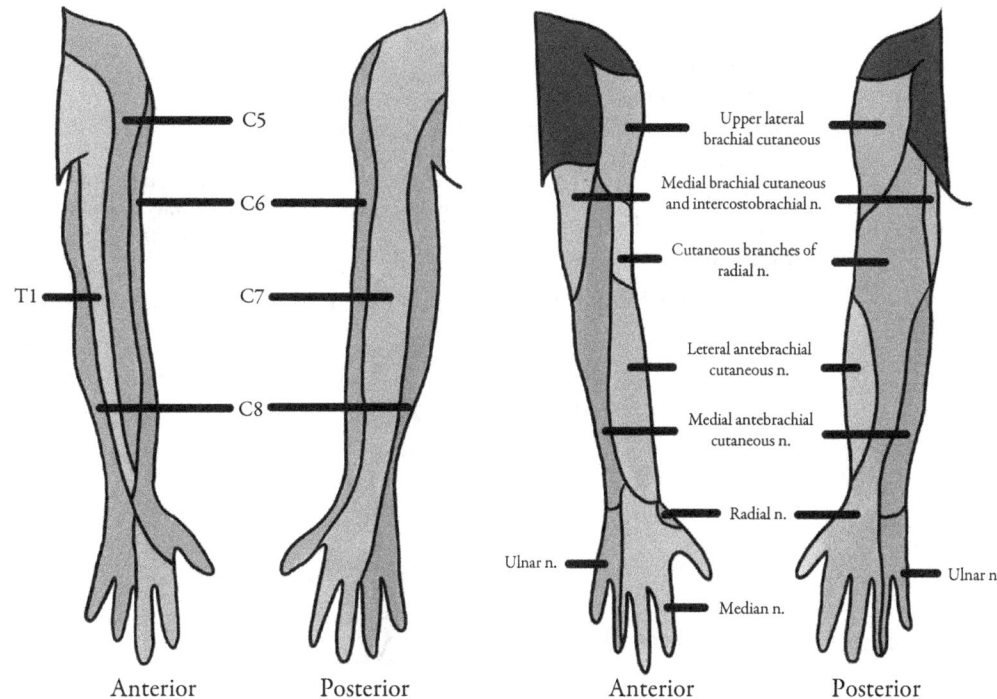

**Figure 11.3.** Distribution of cutaneous nerves of the upper extremity.
Reproduced with permission from Pardo MC, Miller, RD, *Basics of Anesthesia*. 7th ed. Elsevier; 2018.

## INTRAOPERATIVE

- Ulnar nerve injury is the most common peripheral nerve injury, followed by brachial plexus injury.
  - Reduce ulnar nerve pressure by supinating or keeping palms toward body.

- Reduce brachial plexus and axillary vasculature injury by keeping head and neck in neutral position, arms abducted less than 90°, and placing axillary roll if in lateral decubitus position.[2]

*Table 11.2* UPPER EXTREMITY PERIPHERAL NERVE BLOCKS[1]

| NERVE BLOCK | INDICATIONS | ANATOMY | COMPLICATIONS |
|---|---|---|---|
| Interscalene | Surgeries of distal clavicle, shoulder, upper arm | At level of C6, between anterior and middle scalene muscles | Horner syndrome<br>Recurrent laryngeal nerve or phrenic nerve block<br>Epidural or subarachnoid injection<br>Vertebral artery injection<br>Pneumothorax |
| Supraclavicular | Surgeries of lower arm, elbow, forearm, hand | Lateral to clavicle adjacent to subclavian artery | Phrenic nerve block<br>Pneumothorax |
| Infraclavicular | Surgeries of arm below shoulder | 3 cm inferior to midpoint of coracoid process and medial clavicle | Pneumothorax |
| Axillary | Surgeries of elbow, forearm, wrist, and hand | Surrounding axillary artery | Musculocutaneous nerve sparing, may be localized separately while performing axillary block<br>Axillary artery injection |

## POSTOPERATIVE

- Surgeons may need to perform neurovascular exams postoperatively. Discuss with the team if a nerve block would interfere with this critical step.
- Patients with concern for postoperative peripheral neuropathy should be thoroughly evaluated. Findings of sensory loss with intact motor function are usually self-limiting and may be followed by anesthesia team. If motor deficit is encountered, neurologic consultation is advised.

## REFERENCES

1. Schünke M, Schulte E, Schumacher U, et al. Atlas of Anatomy, 2nd ed. Thieme; 2015:274–376.
2. Yap, E., Gray, A. Basics of Anesthesia, 7th ed. Elsevier; 2018: 307–310.
3. NYSORA—The New York School of Regional Anesthesia [Internet]. Available from www.nysora.com/.

# 12.

# LOWER EXTREMITY

*Amit Samba and Alexandria Nickless*

## INTRODUCTION

Millions of surgeries on the lower extremity are performed annually. An anesthetic plan may include general anesthesia, regional block, or a combination of both. Knowledge of the anatomy will allow for formulation of a plan that is beneficial to the patient in the perioperative period and may help decrease postoperative complications.

## BONES

See Figure 12.1 for a depiction of the lower extremity skeleton.

## VASCULATURE

### SMALL SAPHENOUS VEIN

- Starts posterior to lateral malleolus extending posteriorly toward popliteal fossa draining into popliteal vein.

### POPLITEAL VEIN

- In the popliteal fossa, the popliteal vein lies between the popliteal artery and tibial nerve.

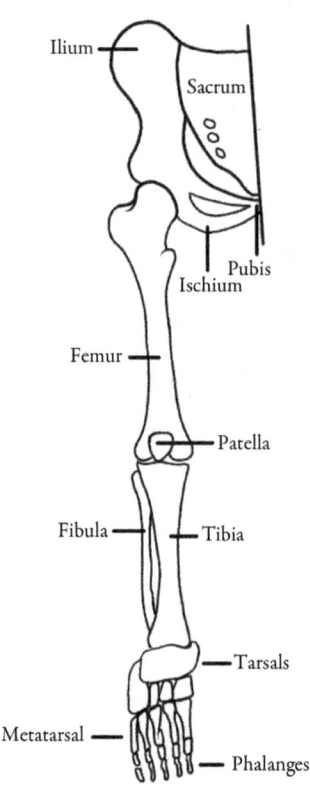

**Figure 12.1.** Anatomy of skeleton.
Reproduced with permission from Schünke M, Schulte E, Schumacher U, eds. *Atlas of Anatomy.* 2nd ed. Thieme; 2015.

- Extends posteriorly through adductor magnus muscle draining into femoral vein.

## GREAT SAPHENOUS VEIN

- Located superficially on dorsum of foot medial to medial malleolus
- Can be used to identify location for saphenous nerve block of ankle
- Extends medially draining into femoral vein near inguinal crease.

## FEMORAL ARTERY

- Lies lateral to femoral vein and medial to femoral nerve
- Extension of external iliac artery; divides into superficial femoral and profunda femoris arteries.

## POPLITEAL ARTERY

- Extension of superficial femoral artery into popliteal artery in popliteal fossa
- Divides into anterior tibial and posterior tibial artery.

## ANTERIOR TIBIAL ARTERY

- Ends as the dorsalis pedis artery

- Pulsatile dorsalis pedis artery used to identify location for deep peroneal nerve block.

## POSTERIOR TIBIAL ARTERY

- Located posterior to medial malleolus
- Pulsatile posterior tibial artery used to identify location for posterior tibial nerve block[1,2] (see Table 12.1 Table 12.2, and Figure 12.2).

## INNERVATION

See Figure 12.2 for a depiction of the innervation of the lower extremity.

## ANESTHETIC CONSIDERATIONS

### PREOPERATIVE

- Assessment of patient's preexisting neurovascular status and risk factors for intraoperative neuropathies should be documented.

*Table 12.1* NERVES OF THE LOWER EXTREMITY

| NERVE | VERTEBRAL LEVELS | MOTOR COMPONENT | SENSORY COMPONENT |
|---|---|---|---|
| Obturator nerve | L2–4 | Hip adduction | Medial thigh |
| Femoral nerve | L2–4 | Hip flexion<br>Knee extension | Anteromedial thigh<br>Lateral knee<br>Medial leg and foot |
| Sciatic nerve (terminal branches: common peroneal and tibial nerves) | L4–S3 | Knee flexion | Dorsum of foot and anterolateral leg (superficial peroneal nerve)<br>Plantar foot (tibial nerve)<br>Posterolateral leg (sural nerve) |
| Common peroneal nerve (terminal branches: deep peroneal and superficial peroneal nerves) | L4–S2 | Knee flexion | Lateral leg at and below knee<br>Dorsum of foot and anterolateral leg (superficial peroneal nerve) |
| Deep peroneal nerve | L4–5 | Ankle dorsiflexion<br>Toe extension | First webspace |
| Superficial peroneal nerve | L4–S1 | Ankle eversion | Anterolateral leg<br>Dorsum of foot except first webspace |
| Tibial nerve | L4–S3 | Ankle plantar flexion<br>Ankle inversion<br>Toe flexion | Plantar aspect of foot (medial and lateral plantar nerves)<br>Posterolateral leg (sural nerve) |
| Superior gluteal nerve | L4–S1 | Hip abduction | |
| Inferior gluteal nerve | L5–S2 | Hip extension | |
| Lateral femoral cutaneous nerve | L2–3 | | Anterolateral thigh |

**Table 12.2** ANESTHETIC CONSIDERATIONS FOR PERIPHERAL NERVE BLOCKS PRIOR TO A SURGERY

| NERVE BLOCK | INDICATIONS | ANATOMY | COMPLICATIONS |
|---|---|---|---|
| Femoral | Surgeries of anterior thigh Analgesia for hip, femur, knee surgeries | Deep into inguinal ligament lateral to femoral artery | Quadriceps weakness Increased risk of falling |
| Adductor canal and saphenous | Surgeries of knee with minimal quadriceps muscle weakness Distally for medial leg, ankle | Deep to sartorius muscle, lateral to femoral artery Distally adjacent to saphenous vein Contains nerve to vastus medialis | |
| Sciatic | Proximal: Surgeries for posterior thigh, lower leg, foot, and ankle Popliteal: Surgeries for foot and ankle | Proximal: Halfway between greater trochanter of femur and ischial tuberosity, deep to gluteus maximus Popliteal: In popliteal fossa, posterior to popliteal vein and artery | Hamstring weakness Foot drop |
| Tibial | Surgeries for heel and plantar foot | Posterior to pulsatile posterior tibial artery | |
| Sural | Surgeries for lateral foot | Adjacent to lateral malleolus and calcaneus next to saphenous vein | |
| Saphenous | Surgeries for medial foot | Anterior to medial malleolus next to saphenous vein | |
| Deep peroneal | Surgeries near webbing between first and second toes | Adjacent to anterior tibial artery, posterior to hallicus longus tendon | |
| Superficial peroneal | Surgeries for dorsum of foot | Superficially from medial to lateral malleoli | |

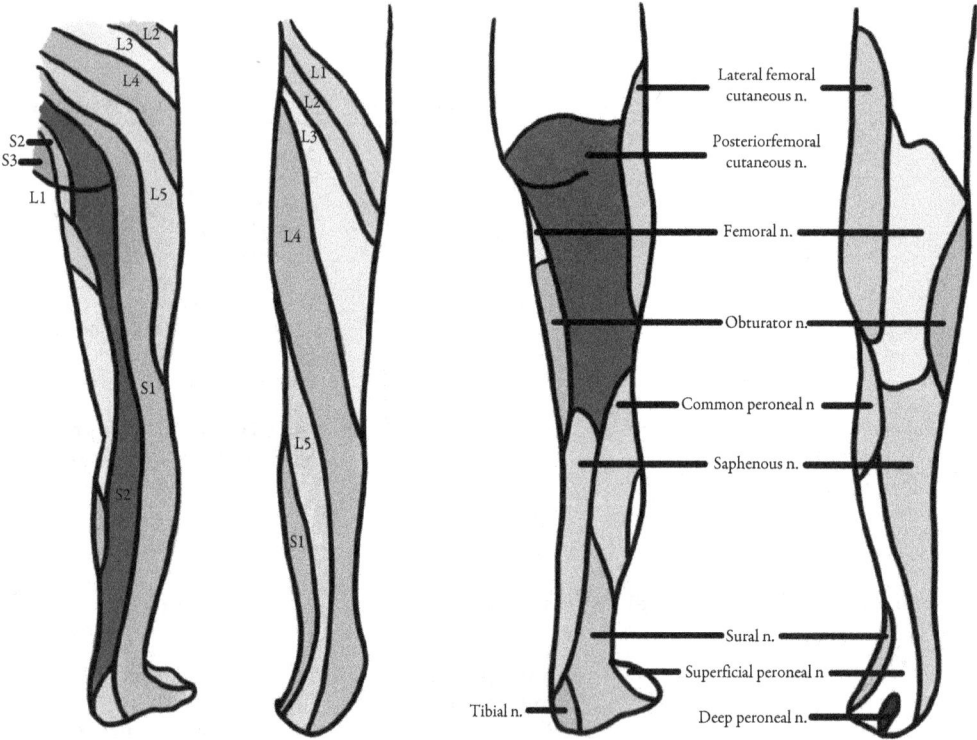

**Figure 12.2.** Distribution of nerves of the lower extremity.
Reproduced with permission from Schünke M, Schulte E, Schumacher U, eds. *Atlas of Anatomy*. 2nd ed. Thieme; 2015.

- Risk factors include: diabetes mellitus, obesity, male gender, alcohol abuse, peripheral vascular disease, preexisting peripheral neuropathy, and arthritis.
- Dislocation or injury to the popliteal fossa can lead to compromise of:
  - Popliteal artery decreasing vascular flow to lower extremity;
  - Tibial nerve leading to muscle weakness and/or atrophy in posterior leg compartment and loss of sensation to sole of foot.
- Fractures of the lower extremity can very frequently lead to compartment syndrome leading to increased pain, paralysis, paresthesia, pallor, decreased temperature distal to the injury, pulselessness. If suspicion of compartment syndrome is present, quick diagnosis is needed and frequently requires decompression emergently.
- Fractures of the femoral neck can lead to avascular necrosis to the femoral head due to compromised vasculature.[1]

## INTRAOPERATIVE

- Injuries to sciatic and common peroneal nerve most commonly occur in lithotomy position. When placing in lithotomy position, it is important to move legs simultaneously to prevent spinal torsion.
- If legs are being placed in padded support, avoid tight compression. This can lead to injury to common peroneal nerve, causing foot drop and in rare instances compartment syndrome of the leg.
- Improper positioning could lead to sciatic and femoral nerves being overstretched. Knee hyperextension could also lead to overstretching of tibial and/or common peroneal nerve.[3]
- Prolonged tourniquet times may put patients at risk for nerve ischemia postoperatively.

## POSTOPERATIVE

- Nerve blockade or injury to the nerves of the lower extremity can put patients at risk for falls. If the patient exhibits signs of quadriceps weakness postoperatively, precautions should be taken.[3]

## REFERENCES

1. Lower limb. In: Schünke M, Schulte E, Schumacher U, eds. *Atlas of Anatomy*. 2nd ed. Thieme; 2015:380–472.
2. NYSORA—The New York School of Regional Anesthesia [Internet] (accessed May 27, 2020). Available from www.nysora.com/.
3. Yap, E., Gray, A. Peripheral nerve blocks. In: Pardo MC, Miller, RD, eds. *Basics of Anesthesia*. 7th ed. Elsevier; 2018:310–317.

# Part II

# MECHANICS

# 13.

# PRESSURE MEASUREMENT OF GASES AND LIQUIDS

*Ben Aquino*

## INTRODUCTION

Pressure, in its simplest terms, is defined as force per unit of area. Gases and liquids exert pressure equally in all directions, but for purposes of measurement, that pressure is quantified as a force that acts in a specific direction. Multiple measures exist for pressure, and a few of the more commonly used ones in anesthesia are millimeters of mercury (mmHg), centimeters of water ($cmH_2O$), and atmospheres (atm).

## MANOMETER

There are multiple devices used in medicine and anesthesia to measure pressures, but one, the manometer, provides an illustration of the principles behind pressure measurement. In its simplest form, a manometer is an open-ended tube, filled with fluid. When a strong enough pressure acts on one end of the tube of fluid, it pushes the entire column of fluid within the tube. The distance the column of fluid travels from baseline is measured as the pressure. The pressure is expressed in terms of the fluid within the manometry tube. If it is water, the pressure is measured in centimeters of water ($cmH_2O$). If the tube is filled with mercury, the pressure is in millimeters of mercury (mmHg).

Atmospheric pressure (at sea level) is a standard reference for pressure units, expressed in atmospheres (atm); 1 atm is most commonly expressed as 760 mmHg. Other measures of atmospheric pressure are: $988\ cm^2\ H_2O$, and 101.3 kiloPascals (kPa). Both are equal to 760 mmHg, or 1 atm.

## PARTIAL PRESSURES

The concept of partial pressures is a key component of understanding and managing the workings of volatile anesthetics. The ideal gas law states that:

$$PV = nRT.$$

P is pressure, V is volume, T is absolute temperature, n is the number of moles present, and R is the ideal gas constant.

Notably, this equation holds true even if n is the sum of multiple numbers (amounts) of gases. This is essentially an illustration of Dalton's Law of partial pressures, which states that each gas in a given mixture exerts a given pressure in proportion to its total amount in that mixture.[1] The quantity of anesthetic gas being given through a vaporizer and into the anesthesia circuit is, instead of being expressed as partial pressures, expressed as a percentage of the mix of gases.

In similar fashion, the partial pressure of a volatile anesthetic in a carrier gas mixture can be calculated. Assuming atmospheric pressure, a 2% mixture of sevoflurane will have a partial pressure of 15.2 mmHg. Variable bypass vaporizers, calibrated for a given agent at a baseline assumed atmospheric pressure, will release anesthetic vapor under a given partial pressure, and not a specific concentration.

## FLOW AND TRANSDUCERS

Pressure is a static measurement, signifying the status of the force per area in one given moment, but pressure can be further quantified. When a gas or liquid under a given pressure encounters an area that contains the same substance, but under a different pressure, it will move from the region of higher pressure to the region with lower pressure, which is defined as flow. Flow can be measured in several ways, but clinically, the arterial line is an example of one of the most useful measuring devices, the transducer.

Transducers convert one form of energy into another—in the case of an arterial line, it receives change in pressure and converts it into changes in electrical resistance or capacitance. The electronic circuit in the transducer that provides the resistance is a Wheatstone bridge. It uses current across three known resistors to determine the fourth unknown resistance, which is the transducer itself. Any signal that is received by the transducer is a series of waves—the fundamental frequency, and a series of harmonic waveforms. A harmonic wave is one that is a frequency that is a positive integer multiple of the original signal wave. The ultimate waveform obtained represents a summation of these waves.

For an arterial line signal, the fundamental frequency is the lowest frequency sine wave and is equal to the pulse rate. The natural frequency of any system is the rate at which it moves or oscillates. When the pulse rate approaches the natural frequency of the measuring system, it is said to be at its resonance frequency, and at this point, the signals will come close to matching and the result with be an increase in the total amplitude of the system and the waveform—an over-exaggeration of the actual systolic blood pressure.

## DAMPING

This undesirable effect of resonance within the system is offset by either (1) making the natural frequency of the measuring system as high as possible, or (2) damping, which is a way of lowering the natural frequency of the system and keeping it from approaching its natural frequency. If natural frequency measures the oscillation of a system, damping coefficients measure how quickly they come to rest.[2] Damping deals mainly with 3 different characteristics—elasticity, mass, and friction.

Clinically, this means that to dampen the pressure transducer system used for invasive arterial monitoring, that is, to lower its effective natural frequency, the tubing would need to be narrow in diameter, low in stiffness, and relatively long. Normal extension tubing will be too compliant and too wide in diameter, and too much damping will take place. If air bubbles are present in the tubing, it decreases the density of the tubing contents and, more notably, it slightly increases the compliance of the liquid in the tubing, both of which contribute to overdamping.

Again, damping *decreases* the natural frequency of a system. See Box 13.1 for a look at factors that increase damping.

The optimal amount of damping is important—an underdamped system has a high natural frequency and exaggerated waveforms, but an overdamped system, with a low natural frequency, will suppress the lower order, higher amplitude harmonic waveforms. This will leave only the higher order, lower amplitude harmonic waveforms, which will be flatter, and underestimate measurement.

Of note, all transducer systems in medical use today are slightly underdamped, and this is done so that there will be a wider range of damping coefficients for which the system will have a good dynamic response, that is, an accurate and precise reading of pressures in a wide numerical range. It is also indicative of the transduction system having a sufficiently high natural frequency.

## ZEROING AND LEVELING

Making sure the transducer is zeroed and placed at the proper level is critically important for accurate measurements. Errors in measurement can mislead anesthesiologists and cause them to make decisions based on incorrectly obtained data. For a transducer to be zeroed, it needs to be opened to air, which means that its reference point is going to be atmospheric pressure. That being done, the transducer needs to be placed at the level that will lead to the most accurate and clinically meaningful measurement. The classic teaching has always been that for a supine patient, the transducer is placed at the level of the midaxillary line. Recent information, though, has shown that this placement overestimates aortic filling pressures, and an even more accurate measurement is obtained by placing the transducer at a height 5 cm posterior to the sternomanubrial junction.[3]

## CHANGES IN WAVEFORMS

A commonly asked question on exams refers to the difference in waveform shapes between the aortic pressure and a more distal site, such as the radial pressure. This difference occurs because of pulse wave reflection. Aortic and radial pressures both have little systemic resistance, but when the wave reaches the distal arteriolar bed, resistance increases markedly, which causes the pulse wave to reverberate back

---

*Box 13.1* PRESSURE MEASUREMENT FACTORS INCREASING DAMPING (DECREASING NATURAL FREQUENCY)

- Long transducer tubing (>1.4 m)
- Highly compliant tubing (<1.5mm)
- Narrow tubing
- Kinks in transducer line
- Air bubbles in transducer line

Most significant factor in affecting damping—tubing diameter.

---

*Box 13.2* DIFFERENCES BETWEEN PERIPHERAL ARTERIAL WAVEFORM AND AORTIC WAVEFORM

Peripheral waveform has a:

1. Steeper systolic upstroke
2. Higher systolic pressure
3. Lower diastolic pressure
4. Wider pulse pressure
5. More delayed systolic upstroke and dicrotic notch
6. Slurred, attenuated dicrotic notch
7. More prominent diastolic waveform
8. Slightly lower MAP.

Pulse wave reflection contributes partially or wholly to most of these (though not to MAP).

toward the arterial waveform. This pulse wave will naturally be more prominent when it is closer to the arterioles, and because of this, the distal waveforms, such as the radial and pedal, will have somewhat greater amplitude, showing a higher systolic, lower diastolic, and wider pulse pressure than the more proximal aortic pressure.

If an aortic and radial waveform are plotted on a graph over time, the radial pulse will have a slightly delayed upstroke on its waveform, as this accounts for the time it takes the energy of the waveform to get from the aorta to the radial artery. The radial pulse will also have a delayed and more slurred dicrotic notch.[4] See Box 13.2 for a summary of the differences between aortic and distal waveforms.

## REFERENCES

1. Szocik J, et al. Fundamental principles of monitoring instrumentation. In: Miller RD, Cohen NH, Erikkson LI, et al., eds. *Miller's Anesthesia*. 8th ed. Philadelphia, PA: Elsevier Saunders; 2015.
2. Mark JB. Technical requirements for blood pressure measurement. In: *Atlas of Cardiovascular Monitoring*. New York, NY: Churchill Livingstone; 1998.
3. Seo JH, et al. Uppermost blood levels of the right and left atria in the supine position: Implication for measuring central venous pressure and pulmonary artery wedge pressure. *Anesthesiology*. 2007;107(2):260–263.
4. Schroeder B, et al. Cardiovascular monitoring. In: Miller RD, Cohen NH, Erikkson LI, et al., eds., *Miller's Anesthesia*. 8th ed. Philadelphia, PA: Elsevier Saunders; 2015.

# 14.

# TRANSDUCERS, REGULATORS, AND MEDICAL GAS CYLINDERS

*Ben Aquino*

## INTRODUCTION

The law of conservation of energy states that energy cannot be created or destroyed, but simply converted from one form of energy to another. This principle underlies transducers and monitoring devices in anesthesia, which convert a signal from one energy form to another. In anesthesia, that transduction is used to take a raw mechanical signal, such as flow from an artery, and convert it into an electrical signal, such as the waveform on an arterial line or the systolic pressure of a blood pressure cuff.

Transduction is complex in that it needs to account for the dynamic changes that can take place in measuring a given parameter. Modern pressure transducers change either resistance or capacitance in response to changes in pressure, all within the same system. The primary setup used in most transducer systems is a Wheatstone bridge, which is a circuit with current flowing through a series of four resistors. Three are of known value, and the fourth is a semiconducting membrane that is in the transducer. With three of the resistances known, it is possible to solve for the fourth, and in doing so, the circuit is able to calculate the change in resistance which comes from the change in pressure. This current is converted into some sort of readable data in the form of an analog or digital signal.

## MEDICAL GAS CYLINDERS

Medical gases are supplied to the anesthesia machine via a central hospital supply, which is usually a cryogenic bulk oxygen storage system. Medical air is compressed on site and stored in holding tanks. The hospital supply pipeline delivers gases at a pressure of 50–55 pounds per square inch (psi). Several safety features exist within this portion of the anesthesia machine. First, the hoses from the anesthesia machine connect to gas inlets at the wall at sites specific for, and unique to, the gas in question. These connections are removable but not interchangeable—that is, the inlet connector for the oxygen hose will connect only with the oxygen outlet on the wall, $N_2O$ will connect only with $N_2O$, and so on. This is referred to as the Diameter Index Safety System (DISS). Second, once gas enters the machine from the central supply, it passes through a one-way valve, which prevents backflow into the central supply, and a pipeline check valve, which monitors the pressure of gases delivered into the machine, and visibly displays those values at the front of the machine.[1]

Should the hospital supply somehow fail, reserve medical gas cylinders attached to the back of the anesthesia machine can supply gases to the patient. Medical gas cylinders come in multiple sizes, ranging from A (small) to M (large), and $N_2O$ central supply usually comes from a bank of large H-type cylinders. However, the reserve tanks attached to the back of an anesthesia machine are usually E-sized cylinders. Oxygen and medical air are stored in these tanks as a compressed gas at 1900–2000 psi, and each full E-cylinder of $O_2$ at 1900 psi contains approximately 660 L of oxygen. Because they are stored as gases, the volume of gas remaining can be calculated if the pressure in the cylinder is known (for example, when it is half empty, it will contain 330 L at a pressure of 950 psi). Nitrous oxide is stored as a liquid at about 745 psi, and a full E-cylinder of $N_2O$ will provide a total of 1800 L of gas. Because $N_2O$ is stored as a liquid, vaporization and release of gas simply causes more vaporization within the cylinder, and the pressure in the cylinder remains the same. Only when all the liquid $N_2O$ has been vaporized (approximately 400 L of $N_2O$ remaining in the cylinder) will the pressure start to fall. Vaporization of a liquid to a gas absorbs heat from the atmosphere and the liquid, which results in cooling of the liquified gas. Frost can form on the outside of the cylinder, causing a decrease in temperature, which in turn will decrease the vapor pressure of the liquid and result in a slight decrease in pressure.

Medical gas E-cylinders attach to the back of the anesthesia machine in yokes that are labeled to accept a specific gas cylinder, and are uniquely designed to fit the tanks of the intended gas. This is facilitated by the Pin Index Safety System (PISS)—there are uniquely positioned, gas-specific pins in each yoke that fit into unique holes in the cylinder head-valve assembly of the tank. The tanks are also color coded—in the United States, $O_2$ tanks are green, $N_2O$ tanks are blue, medical air tanks are yellow, and $CO_2$ is gray.

Incidents involving oxygen supply being switched or mis-attached have happened, though,[2] and the provider always needs to make sure that they are administering the correct gases to the patient.

## PRESSURE REGULATORS

Reserve gas cylinders have their contents at significantly higher pressures than the central hospital supply. It is unsafe to supply such high pressures to the patient circuit, and as such, each cylinder supply source must pass through a high-pressure regulator before reaching the intermediate pressure system within the anesthesia machine.

In physics, pressure can be expressed as:

$$P = F \times A.$$

The pressure of a large force acting on a small area is equivalent to a smaller force acting on a larger area. This can be expressed as:

$$F1 \times A_1 = F_2 \times A_2.$$

Pressure regulators work on this principle. Modern regulators involve gas from a high force system (in this case, compressed gas from a cylinder) acting on a small area (a valve seat in the regulator). That pressure is in equilibrium with a low force (air-filled reservoir of the regulator) acting on a large area (a diaphragm within the regulator). When a downstream stopcock is opened, these two systems engage with each other and, by various mechanisms, gas from the cylinder enters the regulator through the valve seat, and subsequently that same gas from the regulator reservoir exits the regulator, under significantly decreased pressure.[3] The regulators on the gas cylinders are calibrated to reduce these high pressures to lower and more constant pressures, usually between 35 and 45 psi. All such regulators contain a safety valve, through which air exits if the system fails to the point that inner pressure exceeds 4 times the intended delivery pressure.

The tank gases from the high-pressure regulator are calibrated specifically to have psi lower than the hospital pipeline pressure, which means that if both of them are on, the gas from the hospital pipeline, and not from the cylinders, will be delivered to the patient. This means that if gases from the medical gas cylinders are intended to be delivered to the patient, the gas supply line *must* be disconnected from the wall. This is true even when the auxiliary $O^2$ source (where the nasal cannula is often connected) is being used with an $O^2$ tank instead of the wall supply.

## ANESTHETIC CONSIDERATIONS

### PREOPERATIVE

The pin-indexing systems are not fail-proof. Reported instances of failure include excessive seating of pins back into the yoke, bent/broken pins, or multiple washers between cylinder and yoke, overriding the pins. In all of these cases, the wrong gas could have been given to the patient.[4] The anesthesia provider needs to manually inspect the tanks and make sure that the reserve gas cylinders are properly and tightly connected to the proper spots in the rear of the anesthesia machine, and needs to note the pressure gauges

*Table 14.1* GAS CYLINDER SAFETY FEATURES, RATIONALE, AND POSSIBLE COMPLICATIONS

| | SAFETY FEATURE | RATIONALE | POSSIBLE COMPLICATIONS |
|---|---|---|---|
| Wrong gas cylinder attached to anesthesia workstation | Pins on back of yoke fit uniquely into cylinder attachment of the gas in question | Creates tight seal between cylinder and circuit, and ensures match between cylinder and intended gas | Pins can be bent, manipulated to accommodate other cylinders |
| Wrong gas cylinder attached to anesthesia workstation | Cylinder color coded, and yoke on back of anesthesia machine labeled for specific gas | | Incidents have occurred where gas was misfiled at the manufacturer site, or had been refilled by a different gas and painted over[1] |
| Over-pressurized gas | Cylinder gas goes through high-pressure regulator prior to entering the intermediate pressure system of the anesthesia machine. | Cylinder gas at pressures as high as 2200 psi ($O_2$, air) or 745 psi ($N_2O$)—unusable for anesthesia circuit | Failure of regulator |
| Leakage of gas from opened cylinder | Check release valve, either before or after first pressure regulator | Prevents backflow of gas into either a vacant yoke or a second tank under lower pressure | Valve malfunctions and gas escapes through vacant yoke or into another tank. |
| Unknown quantity of gas in cylinder | Pressure gauges of gas cylinders shown on front of machine, either continuously or when cylinder is opened | Amount of gas in air or $O_2$ cylinder can be obtained by knowing the pressure in the cylinder. | Nitrous oxide—exists in cylinder as a liquid—cylinder pressure does not decrease until it is about ¾ depleted, and only 400 L of $N_2O$ gas are left. |
| Unusability of central hospital gas supply | Pressure regulator lowers pressure to a level below hospital pipeline pressure. | Necessitates that hospital pipeline be disconnected from machine in order for cylinder gas to be used | Human error—gas supply line not disconnected from wall; cylinder drains gas that is not being given to the patient |

in the front of the machine, which will display the partial pressures in each of the medical gas cylinders (Table 14.1).

## INTRAOPERATIVE

If a situation arises where the medical gas cylinders need to be opened and used intraoperatively, the anesthesia provider needs to remember that the pressure regulators between the cylinders and the rest of the anesthesia machine reduce source pressure to 35–45 psi, which is less than the baseline of 50–55 psi from the hospital central supply. As a result of this, if the medical gas cylinders are to be used, the following things must happen: (1) the tank needs to be opened, and (2) the anesthesia machine needs to be disconnected from the central air supply. If it is not, the 50+ psi of the central supply will override the lower pressures from the medical gas cylinders, and none of the cylinder supply will be given to the patient.

## POSTOPERATIVE

At the conclusion of any anesthetic—even ones where the cylinders are not used—the provider needs to ensure that the gas cylinder valves are closed, or the supply in the cylinders can silently become depleted.

## REFERENCES

1. Venticinque SG, Andrews JJ. Inhaled anesthetics: Delivery systems. In: Miller RD, Cohen NH, Eriksson LI, et al. *Miller's Anesthesia.* 8th ed. Philadelphia, PA: Elsevier Saunders; 2015.
2. Caplan RA, et al. Adverse anesthetic outcomes arising from gas delivery equipment: A closed claims analysis. *Anesthesiology.* 1997;87(10): 741–748.
3. Dorsch J, Dorsch S. The anesthesia machine. In: Dorsch J, Dorsch S. *Understanding Anesthesia Equipment.* 4th ed. Baltimore, MD: Lippincott Williams & Wilkins; 1999:84–91.
4. Hogg CE. Pin-indexing failures. *Anesthesiology* 1973;38:85–87.

# 15.

# PRINCIPLES OF ULTRASOUND

## *Emily Young and Sherif Zaky*

## INTRODUCTION

Ultrasound is a safe, noninvasive, and relatively inexpensive tool that uses high-frequency sound waves to produce a real-time image of organs and tissues. In anesthesiology, ultrasound plays an important role in both diagnosis and in guiding otherwise blind interventions such as performing peripheral nerve blocks, vascular access, and neuraxial anesthesia. An understanding of the basic principles and techniques of ultrasound is necessary to effectively utilize this modality in practice.

## OBTAINING AN IMAGE

### ULTRASOUND WAVES

Ultrasound imaging relies on high-frequency sound waves to produce an image. Sound waves are longitudinal waves of mechanical energy that propagate in a series of compressions (high pressure) and rarefactions (low pressure). Frequency is the number of cycles, or pressure changes, that occur in 1 second and is measured in Hertz (1 Hz = 1 cycle/sec). The human ear can detect sound waves with a frequency from 20 Hz to 20 000 Hz. Medical ultrasound uses frequencies that are much higher, between 2 000 000 and 15 000 000 Hz (2–15 MHz).[1]

An ultrasound beam is a series of pulsed ultrasound waves that are generated by the transducer in the ultrasound probe. The transducer applies an alternating electrical current to Piezoelectric crystals, which in turn resonate to create ultrasound waves. As the ultrasound beam travels through the body, it is attenuated by the tissues via absorption, reflection, and scattering. The ultrasound waves that are reflected back to the transducer are converted from mechanical energy back into electrical energy, which is interpreted by the receiver to form an image.[2,3]

## ACOUSTIC IMPEDANCE

The degree of reflection of ultrasound waves depends on the acoustic impedance of the tissues it travels through. Acoustic impedance is the product of the density of a substance and the speed that sound waves can travel through this substance. Substances with low impedance (fluids) provide very little resistance to the passage of the ultrasound waves, while substances with high impedance (bones) do not allow the sound waves to penetrate.[4]

The difference in impedance between two substances determines the degree of reflection at their interface. For example, the difference in impedance between air and skin is so large that 99.9% of the ultrasound beam is reflected. This reflection is avoided by the use of a "coupling agent," usually gel, between the probe and skin to match the acoustic impedance of the skin and allow adequate penetration.[2]

## ECHOGENICITY

When an ultrasound beam reflects at the interface between two materials, it creates an "echo" (Figure 15.1) which is

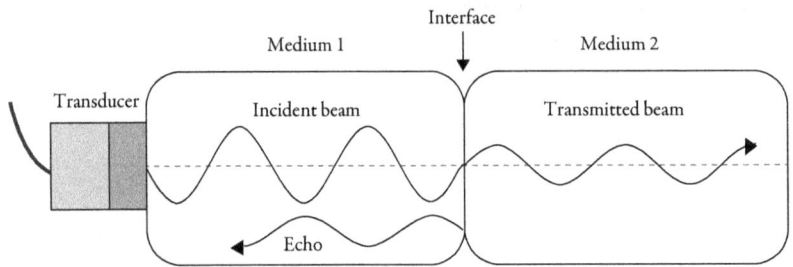

**Figure 15.1.** Echo formation and acoustic impedance.

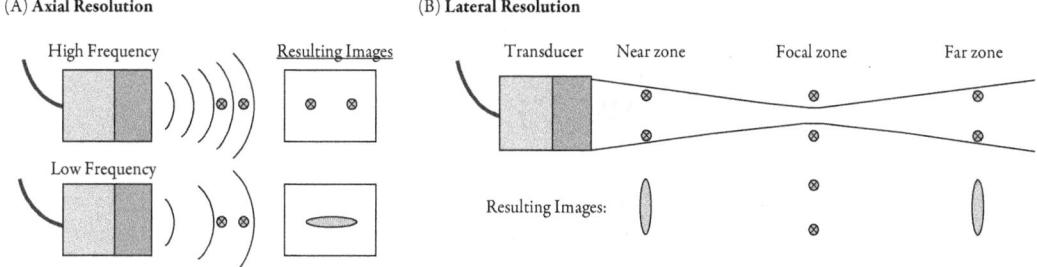

**Figure 15.2.** Axial (A) and lateral (B) resolution.

detected by the probe and appears bright on the resulting image. The following terms are commonly used to describe the appearance of different structures on ultrasound.[4]

i. *Hyperechoic*: Material that produces stronger echoes than the surrounding medium. Caused by large, smooth surfaces that reflect sound, and result in a white or bright signal. For example: diaphragm, bone, pleura, vessel wall, fascial layers.

ii. *Hypoechoic*: Material that gives off fewer echoes than the surrounding medium. Appears gray on the image. For example: most solid organs, soft tissues.

iii. *Anechoic*: Material that produces no echoes. Results in a black signal on the image. For example: fluids (blood, urine, etc.).

## GAIN

Receiver gain, or just "gain," refers to the ability of the ultrasound receiver to amplify returning echoes to increase the brightness of the image. Time gain compensation (TGC) is another feature of most ultrasound machines that allows the operator to adjust the gain at specific depths. This is often useful when imaging deeper structures, which naturally appear darker because the ultrasound beam loses intensity as it travels through tissues.[3]

## IMAGE QUALITY

### RESOLUTION

There are two main types of resolution in ultrasound. *Spatial resolution* (axial and lateral) refers to the ability to distinguish between two objects in space as separate echoes. *Temporal resolution* is the ability to distinguish between two events in time.

i. *Axial resolution*: The ability to distinguish between two objects at different depths along the long axis of the ultrasound beam. In general, the distance between the two points needs to be more than half the wavelength in order to appear separately. This

is why high-frequency waves (short wave lengths) provide the best axial resolution (Figure 15.2A).

ii. *Lateral resolution*: The ability to differentiate between two objects side by side. Lateral resolution is best where the ultrasound beam diameter is smallest. The beam diameter varies with depth and is narrowest in the "focal zone." The lateral resolution is therefore best in this area and is worse in the "near" and "far" zones (Figure 15.2B). The depth of the focal zone can be adjusted by the acoustic lens in the ultrasound probe.

iii. *Temporal resolution*: Needed to visualize a rapidly moving structure. This is determined by the frame rate, which is typically between 15 and 60 frames per second on modern ultrasound. Generally, the frame rate decreases with increasing depth, because it takes more time for the ultrasound beam to travel back to the probe. Thus, temporal resolution is often better when depth is set for the minimum.[2,3]

## PENETRATION

Penetration refers to the ability of ultrasound waves to reach deep structures. The higher the frequency, the more the ultrasound beam is attenuated as it travels, and the less distance it can penetrate. For example, 20 MHz waves can only penetrate about 1.5 cm, while 1 MHz waves can penetrate about 30 cm. Therefore, in order to image deeper structures, a curvilinear low-frequency transducer (4–8 MHz) is often used, and resolution is sacrificed (as discussed earlier). Linear transducers (10–15 MHz) can produce high-resolution images but can only reach more superficial structures.[2,3]

## REFERENCES

1. Terkawi AS, Karakitsos D, Elbarbary M, Blaivas M, Durieux ME. Ultrasound for the anesthesiologists: Present and future. *The Scientific World Journal*, 2013:683–685.
2. Aldrich JE. Basic physics of ultrasound imaging. *Crit Care Med*. 2007;35(5):S131–S137.
3. Shriki J. Ultrasound physics. *Crit Care Clin*. 2014;30(1):1–24.
4. Petra L, et al. *Oxford American Handbook of Radiology*. Oxford: Oxford University Press; 2013:239–245.

# 16.

## FLOW VELOCITY

*Richard Lennertz*

### INTRODUCTION

Anesthesiologists use the basic concepts of fluid dynamics to make clinical decisions. Whether managing a ventilator or vascular access, a common goal is to optimize the flow rate. Laminar flow is an orderly situation in which the layers of a fluid pass along with minimal lateral mixing. Since all the fluid molecules are traveling in the same direction, the resistance to flow is minimized. Turbulent flow is chaotic, and mixing within the fluid creates additional resistance to flow. As a result, turbulent flow deviates from laminar flow as the degree of mixing increases. This chapter reviews factors that determine the rate of flow and factors that influence laminar versus turbulent flow. Understanding the qualitative relationship between these factors is usually sufficient to guide clinical decisions.

### DETERMINANTS OF FLOW

Flow rate is determined by the difference in pressure divided by the resistance to flow: $Q = \dfrac{\Delta P}{R}$. Let us consider an infusion through an intravenous catheter (IV). Raising the IV pole higher above the patient would increase the difference in pressure and increase flow. Decreasing the resistance would also increase flow. However, resistance is determined by several factors, including tubing length, radius, and the viscosity of the fluid: $R = \dfrac{8\eta l}{\pi r^4}$.[1] Viscosity and tubing length are directly proportional to the resistance. For example, packed red blood cells are more viscous than crystalloid solutions and demonstrate a greater resistance to flow. On the other hand, tubing radius is inversely proportional to resistance and directly proportional to flow (Pouiselle's Law): $Q = \dfrac{\Delta P \pi r^4}{8\eta l}$.[1] Radius is raised to the fourth power, making it the single most important factor in determining resistance to flow. Increasing the radius by only 19% will halve the resistance and double the flow rate.

### FLOW AS PATHS CHANGE

Flow does not always proceed down a path of uniform diameter. The cumulative resistance of sequential path segments is additive: $R_{total} = R_1 + R_2 + \ldots$, and the narrowest segment may have a large effect on flow.[1] In an infusion, this is usually the IV catheter itself, but may include narrow segments of tubing used to secure the IV. Therefore, anesthesiologists place large-bore IV catheters when a patient may require rapid resuscitation, especially resuscitation with high-viscosity blood products.

When multiple paths are available, the relative area of each path determines the resistance to flow and the velocity of fluid movement. The total resistance of a system can be calculated according to the equation $\dfrac{1}{R_{total}} = \dfrac{1}{R_1} + \dfrac{1}{R_2} + \ldots$.[1] Importantly, adding parallel paths always decreases the total resistance to flow. Consider blood flow from the heart to the capillaries in the body. These small-diameter blood vessels have a high resistance to blood flow, but the sheer number of paths facilitates a cardiac output of several liters per minute. Adding a low-resistance path to the circulation, such as a large arteriovenous fistula, would reduce R systemic vascular resistance and could precipitate high-output heart failure. Conversely, a loss of capillary density has been associated with systemic hypertension.[2]

At any point along a path, flow rate is proportional to the cross-sectional area times the flow velocity: $Q = Av$. Since the flow rates in and out of a noncompliant system must be equal, flow velocity will vary inversely with the cross-sectional area of the path. For a cylindrical pathway, flow velocity will vary inversely with the radius squared. While physiologic systems are usually compliant, meaning that their volume changes with changes in pressure, assuming noncompliance is a helpful simplification for review.

### TURBULENT FLOW

Turbulence creates additional resistance to fluid flow. It consumes energy as fluid molecules accelerate in directions other than the direction of bulk flow. While tortuous or obstructed paths clearly create turbulence, other factors are important. These are described in the calculation of Reynolds number: $Re = \dfrac{\rho v D}{\mu}$. Reynolds numbers <2000 favor laminar flow, while numbers >4000 favor turbulent flow.[1] Greater density, flow velocity, and path diameter all promote turbulent flow. On the other hand, fluids with greater viscosity tend toward laminar flow. In patients with an airway obstruction, narrowing of the airway and turbulent flow both increase airway resistance. A mixture of helium and oxygen is less dense than air (or pure oxygen) and can be used to promote laminar flow, improving ventilation until the obstruction can be resolved.[3]

A) $Q = \dfrac{\Delta P}{R}$

B) $R = \dfrac{8 n l}{\pi r^4}$

C) $Q = \dfrac{\Delta P \pi r^4}{8 n l}$

D) $R_{total} = R_1 + R_2 + \ldots$

E) $\dfrac{1}{R_{total}} = \dfrac{1}{R_1} + \dfrac{1}{R_2} + \ldots$

F) $Q = Av$

G) $Re = \dfrac{\rho v D}{\mu}$

**Figure 16.1.** Relationships that determine flow rate and resistance.
Q = flow rate; P = pressure; R = resistance; η = viscosity; l = length; r = radius; A = area; v = velocity; Re = Reynolds number; ρ = density; D = diameter; and μ = dynamic viscosity.

## ANESTHETIC CONSIDERATIONS

- Understand the relationships between factors that determine flow and resistance (Figure 16.1).
- Resistance is proportional to $1/r^4$, making diameter the most important determinant of flow.
- Sequential path segments increase resistance, but parallel paths decrease resistance.
- A mixture of helium and oxygen may improve ventilation by promoting laminar flow in the setting of airway obstruction.

## REFERENCES

1. Urone P, Hinrichs R. Fluid dynamics and its biological and medical applications. In: *College Physics*. OpenStax; 2012. https://openstax.org/books/college-physics/pages/12-introduction-to-fluid-dynamics-and-its-biological-and-medical-applications. Accessed July 27, 2020.
2. Cheng C, et al. Capillary rarefaction in treated and untreated hypertensive subjects. *Ther Adv Cardiovasc Dis*. 2008;2(2):79–88.
3. Patel A. Anesthesia for otolaryngologic and head-neck surgery. In: M Gropper, L Eriksson, L Fleisher, J Wiener-Kronish, N Cohen, K Leslie, eds. *Miller's Anesthesia*. 9th ed. Elsevier; 2020: 2210–2235.e4.

# 17.

# FLOWMETERS

*Sohail K. Mahboobi and Mark L. Germani*

## INTRODUCTION

A flowmeter (rotameter) is a glass tube used to gauge the fresh gas flow being delivered to the patient under anesthesia. It is important for providers to understand the structure, functions, and limitations of flowmeters.

## STRUCTURE OF THE FLOWMETER

A traditional flowmeter is a glass tube, also called a Thorpe tube, with variable orifice and a flow measurement scale (graduations) marked on it. Inside there is a floating device, a ball or bobbin, to indicate the flow of gases. Other

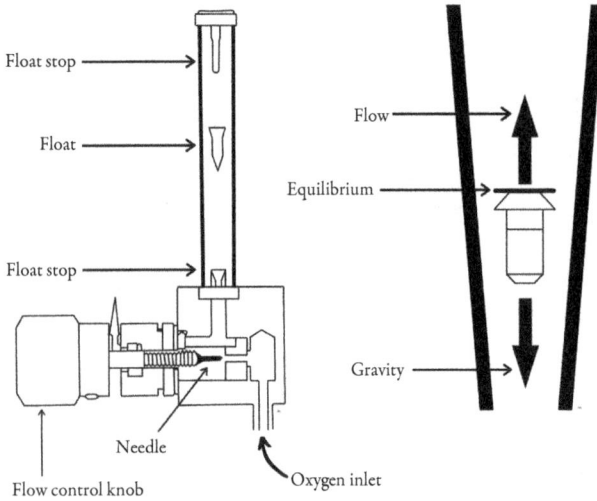

Float stop

Float

Float stop

Needle

Flow control knob

Oxygen inlet

Flow

Equilibrium

Gravity

**Figure 17.1.** Structure of the flowmeter. Note the needle valve shown on left and variable orifice glass tube with bobbin on right. Bobbin floats at level where gravitational force (downward black arrow) is balanced by the gas flow (upward black arrow).
Illustration by Mahad Sohail, Research Fellow, Department of Anesthesiology, Beth Israel Deaconess Medical Center, Boston, MA.

components are a needle valve, knob, and stops (Figure 17.1). The center of the ball and top of the bobbin are used for flow reading. Flowmeters are part of the low-pressure system.[1] The traditional flowmeters are replaced by transitional (hybrid) and electronic flowmeters in newer machines. Transitional flowmeters still have traditional mechanically controlled needle valves, to function in the absence of electric power, but no separate glass tubes are present for individual gases. The flow is electronically displayed as bar graphs and there is a common flowmeter indicating total gas flow, regardless of the type of the gas. The electronic flow display helps record keeping on automated charting. Electronic flowmeters control the flow of all gases electronically as well as the displays on the monitor screen. There is no glass tube in these flowmeters. The principle of specific heat is used to determine gas flow where a specific amount of electronic heat requirement is measured to keep the temperature constant of a known volume of the chamber through which gas is flowing. The operator chooses type of gases, desired fraction of inspired oxygen ($FiO_2$), and total fresh gas flow. The other flowmeters used in anesthesia machines are auxiliary oxygen supply and in the scavenging system to indicate adequate suction.

## PRINCIPLES OF FLOWMETER FUNCTION

The function of flowmeters is based primarily on physical principles. The annular space around the bobbin is tubular at low flow rates and the flow is primarily laminar. The viscosity determines the gas flow (a property independent of

altitude), as described by Poiseuille's law, which states that the flow of a fluid through a tube is directly related to the pressure gradient and diameter and inversely to viscosity and length of tubing. As viscosity increases, flow decreases:

$$Q = \frac{\Delta P \, \pi r^4}{8 \, \eta l}$$

where

$Q$: flow

$\Delta P$: Pressure gradient

$r$: radius

$\eta$: viscosity

$l$: length.

At high flow rates, the annular space simulates an orifice, creating turbulent gas flow. This turbulent flow depends primarily on the density of the gas (a property that is influenced by altitude), following Graham's law, which states that the rate of effusion is inversely proportional to the square root of the density of the gas. When the density of the gases decreases, e.g., at high altitudes, the actual gas flow will be higher than the set flow rate at high flows. Also, the scale on the tube is gas specific and flowmeters cannot be interchanged, because every gas has a different viscosity and density.[2] Two factors that can change the viscosity and density of a gas are temperature and barometric pressure (at higher altitude). If the changes are mild, flowmeter reading is not significantly affected. At high altitude, with a drop in barometric pressure, the density is decreased and flow can be higher than shown.

At pressures below 630 mm, the delivered flow rate will be higher than the set flow rate by 9%–20%. The reverse will be seen at increased pressure, as in a hyperbaric chamber with the delivered flow rate slightly less than the set flow rate.

The reading of gas flows through the flowmeter can be inaccurate if the tube is not vertical, if a downstream obstruction is causing back pressure, and if the float is sticking to the side of the tube due to dirt or static electricity.

Flow across the annular space results in a pressure drop. Restriction of tube diameter with a circular bobbin leads to a corresponding increased speed of gas flow and decreased pressure on the walls of the tube. The pressure drop across the orifice is inversely proportional to the orifice area squared. Since the diameter of the Thorpe tube increases as the bobbin floats upward, the pressure drop decreases. The bobbin reaches a steady state when the pressure drop exactly opposes the gravitational force (Figure 17.1). As gravitational forces are constant, this pressure drop is always the same. However, with increased flow rates, the bobbin will move higher, as the pressure drop will occur over a larger cross-sectional area, causing higher velocity.

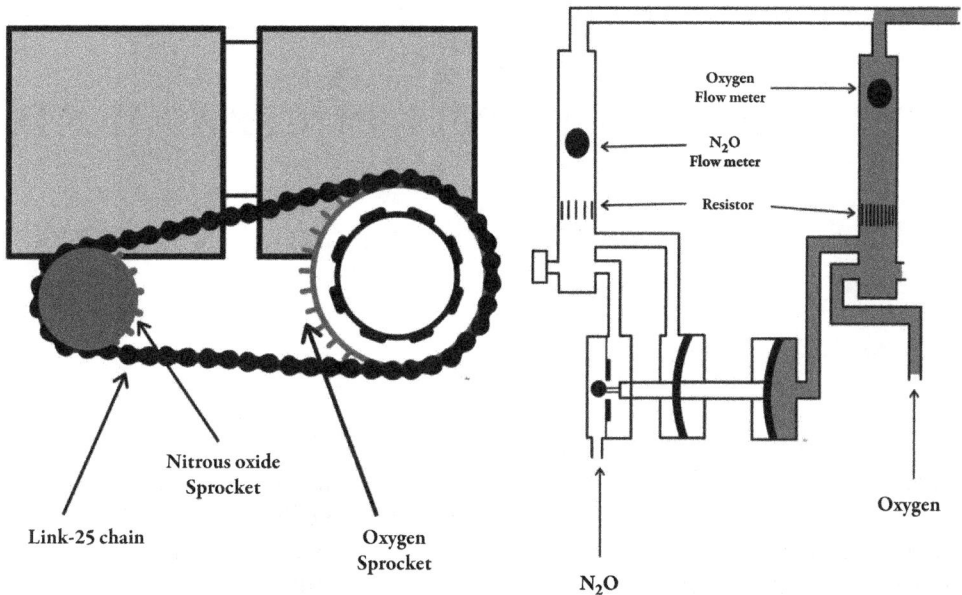

**Figure 17.2.** Oxygen proportioning systems. The mechanical link-25 system is shown at left, where a chain is physically attached to N$_2$O and oxygen knobs. The S-ORC pneumatic system is shown at right, where pressure in the oxygen system opens up valve and flow in N$_2$O flowmeter.
Illustration by Mahad Sohail, Research Fellow, Department of Anesthesiology, Beth Israel Deaconess Medical Center, Boston, MA, USA.

## SAFETY FEATURES OF FLOWMETERS

The traditional and transitional flowmeter control knobs are color- and touch-coded, with oxygen colored green (most prominent), and they have touch-sensitive flutes. Some of the anesthesia machines also have protective guards on the sides of knobs to avoid accidental change in gas flows. The indicator float has ridges also to help it spin constantly and thus avoid sticking to the walls of the tube. The oxygen flowmeter is placed downstream, closer to the patient, to avoid delivery of hypoxic gas mixture in case there is a leak upstream.[3,4] Some of the anesthesia machines have a basal rate of continuous oxygen flow (50–250 ml) through flowmeters even when the knob is in a fully closed position to ensure a continuous supply of oxygen.

Another important safety feature is the hypoxic guard system, also known as a proportioning system. This safety system links nitrous oxide and oxygen flowmeters either electronically, mechanically, or pneumatically. Its function is to prevent delivery of hypoxic breathing mixtures. A mechanical system, also known as Ohmeda "link 25," physically links the control knobs of oxygen and nitrous oxide flowmeters with a chain that turns down nitrous oxide flow when oxygen flow is decreased. The chain link allows oxygen and nitrous oxide flows to be adjusted independently, but automatically interjects to ensure a minimum 1:3 ratio. Drager uses a pneumatic proportioning system called "sensitive oxygen ratio system" (S-ORC). In this system, a resistor present in the oxygen flowmeter generates back pressure on a control diaphragm, which allows nitrous oxide to flow through its flowmeter. This system guarantees a minimum FIO$_2$ of 21% by limiting nitrous oxide flow (Figure 17.2). Electronic flowmeters, as used in Aisys, supply a minimum FIO$_2$ of 25% with nitrous oxide, and 21% with air.

## LIMITATIONS

All proportioning systems cannot sense the type of gas in the oxygen pipeline, and the presence of any gas can allow the flow. The mechanical system function is based only on movement of the knobs, and the pneumatic system senses the pressure created within by any gas. In case of a faulty connection or crossover, when another gas is present in the oxygen system, hypoxic gas mixtures will possibly be delivered to the patient.[5] Although the oxygen flowmeters are located downstream, a leak in the oxygen flowmeter tube can still deliver hypoxic gas to the patient. The presence of an oxygen analyzer in the breathing circuit is required to avoid these catastrophic conditions.

## REFERENCES

1. Loysen P. Flowmeters. *Health Phys.* 1972;22:417.
2. Coppel DL, Wilson J. Oxygen flowmeters. *Anaesthesia.* 1985;40:707.
3. Hay H. Delivery of an hypoxic gas mixture due to a defective rubber seal of a flowmeter control tube. *Eur J Anaesthesiol.* 2000;17: 456–458.
4. Linton RA, et al. A potential hazard of oxygen flowmeters. *Anaesthesia.* 1982;37:606–607.
5. Ishikawa S, et al. Hypoxic gas flow caused by malfunction of the proportioning system of anesthesia machines. *Anesth Analg.* 2002;94:1672.

# 18.

# PRINCIPLES OF DOPPLER ULTRASOUND

*Emily Young and Sherif Zaky*

## INTRODUCTION

Doppler ultrasound is a modality of ultrasound that can be used to examine the direction, velocity, and pattern of blood flow in a vessel. Understanding the Doppler effect, as well as the various types of Doppler ultrasound, is critical for effective clinical application.

## THE DOPPLER EFFECT

When a sound wave reflects off a moving object, its frequency changes based on the direction and speed of the object. This change in frequency is known as the Doppler shift. If the object is moving toward the sound source, the returning frequency will be higher than the original frequency (positive shift). If the object is moving away from the sound source, the returning frequency will be lower than the original (negative shift).[1] The most familiar example of the Doppler effect is the sound of a siren passing. As an ambulance moves toward the observer, the siren sounds high pitched because of the positive frequency shift. Once the ambulance passes, there is negative shift of the frequency, resulting in a lower pitched sound.

In Doppler ultrasound, this shift occurs as ultrasound waves reflect off moving red blood cells (Figure 18.1). The transducer detects these changes in frequency and displays them as a spectral waveform or a color image that we can use to determine the presence or absence of blood flow, the direction of blood flow, and the velocity of blood flow. Notably, Doppler shift cannot occur when the transducer is held perpendicularly to the blood vessel because the frequency of the sound wave will be unchanged.[2]

## CONTINUOUS WAVE DOPPLER

Continuous wave Doppler devices are the simplest Doppler instruments and consist of two transducers: one that emits a continuous sound beam, and one that receives the returning signals. Both transducers are housed in a small portable probe that converts any detected Doppler shift into audible sound waves.[3] This device is often used by vascular surgeons to check for the presence or absence of flow in superficial vessels. Continuous wave Doppler detects all signals along its path and does not provide information of specific depth signals, e.g., blood flow in a specific blood vessel. The returning signal is then displayed in a spectral waveform or as an audible signal (Figure 18.2A).

## PULSED WAVE DOPPLER

Unlike continuous wave Doppler, pulsed wave Doppler sends out a sound beam in short pulses. The time that the

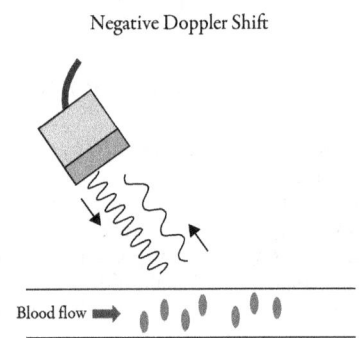
Negative Doppler Shift

Blood flow

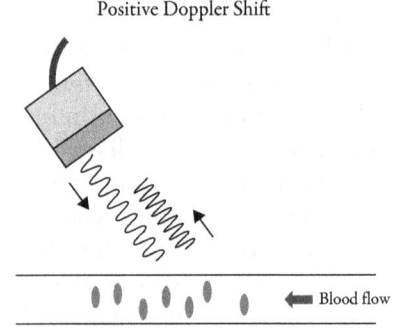
Positive Doppler Shift

Blood flow

**Figure 18.1.** The Doppler effect.

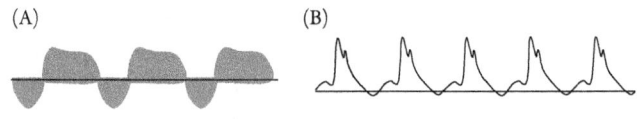

Figure 18.2. Continuous wave (A) and pulsed wave (B) Doppler.

pulse takes to return to the transducer can be used to determine the distance from the transducer to the moving object. An "electronic gate" can be set to evaluate only Doppler signals from a certain target depth. This allows the ultrasound receiver to assess for flow in a specific vessel, even if multiple vessels are in the path of the ultrasound beam.[2] The returning signals are displayed as a spectral waveform, with positive shifts in frequency displayed above the baseline, and negative shifts displayed below the baseline (Figure 18.2B).

## COLOR FLOW DOPPLER

Color flow Doppler assigns a color hue to moving objects based on their direction and speed. Generally, flow toward the transducer is displayed as red, and flow away from the transducer is displayed as blue. It is important to remember that these colors do not necessarily correlate with arterial or venous flow. The higher the velocity of flow, the brighter the color is displayed, with yellow and white representing the highest velocity areas. Turbulent flow appears as a mixture of colors. The color flow image is superimposed on a traditional gray-scale image, allowing for real-time assessment of blood flow within specific anatomical structures.[1]

## POWER DOPPLER

Power Doppler is another way of displaying Doppler ultrasound that is most useful for detecting subtle, low-volume flow. It uses the amplitude of the returning Doppler signals to generate an image without providing information about direction of flow. Areas with a high concentration of moving red blood cells appear brightest. This setting is used when assessing for the presence of blood flow in small vessels or masses, when direction of flow is not of interest.[2]

## REFERENCES

1. Aldrich JE. Basic physics of ultrasound imaging. *Crit Care Med.* 2007;35(5):S131–S137.
2. Sanders RC, Winter TC, eds. *Clinical Sonography: A Practical Guide.* Philadelphia, PA: Lippincott Williams & Wilkins; 2007.
3. Shriki J. Ultrasound physics. *Crit Care Clin.* 2014;30(1):1–24.

# 19.

# PROPERTIES OF LIQUIDS, GASES, AND VAPORS

*Ben Aquino*

## INTRODUCTION

Volatile anesthetics, like any substance, can exist in the gas, liquid, or solid phase. With the delivery of anesthetic gases, the focus is the transition back and forth between the liquid and gas phases. The challenge in administering a volatile agent, in gas form, to the patient is in the fact that most of these agents, at normal temperature and atmospheric pressure, are liquids. Once the gases have reached the body, they redistribute and dissolve in the various bodily compartments and organs. Their movement in and out of the body, as well as within the body, underlie their pharmacokinetics. As a result, knowledge of basic properties of liquids, gases, and vapors is important in understanding the pharmacokinetics of volatile anesthetics.

## CRITICAL TEMPERATURE AND PRESSURE

Every substance can exist in solid, liquid, and gas phases, depending on conditions of temperature and pressure. The temperature above which a substance can only exist as a gas, regardless of the pressure applied to it, is the critical temperature (Tc). The pressure above which a substance can only exist as a liquid, regardless of the temperature, is the critical pressure (Pc). At atmospheric pressure and normal conditions, volatile anesthetics are well below both their critical temperatures and pressures. By definition, this means that under these conditions, the molecules can go back and forth from the liquid to the gas phases. Gas coming out of the liquid phase and into the gas phase is defined as vapor. The vapor form of the volatile anesthetic is what gives it the clinical effect. Notably, vaporization occurs only at the surface of a given liquid. Boiling also results in the formation of gas from liquid, but it occurs when the vapor pressure in the liquid is equal to that of the surrounding air. In that situation, the vaporization takes place within the liquid as well, causing bubbling.

## VAPOR PRESSURE

An anesthetic agent in liquid form, in a sealed container, will have some molecules that evaporate, moving from the liquid to the gas phase. These gas molecules exert pressure on the inside of the container, known as a vapor pressure. Eventually the gas and liquid phases will reach an equilibrium within the container. Assuming a constant temperature, that pressure in the sealed container, exerted by the gas molecules in equilibrium with the liquid molecules, is the saturated vapor pressure. The clinically applicable "vapor pressure" of the anesthetic gases is actually the anesthetic agent's saturated vapor pressure at a temperature of 20°C. Vapor pressure is dependent on only two things: temperature, and the properties of the gas itself.

Dalton's law states that in a mixture of gases, the total pressure exerted by that mixture is equal to the sum of the partial pressures of each individual gas. Saturated vapor pressure can be expressed as absolute partial pressure, or the percentage in volume, in atmospheres, of the substance in question. In anesthesia the potency of the anesthetic agent being delivered is measured in the percentage of volume, although the variable bypass vaporizer delivers the agent at a specific partial pressure in order to get that percent volume of agent in the mixture.

## SOLUBILITY COEFFICIENTS

Once gases enter the alveoli and then the blood, the blood redistributes them to the tissues, and in all three of these locations, the gas dissolves. The ability of a substance to dissolve in a given solute is known as the solubility coefficient. The transfer of gas to the blood and tissues, however, is dependent on the comparative abilities of the gas to dissolve in the solute in question. The solubility difference between two different media is known as a partition coefficient. The clinically applicable coefficients in the delivery of anesthetic gas include the blood-gas partition coefficient (solubility of the substance in blood compared to its solubility in gas) and the oil-gas partition coefficient.[1] Halothane has a higher blood-gas partition coefficient of 2.4, meaning that at equilibrium, blood will contain 2.4 times as much dissolved halothane compared to the amount of dissolved halothane in gas. This means that halothane is more soluble in blood than in gas.

For clinical purposes, the alveolar concentration of a volatile agent equates with the amount of that anesthetic in the central nervous system (CNS). Because halothane, at equilibrium, is 2.4 times as soluble in blood as in gas, the blood needs to take up a significant amount of the gas before it is preferentially taken up by alveolar gas (and the brain). As a result, halothane has a slow onset and slow emergence time.

By contrast, desflurane has a low blood-gas partition coefficient, which means it is relatively insoluble in blood and is taken up more quickly in alveolar gas and in the CNS.

Oil-gas partition coefficients give an idea of the relative movement and solubilities of volatile anesthetic between lipids and gases. Halothane, with an oil-gas coefficient of 224, dissolves and gets stored in lipophilic tissues (such as adipose), which, in an obese patient, increases anesthetic onset and offset time compared to a thinner patient. Desflurane has a relatively low oil-gas coefficient of 18.7, which means it is far less soluble in fat than halothane. This allows for it to have shorter onset and emergence times, and though those times may still be longer in an obese patient than in a thin one, the differences are not nearly as significant as they would be for a more lipophilic drug like halothane.

## DIFFUSION OF GASES

Gases in the respiratory system move by bulk flow, but because of the increase in surface area in each successive generation of airways, gas is moving at almost zero velocity at the alveolar level, and at this point, diffusion is the necessary driving force for gas transport. The movement of gases across the alveolar membrane can be explained by Fick's law of diffusion. It states that the volume of gas per unit time that moves across the alveolar-capillary interface will be directly proportional to the concentration gradient between the two areas, the surface area of the interface, and the diffusivity. It will be inversely proportional to the thickness of the alveolar-capillary layer.

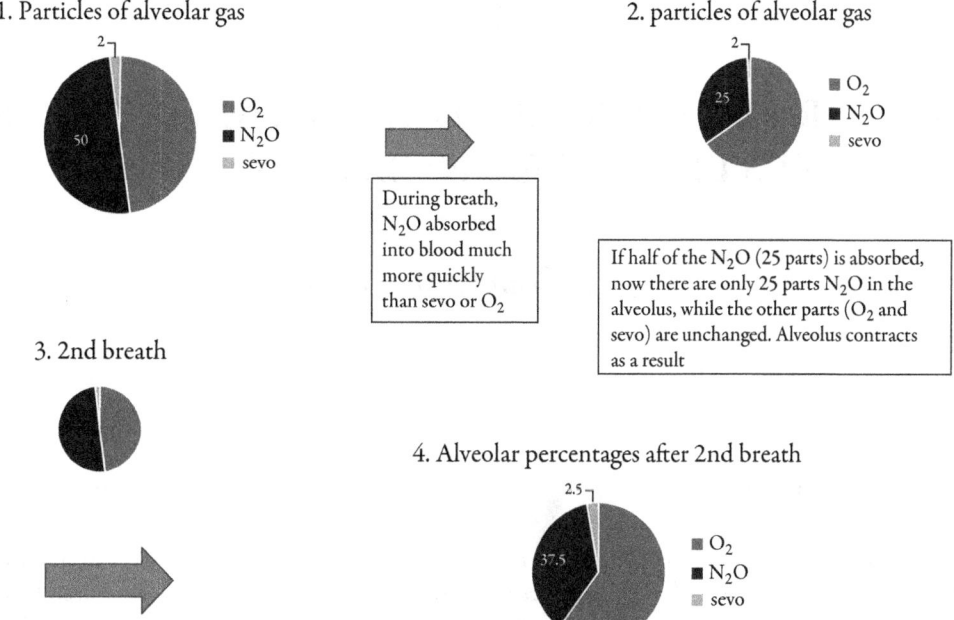

**Figure 19.1.** Second gas effect: illustration with $N_2O$ and 2% sevo.

1. Alveolar mixture: 50 parts $N_2O$, 48 parts $O_2$, 2 parts sevo (50/48/2).

2. Alveolus mixture has contracted because 25 parts of the $N_2O$ are absorbed into the blood before the other gases: now 75 parts total, 25/48/2.

3. Second breath is taken, with the same proportions as the original—50/48/2—but only 25 parts of this mixture enter the alveolus: 12.5 parts $N_2O$, 12 parts $O_2$, 0.5 parts sevo.

4. The two components, added up, are as follows:

    a. 25 + 12.5 = 37.5 parts $N_2O$, i.e., 37.5%

    b. 48 + 12 = 60 parts $O_2$, or 60%

    c. 2 + 0.5 = 2.5 parts sevo, or 2.5%

    d. In one breath, the second gas effect has theoretically increased alveolar concentration from 2.0% to 2.5%, even though the mixture being inspired is only 2%.

## CONCENTRATION EFFECT AND SECOND GAS EFFECT

The concentration gradient is an illustration of Fick's law. It says that as the concentration of a gas increases, the rate of alveolar concentration of a gas approaches the inspired concentration of the gas. The concentration difference between the alveoli and the capillaries becomes greater, and that gradient, according to Fick's law, drives the diffusion of gas through the alveolar-capillary layer and into the blood. This is most applicable clinically to nitrous oxide, because it is administered in a much higher concentration than other inhaled anesthetics. The second gas effect, which is somewhat of a consequence of the concentration effect, occurs with an anesthetic administered at a high concentration, like $N_2O$, facilitates uptake of another co-administered gas.

For example, if $O_2$, sevoflurane, and $N_2O$ are given together, the alveolus expands with the addition of the gas. The $N_2O$ is then rapidly absorbed into the blood, which lowers alveolar $N_2O$ volume and percentage. The lower volume causes the alveolus to contract. Subsequently, the lung gets refilled with more of the mixture containing $O_2$, sevoflurane, and $N_2O$, re-expanding the alveolus. At this point, both the partial pressures of the carrier gas and sevoflurane are increased as a result. This has been postulated to be caused by absorption of large amounts of a soluble gas (like $N_2O$) from the lung, which then results in increased inspiratory inflow of the original mixture.[2] See Figure 19.1 for an illustration of this.

## REFERENCES

1. Forman SA, Ishizawa Y. Inhaled anesthetic pharmacokinetics. Uptake, distribution and toxicty. In: Miller RD, Cohen NH, Eriksson LI, et al. *Miller's Anesthesia*. 8th ed. Philadelphia, PA: Elsevier Saunders; 2015.

2. Epstein RM, et al. Influence of the concentration effect on the uptake of anesthetic mixtures: The second gas effect. *Anesthesiology*. 1964; 25(5):364–371.

# 20.

# VAPOR PRESSURE AND CALCULATION OF ANESTHETIC CONCENTRATIONS

*Ben Aquino and Afshin Heidari*

## INTRODUCTION

Inhaled anesthetics produce immobility via actions on the spinal cord.[1] There is consensus that inhaled anesthetics produce anesthesia by enhancing inhibitory channels and attenuating excitatory channels, but whether or not this occurs through direct binding or membrane alterations is not known.[2]

Since the first publicly performed anesthetic demonstration at Massachusetts General Hospital in 1846, vaporizers have been an essential component of anesthesia equipment.[3] Vaporizers allow a known and reproducible concentration of anesthetic vapor to be delivered in a safe and reliable manner. Modern anesthetic vaporizers have been developed to provide accurate amounts of anesthetic gas while mitigating the effects of temperature and barometric pressure on the evaporation process.

## VAPOR PRESSURE

Vapor pressure is pressure exerted by a vapor when the is in equilibrium with the liquid or solid form, or both, of the same substance—when conditions are such that the substance can exist in both or in all three phases. Vapor pressure is a measure of the tendency of a material to change into the gaseous or vapor state, and increasing temperature will increase the ratio of gas:liquid molecules, thereby increasing vapor pressure. The temperature at which the vapor pressure at the surface of a liquid becomes equal to the pressure exerted by the surroundings is called the boiling point of the liquid.

In a closed container, molecules from a volatile liquid escape the liquid phase and become vapor. Vapor pressure is the force exerted on the container area by these gaseous molecules as they strike the wall of the container.

Equilibrium is the state in which a constant number of molecules jump from the liquid phase to gas phase and vice versa.

## SATURATED VAPOR PRESSURE (SVP)

Saturated vapor pressure is the state at which the gas phase on top of the liquid phase is saturated by the molecules of vapor (i.e., it contains as much vapor as it can handle).

Sevoflurane = 160 mmHg

Enflurane = 175 mmHg

Halothane = 243 mmHg

Isoflurane = 241 mmHg.

## VAPOR CONCENTRATION

Volume % = (saturated partial pressure of volatile anesthetic/atm pressure) × 100.

Sevoflurane = 160/760 = 21%

Enflurane = 175/760 = 23%

Halothane = 243/760 = 32%

Isoflurane = 241/760 = 32%.

In variable bypass vaporizers:
SVP agent (mmHg)/total pressure (mmHg) = volume of volatile anesthetic/total volume leaving vaporizer = volatile anesthetic (ml)/(carrier gas (ml) + volatile anesthetic (ml)).

Thus, if the fresh gas flow is set to 1L and dial is set at 1%, 10 ml/min of sevoflurane gas must exit the vaporizer.

If an agent-specific vaporizer is misfilled with an agent that has a higher SVP than the intended anesthetic, then actual output concentration will be **greater** than the concentration indicated by the dial.

## BOILING POINT

Boiling point is defined as the temperature at which vapor pressure equals atmospheric pressure (760 mmHg).

*Table 20.1* BASIC PROPERTIES OF COMMONLY USED VOLATILE ANESTHETICS

| AGENT | VAPOR PRESSURE MMHG | MAC | BLOOD:GAS PARTITION COEFFICIENT (AT 37°C) | OIL:GAS PARTITION COEFFICIENT (AT 37°C) | BOILING POINT °C | LATENT HEAT OF VAPORIZATION KJ/MOL |
|---|---|---|---|---|---|---|
| Desflurane | 664 | 6.0 | 0.45 | 19 | 22.8 | 24.9 |
| Enflurane | 175 | 1.58 | 1.9 | 175 | 56.5 | 32.7 |
| Halothane | 243 | 0.75 | 2.5 | 197 | 50.2 | 29.8 |
| Isoflurane | 238 | 1.28 | 1.4 | 90.8 | 48.5 | 31.9 |
| Sevoflurane | 157 | 2.05 | 0.65 | 47–54 | 58.6 | 34.1 |

Boiling point (C°):

Sevoflurane: 58.5

Desflurane: 22.8

Isoflurane: 48.5

Enflurane: 56.5

Halothane: 50.2

N20: –88.

## LATENT HEAT OF VAPORIZATION

Energy is required when a molecule changes from liquid to gas, and latent heat of vaporization is the number of calories required to change 1 gram of liquid into vapor without changing temperature. Thus, in the absence of an outside temperature source, volatile liquids will cool significantly, leading to decreasing vaporization. The latent heats of vaporization among the common volatile anesthetic gases are similar. However, desflurane is notable for being less potent than the other agents. Thus, more desflurane molecules are required to achieve a given level of anesthetic depth than with the other agents, leading to greater temperature loss and decreasing vapor pressure.

Modern conventional vaporizers (for halothane, isoflurane, enflurane, sevoflurane) are agent specific, temperature compensated, variable bypass vaporizers. They automatically compensate for changes in altitude because they put out a partial pressure that is determined by the position of the dial. Even though the units on the dial are percentages, the vaporizer is calibrated to release a mixture with a specific partial pressure. The partial pressure of the anesthetic agent is what determines whether a patient is anesthetized, and it does not change at different altitudes. In an anesthetic with isoflurane at high altitude, setting the dial to 1% will have the same effect as it would at sea level.[1–3]

However, if the question relates to volume concentration, then use this equation:

$$VO = (CG \times SVP) / (Pb - SVP)$$

Where VO = vapor output (ml), CG = carrier gas flow(mL/min), SVP = saturated vapor pressure (mm Hg) at room temperature, and Pb is barometric pressure (mmHg)

At a higher altitude where the barometric pressure is one-half that at sea level, the amount of isoflurane vapor output increases due to the lower barometric pressure. Therefore, the settings that delivered 2% isoflurane now deliver 4% isoflurane. However, according to Dalton's law, the partial pressure of isoflurane delivered would be approximately the same at both altitudes since 2% isoflurane at 760 mmHg (15.2 mmHg) is the same as 4% isoflurane at 380 mmHg (15.2 mmHg).

For example, in order to deliver 8.4 mmHg (1 MAC) of isoflurane at 8000 feet, an anesthetic concentration of 1.5% is needed. However, a vaporizer set for 1.1% is actually producing 1.7%, or a partial pressure of 9.9 mmHg. Thus, the vaporizer slightly overcompensates for the reduced atmospheric pressure. Note that this does *not* apply to the desflurane vaporizer.

Alternatively, the desflurane vaporizer is electrically heated to 39°C, which creates a vapor pressure of 2 atmospheres inside the vaporizer, regardless of ambient pressure. The number on the dial reflects the percentage that will be delivered. At any altitude, when the dial is at 5%, it will release a 5% mixture of desflurane. But when that 5% desflurane leaves the vaporizer at high altitude, what is delivered to the patient is 5% of a decreased ambient pressure, so the partial pressure of desflurane in the alveoli will be much less that it would be at sea level. Thus, a **higher** concentration will be needed at high elevation to attain the same clinical effect as at sea level with the desflurane (Tec-9) vaporizer.

See Table 20.1 for some of the basic properties of the more commonly used anesthetic gases.[1,2]

## REFERENCES

1. Campagna JA, Miller KW, Forman SA. Mechanisms of action of inhaled anesthetics. *N Engl J Med*. 2003;348:2110–2124.
2. Forman SA, Ishizawa Y. Inhaled anesthetic pharmacokinetics: Uptake, distribution, metabolism, and toxicity. In: Miller RD, Cohen NH, Eriksson LI, et al. *Miller's Anesthesia*. 8th ed. Philadelphia, PA: Elsevier Saunders; 2015.
3. Robinson DH, Toledo AH. Historical development of modern anesthesia. *J Invest Surg*. 2012 Jun;25(3):141–149.

# 21.

## VAPORIZER TYPES AND SAFETY FEATURES

*Ben Aquino*

### INTRODUCTION

The vaporizer is the key component of any anesthesia machine and any gas-based anesthetic, using oxygen and other carrying gases to safely, predictably, and consistently deliver vaporized volatile anesthetic to the patient via the anesthesia circuit. There are three principal types of vaporizers in modern use—variable bypass, dual circuit, and cassette. Variable-bypass vaporizers are most commonly used, and the dual-circuit vaporizer is primarily for desflurane administration. Cassette vaporizers are much less common but can dispense a variety of anesthetic agents.

### VARIABLE-BYPASS VAPORIZER

This is used for sevoflurane, isoflurane, enflurane, and halothane. Most of the fresh gas flow from the anesthesia machine goes from the flowmeters through the anesthesia machine and into the circle circuit. The variable-bypass vaporizer diverts a small percentage of the fresh gas flow past the vaporizing chamber, where it mixes with vaporized volatile anesthetic and is then remixed downstream with the remainder of the total fresh gas. The amount of the delivered volatile anesthetic is measured as a percentage of the total fresh gas flow. The amount of gas passing through the chamber is controlled by (1) the dial on the vaporizer—as the dial is increased, a greater percentage of the total fresh gas flow is diverted through the vaporizing chamber (splitting ratio); and (2) the temperature-compensation device. Vapor pressure varies with temperature, so the temperature-compensation device is a key element of safe delivery of anesthetic gas, maintaining consistent vaporizer output over a wide range of temperatures. The device, usually a bimetallic strip, directs more flow through the vaporizing chamber in response to decreases in temperature. The splitting ratios needed to create the proper mixture of anesthetic gas and carrier gas are different for each anesthetic agent, and these splitting ratios are what make each vaporizer agent specific. Notably, though the vaporizer is calibrated to deliver anesthetic as a specific percent concentration of the total gas output, it is the anesthetic partial pressure of the gas mixture that reaches the brain which accounts for its clinical effect.

### DUAL-CIRCUIT VAPORIZER

Desflurane presents a unique set of challenges due to its high vapor pressure, which at 660 mmHg closely resembles atmospheric temperature. (1) Desflurane in a variable-bypass vaporizer would need impractically high flows in order to produce output with usable anesthetic concentrations. (2) Its high rate of evaporation would cause significant cooling in a variable-bypass vaporizer, causing progressively less output of gas as the system cooled over time. This would make delivery of gas inconsistent and difficult to control. (3) The desflurane boiling point is 22.8°C, close to room temperature, and boiling of the gas in a variable-bypass vaporizer would also produce unpredictable and uncontrolled outputs.

To allow for these challenges, the desflurane vaporizer has several features. First, the desflurane vaporizer is more a dual gas blender than a "vaporizer"—it contains two parallel circuits, one for fresh gas and the other for desflurane vapor. No variable-bypass mechanism is present. Second, in order to counteract the cooling that would take place with desflurane evaporation at its normal vapor pressure, the desflurane chamber is heated to 39°C, which is warmer than any operating room (OR) room temperature. The chamber in the desflurane vaporizer also pressurizes the vapor to a constant pressure of 1300 mmHg. The heating and pressurization both allow for a more controlled delivery of the desflurane vapor.

At that point, the desflurane is added back to the carrier gas. Instead of splitting ratios, the desflurane vaporizer uses a differential pressure transducer to control anesthetic concentration. The fresh gas flow goes through a restrictor and creates backpressure that is sensed by the differential pressure transducer. The transducer senses the pressure

*Table 21.1* COMPARISON OF VARIABLE-BYPASS AND DUAL CIRCUIT VAPORIZERS

| | NUMBER OF GAS LINES | FRESH GAS FLOW MOVEMENT | METHOD OF MIXTURE | METHOD OF DELIVERY | EFFECTS ON ANESTHETIC DELIVERY AT HIGH ALTITUDE – LOWER ATMOSPHERIC PRESSURE (PATM) |
|---|---|---|---|---|---|
| Variable bypass vaporizer | One | Part of fresh gas flow (FGF) moves through vaporizer, the rest is diverted around it | A percentage of FGF goes through vaporizer according to splitting ratios determined by concentration dial | Calibrated (at atmospheric pressure) to release anesthetic vapor at a specific PARTIAL PRESSURE | Calibrated to release a constant partial pressure – but if Patm is abnormally low, the delivered concentration and partial pressure of gas will be HIGHER than on the vaporizer dial |
| Tec 6 desflurane vaporizer (dual circuit vaporizer) | Two, kept separate until downstream from vaporizer | Fresh gas flow does NOT go through vaporizer | Vaporized desflurane added to FGF, downstream from vaporizer chamber | Differential pressure transducer helps to release the desflurane at a specific CONCENTRATION | Releases gas at a specific concentration, so at lower Patm, a given % of desflurane will have an identical concentration but a LOWER partial pressure that a similar mixture at normal Patm |

difference between the two circuits, which in turn affects a pressure release valve in the vapor circuit. The end result is that when the circuits combine at the vaporizer outlet, the pressures in the vapor circuit and fresh gas flow circuit are equal. See Table 21.1 for a comparison of the basic features of the variable-bypass and dual-circuit vaporizers.

## CASSETTE VAPORIZER

In the early 2000s the Datex-Ohmeda ADU machine was equipped with a unique Aladin Cassette Vaporizer. This electronically controlled vaporizer can deliver 5 different inhaled anesthetics, doing so with interchangeable cassettes that each contained a unique anesthetic liquid. The cassette vaporizer is essentially a computer-controlled variable-bypass vaporizer. The ratio of vaporized flow to bypassed flow is controlled by a throttle valve. This throttle valve is, in turn, affected by five factors: (1) dial setting, (2) cassette temperature, (3) total pressure in the cassette, (4) bypass flow and cassette flow, and (5) carrier gas composition.[1]

## SAFETY FEATURES

Filling a vaporizer with the wrong agent can have dire consequences, most notably in the case of desflurane, where its accidental presence in a variable-bypass vaporizer can cause dangerously high concentrations of gas to be delivered to the patient. A keyed filling system, where a unique bottle nozzle, specific for each agent, adheres to a unique filling port on the vaporizer, prevents this from happening.

Tipping a vaporizer can be dangerous because it can allow the liquid to enter the bypass chamber, causing a dangerously high concentration of agent to be delivered. This is prevented by the vaporizers being securely fastened to a manifold on the anesthesia machine. Newer Drager™ vaporizers have a transport (T) dial setting that isolates the vaporizer chamber from the bypass chamber, eliminating risk of internal overflow.

As part of the mounting mechanism, anesthesia machines contain a vaporizer interlock system, which prevents the administration of more than one agent at a time.

Another potential cause of high gas concentration delivery is from overfilled liquid entering the bypass chamber. Vaporizers that fill from the side and not the top—the maximum fill amount is determined by the level of the filler port—are a necessary part of the design to prevent overfilling. See Table 21.2 for a view of these vaporizer safety features.

In addition to the aforementioned safety features, the desflurane vaporizer has a shut-off valve that closes in the event of major problems, including the following: (1) anesthetic level decreases to less than 20 mL; (2) vaporizer is tilted; (3) power failure occurs (and the vaporizer is no longer heated); and (4) there is a critical disparity between the pressures in the vapor circuit and the fresh gas circuit.[2]

## ANESTHESIA CONSIDERATIONS

### PREOPERATIVE

The anesthesia provider needs to understand the potentially catastrophic consequences of incorrectly filled or overfilled vaporizers, and the fail-safe mechanisms to ensure their safe use. These, however, do not prevent the agent bottles from being filled with impure or incorrect agents. In the event of

*Table 21.2* SUMMARY OF VAPORIZER SAFETY FEATURES

| VAPORIZER RISK | POTENTIAL PROBLEM | SAFETY FEATURE | RATIONALE/ COMMENTS |
|---|---|---|---|
| Overfilling | Extra anesthesia vapor enters bypass chamber – HIGHER than expected anesthetic concentrations | Side port filling | Extent of vaporizer filling is determined by height of side port |
| Tipping | Vapor spills into bypass chamber – HIGHER than expected anesthetic concentrations | "Transport" (T) setting on dial – used when moving vaporizer | Separates bypass and FGF chambers |
| Mixed agents | Unpredictable delivery of gases – potentially ineffectively low, or dangerously high | Vaporizer interlock | Ensures that only one vaporizer at a time can be open |
| Circuit leak | Causes LOWER than expected levels of anesthetic to be delivered. Contamination of operating room air with anesthetic also possible. | Vaporizer locks into manifold system on anesthesia machine | Most common source of vaporizer leak is loose filling cap[a] |
| Filling vaporizer with wrong agent | Unpredictable and potentially dangerous levels of anesthetic gas administered to patient. | 1. Notched, agent-specific interface between agent bottle and dispensing nozzle<br>2. Keyed, agent-specific attachments between dispensing nozzle and vaporizer | |

[a] Dorsch J, Dorsch S. Vaporizers (Anesthetic Agent Delivery Devices). In: Dorsch J. Dorsch S. Understanding Anesthesia Equipment. 4th ed. Baltimore, MD: Lippincott Williams & Wilkins 1999: 172

a vaporizer that has been tipped or overfilled, the general recommendation is to run the vaporizer at high flows for 20–30 minutes. The vaporizer setting and flow time differ between models.[2]

Internal leaks in the vaporizer can only be detected when the vaporizer is turned on (cassette vaporizers are a notable exception to this), and this is true even in machine self-tests. As a result, the provider needs to ensure preoperatively that the vaporizers are functioning properly.

## INTRAOPERATIVE

Once the anesthesia has begun, the anesthesiologist must make sure that the intended anesthetic gas is being administered at its intended concentration. The anesthesiologist also needs to be aware of potential leaks within the vaporizer system, most often from a loose cap on the vaporizer reservoir. Such a leak may cause the gas to be delivered at less than its intended concentration, increasing the likelihood of light anesthesia.

## REFERENCES

1. Hendrickx JF, et al. The ADU vaporizing unit: A new vaporizer. *Anesth Analg.* 2001;93:391–395.
2. Venticinque SG, Andrews JJ. Inhaled anesthetics: Delivery systems. In: Miller RD, Cohen NH, Eriksson LI, et al., eds. *Miller's Anesthesia*. Philadelphia, PA: Elsevier Saunders; 2015.

# 22.

# UPTAKE AND DISTRIBUTION OF INHALATION AGENTS

*Lora B. Levin*

Induction of general anesthesia results when the goal partial pressure of the anesthetic gas is achieved in the central nervous system (CNS). The CNS partial pressure increases as anesthetic gas moves from the vaporizer along a series of concentration/partial pressure gradients until reaching the CNS. Volatile anesthetics gases are delivered from the anesthetic machine vaporizer to the patient's alveoli through the breathing circuit as part of the fresh gas flow delivered to the patient during ventilation. Uptake of the volatile anesthetic occurs when the anesthetic gas diffuses from the alveoli into the patient's pulmonary blood. The volatile anesthetic is then distributed via arterial blood flow to various organ tissues throughout the body, including the brain, where volatile anesthetics act to induce and maintain general anesthesia. The inspired concentration (FI) of anesthetic gas equilibrates with the alveolar gas concentration (FA) which equilibrates with the arterial gas concentration (Fa) which equilibrates with the CNS tissue gas concentration.[1]

The alveolar gas concentration (FA) is easily measurable. Changes in FA correlate with the partial pressure of anesthetic gases in the CNS such that FA can represent the onset and recovery from volatile anesthetics. When FA increases more quickly, induction of anesthesia occurs faster. At any one time, FA is determined by the relative delivery of anesthetic gases to the alveoli (increases FA) versus the uptake of anesthetic gas into the pulmonary circulation (decreases FA).

**Delivery** of gas to the alveoli is determined by the inspired gas concentration (FI) and alveolar ventilation. The FI depends on several factors: gas concentration delivered from the vaporizer, fresh gas flow rate and the amount of rebreathing, the volume of the breathing circuit which can dilute the anesthetic, gas and the absorption of anesthetic gas by the breathing circuit which can lower FI. Using a higher than goal vaporizer setting (overpressure), higher fresh gas flow rates with little to no rebreathing, smaller breathing circuit volumes, and lower circuit absorption materials will speed up the increase of FA and induction times.[1]

Increasing alveolar ventilation, when other factors are constant, will cause an increase in rate of rise of FA as more anesthetic gas is delivered to the alveoli to replace the anesthetic gas taken up into pulmonary blood.[3] This effect is more pronounced in anesthetics with higher blood solubility. Minute ventilation changes have little effect on the least soluble anesthetic gases since uptake into pulmonary blood is minimal.

**Uptake** of gas from the alveoli into the pulmonary circulation is a product of the blood:gas partition coefficient ($\lambda_b$), cardiac output (CO), and the Alveolar-to-venous partial pressure difference (A − v). Uptake $= \lambda_b \times CO \times (A - v)$.

Uptake is most dependent on the blood solubility of the anesthetic gas as reflected by the blood:gas partition coefficient.[3] The blood:gas partition coefficient describes the distribution of anesthetic gas between two states at equilibrium. More soluble gases have higher blood:gas partition coefficients, e.g., halothane, and these gases will have significant uptake into pulmonary blood before equilibrium between FA and Fa is achieved.[2] This results in slower increase of FA and a slower onset of action when compared with anesthetic gases with lower blood solubility, such as desflurane, where minimal uptake into the pulmonary circulation allows for a faster FA increase and equilibrium with Fa, resulting in a faster induction of anesthesia.

Changes in CO also affect the onset of anesthesia. Increases in CO, such as that caused by pain or anxiety, cause increased pulmonary blood flow, resulting in increased uptake of anesthetic gas, which slows the increase of FA leading to a slower induction time. Conversely, decreased CO, such as that caused by hypovolemia or shock, will cause a more rapid induction. The effects of CO on FA and induction time are more pronounced with more soluble than less soluble anesthetics.[2]

The uptake of anesthetic is also affected by the partial pressure difference between the alveoli and pulmonary blood. This pressure gradient drives uptake from the alveoli into the blood, and is affected by tissue uptake. This is especially evident within the first minutes of administering volatile anesthetics.

**Distribution** of volatile anesthetic to various organs results from the delivery and uptake of anesthetic gas from the arterial blood into these tissues. Uptake of anesthetic gas for a particular organ is a product of the tissue:blood partition coefficient ($\lambda_t$), the organ blood flow, i.e., cerebral blood flow (CBF), and the arterial to tissue partial pressure difference (a – t). For example, CNS uptake = $\lambda_{cns}$ × CBF × (a – cns).

The solubility of an anesthetic gas in a particular tissue is represented by the tissue:blood partition coefficient.[2] The tissue:blood partition coefficient is low for all gases for lean tissue such as brain, other vital organs, muscle, and skin. The tissue:blood partition coefficient for all gases, except nitrous, is very high for adipose tissue. Therefore, CNS tissue, with its lower tissue solubility, will have less uptake of anesthetic gas than adipose tissues and will reach equilibrium with arterial anesthetic partial pressure more quickly than adipose tissue, which has much higher tissue:blood partition coefficient.

Blood flow to the various tissues is dependent on tissue vascularity and CO. Vessel rich group (VRG) of organs, such as the brain, heart, kidneys, and liver, receive 75% of CO but represent only 10% of lean body weight.[3] They therefore receive much higher blood flow, approximately 100 ml/minute, than either the muscle group or the adipose group tissues, approximately 2–3ml/minute. As such, VRG will receive more anesthetic gas per unit of time and will reach tissue partial pressure equal to arterial partial pressure much more quickly than either the muscle or adipose groups.

Until the tissue partial pressure of anesthetic gas equals the partial pressure in the blood, uptake of the anesthetic gas into that tissue will occur driven by the difference between the arterial to tissue partial pressures. Uptake into the tissue will decrease over time as the partial pressure of anesthetic gas in the tissue increases and the arterial to tissue partial pressure gradient decreases.

One way to understand the change in anesthetic gas partial pressure for the various tissue groups is to look at the time constant ($\tau$) where $\tau$ = capacity/flow = $\lambda_t$/organ blood flow for anesthetic gases. Therefore, $\tau$ will be much shorter for a lean tissue with low $\lambda_t$ and high perfusion, such as the brain, than for adipose tissue with high $\lambda_t$ and low perfusion. The time constant calculates the speed of change in a particular system where $1\tau$ is the time to 63% change, $2\tau$ is time to 86% change, and $3\tau$ is time to 95% change. Equilibrium is achieved in approximately 3 time constants.[2] VRG tissues such as the brain have low tissue solubility combined with small volumes and high blood

flow, so their tissue partial pressures increase quickly, reaching the arterial partial pressure of an anesthetic and steady state in about 12 minutes. Muscle groups have similar low tissue solubility when compared with VRG, but lower blood flow and a larger volume, so they will have tissue uptake of anesthetic gases for hours. Adipose tissues have very high solubility combined with a larger volume and very reduced blood flow, so uptake into adipose tissue can continue for days.

## ANESTHETIC CONSIDERATIONS

1. Partial pressures equilibrate across the system: FI⇔FA⇔Fa⇔CNS tissue partial pressure:
   - FA is easily measurable and correlates with CNS partial pressure of anesthetic.
   - Induction of anesthesia occurs as FA rises to equal FI.
2. Delivery: Factors that increase delivery of anesthetic gases to the alveoli will speed the increase in FA and hasten the induction of anesthesia. These factors include overpressure, increased FGF to eliminate rebreathing, breathing circuits with less volume and less absorption of anesthetic gases, and increased alveolar ventilation.
3. Uptake = $\lambda_b$ × CO × (A–v).
   Factors that increase the uptake of anesthetic gases will slow the increase in FA and will slow the onset of anesthesia. These factors include higher blood:gas partition coefficient and higher cardiac output.
4. Distribution: CNS has a low tissue:blood coefficient combined with small volume and high blood flow, so time constant for all anesthetics is 1–3 minutes. Therefore, CNS tissue partial pressure of anesthetic gas will equilibrate with Fa and therefore FA in 9–15 minutes.

## REFERENCES

1. Morgan GE, et al. *Clinical Anesthesiology*. New York, NY: Lange Medical Books/McGraw Hill Medical; 2002:127–132.
2. Barash PG, et al. *Clinical Anesthesia*. Philadelphia, PA: Wolters Kluwer; 2017:462–468.
3. Dunn PF, et al. *Clinical Anesthesia Procedures of the Massachusettes General Hospital*. Philadelphia, PA: Wolters Kluwer; 2007:183–187.

# 23.

## UPTAKE AND ELIMINATION CURVES

*Lora B. Levin*

### INTRODUCTION

General anesthesia occurs from the delivery of anesthesia gas to the patient, resulting in a goal partial pressure of the anesthetic gas in the central nervous system (CNS) that induces general anesthesia. Equilibrium between the alveolar concentration of anesthetic gas (FA) and the partial pressure of anesthetic gas in the CNS is relatively quick. Therefore, FA correlates well with the level/dose of inhalational anesthetics. At any one time, FA is determined by the relative delivery of anesthetic gases to the alveoli (increases FA) versus the uptake of anesthetic gas into the pulmonary circulation (decreases FA).

### UPTAKE CURVES

When we look at the rise of FA as compared to the concentration of inspired gas (FI) over time, we can see how quickly anesthesia is induced. All FA/FI uptake curves have a similar shape but different positions on the graph (Figure 23.1).

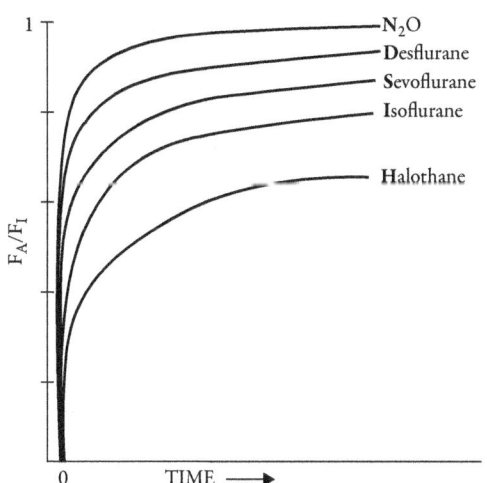

**Figure 23.1** FA/FI uptake curves.

The overall position of anesthetic gases on the graph is determined by the solubility of the anesthetic gas. Keeping ventilation and cardiac output constant, the solubility of the anesthetic as described by its blood:gas partition coefficient is the most important factor determining the rate of rise of FA/FI. Anesthetics with lower blood:gas partition coefficients will have a faster FA/FI rise and therefore a faster induction and onset of general anesthesia.

Although the gases differ in position on the curve as per their blood solubility, they all have similar shapes. In seconds to minutes of gas delivery, FA is low to zero, so there is no uptake into the pulmonary circulation and FA increases quickly and similarly for all gases. As FA rises further and drives uptake into the pulmonary blood, the curves differentiate due to different rates of uptake into the pulmonary circulation. Gases with higher blood:gas partition coefficients, such as halothane, will undergo more uptake into the pulmonary circulation and the rate of rise of FA/FI will slow.

Increased ventilation delivers more anesthetic gas to the alveoli and hastens the rise of FA/FI and thus the onset of anesthesia. This effect is more pronounced for anesthesia gases with higher blood solubility since uptake of lower solubility is minimal. Similarly, changes in cardiac output (CO) will affect the rise of FA/FI. Decreases in CO will decrease uptake of anesthetic and increase the rate of rise of FA/FI, while increases in CO will increase the uptake of anesthetic and decrease the rate of rise of FA/FI. These changes in CO will have little effect on anesthetic gases with low solubility since there is little uptake at baseline. If ventilation and CO are both doubled, you would see a slight increase in FA/FI rise. The increased ventilation would increase FA/FI rise, and the increased CO would decrease FA/FI rise. However, these two changes don't completely cancel each other because the increased CO would also cause faster delivery of the anesthetic to the tissues. Instead of no change, a doubling of ventilation and cardiac output would cause a slight increase in FA/FI rise.

FA/FI rise can also be affected by ventilation/perfusion mismatches as these result in an abnormal FA to Fa (arterial gas concentration) relationship. A right-to-left pulmonary shunt, such as a right mainstem intubation or tetralogy of Fallot, will slow down the rate of induction of anesthesia. The shunted blood will not pick up any anesthetic gas, and this blood will dilute and decrease Fa so it is much less than FA, and less anesthetic will be delivered to the brain. Less soluble agents are most affected as their uptake is minimal and therefore more affected by dilution of the shunted blood. With the more soluble agents, the larger uptake of anesthetic by the ventilated blood helps to offset Fa dilution by the shunted blood.

In a left-to-right shunt such as a patent ductus arteriosus, atrial or ventral septal defect, or an arteriovenous (A-V) fistula, with normal tissue perfusion, you would expect to see less uptake and an increase in rise of FA/FI. This change, however, is minimal and not clinically significant.

The rate of rise of FA/FI is faster in children than adults. This is due to several factors, including higher alveolar ventilation and lower functional residual capacity (FRC) in infants, as well as their greater vessel rich organ perfusion. So, despite having a higher minimum alveolar concentration (MAC), infants will have faster onset of anesthesia.

## ELIMINATION CURVES

There are three routes for elimination of anesthetic gas from the body: exhalation, metabolism, and transcutaneous loss. Transcutaneous loss has a negligible effect. Modern volatile anesthetics undergo minimal metabolism. Thus, recovery from anesthesia is largely the result of a reversal of partial pressure gradients as anesthetic gases move from tissue into the bloodstream, then into the alveoli and exit the body via exhalation. Elimination curves for volatile anesthetics compare FA to FA when gas was turned off (FA0). These curves appear in a reciprocal way when compared to uptake curves (Figure 23.2).

Factors that affect uptake of anesthetic gases will also affect elimination. Recovery from anesthesia most closely relates to the blood:gas partition coefficient for the anesthetic gas, and elimination of less soluble anesthetics is quicker than for more soluble anesthetics. Increasing fresh gas flows to prevent rebreathing, using breathing circuits with less volume and materials with less absorption, and increasing ventilation will more quickly remove anesthetic gas from the alveoli and speed the rate of fall of FA/FA0.

Elimination is also sped up by redistribution. Redistribution occurs when adipose tissue concentration is less than FA, and these tissues continues to uptake

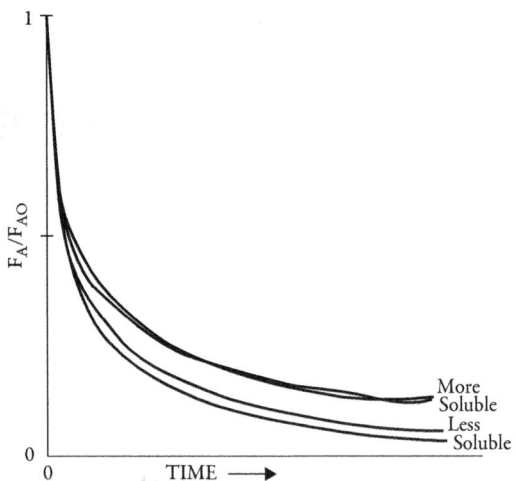

**Figure 23.2** Elimination curves for volatile anesthetics.

anesthesia even while anesthesia is being eliminated by the CNS. This decreases Fa, allowing FA to decrease more quickly. Redistribution causes more of an effect after shorter anesthetics when tissue concentration of adipose tissue is still very low. Longer and deeper anesthetics will result in more uptake of anesthesia by muscle and adipose tissue, which then act as reservoirs. This results in a slower decrease of FA/FA0 as anesthetic gases continue to return to alveoli. Differences in awakening due to length of surgery will be more apparent with more highly soluble anesthetic gases. In shorter anesthetics, the difference in wake-up times between isoflurane and sevoflurane can appear negligible. However, over longer periods of use, wake-up times will be much different.

## ANESTHETIC CONSIDERATIONS

- All uptake curves have a similar shape. All elimination curves have a similar shape.
- Induction and elimination of volatile anesthetics is most rapid for less soluble agents.
- Rate of FA/FI increase and rate of FA/FA0 decrease is most dependent on anesthetic solubility and is fastest for less soluble gases.
- Changes to FA/FI and FA/FA0 due to changes in ventilation and cardiac output have more of an effect with more soluble agents.
- Elimination of volatile anesthetics is also dependent on length and depth of anesthesia, and these changes have more of an effect with more highly soluble agents.
- Changes to FA/FI due to a ventilation perfusion (V/Q) mismatch will have more effect on less soluble agents.
- Rise of FA/FI is faster in infants than adults (Table 23.1).

*Table 23.1* DIFFERENT FACTORS AFFECTING FA/FI AND FA/FA0

| FACTOR | EFFECT | CHANGE TO FA/FI RISE | CHANGE TO FA/FA0 FALL | NOTES |
|---|---|---|---|---|
| Anesthetic solubility as reflected in Blood:gas partition coefficient | Lower solubility results in less uptake into pulmonary blood while higher solubility results in more uptake of anesthetic into blood. | Lower solubility results in faster rate of rise of FA/FI. Higher solubility results in slower rate of rise of FA/FI. | Lower solubility results in faster rate of fall of FA/FA0. Higher solubility results in slower rate of fall of FA/FA0. | Anesthetic gas solubility is the most important factor affecting its speed of onset and elimination. |
| Fresh gas flow | Increased fresh gas flow leads to less rebreathing of gas. | Faster rate of rise of FA/FI | Faster rate of fall of FA/FA0 | |
| Anethestia circuit characteristics | Low volume and less absorbable materials | Faster rate of rise of FA/FI | Faster rate of fall of FA/FA0 | Circuit solubility is more of a factor with more soluble agents. |
| Hyperventilation | More anesthetic delivered alveoli during induction and more anesthetic removed from alveoli during elimination. | Faster rate of rise of FA/FI | Faster rate of fall of FA/FA0 | More pronounced effect with soluble anesthetics. |
| Hypoventilation | Less anesthetic delivered to alveoli during induction and less anesthetic removed from alveoli during elimination. | Slower rate of rise of FA/FI | Slower rate of fall of FA/FA0 | More pronounced effect with soluble anesthetics. |
| Decreased FRC | Less residual air in lungs so quicker dilution of residual air with anesthetic. | Faster rate of rise of FA/FI | | Results in more rapid uptake in pregnancy. |
| increased CO | During induction, more blood travels to lungs so increased uptake removing anesthetic from alveoli. During elimination, more blood brings increased anesthetic to the alveoli. | Slower rate of rise of FA/FI | slower rate of fall of FA/FA0 | More pronounced effect with soluble anesthetics. With most insoluble agents, FA/FI is rapid regardless of CO due to minimal uptake at baseline. |
| Decreased CO | Durning induction, less blood flow to lungs so less anesthetic uptake into the blood. | Faster rate of rise of FA/FI | | More pronounced effect with soluble anesthetics. |
| Increased Ventilation and Increased CO | Increased ventilation causes more gas delivery and increased CO causes more uptake. But, increased CO also causes faster delivery of gas to CNS. | Slightly faster rate of rise of FA/FI | | |
| overpressure | During induction, deliver higher concentration of gas than goal FA. | Faster rate of rise of FA/FI | Not applicable | Cannot set vaporizer to less than zero, so no comparable maneuver to increase rate of fall of FA/FA0 during elimination. |
| Infants vs adults | 1. higher alveolar ventilation 2. lower FRC 3. greater perfusion of VRG in infatnts vs adults | Faster rate of rise of FA/FI | | Although Mac is highest at 6 months, infants have more rapid rise of FA/FI than adults. Neonatal has even faster rise than infants because lower MAC. |

*(continued)*

*Table 23.1* CONTINUED

| FACTOR | EFFECT | CHANGE TO FA/FI RISE | CHANGE TO FA/FA0 FALL | NOTES |
|---|---|---|---|---|
| L to R intracardiac shunt | With normal cerebral blood flow. | No clinical effect | | If CBF is decreased, shunt will slow induction as less anesthetic gas will be delivered to CNS. |
| R to L intracardiac shunt | Shunted blood does not take up any anesthetic gas. When it mixes with blood that passed through lung, it dilutes Fa so Fa<<FA and less anesthetic gas is delivered to CNS | Slower rise of FA/Fi | | Less soluble agents affected most. The slowing of induction is proportional to the degree of the shunt. |
| Mixed intracardiac shunts | | Variable | | L to R shunt attenuates the slowing of the R to L shunt. |
| V/Q mismatch | For example, mainstem intubation. FA increased in ventilated alveoli but Fa diluted by blood that passed through unventilated alveoli. When they mix, Fa<FA so less anesthetic gas is delivered to CNS | Slower rise of FA/Fi | | Less soluble agents affected most as very little anesthetic is taken up by ventilated lung so Fa<<FA. With more soluble agents there is less of a slowing because more blood is taken up by the ventilated lung so Fa<FA. |
| Length of anesthetic | Longer anesthetics lead to more anesthetic uptake by muscle and adipose tissues | Not applicable | Slower rate of fall of FA/FA0 compared with shorter anesthetic | In short anesthetic, awakening times between less soluble and more soluble anesthetics can be mere minutes. In longer anesthetics, there will be more significant differences in wake up times. |
| Redistribution of anesthetic from blood to tissue | Occurs during elimination when tssue concentration is less than FA so anesthesia is taken up into those tissues. | Not applicable | Faster rate of fall of FA/FA0 | This is seen in shorter anesthetics. This effect is lost with longer anesthesia times. |

# REFERENCES

1. Morgan GE, et al. *Clinical Anesthesiology*. New York, NY: Lange Medical Books/McGraw Hill Medical; 2002.

2. Barash PG, et al. *Clinical Anesthesia*. Philadelphia, PA: Wolters Kluwer; 2017.

3. Dunn PF, et al. *Clinical Anesthesia Procedures of the Massachusettes General Hospital*. Philadelphia, PA: Wolters Kluwer; 2007.

# 24.

# CONCENTRATION EFFECT

*Charles Jun and Ned F. Nasr*

## INTRODUCTION

Certain gases have intrinsic properties that allow clinicians to help deliver volatile agents quicker and more efficiently. One such property is the concentration effect. The concentration effect shows how changes in the fraction of inspired anesthetic gas ($F_I$) can either help or hinder the process of achieving the desired fractional alveolar concentration ($F_A$).

## CONCENTRATION EFFECT

The concentration effect can be explained by how $F_I$ influences both the $F_A$ and the rate of saturation at which $F_A$ approaches $F_I$, leading to faster uptake of gas into the body and thus a faster onset of effect.[1]

For gases to exert the concentration effect, gases must be able to relatively easily diffuse across the alveolar membrane into the capillary bloodstream. Nitrous oxide is a

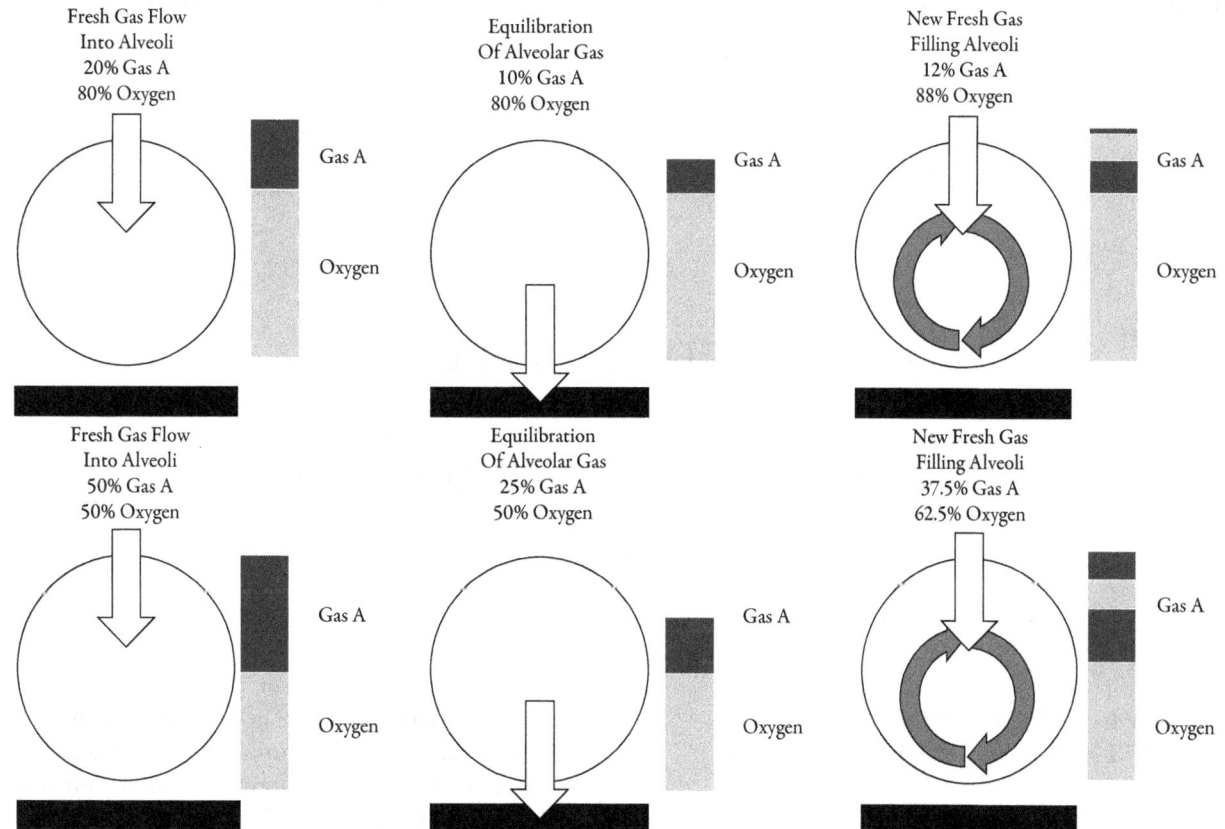

**Figure 24.1.** The concept of the concentration effect.

prime example in which we can quickly see the concentration effect because of its ability to achieve the alveolar partial pressure equilibrium ($F_A/F_I$), the quickest of the volatile anesthetic agents despite its blood:gas coefficient.[1–3] However, other volatile agents also exhibit this property as $F_I$ increases, producing an increase in the $F_A$ and the rate at which alveolar pressure equilibrium is achieved.

### EXAMPLE

To quantify this effect, let's say a flow of gas consists of 80 parts oxygen and 20 parts Gas A with an alveolar capacity of 100 parts, as seen in Figure 24.1. As explained before, the gas needs to have an innate ability to diffuse quickly and efficiently through the alveolar membrane and into the capillaries. For the sake of simplicity, let's assume that half of Gas A is taken up into the blood, leaving the other half in the alveoli, meaning the alveoli now contain 10 parts Gas A and 80 parts oxygen. After a new breath of fresh gas, a new 80:20 fresh gas ratio fills the alveoli. Therefore, the composition of gases is now 12 parts Gas A and 88 parts oxygen in the alveoli ($F_A$).

If we were to now increase the $F_I$ of Gas A by 2.5 times so that the flow of gases so that the composition is now 50 parts Gas A and 50 parts oxygen. After Gas A undergoes exchange equilibrium and mixes with the new 50:50 composition of fresh gas, the final composition of gases would be 62.5 parts oxygen and 37.5 parts Gas A, a 3.125 times increase compared to the initial 2.5 times increase of Gas A. The rise of $F_I$, because of the concentration effect, is reflected with a faster rise of $F_A$.

## INTRAOPERATIVE CONSIDERATION

By increasing $F_I$ by a certain factor, we can expect that $F_A$ will increase by a higher factor. Thus, we can speed up the rate of induction and therefore achieve clinical effect more quickly. However, one must be cautious in terms of the length of time the gas is left on high concentrations as this can lead to toxicity.[3]

## REFERENCES

1. Butterworth JF, et al. Inhalation anesthetics. In: *Morgan and Mikhail's Clinical Anesthesiology*. 6th ed. Columbus, OH: McGraw-Hill Education; 2018:154.
2. McKay, RE. Inhaled anesthetics. In: Pardo M, Miller RD, eds. *Basics of Anesthesia*. 7th ed. Philadelphia, PA: Elsevier, Health Sciences Division; 2017:90.
3. Watcha MF, Seipel CP. Anesthetics: Gases and vapors. In: Williams GW, Williams ES, eds. *Basic Anesthesiology Examination Review*. New York, NY: Oxford University Press; 2016:108–109.

# 25.

# SECOND GAS EFFECT

*Ahmad Reza Parniani and Peggy White*

## ALVEOLAR CONCENTRATION OF INHALED ANESTHETICS

After the uptake of inhaled anesthetics into the blood, the alveolar anesthetic gas concentration (FA) falls behind the inspired gas concentration (FI). The higher the uptake of the inhaled gas, the lower FA:FI ratio.

The alveolar partial pressure of the inhaled anesthetics determines the partial pressure of the anesthetic in the blood and eventually in the brain. The partial pressure of a gas in alveoli or the brain is directly proportional to the concentration of the gas in those tissues. As the uptake of anesthetics increases, the difference between inspired and alveolar concentrations of the gas increases as well.

This results in a reduction in the speed of induction of the inhaled anesthetics.

Uptake of inhaled anesthetics depends mainly on three factors: solubility in blood, alveolar blood flow, and the difference of alveolar and venous blood partial pressure. Solubility of a gas partially determines the speed of induction. For instance, nitrous oxide is a relatively insoluble gas which is taken up in the blood at a slower rate compared to a more soluble gas such as isoflurane. Because of less uptake into the blood, the alveolar concentration of nitrous oxide increases and reaches a steady state faster than isoflurane.[1]

The second factor that affects the uptake of anesthetics by pulmonary circulation is alveolar blood flow, which is the same as cardiac output unless there is pulmonary shunting. As the cardiac output increases, so does the rate of uptake of inhaled gases. This results in a decrease in the rate of the rise in alveolar partial pressure of the gas, which in turn slows down the induction rate. The changes in cardiac output make the highest impact on the rate of induction in gases which are most soluble in blood. It is important to mention the potential for overdose of inhaled gases when there is a combination of low cardiac output and soluble gases.

The third factor that affects the rate of uptake of anesthetics by pulmonary circulation is difference of partial pressure of gas in alveoli and venous blood. This partial pressure gradient is in turn affected by the tissue uptake of inhaled anesthetics. The tissues uptake of gases also depends on three factors: the tissue solubility of the gas, the difference in partial pressure of the gas in the blood versus the tissue, and tissue blood flow.[1] These factors can be summarized as shown in Figure 25.1.

## CONCENTRATION EFFECT AND SECOND GAS EFFECT

Two important factors that also affect the alveolar partial pressure of inhaled gases: the *concentration effect* and the *second gas effect*. A high inspired partial pressure ($P_I$) is needed during the initial delivery of an inhaled anesthetic. This high $P_I$ is needed because there is concurrent uptake of the gas into the blood. The initial high $P_I$ results in a faster induction of anesthesia, as reflected by the faster rate of increase in the gas alveolar pressure ($P_A$). This effect of $P_I$ on the rate of induction of inhaled gases is known as the *concentration effect*.[2,3]

The *second gas effect* is another important phenomenon that impacts the alveolar partial pressure of anesthetics. Second gas effect refers to the ability of large uptake of a gas such as nitrous oxide (first gas) to speed up the rate of increase of the $P_A$ of a simultaneously administered gas such as inhaled anesthetics (second gas). Additionally, the uptake of the first gas results in a reduction of the total gas volume, which results in an increase of the concentration of the second gas (Figure 25.2).[3,4,5]

Both the second gas effect and the concentration effect increase the rate of inhalation inductions of anesthetics. The uptake of large volumes of an anesthetic gas such as nitrous oxide concentrates the remaining gas. The uptake of a large amount of gas also increases the effective alveolar concentration. The combination of the concentrating effect and the increase in effective alveolar ventilation results in an increase in the concentrations of both nitrous oxide and the second gas.[2]

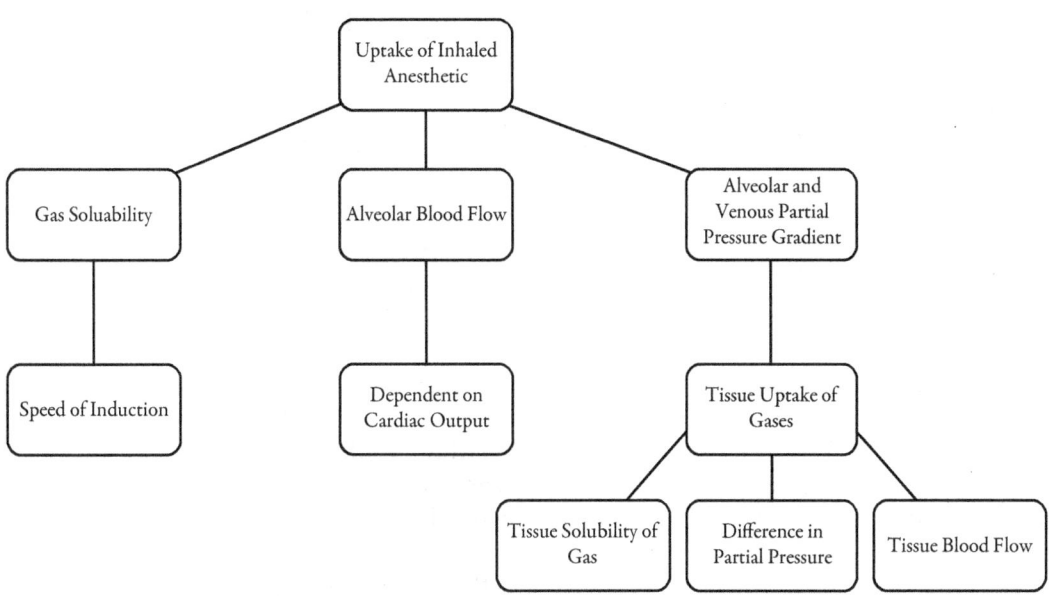

**Figure 25.1.** Factors affecting uptake of inhaled anesthetics.

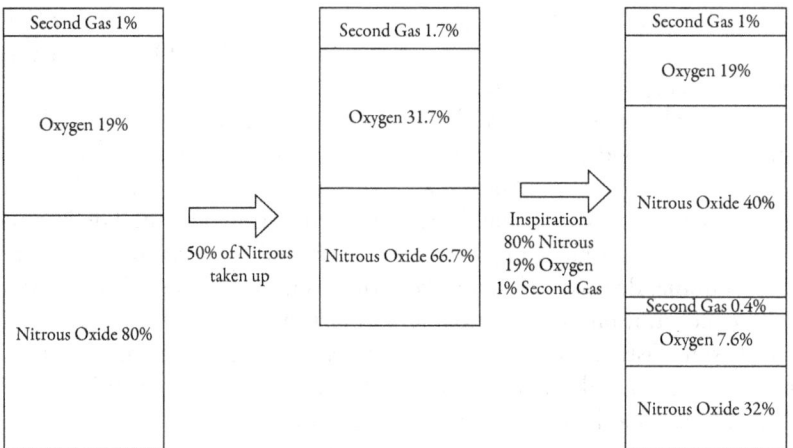

**Figure 25.2.** Second gas effect.

## REFERENCES

1. Morgan & Mikhail's. Inhalation anesthetics. In: *Morgan and Mikhail's Clinical Anesthesiology*. 6th ed. 2018:150–156.
2. Shapiro, DP. Factors affecting anesthetic gas uptake. In: Murray M, ed., *Faust's Anesthesiology Review*. 4th ed. Philadelphia, PA; 2015:142–143.
3. McKay, RE. Factors that determine the alveolar partial pressure. In: Miller RD, ed., *Basics of Anesthesia*. 6th ed. Philadelphia, PA; 2011:84–85.
4. Korman B, Mapleson WW. Concentration and second gas effects: Can the accepted explanation be improved? *Br J Anaesth*. 1997;78:618–625.
5. Kennedy RR. A second look at the second gas effect? *Anesthesiology*. 2018;128:1053–1054.

# 26.

# NITROUS OXIDES AND CLOSED SPACES

*Muhammad Fayyaz Ahmed and Emuejevoke Chuba*

## INTRODUCTION

Nitrous oxide ($N_2O$) is the oldest anesthetic agent in use in anesthesia practice. It is the only inorganic gas used for anesthesia. It is an inflammable, colorless, sweet-smelling, tasteless gas with a boiling point of −88.5°C, a molecular weight of 44, and a density 1.5 times that of air. Although nonflammable, $N_2O$ supports combustion. With a critical temperature of 36.5°C, it can be stored under pressure in a liquid form in a blue color-coded E-cylinder at a maximum capacity of 1590 L and pressure of 745 psi. This pressure in the cylinder is sustained until all liquid is used up. Thus, unlike $O_2$, the volume of the $N_2O$ can be determined by directly weighing the cylinders. It is the least potent inhalational agent with a MAC of 104%; hence it cannot be used as a sole anesthetic, but in combination with other anesthetic agents, as a component of balanced anesthesia. The blood/gas partition coefficient of $N_2O$ is 0.47, and it is poorly soluble in blood. This results in a decreased uptake and a faster equilibration of the alveolar

(Fa) and inspired (Fi) fraction, leading to a faster induction and emergence.[1,3,4]

## CONCENTRATION AND SECOND GAS EFFECT

Increasing the inspired concentration (Fi) of volatile anesthetics increases the alveolar concentration (Fa), which in turn increases Fa/Fi. This is commonly seen with $N_2O$ as it can be used in higher concentrations. The second gas effect is a consequence of the concentration effect. Concomitant administration of a potent inhaled anesthetic and $N_2O$ increases the alveolar concentration of the inhaled anesthetics. Nitrous oxide, with its high partial pressure, moves rapidly from the alveoli into the blood, decreasing the alveolar concentration. This increases the alveolar concentration and rate of uptake of the inhaled anesthetics.[1,2]

## EFFECT OF $N_2O$ ON ORGAN SYSTEMS

### NEUROLOGIC SYSTEM

It increases cerebral blood flow (CBF) and cerebral metabolic rate ($CMRO_2$), leading to an increase in intracranial pressure (ICP); therefore $N_2O$ is used with caution in traumatic brain surgeries and other neurosurgical cases with suspected elevated ICP.

### CARDIOVASCULAR SYSTEM

When used in combination with other volatile anesthetics, $N_2O$ depresses myocardial contractility, and increases the sympathetic nervous system and vascular resistance. $N_2O$ at 40–70% causes a modest increase in heart rate. However, in cases of coronary artery disease, it decreases heart rate when combined with isoflurane. It also causes a slight increase in cardiac output, pulmonary arterial pressure, and pulmonary vascular resistance.

### RESPIRATORY SYSTEM

Like other inhalational agents, $N_2O$ increases respiratory rate and decreases tidal volume, resulting in a minimal change in minute ventilation effect. It also produces a dose-dependent depression of the ventilatory response to hypercarbia.

### GASTROINTESTINAL/HEPATIC SYSTEM

It increases the incidence of postoperative nausea and vomiting. A possible explanation is the activation of the chemoreceptor trigger zone in the medulla. It slightly decreases hepatic blood flow.

### NEUROMUSCULAR SYSTEM

$N_2O$ does not relax skeletal muscles. It does not trigger malignant hyperthermia.

### HEMATOLOGICAL SYSTEM

It inhibits methionine synthetase, a vitamin $B_{12}$ enzyme required for DNA synthesis. It depresses the bone marrow, causing megaloblastic anemia and peripheral neuropathies. The increased plasma level of homocysteine causes impaired endothelial function, enhanced platelet aggregation, and oxidative stress.[1,3,4]

## EFFECT OF NITROUS OXIDE IN CLOSED SPACES

$N_2O$ is 30 times more soluble than nitrogen in the blood. Therefore, the rate at which $N_2O$ diffuses from air-filled cavities is faster than the rate at which nitrogen is absorbed in the bloodstream. This has some potential hazardous effects. In cases of highly compliant cavities, the volume increases, while for less complaint cavities, there is a substantial rise in pressure. Clinical examples include the following:

### PNEUMOTHORAX/BLEBS

Seventy percent $N_2O$ can expand a pneumothorax to double its size in 10 minutes and triple in 30 minutes. In chronic obstructive pulmonary disease (COPD) with significant blebs, diffusion of $N_2O$ into blebs can result in enlargement and rupture.[4]

### AIR EMBOLISM

Expansion in blood occurs rapidly, therefore it should be used with caution during procedures with increased risk of air embolism, including posterior fossa craniotomies and laparoscopy. If air embolism is suspected, nitrous oxide should be discontinued.

### MIDDLE EAR

The middle ear is a noncomplaint cavity. Use of $N_2O$ during tympanoplasty increases the pressure of the middle ear, which can displace the tympanic membrane graft and decrease hearing postoperatively.[1,3]

### BOWEL OBSTRUCTION

The bowel is a highly compliant space, thus diffusion of $N_2O$ increases the volume, causing bowel distension and possible rupture. The increased volume also compresses the blood vessels which supply the bowel, leading to bowel ischemia.

## TUBE CUFFS

$N_2O$ can diffuse into air-filled cuffs of endotracheal tube and pulmonary artery catheter. This causes rapid expansion of the cuff, which in turn increases pressure on the trachea mucosa and pulmonary artery, resulting in tissue damage.

## PNEUMOCEPHALUS

The cranium is a low compliance space; thus the use of $N_2O$ during intracranial surgeries expands the intracranial air space, resulting in pneumocephalus and increased intracranial pressure.[1,3,4]

## EYE SURGERY

In certain eye procedures, gas is injected into the intravitreal space, such as sulfur hexafluoride and/or perfluoropropane. Use of nitrous oxide can increase intraocular pressure, leading to a reduction in ocular perfusion pressure. It is recommended to avoid using $N_2O$ for at least 15 minutes before using the intraocular gas. Once the gas is used, it is recommended to avoid using $N_2O$ for 7 to 45 days for sulfur hexafluoride and at least a month for perfluoropropane.

## ANESTHETIC CONSIDERATION

Nitrous oxide can be used with other inhaled anesthetics during general anesthesia for cesarean section; it provides the benefit of supplement anesthesia without causing uterine relaxation, which can lead to uterine atony. Nitrous oxide should be used with caution in the following scenarios: traumatic brain surgeries and other neurosurgical cases with suspected elevated ICP, COPD with significant blebs, procedures with increased risk of air embolism such as posterior fossa craniotomies and laparoscopy, during middle ear procedures, patients with bowel obstruction, during intracranial procedures, patients with history of PONV or increased risk of nausea and vomiting, patient undergoing eye procedure with intraocular gas, and patients with a recent history of eye procedure with intraocular gas.

## REFERENCES

1. Inhalation anesthetics. In Butterworth JF, Wasnick JD, Mackey DC, eds. *Morgan and Mikhail's Clinical Anesthesiology*. 6th ed. New York, NY: Lange Medical Books/McGraw Hill Medical; 2018:149–170.
2. Kennedy RS. A second look at the second gas effect. *Anesthesiology*. 2018;128(6):1053–1054.
3. Ebert TJ, Naze SA. Inhaled anesthetics. In: Barash PG, Cullen BF, Stoelting RK, Cahalan MK, Stock MC, Ortega R, eds. *Clinical Anesthesia*. 8th ed. Philadelphia, PA: Lippincott Williams & Wilkins; 2017:459–485.
4. Forman SA, Ishizawa Y. Inhaled anesthetic pharmacokinetics: Uptake, distribution, metabolism, and toxicity. In: Miller RD, ed. *Miller's Anesthesia*. 8th ed. New York, NY: Elsevier/Churchill Livingstone; 2015:638–669.

# 27.

# PRINCIPLES

*Lora B. Levin and Mariya Pogrebetskaya*

## RESISTANCE GAS FLOW

When fluid or a gas mixture moves through a tube or circuit, a drop-in pressure occurs. This pressure change is required to overcome resistance to flow and is influenced by the rate at which the gas is flowing as well as the type of flow. Resistance = (peak pressure – plateau pressure)/ flow. The two types of flow are laminar flow and turbulent flow. Laminar flow is smooth and orderly, where gas flows down parallel-sided tubes at a rate less than critical velocity, with the fastest flow of particles in the center of the stream. The Hagen-Poiseulle Law applies to laminar flow and is defined as the pressure drop = (length*viscosity*flow rate)/radius to the fourth power. Turbulent flow is defined as a disorderly flow of particles. This type of flow occurs due to increased resistance, high flow velocities that are greater than critical velocity, and at branch points. Unlike laminar flow, where resistance increases proportional to viscosity of the gas, turbulent flow is proportional to gas density and gas flow rate. Therefore, for patients with airway obstructions, such as tracheal stenosis, where turbulent flow occurs, the use of gases with less density, such as heliox, will help relieve airway obstruction and decrease resistance to flow. Decreasing the gas flow rate and providing slower and larger tidal volumes also helps alleviate airway obstruction.[1] To decrease resistance in a circuit, use appropriately sized endotracheal tubes, eliminate any kinks in the circuit/tube, and use slower flow rates.

## MECHANICAL DEAD SPACE

Dead space refers to the portion of the breathing system where the gas mixture does not participate in gas exchange. Mechanical dead space exists only in intubated individuals, where the fresh gas mixture mixes with exhaled gas. In a circle system, which is most commonly used, this occurs at and beyond the Y-piece, including the endotracheal tube that extends beyond the teeth, humidification management exchangers (HME), and any additional adaptors. Mechanical dead space becomes important when providing anesthesia for small pediatric patients because when dead space increases compared to alveolar ventilation, retention of carbon dioxide ($CO_2$) occurs. If the mechanical dead space volume is equal to or greater than alveolar ventilation volume, then the patient will be unable to clear $CO_2$. In order to minimize dead space, the anesthesiologist must minimize any attachments beyond the Y-piece on a circle system.[2]

## REBREATHING

Breathing circuits can be broadly divided into two main categories based on how they manage the patient's exhaled gases. Rebreathing circuits must use an absorber for $CO_2$ that is able to trap and remove $CO_2$ from the system to allow the patient to rebreathe anesthetic gases without rebreathing $CO_2$. Non-rebreathing circuits use high gas flow rates to remove the exhaled $CO_2$ as well as all other exhaled anesthetic gases from the circuit before the

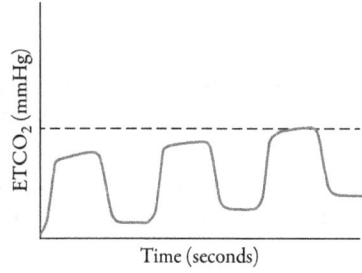

**Figure 27.1.** Capnograph depicting rebreating of $CO_2$.

patient takes the next breath. A hybrid of these two is referred to as a semi-closed system, where some rebreathing occurs, while some of the exhaled gases are vented as waste. Semi-closed systems are most commonly used.[2]

"Low flow" anesthesia technique takes advantage of rebreathing. During this technique, the gas flow rate is less than minute ventilation, allowing the anesthesiologist to save anesthetic gas, decrease environmental pollution, and improve control of patients' temperature and humidity. Disadvantages include the unwanted accumulation of exhaled gases such as $CO_2$, CO, and acetone.[2]

Rebreathing is not always intentional, such as with a "low flow" technique, and can occur from equipment-related problems. Capnography can help determine if rebreathing of $CO_2$ is occurring (Figure 27.1). With rebreathing, there is an elevation of the inspiratory baseline ETCO2. Possible causes include an incompetent expiratory valve, malfunction or channeling of gas through the $CO_2$ absorber, exhaustion of the $CO_2$ absorber, insufficient expiratory time, or inadequate inspiratory flow.[3] Although $CO_2$ can be absorbed during laparoscopic surgeries, this should not increase the inspired $CO_2$.

---

*Box 27.1* SAFEGUARDS AGAINST HYPOXIC GAS MIXTURE AND PROPER ANESTHETIC GAS DELIVERY

Oxygen concentration monitor and alarm (will alarm if FiO2 < 21%)

Low oxygen pressure alarm
    Detects oxygen supply failure at the common gas supply outlet

Vaporizer interlock device which prevent giving multiple anesthetic gases simultaneously

Oxygen/nitrous oxide ratio controller in order to prevent hypoxic gas mixture

Anesthetic gas analyzer which shows inspiratory and expiratory concentration of gases

---

## GAS MIXTURES

Medical gases from central gas supply and volatile anesthetics from vaporizers form the gas mixture that patients receive. There are various safeguards in place to ensure the patient receives a proper combination of gases and prevent a hypoxic gas mixture. Box 27.1 outlines those safeguards.

## LEAKS

Leaks in a breathing circuit are problematic as they can cause issues with anesthesia during induction, maintenance, and wake-up. A leak also increases environmental pollution and exposes the operating theater to anesthetic gases. Leaks can occur anywhere along the breathing circuit. The most common sources include tubing, reservoir bag, points of connection, and the $CO_2$ absorber. The low-pressure circuit is particularly vulnerable to leaks that can result in intraoperative awareness and hypoxic gas mixtures. In order to detect leaks prior to induction, a machine check is performed.[1] However, leaks/disconnections can take place during the course of anesthesia and can be detected in a variety of ways. One of the simplest clues is detecting the odor of anesthetic gas. Others include the inability to deliver a set tidal volume and bellows not filling.[2] Abnormal appearance of capnography may also provide some clues.[3] If a leak has continued for a prolonged amount of time, physiological sensors such as heart rate, blood pressure, and oxygen saturation may be affected as the patient may not be receiving enough anesthetic gas. Even with modern anesthesia machines, it is very important to be diligent when performing an anesthetic in order to make sure that the patient is properly anesthetized and receiving the intended gas mixture.

## HUMIDITY AND HEAT

Humidification and heating of inhaled gases is important. During general anesthesia the nasopharynx is bypassed either with an endotracheal tube or tracheotomy, which allows cold and dry air to be delivered directly to the airway. As a result, the mucous membranes which line and lubricate the airways become dry due to the dry air evaporating liquid from the mucous layer. This evaporation also causes a loss of heat due to the latent heat of vaporization. This heat loss is particularly important in pediatric patients as they have a high minute volume to body surface area, and ventilation for 90 minutes with un-humidified air can lead to a fall in body temperature of 0.75°C.[4] Inadequate humidification of the airway may also thicken sputum, leading to mucous plugging. This can expose patients to increased risk of distal atelectasis, ventilation/perfusion (V/Q) mismatch, and infection. In intensive care unit (ICU) patients, this may present as increased ventilator-associated pneumonia and difficulty weaning from the ventilator.[5]

## REFERENCES

1. Morgan GE, et al. *Clinical Anesthesiology*. New York, NY: Lange Medical Books/McGraw Hill Medical; 2006.
2. Miller RD, Eriksson LI, Fleisher LA, Wiener-Kronish JP, Cohen NH, Young WL. *Miller's anesthesia e-book*. Elsevier Health Sciences; 2014.
3. Capnography. (n.d.). Retrieved August 01, 2020, from https://www.capnography.com/.
4. Tidmarsh M, Lin S. Humidity measurement. In: Smith T, Pinnock C, Lin T, Jones R. (Eds.), *Fundamentals of Anaesthesia*. Cambridge: Cambridge University Press; 2008:824–826.
5. Stoelting RK, Miller RD. *Basics of Anesthesia*. New York, NY: Churchill Livingstone; 2000:286.

# 28.

# COMPONENTS

*Charles Jun and Ned F. Nasr*

## INTRODUCTION

Each component in the anesthesia circuit plays a crucial role in providing safe anesthesia. For providers, a proper understanding of the components behind the mechanics of each component is imperative in providing effective, efficient, and safe anesthesia for patients.

## UNIDIRECTIONAL VALVE (CHECK VALVES)

The unidirectional valve maintains unidirectional flow via a circular ceramic disk, as seen in Figure 28.1. This disk has a larger circumference than its valve seat, which it abuts

in the closed state. On inspiration, gases push against the valve disk, permitting gas to flow through the gap between the valve seat and the valve disk as shown in Figure 28.1. However, when flow is reversed, the backward flow causes the valve disk to push against the valve seat, creating a seal and thus preventing reflux of airflow.[1] These valves help prevent rebreathing of gases.

## INTRAOPERATIVE CONSIDERATIONS

### "Stuck" Valves

These valves may have a hard time with forward flow as disks remain in a "permanently" closed position. Compromised inspiratory valves may hinder delivery of

**Unidirectional Valve (Check Valves)**

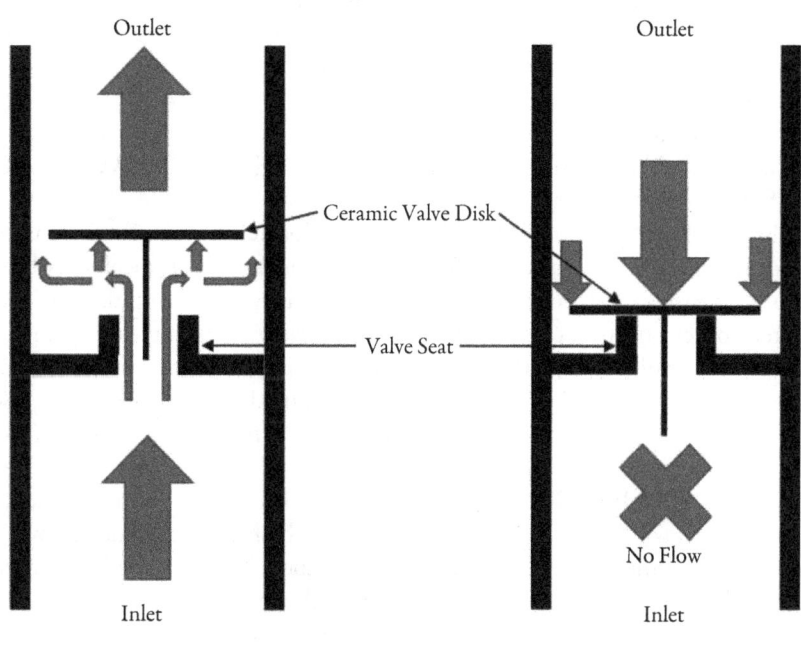

Forward Flow

Reverse Flow

**Figure 28.1.** This figure shows how the unidirectional air flow is maintained via the valve discs, which will occlude against the valve seat when there is backward flow.

gases to patients. Affected expiratory valves can cause barotrauma as air cannot fully escape the lungs during expiration, leading to creation of auto-PEEP (positive end expiratory pressure).

Solution: Visually inspect the valve. Consider switching the machine. However, in the meantime, ventilation can be safely achieved with other modalities such as a portable ventilator like an Ambu-Bag.

### Irregularly Seated Valves

Valves cannot seat properly onto the valve seat to create a proper seal. Conceptually, a closed system can turn into a semi-open system. The system can generate a flow reversal with a risk of rebreathing of gases, which may lead to hypercapnia.

Solution: Inspect the valve. Prevent rebreathing by increasing the fresh gas flows. Consider switching the machine.

### Condensation in Valve

Excess water could compromise the seal between the valve and valve seat leading to flow reversal. Similar to the irregularly seated valves due to warped discs, rebreathing can occur.

Solution: Monitor the condensation and replace the valve as needed. In the meantime, you can increase fresh gas flow rate to accommodate for rebreathing.

## CORRUGATED BREATHING TUBE

The corrugated breathing tube is the interface between the patient and the ventilator, with an accordion-like property designed for easy manipulation. The tubing is typically 1 meter in length with a 22-millimeter diameter bore to allow for minimal resistance, which decreases work of breathing during spontaneous ventilation. The most commonly used plastic tubing has low compliance, allowing for decreased difference between the volume of gas delivered to a circuit by a reservoir bag or a ventilator machine and the volume actually delivered to the patient.[2]

## CONNECTOR/ADAPTOR

Connectors and adaptors allow circuits to be customized for different clinical scenarios. Some connectors allow for various sensors to be placed within the circuit. Adaptors allow connection between different areas and/or connection with an external apparatus (i.e., metered dose inhalers adaptor).

## FACEMASK

The facemask allows for a noninvasive method of controlled ventilation for patients. The mask can be divided into 3 anatomical parts: orifice, body, and seal. The orifice is typically the portion of the mask which allows a tubing or connector to be attached to the mask. The body is transparent and allows the operator to visualize secretions, vomiting, blood, lip color, and exhaled fogging.[2] The seal is usually compliant and the elastic material is designed to create a tight fit around the patient's mouth and nose to provide isolation from gas external to the anesthesia circuit.

## LARYNGEAL MASK AIRWAYS

The laryngeal mask airway is a supraglottic airway device placed superior to the larynx and is less invasive than the endotracheal tubing. At the patient end of the tubing, there is an inflatable boat-shaped rubber cuff designed to overlay the larynx. This rubber cuff creates a seal over the larynx by resting on the hypopharyngeal floor with the sides of the mask lying on the piriform fossae and thus providing isolated airflow into the larynx.[2]

## INTRAOPERATIVE CONSIDERATIONS

The laryngeal mask airway is part of the difficult airway algorithm in emergency situations where neither ventilation nor intubation can be achieved. This device is limited when speak airway pressure on inspiration during mechanical ventilation exceeds 20 cm $H_2O$. Excessive pressure may lead to leakage of air, causing gastric distention and possible gastric aspiration.

## ENDOTRACHEAL TUBES

The endotracheal tube is an invasive airway that is placed within the trachea. Typically made of PVC plastic, it allows for flexibility and manipulation. The hollow circular structure prevents kinking during manipulation. The patient end of the tube is beveled with a circular opening along the proximal end of the tubing, also called the Murphy's eye. The Murphy's eye allows for flow of gases should the tip of the tube become obstructed against the carina or the wall of the trachea. There is a radio-opaque marker along the length of the tube which allows visualization of tubing under chest X-ray to confirm placement and positioning. The inflatable cuff at the patient end of the tubing serves to provide na isolated seal to prevent the contents from entering into the trachea, thus preventing any sort of aspiration. The cuff also prevents gas leak to allow for positive pressure ventilation. Cuff-less tubing is also available, which is important to infants and neonates whose mucosa is friable to the inflated cuff.[2]

## RESERVOIR BAG

The reservoir bag has many functions. Because of the compliance of the reservoir bag, it has the property to increase the compliance and capacitance of the whole system. It can thus act as a buffer to allow time for pressure to slowly build within a closed system.[1] The bags can reach a maximum pressure of 40 to 50 cm $H_2O$. The reservoir bag can also be used to monitor air movement during spontaneous or controlled ventilation and thus assess the adequacy of fresh gas flow and signs of possible leakage in the system. Moreover, the reservoir bag can generate positive pressure within the breathing system.[2]

## AIRWAY PRESSURE RELIEF VALVE

The adjustable pressure-limiting valve (APL) allows the operator to control the amount of pressure that builds up within the breathing system. Figure 28.2 graphically depicts the inner workings of the APL valve. For simplicity, the inner workings of the APL consist of an adjustable knob, which tightens or loosens an internal spring. This spring exerts a specific pressure against the attached valve. Any gas exceeding the preset pressure will flow into the scavenging system. The gas that has not exceeded the set pressure will flow into either the circuit via the absorber or into the reservoir bag.[1,2]

## INTRAOPERATIVE CONSIDERATIONS

During machine-controlled ventilation, gas flow through the APL is bypassed. On spontaneous ventilatory mode, the APL valve should be fully open in an independently ventilating patient to prevent excess work of breathing.

## ABSORBER AND ABSORBENT

The absorbent allows for the filtering of $CO_2$ from the exhaled gas as to prevent hypercapnia. The elimination of $CO_2$ is shown by the involved reactions, as seen in Box 28.1.[1]

## PREOPERATIVE CONSIDERATIONS

The absorbent should be replaced when there is a 50%–70% color change. However, the color can revert to original state with rest, along with its resorptive capacity.

## INTRAOPERATIVE CONSIDERATIONS

Carbon monoxide is a byproduct of the reaction between desflurane (or isoflurane to a lesser extent) and the absorbent (baralyme more so than soda lime) especially when using high concentrations of the volatile anesthetic. Compound A is also seen when using sevoflurane and soda lime absorbent. Nephrotoxicity with the use of sevoflurane, but has only been shown in animal models.[3]

**Airway Pressure Relief Valve**

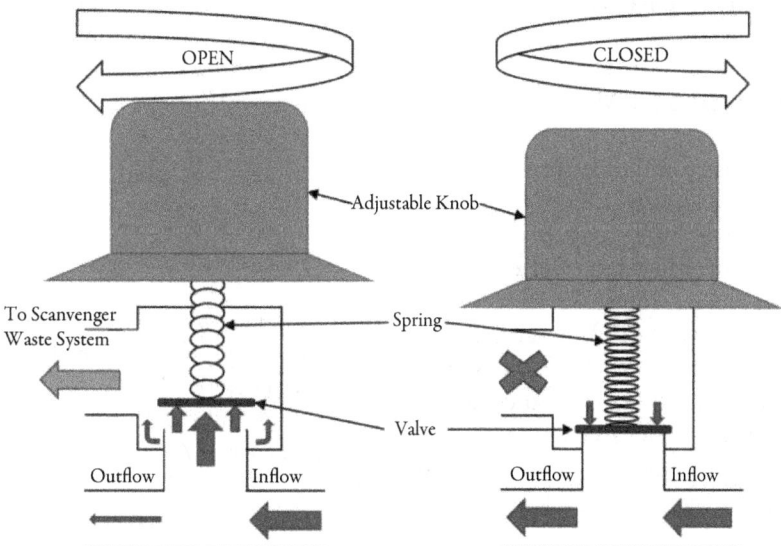

**Figure 28.2.** The schematic layout of the adjustable pressure-limiting valve (APL).

## REFERENCES

1. Butterworth JF, et al. Anesthesia equipment and monitors. In: *Morgan and Mikhail's Clinical Anesthesiology.* 6th ed. Columbus, OH: McGraw-Hill Education; 2018:36–45.
2. Walker SG, et al. Breathing circuits. In: Ehrenwerth J, ed. *Anesthesia Equipment: Principles and Applications.* 2nd ed. Philadelphia, PA: Saunders; 2013:95–124.
3. Kharasch ED, et al. Long-duration low-flow sevoflurane and isoflurane effects on postoperative renal and hepatic function. *Anesth Analg.* 2001;93(6):1511–1520.

# 29.

# CIRCLE SYSTEM

*Charles Jun and Ned F. Nasr*

## INTRODUCTION

Since the innovation of the circle system, it has been commonly adopted in North American operating rooms (ORs) as well as ORs in various countries. The basic structure and components in the typical circle system have largely remained unchanged from the original design.

## CIRCLE SYSTEM

The circle system is the most commonly seen system in the anesthesia machine. Components in the machine are arranged in a circular order. The components seen in the typical system consists of inspiratory and expiratory one-way valves, corrugated breathing tubes, Y piece, adjustable pressure-limiting valve (APL), reservoir bag, $CO_2$ absorbent, and the anesthesia machine, along with the gases (oxygen, nitrous oxide, air, volatile anesthetics). The circle system, depending on the fresh gas flow rate, can be classified as semi-closed or closed.[1,2] For a listing of the advantages and disadvantages of the circle system, see Boxes 29.1 and 29.2.

## CLOSED SYSTEM

The closed system is isolated from the external atmosphere. No fresh gas flow is derived from the external environment; rather, it is drawn from a central source. Fresh gas flow is minimized to equal patient uptake of anesthetic gases and oxygen. The APL valve is completely bypassed or completely closed in a mechanically ventilated patient. $CO_2$ rebreathing is minimized or removed by filtering the exhaled gases through the $CO_2$ absorbent.[1,3]

Box 29.1. ADVANTAGES OF THE CIRCLE SYSTEM

- Constant inspired concentrations of gas;
- Conservation of respiratory heat and humidity (only for closed circuit);
- Useful for all ages (may use down to 10 kg, about 1 year of age or less);
- Allows for closed and low-flow system, decreasing the gas requirements.

## INTRAOPERATIVE CONSIDERATIONS

One should monitor both $FIO_2$ and $FEO_2$ to ensure that adequate oxygen is being administered to the patient to prevent hypoxemia.

## SEMI-CLOSED

The semi-closed system is closed to the external environment. Fresh gas flow is usually derived from a controlled source and is usually greater than the uptake. Excess fresh gas is vented into the scavenging system. Partial rebreathing of exhaled gas may vary depending on the device used. An example of a semi-closed breathing system is the Mapleson system.

## MAPLESON CIRCUITS

This breathing circuit is made up of the face mask, reservoir bag, corrugated tube, fresh gas flow (FGF) inlet, and adjustable pressure-limiting valve (APL). The FGF and APL are located variably along the circuit. However, the reservoir bag, face mask, and corrugated tubing are at fixed locations.[1]

## MAPLESON CLASSIFICATION

See Figure 29.1 and Table 29.1 for details of the Mapleson systems.

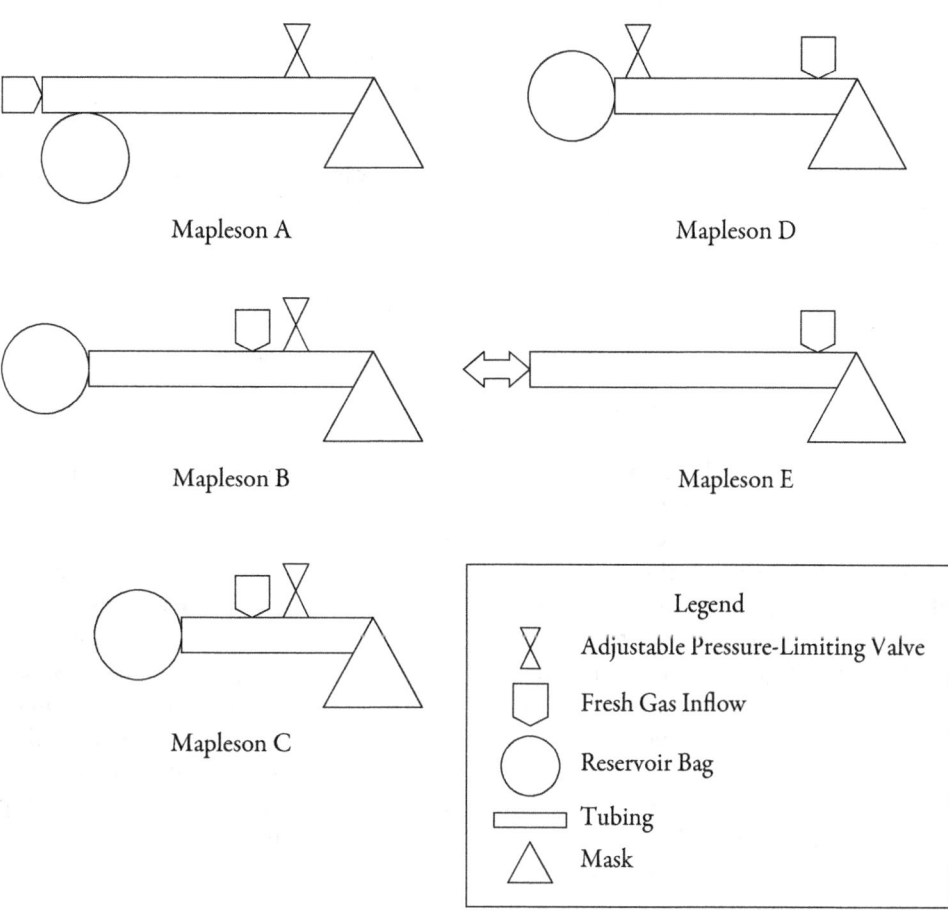

Mapleson A

Mapleson D

Mapleson B

Mapleson E

Mapleson C

Legend
Adjustable Pressure-Limiting Valve
Fresh Gas Inflow
Reservoir Bag
Tubing
Mask

**Figure 29.1.** Graphical representation of the different Mapleson systems.

**Table 29.1** PEARLS OF EACH MAPLESON CIRCUIT

| | |
|---|---|
| Mapleson A (MaGill systems) | Most efficient for spontaneous ventilation, but inefficient for controlled ventilation, as high gas flows will be needed to avoid rebreathing the air that has just left the lungs. |
| Mapleson B and C | Both B and C share a similar layout, but C does not have the reservoir bag. They are both inefficient for both spontaneous and controlled ventilation, as they require high gas flows (>20–25 L/min) to prevent rebreathing. |
| Mapleson D | Highly efficient for controlled ventilation, but not so for spontaneous ventilation as it requires high gas flows to prevent rebreathing. The coaxial modification of the D system is the "Bain" system, which is the most efficient system for controlled ventilation. |
| Mapleson E (Ayre's T-piece) | It has a low resistance system for allowing easier spontaneous ventilation, but inefficient as it requires high gas flows to prevent rebreathing. Consists of a corrugated tubing to act as a reservoir. If the tubing is shortened, then the system functions more like an open system. |

## ADULT VS. PEDIATRIC CIRCLE SYSTEM

In adults, the ribs are mostly ossified, with only a small portion of ribs that remain cartilaginous. The structural rigidity, along with the different directional movements of the ribs during inspiration, allow for effective recruitment of alveoli. Thus, adults can utilize the circle system without worries of fatigue because adults can overcome the work of resistance of the breathing system because of the structural advantages.

In children, the rib cage is oriented horizontally and is highly cartilaginous. There is inward movement during inspiration because the ribs are highly pliable. The underdeveloped anatomy is less efficient at ventilation. This results in a decreased ability to effectively recruit alveoli. Therefore, there is an increased reliance upon accessory muscles and the diaphragm to maintain adequate tidal volumes; however, this creates more work and fatigue to these muscles. In addition, there is structural differences between the pediatric and adult diaphragms. The immature diaphragm in pediatric patients contains fewer type I muscle fibers than the adult counterpart. The lack of type I fibers causes the diaphragm to fatigue much more quickly with increased work of breathing. This often also translates to pediatric patients having a higher metabolic demand (6–8 ml/kg/min of $O_2$ consumption) compared to adults.[2,4] Physiologically, this translates to an increasing requirement of minute ventilation during spontaneous ventilation. The primary compensatory mechanism to increase minute ventilation is to increase the respiratory rate because of the underdeveloped anatomy in pediatric compared to adults, as mentioned previously.[2,4] Thus, tidal volumes, while still important, play a more minute role in minute ventilation in pediatric patients.

The closed circle system should be avoided in neonates and infants due to the increased resistance, leading to increased work of breathing in spontaneous ventilation. The increased resistance in a circle system is primarily contributed by the unidirectional valves, breathing tubes, and $CO_2$ absorbers. For short-term spontaneous ventilation, the circle system can be utilized in healthy older infants.[4] For longer cases requiring spontaneous ventilation, the semi-closed circle system can be used to safely ventilate patients. However, in pediatric patients with severely compromised respiratory function, the resistance in a semi-closed system may also be too much for pediatric patients to overcome. Another option for providing ventilation is the Mapleson D circuit or a Bain system, especially in neonates <10 kg, because of its low airway system resistance. However, if positive pressure ventilation or mechanical ventilation is used, the increased resistance of the circle system may be overcome and thus may be safely used in even the smallest of neonates.

## ANESTHETIC CONSIDERATIONS

### PREOPERATIVE

Peak airway pressure during mask induction of pediatric patients should be carefully monitored for gastric distention, along with impairment of lung expansion.[2] To mitigate this issue, an orogastric or nasogastric tube should be considered to decompress the stomach.

### INTRAOPERATIVE

Use age- and size-appropriate corrugated tubing, mask, and reservoir bag. The pediatric equipment is typically stiffer and less compliant, which decreases the amount of gas lost in the circuit.[2] Older anesthesia machines cannot reliably measure tidal volumes and rapid respiratory rates for neonates and infants. If possible, use circle systems to ventilate the patients.[2] Be very wary of increasing tidal volumes, as this may increase peak airway pressures, leading to possible barotrauma in the alveoli.[2] For children less than 10 kg, adequate tidal volumes can be administered with a peak inspiratory pressure setting between 15 and 18 cm $H_2O$.[2] However, larger children can utilize the typical 6 to 8 mL/kg as seen in adults.[2]

### REFERENCES

1. Butterworth JF, et al. Inhaled anesthetic delivery systems. In: *Morgan and Mikhail's Clinical Anesthesiology.* 6th ed. Columbus, OH: McGraw-Hill Education; 2018:36–45.

2. Butterworth JF, et al. Pediatric anesthesia. In: *Morgan and Mikhail's Clinical Anesthesiology*. 6th ed. Columbus, OH: McGraw-Hill Education; 2018:36–43, 898–899, 914–915.
3. Roth P. Anesthesia delivery systems. In: Pardo M, Miller RD, eds. *Basics of Anesthesia*. 7th ed. Philadelphia, PA: Elsevier, Health Sciences Division; 2017:225–230.
4. Ehrenwerth J. Pediatric anesthesia systems and equipment. *Anesthesia Equipment: Principles and Applications (Expert Consult: Online and Print)*. 2nd ed. Philadelphia, PA: Saunders; 2013:353–376.
5. Dosch MP. Anesthesia gas machine: Breathing circuits. Udmercy. edu. https://healthprofessions.udmercy.edu/academics/na/agm/06.htm.

# 30.

# NON-CIRCLE SYSTEMS

*Charles Jun and Ned F. Nasr*

## INTRODUCTION

With the discovery of anesthetic agents, anesthesia delivery devices were needed in achieving anesthesia in patients. The goal in creating these devices was to create isolated environments where only the desired gases were given to patients.

## OPEN SYSTEM

The open system does not rely on valves, tubing, or a reservoir bag to supply anesthetic gas to patients. It is an indirect way to deliver anesthetic agents to patients. This is the most rudimentary way of delivering anesthetic gases.[1]

## INSUFFLATION

Insufflation is a method to provide general anesthesia via indirect ventilation of gases. Typically, a supine patient is draped with a blanket, or a mask is applied at a distance over the patient's face. Gas is then introduced via the apparatus. If using a blanket-tubing method, a tubing, connected to a machine supplying the various gases, is placed underneath the drape and on top of the patient, which provides a continuous inflow of gases for the patient to spontaneously breathe. While a very crude way of providing gas, it is an invaluable tool for pediatric patients who resist placement of a face mask or an IV line. The obvious downside of this method is the buildup of exhalation gas because of inadequate exchange of fresh gas, which is addressed through the open-air exchange in a form of a hole in the blanket which acts as an exhaust for gas coming from the machine and intake of fresh air from the external environment. However, if there are no holes, exhaled gas accumulation and rebreathing is alleviated by means of high fresh gas flow rates (>10 L/min). The other disadvantage is that the staff confined in the same room as the patient would be susceptible to exposure to the same gases that are experienced by the patient.[1,2]

## OPEN-DROP ANESTHESIA

*Example*: Schimmelbusch mask (open-drop anesthesia). An open-drop technique relies on a Schimmelbusch mask or a rag saturated with anesthetic, typically an ether. This method requires a highly volatile anesthetic. As the piece of fabric soaked in gas is placed over the face, vaporized gas from the highly volatile gas-soaked rag is breathed in by the patient. The vaporization of gas causes a drop in the surrounding temperature, causing the vapors to subsequently condense, leading to a drop in vapor pressure of anesthetic gas. This technique is not used much in the modern day. However, this technique has been modified for use in the present day: draw-over anesthesia.[1,2]

## DRAW-OVER ANESTHESIA

*Equipment*: hose, low resistance vaporizer, supplemental $O_2$, self-inflating bag with a one-way valve.

*Optional equipment*: self-inflating bag, ventilator, non-rebreathing valve, PEEP (positive end expiratory pressure) valve, circuit filter, and/or heat and moisture exchanger.

As mentioned earlier, this technique is a modified version of open-drop anesthesia. In the draw-over anesthesia system, a vaporizer, typically a low-resistance apparatus, is used to supply the anesthetic to the patient; however, this technique requires inspiratory effort to draw from ambient air (or supplied $O_2$) which carries the vaporized gas to the patient. The device can also be fitted to allow intermittent positive pressure ventilation and passive scavenging as well as CPAP (continuous positive airway pressure) and PEEP. Close monitoring of oxygen saturation is required when the patient is not supplemented with auxiliary oxygen, as there is a risk for hypoxia. The supplemental $O_2$ is usually attached to the upstream end of the vaporizer via a T-piece system.[1]

### INTRAOPERATIVE CONSIDERATIONS

When using draw-over anesthesia, the operator must closely monitor oxygen saturation when ventilating patient with ambient air, as it is a risk for hypoxemia in patients. As a solution, the operator can provide intermittent positive pressure ventilation and/or supplemental oxygen attached to the upstream end of the vaporizer via a T-piece system to increase the fractional inspired oxygen concentration.

## SEMI-OPEN SYSTEM

The semi-open system is also known as the non-rebreathing system. This system utilizes high fresh gas flows (80 to 100 mL/kg/min) to eliminate rebreathing. A Mapleson and circle system at high gas flow rates can be considered a semi-open system.[2] A typical semi-open system has a reservoir bag and two one-way valves. The reservoir bag acts to hold fresh gas, which can be administered to the patient via the compression of the bag at the operator's discretion. The one-way valves act to not only minimize apparatus dead space, but also help to set up a pressure gradient for easy switch between spontaneous and controlled ventilation.[3]

### REFERENCES

1. Butterworth JF, et al. Anesthetic equipment and monitors. In: *Morgan and Mikhail's Clinical Anesthesiology*. 6th ed. Columbus, OH: McGraw-Hill Education; 2018:34–36.
2. Sudha V. Circle and noncircle systems. In: Freeman B, Berger J, eds. *Anesthesiology Core Review*. McGraw-Hill Education/Medical; 2014. https://accessanesthesiology.mhmedical.com/content.aspx?bookid=974&sectionid=61586875.
3. Walker SG, et al. Breathing circuits. In: Ehrenwerth J, ed. *Anesthesia Equipment: Principles and Applications (Expert Consult: Online and Print)*. 2nd ed. Philadelphia, PA: Saunders; 2013:95–124.

# 31.

# PORTABLE VENTILATION DEVICES

*Pradeep R. Chawla and Jason Bang*

## INTRODUCTION

Portable ventilation devices have a use in various settings that anesthesiologists might find themselves in. They can be used to provide face mask ventilation for airway management in critical situations. They also are used while transporting patients around the hospital who need mechanical ventilation. These portable devices do not need electricity to function; however, they usually require a constant flow of oxygen to function properly. There are two main classes of portable ventilation devices: self-inflating systems and flow-inflating systems.

## SELF-INFLATING SYSTEMS

Self-inflating portable ventilation devices are regularly used for both in-hospital and out-of-hospital settings. The advantages of self-inflating bags include portability, the ability of the bag to self-inflate, and being able to oxygenate with room air if an oxygen supply is not available.[1,2] Disadvantages include not being able to deliver a fraction of inspired oxygen higher than room air without an external oxygen source and the inability to have a tactile feel of airway resistance and compliance as compared to a circle system.[2] There are numerous self-inflating systems available. The most widely known is an artificial manual breathing unit or AMBU bag; however, they are all composed of similar elements, which are illustrated in Figure 31.1.[1]

### VENTILATION BAG

This bag acts as a reservoir for either oxygen or air that is being delivered to the patient when squeezed, and it self-reinflates during expiration by taking in gas for the next breath.[2] Of note, the bags are latex-free and typically are made of materials such as PVC or rubber, which allow them to be easily compressible in even extremely hot or cold temperatures.[1,2] Adult, pediatric, and neonatal bags all have different volumes. Adult bags range from 1500 to 2000 mL, pediatric bags range from 800 to 1000 mL and neonatal bags range from 300 to 500 mL. Compressing an adult bag with both hands usually will not deliver half of the volume of the ventilation bag. Good bag compressions typically will range from 500 to 800 ml of delivered gas.[1]

### NON-REBREATHING VALVE

Non-rebreathing valves are designed to prevent the mixing of expired gas with fresh inspired gas from the ventilation bag and to release expired gas to the atmosphere. The valve is T-shaped and consists of an inspiratory port that directs gas from the bag to the patient, an expiratory port that directs gas from the patient to the atmosphere, and a patient port that connects with an airway device. The expiratory port is closed by the valve during inspiration, and the inspiratory port is closed during expiration.[2] The valve is visible in a clear plastic housing. The housing has a standard-sized connector which has a 15-mm internal diameter for endotracheal tubes and supraglottic airways, as well as a 22-mm external diameter for facemasks.[1] There are three main classes of valves: spring, duckbill and fishmouth-flap.[1,2]

### OXYGEN RESERVOIR

Oxygen is delivered into the system through an oxygen reservoir, via an oxygen bag (closed reservoir) or tubing (open reservoir). The bag and tubing accumulate oxygen during inspiration and release into the ventilation bag during expiration.[2]

## FLOW-INFLATING SYSTEMS

Flow-inflating systems have bags that do not self-reinflate following a manual compression; they require a continuous flow of gas in order to reinflate. Mapleson D and F are the most commonly used portable flow-inflating circuits.[2] These two Mapleson circuits are portable and have the feel of an anesthesia bag, unlike an AMBU bag.[1] These Mapleson systems require flows 2–3 times higher than the patient's minute ventilation to prevent rebreathing of gases.[2]

## ANESTHETIC CONSIDERATIONS

Portable ventilation devices are commonly used in pre- and postoperative settings when patient transport is required. Self-inflating systems and flow-inflating systems can both

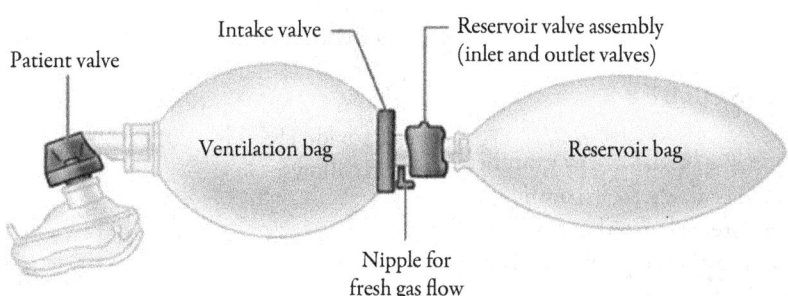

**Figure 31.1.** The components of a self-inflating system.
Reproduced with permission from Butterworth JF, Mackey DC, Wasnick JD, eds. *Morgan and Mikhail's Clinical Anesthesiology.* 5th ed. McGraw-Hill; 2013.

lead to barotrauma secondary to excessive delivered airway pressures.[1,2] Both systems also require a constant flow of oxygen to deliver a $FiO_2$ greater than room air; therefore it is important to check that the oxygen tank you are using has an adequate supply prior to transport and that the oxygen is on while transporting a patient.

## REFERENCES

1. Bag valve mask and Mapleson Circuits. In: Rose G, McLarney J. eds. *Anesthesia Equipment Simplified*. McGraw-Hill; 2013.
2. Breathing Systems. In: Butterworth IV JF, Mackey DC, Wasnick JD, eds. *Morgan & Mikhail's Clinical Anesthesiology*. 5th edition. McGraw-Hill; 2013:1284.

# 32.

# CARBON DIOXIDE ABSORPTION

*Sohail K. Mahboobi and Faraz Mahmood*

## INTRODUCTION

Circle systems are the most commonly used breathing systems due to cost effectiveness and ability to deliver low-flow anesthesia. They function on the principle of alveolar gas rebreathing and conserve heat and humidity. To achieve this, they require a mechanism to remove carbon dioxide ($CO_2$) from the exhaled gases. Rebreathing can be avoided by using higher gas flows, but this is not cost effective or functional. The ideal method is to use a modality that can absorb $CO_2$, and the rest of the gases can be reused with little addition of oxygen and inhalational agent. The $CO_2$ absorbers serve that purpose. Other industries, like mining and diving, also use $CO_2$ absorbers. This chapter will discuss the different types of $CO_2$ absorbers used in anesthetic practice and important clinical considerations.

## CO$_2$ ABSORBERS

The absorbers typically consist of absorbent granules in a clear plastic canister that has a size to accommodate average tidal volume. The canister is located in a way to allow visual inspection by the anesthesia provider. The qualities of an ideal absorber include: inert in reaction with $CO_2$, nontoxic, no resistance to gas flow, has a system to indicate exhaustion, cheap, and easy to install. There are several manufacturers of $CO_2$ absorbents for anesthetic use (Table 32.1). Some of the commonly used absorbers are soda lime, lithium containing (litholyme), lithium based (spiralith), and calcium hydroxide lime without bases (Amsorb). These absorbers vary in their ingredients, safety profile, and capacity to absorb $CO_2$.

## CHEMISTRY OF CO$_2$ ABSORBENTS

Exhaled $CO_2$ chemically combines with water to form carbonic acid. Then, in a series of chemical reactions, the acid (carbonic acid) reacts with and is neutralized by bases (usually calcium hydroxide [$Ca(OH)_2$] to form calcium carbonate ($CaCO_3$), with additional end products being water and heat. Absorbents also typically contain silica, which functions as a hardening agent. This helps produce a harder, more stable pellet while limiting dust production which is an irritant to skin and mucous surfaces.

Soda lime is a commonly used adsorbent that contains 80% $Ca(OH)_2$, sodium hydroxide (NaOH), potassium hydroxide (KOH), water, and silica. The chemical reaction is as follows:

$$CO_2 + H_2O \ H_2CO_3$$

$$H_2CO_3 + 2NaOH \text{ (or KOH)} \ Na_2CO_3 \text{(or } K_2CO_3\text{)} + 2H_2O + hHeat$$

*Table 32.1* COMPONENTS OF COMMONLY USED $CO_2$ ABSORBENTS

| | SODA LIME | LITHOLYME | SPIRALITH | AMSORB |
|---|---|---|---|---|
| $Ca(OH)_2$ | 80% | >75% | — | 83% |
| NaOH | 2%–4% | — | — | — |
| KOH | 1%–3% | — | — | — |
| LiOH | — | — | 95% | — |
| $Li_2CO_3$ | — | — | 3% | — |
| Lithium Chloride | — | <3% | — | — |
| Water Content | 14%–19% | 12%–19% | — | 14.5% |
| Size (Mesh) | 4–8 | 4–8 | — | 4–8 |
| Indicator | Yes | Yes | No | Yes |

*Source:* data from *APSF Newsl.* 2005;2:25–44, https://www.apsf.org/wp-content/uploads/newsletters/2005/summer/pdf/APSF200506.pdf.

$$Na_2CO_3 (or\ K_2CO_3) + Ca\ (OH)_2\ CaCO_2 + 2NaOH\ (or\ KOH) + hHeat$$

NaOH (or KOH) acts as catalyst, and the water and NaOH (or KOH) required initially are regenerated. The catalyst bases react with inhalational agents and can produce degradation products.

The new $CO_2$ absorbents reduce the risk of toxic byproducts formation. Litholyme is a lithium-based $CO_2$ absorbent that contains lithium chloride as catalyst to the formation of calcium carbonate. Litholyme does not contain bases. Spiralith replaces $Ca(OH)_2$ with lithium hydroxide Li(OH). Li(OH) is the alkali hydroxide with the lowest molecular weight and does not require a catalyst to react with $CO_2$.

$$2Li(OH).H_2O + CO2 + hHeat\ Li_2CO3 + 3H_2O$$

Amsorb is another calcium hydroxide–based absorbent that does not contain any base.

Size of the granules is a compromise between absorptive capacity and resistance to airflow. Usually granular size is around 4–8 mesh. Smaller mesh size, despite increased surface area for absorption, also increased the resistance to flow, and larger size can cause channeling and rebreathing. The resistance is <1 cm $H_2O$ at 60 L/min flow through the full canister.

## INDICATORS OF ABSORBENT EXHAUSTION

To show exhaustion, most of the absorbents contain an indicator dye, ethyl violet, that changes color to violet from being colorless when the pH of the absorbent gets lower than 10.3. The color change is not always reliable, as

exposure to fluorescent light can deactivate the color of the dye.[1] Also exhaustion without color change can happen due to channeling through the granules. Newer absorbents, like Amsorb, contain no indicator, and monitored inspired $CO_2$ concentration indicates exhaustion.[2]

## CLINICAL CONSIDERATIONS

Volatile inhalational anesthetic agents react with the bases (NaOH and KOH), usually found in $Ca(OH)_2$ absorbents like soda lime, and form degradation products. Two of the most important products are compound A formation with sevoflurane and carbon monoxide production with use of isoflurane and desflurane.

### COMPOUND A FORMATION

Sevoflurane results in the formation of the trifluoromethyl vinyl ether, also called compound A, after it undergoes base catalyzed degradation. In animal studies, this compound is nephrotoxic at normally occurring concentrations in the breathing circuits. The nephrotoxicity does not occur in humans, even in patients with preexisting renal impairment. It is recommended not to use less than 1 L/m fresh gas flow when using sevoflurane with a catalyst base containing absorbents. Certain conditions are considered to increase compound A production and are as follows:

- Higher sevoflurane concentration
- Higher temperature of absorbents
- Catalyst bases (KOH > NaOH) containing absorbents (baralyme and soda lime)
- Lower fresh gas flow rates (< 1 L/m)
- Fresh absorbent.[3]

## CARBON MONOXIDE GENERATION

Secondly, desflurane, enflurane, and isoflurane are degraded to carbon monoxide (CO) by desiccated and partially desiccated absorbents that contain strong bases. The overall incidence was 0.26%.[4] CO production and exposure is more frequent with desiccated absorbents, especially when the gas flows have been left open for an extended period of time, e.g., Monday mornings after weekends. Routinely, desiccation is unlikely due to production of water and exhaled humidity. Conditions that can increase CO production are as follows:

- Desiccated $CO_2$ absorbent
- Absorbents containing strong bases (NaOH or KOH)
- High concentration of inhalational agents (Desflurane > isoflurane >> sevoflurane = halothane)
- Small absorbent particles
- Higher temperature and low fresh gas flow rate.

The Li(OH) containing and $Ca(OH)_2$ absorbents without NaOH and KOH bases do not generate compound A or CO.

## HEAT PRODUCTION

Desiccated base containing $CO_2$ absorbents can cause exothermic reactions that may result in fire, particularly with the use of sevoflurane. The fire is the result of flammable products like formaldehyde and methanol in the presence of inspired oxygen and very high temperature.[5] To avoid this catastrophic event, it is recommended to change absorbent regularly, turn off gas flows when not in use, and monitor for absorbent exhaustion.

## REFERENCES

1. Pond G, et al. Failure to detect $CO_2$-absorbent exhaustion: Seeing and believing. *Anesthesiology.* 2000 Apr;92:1196–1198.
2. Gerstein N, Rosenberg C. Exhausted Amsorb plus $CO_2$ absorbent recognized only by inspired $CO_2$. *Anesth Analg.* 2007;104:237–238.
3. Struys MMRF, et al. Production of compound A and carbon monoxide in circle systems: An in vitro comparison of two carbon dioxide absorbents. *Anaesthesia.* 2004;59:584–589.
4. Coppens MJ, et al. The mechanisms of carbon monoxide production by inhalational agents. *Anaesthesia.* 2006;61(5):462–468.
5. Marini F, et al. Compound A, formaldehyde and methanol concentrations during low-flow sevoflurane anaesthesia: comparison of three carbon dioxide absorbers. *Acta Anaesthesiol Scand.* 2007;51:625–632.

# 33.

# TOXICITY OF INHALED ANESTHETICS

*Zachary Drennen and Daniel S. Cormican*

## INTRODUCTION

Inhalational anesthetics have been used to administer general anesthesia for over a century, and although their safety profile and ease of use have improved dramatically since the introduction of ether in the 1800s, volatile anesthetics and inhaled gases (nitrous oxide and oxygen) are associated with multiple documented toxicities.

## TOXICITY OF INHALED ANESTHETICS

Volatile anesthetics are halogenated with fluorine, which provides stability to the compound and lowers the risk of toxicity when compared to non-fluorinated agents.[1] Metabolism of these agents can lead to production of intermediate reactive metabolites and fluoride, which can be harmful to patients. Volatile anesthetics can undergo degradation to byproducts in the $CO_2$ absorbers utilized to remove $CO_2$ from anesthetic circuits during mechanical ventilation. $CO_2$ absorbers typically utilize soda lime, which contains a strong base (often calcium hydroxide or sodium hydroxide) as a major component. The reaction between the absorbers and volatile anesthetics can produce harmful byproducts (such as Compound A and carbon monoxide) and can even cause thermal injuries.[2]

Several volatile anesthetics that are no longer used in practice today, including halothane, methoxyflurane, and enflurane, have well-documented toxicities that led to their removal from most anesthesia practices in the United States. Halothane has been linked to fulminant hepatic necrosis. Methoxyflurane metabolism was found to cause renal failure leading to nephrotoxicity caused by production of inorganic fluorides. Enflurane was also found to be metabolized into an inorganic fluoride, which was associated with risk of seizure activity.[1]

Newer volatile anesthetics, including sevoflurane, desflurane, and isoflurane, are commonly used today but are not without toxicity risks of their own. Sevoflurane undergoes metabolism to Compound A in $CO_2$ absorbents. Compound A is a vinyl ether and has been shown to be nephrotoxic in rats; however, this toxicity has not been clinically relevant in humans. Figure 33.1 outlines the reaction scheme for the production of Compound A from sevoflurane. The production of Compound A has been shown to be increased with low fresh gas flows and closed system breathing circuits, as well as with warm or dry $CO_2$ absorbent.[2] Creation of compound A is inversely proportional to inflow rate; therefore it is recommended to avoid inflow rates <1 liter/minute entirely, and use flows of 1 liter/minute for no more than 2 hours with sevoflurane administration.

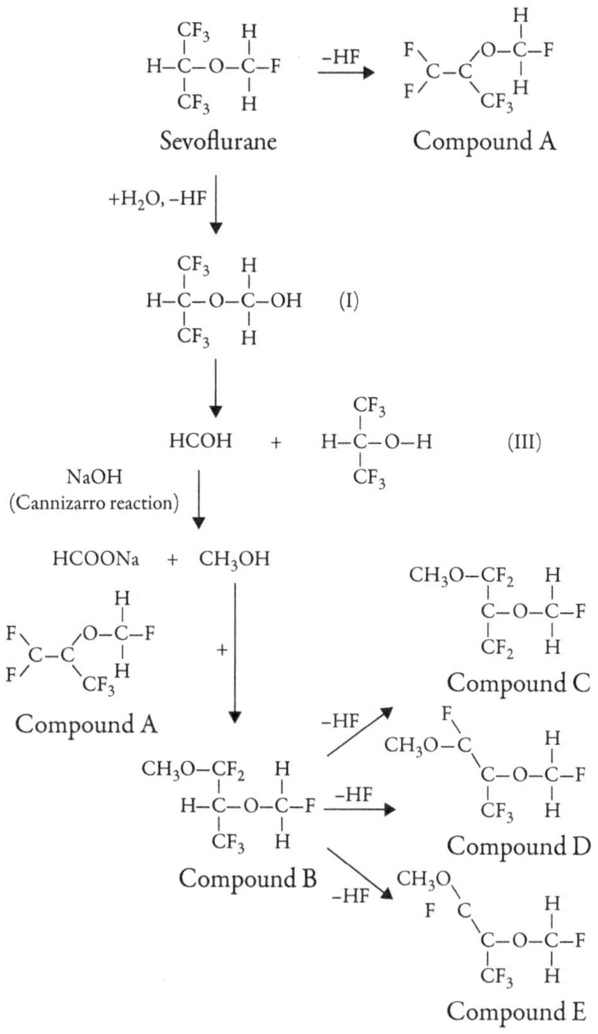

Volatile anesthetic agents can also react with desiccated $CO_2$ absorbers, causing an exothermic reaction and production of carbon monoxide (CO).[3] As temperature rises, CO production also increases. Desflurane is the most likely of the volatile anesthetics to produce CO, followed by isoflurane and sevoflurane.[2] $CO_2$ absorbers no longer use Baralyme as a catalyst, as this agent was associated with increased CO production. CO toxicity can be difficult to diagnose because classic clinical signs and symptoms (headache, dizziness, nausea, vomiting, loss of consciousness, and myocardial ischemia) are somewhat nonspecific, and may go undetected under general anesthesia.

Nitrous oxide ($N_2O$) was discovered over 200 years ago, but still remains commonly used as an anesthetic adjunct. Toxicity is caused by irreversible cobalt oxidation, causing inactivation of the enzyme methionine synthase, which renders vitamin $B_{12}$ inactive. Methionine synthase is an essential enzyme in the process of DNA and RNA synthesis.[4] Figure 33.2 outlines inhibition of methionine synthase by

Figure 33.1. Reaction scheme for sevoflurane in the presence of a base. Reproduced with permission from Cunningham D, Huang S, Webster J, Mayoral J. Sevoflurane degradation to compound A in anaesthesia breathing systems. *Br J Anaesth*. 1996. 77(4):537–543. doi: 10.1093/bja/77.4.537.

nitrous oxide. Megaloblastic anemia—which most commonly occurs in the elderly and those with prolonged vitamin $B_{12}$ deficiency—may occur from inactivation of methionine synthase. Megaloblastic anemia can result in neurologic injury by way of sensory neuropathy, myelopathy, and encephalopathy. These neurologic effects may not be clinically seen for weeks in patients after the toxicity has occurred.

## OXYGEN TOXICITY

Oxygen is vital to human life. Breathing oxygen at higher-than-normal partial pressure can lead to toxicity in the form of central nervous system (CNS), pulmonary, and ocular effects. Toxicity occurs through the generation of reactive oxygen species when oxygen undergoes reduction to form free radicals.[5] The duration and concentration

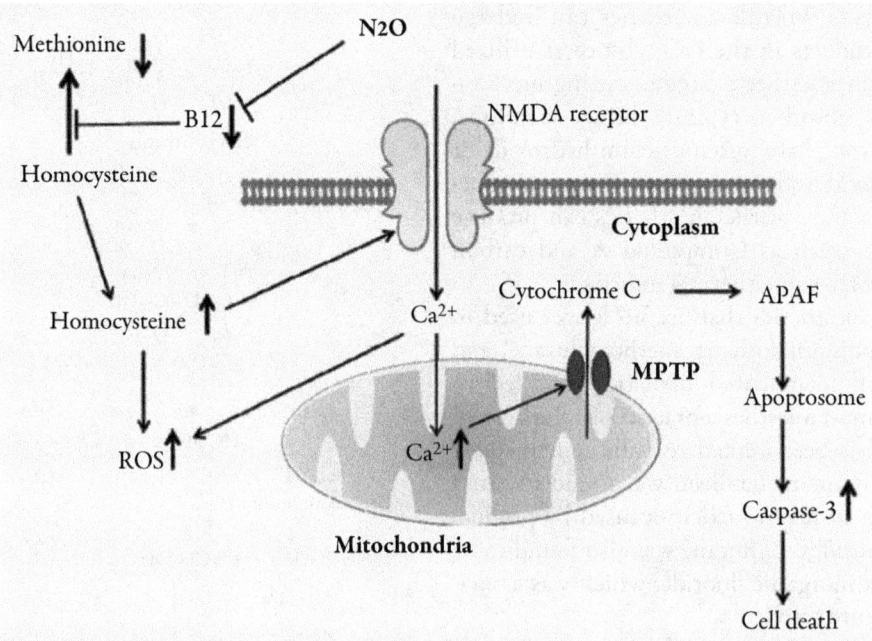

**Figure 33.2.** An overview of the homocysteine-mediated pathway of cell death induced by N₂O exposure.

of oxygen used determine the degree of toxicity. Patients requiring hyperbaric oxygen therapy are at increased risk. CNS toxicity presents with early and late symptoms: early symptoms include perioral and hand muscle twitching; later symptoms include vertigo, nausea, altered mental status, and convulsions. Pulmonary toxicity can be seen as acute lung injury in the form of acute respiratory distress syndrome, which may lead to pulmonary interstitial fibrosis.

Retinopathy of prematurity (ROP) is thought to be caused by uncontrolled oxygen therapy in premature infants.[6] Risk factors for ROP include birth weight, gestational age, anemia, and respiratory distress. It is believed that ROP is caused by disorganized growth of the retinal blood vessel that can result in scarring or retinal detachment. Its incidence has decreased over time due to recognition of ROP, advancements in oxygen regulation, and early detection of the disease.

## APPLICATIONS TO ANESTHESIA PRACTICE

Inhaled anesthetic toxicity can be difficult to prevent and diagnose, but providers can reduce the toxicity risk to patients. Anesthesia personnel should be educated on the risk of exposures to toxic byproducts. Anesthesia machines should have fresh gas flows turned off at the end of each day. If an anesthesia machine has been found with the fresh gas flows on, the $CO_2$ absorber should be changed to avoid its desiccation. Baralyme absorbers have been removed from the market; they should be avoided if older stockpiles exist and newer absorbents used in their place. Care should also be taken to limit inhaled anesthetic use to the minimum amount of time needed. Fresh gas flows should not be used at flow rates <1 liter/minute to minimize exposures to toxic metabolites. Care should be taken to avoid oxygen toxicity, limiting the exposure to the lowest possible concentration for the shortest period of time.

## REFERENCES

1. McKay R. Inhaled anesthetics. In: Pardo M, Miller R, eds. *Basic of Anesthesia.* 7th ed. Philadelphia, PA: Elsevier; 2018:83–103.
2. VanErdewyk, J. Carbon dioxide absorption. In: Murray M, ed. *Faust's Anesthesiology Review.* 4th ed. Philadelphia, PA: Elsevier; 2015:15–16.
3. Ebert T, Naze S. Inhaled anesthetics. In: Barash P, ed. *Clinical Anesthesia.* 8th ed. Philadelphia, PA: Wolters Kluwer; 2017: 459–483.
4. Caswell R. Nitrous oxide. In: Murray M, ed. *Faust's Anesthesiology Review.* 4th ed. Philadelphia, PA: Elsevier; 2015:150–152.
5. Chawla A, Lavania A. Oxygen toxicity. *Med J Armed Forces India.* 2001;57(2):131–133.

# 34.

# OXYGEN SUPPLY SYSTEMS

*David Hutchinson and Chris Giordano*

## CENTRAL OXYGEN SUPPLY/ WALL CONNECTIONS

With multiple types of medical gases available, both from the central supply and through a backup tank, a system to ensure that the correct gas is paired with its associated flowmeter within the anesthesia machine is needed. For the central or wall supply, the Diameter Index Safety System has color-coded hoses with specific diameters of pins for each gas, preventing the incorrect hose from being attached to each flowmeter. In the United States, green, yellow, and blue correspond to oxygen, air, and nitrous oxide, respectively. For reference, the approximate pressure of gases delivered to the anesthesia machine via the wall supply is 50 psig (pounds per square inch gauge, which is pressure relative to ambient atmospheric pressure).[1]

## E-CYLINDERS/BACKUP OXYGEN SUPPLY

In contrast, backup cylinders are mobile, can be exchanged quickly, and require a convenient and quick method to attach to the anesthesia machine. These cylinders often contain medical gases under very high pressures; they must pass through a regulator to reduce these pressures to approximately 45 psig. A full oxygen E-cylinder contains 600 to 660 L and will have a pressure of 1900 to 2200 psig; thus, it requires significant pressure reduction before being supplied to the low-pressure circuit connected to the patient.[1]

While the cylinders are generally color coded in a similar fashion to the central supply hoses, many cylinders are a similar size. In an emergency, they could easily be incorrectly connected. To prevent this, the Pin Index Safety System exists, which typically consists of a pattern of six possible pin locations on the backup tank (Table 34.1).[2]

Pressures contained within the E-cylinders are much higher than allowed within the anesthesia circuit and are stepped down to 45 to 47 psig.[1] This is slightly lower than the pipeline or wall supply pressure of 50 psig, which allows the anesthesia machine to preferentially use the pipeline

supply. Should the pipeline supply fail and the pressure drop below 45 psig, the anesthesia machine will, by default, start using the higher pressure "backup" E-cylinders. This process happens seamlessly; providers should consider closing the backup oxygen supply after verifying adequate pressure to avoid depleting the E-cylinder without realizing that the central supply has failed.[3]

Conversely, there is also protection built into the anesthesia machine should medical gas pressures become too high, which might occur with a pressure regulator failure from an E-cylinder. High-pressure relief valves are built into the anesthesia machines to prevent the delivery of high-pressure gas to the patient, which usually open around 90 to 110 psig.

It is also worth noting that other countries may not abide by the same coloring conventions regarding medical gases. Differences are summarized in Table 34.2.[1]

## OTHER PROTECTIVE MECHANISMS: PHYSICAL AND AUDIBLE

In addition to multiple layers of protection and regulation prior to the medical gases reaching the anesthesia machine, many protective systems are in place to prevent the delivery of hypoxic or inappropriate mixtures or even incorrect medical gas to the patient. Oxygen is supplied directly to its flow-control valve, and it can be delivered to the patient with no other gases present. This oxygen-flow control valve is positioned furthest downstream in the circuit (closest

*Table 34.1* PIN-INDEX SAFETY SYSTEM CONFIGURATIONS OF IMPORTANT MEDICAL GASES

| GAS | PINS | MEMORY TOOL |
| --- | --- | --- |
| Air | 1,5 | A is first letter (1) |
| Oxygen | 2,5 | O2 has (2) atoms |
| N2O | 3,5 | N2O has (3) atoms |

**Table 34.2** MEDICAL GAS CYLINDER COLOR DIFFERENCES BETWEEN USA AND INTERNATIONAL

| MEDICAL GAS | USA | INTERNATIONAL |
|---|---|---|
| Oxygen | Green | White |
| Carbon Dioxide | Gray | Gray |
| Nitrous Oxide | Blue | Blue |
| Helium | Brown | Brown |
| Nitrogen | Black | Black |
| Air | Yellow | Black & White |

to the patient) to provide protection against an upstream circuit leak. In the event an upstream component such as a flow-control valve, vaporizer, or other part of the system fails, oxygen will still be delivered to the patient.[2] Finally, most anesthesia machines have a minimum oxygen flow within the circuit to prevent delivery of an anoxic mixture. This minimum flow rate differs among manufacturers, with older machines delivering 200 mL/min and some newer machines as little as 50 mL/min or even none in the case of some new Dräger and Apollo models. An alarm on these machines prevents beginning a case with no flow.[4]

Gases such as nitrous oxide can cause profound hypoxia if they are not administered concurrently with oxygen; several safety mechanisms prevent its sole administration. Nitrous oxide is usually administered with oxygen, and systems within the anesthesia machine will allow only nitrous oxide to be delivered if a sufficient pressure of oxygen within the circuit is detected. Furthermore, the anesthesia machine will have a mechanism for linking or "coupling" the oxygen/nitrous oxide ratio to ensure that a minimum concentration of 25% oxygen is delivered with nitrous oxide.

With the advent of digital anesthesia machine interfaces, one of the inherent physical safety mechanisms has been phased out. Oxygen-flow control knobs on analog machines are usually fluted, protrude further, or contain a feature that makes them readily identifiable by feel.[1] Digital interfaces may lack this tactile feedback, but they are clearly labeled and color coded to prevent inadvertent administration of an undesirable concentration or mixture.

Should the oxygen supply pressure drop below 20 to 30 psig (varies by manufacturer), an alarm will sound.[3] However, this is simply a pressure alarm and does not discriminate which gas is flowing in the system. If an E-cylinder or wall supply is incorrectly connected, this alarm will not provide any warning of an incorrect gas. Additionally, there are alarms for delivery of hypoxic mixtures and delivery of inadequate oxygen flows to the patient.

## ANESTHETIC CONSIDERATIONS

- Thirty minutes into a surgery, a patient's oxygen saturation begins to decline and continues to fall slowly. The low-oxygen pressure alarm sounds and a decision to turn on the backup oxygen supply is made. Unfortunately, while trying to open the cylinder, it is noted that the valve was already open, and the tank is now empty. This necessitates ventilation with air from the low- or high-pressure circuits or connection of an auxiliary oxygen tank to an Ambu bag to maintain adequate oxygenation. Under normal circumstances, if the backup low-pressure system oxygen tank had remained closed, failure of the high-pressure system would not have automatically begun exhausting the backup supply. It is important during machine checks to ensure that after the pressure in the backup oxygen supply is verified, the valve is closed to prevent masking of a failed high-pressure system.

- A patient requires supplemental oxygen for transport directly to an intensive care unit. A green E-cylinder under the patient stretcher is connected to a nasal cannula and set to 6 L/min of flow. A quick check of the pressure gauge before leaving the operating room indicates the tank is approximately half full or approximately 1100 psig (330 L). With this information, the maximum allowable transport time can be accounted for at the set flow of 6 L/min. Using the formula: time remaining = (psig)/[200 × flow rate (L/min)] or (1100)/(200 × 6), the time is 0.91 hours or 55 minutes. Alternatively, the volume can be used in the following way: time remaining = cylinder volume (L)/flow rate (L/min). This would yield the following calculation: time remaining = (330 L)/(6 L/min), which is 55 minutes.

## REFERENCES

1. Butterworth JF, et al., eds. *Morgan & Mikhail's Clinical Anesthesiology.* 6th ed. McGraw-Hill Education; 2018.
1. Barash PG, et al., eds. *Clinical Anesthesia.* 6th ed. Philadelphia, PA: Lippincott Williams & Wilkins; 2009.
2. Murray MJ, et al. *Faust's Anesthesiology Review.* 4th ed. Philadelphia, PA: Elsevier Saunders; 2014.
3. Anesthesia Patient Safety Foundation. Reader questions. Apsf.org. https://www.apsf.org/article/reader-questions-why-some-anesthesia-machines-allow-o2-flow-below-basal-metabolic-needs/.

# 35.

# WASTE GAS EVACUATION SYSTEMS

*David E. Swanson*

## INTRODUCTION

Currently available studies indicate no association between occupational exposure to trace levels of waste anesthetic vapors in scavenged operating rooms and adverse health effects. However, it is desirable to vent out the exhaled anesthetic vapors and maintain a vapor-free environment. A prudent plan for minimizing exposure includes maintaining equipment, training personnel, and monitoring exposure routinely.[1] The opinion of Al-Shaikh on the lack of health effects of trace gases is not accepted by many, in particular concerning the effects on pregnant women.

Operating rooms (ORs) in developed countries have waste anesthetic gas (WAG) evacuation systems built in and are effective in lowering the concentration of volatile anesthetics in the OR. A study from Brazil demonstrated about a fourfold reduction in the anesthetic concentrations in 6 ORs with a scavenging system, compared to 7 ORs without, although not to the internationally recommended values.[2] This study also shows the importance of ventilation standards, with 7 rather than the 15 air changes per hour recommended for ORs by the American Institute of Architects guidelines. This correlates very well with Al-Shaikh's assessment that unventilated ORs are four times as contaminated with anesthetic gases compared to those with proper ventilation.[1]

Anesthesia machines have active WAG scavenging systems. When connected to the suction of the WAG evacuation system, the anesthetic gases that are no longer usable in the anesthesia machine are transported out of the hospital and released into the atmosphere (see Figure 35.1). Active scavenging is required by the Joint Commission.

A WAGD system has 4 parts, as shown in Figure 35.2: the relief valves by which the anesthesia gas leaves the machine, the tubing, the interface, and the disposal line. A passive WAGD system has a disposal line that exits the

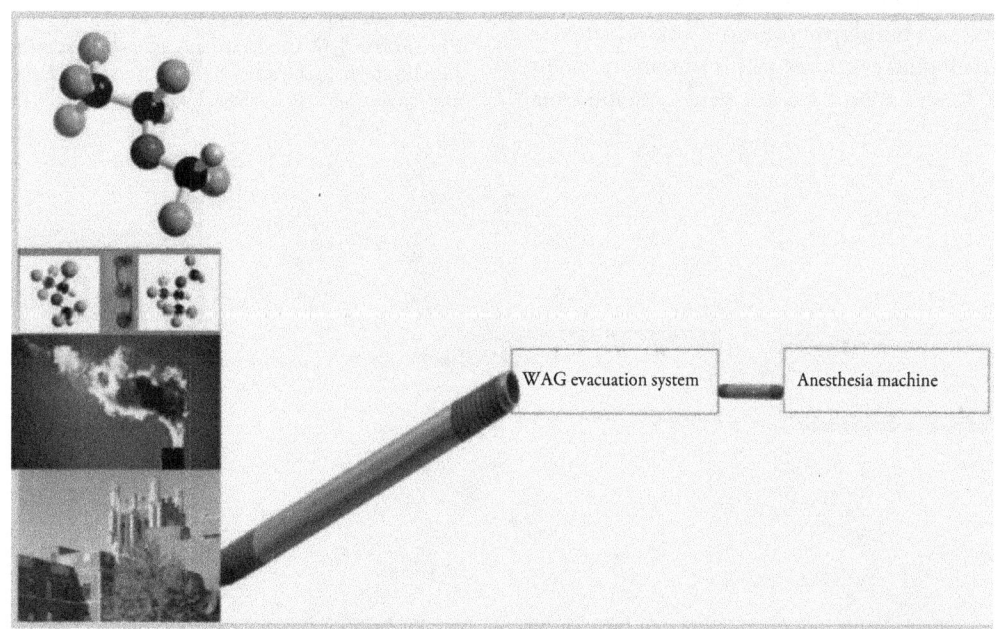

**Figure 35.1.** Waste anesthetic gas (WAG) is piped out of the anesthesia machine via the active suction of the WAG evacuation system and exhausted outside the hospital into the environment. The molecules shown are nitrous oxide, isoflurane, sevoflurane, and desflurane.

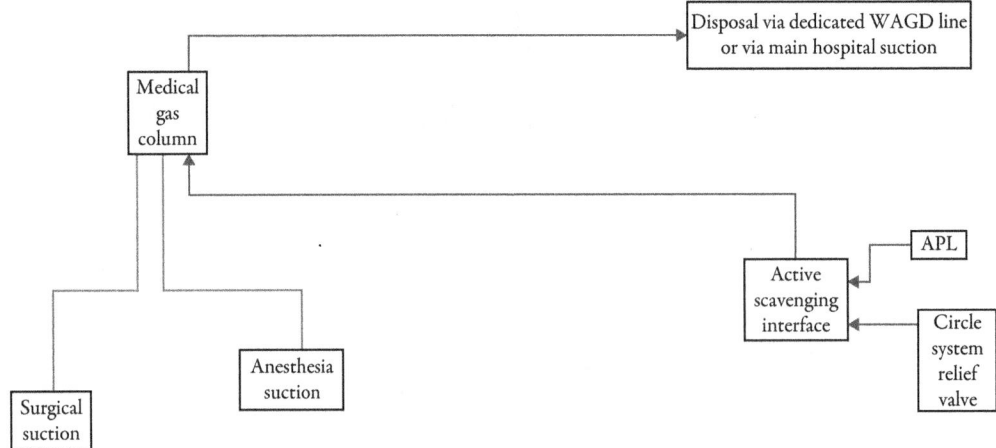

**Figure 35.2.** The 4 parts of a waste anesthetic gas disposal (WAGD) system: (1) Relief valve of the circle system and the adjustable pressure-limiting (APL) valve by which the anesthesia gas leaves the machine, (2) Tubing, (3) Interface, (4) Disposal line.

room or empties into the OR ventilation exhaust, whereas an active system disposal line can have a dedicated vacuum (preferred) or empty into the hospital vacuum system.

Closed reservoir interface systems involve a collection bag which should fill with exhalation and then empty during inhalation. For safety, a closed system should have a negative pressure relief valve. An open reservoir interface system has holes allowing for overflow, and appropriate suction can be checked by seeing the ball floating between the markers.

Engineering connection safety measures include the use of 19 and 30mm tubing to avoid connection to the circuit and purple and yellow pipelines and connections with diameter index safety system fittings.

Risks increase with the complexity of the machine, and scavenging can potentially lead to negative pressure within the circuit or a buildup of pressure. This is primarily a problem in developing countries and is important to understand if one does mission trips, but whenever abnormal pressure exists in the breathing circuit, the scavenging system should be checked for possible malfunction.[3]

A low-flow scavenger interface is commercially available that is more energy efficient. An estimated 500,000 gallons of anesthetic agents are used annually in the United States. Reclamation of these agents would be of environmental benefit but is currently cost prohibitive.

## REFERENCES

1. Al-Shaikh B, Stacey S. Pollution in theatre and scavenging. In: *Essentials of Equipment in Anaesthesia, Critical Care and Peri-Operative Medicine.* Edinburgh, Scotland; New York: Elsevier; 2019:43–52.
2. Braz LG, Braz JRC, et al. Comparison of waste anesthetic gases in operating rooms with or without a scavenging system in a Brazilian University Hospital. *Rev Bras Anestesiol.* 2017 Sep–Oct;67(5):516–520.
3. Ehrenwerth J. Waste anesthetic gases and scavenging systems. In: Eisenkraft JB, McGregor DG, eds., *Anesthesia Equipment: Principles and Applications.* 2nd ed. St. Louis: Saunders; 2013:125–147.

# 36.

# SAFETY FEATURES

*Meghan Brennan and Chris Giordano*

## PREOPERATIVE SAFETY FEATURES

As part of the American Society of Anesthesiologists' basic standards for anesthetic monitoring, an alarm capable of detecting a disconnect of the components of the system must be present when using mechanical ventilation.[1] Problem-solving a ventilator disconnection alarm or malfunction in a ventilator involves a combination of information from multiple monitors, such as capnography and low-pressure alarms. The low-pressure alarm can indicate ventilator disconnections from the patient, leaks in the circuit, fresh gas flow system failures, and scavenging system failures. Pressure monitors and the low-pressure alarm, which are part of the anesthesia circuit and typically are located near the unidirectional inspiratory valves, are set to alarm if the circuit pressure does not exceed a set limit within a certain time period. Older anesthesia machines may not have these built-in alarms and may require a separate external alarm. Preoperatively, it is important to conduct a machine check to verify that the high- and low-pressures systems, scavenging system, and oxygen analyzer are functioning appropriately (Table 36.1).

## INTRAOPERATIVE SAFETY FEATURES

Intraoperative ventilator alarm settings are important to immediately detect ventilator errors and circuit disconnections. It is recommended that the low-pressure alarm be set to just below the peak inspiratory pressure to avoid missing possible ventilator disconnections. If the alarm is set too low, it is at risk of failing to alert to circuit disconnection. If the alarm does activate, it is important to evaluate the patient and circuit for obvious signs of a ventilator disconnection or an incompetent endotracheal tube cuff and correlate with other monitors, such as capnography

and peak pressures. Next, one should switch to manual ventilation, recheck the circuit for leaks and loose connections, and evaluate fresh gas flows and flow meters. A systematic approach to troubleshooting this alarm is important to avoid patient injury.

## INTRAOPERATIVE ELECTRICAL SYSTEMS

Ohm's law describes the relationship of voltage (V), current (I), and resistance (R):[2]

$$V = I \times R$$

A basic electric circuit consists of current, made up of electrons flowing between two points of different voltage. All electrical circuits and electrical equipment risk current leakage between conductors, which are the materials that transmit the electric charge. If a patient or provider

*Table 36.1* ALARMS THAT TRIGGER AS PATIENT SAFETY FEATURES

| PREOPERATIVE SAFETY FEATURES | INTRAOPERATIVE SAFETY FEATURES |
|---|---|
| Machine check | High-pressure alarm—ventilator |
| High-pressure system alarm | Low-pressure alarm—ventilator |
| Low-pressure system alarm | Vital sign alarms: pulse oximeter, EKG, blood pressure, temperature |
| Line isolation monitor alarm | $CO_2$ alarm |
| | Inspired oxygen alarm |
| | Line isolation monitor alarm |

$CO_2$, carbon dioxide; EKG, electrocardiogram.

**Table 36.2** ELECTRICITY LEAK AND RESULTING CONTACT EFFECT

| | CURRENT | EFFECT WITH 1-SECOND CONTACT |
|---|---|---|
| **Microshocks** | 10 uA | Allowable maximum current leakage |
| | 20–100 uA | Ventricular fibrillation |
| **Macroshocks** | 1 mA | Perceptible electric current |
| | 5 mA | Maximum current not causing injury |
| | 10–20 mA | "Let-go" current before sustained muscle contraction |
| | 50 mA | Pain and mechanical injury |
| | 100–300 mA | Ventricular fibrillation |

contacts part of the circuit in two places, a serious electric shock may result. Equipment is often insulated to limit current leakage, and parts of electrical equipment in contact with the patient may be doubly insulated to reduce the risk of shock. In the operating room (OR), two separate electrical systems may be present to help reduce the risk of shock: a grounded system containing ground fault circuit interrupters (GFCIs) and line isolation monitor (LIM) systems.

Grounded systems are used in most locations, such as homes, commercial buildings, and ORs, to reduce the risk of macroshocks, or large shocks greater than 1 mA. An electrical ground is a wire or object that is connected to a circuit that can conduct large amounts of current, which may disperse the electricity into the earth or into

an electrical charge reservoir. In the three-pronged plugs typically found in ORs, one prong supplies a high voltage. In the United States, this is typically 120 V. The second is typically neutral to allow for current flow, and the third prong is connected to a ground wire. In the OR, if a person becomes grounded by touching the ground wire and comes into contact with two conductive materials of different voltages that are not grounded, an electrical current can pass through them to complete the circuit and cause an electrical shock. The severity of the electric shock is based on the amount of current and the time that current contacts a person. It can cause significant tissue injury, burns, and even death. The maximum amount of "harmless" current intensity is 5 mA; anything greater than that risks tissue damage (Table 36.2).

Grounded systems contain GFCIs designed to prevent or reduce the risk of electric shock. A GFCI detects current leakage, typically of 5 mA or more, as this is the maximum amount of harmless current and it stops current to that circuit. By shutting off power to the circuit, it reduces the risk of shock.

In an isolated system, power from the main power supply is connected to an isolation transformer, which creates a separate, isolated, ungrounded system from the wall outlet power supply (Figure 36.1). To deliver a shock to a person within an isolated system, two faults must occur. First, the system must be connected to the ground, and a person must come into contact with two points of that circuit of different voltage (Figure 36.1). Isolated systems must contain an LIM to alert for leakage current to the ground or short circuits. The LIM determines the amount of current that is flowing through the system to the ground and is designed to alarm at a current leakage of 2 to 5 mA. The LIM is only an alarm that indicates

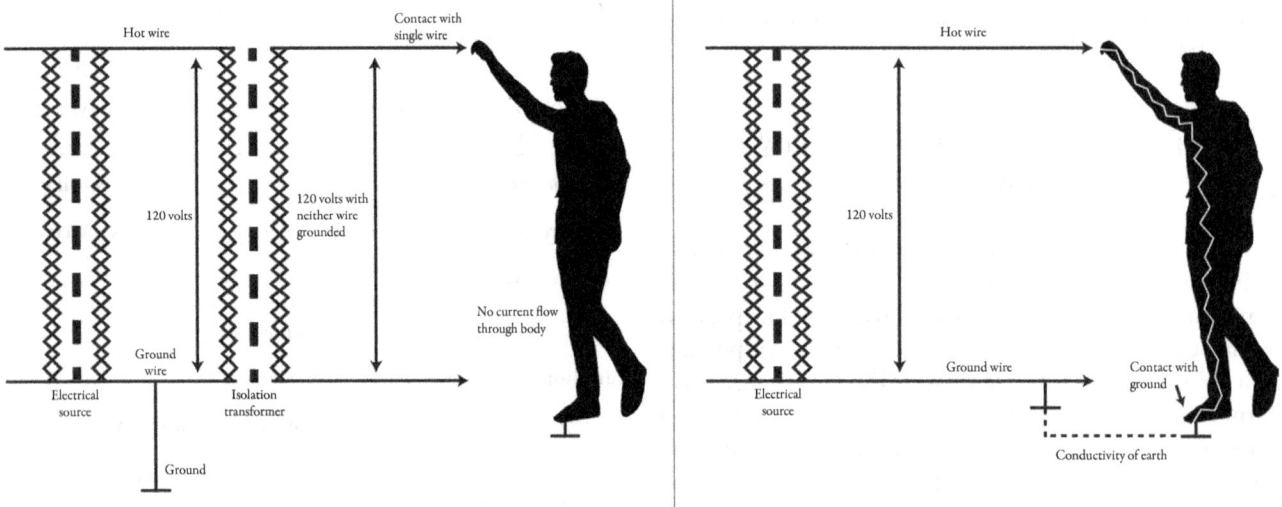

**Figure 36.1.** Illustration of a line isoloation monitor and the requisite need to experience an electrical shock.

current leakage; it does not stop power to the circuit, as the GFCI does. Once the LIM alarms, equipment must be unplugged individually, typically in the order it was plugged in so that the defective equipment that created the current leakage can be found. Because of this, isolated power systems and LIMs are more commonly used with equipment that cannot be safely turned off during a procedure. LIMs alarm if they detect the risk of macroshocks only; the amount of current that causes microshocks is too low to be detected with an LIM.

## REFERENCES

1. *Standards for Basic Anesthetic Monitoring.* Committee of Origin: Standards and Practice Parameters (Approved by the ASA House of Delegates on October 21, 1986, last amended on October 20, 2010, and last affirmed on October 28, 2016) https://www.asahq.org/~/media/Sites/ASAHQ/Files/Public/Resources/standards-guidelines/standards-for-basic-anesthetic-monitoring.pdf
2. Singh SK, et al. Basics of electricity for anaesthetists. *Cont Educ Anaesthes Crit Care Pain.* 2011;11(6):224–228.
3. Barker SJ, Doyle DJ. Electrical safety in the operating room: Dry versus wet. *Anesth Analg.* 2010;110(6):1517–1518.

# 37.

# MONITORING METHODS

*Santiago Luis and Snehal Raut*

## BASIC ANESTHETIC MONITORING

Standard I: Qualified anesthesia personnel
Standard II: Ventilation: End tidal $CO_2$, inspired anesthetic gases

Oxygenation: $SpO_2$ and inspired $O_2$ (with an alarm)
Temperature
Circulation: Heart rate, EKG, noninvasive blood pressure (BP) at least every 5 minutes.[1]

## CAPNOGRAPHY

Capnography, the monitoring of $CO_2$ in respiratory gases, has become an integral part of anesthesia monitoring. Capnography provides information about $CO_2$ production, pulmonary perfusion, alveolar ventilation, respiratory patterns, and elimination of $CO_2$ from the anesthesia circuit and ventilator.

## TERMINOLOGY

*Capnography*: graphic display of $CO_2$ concentration during a respiratory cycle

*Capnograph*: the machine that generates a waveform; or the waveform itself.

*Capnometry*: the measurement and numerical display of maximum inspiratory and expiratory $CO_2$ concentrations during a respiratory cycle.

*Capnometer*: the device that performs the measurement and displays the reading.

## METHODS

Methods include infrared spectrography, Raman spectrography, mass spectrography, photoacoustic spectrography, and chemical colorimetric analysis.

The infrared method is most widely used. The intensity of IR radiation projected through a gas mixture containing $CO_2$ is diminished by absorption; this allows the $CO_2$

absorption band to be identified and is proportional to the amount of $CO_2$ in the mixture.

The colorimetric method of measuring $CO_2$ employs a chemically treated pH-sensitive indicator contained in a plastic housing that functions as an endotracheal tube elbow adapter.

## CAPNOGRAPHS: SIDE STREAM AND MAIN STREAM CAPNOGRAPHS

In side stream capnography, the $CO_2$ sensor is located in the main unit itself, and a pump draws gas samples from the patient's airway. The optimal gas flow is 50–250 ml/min. The side stream capnographs allow monitoring of spontaneously breathing non-intubated subjects.

In the main stream capnograph, a device containing the $CO_2$ sensor is inserted between the breathing circuit and the endotracheal tube, with all of the inhaled and exhaled gas flowing through this measuring system.

*Capnograms* are the graphic display of $CO_2$ concentration versus time (time capnogram) or expired volume (volume capnogram) during a respiratory cycle.

The time capnogram (Figure 37.1) is the most commonly used, but the volume capnogram helps in assessment of dead space and the V/Q status of the lungs.

Phase I: anatomical and apparatus dead space gas is exhaled which contains no $CO_2$.

Phase II: a rapid upstroke due to mixing of dead space gas with alveolar gas.

Phase III: the alveolar plateau represents the $CO_2$ rich gas from the alveoli.

Phase IV: the inspiratory phase during which the fresh gases (CO2 free) are inhaled and CO2 concentration falls rapidly to zero.[1,2]

A sudden drop in $ETCO_2$ followed by the absence of a $CO_2$ waveform can occur in a potentially life-threatening event that could indicate malposition of an endotracheal tube into the pharynx or esophagus, sudden severe hypotension, massive pulmonary embolism, a cardiac arrest, or a disconnection or disruption of sampling lines (Figure 37.2).

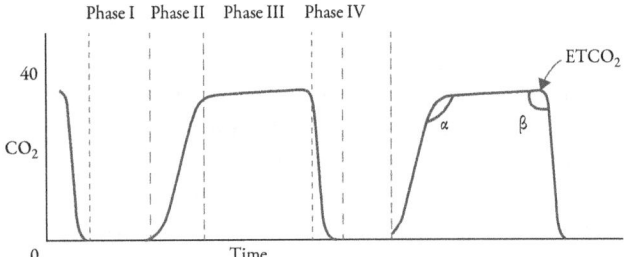

**Figure 37.1.** Normal time capnogram.

During life-saving cardiopulmonary resuscitation, the generation of adequate circulation can be assessed by the restoration of the $CO_2$ waveform.

## PULSE OXIMETRY

Pulse oximetry is a noninvasive method of assessing oxygen saturation of hemoglobin by spectrophotometry. It is based on the Lambert-Beer law, which relates the concentration of a solute to the intensity of light transmitted through a solution.

The reduced hemoglobin (HHb) has a peak absorption at 660 nm (red light), and oxygenated hemoglobin (HbO2) at 940 nm (near infrared light).[3]

### PRINCIPLE OF PULSE OXIMETRY

Each pulse oximeter probe contains LEDs, which emit two wavelengths of light (red and near infrared) through a cutaneous vascular bed. The probe is commonly placed on the digits or earlobe. A photodetector on the other side measures the intensity of transmitted light at each wavelength from which oxygen saturation is derived.

Pulse oximetry is based upon two physical principles:

1. Spectrophotometry, used to calculate $SpO_2$
2. Optical plethysmography, used to measure pulsatile changes in arterial blood volume.

The advanced analysis of pleth waveform using algorithms helps to determine the plethysmographic variability index (PVI), which is a measure of the dynamic changes in the perfusion index over respiratory cycle, with the goal of predicting fluid responsiveness.

### PITFALLS AND LIMITATIONS

1. Dyshemoglobinemias: If carboxyhemoglobin or methemoglobin are present in appreciable amounts, the accuracy is suspected. As metHb increases, $SpO_2$ approaches 85%, regardless of the true level of $HbO_2$. Also, the pulse oximeter interprets COHb as a mixture of approximately 90% $HbO_2$ and 10% HHb.
2. The pulse oximeter fails to give accurate readings whenever the peripheral pulsations are poor.
3. Delayed detection of hypoxic events: Most pulse oximeters average pulse data over 5 to 8 seconds before displaying a value.
4. Nail polish and coverings: Some shades of black, blue, and green nail polish may cause significantly lower saturation readings.
5. Dyes and pigments: Injections of dyes like methylene blue, indocyanine green, and indigo carmine .

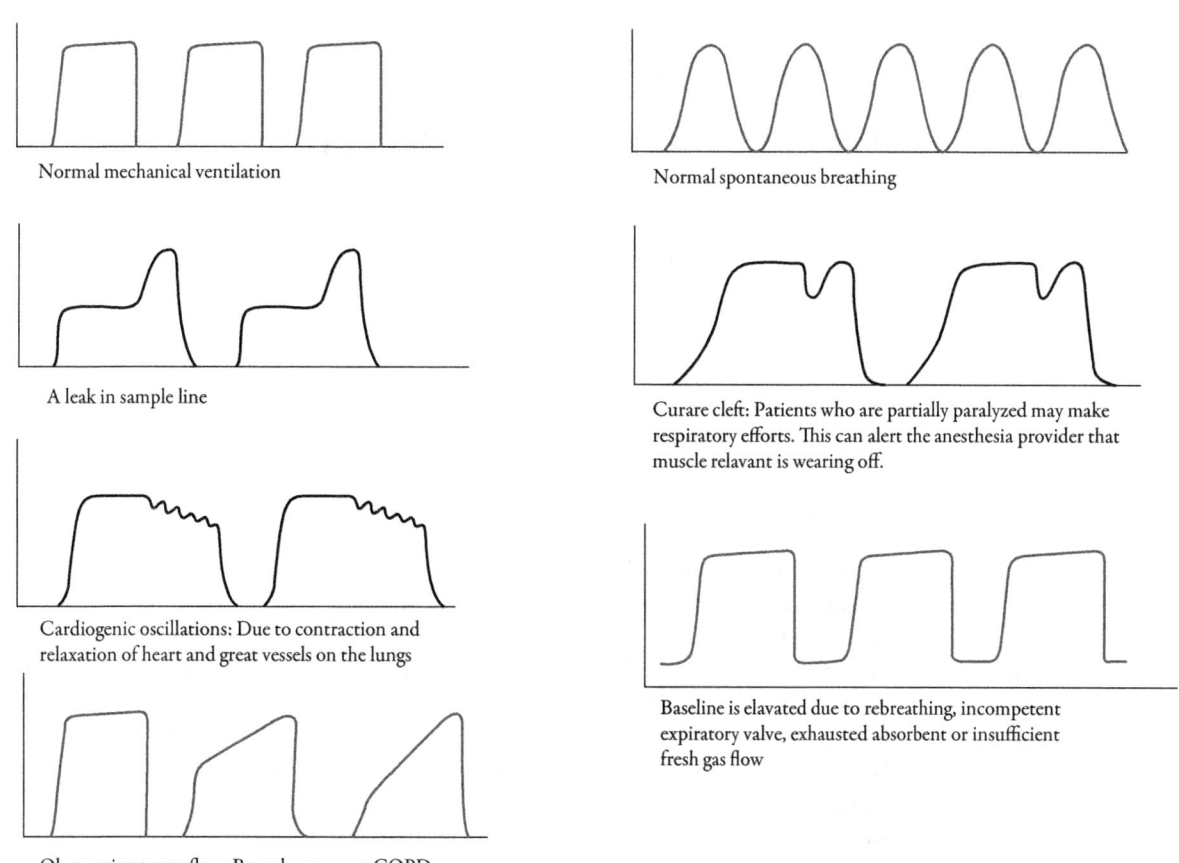

**Figure 37.2.** Various waveforms of capnogram and how they correspond to disease patterns or device malfunction.

Labels within figure:

Normal mechanical ventilation

Normal spontaneous breathing

A leak in sample line

Curare cleft: Patients who are partially paralyzed may make respiratory efforts. This can alert the anesthesia provider that muscle relavant is wearing off.

Cardiogenic oscillations: Due to contraction and relaxation of heart and great vessels on the lungs

Baseline is elavated due to rebreathing, incompetent expiratory valve, exhausted absorbent or insufficient fresh gas flow

Obstruction to gas flow: Bronchospasm or COPD

6. Electrocautery: Electrocautery can cause interference.
7. Ambient light: Surgical lamps, fluorescent lights, infrared light-emitting devices, and fiberoptic light sources can lead to inaccurate SpO$_2$ readings.
8. Arrhythmias.
9. Motion artifacts: Motion of the sensor relative to the skin can cause an artifact that the pulse oximeter is unable to differentiate from normal arterial pulsations.

## REFERENCES

1. *Standards for Basic Anesthetic Monitoring.* https://www.asahq.org/standards-and-guidelines/standards-for-basic-anesthetic-monitoring.
2. Dorsch JA, Dorsch SE. Gas monitoring. In: Dorsch JA, Dorsch SE. *Understanding Anesthesia Equipment.* 5th ed. Philadelphia, PA: Lippincott Williams & Wilkins; 2007:686–727.
3. Dorsch JA, Dorsch SE. Pulse oximetry. In: Dorsch JA, Dorsch SE. *Understanding Anesthesia Equipment.* 5th ed. Philadelphia, PA: Lippincott Williams & Wilkins; 2007:776–795.

# 38.

# NEUROMUSCULAR FUNCTION

*Nimit K. Shah and Chike Gwam*

## INTRODUCTION

Postoperative residual neuromuscular blockade or curarization (PORC), though a misnomer as curare is no longer used, remains a frequent occurrence after administration of NMBA (neuromuscular blocking agent), even after a single dose of intermediate acting NMBAs.[1–4] Several studies have shown that 20%–40% of patients who receive NMBAs have significant PORC even after reversal. This can lead to various airway and respiratory adverse events in the postanesthesia care unit (PACU) and postoperative pulmonary complications which significantly increase postoperative morbidity and mortality.[4]

## ASSESSMENT OF NEUROMUSCULAR BLOCKADE

(1) *Clinical evaluation for signs of muscular weakness*: Various tests of muscle strength, such as 5 s head lift, sustained hand grip, etc., have traditionally been used to evaluate recovery of neuromuscular function at the end of surgery. However, they are unreliable indicators of adequate neuromuscular function recovery,[7] as none of them has a sensitivity of >0.35 or a PPV of >0.52.

(2) *Qualitative neuromuscular monitoring*: Degree of neuromuscular block (NMB) is subjectively assessed by evaluating visually or tactilely the strength of a muscle contraction following a nerve stimulus given by a peripheral nerve stimulator (PNS).

(3) *Quantitative neuromuscular monitoring*: Degree of NMB is objectively assessed by monitors which are capable of both giving a nerve stimulus like a PNS and measuring the evoked response by various techniques and displaying a numerical value for the evoked response.

In both qualitative and quantitative neuromuscular monitoring, the principle of peripheral nerve stimulation is used. A stimulus in the form of electrical current is applied by the PNS over a peripheral nerve, which evokes a contraction of the innervated muscle. The stimulus mimics an action potential and is a supramaximal monophasic current with a rapid rise and fall, applied for a duration of 0.2–0.3 ms.

The response of a single muscle fiber to a stimulus obeys the *all or none phenomenon*.[5] The current which generates a response from all nerve fibers in a nerve and hence a maximal muscle contraction is termed a *maximal current*. This maximal current delivered will depend on the skin impedance or resistance, which can increase up to 5 kΩ intraoperatively due to hypothermia. Traditionally, a current of 25% above the maximal stimulus is applied when stimulating a peripheral nerve to ensure stimulation of all muscle fibers despite skin resistance changes, and this is called *supramaximal current*.

## DIFFERENTIAL MUSCLE SENSITIVITY

The diaphragm is the most resistant muscle to both nondepolarizing and depolarizing muscle relaxant as it has highest density of nAch receptors. Airway (laryngeal) muscles are the second most resistant. However, these are also central muscle groups with greater blood supply (and hence greater drug supply) than peripheral muscle groups. Hence with a large dose like an intubating dose, diaphragm and airway muscles are paralyzed faster than APM, and they also recover faster than APM. Corrugator supercilii muscle behaves like a central muscle like the diaphragm[7] and larynx, whereas Orbicularis oculi behaves like a peripheral muscle like APM.[7] However, practically it is difficult to separate the responses of these two muscles on facial nerve stimulation and hence facial nerve stimulation is not reliable for assessing the degree of NMB.

## PATTERNS OF STIMULATION

### SINGLE TWITCH STIMULATION

Single monophasic and square wave electrical stimulus of supramaximal intensity is applied transcutaneously to a peripheral motor nerve at a frequency of 0.1 to 1 Hz[1,5] for a duration of 0.2 ms and the subsequent evoked muscle response is observed. Twitch response will start diminishing after administration of NMB when more than 70% of Ach receptors are occupied and completely disappear when 90%–95% of Ach receptors are occupied by NMBA. It may be used to evaluate the time to onset of NMB (both depolarizing and nondepolarizing); however, it cannot be used to quantify the level of NMB or estimate the recovery from the NMB.

## TRAIN-OF-FOUR (TOF) STIMULATION

Four supramaximal stimuli are given at a frequency of 2 Hz, and 4 corresponding evoked muscle responses are evaluated. Ratio of the fourth response to the first response (T4/T1) is called TOF ratio (TOFR).[1,5] T1 acts as a control.

TOFR before administration of NMBA is 1.0. With the onset of nondepolarizing block, height of T4 decreases more than T3, which decreases more than T2, which decreases more than T1 (the higher the degree of NMB, the lower the TOFR). Successive decrement in twitch heights is known as fade, which is thought to be due to presynaptic blockade by the nondepolarizing blockade in addition to the postsynaptic blockade, and prevents the positive feedback action of Ach on the presynaptic Ach receptors to release more Ach with subsequent stimuli. With the onset of depolarizing block, all four twitches are decreased equally in heights until they disappear and there is no fade, as depolarizing muscle relaxants don't inhibit the positive feedback of Ach on the presynaptic receptors. This is also observed during recovery.

As the nondepolarizing blockade becomes more intense, T4 disappears first, followed by T3, T2, and lastly T1. During recovery from nondepolarizing block, T1 reappearance of responses is in reverse, from T1 followed by T2, T3, and lastly T4.

All twitches are present when <70% receptor sites blocked, T4 lost >70% receptor sites blocked, T3 lost >80%, T2 lost >90%, T1 lost >95%–100%.

TOF is most commonly used for NM monitoring. The advantages are that there is no control needed as T1 response acts as a control and is less painful. **Onset, degree of NMB, and recovery can all be monitored.** The disadvantage is that visual or tactile estimate of fade is only accurate until TOFR <0.4. Between TOFR of 0.4–0.9, fade cannot be reliably estimated visually or tactilely.

Traditionally, TOFR >0.7 was accepted for adequate reversal, but now TOFR ≥0.9 should be achieved before tracheal extubation.[5]

## DOUBLE-BURST STIMULATION

Double-burst stimulation (DBS) was developed as an alternative to TOF as the fade is not appreciable both visually and tactilely above TOFR >0.4. In DBS, two short tetanic bursts of three 0.2 ms stimuli of supramaximal current at 50 Hz delivered over 20 ms followed 750 ms with an identical burst consisting of either 3 or 2 stimuli (DBS 3,3 or DBS 3,2).[1,5] In normal nonparalyzed muscle, DBS 3,3 will evoke 2 separate muscle contractions of equal intensity. In partially paralyzed muscle with a nondepolarizing muscle relaxant, the evoked response to the second stimuli will be of lesser amplitude due to fade. The ratio of the amplitude of the second response to the first is called DBS ratio similar to TOFR. The responses to the 2 bursts will be fused muscle contractions to each stimuli in the burst due to tetanic frequency and hence this response will be greater compared to single response of ST or TOF stimuli. This allows improved subjective evaluation of the fade and it improves detection over TOF from TOFR of 0.4 to 0.6; however, it still cannot detect the fade between TOFR of 0.6 and 0.9.[5]

## TETANIC STIMULATION

High frequency of supramaximal current at a frequency of 50–100 Hz is applied for 5 seconds.[1,5] This will evoke a strong sustained muscle contraction in normal nonparalyzed muscle, but in a muscle partially paralyzed with nondepolarizing muscle relaxant there will be fade. As the response is a strong muscle contraction with a fade, even a small degree of NMB can be assessed. It is painful in non-anesthetized patients and hence is only used clinically as a component of PTC mode in anesthetized patients.

## POST-TETANIC COUNT (PTC)

During intense nondepolarizing block, TOF or ST may not evoke any response. PTC is used in these cases to allow assessment of an intense or deep neuromuscular blockade. It is a composite stimulation mode consisting of a tetanic stimulation (50 Hz applied for 5 seconds), followed 3 seconds after with 10–15 single twitches at 1 Hz.[1,5] It is based on *post-tetanic potentiation*[5] in which a tetanic stimulus leads to significantly increased Ach in the NM Jn, and single twitches applied after will elicit increased height of twitch response. The number of twitch responses are counted, and this number is inversely proportional to the degree of NMB. PTC is 0 during intense NMB, and as the intense NMB wears off, the first twitch response will be elicited and will herald onset of deep level of block. PTC is mainly used in surgeries which require intense or deep level of NMB to prevent any diaphragmatic movements, as during certain laparoscopic surgeries and to prevent bucking or coughing during tracheal stimulation in open globe surgeries or certain intracranial surgeries (Figure 38.1).

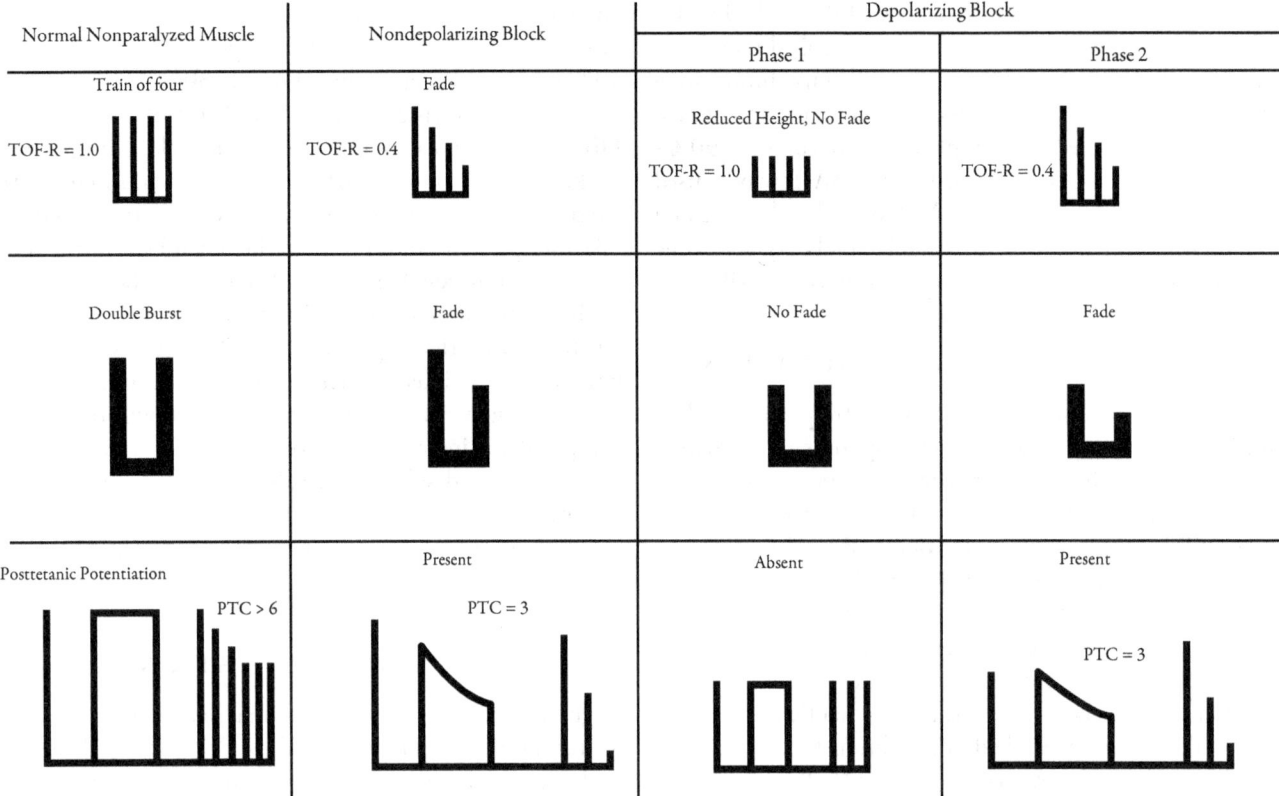

| Normal Nonparalyzed Muscle | Nondepolarizing Block | Depolarizing Block | |
| --- | --- | --- | --- |
| | | Phase 1 | Phase 2 |
| Train of four <br> TOF-R = 1.0 | Fade <br> TOF-R = 0.4 | Reduced Height, No Fade <br> TOF-R = 1.0 | TOF-R = 0.4 |
| Double Burst | Fade | No Fade | Fade |
| Posttetanic Potentiation <br> PTC > 6 | Present <br> PTC = 3 | Absent | Present <br> PTC = 3 |

**Figure 38.1.** Patterns of response to depolarizing and nondepolarizing blocks.

## QUANTITATIVE NEUROMUSCULAR MONITORING

These employ techniques such as MMG, EMG, AMG, KMG.

### MECHANOMYOGRAPHY (MMG)

This involves measurement of evoked muscle tension after an isometric contraction of a muscle (muscle not allowed to move), most commonly adductor pollicis muscle after ulnar nerve stimulation at the wrist. This technique can be used for assessment of any pattern of nerve stimulation and is the gold standard.[5] However, it will require a control recording first, which may take up to 15 mins, and the setup is cumbersome and impractical for use in the operating theater.

### ELECTROMYOGRAPHY (EMG)

This involves measurement of electrical activity (compound action potentials) during contraction of muscles when peripheral nerve innervating the muscles is stimulated (it is assumed that these are equivalent to the muscular contraction, i.e., mechanical events that occur after excitation-contraction coupling). It is the most physiologic and most precise method of measuring NMB. Control is obtained before administration of NMBA, and the ratio of response over control will give measurement of residual NMB. Ulnar nerve and APM are the most commonly used nerve-muscle unit. Stimulating electrodes are placed over the ulnar nerve and recording electrodes are placed in the thenar eminence (APM), hypothenar eminence (abductor digiti minimii muscle), and first dorsal interosseous muscle. This gives compound action potentials in muscles supplied by ulnar nerve. It can record compound MAPs from virtually any muscle, including the diaphragm and laryngeal muscles. It is easier to set up, and arm and hand do not need to be fixed as rigidly as in the case of MMG. Results obtained from EMG are comparable to those from MMG. Interference from electrical devices, especially from diathermy and hand temperature and movement, will affect the recordings.[1]

### ACCELEROMYOGRAPHY (AMG)

AMG is the commonly used quantitative monitor. It is based on the Newton's second law of motion (i.e., force = mass × acceleration). An accelerometer (piezoelectric ceramic wafer with electrodes on both sides) is mounted to the thumb. Ulnar nerve is stimulated and acceleration of the evoked isotonic APM contraction is measured. Since the mass of the thumb is constant, the force generated by the thumb contraction is derived. This force generates a voltage which is converted into an electrical signal and displayed as twitch response. The most common pattern used is TOF, and 4 twitches will be recorded, thus enabling a TOFR to be measured. TOFR measured in a normal nonparalyzed muscle is often 110%–140%. This high control baseline value TOFR means TOFR necessary for excluding residual neuromuscular blockade is equally higher. The TOFR obtained during recovery should be normalized with the baseline control TOFR. Currently available monitors do not offer normalizations of TOFR during recovery with control TOFR. Hence control TOFR becomes necessary, and to add a safety factor, TOFR of 1.0 instead of 0.9 (control TOFR = recovery TOFR) is used to indicate adequate recovery of neuromuscular function.[5] AMG requires unrestricted movement of thumb for accurate measurements. Any change in arm position during surgery requires recalibration. Newer models have tri-axial accelerometry (Stimpod NMS X 450) which measures thumb movements in 3 dimensions and negates the need for calibration. Other patterns used are PTC and DBS. Results are comparable to MMG.[1]

## KINEMYOGRAPHY (KMG)

It is based on the principle that deformation of piezoelectric wafer leads to development of voltage which can be converted into an electrical signal and measured. On stimulation of the ulnar nerve, thumb movement distorts a piezoelectric sensor pad embedded in a bending strip between thumb and index finger, which leads to a voltage proportional to the thumb movement. Currently it is available for only ulnar nerve–APM unit. Results are comparable to MMG and AMG.[5]

## REFERENCES

1. McGrath CD, Hunter JM. Monitoring of neuromuscular block. *Cont Ed Anaesth Crit Care Pain.* 2006;6(1).
2. Debaene B, et al. Residual paralysis in the PACU after a single intubating dose of nondepolarizing muscle relaxant with an intermediate duration of action. *Anesthesiology.* 2003;98:1042–1048.
3. Baillard C, et al. Residual curarization in the recovery room after vecuronium. *Br J Anaesth.* 2000;84:394–395.
4. Berg H, et al. Residual neuromuscular block is a risk factor for postoperative pulmonary complications: A prospective, randomised, and blinded study of postoperative pulmonary complications after atracurium, vecuronium and pancuronium. *Acta Anaesthesiol Scand.* 1997;41:1095–1103.
5. Claudius C, Fuchs-Buder T. Neuromuscular monitoring. In Miller RD, ed. *Anesthesia,* 9th ed. Elsevier 2020;1354–72e4.
6. Checketts MR et al. Recommendations for standards of monitoring during anaesthesia and recovery 2015: Association of Anaesthetists of Great Britain and Ireland. *Anaesthesia.* 2016; 71:85.
7. Plaud B, et al. Guidelines on muscle relaxants and reversal in anaesthesia. *Anaesth Crit Care Pain Med.* 2020;39:125.

# 39.

# MECHANISM OF PULMONARY VENTILATION

*Brook Girma and Alan D. Kaye*

## INTRODUCTION

Ventilation is the process of the exchange of air and other gases between the atmosphere and the lungs, commonly referred to as breathing. There are several factors that play a role in the movement of air to and from the lungs and that vary when comparing the two forms of ventilation, spontaneous versus mechanical. During spontaneous ventilation, the changes in intrathoracic pressure generate a gradient for the natural flow of air. In contrast, mechanical ventilation uses positive pressure to facilitate the transfer of air to the lungs. Each breath starts with pressure applied by the respiratory muscles (negative pressure) or by a ventilator (positive pressure), generating a flow of gas through the airways that expands the volume of the lung and surrounding structures.[1] Pressure, volume, flow, resistance, and compliance are important variables involved in the mechanical process of breathing, whether spontaneous or provided by a ventilator. In terms of hypoxia, it is important to consider ventilation, or the movement of air, as one of the factors limiting oxygenation.

## SPONTANEOUS VENTILATION

The external forces produced by the ventilatory muscles drive inspiration. The diaphragm, the major contributor, and to a lesser extent the intercostal muscles are involved in quiet breathing. Other muscles that assist but do not play a primary role include but are not limited to the sternocleidomastoid and the anterior, middle, and posterior scalenes. Expiration at rest is normally passive, secondary to the natural tendency of the lungs and alveoli to collapse because of elastic recoil due to their high content of elastin fibers as well as surface tension forces. The difference between intrapleural and alveolar pressure, or transpulmonary pressure, is directly proportional to lung volume and is used as a measure of intrathoracic pressure or alveolar transmural pressure gradient, normally +5 cm $H_2O$ when no flow is present.

$$P_{transpulmonary} = P_{alveolar} - P_{intrapleural}$$

These changes in intrepleural and alveolar pressures dictate the gradient and flow during inspiration and expiration (Figure 39.1). Alveolar pressure is normally atmospheric at end inspiration and end expiration. During inspiration, intrapleural pressure and alveolar pressure become more negative, typically –8 cm $H_2O$ and –1 cm $H_2O$, respectively. This decrease in pressure is directed by muscle activation of the diaphragm and intercostal muscles, as a result decreasing alveolar pressure and creating a gradient for airflow. During expiration, the diaphragm relaxes, increasing intrapleural and alveolar pressure to –5 cm $H_2O$ and +1

cm $H_2O$, respectively. As a result, the transpulmonary pressure is unable to support the lung volume; therefore elastic recoil reverses the gradient of airflow until the original lung volume is restored. This volume at end expiration is represented as FRC, when the outward force and inward force on the lung are equal.

## MECHANICAL VENTILATION

Most ventilators achieve the process of breathing primarily by applying intermittent or continuous positive airway pressure. By administering positive pressure at the upper airways, gas flows along the gradient toward the alveoli until the pressure in the alveoli reaches that in the upper airway. Utilizing the same concept of transpulmonary pressure, the alveoli pressure increases enough to provide a similar transmural pressure to allow ventilation and oxygen exchange.

## METHODS OF VENTILATION DELIVERY WITH ANESTHESIA MACHINE

Modern ventilators have become more complex since being invented in the 1920s and becoming widely used in the 1950s. Mechanical ventilators utilize two primary methods of delivering positive pressure, by controlling pressure or volume. These modes have changed over the years and vary by manufacturers, allowing more precise delivery and maintenance of ventilation. Utilizing the pressure-regulated modes allows an open lung strategy with the lung distended open at a high continuous positive airway pressure (CPAP) most of the time, with the occasional release to a low airway pressure for a brief period.[2] Volume controlled mode's primary function is to deliver a specific volume. By setting

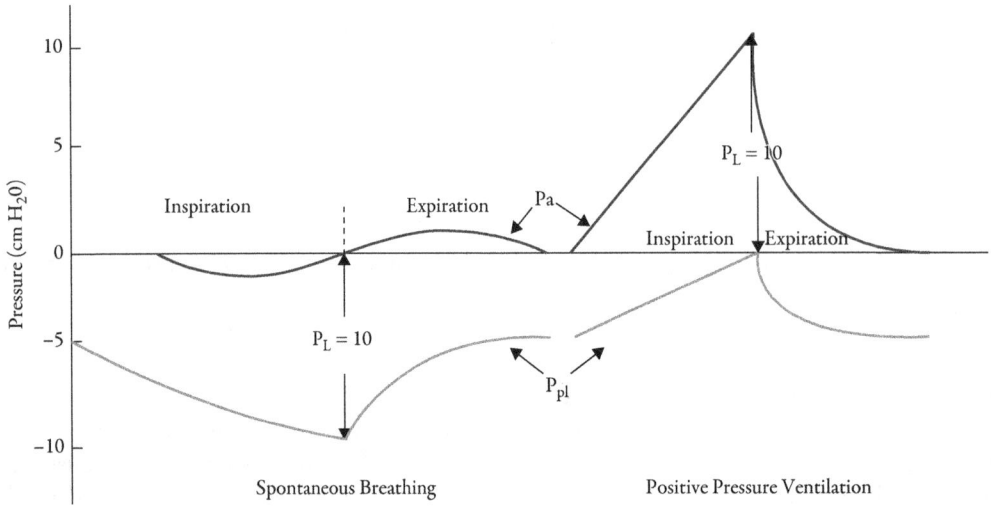

**Figure 39.1.** Effect of intrepleural and alveolar pressures on the gradient and flow during inspiration and expiration

certain variables in these specific modes, adequate ventilation can be achieved in patients, even if the patient is spontaneously breathing. Generally, mechanical ventilators also have on-board monitoring of peak inspiratory pressure (cm $H_2O$), flow (L/min), and volume (mL) to allow the provider to adjust settings to reach desired effect.

## CONTROL MECHANICAL VENTILATION (CMV)

CMV mode delivers a set tidal volume at a set respiratory rate. CMV does not allow any assistance with spontaneous breathing, nor does it allow spontaneous breaths in between. The ventilator works independently of the patient's efforts and if used may cause hyperinflation or respiratory alkalosis. This mode is rarely used, and generally is reserved for organ donors or patients with muscle relaxation. This can utilize pressure control to use certain pressure or volume control to deliver certain volume.

## ASSIST CONTROLLED VENTILATION (ACV)

In this particular mode, the ventilator has a preset backup rate, or number of mandatory respirations per minute, and can sense decreased airway pressures, which triggers a breath. Its advantages include full ventilatory support and ability to respond to changing patient needs, such as in sepsis or fever, and it appears to be more advantageous in awake patients with an intact respiratory drive.[3] Since this mode provides predetermined tidal volumes and can vary to the rate of patient's breathing, it has the tendency to cause hyperventilation, resulting in respiratory alkalosis and generation of auto intrinsic positive end expiratory pressure due to shortened expiratory times.

## SYNCHRONIZED INTERMITTENT MANDATORY VENTILATION (SIMV)

This commonly used mode allows a patient to spontaneously breathe through the vent as well as delivering a mandatory preset amount of breaths per minute. This mode allows better matching of a patient's physiologic needs, as it allows setting of both the rate and tidal volume of spontaneous breathing as well, which is beneficial in COPD (chronic obstructive pulmonary disease) patients, as it allows more time for expiration decreasing the risk of respiratory alkalosis. Some claim that this mode of ventilation is superior to A/C mode due to decreased barotrauma, less need for patient sedation, less ventilation/perfusion mismatch, and improved patient synchrony with the ventilator.[3] As the patient begins to spontaneously breathe, the ventilator begins to sense the patient's efforts and delivers and begins to assist in respirations at the predetermined pressure, rate, and volume. If a patient does not attempt to breathe, the patient will deliver positive pressure at the preset rate and volume as well. Disadvantages to SIMV are that it may cause respiratory muscle fatigue if patient as respiratory muscle atrophy, prolongation of weaning as it may cause dependency, or risk of inadequate ventilation leading to hypercarbia.

## PRESSURE REGULATED VOLUME CONTROL (PRVC)

This mode is considered a dual mode, as it allows regulation of the delivered pressure and volume. Adjusting a preset volume guarantee and setting a pressure limit modulates the flow to achieve delivery of both the volume guarantee without surpassing the designated pressure limit. This is described as a pressure assist-control mode with a volume target backup.

## PRESSURE SUPPORT VENTILATION (PSV)

During PSV, the ventilator augments spontaneous breathing or is used to overcome ventilator tubing by providing pressure support. This mode only allows adjustment of inflation volume and therefore requires spontaneous breathing for it to trigger.

## MAIN CONTROLS

Common controls seen on vents are fraction of inspired oxygen ($FiO_2$), tidal volume (TV), respiratory rate (RR), flow trigger, pressure support, inspiratory/expiratory ratio (I:E), rise time, positive end expiration pressure (PEEP).

## FRACTION OF INSPIRED OXYGEN ($FIO_2$)

$FiO_2$ is the concentration of oxygen; when increased, the higher concentration can improve oxygenation and displace nitrogen in the alveoli, also called denitrogenation.

## TIDAL VOLUME (TV)

TV is the desired amount of volume to be delivered. TV is only available in volume-controlled modes and can assist in delivering the appropriate volume. Pressure controlled modes may not deliver the appropriate volumes as they are driven by inspiratory pressures. Higher TV increases the risk of barotrauma.

## FLOW TRIGGER

This determines the sensitivity and ease for a patient to trigger the ventilator to deliver a breath. Once the set amount of flow is sensed in the circuit, the ventilator is notified that the patient wants a breath. Increased sensitivity is preferred to improve patient-ventilator synchrony.

## PRESSURE SUPPORT

For a spontaneously breathing patient, pressure support provides assistance in each breath to decrease the work of breathing. Pressure support is commonly used in weaning from the vent as well as overcoming ventilator circuit resistance

## INSPIRATORY/EXPIRATORY RATIO (I:E)

This ratio is defined as the inspiratory time plus inspiratory pause compared to expiration. Generally, the I:E ratio is 1:2 to mimic usual pattern of breathing. A 1:1 ratio increases the risk of hyperinflation.

## RISE TIME

This determines the speed of rise of flow or pressure during inspiration. Short rise times may cause patient discomfort and long rise times may result in lower tidal volumes delivered

## POSITIVE END EXPIRATORY PRESSURE (PEEP)

PEEP is the pressure in the lungs above atmospheric pressure that exists at the end of expiration. This pressure prevents

alveoli from collapsing as it reopens or splints alveoli. Increasing this setting could improve recruitment of alveoli and may be need to be adjusted in patients with low lung compliance or body habitus.

## ANESTHETIC CONSIDERATIONS

It is important to thoroughly examine the past medical history and current diagnosis of a patient, as it may provide important clues that can be critical in determining not only the anesthesia plan but also ventilation support strategies. Taking any patient from the intensive care unit requires a careful review of peak pressures, oxygen delivery, ventilatory mode, and other settings.

## REFERENCES

1. Culley DJ, et al. Vol. 130, This Month in Anesthesiology. 2019.
2. Lumb PD, Wright LD. Ventilator management. In: Wylie and Churchill-Davidsons, eds. *A Practice of Anesthesia*. 7th ed. CRC Press; 2003:1079–1090.
3. Chen K, et al. Mechanical ventilation: Past and present. *J Emerg Med*. 1998;16(3):453–460.

# 40.

# METHODS OF MONITORING OXYGEN

*Shivani Varshney and Tina Nowak*

## PULSE OXIMETRY

A pulse oximeter consists of a monitor and probe. The monitor is connected to the patient via the probe. Pulse oximeter probes are designed for use on the finger, toe, or ear lobe. Ear probes are lightweight and are useful in children or if the patient is very vasoconstricted. The probe consists of two light emitting diodes (LEDs) and a light photodetector. The light-emitting diodes produce beams at red and infrared frequencies (660 nm and 940 nm, respectively).[1-3]

Oxygen saturation is estimated using spectrophotometry and based on the Beer-Lambert law. This is a combination of two laws describing absorption of monochromatic light by a transparent substance through which it passes. The Beer law states that the concentration of a given solute in a solvent is determined by the amount of light that is absorbed by the solute at a specific wavelength.[1,4] Deoxyhemoglobin has a greater absorbance of red (660 nm) light than oxyhemoglobin. Oxyhemoglobin has a greater absorbance of infrared (940 nm) light than deoxyhemoglobin. Thus, the relative absorbance at each wavelength allows determination of the proportions of oxygenated and deoxygenated hemoglobin. According to Lambert's law, the intensity of transmitted light decreases exponentially as the distance traveled through the substance increases.[1] When the arteries pulsate, the distance traveled by light though them changes. This fact enables the selective determination of oxygenation in arterial blood.

An important tool for validating any $SpO_2$ reading is the plethysmography tracing, or "pleth," which measures volumetric changes associated with pulsatile arterial blood flow.

## USE OF PULSE OXIMETER

Pulse oximeter measures the oxygen saturation in the arterial blood ($SaO_2$). $SaO_2$ is read by pulse oximetry as $SpO_2$. The oxygen saturation is the ratio of the oxygenated hemoglobin to the total concentration of hemoglobin present in the blood (i.e., oxyhemoglobin + reduced hemoglobin). It is primarily dependent on partial pressure of the oxygen in the blood ($PaO_2$). The higher the $PaO_2$, the more readily oxygen binds to hemoglobin.

## OXYHEMOGLOBIN DISSOCIATION CURVE (OHDC)

The OHDC is a graph that plots the relation between oxygen saturation of hemoglobin ($SaO_2$) on the vertical axis and the partial pressure of arterial oxygen $PaO_2$ on the horizontal axis (see Figure 40.1). However, the plot is not linear but sigmoidal.[5]

The sigmoid shape reflects the cooperative interaction between hemoglobin and oxygen molecules. Each hemoglobin molecule is made up of four strands of amino acids, each of which are able to bind to one molecule of oxygen. As each $O_2$ molecule binds, it alters the conformation of hemoglobin, making subsequent binding easier, described

as cooperative binding. This means hemoglobin will have a higher affinity for $O_2$ in oxygen-rich areas (like the lung), promoting oxygen loading, and will have a lower affinity for $O_2$ in oxygen-starved areas (like muscles), promoting oxygen unloading.

The most important clinical aspect of the oxygen dissociation curve with regard to pulse oximeter is that, at very high $SpO_2$ levels, $PaO_2$ values can vary widely without producing a significant change in $SpO_2$ levels, but as the oximeter reading falls below 90%, the partial pressure of oxygen in the blood drops very rapidly and oxygen delivery to the tissues is sharply reduced. A $SaO_2$ value of 90% correlates to a $PaO_2$ level of 60 mmHg. A pulse oximetry value of 90% or lower is a red flag and requires immediate attention.[2]

## LIMITATIONS OF PULSE OXIMETRY

(1) A pulse oximeter detects only hypoxemia. It cannot detect hypercapnia.
(2) Nail polish paint, motion artifacts, shivering, and operating theater light directly on the probe can interfere with the correct working of a pulse oximeter.
(3) Pulse oximetry may be less effective in critically ill patients with poor tissue perfusion.[5] Application of a pediatric probe to an oropharyngeal airway can be tried in such cases.
(4) Pulse oximetry does not distinguish among the different types of hemoglobins.[5]

## CO-OXIMETRY

A co-oximeter is a blood gas analyzer that measures actual concentrations of oxygenated hemoglobin (oxyHb), deoxygenated hemoglobin (deoxyHb or reduced Hb), carboxyhemoglobin (COHb), and methemoglobin (MetHb) as a percentage of the total hemoglobin concentration in the blood sample. It follows the same principle of spectrophotometry as with pulse oximetry. However, it uses more than two to three wavelengths of light waves to identify different hemoglobin concentrations.

It is invasive and requires a blood sample to measure $SaO_2$. It is indicated when there is a discrepancy between the $PaO_2$ on a blood gas determination and the oxygen saturation on pulse oximetry ($SpO_2$), or the clinician suspects dyshemaglobinemias.

In carbon monoxide poisoning, pulse oximetry shows high $SpO_2$ saturation despite arterial hypoxemia. Methemoglobinemia typically causes the pulse oximeter to report a saturation of ~82%–86% even if the $PaO_2$ is very high. Direct measurement of suspected dyshemaglobin by the co-oximeter would confirm the diagnosis.

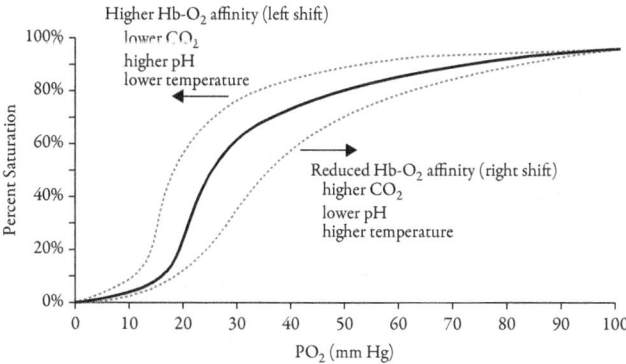

**Figure 40.1.** Oxyhemoglobin dissociation curve (OHDC).

## REFERENCES

1. Anaesthesia UK. Principles of pulse oximetry. Available at: https://www.frca.co.uk/article.aspx?articleid=332.
2. *Standards for Basic Anesthetic Monitoring* (amended by ASA House of Delegates October 25, 2005). Available at: https://www.asahq. org/standards-and-guidelines/standards-for-basic-anesthetic-monitoring. Accessed June 30, 2020.
3. Nitzan M, et al. Pulse oximetry: Fundamentals and technology update. *Med Devices (Auckl)*. 2014;7:231–239.
4. Jubran A. Pulse oximetry. *Crit Care*. 2015;19(1):272.
5. Hill E, et al. Practical applications of pulse oximetry. *Update Anaesth*. 2008;24:156–159.

# 41.

# BLOOD PRESSURE MONITORING METHODS

*Candice C. Hithe and Jerome B. Huebsch*

## INTRODUCTION

Blood pressure monitoring plays a significant role in the decision-making process during the delivery of every anesthetic. According to the American Society of Anesthesiologists, every patient receiving anesthesia should have arterial blood pressure measured at least once every 5 minutes. Blood pressure is measured noninvasively via indirect cuff devices or invasively by direct arterial cannulation. There are several noninvasive methods of measurement, including the palpatory technique, auscultatory method, intermittent noninvasive, and continuous noninvasive techniques.

## NONINVASIVE BLOOD PRESSURE MONITORING

### PALPATORY METHOD

In 1896, Scipione Riva-Rocci introduced the first easy-to-use sphygmomanometer to measure blood pressure.[1] This method required an inflatable cuff placed around the arm, a rubber bulb, and a mercury manometer to measure cuff pressure. While the pulse of the radial artery was palpated, the pressure in the cuff was increased until the pulse disappeared. This was identified as the systolic blood pressure, and hence, the palpatory method of arterial blood pressure monitoring was discovered.[2] This technique underestimates systolic blood pressure by 25%, whereas diastolic and mean arterial pressure cannot be determined.[3]

## AUSCULTATORY METHOD

In 1905, Nikolai Korotkov, a Russian surgeon, discovered that the sounds heard distal to the Riva-Rocci cuff during measurement of blood pressure were not the same as the heart sounds associated with the closing of valves in the heart.[1,3,4] These sounds, known today as Korotkov sounds, would allow both systolic and diastolic blood pressure to be identified.[1,2] Korotkov sounds, which are audible frequencies produced by turbulent flow distal to the partially occluding cuff, have five distinct phases.[2,5] Each phase is described in Table 41.1.[5] Mean arterial pressure can be calculated via the following equation once the systolic and diastolic pressures are obtained: MAP = [SBP + (2 × DBP)]/3.[3] The major limitation of this technique is the requirement of enough blood flow to produce the turbulence needed to auscultate. In obese patients and patients with stiff arteries, it may be difficult for the cuff to occlude the vessel.[4]

## DOPPLER METHOD

The Doppler method is similar to the palpatory and auscultatory methods in that a cuff is inflated to occlude arterial blood. Instead of palpation or use of a stethoscope,

## Table 41.1 KOROTKOV PHASES

| | |
|---|---|
| Phase 1 | Appearance of faint tapping = systolic blood pressure |
| Phase II | Soft and swishing sounds |
| Auscultatory Gap | Disappearance of sounds for a short time |
| Phase III | Reappearance of sounds which are sharper, crisper, and more intense |
| Phase IV | Distinct abrupt muffling of sounds; soft, blowing |
| Phase V | Sounds disappear = diastolic blood pressure |

a Doppler ultrasound probe is used to detect flow through the artery as the cuff is deflated. Blood flow in either direction of the ultrasound probe reflects sound waves that cause a change in frequency that is detected by the Doppler probe. When the pressure in the cuff is just below the systolic pressure, blood flow can pass, and the systolic blood pressure can be recorded.[3]

### INTERMITTENT NONINVASIVE BLOOD PRESSURE MONITORING

Adapted from the Korotkov technique, the oscillometric method serves as the basis for intermittent noninvasive blood pressure monitoring used today.[1] A cuff is placed around an extremity and inflated to a pressure above the systolic pressure. Instead of listening for Korotkoff sounds during deflation, a pressure sensor in the cuff detects small changes (oscillations) in the cuff pressure with arterial pulsation.[2] As the cuff deflates, oscillations in cuff pressure increase in amplitude, then decrease in amplitude. The occluding pressure that resulted in the maximum oscillations closely estimates the mean arterial pressure (see Figure 41.1). The

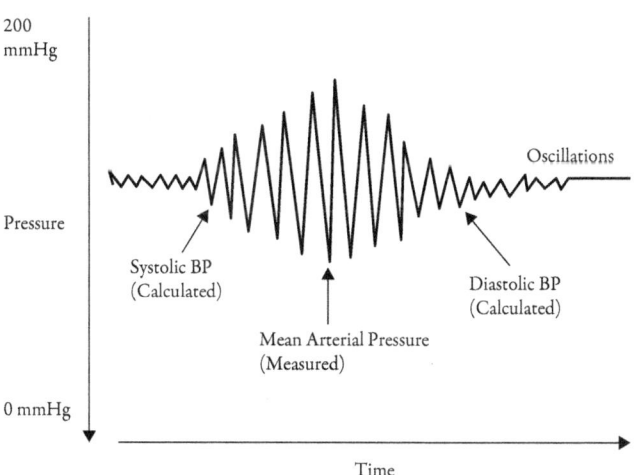

**Figure 41.1.** Oscillometry.

mean arterial pressure is directly measured, and systolic and diastolic blood pressures are calculated based on complex algorithms.[1] Systolic blood pressure is typically found at about 25%–50% of the maximum amplitude during the rising phase. Diastolic blood pressure is the most unreliable pressure calculated from the oscillometric technique and is identified when the pulse amplitude is a small fraction of its peak value.[2]

The accuracy of oscillometry is dependent on an appropriately sized cuff. The cuff should be 80% the length of the arm and 40% the width of the arm.[1] The limitations of this technique also rely on the ability of the cuff to occlude the vessel. The disadvantages of this technique include: no arterial waveform analysis to estimate pulse pressure variation or stroke volume; poor performance in obese patients, patients with peripheral vascular disease, or patients unable to hold still (children); and inaccuracy in patients who are hypertensive, hypotensive, or those with arrhythmias.[1,4] The measured blood pressure is most accurate when the mean arterial pressure is 75 mmHg.[4]

### CONTINUOUS NONINVASIVE BLOOD PRESSURE MONITORING

#### Volume Clamp Technique

This technique measures blood pressure using the Penaz principle, which states, "a force exerted by a body can be determined by measuring an opposing force that prevents physical disruption."[1,4] A small cuff is placed around the finger at the middle phalanx. A light-emitting diode within the cuff shines light through the finger and is detected on the other side (photoplethysmography).[1,3] The volume of blood within the finger and the light absorbed vary with each cardiac cycle. Pressure is applied to the finger to keep both constant. The applied pressure waveform correlates to the waveform of the arterial supply to the finger. The information can recreate the shape of the arterial blood pressure tracing. This technique can only approximate blood pressure and requires an additional calibration step.[3] The limitations are related to the use of photoplethysmography. Conditions that change peripheral blood flow and perfusion also alter photoplethysmography. Consequently, hypothermia, high dose vasopressors, and obesity will decrease the accuracy of this method.[1]

#### Applanation Tonometry

The limitations of other noninvasive blood pressure techniques have led to the need for further development of additional methods. Radial artery applanation tonometry (RAAT) is a newer technique that has not gained widespread use in clinical practice.[1] The radial artery is compressed with the tonometer, and the arterial pressure is transmitted to a strain gauge. The central pressure is estimated using a mathematical formula. The radial pressure waveform is analyzed, and the brachial blood pressure is measured simultaneously.[1] A meta-analysis has suggested that tonometric devices outperform volume clamp devices. However, no three-way studies have analyzed the accuracy of oscillometry and tonometry using arterial cannulation as a reference.[1]

## INVASIVE BLOOD PRESSURE MONITORING

### Arterial Cannulation

Arterial cannulation is considered the gold standard of blood pressure measurement and gives a near-instantaneous measure of systolic, diastolic, and mean arterial pressures.[3,4] Arterial catheters are placed directly into a peripheral artery (radial, brachial, axillary, femoral, dorsalis pedis) and require the following components: intra-arterial cannula, crystalloid fluid within a noncompliant tubing system, bag pressurized to 300 mmHg (counteracts systemic arterial pressure), transducer, microprocessor, display monitor, and a mechanism for zeroing.[3] The transmitted pressure from the heart displaces fluid within the infusion tubing, which is in contact with the diaphragm of the transducer. The diaphragm moves a small plate that is connected to four strain gauges, which form a Wheatstone bridge. This movement is then converted into an electrical signal and viewed as a waveform.[3,4]

The transducer must be leveled and zeroed for accuracy. To level, the transducer should be placed at the phlebostatic axis (fourth intercostal space along the mid-axillary line) to measure pressures in the right atrium. Raising or lowering the transducer in relation to this point will change the pressure reading based on the height the transducer moves. For every 10-cm change in height, the pressure will change by 7.5 mmHg. Raising the transducer will falsely lower the blood pressure, and lowering will falsely elevate the pressure. The microprocessor provides a graphical display of the arterial waveform, which allows a beat-to-beat measurement of blood pressure, as well as analysis of the waveform. To zero the system, the transducer must be opened to atmospheric pressure.[3] The limitations of intra-arterial monitoring relate directly to its invasiveness. Patients are at risk of nerve injury, pseudoaneurysm and hematoma formation, permanent arterial occlusion, and infection. The use of chlorhexidine-impregnated sponges lowers this risk.[1] Of note, frequency and damping are two important principles that must be understood when discussing intra-arterial blood pressure monitoring.[1] These topics will be covered in other chapters.

## REFERENCES

1. Roach J, Thiele R. Perioperative blood pressure monitoring. *Best Pract Res Clin Anaesthesiol.* 2019;33(2):127–138.
2. Schroeder B, et al. Cardiovascular monitoring. In: Miller R, ed. *Miller's Anesthesia.* 7th ed. Elsevier; 2009:1345–1361.
3. Ward M, Langton J. Blood pressure measurement. *Cont Educ Anaesth Crit Care Pain.* 2007;7(4):122–126.
4. Bartels K, et al. Blood pressure monitoring for the anesthesiologist. *Anesth Analg.* 2016;122(6):1866–1879.
5. Beevers G. ABC of hypertension: Blood pressure measurement. *BMJ.* 2001;322(7293):1043–1047.

# 42.

# HEART FUNCTIONS

*Nazir Noor and Omar Viswanath*

## INTRODUCTION

The American Society of Anesthesiologists (ASA) recommends a standard 5 monitors as the bare minimum of any case requiring anesthesia services. These include both direct and indirect monitoring of heart function. The common approach to describing heart function involves movements that adhere to conventional topographical separation of the cardiac muscle into the right and left sides of the heart, including the right and left atria and ventricles, respectively.[1] The first approach in assessing and monitoring heart function involves using a stethoscope for auscultation of the different heart tones, S1 and S2, and if applicable, S3 and S4.[2] At minimum, this should be done preoperatively for every patient. Next would be the electrocardiogram (EKG), one of the standard ASA monitors. Invented in 1902 by William Einthoven, a Dutch physician, the EKG is an essential component of heart function monitoring not only during anesthesia, but in all aspects of medicine.[3] It is arguably one of the most vital monitors used by physicians in all specialties. With knowledge of the different waves and segments, supplemented by other monitoring techniques and clinical judgment, the different phases of heart function can be determined relative to time, such as systole, diastole, mitral valve closure, aortic valve opening, and so on. With this, physiologic responses of the heart, hemodynamic effects of medications, and cardiac pathologies are more efficiently recognizable, allowing for a more accurate and efficient diagnosis. The final tool discussed for assessing heart function is echocardiography, which provides a visual representation of actual movement of cardiac muscle via sonogram images and real-time video.

Few, if any, specialties have such a direct influence on a patient's hemodynamics as anesthesiology. For this reason, close monitoring is essential in providing proper and safe care. A thorough history and physical exam are crucial in devising a proper preoperative plan for patients. And a vital component of the physical exam is assessing the heart via auscultation of the different heart sounds or tones. First of the heart tones is S1, best auscultated at the midclavicular line in the fifth intercostal space. It represents the closure of the right and left atrioventricular valves, which are the tricuspid and mitral valves, respectively. This occurs at the beginning of systole as isovolumetric contraction begins. S2, the second heart tone, results as the aortic and pulmonary valves close, signifying the end of systole and beginning of diastole. It represents the start of isovolumetric relaxation. The aortic valve is best auscultated at the upper-right sternal border, and the pulmonary valve is best heard at the upper-left sternal border. Two other heart tones that may be heard during auscultation in the perioperative period are S3 and S4, both of which are diastolic heart sounds. The S3 heart sound may be a physiologic finding in pediatric patients and athletes, while the S4 heart sound is always considered to be pathologic. The S3 heart sound is a result of increased filling pressures, such as in congestive heart failure. S4 heart sound occurs toward the end of diastole, right before S1 and the beginning of systole. Clinically, it signifies poor ventricular compliance, which can be seen in patients with long-standing left ventricular hypertrophy.

In addition to the physical exam, the EKG is a monitor that is used throughout the entire perioperative course. In patients with cardiovascular disease history, a 12-lead EKG may be recorded as a baseline reference during their perioperative period. During their immediate preoperative, intraoperative, and postoperative times they usually have a 3- to 5-lead EKG providing beat-to-beat monitoring. London et al. calculated optimal leads for detecting intraoperative myocardial ischemia, concluding that use of leads V4 and V5 together provided a sensitivity of 90% in diagnosing myocardial ischemia.[4] EKG monitoring with only V5 had a 75% sensitivity, and V4 alone had a 61% sensitivity.[4] A combination of the three leads, II, V4, and V5, improved the sensitivity to 96%.[4] The importance of this is appreciated during intraoperative management, especially under general anesthesia, when clinical presentation and symptomatology are nonexistent. As mentioned before, the EKG is used in the preoperative and postoperative periods, as well. However, it is hard to neglect its heightened importance for an anesthetized patient because the patient cannot express what they are feeling and the physician is unable to perform a complete clinical assessment.

The last monitor of heart function that will be discussed is echocardiography. Simply put, it is an ultrasound of the heart done either via the transthoracic (TTE) or transesophageal (TEE) method. TEE is the preferred intraoperative route of monitoring. The three major methods of monitoring for perioperative heart function and ischemia are the TEE, pulmonary artery catheterization, and EKG. Of these three, TEE is the most sensitive method for detecting ischemia, and it is predominantly characterized by left ventricular (LV) systolic dysfunction that is defined as a new or reversible LV segmental wall-motion abnormality.[5]

Three methods of evaluating heart function have been discussed. It cannot be emphasized enough that it is unjustifiable to only opt to use the most sensitive or most specific one of these methods. Each of the techniques was developed to further the advancements of efficient and accurate diagnoses involving the heart. They must be used as supplements to one another if the anesthesiologist hopes to gain full advantage of these technologies.

## REFERENCES

1. Buckberg GD, et al. What is the heart? Anatomy, function, pathophysiology, and misconceptions. *J Cardiovasc Dev Dis*. 2018; 5(2):33.
2. Spodick DH. Heart sounds: Important and neglected. *Am J Cardiol*. 2010;105(7):1040.
3. Sattar Y, Chhabra L. Electrocardiogram. *StatPearls*. 2020. https://www.ncbi.nlm.nih.gov/books/NBK549803/.
4. London MJ, et al. Intraoperative myocardial ischemia: Localization by continuous 12-lead electrocardiography. *Anesthesiology*. 1988;69(2):232–241.
5. Mark JB, Nussmeier NA. Multimodal detection of perioperative myocardial ischemia. *Cardiovasc Anesthesiol*. 2005;32(4):461–466.

# 43.

# ECHOCARDIOGRAPHY

*Benjamin B. G. Mori and Piotr Al Jindi*

## INTRODUCTION

Echocardiography uses standard 2-D, 3-D, and Doppler ultrasound to evaluate the integrity and dynamics of the heart's valves, chambers, pericardium, and major blood vessels, along with blood flow within these structures. Transthoracic echocardiography (TTE) is a noninvasive technique where the transducer is placed over the chest wall. Transesophageal echocardiography (TEE), by contrast, is an invasive test where the transducer is located in a specialized probe that is placed in the esophagus and provides better visualization of most heart structures and major vessels, especially those located posteriorly.

The introduction of high-quality portable platforms has allowed echocardiography to become widely used in a variety of settings, including the emergency room, intensive care unit (ICU), and operating room. Perioperatively, it has become an essential tool in the anesthetic management of those patients with suspected or known cardiac pathology undergoing both cardiac and noncardiac surgery. The limiting factor of echocardiography is the availability of trained operators.[1] Refer to Table 43.1 for the general indications for TEE.

TEE is relatively safe, with a mortality and morbidity of <1/10,000 and 2–5/1,000 patients, respectively.[2] Observational findings and case reports illustrate potential complications of TEE, including esophageal injury/perforation, hematoma, laryngeal palsy, dysphagia, dental injury, and death. The only widely accepted absolute contraindications to TEE are esophageal stricture, fistula,

*Table 43.1* TABLE OF GENERAL INDICATIONS FOR TEE

| GENERAL INDICATION | SPECIFIC EXAMPLES |
| --- | --- |
| Evaluation of cardiac and aortic structure and function (TTE is nondiagnostic or deferred and findings will change management) | Evaluation of structures in far field (e.g., aorta, left atrial appendage) <br> Evaluation of prosthetic heart valves <br> Evaluation of paravalvular abscesses <br> Patients on ventilators or chest wall injury <br> Body habitus prevents adequate TTE <br> Patients unable to move into left lateral decubitus position |
| Intraoperative TEE | All open-heart and thoracic aortic procedure <br> Use in some coronary artery bypass graft surgeries <br> Noncardiac surgery with known/ suspected cardiovascular pathology |
| Guidance of transcatheter procedures | Guiding management of catheter-based intracardiac procedures |
| Critically ill patients | Information not obtainable by TTE and is expected to alter management |

trauma, or prior esophageal surgery. TEE can be used in oral, esophageal (e.g., esophageal varices), or gastric disease if the expected benefit outweighs the potential risk.[3]

## STANDARD TEE EXAMINATION

The TEE exam begins with the patient supine in the anatomic position; the imaging plane is directed anteriorly from the esophagus through the heart. (Superior means toward the head, inferior toward the feet, posterior toward the spine, anterior toward the sternum, right and left denote the patient's right and left sides, respectively.) Pushing the probe distally, toward the stomach, is called advancing the transducer, while pulling the tip more proximally is called withdrawing. The tip of the probe can be flexed anteriorly (anteflexing) and posteriorly (retroflexing). The probe can also be rotated (clockwise/counterclockwise) and flexed to the left and right sides. Aside from the physical manipulation of the probe, the imaging plane can itself be rotated forward from 0° to 180°. The degree of this rotation is termed the multiplane angle. At a multiplane angle of 0° the image is in the horizontal/transverse plane. At a multiplane angle of 90° the image is in the vertical/longitudinal plane (i.e., moves to the left side of the display inferiorly, toward the patient's feet).[4]

TEE views follow a standardized nomenclature system utilizing the acoustic windows, the structure(s) visualized,

and the multiplane angle.[4] For example, an image of the 4 chambers of the heart from the mid-esophageal (ME) acoustic window will be called an ME 4 Chamber View image. The comprehensive, intraoperative TEE examination consists of a series of 20 cross-sectional views of the heart and great vessels. These images are shown in Figure 43.1.

## ANESTHETIC CONSIDERATIONS

### PREOPERATIVE

Heart murmurs are commonly encountered during the preoperative assessment, and valvular disease is a known independent risk factor for perioperative mortality and morbidity. As such, preoperative TTE is recommended in patients with known or suspected valvular disease to assess its severity and hemodynamic consequences. The benefit of preoperative TTE for the assessment of ventricular function is debated. A resting TTE is unlikely to reliably detect coronary artery disease and inducible ischemia. Furthermore, there are limited therapeutic options for patients with poor systolic/diastolic function, once detected, to better prepare them for surgery.[1] TTE may, however, help better risk-stratify those patients with severe cardiopulmonary disease, such as pulmonary hypertension. Additionally, preoperative TTE has been shown to influence anesthetic management with respect to delaying/ canceling nonessential surgery, escalation/de-escalation of management, guiding the choice of vasopressors intraoperatively, and helping with the decision to use or forgo invasive hemodynamic monitoring.[1]

### INTRAOPERATIVE

Intraoperative TEE (IOTEE) is widely used in cardiac surgery, where it serves to confirm the preoperative diagnosis, enhance/adjust surgical and anesthetic planning, identify incidental abnormalities that may require attention at the time of surgery, provide a timely assessment of the surgical result, and identify surgical complications.[3,5] For adults without contraindications, TEE should be used in all open heart, transcatheter intracardiac procedures under general anesthesia without intracardiac ultrasound, septal defect closure, atrial appendage obliteration, catheter-based valve replacement/repair, thoracic aortic procedures, and should be considered in coronary artery bypass graft surgeries. IOTEE is also recommended in certain noncardiac surgeries, such as lung transplantation or major thoracoabdominal trauma. IOTEE can also be considered during open abdominal aortic procedures, liver transplantation, endovascular aortic procedures, seated neurosurgical procedures, and percutaneous cardiovascular interventions (e.g., femoral artery stenting).[3] Again, refer to Table 43.1 in

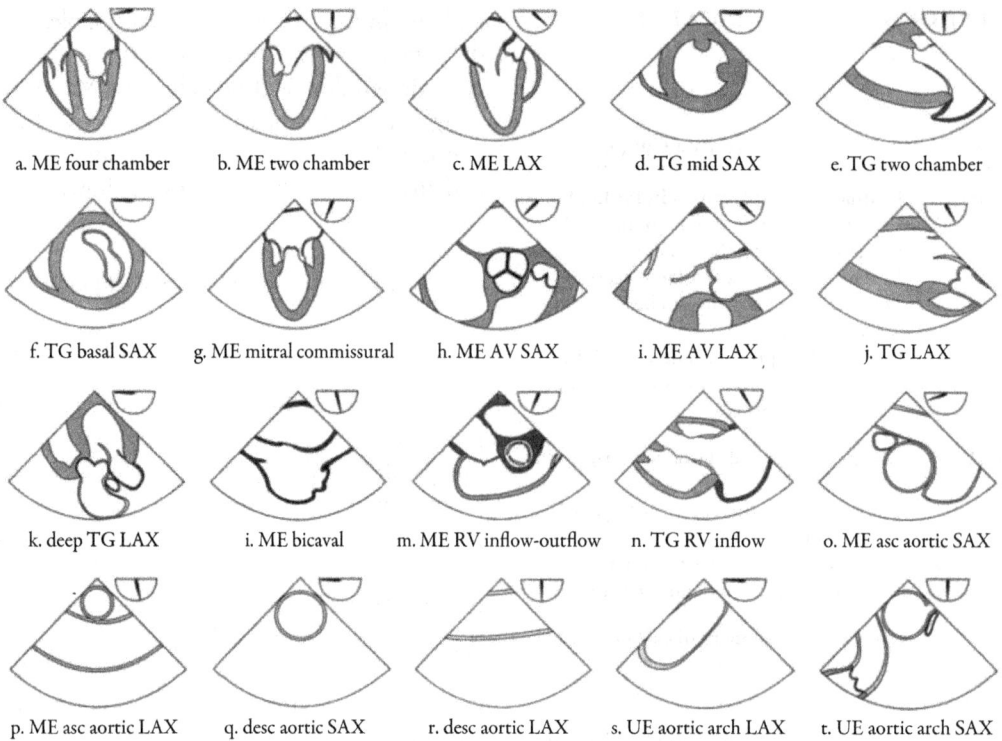

**Figure 43.1.** Twenty cross-sectional views composing the recommended comprehensive transesophageal echocardiographic examination. Approximate multiplane angle is indicated by the icon adjacent to each view.

ME, mid esophageal; LAX, long axis; TG, transgastric; SAX, short axis; AV, aortic valve; RV, right ventricle; asc, ascending; desc, descending; UE, upper esophageal.

a. ME four chamber (4C) view (0°) with the plane is directed through the LA, center of the MV, and apex of the LV. A snapshot of the heart is obtained that includes all 4 chambers (LA, RA, LV, RV), 2 valves (MV, TV), the septums (IAS, IVS), and the inferoseptal and anterolateral LV walls. Segments of the anterior (A2) and posterior (P2) mitral valve leaflets are typically imaged in this view. b. In the ME 2 chamber (2C) view (90°) the imaging plane is directed through the LA to image the LA, MV, and LV apex. This view is orthogonal to the ME4C view. The image is displayed with the anterior left ventricular wall to the right and the inferior left ventricular wall to the left. The anterior (A1 & A2) and posterior (P3) segments of the mitral valve are seen in this view. c. In the ME LAX view (120°) the imaging plane is directed through the LA to image the aortic root in LAX and the entire LV. The more cephalad structures are lined up on the display right. Segments of the anterior (A2) and posterior (P2) are reliably imaged in this view. d. In the TG mid SAX view (0°) the imaging plane is directed transversely through the mid inferior wall of the LV with all 6 mid LV segments viewed at once from the stomach. e. In the TG two chamber view (90°), the imaging plane is directed transversely through the inferior wall of the LV and subvalvular structures of the mitral valve from the stomach. This view is similar to the ME 2 Chamber view now turned 90° with the probe closest to the inferior wall of the LV (apex of sector). f. In the TG basal SAX view (0°), the imaging plane is directed longitudinally through the basal inferior wall of the LV with all 6 basal LV segments viewed at once from the stomach. This permits a view of the MV that is parallel to the annulus with the posterior segments of the anterior (A3) leaflets and the posterior commissure closest to the probe. g. In the ME mitral commissural view (60°) the imaging plane is directed through the LA to image the LA, MV, and LV apex. The MV is imaged with the P3 scallop (left), P1 scallop (right) and AMVL (usually A2) in the middle, forming the intermittently seen "trap door." The left ventricle is seen with both the posteromedial and anterolateral papillary muscles and LV apex. h. In the ME AV SAX view (30°–45°) the image plane is directed through the LA and aligned parallel to the AV annulus. All three aortic cusps should appear symmetrical. The non-coronary cusp of the aortic valve is adjacent to the inter atrial septum, the right coronary cusp is most anterior, and the left coronary cusp is adjacent to the pulmonary artery. i. in the ME AV LAX view (120°) the imaging plane is directed through the LA to image the aortic root in LAX. The LVOT, part of the AV, proximal ascending aorta (1 cm distal to the sino-tubular junction) are lined up on the right side of the display, while the MV and LV are eliminated from the image. j. In the TG LAX view (110°–120°) the imaging plane is directed longitudinally through the LV to image the aortic root in LAX. The LVOT and AV appear on the display right, depending on the depth settings. This view is similar to the ME AV LAX view and permits better spectral doppler alignment. k. In the deep TG LAX view (0°) the imaging plane is directed back through the base of the heart from the LV apex. This view is similar to the ME 5C view (only upside down). Leftward flexion may be necessary to place the LVOT and AV in the center of the screen. This image may be used to measure the Doppler derived velocity of flow across the LVOT or AV. l. in the ME Bicaval view (90°) the imaging plane is directed in LAX through the LA, RA, IVC, and SVC. The structures are displayed with the LA at the sector apex (closest to probe), RA in the far field, caudad IVC (left) and cephalad SVC (right). m. In the RV Inflow-Outflow view (60°–75°) the imaging plane is directed through the LA to image the RV inflow from the tricuspid valve (display left) and RV outflow through the pulmonic valve (display right) in a single view. An off-axis image of the AV is displayed centrally. n. in the TG RV inflow view (90°) the imaging plane is directed longitudinally through the posterior RV wall to reveal a long axis view of the RV, with the apex of the RV to the display left and the anterior free wall in the far field. o. In the ME Ascending Aorta SAX view (0°) the imaging plane is directed slightly above the aortic valve through the right pulmonary artery (seen in LAX), ascending aorta (seen in SAX), and superior vena cava (seen in SAX). p. in the ME Ascending Aorta LAX view (90°) the imaging plane is directed through the right pulmonary artery to image the proximal ascending aorta in LAX. q. In the Descending Aorta SAX view (0°) the imaging plane is directed through the transverse axis of the descending aorta. The near field image of the circular aorta represents the right anterior wall of the aorta. Advance and withdraw the probe to image all of descending aorta. r. In the Descending Aorta LAX view (90°) the imaging plane is directed through the longitudinal axis of the descending aorta. The distal aorta is to the display right and the proximal aorta to the display left. s. In the UE Aortic Arch LAX view (0°) the imaging plane is directed through the longitudinal axis of the transverse aortic arch. The circular shape of the descending thoracic aorta changes to an oblong shape of the transverse aortic arch (0°). The proximal aortic arch is to the display left and the distal arch to the right. Further withdrawal may image the great vessels of the head and neck. t. In the UE Aortic Arch SAX view (60°–90°) the imaging plane is directed through the transverse aortic arch in SAX and the pulmonary artery in LAX. The display shows the proximal origin of the left subclavian artery and innominate vein in the upper right. The pulmonic valve and main pulmonary artery in LAX are seen in the lower left of the display.

the "Introduction" section of this chapter for a summary of the indications for TEE.

## POSTOPERATIVE

Echocardiography has utility postoperatively, in the critically ill, when diagnostic information is expected to alter management and cannot be obtained via other diagnostic modalities.[3] Critically ill patients often exhibit deranged physiology, which is continuously being influenced by interventions, such as fluid infusion and vasoactive drug administration.[1] Furthermore, heart–lung interactions are complex and traditional physical exam/monitors (e.g., CVP, pule-pressure) offer nonspecific findings, which can make therapeutic decision-making challenging. As such, postoperative echocardiography is indicated with unexplained persistent hypotension or hypoxemia.[3] This can be helpful in the detection of regurgitant valvular lesions, aortic/mitral valve vegetation, dynamic left ventricular outflow tract obstruction, aortic dissection, intracardiac masses, pericardial hematoma, tamponade, ventricular failure, aortic root abscess, hypovolemia and signs/complications of myocardial infarction (e.g., wall motion abnormalities, papillary muscle rupture).[1,3] Moreover, right ventricular dysfunction and pulmonary hypertension are underdiagnosed conditions commonly encountered in critically ill patients with lung injury and sepsis.[1]

Echocardiography has been shown to alter the management of critically ill patients significantly. Echocardiography can readily identify the causes of shock and predict fluid responsiveness. For hypotensive patients who are unresponsive to fluids, it can help guide pharmacological and mechanical support of the cardiovascular system.[1]

## REFERENCES

1. Barber RL, Fletcher SN. A review of echocardiography in anaesthetic and peri-operative practice. Part 1: Impact and utility. *Anaesthesia.* 2014;69(7):764–776.
2. Reeves ST, et al. Basic perioperative transesophageal echocardiography examination: A consensus statement of the American Society of Echocardiography and the Society of Cardiovascular Anesthesiologists. *J Am Soc Echocardiogr.* 2013;26(5):443–456.
3. Practice guidelines for perioperative transesophageal echocardiography. *Anesthesiology.* 2010;112(5):1084–1096.
4. Shanewise JS, et al. ASE/SCA guidelines for performing a comprehensive intraoperative multiplane transesophageal echocardiography examination: Recommendations of the American Society of Echocardiography Council for Intraoperative Echocardiography and the Society of Cardiovascular Anesthesiologists Task Force for Certification in Perioperative Transesophageal Echocardiography. *Anesth Analg.* 1999 Oct;89(4):870–884.
5. Thaden JJ, et al. Adult intraoperative echocardiography: A comprehensive review of current practice. *J Am Soc Echocardiogr.* 2020; 33(6):735–755.e11.

# Part III

# INSTRUMENTATION

# 44.

# GAS CONCENTRATIONS

*Samiya L. Saklayen and Joseph Cody*

## INTRODUCTION

Basic anesthetic monitoring standards include measurements of oxygenation and ventilation. In order to ensure appropriate oxygen delivery to patients under general anesthesia, an oxygen analyzer is used to measure inspired oxygen concentration in the breathing circuit. Likewise, quantitative end-tidal carbon dioxide measurements are obtained continually in intubated patients to assess the adequacy of ventilation.[1] Although measurements of inhaled anesthetic agents are not a standard for monitoring, this is valuable information that aids in the delivery of safe anesthetic care. The technology used to obtain these data has evolved over time. This chapter will review how clinically important gases (oxygen, carbon dioxide, and inhaled anesthetic agents) are identified and measured.

## OXYGEN ANALYSIS

All anesthesia machines include an oxygen analyzer by regulation, either built into the inspiratory limb of the ventilator or connected to a monitor that measures other gases. Oxygen analyzers are also utilized in blood gas analysis. There are three types of sensors used to measure oxygen in the operating room: paramagnetic, electrogalvanic, and polarographic.

The most common technology used to measure oxygen concentration in the operating room is the paramagnetic oxygen analyzer.[2] The distinctive paramagnetic properties of oxygen arise from unpaired electrons in the molecule's outer ring, making it attracted to a magnetic field. Consequently, when a sample gas is exposed to an electromagnetic field within the paramagnetic analyzer, a pressure difference is created between the sample gas and a reference sample in proportion to the concentration of oxygen in the sample.[2,3] The transduced pressure difference is

converted to an electrical signal and ultimately displayed as a numerical value for oxygen concentration on the monitor.[2,3] Alternatively, many modern devices may measure the difference in thermal conductivity (proportional to oxygen content) that results from the magnetic field exposure. The accuracy and rapid readout of these oxygen sensors allow for breath-to-breath analysis, making them practical for use in the operating room. The use of a water trap helps reduce measurement errors from the presence of water vapor. Measurement errors may also be introduced by the presence of other paramagnetic gases, such as nitric oxide, though the effect tends to be minimal.[4]

Another instrument used to measure oxygen concentration is the electrogalvanic fuel cell (also known as a Hersch cell), sometimes found on the inspiratory limb of the ventilator. The cell contains a gold or silver cathode and lead anode in a potassium hydroxide buffer surrounded by a membrane. When oxygen crosses this membrane, a chemical reaction occurs, resulting in an electrical current between the electrodes that is proportional to the oxygen content in the sample. While these devices are accurate, low-cost, and small enough to fit within the inspiratory limb of the ventilator, they are too slow to allow for breath-to-breath analysis of oxygen concentration, and they require regular calibration to work properly.[2] Additionally, the fuel cells degrade easily and therefore have a short shelf life (6–12 months).

Polarographic oxygen sensors (also known as Clarke sensors) similarly measure a current that is produced proportional to the oxygen content in an electrolyte solution. Unlike electrogalvanic sensors, which do not require an external power source, polarographic oxygen sensors require an external current to drive the cathode reaction.[3] Polarographic oxygen sensors must also undergo regular calibration and replacement. This technology is commonly used to measure oxygen levels in blood gas samples and may also be found in the inspiratory limb of the ventilator.

# ANALYSIS OF CARBON DIOXIDE AND INHALED ANESTHETICS

Other gases of interest in anesthesia, including carbon dioxide, nitrous oxide, and volatile agents, can be measured in a variety of ways, including infrared absorption spectroscopy, Raman scattering, and mass spectrometry.

## INFRARED ANALYSIS

Infrared absorption spectroscopy is the most common method of analyzing carbon dioxide and anesthetic gases. When infrared light is passed through a sample gas containing polyatomic molecules, light absorption will occur proportional to the concentration of gas in accordance with the Beer-Lambert law. The amount of light absorbed also depends on the absorption spectrum of the molecules; because different molecules have absorption peaks at different wavelengths, the use of narrowband filters to select for these wavelengths can help differentiate the sampled gases.[3] Advantages of infrared analysis include low-cost and rapid results, allowing for breath-to-breath analysis of inspired and expired gas concentrations. Diatomic molecules such as oxygen and nitrogen do not absorb infrared radiation and therefore cannot be analyzed using this technology.

## RAMAN SCATTERING

When a single photon of light encounters a molecule, the photon may be absorbed or scattered. The most common type of scattering is elastic and produces no change in energy of the photon; this is termed Rayleigh scattering and is the reason the sky looks blue. In contrast, Raman scattering is inelastic, and the scattered photon emerges with a different wavelength than the original light.[3] The value and intensity of the new wavelength can be compared to a set of known values to identify the compound and its concentration.[2] Advantages of Raman spectroscopy include greater accuracy than infrared analysis, ability to identify multiple gases, fast response time, and small size.[3] Because this technology is more expensive than infrared analysis, it is no longer commonly used in clinical anesthesia.[2]

## MASS SPECTROMETRY

Mass spectrometry refers to the identification of molecules based on their mass-to-charge ratio. Sample molecules are ionized in a vacuum and then deflected; the amount of deflection is relative to their mass-to-charge ratio and can be compared to a set of known values for identification.[2] Advantages of mass spectrometers include their ability to identify a variety of substances with a high degree of accuracy, as well as a small sample volume requirement. However, several limitations have rendered this technology impractical for use in the operating room. Because the machines are very large and costly, they typically would serve multiple operating rooms from a central location; therefore, gas analysis would only be updated periodically.[5] Despite being one of the first clinical gas analyzers, these powerful machines are no longer produced for use in clinical anesthesia.

## REFERENCES

1. *Standards for Basic Anesthetic Monitoring.* American Society of Anesthesiologists (ASA). https://www.asahq.org/standards-and-guidelines/standards-for-basic-anesthetic-monitoring. Accessed August 29, 2020.
2. Rose G, McLarney JT. Capnography and gas monitoring. In: Brian Belval, Christina Thomas, eds. *Anesthesia Equipment Simplified.* New York, NY: McGraw-Hill Education Medical; 2014:147–157.
3. Langton JA, Hutton A. Respiratory gas analysis. *Cont Educ Anaesth Crit Care Pain.* 2009;9(1):19–23.
4. Aston D, Rivers A, Dharmadasa A. *Equipment in Anaesthesia and Critical Care: A Complete Guide for the FRCA.* Banbury: Scion; 2014.
5. Gravenstein JS, et al. Pitfalls with mass spectrometry in clinical anesthesia. *Int J Clin Monit Comput.* 1984;1(1):27–34.

# 45.

# PRESSURE TRANSDUCERS

*Kathy D. Schlecht*

## INTRODUCTION

When setting up an atrial line, a catheter in an artery is connected to high-pressure tubing flushed with fluid entering a pressure transducer (encased in clear plastic for protection), and exiting the pressure transducer is an electrical cable that we connect to see a pressure waveform appear on a display monitor. A *transducer* is any device that converts something (like energy) into another form. *Pressure transducers* are aptly named, as they *convert mechanical energy* (the pressures in the fluid tubing) *into electrical energy* (the electrical signal displayed as a pressure waveform).[1,2]

## COMPONENTS OF A PRESSURE TRANSDUCER

The steps in this conversion process are as follows: pressure pulse waves are transmitted along pressurized fluid-filled tubing, causing a diaphragm (located in the pressure transducer) to oscillate and change shape. The deflection of the diaphragm is measured using a *strain gauge*. Originally, a resistance-wire strain gauge was a metal wire bonded to the diaphragm that became stretched or "strained" by the movement of the diaphragm; when the wire stretched longer, its electrical resistance would increase. The strain gauge resistor is attached to a side of a Wheatstone bridge configuration (a four sided diamond shape with resistors on each side). As electricity passes through the Wheatstone bridge configuration, the resistance will vary (based upon the stretch placed on the strain guage from the movement of the diaphragm), which produces the final electrical signal that is transmitted via a cable to a *processor box* to be filtered, amplified, and displayed as a pressure waveform with corresponding digital numbers on the monitor.[1,2] The technological development of semiconductors has impacted pressure transducers. The diaphragm is now made of silicon that alters its crystalline structure to applied pressure. creating varying resistance and change of voltage across the Wheatstone bridge.[1]

## NATURAL FREQUENCY, RESONANCE, AND DAMPING

The arterial pressure waveform displayed is constructed via Fourier analysis on a summation of multiple propagated sine waves of successively higher frequencies.[1,3] The sine wave occurring at the pulse rate is referred to as the *fundamental frequency* or first harmonic.[3,4] Subsequent reflected sine waves in the tubing are harmonics or multiples of the original (like octaves on a musical scale).[4] Adding the second sine wave (second harmonic) to the first systolic sine wave (first harmonic) will create the dicrotic notch;[2,3] however, analysis of 6–10 harmonics are considered necessary to produce an accurate waveform.[3,4] Transducing systems oscillate based on their own "natural frequency," which is determined by the mass of fluid in the column, the elasticity of the transducer diaphragm, the density of the fluid, and the length and radius of the tubing.[1] Think of a cowboy lasso requiring oscillating hand movements to create a larger noose in the air. The frequency of the oscillating hand movements is adjusted to match the properties of the rope (elasticity, length, thickness) to keep it in the air. When the frequencies of the arterial pressure wave match the natural frequency of the transducing system, the wave becomes augmented, exaggerating the signal amplitude displayed on the monitor (referred to as ringing, resonance, or underdamping), overshooting the systolic pressure, decreasing diastolic readings, and minor impact of the mean arterial pressure; extra non-physiologic "resonant" waveforms make it difficult to discern the dicrotic notch.[1-5] Resonance often occurs when the natural frequency of the system is low and the heart rate is high. Diastolic pressure and central venous pressure (CVP) are not usually distorted by resonance as they have lower frequency components.[4]

Damping (or overdamping) is caused by anything that dissipates the pressure waveform energy before it hits the diaphragm in the pressure transducer.[2,4] The resulting waveform on the monitor has decreased amplitude, a slow uptake, and an absent dicrotic notch, that depicts an artifactually decreased systolic pressure, increased diastolic pressure, with a relatively accurate mean arterial pressure.[3]

Poiseuille's law calculates flow in the fluid column and is incorporated into a formula to calculate the *damping coefficient* of the system.[1] Factors contributing to damping include: lengthening the tubing, which increases the surface area available to absorb the pressure wave and increases the amount of fluid through which the pressure wave must traverse; increasing the elasticity of the tubing, which adds compliance and absorbs more energy of the pressure wave; increasing the viscosity of the fluid, which will increase the friction to flow of fluid in the column; air bubbles in the line, which will compress and absorb the energy of the pressure wave; and a blood clot in the line.[1,2]

## ANESTHETIC CONSIDERATIONS

### FAST-FLUSH TEST

A fast-flush test is used clinically to determine the natural frequency and damping of a transducing system. The flush is pulled to create a square wave on the display monitor. When the flush is released and the waveforms return slowly to the zero line, the system is damped. If the waveform overshoots zero and then has numerous extra small pressure waveforms before returning to the zero, the system is underdamped. It is normal if there are four or five small resonant waves recorded before returning to the zero line. If the fast flush is recorded with a paper strip, the natural frequency of the system can be calculated (in Hz) by dividing the speed of the paper strip (in mm/sec) by the distance between waveform cycles (in mm).[2,3,4]

### ZEROING, LEVELING, AND ZERO DRIFT

A pressure transducer needs to be "zeroed" to ambient atmospheric pressure to establish a reference point and "leveled" to align the "zero" reference point to a point on the patient's body.[3] Zeroing is performed by opening a stopcock to the air and exposing the pressure transducer to ambient atmospheric pressure so no current flows across the Wheatstone bridge and then pushing the "zero button" to calibrate it on the monitor (eliminating the effect of atmospheric pressure on the body).[2–4] Pressure transducers are leveled at 5 cm posterior to the sternal border to reflect aortic root pressures and at the ear to reflect cerebral perfusion pressures at the Circle of Willis.[3,4,5] When submerged underwater, you can sense the water pressure (hydrostatic pressure). If a pressure transducer falls on the floor, it is (essentially) under a column of fluid contained in the pressure tubing, causing it to sense the hydrostatic pressure in addition to the patient's blood pressure. Every 10-cm change in vertical height (from where the transducer was zeroed and aligned with the body) will alter the hydrostatic pressure in the tubing by 7.5 mmHg (adding 7.5 mmHg for every 10 cm that the transducer is lower than its alignment level to the body, and subtracting 7.5 mmHg for every 10 cm it is above its alignment level to the body).[3,5] It does not matter if the change in alignment is due to moving the transducer or changing the height of the operating room (OR) table. Therefore, every time the OR table height is changed, the pressure transducer must be re-leveled and re-zeroed to create a new "zero" reference point to eliminate the false effect of hydrostatic pressure on the accuracy of the blood pressure reading. *Zero drift* is a phenomenon that occurs over time and can be ascertained by opening the stopcock to air and checking to see if the baseline on the monitor is still at zero or if it has "drifted off," indicating the pressure transducer needs to be re-zeroed.[2]

## REFERENCES

1. Gilbert M. Prinicples of pressure transducers, resonance, damping and frequency response. *Anaesth Intens Care Med* 2011;13:1–6.
2. Hemodynamic monitoring. In: Rose G, McLarney J. eds. *Anesthesia Equipment Simplified*. https://accessanesthesiology-mh-medical-com/content.aspx?bookid=871&sectionid=51860134. Accessed August 11, 2020.
3. Schroeder B, et al. Cardiovascular monitoring. In: Gropper MA, ed. *Miller's Anesthesia*. 9th ed. Philadelphia, PA: Elsevier; 2020:1145–1193.
4. Barbeito A, Mark JB. Arterial and central venous pressure monitoring. *Anesthesiol Clin*. 2006;24:717–735.
5. Alexander B, et al. Blood pressure monitoring. In: Ehrenwerth J, Eisenkraft JB, Berry JM, eds. *Anesthesia Equipment: Principles and Application*. 2nd ed. Philadelphia, PA: Saunders; 2013:273–282.

# 46.

# NEUROLOGIC FUNCTION MONITORS

*Dustin Latimer and Alan D. Kaye*

## INTRODUCTION

Neuromonitoring is used to assess the functional neurologic integrity of a patient during surgery by a variety of different monitoring modalities. The brain, brainstem, spinal cord, and peripheral nerve function are able to be monitored intraoperatively and have commonly replaced the intraoperative wake-up testing. Electrophysiologic monitoring of neurologic function requires a team with expertise in the appropriate neuromonitoring technique. This chapter will expand on a few of the most popular neuromonitoring techniques in modern times.

## ELECTROENCEPHALOGRAPHY

Electroencephalography (EEG) is a neuromonitoring technique that records the electrical activity in the cerebral cortex. Electrodes are most commonly placed on the scaled prior to surgery and each electrode is used to monitor a 2- to 3-centimeter region for ischemia or seizure activity. Electrodes are occasionally placed intraoperatively if a patient is undergoing seizure surgery, brain mapping, or select tumor resections.[1] Continuous monitoring of cerebral activity measures any reductions in cerebral blood flow. During a decrease in cerebral blood flow, cerebral electrical activity slows, resulting in a loss of high-frequency activity and ultimately, cerebral electrical silence. EEG is a very popular technique to use during carotid endarterectomy because of the reduction of cerebral blood flow seen during carotid cross clamping.[1] A cardiopulmonary bypass would also prove to be a viable surgery for EEG to monitor for areas of ischemia due to possible embolization, low arterial pressure, or any initiation of nonpulsatile blood flow.[2] If there is a high possibility of reduced cerebral blood flow, ischemia, or seizure activity, an EEG will provide reliable monitoring to limit complications attributable to those situations (see Figure 46.1).

## ELECTROMYOGRAPHY

Electromyography (EMG) is a neuromonitoring modality used to monitor muscle activity innervated by spinal or cranial nerves at risk of damage during surgery. EMG is not limited to the surgical setting; it can be used in a variety of settings to access the health of muscle and motor neurons or to diagnose dysfunction within the muscle or neuromuscular junction. EMG can by monitored by spontaneous or evoked compound muscle action potentials. Spontaneous EMG are continually running EMGs used to identify stretch or blunt mechanical trauma by high-frequency trains of electrical activity in nerves that should otherwise be null on EMG.[1] Stimulus-triggered EMG differs from spontaneous EMG because there is an intentional electrical stimulus to evoke a compound action potential upon a specific nerve to assess the function so as to avoid cutting or coagulating the nerve. A stimulus-triggered EMG uses a mono- or bipolar stimulator to record electrical activity within the confines of the surgical site, and any increase in latency of the action potential between the two recording electrodes may indicate a neuronal compromise. This technique is commonly used during spine surgery to access for nerve irritation, prevent

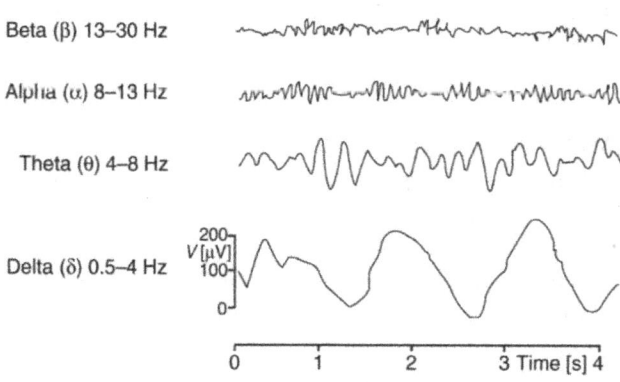

**Figure 46.1.** Clinically relevant electroencephalographic frequencies.

postoperative radiculopathy, and identify malposition of pilot holes or pedicle screws. Stimulus-triggered EMG can also be used to monitor cranial nerves with a motor component (III, IV, V, VI, VII, IX, X, XI, XII) and for brainstem and motor-strip mapping for surgeries with abnormal anatomy due to a tumor.[1]

## EVOKED POTENTIALS

Evoked potential monitoring comprises somatosensory evoked potentials (SSEP), brainstem auditory evoked potentials (BAEP), visual evoked potentials (VEP), and motor evoked potentials (MEP). All of these techniques are used to assess the integrity of a specific neural pathway[1] (see Box 46.1).

## ANESTHESIA DEPTH AND NEUROMONITORING

Depression of synaptic activity in a dose-dependent fashion is something to be aware of when using neuromonitoring and anesthetic agents. MEP and cortical potentials are the most susceptible to decrease in potential amplitude[1], and an emphasis on maintaining anesthetic agent levels during crucial monitoring periods is paramount for achieving desired results (e.g., 0.5 inhalational agent dosing). Finally, a variety of integrated EEG machines are utilized to measure depth of anesthesia, including the most popular unit known as BIS. These monitors add science to dosing of anesthetics to ensure for amnesia and to limit overdosage of anesthetic delivery intraoperatively (see Figure 46.2).

---

**Box 46.1** EFFECTS AND BEST PRACTICES OF GENERAL ANESTHETICS ON COMMON NEUROPHYSIOLOGIC TESTS.

**EEG:** General anesthesia results in generalized slowing of the EEG pattern in a dose-dependent manner.
**SSEP:** No more than 0.5 MAC of inhalational agent is recommended.
**MEP:** Neuromuscular blocker agents must be avoided.
**Integrated EEG Depth of Anesthesia (BIS, etc.):** Studies show that brainwave scores below 40 are correlated with no intraoperative recall.
**Electromyography:** Neuromuscular blocker agents must be avoided.
**Brainstem Auditory Response:** Latency is progressively increased with increasing doses of general anesthesia.

---

## NARCOTICS

### FENTANYL

EEG changes produced by fentanyl are consistent. The alpha rhythm slows 1 minute after induction. Diffuse theta waves are seen in 1–2 minutes, followed by slow diffuse alpha waves, which can become more synchronized. Low doses of fentanyl produce significantly faster brain wave activity. As doses increase, patients display sharp wave activity in the frontotemporal region (20% at 30 ug/kg and 60% at 50 ug/kg).[3]

### KETAMINE

Intravenous doses of 0.25–0.5 mg/kg ketamine produces a dissociative state and 1–2 mg/kg produces an unconscious state. This presents on the EEG hypersynchronous delta waves with activity in the thalamic and limbic regions of the brain.[3]

### BENZODIAZEPINES

Dose-related EEG changes are produced by midazolam. Initially the delta waves have increased amplitude with decreased frequency (4–8 Hz). When the dose is increased, it produces high amplitude activity below 8 Hz. Burst suppression does not occur and the EEG does not become isoelectric.[3]

### BARBITURATES

Initially barbiturates produce fast EEG waves of 20–30 Hz, which is known as the initial rapid response. This activity begins in the frontal lobe and spreads toward the occipital lobe. As the total cumulative dose increases, the frequency of the fast waves decreases. Barbiturates increase the amplitude and frequency of beta activity in sub-minimum alveolar concentration (MAC) doses. As the dose of barbiturates increases, there is increased beta, theta, and delta activities with decreasing levels and frequency of alpha rhythm. Loss of consciousness is associated with 5–12 Hz activity occurring in spindle-shaped bursts, called barbiturate spindles. This burst suppression activity is associated with high doses of barbiturates. A further increase in the dose causes a decline in spindle bursts and the presence of 1–3 Hz polymorphic waves. Rapid injection of barbiturates produces slow-wave activity, and when this activity becomes dominant the patient will tolerate skin incision. Each of these periods is followed by a burst of renewed activity with high-frequency components. This burst will subside, and the next period of suppression will follow, with the burst starting at the 8 Hz range and decelerating to 2–6 Hz (see Figure 46.3).[3]

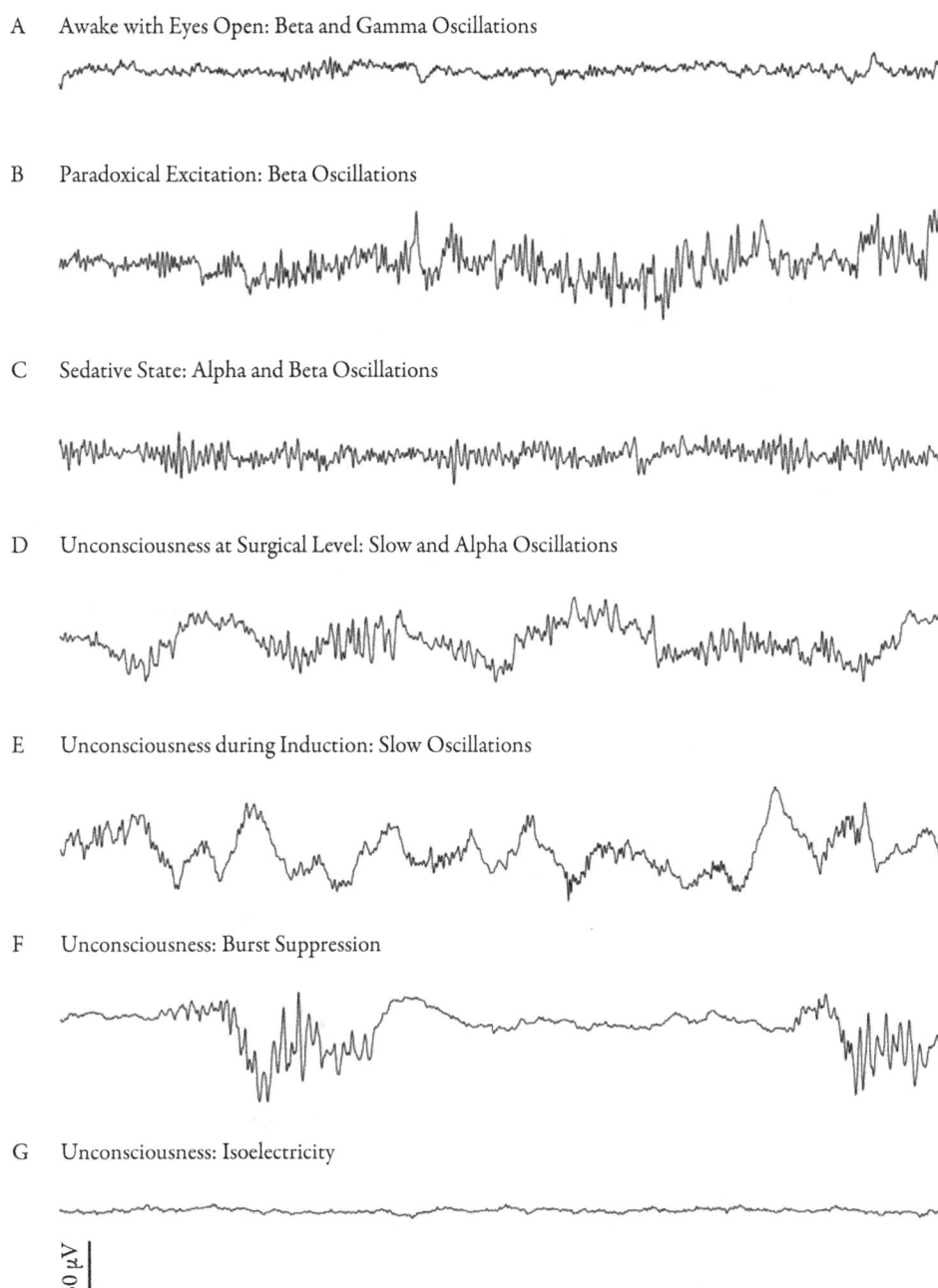

A   Awake with Eyes Open: Beta and Gamma Oscillations

B   Paradoxical Excitation: Beta Oscillations

C   Sedative State: Alpha and Beta Oscillations

D   Unconsciousness at Surgical Level: Slow and Alpha Oscillations

E   Unconsciousness during Induction: Slow Oscillations

F   Unconsciousness: Burst Suppression

G   Unconsciousness: Isoelectricity

50 μV

1 s

**Figure 46.2.** EEG progression from sedation to general anesthesia.

## INHALED ANESTHETICS

### ISOFLURANE

At subanesthetic concentrations, isoflurane yields 15–30 Hz wave activity in the frontal area of the brain; 1.0 MAC yields wave activity of 4–8 Hz. At 1.5 MAC the waves increase in amplitude and slow to 1–4 Hz. The suppressions also become longer until electrical silence occurs at 2–2.5 MAC.[3]

### ENFLURANE

Subanesthetic concentrations of enflurane yield rapid EEG activity during which the patient will lose consciousness. At 1 MAC large waves appear (7–12 Hz). At 1.5 MAC spikes and spike waves appear, followed by a burst suppression. At 2–3 MAC there are groups of 400–800 V spike and wave discharges which are separated by 5–15 seconds of isoelectricity. EEG seizures can be seen with end-tidal concentrations of 3% enflurane with hypocapnia.[3]

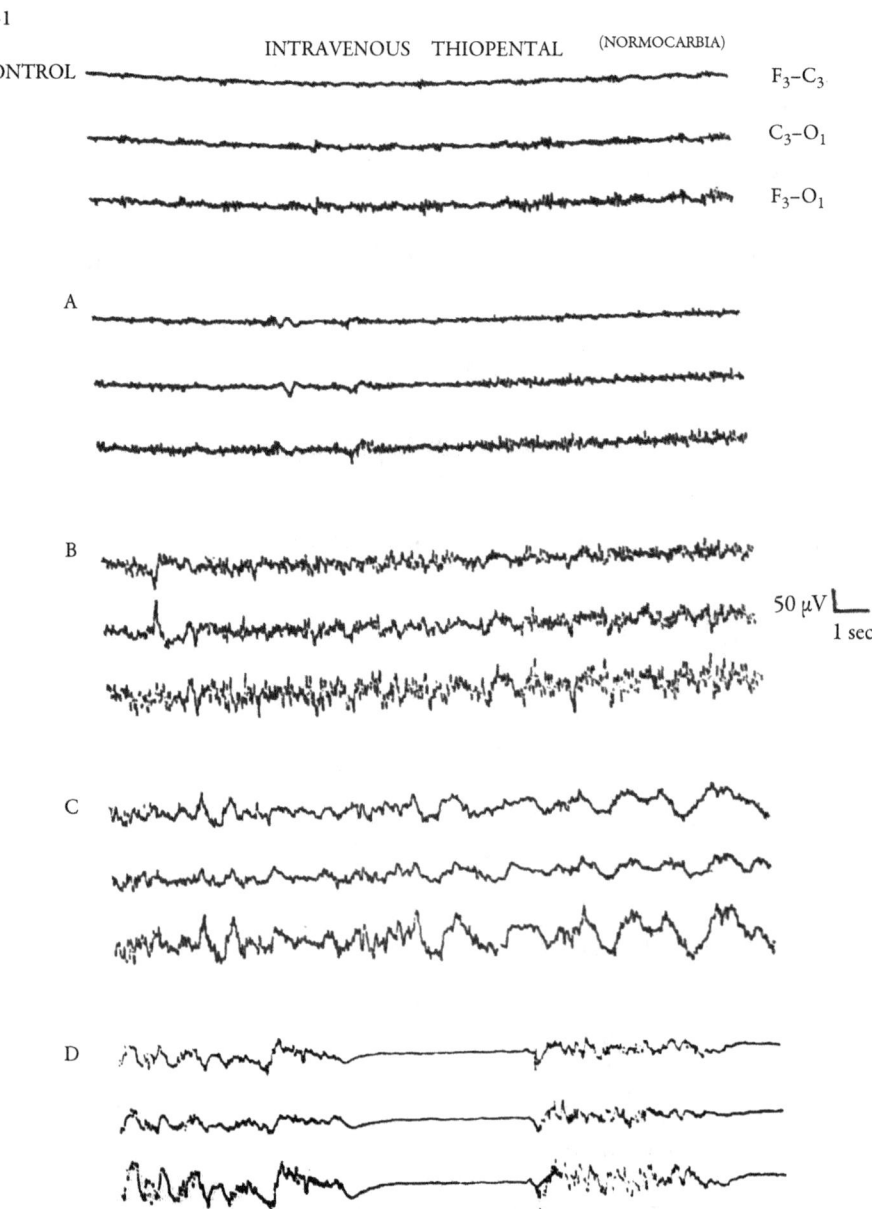

**Figure 46.3.** EEG effects of intravenous administration of thiopental in humans. A: Rapid Activity, B: Barbiturate Spindles, C: Slow Waves, D: Burst Suppression.

## HALOTHANE

Subanesthetic concentrations produce fast sinusoidal activity. Halothane is associated with an initial suppression of alpha EEG activity and the development of fast activity of 20–28 Hz which indicates a loss of consciousness. This is followed by a progressive increase in amplitude and slowing in frequency and the appearance of typical spindle activity. At 1 MAC the EEG frequencies are 10–15 Hz; at 2 MAC, 7.5 Hz; and at 2.5 MAC, 6 Hz. At 4 MAC almost all activity is in the 0.5 Hz range.[3]

## SEVOFLURANE

Some cases of seizure-like movements have been reported with sevoflurane; however, it is unclear whether these movements are akathisia or true seizures. Increasing sevoflurane from 2% to 5% yields high amplitude slow waves, then burst suppression, then isoelectric, then spikes interspersed with isoelectricity, similar to enflurane. At 1.5 MAC sevoflurane is similar to isoflurane in that it protects against lidocaine and penicillin-induced seizures and against bupivacaine-induced seizures.[3]

## NITROUS OXIDE

Nitrous oxide ($N_2O$) yields dose-dependent changes in EEG patterns. Even concentrations of up to 30% rarely alter EEG patterns. The initial change in EEG presents as a progressive loss of alpha rhythm (8–13 Hz). As the patient loses consciousness, the alpha waves will disappear. Then theta waves will appear (4–8 Hz) with superimposed fast activity, especially in the frontal regions. The 4–8 Hz range waves will increase in number and grow larger in the temporal region.[3]

## REFERENCES

1. A. Koht T, et al., Neuromonitoring in surgery and anesthesia. In: *UpToDate*, 2020.
2. McMeniman WJ, Purcell GJ. Neurological monitoring during anaesthesia and surgery. *Anaesth Intensive Care*. 1988.
3. The Mayo Foundation for Medical Education, *Faust's Anesthesiology Review*. 5th ed. Elsevier; 2020.

# 47.

# FLUID WARMERS AND AUTOTRANSFUSION DEVICES

*Jayakar Guruswamy and Akshatha Gururaja Rao*

## INTRODUCTION

Maintenance of normothermia is fundamental to prevent complications in the perioperative period. Redistribution of blood from the core to periphery decreases temperature by 0.5–1.5°C during general and neuraxial anesthesia. Administration of one liter (L) of crystalloid solution or a unit of refrigerated packed red blood cells (stored at 4°C) at room temperature decreases mean body temperature by approximately 0.25°C.[1] Warmed intravenous (IV) fluids keep core temperature warmer by 0.5°C and help prevent shivering.[2] Thus, IV fluids and blood products (>500 milliliters/hour (ml/h)) should be actively warmed using fluid warmers. Administration of platelets, cryoprecipitate, or granulocyte suspensions do not require warmers, as warming may render these products less effective.

Fluid warmers can be broadly classified into the following: dry warming system, countercurrent heat exchanger, water bath system, convective air system, and insulators. The ability of devices to deliver heated fluid depends on the warming method, flow rate, and length of tubing between warmer and patient. Clinical studies examining warmer performance have shown that Hotline (a countercurrent system circulating warmed water around a central delivery channel) and Level 1 infuser (a countercurrent system with

thermally conductive aluminum tube interface) deliver the highest temperature at low (<0.5L/h) and high (>9L/h) flow rates, respectively. Significant heat loss between warmer and patient at low flow and limited time, surface area for heat exchange, and resistance at high flow are some drawbacks of warmers.[3]

The Ranger blood/fluid warming system (3M, St. Paul, MN) is most commonly used (Figure 47.1). It has a disposable set with a fluid pathway that fits into warming dock. It uses dry heat, and can warm fluids at flow rates up to 500 ml/minute. Belmont Rapid Infuser and Hyperthermia Pump (large-volume warmers) use electromagnetic induction heating. Some concerns include risk of contamination and electrolyte disturbance from leak in coaxial counter current system, risk of thermal damage, and hemolysis of red cells, with reduced oxygen-carrying capacity if distal temperature >43°C and air embolus during rapid infusion of warm fluid.

## WARMING CABINETS

Warming cabinets are simple, cheap, and are used to prewarm fluids for administration through conventional infusion lines. If the fluid bag is insulated, distal temperature is

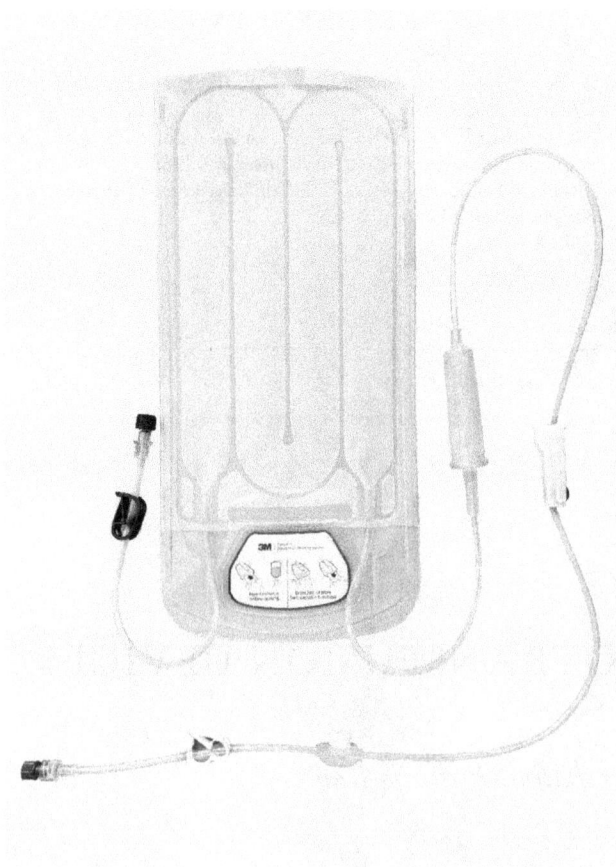

Figure 47.1. Ranger blood/fluid warming system.

comparable to warming devices and prevents perioperative hypothermia, especially for short surgical procedures.

## AUTOTRANSFUSION DEVICES

Autologous blood transfusion is the collection and reinfusion of patient's own blood for volume replacement. Autotransfusion reduces or avoids the need for allogenic red cell transfusion and its associated cost and risk. Intraoperative cell salvage (ICS) is an important blood-conservation technique. It can be considered in any surgical procedure with high expected blood loss, such as cardiac, major vascular, urological, spinal, abdominal, obstetric, and orthopedic surgeries. The term *cell saver* was introduced in 1974 when Haemonetics (Braintree, MA, USA) marketed the first device to collect, wash, and concentrate autologous blood.

## INTRAOPERATIVE CELL SALVAGE (ICS)

It is useful in patients with rare blood types and antibodies, restricted blood availability, trauma surgeries, severe anemia with high bleeding risk, and may be considered by Jehovah's Witness patients. Association of Anesthetists guidelines recommend its use when expected loss is >500 ml (or 10% of total blood volume) in adults and >8ml/kg (or 10% of total blood volume) in children over 10 kg.[4] A notable advantage of autotransfusion is quick availability of functionally superior normothermic red cells, with high 2,3 DPG (diphosphoglycerate) and hematocrit (55%–70%). Relative contraindications to ICS are contamination of blood by bacteria, bowel content, tumor cells, or amniotic fluid. The safety of autotransfusion can be increased with the use of leukoreduction filters. Sickle cell disease, medical contaminants like prep solutions, hemostatic agents, and bone cement are other contraindications. Acid citrate dextrose (ACD) containing solution can be used instead of heparin in heparin-induced thrombocytopenia. Transfusion of red cell concentrate should occur within 4 hours of processing for ICS and 6 hours for postoperative blood salvage.

The steps of cell salvage include collection of blood from the surgical field in a reservoir using a low-pressure suction while mixing with an anticoagulant like heparinized saline or ACD. Red blood cells (RBC) are then separated by centrifugation, washed with 0.9% saline, and collected in a bag ready for transfusion (see Figure 47.2). A standard blood administration tubing with filter should be used to transfuse. Most modern devices have a double lumen suction tube that allows the flow of anticoagulant to the tip of the suction catheter, thus preventing clotting of suctioned blood. Vacuum pressures of –100 to –150 are typically used to prevent hemolysis. This anticoagulated blood then collects in a reservoir until enough is available for processing. Blood

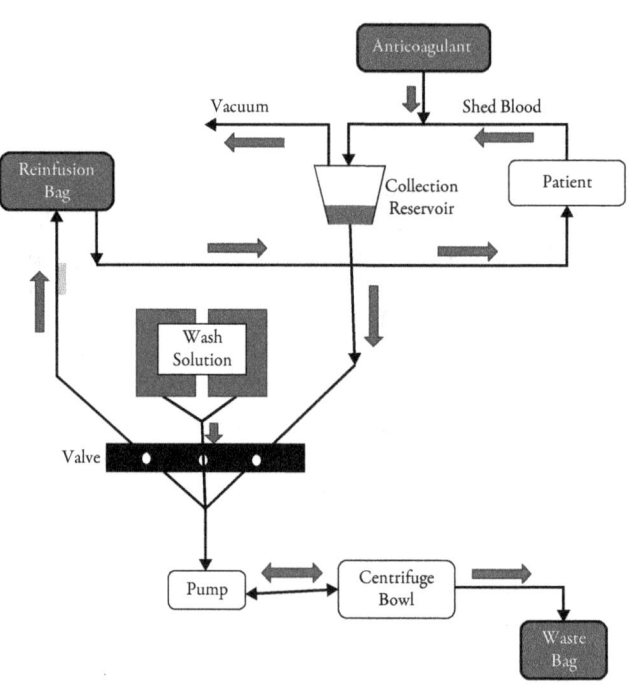

Figure 47.2. Schematic representation of the autotransfusion process.

then enters the bottom of a conical/cylindrical centrifugal bowl where centrifugal forces of approximately 5000 rpm result in red cell concentrate to separate and remain in the bowl. Low-density plasma spills over. Collected blood volume should be at least twice that of bowl volume for processing to occur. Concentrated RBCs are subsequently washed with thrice the volume of saline, and processed RBCs are pumped into a bag, ready to reinfuse.[5] The effluent line going to the waste bag should be clear. Inadvertent use of sterile water for washing can result in severe hemolysis. Minimal data on reinfusion bag and reservoir should include patient's name, date of birth, unique identification number, expiry date, and time of salvaged blood.

## POSTOPERATIVE AUTOTRANSFUSION

Postoperative autotransfusion includes the reinfusion of blood collected from surgical drains in the early postoperative period. This involves either reinfusing red cell concentrate that is centrifuged and washed, or unwashed/filtered red cells that are not centrifuged. The latter is associated with febrile reactions, hypotension, possible thromboembolism, and renal failure from free hemoglobin. OrthoPAT and CardioPAT are small cell-salvage devices manufactured by Haemonetics for bedside use, to obtain centrifuged and washed blood. Postoperative blood salvage is, however, a less commonly used blood management strategy. Availability of equipment and trained personnel 24 hours/day limits the use of ICS.

## REFERENCES

1. Bindu B, et al. Temperature management under general anesthesia: Compulsion or option. *J Anaesthesiol Clin Pharmacol.* 2017;33(3):306–316.
2. Campbell G, et al. Warming of intravenous and irrigation fluids for preventing inadvertent perioperative hypothermia. *Cochrane Database Syst Rev.* 2015;2015(4):CD009891.
3. John M, et al. Peri-operative warming devices: Performance and clinical application. *Anaesthesia.* 2014;69(6):623–638.
4. Klein AA, et al. Association of Anaesthetists guidelines: Cell salvage for peri-operative blood conservation 2018. *Anaesthesia.* 2018;73(9):1141–1150.
5. Sikorski RA, et al. Autologous blood salvage in the era of patient blood management. *Vox Sang.* 2017;112(6):499–510.

# 48.

# WARMING DEVICES AND TECHNIQUES

*Jayakar Guruswamy and Akshatha Gururaja Rao*

## INTRODUCTION

Mean core body temperature is normally around 36.5°–37.3°C, with hypothalamus being the site of thermoregulation. In unanesthetized humans, threshold temperature for vasoconstriction and shivering are 36.5°C and 36°C, respectively. Perioperative hypothermia (PH) is defined as core temperature <36°C and is common due to anesthetic induced inhibition of thermoregulation, 20%–30% reduction of metabolic heat production, and heat loss due to exposure of body surface to cold environments. Heat transfer from the human body occurs in four ways: conduction, convection, radiation, and evaporation.[1] Radiation (50%–70%) and convection (15%–25%) are the predominant mechanisms, and active body surface warming during the perioperative period helps prevent inadvertent hypothermia. Since PH is associated with complications like coagulopathy, increased transfusion requirements, poor wound healing, adverse cardiac events, etc., the National Institute for Clinical and Health Excellence (NICE) guidelines have recommendations for its prevention, including preoperative hypothermia risk assessment, regular temperature monitoring, and active and passive warming strategies.[2] Cutaneous warming is achieved by active warming or passive insulation.

## ACTIVE WARMING

Active warming devices include forced air warmers, resistive heating devices, circulating water mattresses/garments, negative pressure water warming systems, and radiant warmers.

### FORCED AIR WARMING (FAW) DEVICE

These are the most used systems. They supply heated air by convection via special blankets covering the body. They prevent heat loss by radiation and are superior to passive insulation/resistive heating for the prevention and treatment of hypothermia.[3] They can increase core temperature by approximately 0.75°C per hour. Various varieties of disposable blankets are available, and their efficacy is dependent on type of blanket, its ability to distribute heat evenly, and body surface area covered (lower body is better than upper body). An example is the Bair Hugger normothermia system (3M, St. Paul, MN). These devices are associated with a potential for microbial contamination of the operation theater by convection current and disruption of laminar air flow. This can be prevented by the use of filters. Rarely, thermal injuries can occur secondary to "hosing"—when hot air is blown onto the skin due to incorrect assembly/accidental disconnection.

### RESISTIVE WARMING DEVICE

Heat transfer occurs via conduction, where heat is generated by passing low voltage electric current through semiconductive polymer/carbon fiber underbody mattresses. These are reusable, cost effective, are not affected by surgical draping/skin preparation, and have no risk of operating room (OR) contamination.[1] Some drawbacks include lower final temperatures compared to forced air warming, limited posterior heat transfer due to reduced perfusion in dependent areas, risk of thermal injury at temperature >39°C from a combination of local heat and hypoperfusion, and efficacy depends on surface area covered. The VitaHEAT UB3 underbody heating mattress (VitaHEAT Medical, Deer Park, IL) works on AC and battery. The HotDog Patient Warming System (Augustine Surgical Inc, Eden Prairie, MN) utilizes reusable electric blankets to simultaneously warm patients from above and below, with no risk of OR contamination.

## CIRCULATING WATER MATTRESS/GARMENTS

Heat transfer occurs via conduction. Heated water is passed through blankets/garments/mattresses that are placed in contact with patient. They can also be used to cool the patient. They do not cause ambient warming, have low risk of burns, and anterior garments are more effective at transferring a large amount of heat. However, they have long warm-up time, risk of pressure point ischemia/burns, ineffective warming in lateral or lithotomy positions and with posterior mattress due to decreased perfusion.[1,3] The Kimberly-Clark patient warming system (Kimberly-Clark Corp, Roswell, GA) has thermal pads connected to fluid delivery lines from the control unit. Circulating mattress can be used for warming in pre-bypass period as well.

### NEGATIVE PRESSURE WATER WARMING SYSTEM

The principle is to apply sub-atmospheric pressure with thermal load to extremities to improve subcutaneous perfusion and open arteriovenous shunts. This results in heat transfer from periphery to core. An example is the vitalHEAT (Aquarius Medical Corp, Phoenix, AZ). The effectiveness of this system in the presence of anesthesia-induced vasodilation is questionable.[3]

### RADIANT WARMERS

Radiant heaters are electric heaters that transfer heat by radiation. Heat transfer depends on the emissivity of source, absorptivity of receiver, temperature gradient, and distance between them. They have quick warm-up time, are useful in pre- and postoperative holding areas, for pediatric patients, and in trauma resuscitation. Drawbacks include ambient warming, bulky size, and potential for burns.[1] Warming lights focused on the face and torso help reduce shivering in patients.

## PASSIVE WARMING

Passive warming includes cotton blankets, surgical drapes, sleeping blankets, and reflective composites. Trapped air beneath a single layer of blankets prevents radiant heat loss by 30% depending on body surface area covered.[1] They do not increase body temperature. Cotton blankets are simple, inexpensive, and can be readily available in warming cabinets. Temperature can be set from 32°C to 60°C (90°–140°F). "Space blankets" are a lightweight, nonpermeable material with a reflective layer made from Mylar foil that reduce radiant and convective heat loss.

## INVASIVE TEMPERATURE MANAGEMENT SYSTEMS

The Thermogard XP Temperature Management System (Zoll Medical Corporation, Chelmsford, MA) utilizes a heat exchanging, multi-balloon catheter inserted into a central vein, through which saline is infused. Heat exchange occurs as blood passes over each balloon. Use is restricted to trauma, critically ill patients undergoing major surgery, and in coronary artery bypass surgery. The cardiopulmonary bypass pump oxygenator can warm blood passing through a heat exchanger of bypass circuit. It can reverse profound hypothermia. Both systems can actively warm and cool blood.

## ANESTHETIC CONSIDERATIONS

Maintaining normothermia in the perioperative period is of paramount importance. Operating room temperature should be at least 21°C and 24°C for adult and pediatric patients, respectively. Any infusions and blood transfusions at rates of >500 milliliters/hour should be warmed. In addition, patients should be actively warmed if expected anesthesia duration is longer than 60 minutes (30 minutes, without prewarming).[4] Active "prewarming" for 10–30 minutes before induction of general anesthesia prevents PH. It reduces the redistribution of heat from core to periphery.[3,4] Convective warming with FAW is an effective method in the perioperative period.[3]

## REFERENCES

1. Bindu B, Bindra A, Rath G. Temperature management under general anesthesia: Compulsion or option. *J Anaesthesiol Clin Pharmacol*. 2017;33(3):306–316.
2. Duff J, et al. Effect of a thermal care bundle on the prevention, detection and treatment of perioperative inadvertent hypothermia. *J Clin Nurs*. 2018;27(5–6):1239–1249.
3. John M, et al. Peri-operative warming devices: Performance and clinical application. *Anaesthesia*. 2014;69(6):623–638.
4. Torossian A, et al. Preventing inadvertent perioperative hypothermia. *Dtsch Arztebl Int*. 2015;112(10):166–172.

# 49.

# MECHANICAL VENTILATORS

*Peggy White and Chris Giordano*

## INTRODUCTION

Operating room anesthesia machine ventilators contain the same basic features as intensive care unit (ICU) ventilators. However, the ventilators that equip the anesthesia machine typically do not have the ability to deliver advanced modes like airway pressure release ventilation (APRV) or bilevel. Furthermore, the microprocessor does not allow for advanced modes used for weaning, such as adaptive-support ventilation or proportional-assist ventilation. More modern anesthesia ventilators do have the capacity to give flow volume loops.

Transport ventilators are miniature ventilators that operate off battery packs and an E-cylinder oxygen tank. The use of transport ventilators decreases the variability in breath delivery during transport while delivering 100% oxygen. However, it remains important to monitor the patient's vital signs as well as work of breathing, skin color, and chest rise and fall. End-tidal carbon dioxide monitoring is not mandatory, but it is suggested, especially when transporting neurologically impaired patients.[1]

## LUNG PRESSURES

### STATIC PRESSURE

Total lung static pressure comprises alveoli, intrapleural, transpulmonary, and chest wall/diaphragm pressures.

Static pressure is measured at the mouth with no air movement at a certain volume. This is representative of the alveolar pressure. For a graphical representation of these pressures, volume and pressure measurements are plotted to yield the compliance curve, with pressure on the *x*-axis and volume (as a percentage of total lung capacity) on the *y*-axis. Compliance is the amount of volume change with a given pressure. The inverse of this relationship is elastance, which is the opposing force of recoil. Two lung disorders, emphysema and acute respiratory distress syndrome (ARDS), are at opposite ends of the spectrum. An emphysematous lung has a high compliance and low elastance, whereas a lung with ARDS has a low compliance and high elastance.[2]

## DYNAMIC PRESSURE

Dynamic pressure is the flow of gas from the mouth and nose to the alveoli. Factors that affect resistance and hence dynamic pressure are the laminar versus turbulent flow, the viscosity of the gas, and, most importantly, the radius of the tube. Any factor that decreases the radius of the conducting airways will increase the resistance by a factor of four; these factors include mucus plugging, small endotracheal tube, and bronchospasm.[2]

## COMPLIANCE CURVE

When receiving positive-pressure ventilation, the compliance and elastance can be visualized with the compliance curve (Figure 49.1). Inflating the lungs with positive pressure is like blowing up a balloon. It takes significant pressure to start the

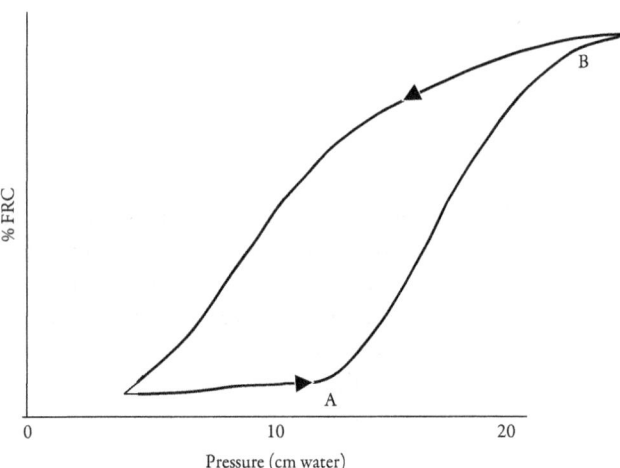

**Figure 49.1.** The normal compliance curve with positive pressure ventilation. The curve starts at 5 cm H$_2$O, accounting for normal intrinsic PEEP. Point A is the lower inflection point, and point B is the upper inflection point. On the ventilator, PEEP should be sent between the upper and lower inflection points.

insufflation, but once alveoli are recruited, it becomes easier to expand; the point at which this occurs is considered the lower inflection point. The balloon will expand with minimal pressure until it reaches maximum capacity and becomes overdistended. At that point, increased pressure is required to cause the same volume change. This is considered the upper inflection point and occurs as the lungs approach total lung capacity. To minimize the amount of pressure required to insufflate the lungs during mechanical ventilation, the positive end-expiratory pressure (PEEP) is set between the lower and upper inflection points on the compliance curve.

When the pressure is released from the lungs and gas escapes the alveoli, the plotted expiratory curve is different than the insufflation curve and is representative of the resistance caused by surfactant and lung. This is termed *hysteresis*.

## POSITIVE-PRESSURE VENTILATION

The equation of motion is the mathematical representation of the forces causing gas flow during mechanical ventilation. It has three components that comprise the ventilator breath: pressure, volume, and flow.[3-5]

$$\text{Ptot} = \text{Pvent} + \text{Pmus} = \frac{Vt}{C} + \dot{V} \times R$$

where Ptot = total pressure, Pvent = pressure measured at the circuit, Pmus = pressure of the respiratory muscles, $Vt$ = total volume, $C$ = compliance, $\dot{V}$ = flow, R = resistance of the conducting airways (including endotracheal tube).

When initiating mechanical ventilation, it is important to consider variables that affect delivery of the breath, including a trigger, target variable, and breath termination.[6] A trigger is the parameter that tells the ventilator to deliver a breath. A trigger can be ventilator driven, time driven (e.g., every 10 seconds to give 6 breaths per minute), or patient driven, based on patient effort from negative pressure or flow generated by the patient. The target variable is either flow, volume, or pressure. The target variable is "dialed" into the ventilator when attaching the patient to the ventilator. This is the independent variable and determines the mode of ventilation: pressure controlled, pressure support, or volume controlled. Breath termination is determined by inspiratory time, volume, or flow.[3-5]

## SCALARS

The volume-time scalar is the amount of volume measured at the expiratory limb of the circuit (Figure 49.2). In pressure-controlled and pressure-support ventilation, it is important to evaluate this scalar to identify the patient's tidal volume. The graph should start and end at zero. A graph that does not return to zero is indicative of an air leak around the endotracheal tube or from the circuit.[3,4]

The flow-time scalar provides information about the inspiratory and expiratory cycle (Figure 49.2). The shape of the graph is determined by respiratory mechanics, patient effort, and parameters set on the ventilator (e.g., inspiratory time, flow, continuous, or decelerating). This scalar provides a significant amount of information by identifying Tau, decelerating or constant flow, air trapping, and airway obstruction.[3,4]

In volume-control ventilation, the pressure-time scalar provides information about patient compliance, resistance, PEEP, and patient effort (Figure 49.2). The peak inspiratory pressure is determined by flow and resistance (i.e., dynamic pressure). Plateau pressure is representative of lung compliance. A high peak inspiratory pressure with normal plateau pressure during an inspiratory pause indicates increased resistance. This can be caused by bronchoconstriction, mucus plug, or mainstem intubation. On the contrary, a high peak inspiratory pressure and plateau pressure is indicative of low compliance, as seen in ARDS. To assess the static pressure, the patient must be completely relaxed, with no respiratory effort permitted. To assess the amount of intrinsic PEEP, an expiratory pause is used. This is important to assess for air trapping (auto-PEEP or intrinsic PEEP). Excessive air trapping can cause a systematic increase in TLC and associated decrease in preload and barotrauma. Other parameters that can be assessed by examining this waveform include driving pressures and stress index. These advanced topics are beyond the scope of this chapter.[3,4]

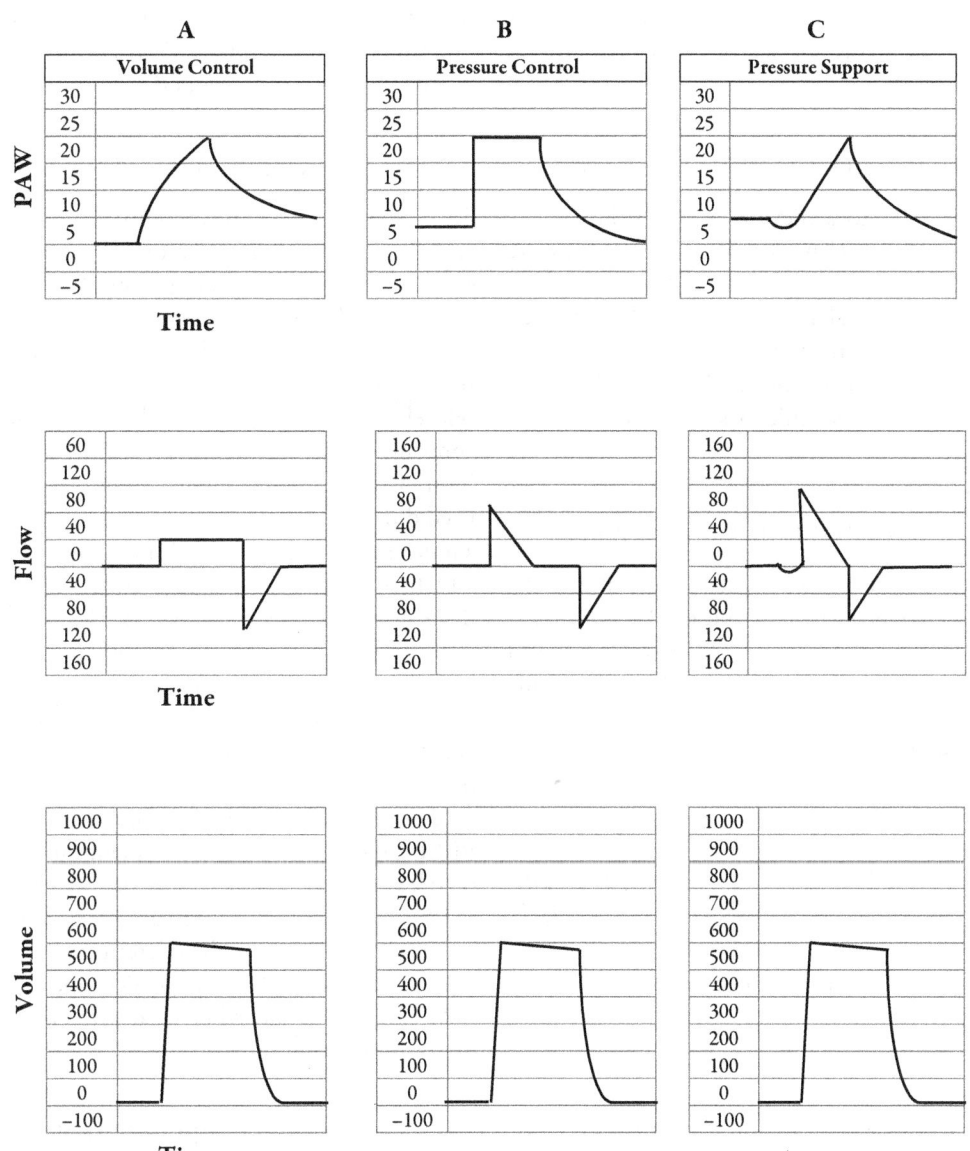

Figure 49.2. Ventilator scalars. A: volume-controlled ventilation; B: pressure-controlled ventilation; C: pressure-support ventilation. The negative deflections on the pressure and flow waveforms denote spontaneous breaths.

# MECHANICAL VENTILATION MODES

Mechanical ventilators, used in all areas of the hospital, provide different options for modes of ventilation. The most sophisticated software, and thus modes of ventilation, are found in the ICU ventilators. These ICU ventilators can provide all possible modes of ventilation. The next level of ventilator complexity can be found in the operating room, where software has enabled mechanical ventilation to evolve from only volume-controlled mode dictated by prescribed minute ventilation settings to all of the modes listed in the following. Furthermore, many of those settings can be volume guaranteed or pressure limited to assist dynamic events in the operating room. Transport ventilators, which are much more limited but still useful, permit various levels of PEEP, pressure, and volume to facilitate the transfer of patients throughout the hospital. The following subsections will elaborate on these options.

## VOLUME-CONTROLLED VENTILATION

The desired flow is set to achieve a certain volume. The ventilator delivers that volume regardless of the pressure encountered while delivering the volume; however, a programmed airway pressure alarm will restrict the delivered breath to prevent barotrauma if a threshold pressure is reached. Pressure is the dependent variable and will change according to pulmonary mechanics based on resistance and compliance.

## PRESSURE-CONTROLLED VENTILATION

A driving pressure is set on the ventilator, which is delivered to the patient, resulting in a variable tidal volume. This resulting tidal volume will depend on the compliance and resistance of the respiratory system. An established volume alarm will turn the pressure delivery off to prevent barotrauma if a threshold volume is reached.

## PRESSURE-SUPPORT VENTILATION

In this patient-triggered mode of ventilation, all breaths are initiated by the patient. Once triggered, the ventilator delivers a programmed pressure and the patient receives the pressure flow based on their inspiratory effort. When the ventilator senses a reduction in flow, it will stop the flow, allowing for exhalation.

## ASSIST-CONTROL VENTILATION

This mode of ventilation can be pressure controlled or volume controlled. A programmed rate and pressure (or volume) is dialed, and the patient receives a rate-based ventilator breath. If the patient makes respiratory efforts during the mechanical cycle, the ventilator will assist the patient by delivering additional breaths according to the preset architecture. Each assisted or controlled breath delivered is the same, and the patient is susceptible to hyperventilation as well as breath-stacking if additional respiratory efforts are made prior to full exhalation.

## SYNCHRONIZED INTERMITTENT MANDATORY VENTILATION (SIMV)

The patient is given a set number of mandatory ventilator breaths with a preset architecture, which can be pressure- or volume-based breaths. Spontaneous respiratory efforts are permitted in between the mandatory breaths, and the ventilator attempts to synchronize spontaneous effort to a mandatory breath based on the patient's initiation of a breath during a timed window. All spontaneous breaths taken are pressure-supported breaths with respiratory flow based on the patient's demand.

## INVERSE RATIO VENTILATION

This mode of mechanical ventilation promotes lung recruitment by allowing prolonged inspiratory times and continuous positive airway pressure with release times. In a more traditional form of ventilation, this can be done using pressure-controlled ventilation and programming a prolonged inspiratory time. In specialized modes, such as bilevel and airway pressure release ventilation (APRV), a "pressure high" is set for a prolonged period. The "pressure high" is typically the same airway plateau pressure measured during conventional ventilation. The "pressure low" is a much shorter time, typically between 0.6 and 0.8 seconds, which is dependent on the patient's lung physiology and disease state. For both APRV and bilevel, the patient can initiate their own breaths at any time during the cycle, and the main difference is the time period and "pressure low" settings. In APRV, the "pressure low" is set at 0 to 5 $cmH_2O$ and the "time low" is determined by the reversal of flow (typically set at 75% of the expiratory phase) through analysis of the expiratory flow-time scalar. APRV uses auto-PEEP to maintain lung recruitment during the exhalation or release phase. In bilevel ventilation, the ventilator is set to alternate between a "pressure high" and "pressure low." The time at pressure high is determined by the breaths per minute, and bilevel has been described as "upside-down SIMV." Caution should be used with these modes because hypercarbia easily occurs.[7]

## ADAPTIVE-SUPPORT VENTILATION

Adaptive-support and proportional-assist ventilation are more complex modes of ventilation based on an integrated feedback system. The minute ventilation is set through a microprocessor and the ventilator delivers support according to a preset work of breathing. These are advanced modes and are beyond the scope of this chapter.

## REFERENCES

1. Pham T, et al. Mechanical ventilation: State of the art. *Mayo Clin Proc.* 2017;92(9):1382–1400.
2. Henderson W, et al. Respiratory system mechanics and energetics. In: Broaddus VC, Mason RJ, Gotway MB, eds. *Murray & Nadel's Textbook of Respiratory Medicine*, 6th ed. Elsevier Saunders; 2016:Vol. 1, 76–91.e2.
3. Dexter AM, Clark K. Ventilator graphics: Scalars, loops and secondary measures. *Respir Care.* 2020;65(6):739–759.
4. Georgopoulos D, et al. Bedside waveforms interpretation as a tool to identify patient-ventilator asynchronies. *Intensive Care Med.* 2006;32(1):34–47.
5. MacIntyre NR. Mechanical ventilation. In: Broaddus VC, Mason RJ, Gotway MB, eds. *Murray & Nadel's Textbook of Respiratory Medicine.* 6th ed. Elsevier Saunders; 2016:Vol. 2, 1761–1777.e4.
6. Gilstrap D, MacIntyre N. Patient-ventilator interactions: Implications for clinical management. *Am J Respir Crit Care Med.* 2013;188(9):1058–1068.
7. Stawicki SP, et al. High-frequency oscillatory ventilation (HFOV) and airway pressure release ventilation (APRV): A practical guide. *Intensive Care Med.* 2009;24(4):215–229.

# 50.

# DEFIBRILLATORS

## *Peggy White and Chris Giordano*

## INTRODUCTION

A defibrillator includes a power supply, capacitor, inducer, rectifier, and transformer. The capacitor consists of two conductors separated by an insulator. Potential energy is stored between the two. The power supply is plugged into the wall or stored in a battery. The capacitor is charged by the rectifier converting alternating current to direct current. The energy delivered with capacitor discharge is prolonged by the inducer, improving shock effectiveness. The inducer is a wire coil that causes a magnetic field flowing in the opposite direction. The magnitude of energy required differs based on the underlying pathological rhythm, according to the American Heart Association (AHA) guidelines.[1] The delivery of a shock depends on the type of defibrillator used and the transthoracic impedance (TTI) incurred.

TTI differs based on the patient's body habitus, paddle size, and pad placement. The anterior-posterior position is typically the most effective for placement of adhesive hands-off pads; alternatively, the right anterior and left lateral positions are acceptable. To further decrease the TTI, 8 kg of pressure can be placed over the self-adhesive pads.

When using manual paddles, it is best to use gel pads to improve conductance, but a water-soluble jelly is considered acceptable.[2]

## MONOPHASIC VS. BIPHASIC

Monophasic defibrillators deliver current in one direction between the paddles, and a higher charge is required to obtain the desired effect. Regardless, biphasic defibrillators are the preferred method because of their improved first shock success rate.[2] Biphasic defibrillators deliver current in both directions, which allows for a smaller amount of electricity to achieve the same therapeutic effect. As a result, an organized rhythm is restored with fewer shocks, and the delivery of fewer and smaller shocks results in less damage. Biphasic defibrillators can further be described by the type of waveform delivered. Some studies support the use of biphasic truncated exponential or rectilinear biphasic above pulsed biphasic waveform. Each type of biphasic defibrillator delivers the same programmed energy at peak currents, but the adjustment to patient TTI differs.[2]

Electrical shocks can be delivered as unsynchronized or synchronized. Defibrillation refers to successful cessation of ventricular fibrillation or ventricular tachycardia for more than 5 seconds after delivery of the shock. Synchronized cardioversion is a timed shock that avoids delivery of energy during the absolute refractory period, which would put the patient at risk for developing ventricular fibrillation. Synchronized cardioversion is used for supraventricular rhythms or monomorphic ventricular tachycardia. In adults, the initial dose of biphasic cardioversion should be 120 to 200 J. If the rhythm does not convert, subsequent shocks should be at increasing doses. For children, the initial dose is 0.5 to 1 J/kg. If unsuccessful, the dose should be increased to 2 J/kg with a maximum dose of 200 J/kg.[3]

Recommendations for ventricular fibrillation and pulseless ventricular tachycardia support the use of single biphasic shock at peak current according to manufacturer recommendations (typically 150–200 J). For pediatric patients, it is reasonable to start with 2 to 4 J/kg and increase up to 10 or 200 J maximum.[3] It is reasonable to increase the dose up to the maximum according to the device, and the AHA recommends following manufacturer's recommendations on the dose of subsequent shocks in ventricular fibrillation/pulseless ventricular tachycardia.[2] There is also no evidence to support the use of stacked shocks; rather, the emphasis is placed on maximizing chest compressions while charging the device.

Automatic implantable cardiac defibrillators (AICDs) are the gold standard for primary and secondary prevention of sudden cardiac death in patients with systolic heart failure (left ventricular ejection fraction <35%), arrhythmogenic conditions, or previous cardiac arrest. AICD units have three main functions: therapeutic delivery of a shock, sensing of cardiac electrical depolarization/repolarization, and recording of AICD activity. The device is typically implanted in the subcutaneous tissue over the pectoralis muscle, and it has electrical wires that course transvenously through the subclavian vein into the right atrium, landing in the apex of the right ventricle. The defibrillator wire can be differentiated from pacing wires by the presence of an insulated covering, making it larger in diameter, which can be seen on a chest X-ray.[4,5]

## ANESTHETIC CONSIDERATIONS

### PREOPERATIVE

Patients with an AICD warrant considerable investigation into the underlying cardiac condition, device manufacturer, settings, and interrogation history. If the surgical procedure is considered an emergency, a chest X-ray should be done to identify a defibrillating wire. Application of a magnet over the pulse generator to disarm the defibrillation component can be performed by the anesthesiologist, but this

is recommended only in emergency circumstances.[5] When changing AICD functionality, it is important that the patient has continued telemetry, pulse oximeter, and blood pressure monitoring in place at all times. In addition, an external defibrillator should remain readily available.

### INTRAOPERATIVE

Patient conditions or surgical procedures that pose an increased risk for a sudden cardiac event warrant placement of self-adhesive defibrillator pads. This allows for decreased time to electrical discharge with minimal disruption to the sterile field if an event were to occur intraoperatively.

For patients with an AICD, the defibrillating function should be disabled prior to operative procedures that pose a high risk for electromagnetic interference, such as monopolar Bovie, magnetic resonance imaging, electroconvulsive therapy, lithotripsy, and radiofrequency ablation. An external defibrillator should remain readily available throughout the procedure.[5] All patients should be monitored with telemetry, pulse oximeter, and blood pressure until AICD functionality is returned to preoperative settings. Until then, an external defibrillator should remain readily available. The patient should be evaluated by their electrophysiology cardiologist in the immediate postoperative period.

### ANESTHETIC MANAGEMENT

A spark can be generated from poor adherence to the skin. This can be minimized with self-adhesive pads or gel pads when using paddles. Care should be taken to ensure there is an occlusive seal between the paddles and the patient. In addition, an oxygen-rich source may increase the risk of a fire if a spark were to occur.

## REFERENCES

1. Braga A, Cooper R. Physical principles of defibrillators. *Anaesth Intensive Care Med.* 2015;16(5):235–245.
2. Link MS, et al. Part 7: Adult advanced cardiovascular life support: 2015 American Heart Association Guidelines update for cardiopulmonary resuscitation and emergency cardiovascular care. *Circulation.* 2015;132(18 Suppl 2):S444–464.
3. Link MS, et al. Part 6: Electrical therapies: Automated external defibrillators, defibrillation, cardioversion, and pacing: 2010 American Heart Association Guidelines for cardiopulmonary resuscitation and emergency cardiovascular care. *Circulation.* 2010;122(18 Suppl 3):S706–719.
4. Goldberger Z, Lampert R. Implantable cardioverter-defibrillators: Expanding indications and technologies. *JAMA.* 2006;295(7):809–818.
5. Practice advisory for the perioperative management of patients with cardiac implantable electronic devise: Pacemakers and implantable cardioverter-defibrillators 2020: An updated report by the American Society of Anesthesiologists Task Force on Perioperative Management of Patients with Cardiac Implantable Electronic Devises: Erratum. *Anesthesiology.* 2020;132(4):938.

# 51.

# ELECTRICAL, FIRE, AND EXPLOSION HAZARDS

*Amanda Frantz and Chris Giordano*

## INTRODUCTION

Fires are uncommon in the operating environment, but they can be deadly. As a result, it is imperative that anesthesiologists remain alert in their everyday practice for impending hazards and acknowledge alarms when equipment malfunctions. Literature involving case series and expert opinions are the basis for guidelines on how to prevent and manage fires, which happen up to 650 times per year and result in two to three patient deaths annually.[1] Various groups have created operating room (OR) algorithms for fire prevention and management. For example, the anesthesiologist should know the location and type of fire extinguishers in the OR and the location of the emergency oxygen shutoff valves.[2]

## FIRE PREVENTION AND MANAGEMENT

Three elements make up every fire: a source of ignition, fuel, and an oxidizer.[3] The oxidizer present could include supplemental oxygen gas or nitrous oxide. Examples of an ignition source are an electrosurgery unit (ESU), more commonly known as a "Bovie" or monopolar cautery, lasers, or static. Sources of fuel include surgical drapes and gowns, OR equipment, and alcohol-based preparation on the patient, especially if the preparation is not allowed the proper time to dry. These components are present in most surgical procedures, leading institutions to use a fire risk assessment during the surgical time-out to identify procedures that are high risk. This assessment includes the use of oxygen concentration >30%, use of an ESU above the xiphoid, appropriate time for skin preparation to dry prior to draping (3 minutes for hairless areas and up to 1 hour for untrimmed areas), and use of wet gauze and sponges near any ignition source.[1,3]

When using 100% fraction of inspired oxygen ($FiO_2$) during intubation, significant time is needed to allow the patient's expired oxygen to reach a safe concentration once the $FiO_2$ is decreased to 30%, which is approximately 1–2 minutes based on flow rates.

If a fire occurs, the following actions need to be performed simultaneously: stop the flow of all gases, remove the endotracheal tube if the fire is in the airway, withdraw all flammable and burning materials, and extinguish the remaining fire by dousing it with saline and using fire extinguishers.[1,3] It is important to note that there are many different types of fire extinguishers, and not all can be used on every type of fire. For example, water extinguishers should not be used on electrical and chemical fires; carbon dioxide should be used instead.

## BASICS OF ELECTRICAL SHOCK

The basic electrical circuit operates under Ohm's Law, represented in the equation $V = I \times R$. The components are defined as follows: V is the voltage supplied to the circuit, which equals the resistance, noted by ohms, multiplied by the current, measured in amperes. These circuits are basic pathways for currents to run to and from a voltage source with electrons running on a hot wire away from the source to provide power to a piece of equipment and returning on a neutral wire or grounding wire following the path of least resistance.

Electrical shock occurs when a person completes, or becomes part of, an electrical circuit. The result is the release of thermal energy. With the assistance of clinical bioengineers, the anesthesiologist has the responsibility to maintain all equipment operations to the standards of the National Fire Protection Association (NFPA).[1]

To prevent electrical shocks and burns, all OR equipment needs to have a grounding prong (i.e., three prongs), including a grounding pad connected to the patient when an ESU is in use. As defined by the NFPA, grounding is the process of bonding one or more objects to the earth so that there is no electrical potential.[4] When an object is not

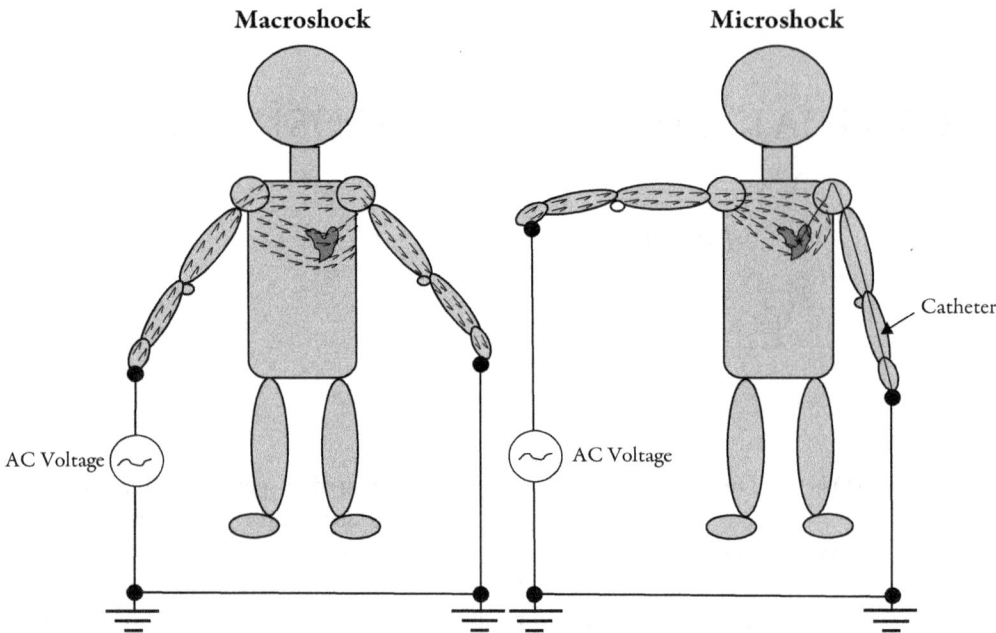

**Figure 51.1.** Mechanism of Macroshock and microshock.

grounded appropriately, an alarm will sound; in the OR, this alarms emits from the line isolation monitor (LIM).[1] NFPA requirements in wet environments, such as the OR, include the use of a ground fault current interrupter (GFCI), which is a safety mechanism to verify that the equipment is appropriately grounded.[1] These safety features have two mechanisms of action when they sound. If there is a fault in the circuit, such as when a power line is accidently grounded, the GFCI will cut the power to the outlet. Meanwhile, the LIM will sound an alarm but will not eliminate the power from the outlet (Figure 51.1).

## Table 51.1 ELECTRICITY LEAK AND RESULTING CONTACT EFFECT

| | CURRENT | EFFECT WITH 1-SECOND CONTACT |
|---|---|---|
| Microshocks | 10 uA | Allowable maximum current leakage |
| | 20–100 uA | Ventricular fibrillation |
| Macroshocks | 1 mA | Perceptible electric current |
| | 5 mA | Maximum current not causing injury |
| | 10–20 mA | "Let-go" current before sustained muscle contraction |
| | 50 mA | Pain and mechanical injury |
| | 100–300 mA | Ventricular fibrillation |

If there is accidental contact with a voltage terminal, the resultant burn or shock will depend on the amount of current that runs through the person. The type of shock also depends on the source of contact, not just the current. For example, a macroshock describes a disturbance in the nervous and musculoskeletal systems that results from high voltage or current traveling through the skin across the chest, whereas a microshock occurs when the current travels directly through the cardiac tissue (Figure 51.1). There are different physical effects of microshocks and macroshocks with varying currents. For example, at 10–20 mA, known as the let-go current, involuntary muscle contraction sets in and the person is unable to release an object (Table 51.1).

The most common implanted medical devices associated with microshocks are pacemakers and automated implanted cardioverter defibrillators, but microshocks also occur through temporary indwelling venous lines such as pulmonary artery catheters. A current as low as 100 μA can induce ventricular fibrillation because of the proximity to the heart. Preoperative interrogation to ensure proper functioning of pacemakers is helpful, and these devices can be reprogrammed by an experienced provider to turn off the tachydysrhythmia functions. When using an ESU, it is important to turn off this feature to prohibit pacemaker interference, which can result in inadvertent defibrillation. The surgical team can also be encouraged to use bipolar in place of monopolar cautery to decrease ESU interference.[1] It is important to note that the LIM detects currents greater than 2 mA; therefore, it does not protect against microshocks, which occur at 20μA.[1]

## REFERENCES

1. Jones TS, et al. Operating room fires. *Anesthesiology*. 2019;130: 492–501.
2. Miller RD, et al. *Miller's Anesthesia*. 8th ed. Philadelphia, PA: Elsevier; 2014.
3. Apfelbaum JL. Updated by the Committee on Standards and Practice Parameters. The original document was developed by the American Society of Anesthesiologists Task Force on Operating Room Fires: Caplan RA, et al. *Anesthesiology*. 2013;118:271–290.
4. *NFPA Glossary of Terms*, 2019 edition. Available at: https://www.nfpa.org/-/media/Files/Codes-and-standards/Glossary-of-terms/glossary_of_terms_2019.ashx.

# 52.

# INTRAVASCULAR PUMPS

*Jack Hagan and Chris Giordano*

## INTRODUCTION

Intravenous (IV) infusion has been accomplished by a variety of tools since the 1600s. Modern devices fall into three main categories: manual resistance, syringe pump, and IV pump. Whether powered by gravity, pressure bag, or elastomeric pouch, manually adjusting the drop rate via a resistance dial or roller clamp is perioperatively ubiquitous. Electronic pump devices have developed from simple volume over time delivery devices to present-day "smart" pumps with programmed medication libraries, pressure and air bubble detection, closed- or open-loop dose control mechanisms (Table 52.1), and even wireless connection to the health record. Perioperatively, these devices are used to deliver total intravenous anesthesia (TIVA) or as part of a balanced anesthetic technique between IV and inhalational medications, infusion of other specific medication such as analgesics, vasoactive agents, and antibiotics, and when tight control of IV fluids is required (e.g., neonatal care, end-stage renal disease requiring dialysis).[1]

## INTRAOPERATIVE

The starting point for most cases is simply a gravity powered IV line with a "thumb roller" resistance device. From there, based on availability and anesthetic goals, the provider can design an optimal layout to meet anesthetic goals (Table 52.2).

## SPECIAL ANESTHESIOLOGY CONSIDERATIONS

### DISCONNECT

Modern pumps have a high-pressure alarm to detect occlusion; however, there is no way to electronically detect a line disconnect. If an IV line becomes disconnected or broken

*Table 52.1* COMPARISON BETWEEN OPEN AND CLOSED CONTROL LOOP DEVICES

| OPEN CONTROL LOOP DEVICE | CLOSED CONTROL LOOP DEVICE |
|---|---|
| • Non-Feedback System<br>• Output does not depend on sensor data<br>• Dose adjustment requires user intervention or follows a fixed time/formula<br>• Example: Target Controlled Infusion Pump, adjusts dose based on time, weight, and formula to achieve an estimated blood concentration | • Feedback System<br>• Output changes based on sensor data<br>• No user intervention needed to change dose<br>• Example: Insulin pump, samples blood glucose and adjusts dose on results. |

*Table 52.2* DIFFERENT INFUSION DEVICES

| TYPE | DESIRED GOAL | EXAMPLES |
|---|---|---|
| Syringe Pump | • Delivery of small & precise volumes<br>• Convenient, readily available in OR environment | • Neonatal infusions<br>• High Potency Opioids (i.e., Remifentanil)<br>• Medications reconstituted in OR (i.e., Vasopressin, Dexmedetomidine) |
| IV Pump/ "Smart Pump" | • Delivery of "high alert" medications of higher clinical risk<br>• Delivery of fluids or medications not continuously monitored (i.e., Floor patient) | • Insulin, vasopressors, inotropes, sedation, IV fluids |
| Elastomeric Pump | • Outpatient administration, simple use, disposable | • Continuous peripheral nerve catheter for postop pain control |
| Manual flow regulator, gravity powered infusion | • Simplicity, readily available, low cost, no electricity required<br>• When continuous observation is possible | • Monitored Anesthesia Care<br>• Preop, PACU<br>• Austere environment or shortage |

under the drapes, such as after tucking an arm, the infusion may appear to be running but is going into the sheets.

## INFILTRATION

The pump cannot detect IV infiltration from the vein into subcutaneous tissues. This can be potentially harmful to surrounding tissues (e.g., calcium chloride) or harmful if the infusion had a specific condition to correct (e.g., antibiotics in sepsis). However, many pumps have pressure gauges and corresponding thresholds that are user adjustable and visible on the device. This permits the user to view occlusions (e.g., clamped line or blood pressure cuff inflation) even prior to the alarm sounding. This feature may help detect pressure buildup in an infiltrated limb; however, soft tissue can often absorb liters of fluid prior to developing enough back pressure to trigger the alarm. This feature makes detecting infiltration helpful but unreliable.[2]

## BODY WEIGHT

Medication library and pump software do not account for differences in volumes of distribution. Depending on the medication, ideal, lean, or total body weight may be more

appropriate. This becomes particularly important when programing infusion rates for obese patients.

## MANUAL PROGRAMMING

"Anesthesia mode" allows manual programming outside a pharmacy-approved, loaded medication library and associated limits of infusion rates. This requires extreme care and vigilance. Delivery of 0.2 mcg/kg/hr of dexmedetomidine versus 0.2 mcg/kg/min would lead to a 60-fold dosing error.[3]

## INABILITY TO DETECT INFUSION

The medication library anticipates that a standardized dilution of medication will be hung and the anesthesia professional is routinely required to create an infusion from a vial. The pump cannot sense the concentration running in the line—it assumes a correct and anticipated reconstituted concentration when calculating infusion rates. Additionally, some medications come in various pre-mixed concentrations. Providers must be vigilant in their selection from the medication library. For example, mistaking 40 mg/mL of double-strength (DS) esmolol for 20 mg/mL of regular esmolol could have profound adverse side effects.

## MULTIPLE LINES

A complex patient can have an array of infusions running, with multiple crisscrossing lines. Improper labeling can lead to adjustment of the wrong pump and potentially harm the patient (e.g., vasopressin and insulin, both pumps in units per hour). Or perhaps flushing a line full of a potent medication when it was thought to be simple IV fluid.

## NUISANCE AND DISTRACTION

Distraction is a serious risk to patient safety. Infusion pumps add a potential alarm to redirect attention, such as an overly sensitive bubble detection. Finally, there is no standardized user interface among manufacturers. Each new pump requires training and practice on programming, indicators that the pump is actually running and not paused, line-pressure meters, ways to override drug library limits, and engaging anesthesia mode.

## REFERENCES

1. Schlotterbeck, D. Infusion pumps and their safety in OR. *APSF Newsletter.* 2000;15(4).
2. Ball RD, et al. Peripheral intravenous catheter infiltration: Anesthesia providers do not adhere to their own ideas of best practice. *J Clin Anesth.* 2013;25(2):115–120.
3. Ohashi K, et al. Benefits and risks of using smart pumps to reduce medication error rates: A systematic review. *Drug Saf.* 2014 Dec;37(12):1011–1120.

# Part IV

# MATHEMATICS

# 53.

# STATISTICS AND SIMPLE MATH IN ANESTHESIA PRACTICE

*R. Scott Stayner and Kris Ferguson*

## DATA TYPES

The types of data collected in medical research are broadly categorized into interval and categorical data. Interval data have two subtypes: discrete and continuous. Categorical data have three subtypes: dichotomous, nominal, and ordinal. These are described in Table 53.1.[1]

## NULL HYPOTHESIS

In the simplest study design, two groups are examined with a control and experimental group, with a simple positive or negative outcome measured. The control is not subjected to the proposed intervention, whereas the experimental group is administered the proposed intervention. The default hypothesis, termed the null hypothesis, is that there is no difference in the measured result between the two groups.[2]

*Table 53.1* DATA TYPES AND SUBTYPES USED IN MEDICAL RESEARCH[1]

| DATA TYPE | DEFINITION | EXAMPLES |
|---|---|---|
| Interval | | |
| Discrete | Data measured with an integer only scale | Number of fingers |
| Continuous | Non-integral but numeric data | Fluid volume |
| Categorical | | |
| Dichotomous | Binary data | Yes/No, gender |
| Nominal | Qualitative data without order or rank | Blood type, hair color |
| Ordinal | Data that are ordered or ranked or measured without a constant scale interval | Mallampati score, pain score |

For example, a study could be done to determine if patients with a pain score greater than 8 who receive 50 mcg of fentanyl in the recovery room after surgery report pain reduction compared to those who receive 1 mL of saline. The experimental group would be the group that receives the fentanyl and the control group would receive saline. The null hypothesis would be that the group that receives fentanyl would report the same pain score as the group that receives saline. The alternative hypothesis is that the experimental group (fentanyl) reports a different pain score, demonstrating that the intervention is effective.

## P VALUE

A P value is an estimate of the probability that the conclusion drawn from the statistical analysis occurred simply by chance rather than due to the intervention proposed in a study. In the preceding example, if 80% of the patients who received fentanyl for post-surgical pain reported a pain reduction, the P value would indicate the probability that the observed pain reduction is due to chance. For example, a P value of 0.05 indicates that in the patients who reported pain reduction with fentanyl, there is a 5% chance that the pain reduction was due to chance rather than the administration of fentanyl. The P value is used to accept or reject the null hypothesis if it is less than a certain threshold. The accepted threshold is usually 0.05 or 0.04. In the preceding experiment, a P value of 0.05 would generally be used to reject the null hypothesis that patients report the same pain reduction for fentanyl administration and saline administration, i.e., that fentanyl is effective in treating post-surgical pain.

## TYPE 1 AND TYPE 2 ERRORS AND THE NULL HYPOTHESIS

Statistics is based on probability, so it is possible that even when the P value is set at 0.05, the decision to accept or reject the null hypothesis is erroneous. The error of wrongly accepting the null hypothesis is called a Type 1 or α error. In the preceding example, this would mean that the positive result of pain reduction with administration of fentanyl is false, therefore a false positive. Alternatively, if the null hypothesis is wrongly accepted, this is termed a Type 2 error or β error.

## CONFIDENCE INTERVAL

The confidence interval can provide more information than the binary "yes/no" result given by accepting or rejecting the null hypothesis using a P value threshold. The confidence interval is the probability that mean value reported will be found within the range of the confidence interval. A higher confidence interval suggests that the evidence supporting the conclusion is stronger than a lower confidence interval. A confidence interval of 90%–95% is generally considered a quality result. In the preceding example, suppose the mean pain score reported after administration of fentanyl was 3 with a 95% confidence interval. This means that if the experiment were performed 100 times, the true average pain score of 3 would be observed in 95 of the 100 iterations of the study.[2]

## DATA CENTRALITY: MEAN, MEDIAN, MODE

Interval data are usually reported in summary using the mean, median, and mode. The mean is calculated by summing the numbers in the data set and dividing by the number of data points. The median is the value that divides the data set into two. The mode is the most value that occurs most frequently in the data set.[1]

For the following data set:

1, 3, 5, 5, 6,7, 8, 9, 9, 9, 9

Mean = $(1 + 3 + 5 + 5 + 6 + 7 + 8 + 9 + 9 + 9)/11$
$= 5.64$

Median = 7

Mode = 9

## VARIABILITY AROUND THE MEAN: STANDARD DEVIATION

The mean is usually reported with a value of standard deviation. The value for standard deviation gives an indication for how similar most data points measured are to the calculated mean. If all data points are the same value, then the standard deviation would be 0. However, this is generally not the case. If the assumption is made that the data are symmetric with a normal, bell-shaped curve distribution, then 68% of the data

will fall within 1 standard deviation interval, 95% of the data will fall within 2 standard deviation intervals, and 99% of the data will fall within 3 standard deviation intervals.[3]

## STATISTICAL TESTS

The decision regarding which type of statistical test to use in data analysis is driven by the variable type, number of variables to be analyzed, and whether the data follow a normal bell curve distribution. The most important factor in deciding which statistical test to apply to a data set is whether a parametric or nonparametric test should be used.

### PARAMETRIC STATISTICAL TESTS

When a parametric test is used, the interval (discrete or continuous) data are assumed to be normally distributed with equal variance between the groups tested. The classic parametric test is the *Student's t test*. This test is used for comparing the outcome of a control and experimental group (unpaired) or if the outcome of one group is compared before and after an intervention (paired). If interval data from more than two groups are analyzed, the ANOVA (analysis of variance) test is used.[1]

### NONPARAMETRIC STATISTICAL TESTS

Nonparametric tests are used to analyze categorical data (ordinal, binary, or nominal) or interval data (continuous or discrete) that does not have a normal distribution. For categorical data, the chi-square test can generally be used. The *Fisher's Exact test* can be used for two sample sets.

For interval data that cannot be assumed to have a normal distribution with equal variance, special nonparametric tests must be utilized for analysis. The *sign test* is the equivalent of the paired *Student's t test*. The *Whitney rank-sum test (Mann-Whitney rank-sum test)* is the equivalent of the unpaired *Student's t test*. The *Kruskal-Wallis test* is the equivalent of the ANOVA test.[1]

A summary of the various tests, parametric and nonparametric, that can be used to analyze specific types of data is outlined in Table 53.2.

## DIAGNOSTIC TEST SENSITIVITY AND SPECIFICITY

Predictive or diagnostic tests have profound importance in medicine. Such tests influence which interventions are selected by physicians to treat patients. The sensitivity and specificity are used to help determine the reliability of a test result. Sensitivity is a measure of the false negative rate, or the ability of the test to detect a disease. Specificity is a measure of the false positive rate or the chance that the test

*Table 53.2* SUMMARY OF APPROPRIATE TESTS FOR STATISTICAL ANALYSIS OF MEDICAL DATA[1-3]

| INTERVAL DATA | ONE SAMPLE TESTS | TWO-SAMPLE TESTS | MULTIPLE SAMPLE TESTS |
|---|---|---|---|
| Parametric Continuous or discrete | Student's t-test | Student's t-test, (paired/unpaired) | ANOVA |
| Nonparametric Continuous or discrete | Sign test | Mann-Whitney rank test | Kruskal-Wallace test |
| **CATEGORICAL DATA** | | | |
| Nominal or dichotomous | Binomial distribution | Chi-square test, Fisher's Exact test | Chi-square test |
| Ordinal | Chi-square test | Chi-square test | Chi-square test |

will falsely return a positive result for a condition that does not exist. Sensitivity and specificity are calculated using the following parameters:[3]

True positive (TP): The patient has the disease and the test is positive.

False positive (FP): The patient does not have the disease and the test is positive.

True negative (TN): The patient does not have the disease and the test is negative.

False negative (FN): The patient does have the disease and the test is negative.

Mathematically, sensitivity and specificity are expressed using the following equations:

$$\text{Sensitivity} = TP/(TP+FN) \quad \text{Specificity} = TN/(TN+FP)$$

The ideal test would have no false negative and no false positive results. The sensitivity and specificity of such a test would both be 1.

$$\text{Sensitivity} = TP/(TP + 0) = TP/TP = 1$$
$$\text{Specificity} = TN/(TN+0) = TN/TN = 1$$

## DIAGNOSTIC TEST POSITIVE PREDICTIVE VALUE (PPV) AND NEGATIVE PREDICTIVE VALUE (NPV)

Just as sensitivity and specificity can be useful measures to ascertain the reliability of a test, it is often useful to know the positive predictive value (PPV) and negative predictive value (NPV) of a diagnostic test. These are also calculated as follows:

$$PPV = TP/(TP+FP) \quad NPV = TN/(TN+FN)$$

PPV and NPV are limited by the prevalence of a disease in the population and should be used with caution in populations where the disease is nearly ubiquitous or nearly absent.[3]

## REFERENCES

1. Pace N. Experimental design and statistics. In: *Clinical Anesthesia*. 5th ed. Philadelphia, PA: Lippincott Williams & Wilkins; 2006:63–75.
2. Hulley S. *Designing Clinical Research*. Philadelphia, PA: Lippincott Williams & Wilkins; 2013.
3. Rosenbaum S. Statistical methods in anesthesia. In: *Miller's Anesthesia*. Vol 1. 6th ed. Elsevier Churchill Livingstone; 2005:881–890.

# Part V

# PHARMACOLOGY

# 54.

# PHARMACOKINETICS AND PHARMACODYNAMICS

*Nicholas M. Parker and Syed Waqar*

## INTRODUCTION

*Pharmacology* is a broad term that refers to the study of how drugs work, and is a key area of focus in a pharmacist's training. Pharmacology may be split conceptually into pharmacokinetics and pharmacodynamics. *Pharmacokinetics* refers to the ways drugs are moved through and processed by the body, or "what the body does to the drug."[1] *Pharmacodynamics*, in contrast, refers to the ways drugs interact with the body at the site of action to cause physiologic effects, that is, "what the drug does to the body."[1] These concepts are essential when selecting a drug, dose, route, and frequency for a given patient, and for understanding drug interactions.

## PHARMACOKINETICS

Pharmacokinetics is often subdivided into *absorption, distribution, metabolism,* and *excretion.*[1,2]

### ABSORPTION

*Absorption* is the process of moving drugs from outside the body to the bloodstream.[1,2] The speed and efficiency of this process vary widely, depending on the drug and the route of administration. *Bioavailability* refers to the proportion of drug that reaches the bloodstream intact compared to the dose administered.[1]

The rate and extent of absorption vary widely, and depend on the route of administration, physical and chemical characteristics of the drug, hemodynamics, enzyme function, and other factors.[1] Intravenous administration is the most rapid and efficient method of drug administration because it bypasses every barrier to absorption and delivers the drug directly to the bloodstream.

### DISTRIBUTION

After being absorbed into the blood, the drug must then travel to the site of action. Perfusion of the tissue is necessary,

which can be impaired by shock or vascular disease. Water-soluble drugs tend to dissolve freely in the blood but may have difficulty crossing the blood-brain barrier.[1,2] Fat-soluble drugs, on the other hand, can accumulate in adipose tissue to concentrations orders of magnitude higher than in the blood. Some drugs travel through the blood bound to proteins like albumin, which increases the blood's capacity to carry drugs that are otherwise not very soluble in water.

### METABOLISM

*Metabolism* of drugs refers to enzymes in the body making a change to the chemical structure of the drug.[1,2] Importantly, no part of the drug leaves the body at this step (that would be excretion; see later discussion). The effects of drug metabolism may be complex and depend on the specific drug, enzyme, and environment. Metabolism of a drug usually inactivates it and promotes its elimination from the body.[1] In some cases, however, metabolism is necessary to activate the drug, and some drugs are metabolized to compounds that are themselves pharmacologically active or toxic.[1] Drug-drug interactions and genetic variants can result in drastic changes to the rate at which certain drugs are metabolized, necessitating individualized dosing or use of alternative agents.[1,2]

### EXCRETION

*Excretion* refers to drug molecules (and/or drug metabolites) actually leaving the body. Most drugs are excreted by the kidneys into the urine, either as unchanged drug or after metabolism (or both).[1,2] Renal clearance depends foremost on adequate perfusion of functioning kidneys. Many drugs require dose reductions in patients with renal impairment since elimination of the drug is diminished.[3]

## PHARMACODYNAMICS

*Pharmacodynamics* refers to how drugs interact with the body to cause a clinical effect.

## RECEPTOR ACTION

Many drugs act by binding to enzymes or other proteins responsible for transport, signaling, or other functions.

### Agonists

Receptor agonists are recognized by the receptor as the endogenous ligand, and the protein performs its normal function as if being stimulated in the physiologically normal way.[1,4] Phenylephrine binds to adrenergic receptors on arterioles, causing vasoconstriction just as endogenous epinephrine would.[3,5]

### Antagonists

Drugs usually do not have the same effect as the endogenous ligand when they bind to the target protein. A receptor antagonist, or inhibitor, is a drug that decreases the function of the protein to which it binds.[1,4] Metoprolol is an antagonist of adrenergic receptors on the heart, causing the opposite effect of the usual ligand epinephrine.[3]

### Partial Agonists/Partial Antagonists

A few drugs bind to receptors tightly, thereby blocking the usual ligand, but still cause some of the same downstream signaling.[1,4] These are sometimes called *partial agonists* and sometimes called *partial antagonists*; both names refer to the same thing. An important partial agonist is buprenorphine, which mildly stimulates opioid receptors while blocking other opioids from binding.[3] Patients using buprenorphine who become injured or need surgery will usually need higher doses of opioids to overcome the antagonist effect of buprenorphine.[3]

## CHEMICAL AND PHYSICAL ACTION

A few drugs don't bind to proteins at all, and are simply involved in chemical reactions. Antacids like calcium carbonate neutralize acid in the stomach but don't inhibit its production in any way.[3] Other drugs simply have some bulk effect in the body, such as adsorption of another substance. For example, polyethylene glycol 3350 softens stool by attracting water, and idarucizumab sequesters dabigatran to reverse its anticoagulant effect.[3]

## ANESTHETIC CONSIDERATIONS

### PREOPERATIVE

The patient should be assessed carefully preoperatively to determine if special drug selection or drug dosing is needed. Does the patient have very high or very low body weight? Do they have renal or hepatic impairment? Do they take medications at home that may interact with medications that might be given in the operating room, or interact with the procedure itself? For an elective procedure, how long should these medications be held beforehand? If impossible to hold the medications that long, what must be done to overcome the interaction?

### INTRAOPERATIVE

How should medications be administered based on the drug and the patient's current condition? Do they have adequate perfusion of their gut or skin to rely on these sites for drug absorption? How long will each drug take to start working? How long to stop working? How often do medications need to be re-dosed?

### POSTOPERATIVE

Were any medications given intraoperatively that may have long-lasting effects? What medications should the patient avoid during that time? When is it safe for the patient to restart their home medications?

## REFERENCES

1. Rowland M, Tozer TN. *Clinical Pharmacokinetics and Pharmacodynamics*. 4th ed. Philadelphia, PA: Lippincott Williams and Wilkins; 2011.
2. Holford NHG. Pharmacokinetics and pharmacodynamics: Rational dosing and the time course of drug action. In: Katzung BG, ed. *Basic and Clinical Pharmacology*. 14th ed. New York: McGraw-Hill; 2018:42–56.
3. *Lexicomp*. Wolters Kluwer; 2020. http://online.lexi.com. Accessed August 23, 2020.
4. von Zastrow M. Drug receptors and pharmacodynamics. In: Katzung BG, ed. *Basic and Clinical Pharmacology*. 14th ed. New York: McGraw-Hill; 2018:21–41.
5. Biaggioni I, Robertson D. Adrenoreceptor agonists and sympathomimetic drugs. In: Katzung BG, ed. *Basic and Clinical Pharmacology*. 14th ed. New York: McGraw-Hill; 2018:142–160.

# 55.

# DRUG ABSORPTION AND DISTRIBUTION

*Nicholas M. Parker*

## INTRODUCTION

For a drug to have an effect, it must reach the site of action. In pharmacokinetics, this journey is comprised of absorption from outside the body to the bloodstream, followed by distribution from the bloodstream to the target tissues.

## ABSORPTION

Absorption is the process of moving drugs from outside the body to the bloodstream. The speed and efficiency of this process vary widely, depending on the drug and the route of administration. *Bioavailability* refers to the proportion of drug that reaches the bloodstream intact compared to the dose administered. $T_{max}$ is the time from administration to the peak concentration of the drug in the patient's blood.[1,2]

### INTRAVENOUS ADMINISTRATION

Many drugs given in the operating room are administered intravenously. In this case, absorption is complete and instantaneous—all the body's barriers are bypassed and the drug is delivered directly to the bloodstream. Bioavailability is 100%, and $T_{max}$ occurs at the end of the infusion.[1]

### SUBCUTANEOUS AND INTRAMUSCULAR ADMINISTRATION

Injections given into the muscle or subcutaneous tissue still enjoy 100% bioavailability, but the drug must still diffuse away from the injection site to reach the bloodstream.[1,2] This may occur over the course of minutes or months, depending on the drug's formulation. The many forms of insulin differ only in the rate of absorption out of the subcutaneous tissue. Hypotensive patients requiring vasopressors will likely have decreased blood flow to the skin, resulting in delayed absorption of drugs given subcutaneously.

### ENTERAL ADMINISTRATION

The most harrowing journey a drug may take to reach the bloodstream is through the stomach. Solid dosage forms such as tablets must disintegrate into small particles, dissolve in water, survive acidic and basic environments, migrate through the greasy lipid bilayer, and avoid being kicked back into the gut lumen by efflux pumps. Even when this drug has reached the bloodstream, it still must face the liver and its tremendous capacity to modify and inactivate all manner of foreign molecules.[1,2] Medications taken orally may have 100% bioavailability or nearly zero, depending on a multitude of factors. $T_{max}$ ranges from at least 20 to 30 minutes to several hours.

### PARTITION COEFFICIENTS

One of the factors affecting bioavailability is the solubility of the drug in water compared to its solubility in octanol, which is an oily organic solvent.[1] Water in this case represents blood, the gut lumen, and water-rich tissues like skeletal muscle. Octanol represents the lipid bilayer through which drugs must diffuse to exit the gut lumen, as well as lipophilic tissues like the blood-brain barrier and adipose tissue. Drugs must dissolve in water to some extent to allow a tablet to dissolve or to make an acceptable solution for injection, but must also be adequately lipophilic if absorption through hydrophobic barriers is needed to reach the site of action.

## DISTRIBUTION

After an absorption process that may be simple or arduous, the drug must now reach the site of action.

### PERFUSION

Richly perfused organs such as the heart, lungs, brain, gut, liver, and kidneys will usually receive an adequate supply of drug for as long as the drug is present in the bloodstream.[1]

For some targets, seeping out of the capillaries into the interstitium completes the journey. Some peripheral tissues may have severely impaired blood flow (such as a diabetic foot), which can hinder drug delivery to that site.

## BLOOD-BRAIN BARRIER

Other targets, most notably within the central nervous system (CNS), are significantly protected from foreign molecules in the bloodstream. The blood-brain barrier (BBB) allows only specific pre-approved compounds to pass through dedicated transporters, and actively pumps out potentially threatening molecules using efflux pumps like P-glycoprotein (PGP).[1,2] Drugs intended to reach the CNS typically must be quite lipophilic to cross the BBB.

## PROTEIN BINDING

Some drugs travel through the bloodstream bound to plasma proteins like albumin and alpha-1-acid glycoprotein.[1] This increases the blood's total capacity to contain that drug, just as hemoglobin increases the blood's capacity to carry oxygen.

## VOLUME OF DISTRIBUTION

The volume of distribution ($V_d$) is an imaginary amount of solution in which the dose of a drug seems to dissolve, based on measured blood concentrations.[1,2] Lipophilic drugs will tend to accumulate in adipose tissue, leaving only a small amount of drug in the blood. In this case, the drug can appear to have dissolved in many hundreds of liters of blood! Drugs that accumulate in this way may require loading doses to fill this reservoir before a high enough drug level can be maintained in the blood. Conversely, some medications take longer than expected to wear off if significant accumulation has occurred.

## ANESTHETIC CONSIDERATIONS

### PREOPERATIVE

Review the patient's labs, anthropometrics, vitals, and medical/surgical history. Does the patient have impaired gut function? Severe hypotension? Extreme body weight? Low serum albumin? Based on this review, are any modifications needed to the plan for drug selection, dosing, or route of administration?

### INTRAOPERATIVE

Administer most drugs intravenously to ensure a rapid and complete response. Epidural, intrathecal, or local injections are also reliable routes during surgery. Subcutaneous and intramuscular injections may be less effective if the patient is hypotensive. Give each medication enough time to start working before re-dosing.

### POSTOPERATIVE

Consider whether excessive drug accumulation has occurred if a patient has delayed recovery from anesthesia. Note that reversal agents like naloxone may wear off before this reservoir has been emptied.

## REFERENCES

1. Rowland M, Tozer TN. *Clinical Pharmacokinetics and Pharmacodynamics.* 4th ed. Philadelphia, PA: Lippincott Williams & Wilkins; 2011.
2. Katzung BG, ed. *Basic and Clinical Pharmacology.* 14th ed. New York: McGraw-Hill; https://accessmedicine-mhmedical-com.ezproxy.library.wisc.edu/content.aspx?bookid=2249&sectionid=175220393. Accessed August 23, 2020.

# 56.

# PHARMACOKINETICS OF NEURAXIAL ANESTHESIA

*Nimesh Patel and Mohamed Fayed*

## INTRODUCTION

In both spinal and epidural anesthesia, the target receptors for local anesthetics are found at the spinal nerve roots and dorsal root ganglia. The onset of action of local anesthetics depends on the size of the nerve, the degree of myelination, and the surface area of the nerve that is exposed to the medication. Therefore, the sympathetic and parasympathetic nerve fibers are blocked first, as they contain minimally myelinated B fibers that are 1–3 micrometer in diameter. Blockade of C fibers that are 0.3–1 micrometer unmyelinated sensory nerves that convey temperature occurs shortly after, which is then followed by A-delta fibers that are 1–4 micrometers, myelinated, and carry pinprick sensation. A-beta fibers are 5–12 micrometers, myelinated, convey touch sensation, and are the last sensory nerve fibers that are blocked. Motor fibers, A-alpha, are the last nerve fibers to be blocked, which are 12–20 micrometers and myelinated. Recovery of blockade occurs in the opposite direction, with motor activity returning first, followed by touch, pinprick, and temperature.[1] Furthermore, due to differences in sensitivity to nerve fibers, autonomic nerve blockade occurs most cephalad, which is 2 or more dermatomes higher than sensory blockade, which is 2 or more nerve segments higher than motor fiber blockade.[2]

## SPINAL ANESTHESIA

The local anesthetic distribution in spinal anesthesia is determined by baricity, patient positioning, as well as local anesthetic dosage. Baricity is defined as the ratio of density of the local anesthetic to the density of cerebral spinal fluid (CSF).[3] Local anesthetics that have the same density as CSF are referred to as isobaric solutions and remain at the injection level. Hyperbaric solutions are made by adding 5% or 8% dextrose to local anesthetic and will sink with gravity, compared to hypobaric solutions, which are made by the addition of distilled water to local anesthetic and will rise against gravity.[2]

Patient positioning will also affect the spread of anesthetic. Trendelenburg position will cause the anesthetic to travel cephalad, and reverse-Trendelenburg will cause it to travel caudal. By incorporating baricity of the local anesthetic, the distribution of local anesthetic is further influenced. For instance, placing a patient in lateral decubitus will cause the anesthetic to move into the dependent side for a hyperbaric solution and non-dependent side for a hypobaric solution.[3] Attention should also be placed on the natural curvature of the spine, which has a posterior curvature at T4–T8 and can cause hyperbaric solutions to be moved on the dependent side in the supine position.

Local anesthetic dose is also an important determinant of spinal anesthesia spread. Dose is calculated by multiplying volume and concentration. For isobaric and hypobaric solutions, dosage is a reliable indicator of spread, compared with baricity for hyperbaric solutions. In addition, patient factors can also influence block height, such as height, pregnancy, age, sex, and spine variations.[1]

In the past, lidocaine was commonly used for spinal anesthesia. It is a hydrophilic amide local anesthetic compound with duration of action of 60–90 minutes with excellent sensory and motor blockade. However, reported cases of transient neurologic symptoms (TNS) and nerve injuries, even at reduced doses, have led to its decreased use.[3] Alternatively, bupivacaine is an amide local anesthetic that can be prepared as a 0.25%, 0.5%, 0.75% isobaric solution, or 0.5% and 0.75% hyperbaric solution. It is widely used with doses of 5–20 mg with duration of action of up to 120 minutes. Its recovery is similar to lidocaine; however, it has less incidence of TNS and is now commonly favored.[1]

## SPINAL ADJUVANTS

Adjuvants are molecules that improve the efficacy or potency of another compound while reducing any adverse effects. Commonly used spinal adjuvants are vasoconstrictors, opioids, and a2-agonists. Epinephrine (0.1–0.2 mg) or phenylephrine (2–5 mg) causes the sensory and motor blockade of local anesthetics to be extended by vasoconstriction of spinal vessels and further reduces the risk of local anesthetic systemic toxicity.[3] Fentanyl (25 mcg), sufentanil (2–10 mcg), or morphine (0.1–0.5 mg) can enhance analgesia by binding to opioid receptors primarily located at the dorsal horn.[2] Particular attention should be placed on hydrophilic opioids as these compounds have a greater propensity to spread and may cause late-onset respiratory depression (6–18 hr).[1,4] Clonidine (15–225 mcg) and dexmedetomidine (3 mcg), modulates a2-receptors located in the dorsal horn, prolonging sensory and motor blockade, but with an increased risk of hypotension seen in clonidine.[1,5]

## EPIDURAL ANESTHESIA

Local anesthetics placed into the epidural space can have a wide drug distribution. It can cross into the subarachnoid space through the dura mater, can spread within the epidural space superiorly or inferior, can move around circumferentially within the epidural space, travel through the intervertebral foramina to affect the spinal nerve roots, and can be absorbed into epidural fat and vessels. Distribution into epidural fat allows for a reservoir to form, which then slowly redistributes, allowing for a longer medication effect. Furthermore, systemic absorption of local anesthetic from the epidural space follows the two-compartment model, where the first fast phase is absorption into epidural veins and the second slower phase may be due to redistribution of local anesthetic from the epidural fat.[1] Systemic absorption may also be influenced by pH, pKa, and protein binding of the local anesthetic solution.

Level of injection also has an important effect on spread, as a low thoracic or lumbar injection may result in rostral spread, and a cervical and high thoracic injection can result in a caudal spread.[3] Block height is also affected by drug factors, such as volume and dose.[1] Additives, such as sodium bicarbonate and opioids, will have less effect on local anesthetic distribution and block height, but will influence onset and duration of anesthesia. Increased age can cause a high block, since there is less leakage of local anesthetic through the intervertebral foramina and decreased compliance of the epidural space.[1,3] Pregnancy causes an increase in epidural pressure due to engorgement of epidural veins, which can cause a high thoracic epidural block.[1] Furthermore, patient positioning has been shown to affect

spread, as the dependent side in the lateral decubitus position is primarily affected in a lumbar epidural injection, as seen in pregnancy.[3]

The type of local anesthetic used influences the duration of action of an epidural. Chloroprocaine is an ultra-short-acting ester with TNS at high doses. Lidocaine and mepivacaine have similar onset time, as well as intermediate duration of action. Compared to spinal, epidural lidocaine has TNS.[3] Bupivacaine, levobupivacaine, and ropivacaine are long-acting local anesthetics. Levobupivacaine and ropivacaine have an improved safety profile compared to bupivacaine, as they are less cardiotoxic.[1] Generally, a local anesthetic should be selected based on how quickly anesthesia is required, duration of the surgery, and whether sensory and/or motor blockade is required.[2]

## EPIDURAL ADJUVANTS

Similar to spinal adjuvants, epidural additives should be considered. Epinephrine in an epidural is used as an indicator for intravascular injection. It also prolongs anesthesia by decreasing local anesthetic vascular absorption from the epidural space.[5] Lipophilic epidural opioids are more readily absorbed into the vascular system and into epidural fat, resulting in less medication diffusing into the intrathecal space and reaching the dorsal horn.[1,3] Alternatively, hydrophilic opioids can provide thoracic analgesia from a lumbar epidural if desired, by diffusion into subarachnoid space and traveling rostral.[1,4] Sodium bicarbonate is added to local anesthetics to increase the proportion of the non-ionized molecule, which has an overall effect of decreasing onset time for the local anesthetic.[5] Care should be taken that sodium bicarbonate not be added with bupivacaine as it can lead to precipitation at high pH.[3]

## REFERENCES

1. Gropper MA. *Miller's Anesthesia*. Amsterdam: Elsevier; 2019.
2. Faust R. *Faust's Anesthesiology Review*. Elsevier; 2015.
3. Miller RD, et al. *Basics of Anesthesia*. Philadelphia, PA: Elsevier/Saunders; 2011.
4. Bernards CM. Understanding the physiology and pharmacology of epidural and intrathecal opioids. *Best Pract Res Clin Anaesthesiol*. 2002;16(4):489–505.
5. Farag E, et al. *Basic Sciences in Anesthesia*. Cham, Switzerland: Springer; 2018.

# 57.

# TOLERANCE AND TACHYPHYLAXIS

*Sherif Zaky and Nicholas Hozian*

## INTRODUCTION

Drug tolerance and tachyphylaxis are two constructs with great importance in the field of anesthesiology. *Tolerance* is defined as a state of adaptation in which exposure to a certain dose of a drug for a long duration of time leads to diminished drug effects, thus requiring an increase in dosage on subsequent administrations to achieve the same effect. *Tachyphylaxis* is a type of tolerance that develops acutely within only a few doses of a drug.[1] Understanding both these concepts is imperative for a physician to be able to surmount them properly when they arise in a patient setting.

## CELLULAR MECHANISMS OF TOLERANCE AND TACHYPHYLAXIS

*Pharmacokinetic tolerance* is a type of tolerance that develops as a result of bodily adaptations to an administered drug, as a means to alter drug effectiveness. These adaptations are mapped by four phases: absorption, distribution, metabolism, and elimination. Enzyme induction is a common cause of pharmacokinetic tolerance.

*Pharmacodynamic tolerance* refers to the body's biological responses to certain drug stimuli. This involves either adaptive changes at the receptor level or the recruitment of processes that limit or oppose the effects of the drug on receptor-mediated signaling pathways. These mechanisms explain why tolerance can occur at such a quick rate, as seen in tachyphylaxis.

## CLINICAL EXAMPLES OF TOLERANCE AND TACHYPHYLAXIS

Tolerance is a common phenomenon with prolonged use of all opioid agonists. Tolerance develops to analgesic, sedative, euphoric, and respiratory depressive effects, but not to miosis and constipation with chronic opioid use. Different mechanisms have been described to explain tolerance to opioids. Neuroadaptive changes at the receptor level in the

forms of receptor desensitization and downregulation of the number of receptors on the cell membrane are a widely accepted theory. Prolonged exposure to opioids activates NMDA receptors through a second messenger mechanism. It also downregulates spinal glutamate transporters, leading to high synaptic concentration of glutamate. These mechanisms lead to abnormal pain sensitivity, resulting in tolerance to opioids.[2]

Tolerance to other drugs, such as dobutamine, happens as a result of β adrenergic receptor downregulation with infusions lasting more than 24 hours.[3]

Tachyphylaxis occurs commonly with indirect acting sympathomimetics such as ephedrine and may reflect depletion of norepinephrine stores with repetitive administration.[4] Similarly, resistance to the hypotensive effect of sodium nitroprusside (SNP) may reflect tachyphylaxis to the drug due to cyanide toxicity or secondary to an increase in plasma renin activity. Tachyphylaxis to local anesthetics could be due to local acidosis and can be corrected by adding sodium bicarbonate to the solution.[5]

## DRUG DEPENDENCY AND TOLERANCE

Drug dependence is defined as: "[a] state of adaptation in which an individual will experience withdrawal symptoms if they stop or decrease the dose of a drug that has been used chronically." Tolerance differs from drug dependency in that drug tolerance is the need for an added dosage of a drug in order that the desired effect be reached; it has little to do with the individual's inherent need for the drug, as seen with dependency.

## MANAGEMENT OF TOLERANCE AND TACHYPHYLAXIS

### DRUG ROTATION

Rotating between similar drugs that can achieve the same desired effect, the physician can continue to produce the same desired effect for treatment without causing the patient to build up tolerance to a singular drug.

## INCREASING DOSE AND INCREASING FREQUENCY

As the body becomes more effective in overcoming the effects of the drug, increased dose and frequency might be required to achieve the desired effect again in all cases other than those involving tachyphylaxis. However, as the body continues to adapt to new doses, the physician must find a balance between increasing dosage to increase effectiveness and the subsequent side effects of an increased dosage.

## GRADUAL DOSAGE REDUCTION

In reducing dosage for a patient suffering from either tachyphylaxis or tolerance, it is crucial to do so in a gradual and progressive manner. These two problems cannot be resolved with immediate discontinuation of the administered drug. This will only cause withdrawal symptoms and serve to further exacerbate the issue. A physician must wean their patient off of the specific drug in order that the body be given enough time to normalize receptor amounts and proper homeostatic conditions. Drug weaning or tapering is important in properly quelling the symptoms of both tolerance and tachyphylaxis and is widely used throughout the medical field.

## REFERENCES

1. Robert K, et al. Pharmacokinetics and pharmacodynamics of injected and inhaled drugs. In: *Pharmacology and Physiology in Anesthetic Practice*. 4th ed. Philadelphia, PA: Lippincott Williams & Wilkins; 2006:5.
2. Mitra S, Sinatra RS. Perioperative management of acute pain in the opioid-dependent patient. *Anesthesiology*. 2004;101:212–227.
3. Parrillo, Dellinger: Severe heart failure. In: *Critical Care Medicine*. 3rd ed. 2007:1345.
4. Stoelting R, et al. Sympathomimetics. In: *Pharmacology and Physiology in Anesthetic Practice*. 4th Edition. Philadelphia, PA: Lippincott Williams & Wilkins; 2006:303.
5. Chestnut DH, et al. The influence of pH adjusted 2-chloroprocaine on the quality and duration of subsequent epidural bupivacaine analgesia during labor: A randomized, double blind study. *Anesthesiology*. 1989;70:437–441.

# 58.

# TERMINATION OF DRUG ACTION

*Nicholas M. Parker*

## INTRODUCTION

The primary process that allows the effects of a drug to wear off is removing the drug from the site of action. Removing a drug from the target tissue most often starts with removing the drug from the blood; this creates a concentration gradient that pulls the drug from the site of action back into the bloodstream. Removing a drug from the blood, however, is more complex. Pharmacodynamic factors such as irreversible inhibition, tolerance, and tachyphylaxis can also prolong a drug's effects. See Table 58.1 for examples of each mechanism discussed in this chapter.

## CHEMICAL CHANGE: BIOTRANSFORMATION

*Biotransformation* refers to enzymatic alteration of an active drug to an inactive metabolite.[1] None of the drug's atoms exits the body at this step, but the concentration of active drug steadily drops as it is converted to inactive forms. The enzyme family most often responsible for biotransformation is cytochrome P450 (CYP450), which oxidizes or reduces drug molecules in preparation for further metabolism and clearance. Other deactivation reactions include hydrolysis and conjugation.[1]

*Table 58.1* DRUG EXAMPLES WITH VARIOUS MECHANISMS LEADING TO TERMINATION OF ACTION

| DRUG | TYPICAL USE | FACTORS DETERMINING RATE OF TERMINATION OF ACTION |
|---|---|---|
| Ondansetron (Zofran®) | Antiemetic | Oxidation by CYP1A2, CYP2D6, and CYP3A4 in the liver |
| Hydromorphone (Dilaudid®) | Analgesic | Glucuronidation (a form of conjugation) in the liver |
| Remifentanil (Ultiva®) | Surgical anesthesia | Hydrolysis by tissue and plasma esterases |
| Atracurium (Tracrium®) | Paralytic | Hoffman elimination (non-enzymatic chemical degradation) in the tissue/plasma |
| Cefotaxime (Claforan®) | Antibiotic | Active secretion into urine by the OAT3 efflux pump in the kidneys |
| Vancomycin (Vancocin®) | Antibiotic | Passive glomerular filtration into the urine |
| Ursodiol (Actigall®) | Gallstone dissolution/prevention | Excreted into the bile; undergoes enterohepatic circulation; ultimately eliminated in the feces |
| Polyethylene glycol 3350 (Miralax®, GoLytely®) | Laxative/stool softener | Not absorbed from the gut; given enterally and eliminated in feces |
| Isoflurane (Forane®, Terrell®) | Surgical anesthesia | Eliminated as gas through the lungs |
| Fentanyl (Sublimaze®) | Analgesia, surgical anesthesia | Demethylated by CYP3A4 in the liver; context-sensitive half-time due to extensive accumulation in adipose tissue |

Reproduced with permission from *Lexicomp*. Wolters Kluwer; 2020. http://online.lexi.com. Accessed August 30, 2020.

Biotransformation occurs primarily in the liver, so blood flow through the liver may define the rate of biotransformation. Drugs that are tightly bound to serum proteins like albumin undergo slower biotransformation. Metabolic enzymes usually have excess capacity, so drug concentration will decay exponentially, and the familiar concept of half-life applies.[1] If the enzymes are saturated, however, decay becomes linear until no longer saturated (Figure 58.1).

Metabolism may also occur outside the liver—the gut and kidneys are also rich in CYP450 and other enzymes.[1] A few drugs are deactivated via hydrolysis by plasma or tissue esterases, which is usually a rapid process since the whole body's store of that drug can be degraded simultaneously without needing to travel to a specific organ. Some drugs decompose spontaneously through chemical reactions without help from enzymes.[2]

## ACTIVE REMOVAL: EFFLUX PUMPS

Another tactic the body employs to remove foreign molecules (i.e., drugs) is to pump them across membranes toward the two waste streams: urine and feces. Examples of these proteins are P-glycoprotein (P-gp), organic cation/anion transporters (OCTs and OATs), and multidrug resistance-associated proteins (MRPs).[1] These efflux pumps are present in the gut, liver, kidneys, and the blood-brain barrier and accelerate the termination of drug action by drawing the drug away from target tissues.

## PASSIVE REMOVAL: ELIMINATION

Drugs and drug metabolites eventually leave the body through the urine, stool, or exhaled breath. For the roughly 25% of drugs that do *not* undergo biotransformation, termination of action depends on this final elimination step.[1]

Renal elimination into the urine is the most common, and depends on adequate blood flow to the kidneys (as well as intrinsic kidney function). Since renal perfusion is very sensitive to hemodynamic changes, and hemodynamics may vary greatly during surgery, urine output must be

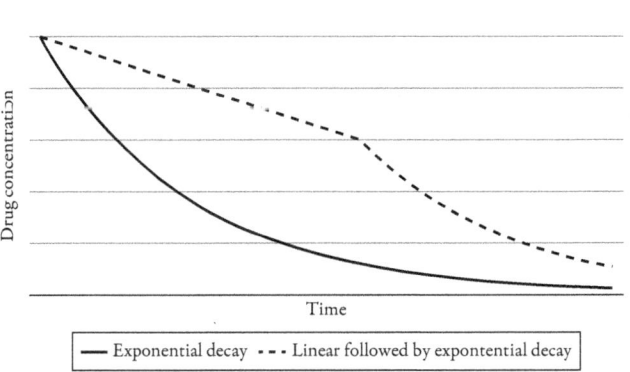

**Figure 58.1.** Comparison of drug clearance with excess enzyme capacity (solid line) resulting in exponential decay and saturated enzyme capacity (dashed line) resulting in linear decay followed by exponential decay.
Credit: Parker NM. 2020.

monitored closely when using drugs that rely on renal elimination for termination of action.

Enterally administered drugs may be eliminated through the stool because they were never absorbed in the first place; otherwise, drugs most often reach the stool via biliary excretion from the liver.[1,2] If drugs excreted in the bile are reabsorbed in the gut, this is known as enterohepatic cycling and will prolong the elimination of the drug.[1]

Inhaled anesthetics are unique in their elimination as gas exhaled through the lungs.[2] This type of elimination is quite reliable since it does not rely on biochemical activity and only on pulmonary blood flow and adequate ventilation.

## DISTRIBUTION AND THE CONTEXT-SENSITIVE HALF-TIME

One more variable may affect how quickly active drug is removed from the site of action: gradual accumulation of the drug in a reservoir, most often adipose tissue.[1] If a highly lipophilic drug is given only briefly, at the end of the infusion, the blood concentration will be greater than the adipose concentration. The drug will be removed from the blood using the previously described methods, but will simultaneously diffuse into the adipose tissue—in this case, the reservoir effect hastens the termination of action by helping to remove the drug from the blood.

However, after a prolonged infusion of the same drug, the reservoir can accumulate a substantial amount of drug before reaching equilibrium with the blood.[1,2] When the infusion is stopped, the reservoir will push the drug back into the bloodstream. This redistribution can profoundly extend the duration of a drug's effect. Drugs that behave in this way are said to have a context-sensitive half-time because the duration of action depends on the dose administered, dosing frequency, or duration of infusion, and the patient's body size and composition.[1,2]

## ANESTHETIC CONSIDERATIONS

### PREOPERATIVE

Review the patient's chart for organ dysfunction or use of medications that may increase or decrease the rate of metabolism of anesthetics.

### INTRAOPERATIVE

Maintain normal hemodynamics to allow adequate blood flow to the liver and kidneys. For drugs with a context-sensitive half-time, consider using bolus doses and titrate to effect, rather than prolonged continuous infusions.

### POSTOPERATIVE

Keep in mind that most reversal agents have a short duration of action, and could wear off before a drug reservoir is adequately depleted.

## REFERENCES

1. Rowland M, Tozer TN. *Clinical Pharmacokinetics and Pharmacodynamics*. 4th ed. Philadelphia, PA: Lippincott Williams & Wilkins; 2011.
2. *Lexicomp*. Wolters Kluwer; 2020. http://online.lexi.com. Accessed August 30, 2020.

# 59.

# IMPACT OF RENAL DISEASE

*Eileen Bui and Aladino De Ranieri*

## INTRODUCTION

Perioperative renal function is an important aspect to consider for anesthesiologists, as the kidneys are responsible for or are involved in a number of essential functions. These include solute regulation and transport, intravascular osmolality and water balance, excretion of the end products of metabolism and drugs, neurohumoral functions, hematopoiesis, and bone remodeling.[1-3]

## PREOPERATIVE CONSIDERATIONS

Preoperative renal function should be assessed to determine the cause and severity of disease as it may impact anesthetic management. Additionally, patients with preexisting renal insufficiency are at risk for acute kidney injury in the perioperative period. Kidney disease is a health problem globally, and in the United States, chronic kidney disease (CKD) affects approximately 10% of the population. Of those affected, there are three groups that require different preoperative preparation: those with functioning kidneys; those with end-stage renal disease on dialysis; and those with a transplanted kidney. Diagnostically, renal disease can also be categorized anatomically as prerenal disease, intrinsic renal disease, and postrenal disease.[3]

There are a few lab values that are considered the gold standards for the diagnosis and monitoring of kidney injury; they reflect glomerular filtration rate (GFR) and renal tubular function. GFR measures one of the key roles of the kidney. It can be measured provided a substance is freely filtered at the glomerulus and is neither reabsorbed nor secreted. An absolute GFR is generally not needed for most clinical settings and is time-consuming to obtain; thus an estimated GFR (eGFR) is used. Various equations exist to calculate eGFR based on the serum concentration of a filtration marker with other characteristics factored in, such as sex, weight, and ethnicity. Normal GFR is proportional to body surface area and is $>90$ mL/min/1.73 m$^2$, which in a healthy adult GFR is approximately 120 to 130 mL/min/1.73 m$^2$.

(1) Under steady-state conditions, creatinine (Cr) is the most reliable biomarker to calculate eGFR. Normal values are dependent on muscle mass and diet, and range from 0.6 to 1.0 mg/dL in women and 0.8 to 1.3 mg/dL in men.

(2) As it is independent of steady state and age, creatinine clearance from a 24-hour urine sample best correlates with GFR. Normal values for males are 107–139 mL/min and for females are 87–107 mL/min.

(3) Blood urea nitrogen (BUN) will be more likely to vary based on extrarenal factors including protein intake, gastrointestinal bleeding, catabolic states, malnutrition, and hypoperfusion. BUN concentrations greater than 50 mg/dL usually reflect a decreased GFR. Approximate normal values range from 7 to 20 mg/dL.

(4) Tests to evaluate renal tubular function and integrity examine urine concentrating ability through urine specific gravity, presense of persistent proteinuria, fractional excretion of urine sodium, and a urinalysis.

(5) Cystatin C is a relatively novel biomarker of GFR. It is produced at a constant rate by all nucleated cells and is freely filtered by the glomerulus and not secreted by the tubules. Its levels are less influenced by muscle mass when compared to Cr. Blood levels of cystatin C equilibrate faster than Cr and may be a more accurate measure of acute changes in kidney function.[2]

Kidney disease is classified according to duration, severity, cause, and prognosis. Acute kidney disease (AKD) is defined by duration of ≤3 months, which includes the subset of acute kidney injury (AKI) occurring ≤1 week. AKI is defined by any one of the following: increase in serum creatinine (SCr) by ≥0.3 mg/dl (≥26.5 μmol/l) within 48 hours; or increase in SCr to ≥1.5 times baseline, which is known or presumed to have occurred within the prior 7 days; or urine volume < 0.5 ml/kg/h for 6 hours. Based on the Kidney Disease Improving Global Outcomes guidelines, severity is then staged based on SCr and urine output. Duration of kidney disease longer than 3 months is then defined as chronic kidney disease.[4]

Kidney disease is most easily categorized by anatomical etiology as prerenal, intrinsic renal, or postrenal. Intrinsic disease is then subcategorized according to the site of injury: glomerular, tubular, interstitial, and vascular. A few common causes of kidney diseases in each category include: intrarenal vasoconstriction from nonsteroidal anti-inflammatory drugs/angiotensin-converting enzyme inhibitors; systemic vasodilation from sepsis; volume depletion; glomerulonephritis; tubular necrosis; interstitial nephritis from nephrotoxic medications; renal atheroembolic disease; and prostatic hypertrophy.

Important pathophysiological manifestations of chronic renal failure to consider include hypervolemia, acidemia, hyperkalemia, hypertension, pulmonary edema, restrictive pulmonary dysfunction, and anemia.

## INTRAOPERATIVE CONSIDERATIONS

A simple and traditional evaluation of intraoperative (and postoperative) kidney function in the absence of laboratory studies is the measurement of urine output (UOP). While low urine output is an indicator used by many anesthesiologists to prompt intravenous fluid administration, perioperative low UOP is not always associated with renal failure. Oliguria, defined as output <0.5 mL/kg/h, in the perioperative period is a common appropriate response to hypovolemia or surgical stress. It is not necessarily associated with postoperative renal dysfunction, especially without other signs of hypoperfusion. Intraoperative oliguria is typically transient and should resolve when arterial blood pressure and intravascular volume are restored to normal levels. Anuria would likely be caused by a postrenal obstruction and can be caused by obstruction of an indwelling catheter or from the surgical field.[3]

A small change in UOP itself is not an independent risk factor for mortality, unlike a change serum creatinine indicating AKI. Thus, maintenance of hemodynamics and prevention of intraoperative hypotension can reduce the incidence of AKI. A retrospective study found that the odds of developing AKI increased greatly as the duration increased with a mean arterial pressure (MAP) less than 55 mmHg.[5]

Careful consideration of anesthetic pharmacology must be taken in patients with renal failure as they are at a higher risk for adverse drug reactions. Patients with renal azotemia can have excessive pharmacological drug effects due to uremic-induced physiologic changes in the tissue. Additionally, accumulation of drugs and their metabolites can occur for those that rely on renal excretion for elimination.

*Table 59.1* MEDICATIONS WITH PROLONGED AFFECTS IN RENAL DYSFUNCTION

| CLASS | MEDICATIONS (ACCUMULATED METABOLITES) |
| --- | --- |
| Opioids | Morphine (Morphine-6-glucuronide) |
| | Meperidine (Normeperidine) |
| | Hydromorphone (Hydromorphone-3-glucuronide) |
| | Pancuronium |
| | Vecuronium |
| | Rocuronium |
| Muscle Relaxants and Antagonists | Mivacurium |
| | Neostigmine |
| | Pyridostigmine |
| | Edrophonium |
| | Sugammadex-neuromuscular blocker complex |
| Vasopressors and Antihypertensives | Thiazide diuretics |
| | Furosemide |
| | Hydralazine |

Lipid insoluble drugs or drugs that are highly ionized in physiologic pH are eliminated unchanged in urine. For these drugs and others, effects can be prolonged due to accumulation of the drug (Table 59.1). Some neuromuscular blockers, cholinesterase inhibitors, and many antibiotics fall into this category and the action of these drugs can be prolonged secondary to impaired excretion. Although hydromorphone has an active metabolite that can accumulate, with monitoring it can be used with an adjusted dose.[1,3]

In contrast, the termination of action of most anesthetic drugs does not depend on renal excretion; this is accomplished by redistribution and metabolism and later excretion in the urine in a water-soluble, polar form of the parent compound. Thus, drugs are not dependent on renal function for termination of effect (Table 59.2). Examples of such medications include most narcotics (fentanyl and its derivatives), barbituates, phenothiazines, antipsychotics, butyrophenone derivatives, benzodiazepines, ketamine, and local anesthetics. Special consideration should be taken despite route of metabolism for drugs that are affected by uremia or decreased enzyme activity; for short-acting barbituates, thiopental and methohexital, the concentration of protein binding can be reduced, which allows

**Table 59.2** MEDICATIONS NOT DEPENDENT ON RENAL FUNCTION FOR TERMINATION OF EFFECT

| CLASS | MEDICATIONS |
|---|---|
| Inhaled Anesthetics | Sevoflurane |
| | Desflurane |
| | Isoflurane |
| Opioids | Fentanyl |
| | Sufentanil |
| | Remifentanil |
| Intravenous Anesthetics | Barbituates: Thiopental, Methohexital |
| | Propofol |
| Muscle Relaxants and Antagonists | Succinylcholine |
| | Atracurium |
| | Cisatracurium |
| Vasopressors and Antihypertensives | Phenylephrine |
| | Propanolol |
| | Esmolol |
| | Labetalol |
| | Nifedipine |
| | Verapamil |
| | Diltiazem |
| | Nitroglycerine |

for a higher free fraction of drug. While benzodiazepines are metabolized by the liver, long-acting benzodiazepines such as diazepam can accumulate and thus dosing should be reduced. Mivacurium metabolism is reduced due to decreased plasma pseudocholinesterase activity associated with uremia and hemodialysis.

## POSTOPERATIVE CONSIDERATIONS

The etiologies of postoperative renal dysfunction can be again broken down into the anatomical prerenal, intrarenal, and postrenal causes (due to obstruction of an indwelling catheter or intraoperative surgical injury). Typically, postoperative renal injury is due to an intraoperative exacerbation of preexisting kidney insufficiency. In the postanesthesia care unit (PACU), oliguria will be an early sign of renal dysfunction. The most common cause of oliguria is due to hypovolemia. Other prerenal causes are due to hepatorenal syndrome, low cardiac output, renal vascular obstruction, and intra-abdominal hypertension (abdominal compartment syndrome). Intrarenal etiologies include ischemia, hemolysis, tumor lysis, contrast nephropathy (patients who have undergone angiography), and rhabdomyolysis (from crush or thermal injury).

Postoperative urinary retention must be ruled out in the differential for oliguria. Ultrasonography can be used to measure bladder volume to diagnose urinary retention.

In patients with preexisting renal disease, again, pharmacology of neuromuscular blocking agents must be considered. Upper airway obstruction in the PACU may be due to residual neuromuscular blockade. Renal failure is among the many factors that contribute to prolonged blockade.

## REFERENCES

1. Miller RD, et al. *Basics of Anesthesia*. 6th ed. Philadelphia, PA: Elsevier/Saunders; 2011.
2. Stoelting RK, Dierdorf SF. *Handbook for Anesthesia and Co-existing Disease*. New York, NY: Churchill Livingstone; 1993.
3. Gropper MA. *Miller's Anesthesia*. 9th ed. Philadelphia, PA: Elsevier; 2019.
4. Yu AS. *Brenner & Rector's The Kidney*. 11th ed. St. Louis, MO: Elsevier; 2019.
5. Walsh M, et al. Relationship between intraoperative mean arterial pressure and clinical outcomes after noncardiac surgery: Toward an empirical definition of hypotension. *Anesthesiology*. 2013;119:507–515.

# 60.

# IMPACT OF HEPATIC DISEASE

*Muhammad Haseeb Zubair and Aladino De Ranieri*

## INTRODUCTION

The liver is involved in drug and glucose metabolism, protein synthesis, and production of coagulation factors. Consequently, screening for liver disease is of paramount importance. Preoperative history and physical examination findings should include alcohol and illicit drug use, transfusion history, sexual history, ascites, hemolysis, hemoptysis, cirrhosis and presence of jaundice, spider angiomata, and palmer erythematic. Laboratory studies include PT/INR, liver function tests, albumin, pre-albumin, LDH, direct and indirect bilirubin, and in special cases genetic testing for anti-trypsin deficiency and Wilson's disease. The spectrum of liver dysfunction ranges from fatty liver disease to cirrhosis. The preoperative optimization depends upon severity of the liver disease, nature of surgery, timing of surgery, and presence of other comorbidities. Since most surgeries are elective, there is sufficient time available for medical optimization.

Elective surgery is contraindicated in the following population: acute hepatitis, acute liver failure, alcoholic hepatitis. Patients with chronic liver disease including hepatitis pose a significant risk and should be medically optimized, especially with biopsy-proven portal hypertension and multi-lobular necrosis.[1] Child Pugh score previously and model of end stage liver disease (MELD) score recently have shown prognostic value in liver surgery.[2] The acute physiology and chronic health evaluation (APACHE) score can be used predict survival in intensive care unit (ICU) patients with existing cirrhosis.[3]

## DRUG METABOLISM AND INTERACTIONS

The hepatic system is responsible for the selective uptake, concentration, metabolism, and excretion of majority of the drugs by the body. Drug metabolites are mostly responsible for their effects. The compounds undergo the extensive process and ultimately are processed by a variety of soluble, membrane-bound enzymes. Every class of drug has its own biotransformation pathway involving one or multiple enzyme systems. Alcohol has also been shown to alter the pathways of drug metabolism. Most of the drugs absorbed from the gastrointestinal tract are water insoluble or lipophilic and undergo a biotransformation to be water-soluble compounds that can be easily excreted. Exogenous products are hepatic ally metabolized predominantly through two mechanisms: phase I and phase II reactions.

## PHASE I REACTIONS

Phase I reactions transform lipophilic molecules into more polar, hydrophilic molecules via oxidation, reduction, or hydrolysis which is catalyzed by the membrane-bound cytochrome P450 superfamily of mixed-function oxidases (CYP), which consist of apoprotein and a heme prosthetic group which function as an oxidizing center. Enzyme inducers are substances that stimulate the synthesis of additional enzyme, increase clearance of anesthetic medications, decrease their half-life, and decrease plasma levels. Examples include tobacco smoke, ethanol, barbiturates, phenytoin, rifampin, carbamazepine. Enzyme inhibitors compete for the binding site on an enzyme, decrease the clearance, increase the half-life, and increase plasma levels. Examples include SSRIs, grapefruit juice, omeprazole, isoniazid, erythromycin, ketoconazole, and cimetidine.

The following is the list of common CYP isoforms and their *inducers* and *inhibitors*.

**CYP3A4**: Metabolizes acetaminophen, alfentanyl, dexamethasone, fentanyl, lidocaine, methadone, midazolam, sufentanyl.
*Inducers*: Rifampin, rifabutin, tamoxifen, carbamazepine, barbiturates, St. John's wort.
*Inhibitors*: Grapefruit juice, anti-fungal, protease inhibitors, mycin, and SSRI.
**CYP2B6**: Propofol, verapamil, seligelline, bupropion, ketamine, etc.

*Inducers*: Phenytoin, phenobarbital, rifampicin, and carbamazepine.

*Inhibitors*: Ketaconazole, fluoxetine, sertraline.

**CYP2D6**: Codeine, tramadol, fluoxetine, hydrocodone, mirtazapine.

*Inducers*: Glutethemide, rifampicin, dexamethasone.

*Inhibitors*: SSRI, quinidine, ritonavir, and cannabinoids.

**CYP2C19**: TCAs, SSRIs, bupropion, diazepam, PPIs, clopidogrel, warfarin, and progesterone.

*Inducers*: Rifampin, carbamazepine, prednisone, aspirin in low doses.

*Inhibitors*: fluconazole, fluvoxamine, and ticlopidine.

## INHALATION AGENTS AND METABOLISM

Less than 5% of inhaled anesthetic is metabolized by the body, and the elimination is through the alveolus. Methoxyflurane is an exception, which is metabolized by enzymatic transformation. Small doses of opioids result in marked reduction in the minimum alveolar concentration (MAC) values of volatile anesthetic. That will prevent a purposeful response in 50% of the population at skin incision. Further increases in opioid concentration may produce a ceiling effect. Benzodiazepines have been known to induce cytochrome oxidase systems and to synergistically work with inhalation agents.

## PHASE II REACTIONS

Phase II reactions occur either directly with a parent compound (rare) or with a metabolite formed by a phase I reaction. These reactions conjugate the drug or metabolic byproducts to polar molecules such as glucoronate, sulfate, acetate, glycine, glutathione, or a methyl group. Mostly, phase II reactions result in the formation of readily excreted, nontoxic substances.[10] Phase II reactions occur predominantly within the hepatocyte cytoplasm via the uridine diphospho (UDP)-glucuronyl transferases (UGT), sulfotransferases, and glutathione S-transferases. Conjugation mostly leads to a decrease in pharmacologic activity with enhanced clearance of the compound (e.g., acetaminophen, furosemide, and bilirubin), and these enzymes are rarely responsible for toxic metabolite formation. However, exceptions do occur. In some cases, conjugation leads to increased pharmacologic activity. For example, glucuronidation of morphine leads to increased analgesic potency, and sulfation of minoxidil is required for its antihypertensive effect. Lorazepam is also metabolized by phase II reactions.

## PHASE III: FURTHER MODIFICATION AND EXCRETION

After phase II reactions, the xenobiotic conjugates may be further metabolized. A common example is the processing of glutathione conjugates to acetyl cysteine (mercapturic acid) conjugates.

## REFERENCES

1. Hargrove MD Jr. Chronic active hepatitis: Possible adverse effect of exploratory laparotomy. *Surgery*. 1970;68:771.
2. O'Leary JG, Friedman LS. Predicting surgical risk in patients with cirrhosis: From art to science. *Gastroenterology*. 2007;132:1609.
3. Zimmerman JE, et al. Intensive care unit admissions with cirrhosis: Risk-stratifying patient groups and predicting individual survival. *Hepatology*. 1996;23:1393.
4. Nelson DR, et al. The P450 superfamily: Update on new sequences, gene mapping, accession numbers, early trivial names of enzymes, and nomenclature. *DNA Cell Biol*. 1993;12(1):1.

# 61.

# DRUG INTERACTIONS

*Michelle A. Carroll Turpin and Elyse M. Cornett*

## INTRODUCTION

The nature of drug interactions can be categorized in three ways: pharmacodynamic, pharmacokinetic, or pharmaceutical. Pharmacodynamic and pharmacokinetic interactions are related to the pharmacological properties of the drugs and occur within the body. Pharmaceutical interactions are due to the chemical or physical properties of the drugs and occur outside the body.

## PHARMACODYNAMIC INTERACTIONS

Pharmacodynamic interactions refer to an agent's site of activity. Thus, the most straightforward pharmacodynamic drug interaction occurs when two agents bind the same site and so each impacts the other's inability to elicit, or block, a response. This relationship is most obvious when administering both an agonist and an antagonist for the same receptor, such as when the opioid antagonist naloxone is administered to reverse the effects of acute opioid overdose. Similarly, drugs that act at different sites may alter the action of the other, depending on how the affected signal transduction pathways interact with one another. During the reversal of neuromuscular blockade, an anti-acetylcholinesterase such as neostigmine will increase desired acetylcholine action at nicotinic receptors. Meanwhile, unwanted muscarinic receptor activation can be avoided by the coadministration of a selective muscarinic antagonist, such as glycopyrrolate.

Pharmacodynamic drug interactions can produce synergetic responses that can have therapeutic benefits. *Synergism* occurs when the response produced by the combination of two drugs is more than the expected if both responses were simply added together. This can be very useful in the clinical setting, as synergism typically allows for the doses of the individual medications to be reduced, thus decreasing the side effect profile. For example, the combination of the benzodiazepine midazolam with intravenous agents such as thiopentone or propofol produces desired sedative and anesthetic effects at doses significantly lower than would

be necessary if either agent were used alone. Generally, intravenous (IV) anesthetics (except ketamine) display synergy when combined with other IV anesthetics (that act at different sites), or inhaled anesthetics. However, inhaled anesthetics do not demonstrate synergism with one another.

When the elicited response is equal to the expected sum, it is referred to as an *additive response*, such as that which occurs with nitrous oxide and volatile inhaled anesthetics. The combination of a 50% minimum alveolar concentration (MAC) of each will produce an anesthetic effect equal to that which could be generated by 100% MAC of either agent alone.

## PHARMACOKINETIC INTERACTIONS

Pharmacokinetic interactions occur when one agent influences the absorption, distribution, metabolism, and/or elimination of another agent.

### ABSORPTION

Intravenous administration bypasses the challenges of absorption by introducing the agent directly to the bloodstream. Otherwise, a drug must leave its site of administration and pass through at least one barrier to enter the circulation.

The absorption of orally administered medications is often dependent on the pH of the gastrointestinal tract. Weak acids are easily absorbed in strongly acidic environments; similarly, weak bases are absorbed in strongly basic environments. Thus, agents that change gastric pH, such as antacids and proton pump inhibitors, can alter absorption. Food can also influence gastric pH. Drugs that are to be taken on an empty stomach are often those better absorbed in low pH.

Other agents alter gastric motility, which can also impact absorption. Agents that enhance gastric motility, such as the antiemetic metoclopramide, can hinder absorption of other agents present in the gastrointestinal (GI) tract because they are moved through too quickly and do not have adequate time to be absorbed. Conversely, when gastric motility is slowed, such as that which occurs as a side effect of opioid medications, drugs remain within the GI tract for an extended period of time, allowing for increased absorption.

The absorption of some agents is related to transmembrane p-glycoprotein (also known as multidrug resistance protein, or MDR1) efflux activity. P-glycoprotein is expressed in numerous tissues throughout the body and plays a protective role by reducing intestinal absorption and enhancing excretion of drugs. A wide variety of medications and/or metabolites are substrates of p-glycoprotein and can compete with one another for binding to the transporter, in addition to being affected by agents that can inhibit or induce transporter activity. Medications which inhibit p-glycoprotein activity, such as amiodarone, atorvastatin, captopril, carvedilol, diltiazem, lovastatin, macrolide antibiotics, meperidine, methadone, propafenone, quercetin, ranolazine, ritonavir, tamoxifen, ticagrelor, and verapamil, slow removal from the GI tract and reduce excretion, increasing the likelihood that any agents present will be absorbed. Alternatively, drugs which stimulate p-glycoprotein activity, such as carbamazepine, morphine, phenobarbital, phenytoin, prazosin, rifampin, and St. John's wort, reduce the absorption rates of some drugs and hasten the rate of excretion.

Agents can also impact the absorption of other agents if the two form a complex when combined. Often the product of such an interaction is poorly absorbed when compared to the individual agents. This type of interaction is the basis of the use of activated charcoal in some cases of drug overdose. Activated charcoal adsorbs to some agents, such as barbiturates, producing a complex that is not easily absorbed, thereby accelerating excretion.

Finally, interactions influencing absorption are not confined to the GI tract. Absorption of an inhaled agent can be hastened by the presence of the second agent. Known as the "second gas effect," this occurs when the first agent quickly passes from the lungs to the bloodstream, causing the concentration of the second gas to rise quickly in the alveoli. This in turn, results in rapid absorption of the second agent.

## DISTRIBUTION

Once a drug is absorbed, it is distributed throughout the body via the circulation. A major factor governing distribution is protein binding in the plasma or tissue. Only unbound drug is capable of exerting pharmacological effects. Some agents are highly protein bound, leaving a comparatively small proportion of drug available to bind its therapeutic target. If multiple highly protein-bound agents are administered concurrently they will compete for protein binding, resulting in a relative increase in the unbound proportion of each, leading to increasing pharmacological activity. This interaction is often most apparent

following the addition or removal of a drug from a treatment regimen.

Changes in blood flow also impact distribution. Vasoconstriction will slow distribution, while vasodilation can enhance it. This is particularly pertinent with the administration of subcutaneous and intramuscular injection, as local vasoconstriction will slow the dispersion from the injection site. This can be very useful when administering local anesthesia; vasoconstriction induced by epinephrine will help prolong therapeutic action at the site of application.

Despite receiving generous blood flow, the distribution of drugs into the central nervous system (CNS) is limited by the blood-brain barrier (BBB). The p-glycoprotein transporter, mentioned earlier, provides additional protection to the CNS by actively pumping drugs out. Inhibition or blockade of this transport can allow for enhanced CNS distribution of p-glycoprotein substrates, such as is the case with the anti-diarrheal agent loperamide. Although it is a potent opioid, loperamide does not produce any CNS effects at usual doses due to its high affinity to p-glycoprotein, which prevents it from crossing the BBB. Combination with strong p-glycoprotein inhibitors has the potential to produce opioid-related side effects, such as respiratory depression.

## METABOLISM

Drug metabolism in particular is a common point at which interactions occur. Inhibition or induction of drug metabolism may occur incidentally or be an intentional part of a treatment regimen.

Because the majority of drug metabolism occurs in the liver, hepatic blood flow is a factor in determining the metabolic rate of many agents, especially those subject to extensive first-pass metabolism, such as lidocaine. Most anesthetics cause a reduction in hepatic blood flow, as a result of decreased cardiac output. Reduced hepatic blood flow slows the delivery of drugs to the liver, which in turn slows drug metabolism, without directly impacting metabolic enzymes.

Metabolic enzymes are the source of most metabolism-related drug interactions, which are caused by the ability of certain agents to induce or inhibit enzyme activity, and/or compete for binding. Cytochrome P450 (CYP450) enzymes are responsible for the vast majority of all oxidative biotransformation of xenobiotics—including drugs—and about 90% of therapeutic agents are subjected to CYP450 metabolism.[1] Thus, any changes in CYP450 activity mediated by one agent will impact the metabolism of any other agents present that are CYP450 substrates. Those CYP450 enzymes most often involved in drug metabolism are listed in Table 61.1 with notable substrates, inhibitors, and inducers.

The isoforms CYP3A4 and CYP2D6 in particular mediate the metabolism of over half of all clinically relevant

**Table 61.1** NOTABLE SUBSTRATES, INHIBITORS, AND INDUCERS OF CYP450 ENZYMES TYPICALLY INVOLVED WITH DRUG METABOLISM

| CYTOCHROME P450 | NOTABLE SUBSTRATES | NOTABLE INHIBITORS | NOTABLE INDUCERS |
|---|---|---|---|
| CYP1A2 | Caffeine, clozapine, haloperidol, R-warfarin, theophylline, tizanidine | Amiodarone, cimetidine, ciprofloxacin, fluvoxamine | Barbiturates, carbamazepine, omeprazole, rifampin, phenytoin, tobacco |
| CYP2B6 | Bupropion, diazepam, ketamine, lidocaine, methadone, methobarbital, midazolam, pentobarbital, propofol, selegiline, sevoflurane, valproic acid | Clopidogrel, ticlopidine | Carbamazepine, rifampin |
| CYP2C9 | Carvedilol, celecoxib, diclofenac, fluvastatin, glipizide, ibuprofen, losartan, naproxen, phenytoin, S-warfarin | Amiodarone, "azole" antifungals, fluoxetine, ritonavir | Carbamazepine, phenobarbital, rifampin |
| CYP2D6 | Amitriptyline, carvedilol, codeine, desipramine, dextromethorphan, fluoxetine, haloperidol, metoprolol, oxycodone, propafenone, risperidone, tramadol | Bupropion, cimetidine, diphenhydramine, fluoxetine, mirabegron, terbinafine | None of significance |
| CYP3A4 & 3A5 | Alfentanil, alprazolam, amlodipine, atorvastatin, carbamazepine, cyclosporin, diazepam, estradiol, fentanyl, lidocaine, midazolam, nifedipine, propofol, sildenafil, simvastatin, sufentanil, tadalafil, ticagrelor, zolpidem | "Azole" antifungals, diltiazem, grapefruit juice, HIV protease inhibitors, macrolide antibiotics, propofol, verapamil | Barbiturates, carbamazepine, glucocorticoids, St. John's wort, phenobarbital, phenytoin, rifampin |

agents, which makes it not unlikely that two or more substrates for CYP3A4 and/or CYP2D6 might be present in a drug regimen. In such a case where multiple agents are substrates for the same enzymes, competition for binding would negatively impact the metabolic rate of all agents. This nature of interaction is particularly relevant when using opioid analgesics; for example, fentanyl, alfentanil, sufentanil, and methadone are all metabolized by CYP3A4. These agents have the potential to interfere with each other's metabolism or to be influenced by additional medications the patient may be taking which themselves are substrates for the same enzymes.

Not all drugs may bind an enzyme at the same site. Some agents may inhibit an enzyme, not by competing for the same binding site as another agent, but by binding an alternative, allosteric site. Allosteric binding initiates a conformational change of the enzyme protein which alters the active site, preventing a substrate from binding.

Some drug-enzyme interactions result in irreversible binding, rendering the enzyme unable to facilitate any further metabolic reactions. The synthesis of new enzyme proteins is often necessary to overcome the effects of irreversible binding.

Beyond binding, drugs can inhibit enzyme activity in other ways. Gene transcription and/or protein enzyme translation may be downregulated. Alternatively, the rate of enzyme degradation or turnover may increase.

Rarely, an agent has a particular affinity for an enzyme-substrate complex and will bind, interfering with the creation and/or release of the product.

In all instances of inhibition, there is less enzyme present capable of facilitating metabolism. In most cases, metabolism terminates pharmacological activity, so enzyme inhibition would prolong the presence of active drug and potentially lead to toxic side effects.

Enzyme activity can be induced as well. Gene transcription may be upregulated and/or enzyme protein translation stimulated. Alternatively, the rate of enzyme degradation or turnover may be decreased. In either case, the result is more enzyme available, leading to increased drug metabolism. In most cases, an uptick in metabolic enzyme activity will reduce the amount of therapeutically available drug. However, sometimes, Phase I metabolism is responsible for the transformation of an inactive prodrug to a pharmacologically active product, or, rarely, may produce a reactive or toxic intermediate. If metabolism is stimulated, the production of intermediate compounds might outpace subsequent downstream metabolic processes, causing a buildup of intermediates that may be responsible for producing adverse side effects.

## EXCRETION

Most drugs and/or their metabolites are excreted from the body in the urine or bile. The resulting products of most metabolic processes are more hydrophilic than their parent compounds, to more easily facilitate water solubility and, ultimately, renal elimination. Water solubility is also dependent upon ionization, thus the pH in the lumen of the collecting duct influences how much drug/metabolite is eliminated. Basic urine pH means weak acids, such as barbiturates, will be ionized upon entering the collecting duct, preventing them from returning to the surrounding tissue. Thus, an increase in urine pH will result in enhanced excretion of weakly acidic agents.

Some agents impact renal elimination of other agents by impairing renal function. For example, the major route of elimination for the nondepolarizing neuromuscular blocking drugs (NMBDs) doxacurium, pancuronium, and pipecuronium is via the kidneys; thus these agents are contraindicated in cases of renal dysfunction and should not be used with agents known to cause nephrotoxicity, such as aminoglycoside antibiotics.

In the case of biliary excretion, some drugs that arrive in the liver end up in the bile, as in the case of the NMBDs vecuronium and rocuronium, and are delivered to the GI tract, to be subsequently removed from the body. Liver dysfunction or extrahepatic biliary obstruction can impede this route of elimination.

Inhaled agents are excreted primarily via the lungs. Therefore, drugs that alter cardiac output or respiratory rate can impact this route of elimination. Opioids, benzodiazepines, and other depressants will slow the elimination of inhaled anesthetics in a spontaneously breathing patient due to their negative effects on respiration and heart rate.

## PHARMACEUTICAL INTERACTIONS

Pharmaceutical interactions are not related to the pharmacological properties of the interacting drugs but are the result of chemical or physical incompatibilities. This is a particularly significant consideration in intravenous drug administration, where the combination of agents could result in the formation of a precipitate, or an agent(s) may adsorb to the IV materials. For example, the combination of thiopentone and NMBDs can result in a crystalline precipitate in the IV line, with the most precipitate produced by rocuronium.[2]

Sometimes, a chemical interaction may occur that produces a toxic product, such as what can occur when the halogenated anesthetics desflurane, isoflurane, and enflurane interact with barium hydroxide lime or soda lime to produce carbon monoxide.

## REFERENCES

1. Lynch T, Price A. The effect of cytochrome P450 metabolism on drug response, interactions, and adverse effects. *Am Fam Physician.* 2007;76(3):391–396.
2. Torri G, et al. Interazioni tra calce sodata ed anestetici alogenati [Interaction of soda lime and halogenated anesthetics]. *Minerva Anestesiol.* 1997;63(5):159–165.

# 62.

# HEPATIC BLOOD FLOW

*Courtney R. Jones*

## INTRODUCTION

The liver is a highly vascular organ and receives 20%–25% of the cardiac output under normal circumstances. This equates to approximately 1500 mL of blood that flows through the liver every minute in a healthy individual. Seventy-five percent of the hepatic blood flow originates in the portal vein, with the remaining 25% coming from the hepatic artery.[1] The portal vein drains blood from the stomach, intestines, spleen, pancreas, and visceral fat and then flows into the liver.[2] The common hepatic artery arises from the celiac trunk off the aorta and continues as the proper hepatic artery before branching into the right hepatic artery and the left hepatic artery, supplying the right and left lobe of the liver, respectively. Fifty-five percent of the liver's oxygen needs are supplied by the portal vein, with the remaining oxygen coming from the hepatic artery.[3]

In a healthy liver, blood circulates through a low resistance system in the vascular bed. The portal vein has the highest pressure in the healthy liver, which directs flow through a vascular network with progressive drops in pressure back to the right atrium. The physiologic flow through the liver is from the portal vein, to the hepatic sinusoids, to the hepatic veins, back to the inferior vena cava, and then ultimately to the right atrium.[1]

The hepatic venous pressure gradient (HVPD) is defined as the pressure difference between the portal vein and the hepatic veins and is normally 1–5 mmHg. In portal hypertension, the pressure gradient increases to greater than 10–12 mmHg. Higher pressure gradients will cause more significant portosystemic shunting.[1]

## HEPATIC ARTERIAL BUFFER RESPONSE

Although the hepatic artery contribution to hepatic blood flow is relatively minor, it has important implications for drug metabolism and for the synthetic function of the liver. Portal venous flow and hepatic arterial flow exist in a reciprocal relationship in order to maintain constant hepatic blood flow: when portal flow decreases, the hepatic arterial flow increases; and when the portal flow increases, the hepatic arterial flow decreases through modulation in hepatic arterial tone. Portal flow does not modulate based on the hepatic artery flow, however. This physiologic adaptation is known as the hepatic arterial buffer response.[1]

Unlike other organs, the liver does not appear to respond to changes in $pO_2$ or $pCO_2$ to modulate the arterial tone. Hepatic arterial tone is instead regulated by adenosine through its vasodilatory effects.[1] Smooth muscle and other tissue in the space of Mall produce adenosine at nearly constant levels, allowing it to modulate local blood flow.[1,2] When portal venous flow increases, it dilutes the adenosine, which then results in less hepatic arterial vasodilation and ultimately less hepatic artery blood flow. This same principle works in reverse; when portal venous flow decreases, there is less washout of locally produced adenosine with subsequent hepatic artery vasodilation and increased hepatic artery blood flow.[1]

## OTHER MECHANISMS FOR MAINTAINING HEPATIC BLOOD FLOW

The liver has several other acute and chronic adaptations to maintain a steady rate of hepatic blood flow. The liver provides a large reservoir of blood for the body as a result of its high capacitance and compliant vessels. One mechanism for maintaining hepatic blood flow is by increasing cardiac preload when the portal flow decreases; the decrease flow leads to lower intrahepatic pressure and subsequent emptying of the hepatic blood into the inferior vena cava. This increases preload and subsequently cardiac output. A higher cardiac output increases flow to the splanchnic arteries that then lead to higher portal flow to the liver.[2]

An additional mechanism the liver uses to maintain hepatic blood flow is the hepatorenal reflex. When portal blood flow decreases and adenosine accumulates, it also initiates the hepatorenal reflex via hepatic sensory nerves in addition to the hepatic arterial buffer response. This reflex rapidly results in fluid retention by increasing sodium reabsorption and decreasing urine production, which then causes a higher circulating blood volume → higher preload → higher cardiac output → increased splanchnic artery flow → increased portal flow.[2]

The preceding mechanisms are rapid adaptations the liver has in place to modulate hepatic flow, but the liver also has chronic adaptations. The liver will adjust the mass of the hepatocytes to match the average hepatic blood flow over time through hepatocyte proliferation or apoptosis.[2]

## SPECIAL OPERATIVE CIRCUMSTANCE

### ANESTHETICS

All inhaled anesthetics can decrease the hepatic blood flow, but the older anesthetic halothane has the greatest decrease on the hepatic blood flow. Propofol increases hepatic blood flow, ketamine has little effect, and barbiturates can decrease hepatic blood flow. Spinal, epidural, and general anesthesia can also decrease hepatic blood flow, but it is generally mediated through hypotension and reduced cardiac output.[3]

### LIVER TRANSPLANTATION

Liver transplantation presents a unique circumstance in which the understanding of hepatic blood flow is important. Excessive portal blood flow in a newly transplanted liver can cause hepatic congestion, shear stress, graft dysfunction, and reduced hepatic arterial flow. This effect can be more pronounced in living donor liver transplants, split liver transplants, or grafts that are relatively small for the size of the recipient. Techniques to reduce portal blood flow in these situations and improve graft outcome include splenic artery ligation, portocaval shunt, and splenectomy.[4]

## REFERENCES

1. Wagener G. *Liver Anesthesiology and Critical Care Medicine*. New York, NY: Springer Science; 2012.
2. Lautt WW. Regulatory processes interacting to maintain hepatic blood flow constancy: Vascular compliance, hepatic arterial buffer response, hepatorenal reflex, liver regeneration, escape from vasoconstriction. *Hepatol Res*. 2007;37(11):891–903.
3. Morgan GE, et al. *Clinical Anesthesiology*. New York, NY: Lange Medical Books/McGraw Hill Medical; 2006.
4. Yoshizumi T, Mori M. Correction to: Portal flow modulation in living donor liver transplantation: Review with a focus on splenectomy. *Surg Today*. 2020 Apr;50(4):423]. Erratum for: *Surg Today*. 2020;50(1):21–29.

# 63.

# DRUG-DRUG BINDING

*John Ozinga and Nebojsa Nick Knezevic*

## INTRODUCTION

Understanding the concepts of drug-drug binding is an essential part of anesthesia practice. By understanding these concepts, anesthesiologists can better predict adverse medication effects and provide a better quality of anesthesia care.[1]

## DRUG-DRUG BINDING BASIC PHARMACOLOGIC DEFINITIONS AND PRINCIPLES

- An **agonist** is a medication that mimics the action of the signal ligand by binding to and activating a receptor.
- An **inverse agonist** produces an effect opposite to that of an agonist, yet binds to the same receptor binding site as an agonist.
- A **partial agonist** has lower efficacy than a full agonist. It cannot produce the maximal response, irrespective of the concentration applied, therefore produces submaximal activation even when occupying the total receptor population. By binding to one of the receptor's secondary sites, a partial agonist has the same effect as the main drug, although with a lower intensity (e.g., buprenorphine is an opioid partial agonist that has less of an effect on the μ receptors than a pure opioid agonist like morphine) (Figure 63.1).
- An **antagonist** is a medication that typically binds to a receptor without activating them, but instead decreases the receptor's ability to be activated by an agonist.
- A **competitive antagonist** binds to the same site as the agonist but does not activate it, thus blocking the agonist's action. The amount of antagonist or main drug that binds with the receptor depends on the concentrations of each one in the plasma.
- A **noncompetitive antagonist** binds to an allosteric (non-agonist) secondary site on the receptor to prevent activation of the receptor. Since the noncompetitive agonist binds to a secondary site, binding of the agonist

to the primary site of the receptor will no longer cause a response, and increasing the concentration of the agonist will not cause a physiologic effect.
- A **reversible antagonist** binds noncovalently to the receptor and can therefore have its effect diminished by competing ligands or by increasing the concentration of the agonist.
- An **irreversible antagonist** binds covalently to the receptor and cannot be displaced by either competing ligands or increasing the concentration of the agonist.
- An **allosteric modulation** is a drug that binds to a receptor at a site distinct from the active site. It induces a conformational change in the receptor, which alters the affinity of the receptor for the endogenous ligand. Positive allosteric modulators increase the affinity, while *negative allosteric modulators* decrease the affinity.

As an anesthesia clinical example, benzodiazepine binding acts as a positive allosteric modulator by increasing the total conduction of chloride ions across the neuronal cell membrane when gamma-aminobutyric acid (GABA) is bound to its receptor. This increased chloride ion influx hyperpolarizes the neuron's membrane potential.

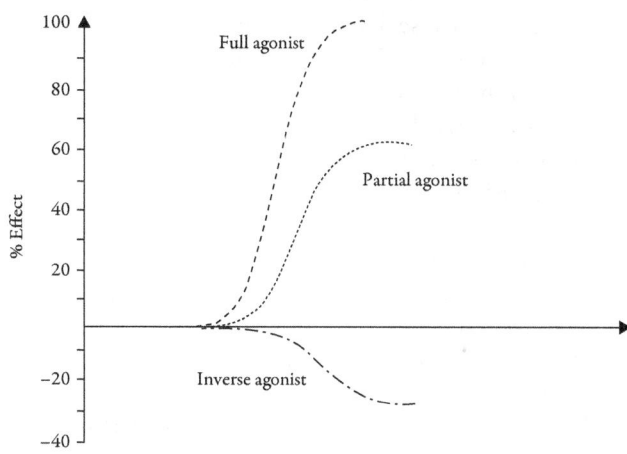

**Figure 63.1.** Modulation of receptor response by increasing concentrations of full, partial and inverse agonists.

As a result, the difference between resting potential and threshold potential is increased and the firing is less likely. This produces the sedative effects.

## ANESTHESIA CLINICAL EXAMPLES OF AGONIST AND ANTAGONISTS

- Fentanyl is a direct μ opioid receptor **agonist** that produces its analgesic effect by directly binding to the μ opioid receptors.[2]
- Naloxone is an opioid receptor **competitive antagonist**. It directly binds to the opioid receptors, but does not cause a physiologic response. It instead blocks the binding site of the agonist so the effect can be reversed.
- Ketamine is a **noncompetitive** N-methyl-D-aspartate (NMDA) receptor antagonist that binds in the receptor channel pore, whereas the NMDA receptor agonist, glutamate, binds to the extracellular surface of the receptor.
- **Pharmacodynamic drug-drug interactions** take place by a direct additive or opposed effect at the receptors of the effector organ. They can also occur by an upstream or downstream effect on a physiological process by one drug that alters the effect of the other drug.
- **Synergy** is an interaction between two or more drugs that causes the total effect of the drugs to be greater than the sum of the individual effects of each drug. A synergistic effect can be beneficial or possibly harmful for the patient (e.g., concomitant use of opioids and benzodiazepines [BNZ] may produce a number of adverse events, including profound sedation, slowed response time, difficulty breathing, and death).
- Another example of synergism, from another perspective, is the effect of different drugs on the binding sites of another drug. Local anesthetics, volatile anesthetics, calcium channel blockers, and certain classes of antibiotics (aminoglycosides, clindamycin) cause desensitization of acetylcholine (Ach) receptors (AChRs). Desensitized AChRs do not open their ion channels in response to an agonist binding and are therefore unable to contribute to neuromuscular transmission. As the number of desensitized AChRs increase, neuromuscular transmission becomes less efficient and skeletal muscle becomes more susceptible to neuromuscular block by nondepolarizing neuromuscular blocking drugs (NDNMBD).
- **Affinity** is defined as the strength of binding of the ligand (drug) and its corresponding receptor.
- **Efficacy** represents the maximum response that an applied ligand is able to produce. Collectively, **potency** of a drug integrates both its affinity and efficacy to

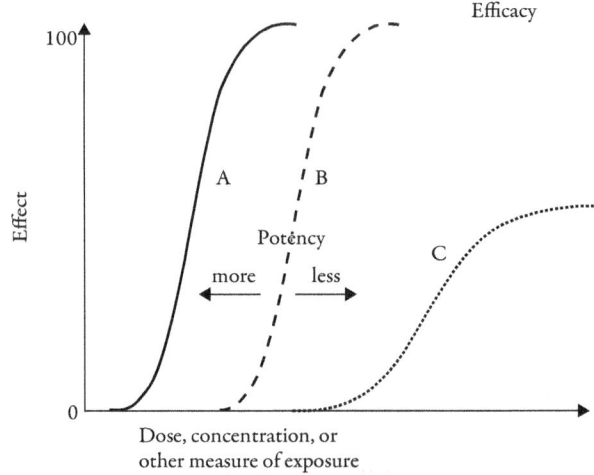

Figure 63.2. Effect of ligand potency and efficacy on the dose-response curve.

express the amount of drug necessary to produce a specific effect.

- A **dose-response curve** depicts the relationship between the amplitude of a stimulus and the feedback of a receptor. Increased affinity of a drug for a particular receptor causes a shift of the dose-response curve to the left (e.g., as seen in Figure 63.2, drugs A and B exhibit the same maximum efficacy; however, drug A is more potent than drug B as it requires lower drug concentration). Drug C is not able to produce the maximum efficacy. Furthermore, the slope of curves A and B are different than that of curve C. The reason behind this observation is that if a drug must occupy the majority of receptors before an effect can occur, the slope of the curve will be steep. *Steeper curves* mean that small increases in drug dose evoke large increases in drug effects. This is seen with volatile anesthetics, where 1 minimum alveolar concentration (MAC) of this agent prevents muscle movement following skin incision in 50% of patients, in contrast to 95% patients seen with 1.3 MAC. However, with steep dose-response curves, the difference between the doses that produce therapeutic and toxic effects may be small.

## DRUG-DRUG BINDING IN REVERSAL OF NEUROMUSCULAR BLOCKADE

Sugammadex antagonizes steroidal neuromuscular blocking drugs, especially rocuronium and vecuronium. It accomplishes this action by encapsulating the molecules of the neuromuscular-blocking drug and thus prevents them from binding to the AChR sites. This allows for rapid and complete reversal of neuromuscular blockade with no cardiovascular side effects.

## REFERENCES

1. Zastrow M. Drug rec eptors and pharmacodynamics. In: Bertram G. Katzung, ed. Katzung & Trevor *Basic and Clinical Pharmacology*. 14th ed. New York, NY: McGraw-Hill Education; 2017:20–40.

2. Kim TK, Obara S, Johnson KB. Basic principles of pharmacology. In: Michael A. Gropper, Ronald D. Miller, Lars I. Eriksson, Lee A. Fleisher, Jeanine P. Wiener-Kronish, Neal H Cohen, Kate Leslie, eds. *Miller's Anesthesia*. 9th ed. Philadelphia, PA: Elsevier Health Sciences; 2019:462–486.

# 64.

# ALTERNATIVE AND HERBAL MEDICINES

## *Muhammad Haseeb Zubair and Aladino De Ranieri*

Herbal supplements have been used for centuries in the Western and Eastern world. The World Health Organization (WHO) estimates that 80% of the world population utilizes herbal medications. Due to an increase in interest, the National Institute of Health (NIH) Office of Alternative Medicine was established in 1992.[1,2] The NCCIH has been instrumental in prioritizing in regulating and evaluating the mechanisms, efficacy, and safety of these herbal medicines.[3] The use of herbal medicines in the United States has followed a very interesting trend, with use declining in the early 1900s and then later rising in the 1960s and 1970s.[4] The Dietary Supplement Health and Education Act (DHSEA) in 1994 allowed the marketing of herbal products without prior demonstration of their safety and efficacy. A 1990 telephonic survey reported that 2.5% of the respondents used herbal medicines. This increased fivefold by 1997. Total sales for herbal supplements were estimated to be $8.8 billion for 2018.[5]

Numerous dietary and herbal supplements have prompted therapeutic value. Patients' hesitation to report their use limits management strategies that then can be applied to provide anesthesia care of patients using herbal supplements. Our knowledge is anecdotal; there are some case reports and trials, but due to the evolving regulatory structure, there is extensive variability in the quality of these studies, which in turn affects the safety, efficacy, and clinical usefulness.

What follows is a list of common herbal medications, their *common clinical usage*, side effects, and/or anecdotal implications.

- **Black Cohosh**: *Management of hot flashes*; contains anti-inflammatory compounds including salicylic acid and could have antiplatelet activity and increase bleeding.
- **Capsicum pepper**: *Alternative therapy used for the management of allergic rhinitis, conjunctivitis, chronic neuropathic pain*; may cause bleeding, local burning, flushing, abdominal irritation, and liver damage.
- **Chamomile**: *Relieves infantile colic, reduces inflammation, fever, sedative*; causes increased bleeding due to the presence of phytocoumarins which are hepatotoxic and interfere with the coagulation cascade.
- **Coenzyme Q10**: *Enhances insulin sensitivity and acts as an antioxidant, in turn helping as an anti-cancer medication*; decreases the response to warfarin.
- **Creatine**: *Used for the management of unipolar depression and muscle strength*; risk of stroke, kidney stones, nausea, diarrhea, and dermatosis.
- **DHEA (dehydroepiandrosterone)**: *Used for adrenal insufficiency in adults*; may cause hair loss, stomach upset, high blood pressure, alteration of menstrual cycle, hirsutism, and fatigue.

- **Echinacea**: *Augments the immunological system via modulation of cytokines and via stimulation of NK cells and macrophages and is commonly used to treat respiratory tract infections*; causes GI disturbance, headache and dizziness, hepatotoxicity.
- **Ephedra**: *This compound is a CNS stimulant and has significant adrenergic activity and is used for weight loss and asthma.* It has to be used with caution and is associated with arrhythmia when used with other sympathomimetic drugs.
- **Evening primrose oil (Oenotherabiennis)**: *Used for atopic dermatitis, eczema, rheumatoid arthritis, and postmenopausal hot flashes*; may cause stomach upset, headache, nausea, and diarrhea.
- **Feverfew (Tan acetum parthenium)**: *Helps with migraine headaches*; may cause rebound headaches, contact dermatitis, increased risk of bleeding, and in pregnant women may cause miscarriage.
- **Fish Oil**: *Omega-3-fatty acids in fish oil have been shown to provide benefit against hyperlipidemia, prevent or treat sclerotic cardiovascular disease, and decrease triglycerides*; increased bleeding risk with doses greater than 3 grams per day.
- **Garlic (Allium Sativum)**: *Anti-platelet activity have been shown to be beneficial in HTN, DM, and atherosclerosis*; associated with significant risk of bleeding.
- **Ginger**: *Its anti-inflammatory and anti-emetic properties are due to its effect on the serotonergic and dopamine pathways.* It has been known to cause bleeding due to its anti-platelet effects and should be avoided in people on anti-coagulants.
- **Ginkgo biloba**: *Used in peripheral vascular disease, age-related macular degeneration, cognitive disorders, tinnitus, vertigo*; anti-platelet activity associated with risk of bleeding, should be discontinued 36 hours before surgery.
- **Ginseng**: *Due to its sympathomimetic properties it has been shown to be a mood enhancer and aphrodisiac, cognitive function, diabetes, impotence, and viral infections*; inhibits platelet aggregation in vitro and prolongs the PTT and PT. Also decreases post-prandial blood glucose in type 2 diabetes. We recommend discontinuation 7 days before surgery.
- **Grapefruit**: *Treats high cholesterol, asthma, increases red blood count (RBC) level, weight loss, and psoriasis*; increased risk of hormone sensitive cancers and tachy arrythmias, increases the effects of anti-seizure medications and increases metabolism, increases carbamazepine metabolization.
- **Green tea**: *Has anti-microbial properties, anti-aging, prevents type II diabetes, cardiovascular disease and is protective to the skin*; may cause headache, diarrhea, vomiting, irritability, tremors, GERD, and convulsions.
- **Hawthorn**: *Investigational for the management of heart failure patients, heart failure, anxiety, angina*; may cause nausea, stomach upset, dizziness, palpitations, epistaxis, insomnia.
- **Horse chestnut seed extract**: *Used in the management of lower extremity venous insufficiency*; associated with kidney stones, muscle weakness, depression, diarrhea, stupor, hypoglycemia, and decreases blood clotting.
- **Kava**: *Treatment of anxiety disorders, benzodiazepine withdrawal, migraines, and insomnia*; may cause headache, liver damage, dizziness, and allergic skin reactions due to its effect on GABA receptors; has sedative hypnotic properties and is known to augment induction.
- **Melatonin**: *Used as a sleep aid*; may cause depression, hyperglycemia, hypertension, and seizure disorders.
- **Milk thistle (Silymarin)**: *One of the emerging therapies for hepatic fibrosis and non-alcoholic fatty liver disease*; may cause abdominal bloating and diarrhea.
- **S-adenosylmethionine (SAMe)**: *Management of alcohol-based steatosis, alcohol-associated cirrhosis, depression, osteoarthritis, and AIDs-related neuropathy*; confusion, dizziness, anorexia, headache, dry mouth, and worsens parkinsonism symptoms. We recommend discontinuation 2 weeks before surgery.
- **Saw palmetto**: *Used in benign prostate hypertrophy, inhibit estrogen receptors, induction of apoptosis, blocking prolactin receptor signal and anti-inflammatory*; platelet dysfunction secondary to cyclo-oxygenase inhibition.
- **Soy isoflavones (Glycine max)**: *Used in the management of osteoporosis in postmenopausal women*; itching, swelling of tongue and face.
- **St. John's wort**: *Inhibits MAOI and induces cytochrome p450 and works as an anti-depressant for mild to moderate depression and is also implicated in serotoninergic crisis*; increases risk of thromboembolism by decreasing warfarin levels in the blood.
- **Valerian**: *Potentiates GABA receptors, anxiolysis, and sedation*; may cause drowsiness and often insomnia.

## REFERENCES

1. American Society of Anesthesiology. What you should know about herbal and dietary supplement use and anesthesia, 2003. Patient information leaflet.
2. Skinner CM, Rangasami. Preoperative use of herbal medicines: A patient survey. *Br J Anaesth.* 2002;89:792–795.

3. National Center for Complementary and Integrative Health. 2016 strategic plan: Exploring the science of complementary and integrative health. US Department of Health and Human Services 2016. https://nccih.nih.gov/sites/nccam.nih.gov/files/NCCIH_2016_Strategic_Plan.pdf.

4. Eisenberg DM, et al. Unconventional medicine in the United States: Prevalence, costs, and patterns of use. *N Engl J Med*. 1993; 328:246.

5. Smith T, Gillespie M, Eckl V, Knepper J, Morton-Reynolds C. Herbal supplement sales in US increase by 9.4% in 2018. American Botanical Council. Press release: US retail sales of herbal supplements increase by 9.4% in 2018. Accessed on November 17, 2019.

# 65.

# DRUG REACTIONS

*Daniel Gonzalez Kapp*

## INTRODUCTION

Adverse drug reactions are any undesirable effects of a drug, which primarily arise in one of two ways: as a consequence of the drug's underlying pharmacology (e.g., opioid-induced respiratory depression, opioid-induced nausea), or as an unpredictable occurrence (e.g., anaphylactoid reactions to morphine, malignant hyperthermia from succinylcholine).[1] Reactions may include specific signs and symptoms or changes in laboratory parameters. The severity of adverse drug reactions ranges from relatively minor to serious and life-threatening. Historically, these reactions are classified as either:

(1) Type A, when the reaction is reasonably associated with the drug's mechanism of action and is usually dose related; or
(2) Type B, when the reaction is idiosyncratic.

The risk of dose-related adverse events is dependent on inter-patient variability in the underlying pharmacokinetic and pharmacodynamic drug properties, and while dose-related adverse reactions are more common than idiosyncratic reactions, particularly for anesthetics, the idiosyncratic-type reactions can be more serious and/or life-threatening.[2]

## KEY TERMINOLOGY

### IDIOSYNCRATIC REACTIONS

Idiosyncratic adverse drug reactions are an abnormal response to a drug that is:[3]

- unique to a given individual; and
- does not correlate with drug dose; and
- is not considered an allergic-type reaction.

These adverse events are usually rare and therefore difficult to study; however, most idiosyncratic reactions are hypothesized to arise from underlying genetic variation in the individual.

### ANAPHYLAXIS

Allergic-type hypersensitivity reactions are heightened immunologic responses that are triggered by an allergen or antigen in a previously sensitized individual.[4] Hypersensitivity reactions can be classified into 4 types based on the underlying immune response (see Table 65.1).

Anaphylactic and immediate hypersensitivity reactions are Type I reactions; in these cases, antigens interact with immunoglobin E (IgE) antibodies, leading to mast cell

**Table 65.1** HYPERSENSITIVITY REACTIONS

| TYPE | IMMUNE RESPONSE |
|---|---|
| Type I | Immediate |
| Type II | Cytotoxic |
| Type III | Immune complex-mediated |
| Type IV | Cell-mediated (delayed) |

**Table 65.3** CAUSES OF ANAPHYLAXIS

| | |
|---|---|
| Anaphylactic reactions | Antibiotics (penicillins, cephalosporins, sulfa drugs), local anesthetics<br>Latex<br>Disinfectants (chlorhexidine), enzymes (trypsin, streptokinase), human proteins (insulin, corticotrophin) |
| Anaphylactoid reactions | Muscle relaxants (succinylcholine, rocuronium)<br>Opioids (morphine, meperidine), radio contrast dye<br>Anesthetics (propofol, thiopental), NSAIDs<br>Protamine<br>Dextran<br>Preservatives (sulfites) |

activation and the release of inflammatory mediators.[5] In these cases, prior antigen exposure results in B cell creation of peptide-specific IgE and subsequent fixation on mast cells and basophils. Secondary antigen exposure leads to rapid degranulation and release of inflammatory mediators (e.g., histamine, prostaglandins), resulting in varying degrees of bronchial smooth muscle constriction, increased vasodilation, and increased vascular permeability (see Table 65.2). Anaphylaxis is a severe form of this immunologic response that presents as life-threatening alterations of cardiovascular, dermatologic, and respiratory systems (see Table 65.3).

In practice, allergic reactions are more likely to occur with antibiotics, blood products, colloids, or nonsteroidal anti-inflammatory drugs (NSAIDs), but may be elicited by any substance (Tables 65.2 and 65.3). The antibiotics most correlated with anaphylactic reactions are β-lactam antibiotics (e.g., penicillins, cephalosporins), and cross-reactivity with a penicillin allergy is seen with carbapenems and cephalosporins.

## ANAPHYLACTOID REACTIONS

Anaphylactoid reactions may present similarly to anaphylaxis, as they too are mediated by mast cell and basophil responses; however, these reactions are not caused by an immune response subsequent to cell surface antibody activation, as seen in a true Type I hypersensitivity reaction.[1]

Anaphylactoid reactions are primarily caused by drug- or substance P-induced release of histamines. Drugs associated with anaphylactoid reactions include antibiotics (classic

**Table 65.2** HYPERSENSITIVITY REACTIONS BY SYSTEM

| SYSTEM | PRESENTATION |
|---|---|
| Cardiovascular | Hypotension, tachycardia |
| Dermatologic | Rash, edema |
| Respiratory | Dyspnea, bronchospasm, laryngeal edema |

example is the "red man" syndrome from vancomycin), barbiturates, hyperosmotic agents, muscle relaxants, and opioids.[4] Despite the difference in underlying mechanism between anaphylaxis and anaphylactoid reactions, patients can have identical signs and symptoms to an allergic-type response, including severe cardiovascular or respiratory compromise.

## ANESTHETIC CONSIDERATIONS

### PREOPERATIVE

Anaphylaxis is a serious but rare complication; for penicillin, approximately 2% of the general population has an allergy, but only 0.01% of administrations result in anaphylaxis. Despite the rarity of anaphylaxis, clinicians should evaluate the patient's history for preexisting conditions associated with an increased risk of anaphylaxis (e.g., asthma, allergies) when high-risk medications will be used perioperatively. Further investigation is warranted when there is a history of anaphylaxis (or any severe-type drug reaction) and the triggering agent is unknown; when the trigger is known, alternative treatment should be chosen.

### INTRAOPERATIVE

Features of hypersensitivity-type reactions are variable, but typically include bronchospasm, hypotension, and tachycardia. An example of an intraoperative allergen is latex. Clinicians should evaluate the timing between administration of a potential trigger and possible signs of a hypersensitivity reaction; anaphylaxis generally occurs with 2–20 minutes of antigen exposure. Treatment begins with discontinuation of the suspected trigger and stabilization of the patient's airway. The primary drug treatment for anaphylaxis is epinephrine, as it is critical for the reversal of bronchospasm and management of laryngeal edema, cardiovascular compromise, and severe hypotension.

## POSTOPERATIVE

Cases of anaphylaxis require at least 24 hours of intensive monitoring due to the risk of recurrence after the initial treatment phase. Post-incident documentation should include a detailed account of the reaction and triggering agent, as future administration of the triggering agent is contraindicated.

## REFERENCES

1. Patton K, Borshoff DC. Adverse drug reactions. *Anaesthesia.* 2018;73:76–84.
2. Butterworth IV JF, Mackey DC, Wasnick JD. Anesthetic complications. In: *Morgan & Mikhail's Clinical Anesthesiology.* 6th ed. McGraw-Hill Education; 2018. http://accessanesthesiology.mhmedical.com/content.aspx?aid=1161433773.
3. Reddy SK. Drug reactions. In: Freeman BS, Berger JS, eds. *Anesthesiology Core Review: Part One Basic Exam.* McGraw-Hill Education; 2014. http://accessanesthesiology.mhmedical.com/content.aspx?aid=1102566874.
4. Holzman RS, Tinch BT. Anaphylactic reactions and anesthesia. In: Longnecker DE, Mackey SC, Newman MF, Sandberg WS, Zapol WM, eds. *Anesthesiology.* 3rd ed. McGraw-Hill Education; 2017. http://accessanesthesiology.mhmedical.com/content.aspx?aid=1144136463.
5. Kim BA, Yang SW. Anaphylaxis. In: Freeman BS, Berger JS, eds. *Anesthesiology Core Review: Part One Basic Exam.* McGraw-Hill Education; 2014. http://accessanesthesiology.mhmedical.com/content.aspx?aid=1102568317.

# 66.

# ANESTHETIC GASES AND VAPORS

*Rhett Reynolds and Elyse M. Cornett*

## INTRODUCTION

The inhalation agents commonly used in anesthesia include nitrous oxide (nonvolatile) and the volatile agents (desflurane, halothane, isoflurane, sevoflurane). Overall, inhaled anesthetics work to decrease the neurotransmission of the excitatory pathways and augment the neurotransmission of the inhibitory pathways. However, the precise mechanism of action of these agents is not completely understood. It is believed that the volatile agents act on a combination of receptors in the central nervous system including the gamma-aminobutyric acid$_A$ (GABA$_A$), glycine, and glutamate receptors;[1] whereas nitrous oxide acts as both an agonist and antagonist on the GABA$_A$ and NMDA receptors, respectively.

## PHYSICAL PROPERTIES

One of the main differences between nitrous oxide and the volatile anesthetics are their respective physical properties.

The volatile agents exist as liquids at room temperature because they have low vapor pressures and high boiling points. Therefore, these agents require the use of a vaporizer to convert them into gas form in order to be inhaled. On the other hand, nitrous oxide has a high vapor pressure and low boiling point; therefore, it exists as a gas at room temperature.

## EFFECTS ON THE CENTRAL NERVOUS SYSTEM

The volatile anesthetic agents all cause dose-dependent cerebral vasodilation. They decrease the cerebral metabolic rate as well as oxygen consumption. In addition, they uncouple the autoregulation of cerebral blood flow to $CO_2$.[2] These factors can lead to an unwanted increase in intracranial pressure. With that being said, studies have shown that at minimum alveolar concentration (MAC) values <1, these effects are modest, and responsiveness to $CO_2$ and intracranial pressure remain normal. However, at MAC values >1, cerebral blood flow and intracranial pressure can rise significantly. Nitrous oxide also causes an increase in cerebral blood flow and intracranial pressures, but generally preserves $CO_2$ responsiveness.

## EFFECTS ON THE CARDIOVASCULAR SYSTEM

Although the mechanism may differ, all of the volatile anesthetics can cause myocardial depression with dose-dependent reductions in blood pressure and cardiac output. Desflurane, isoflurane, and sevoflurane are vasodilators and cause a decrease in systemic vascular resistance with little influence on the myocardial contractility itself.[2] On the contrary, halothane reduces blood pressure by its negative inotropic effect with decrease in myocardial contractility and heart rate, but it has little effect on the systemic vascular resistance. At higher doses, halothane has been shown to be a negative chronotropic agent as well and can cause bradycardia and asystole, particularly in younger children. In addition, one of the most feared outcomes while using volatile anesthetics is ventricular dysrhythmia. This is due to the fact that they can sensitize the myocardium to the effect of catecholamines. Therefore, extreme caution must be taken to know which other drugs are given perioperatively. Although nitrous oxide has been shown to cause mild myocardial depression and sympathetic nervous system stimulation, the effects are much milder compared to the volatile agents. Heart rate may increase with isoflurane, desflurane, and enflurane, while halothane may cause no change; this can be explained by the impairment of baroceptors function under halothane anesthesia. The depression of cardiac contractility may be attributed to alteration in intracellular calcium homeostasis.

## EFFECTS ON RESPIRATION

The volatile agents all cause a dose-dependent decease in tidal volume with a reflexive increase in the respiratory rate. The increase in respiratory rate is not sufficient; therefore, mechanical ventilation is required. In addition, the volatile agents are all bronchodilators. They act on beta 2 receptors and cause bronchial smooth muscle relaxation. Some reports show that these agents could even be used to treat status asthmaticus. Finally, volatile agents, particularly desflurane and isoflurane, can cause extensive airway irritation (coughing, laryngospasm).[3] Therefore, these agents should be avoided in patients who smoke or who have reactive airway diseases. Nitrous oxide has little effect on the airways or respiration. It does not affect tidal volume, nor is it a bronchodilator or irritant.

## EFFECTS ON NEUROMUSCULAR FUNCTION

By inhibiting excitatory nicotinic acetylcholine receptors, the volatile anesthetics induce dose-dependent skeletal and smooth muscle relaxation. These agents are not powerful enough to get the job done on their own, but they potentiate the effects of the neuromuscular blocking agents. The strength of each agent in inducing potentiation from highest to lowest is desflurane > sevoflurane > isoflurane > halothane > nitrous oxide.

## EFFECTS ON RENAL FUNCTION

The never inhaled anesthetics have little effect on renal blood flow or glomerular filtration, but can lead to decreased renal blood flow secondary to decreased cardiac output; however, nephrotoxicity can take place with all the volatile anesthetics. The metabolism of the halogenated agents produces fluoride, which is believed to cause renal toxicity.[2] Sevoflurane in particular is metabolized the quickest and produces the highest levels of fluoride, whereas halothane and desflurane produce very little. Fluoride toxicity impairs the ability to concentrate urine, resulting in polyuria, hypernatremia, and increased serum osmolarity. This can happen as fluoride-induced inhibition of adenylate cyclase can prevent normal response to antidiuretic hormone, and it can also cause intrarenal vasodilation with shunting of blood from cortical to medullary nephrons interfering with the countercurrent multiplier mechanism.

## EFFECTS ON HEPATIC FUNCTION

Hepatic blood flow is slightly decreased by all inhaled anesthetics. However, the main issue is with halothane. While the rest of the volatile agents are only metabolized 2%–5% and mostly are excreted unchanged, halothane is metabolized 25% by the hepatic CYP450 system. Halothane's chief breakdown product is trifluoroacetic acid (TFA).[2] TFA is protein bound, and this complex has the capability to stimulate a T-cell–mediated immune response, resulting in fulminant hepatic failure. It is important to note that surgery near the liver causes a greater decrease in total hepatic blood flow than surgery far from the liver; in addition, the site of surgery has a greater effect on liver function than the type of anesthetic.

## EFFECTS ON THE HEMATOLOGIC SYSTEM

Nitrous oxide in particular has been associated with vitamin $B_{12}$ deficiency. Nitrous oxide reduces the activity of methionine synthase, which is a crucial enzyme in the production of vitamin $B_{12}$. $B_{12}$ deficiency can lead to numerous problems, including megaloblastic anemia and subacute combined degeneration of the spinal cord.

## TOXICITY

In addition to the potential problems discussed in the preceding sections, including nephrotoxicity, hepatotoxicity, and vitamin $B_{12}$ deficiency, one of the most severe complications involving the volatile anesthetics is malignant hyperthermia. Malignant hyperthermia can take place during the induction of anesthesia or any time during the maintenance phase. Clinical signs include hyperthermia, hypercarbia, and generalized muscle rigidity. Treatment with dantrolene must be initiated emergently because the mortality rate can be quite high.

To continue, there has also been fear about operating room personnel, particularly pregnant women, who are chronically exposed to trace concentrations of anesthetic gases. Studies have not provided clear-cut evidence showing whether or not chronic exposure leads to fetal loss or congenital malformation.[4]

## COMPARING AGENTS

Although the volatile anesthetics as a class are similar, each agent is unique. To begin, sevoflurane is the most commonly used inhalation induction agent due to its minimal odor and powerful bronchodilation. In addition, sevoflurane has a quick onset of action due to its low blood:gas solubility.[5] Next, desflurane which has the quickest onset and offset of action, is most commonly used as a maintenance agent during short procedures due to rapid recovery during emergence. In addition, desflurane has a low oil:gas partition coefficient, meaning it is not taken up into adipose tissue well; therefore, it is a preferred agent for obese patients. The disadvantages of desflurane are that it is very pungent, and it causes airway irritation (coughing, laryngospasm).

Therefore, it is not a first-line option for induction or for patients who smoke or who have reactive airway diseases. To continue, isoflurane is another agent commonly used for maintenance (particularly during long procedures) due to its high potency and low cost. The disadvantages of isoflurane are that it is very pungent and that it has a high blood:gas solubility and therefore a very slow onset and offset of action. Furthermore, isoflurane has high fat solubility, which leads to a delayed emergence from anesthesia because the agent can accumulate in the body tissues. Finally, halothane is no longer used in the United States due to adverse effects such as negative ionotropy and chronotropy, high incidence of ventricular arrhythmias, and significant hepatotoxicity.

Nitrous oxide is a sweet-smelling gas with a very low blood:gas partition coefficient and rapid onset and offset of action. Due to its low potency, it is frequently used as an adjunct to another agent in both induction and maintenance. The addition of nitrous oxide to another volatile inhalation agent can increase the speed of anesthetic onset and offset due to the "second gas effect." One study showed that the addition of nitrous oxide during the last 30 minutes of surgery reduced time to extubation by about 2 minutes. Some of the disadvantages of nitrous oxide are that it diffuses into air-filled cavities, and that it has been associated with a possible increase in postoperative atelectasis. Therefore, nitrous oxide is contraindicated in patients with preexisting bowel distention, increased middle ear pressure, pneumothorax, pneumoperitoneum, and poor pulmonary function.

## REFERENCES

1. Franks NP. General anaesthesia: From molecular targets to neuronal pathways of sleep and arousal. *Nat Rev Neurosci*. 2008.
2. Khan KS et al. Pharmacology of anaesthetic agents II: Inhalation anaesthetic agents. *Contin Educ Anaesthes Crit Care Pain*. 2014.
3. Nyktari V et al. Respiratory resistance during anaesthesia with isoflurane, sevoflurane, and desflurane: A randomized clinical trial. *Br J Anaesth*. 2011.
4. Burm AGL. Occupational hazards of inhalational anaesthetics. *Best Pract Res Clin Anaesthesiol*. 2003.
5. Thwaites A et al. Inhalation induction with sevoflurane: A double-blind comparison with propofol. *Br J Anaesth*. 1997.

# 67.

# MINIMUM ALVEOLAR CONCENTRATION (MAC)

*Hao Hua and Daniel S. Cormican*

## INTRODUCTION

The concept of minimum alveolar concentration (MAC) was first introduced by Eger and Merkel in an animal study comparing halothane and halopropane in 1963.[1] MAC was later extended to halothanes in human beings in 1964. Finally, in 1965, it was used to measure potency for different volatile anesthetic agents.[2] Previous measurements used to determine anesthetic dosing were qualitative measurements that varied depending on different inhaled anesthetics. MAC is defined as the concentration of an anesthetic gas at 1 ATM which prevents motor response in 50% of people from surgical stimulation. Abolition of the reflex arcs in the spinal cord (sensory neurons in the dorsal root ganglion and motor efferent neurons) is thought to be the primary mechanism for absence of movement, but whether this occurs through direct binding or membrane alterations is not known.[3] MAC uses end-tidal anesthetic gas as a measurement of the level of anesthetic within the alveoli, which is equivalent to the level of anesthetic at the central nervous system. Compared to previous methods of anesthetic measurements, it is a more useful quantitative measure that is reproducible in both animals and humans across different volatile agents. Despite some imperfections and limitations, MAC remains the standard for comparing the potency of different volatile anesthetic agents (see Table 67.1).

## MAC VALUES AND CLINICAL SIGNIFICANCE

Different MAC values are used to evaluate different responses in the patient. For example, the MAC-awake (or MAC-aware) value is the concentration of volatile anesthetic agent at the alveoli in which 50% of people will respond to a verbal or non-noxious tactile stimulus. In other words, MAC-aware is the ED50 for awareness and recall, and it varies between 0.15 MAC to 0.5 MAC. The mechanism responsible for response to voice or light touch is thought to be suppressed by anesthetic agents at brainstem

and cortical regions involved in consciousness, in particular the involvement of the reticular activating system.[3]

MAC-BAR value is the concentration of volatile anesthetic agent at the alveoli which blunts adrenergic responses to noxious stimuli in 50% of people. MAC-BAR has been approximated to be 50% higher than standard MAC.[4] MAC values have also been established for different EEG values such as burst suppression and isoelectricity.[3]

## FACTORS THAT AFFECT MAC

Standard MAC values of anesthetic gasses are additive. For example, the additive effect of 0.5 MAC of sevoflurane plus 0.5 Mac of $N_2O$ is equivalent to 1.0 MAC. Other parameters of MAC—such as cardiovascular effects—are not necessarily additive. For example, 0.5 MAC of $N_2O$ plus 0.5 MAC of isoflurane will result in less hypotension compared to 1.0 MAC of isoflurane alone because isoflurane is a more potent vasodilator compared to $N_2O$.[3] Various factors will

*Table 67.1* MAC OF COMMON VOLATILE ANESTHETICS

| ANESTHETIC GAS | 1 MAC AT 1 ATM (% IN VOLUME) |
|---|---|
| Nitrous oxide | 104 |
| Desflurane | 6.6 |
| Sevoflurane | 2 |
| Enflurane | 1.7 |
| Isoflurane | 1.17 |
| Halothane | 0.75 |

MAC values standardized for 40-year-old patient. MAC values differ for each inhalation anesthetic agent. Notice only nitrous oxide (N2O) gas has a MAC value >100 (104% at standard pressure and temperature). Thus, N2O has very low potency, and 1 MAC cannot be achieved when N2O is delivered under standard conditions.

Reproduced with permission from Ebert TJ, Schmid PG. Inhaled anesthetics. In: Barash PG, Cullen BF, Stoelting RK, et al., eds. Clinical Anesthesia. 6th ed. Philadelphia, PA: Lippincott Williams & Wilkins; 2009:413–443.

*Table 67.2* FACTORS THAT INFLUENCE MAC

| FACTORS THAT INCREASE MAC | FACTORS THAT DECREASE MAC |
|---|---|
| Chronic alcohol use | Acute alcohol use |
| Amphetamines | IV lidocaine |
| Anxiety | Alpha 2 agonists |
| Cocaine | Propofol |
| Ephedrine | Benzodiazepine |
| Hypernatremia | Opioids |
| Hyperthermia | Lithium |
| Monoamine oxidase inhibitors | Hypo-osmolality |
| Levodopa | Ketamine |
| Infancy (highest MAC at 6 months) | Barbiturates |
| | Verpamil |
| | THC |
| | Nitrous oxide |
| | Pregnancy |
| | Metabolic acidosis |
| | Hypoxia |
| | Hypotension |
| | Hypercarbia |
| | Anemia |
| | Hypothermia |
| | Hyponatremia |
| | Increased age |

Reproduced with permission from Ebert TJ, Schmid PG. Inhaled anesthetics. In: Barash PG, Cullen BF, Stoelting RK, et al., eds. *Clinical Anesthesia*. 6th ed. Philadelphia, PA: Lippincott Williams & Wilkins; 2009:413–443.

alter the predicted MAC (see Table 67.2). Currently, there is no single mechanism to explain the alterations in MAC.

The MAC requirement to prevent movement to surgical stimulus and/or blunt sympathetic response for any volatile anesthetic agent is decreased by administration of any IV anesthetic, sedative, or analgesic agents. MAC is decreased by acute alcohol use due to its sedative effects. On the other hand, MAC is increased by chronic alcohol intake and by recent use of amphetamines, cocaine, or ephedrine because these drugs will acutely increase catecholamine levels in the CNS, increasing focused consciousness.[3]

MAC values are also influenced by patient-related factors. In general, MAC decreases with age and is decreased in premature infants. MAC rises until at 6 months of age before decreasing. Pregnancy and hypothyroidism also decrease MAC. Other factors that markedly decrease MAC in patients include acute conditions including severe anemia, electrolyte abnormalities, shock, metabolic acidosis, hypoxia, hypercarbia, and hypothermia.[3] Patient conditions associated with increased psychomotor activity increase MAC (i.e., hyperthermia, hyperthyroidism, or anxiety). Awareness of these factors is critical to avoid inadequate anesthesia and anesthetic overdose.

## MONITORING MAC

End-tidal anesthetic concentration (ETAC) is used for continuous monitoring of an inhaled anesthetic agent. ETAC close to MAC value for the desired effect is used to target the depth of anesthesia and avoid intraoperative awareness. Electroencephalogram-derived bispectral index (BIS) can be used in addition to ETAC to prevent excessive anesthetic depth in older patients and to monitor patients undergoing neurosurgical procedures. However, BIS alone is not superior to ETAC in the prevention of intraoperative awareness. In the landmark BAG-RECALL trial, fewer patients in the ETAC group experienced intraoperative awareness compared to the BIS group.[5]

## REFERENCES

1. Merkel G, Eger EI. A comparative study of halothane and halopropane anaesthesia. *Anesthesiology*. 1963;24:346–357.
2. Eger EI, et al. Minimum alveolar anesthetic concentration: A standard of anesthetic potency. *Anesthesiology*. 1965;26:756–763.
3. Ebert TJ, Schmid PG. Inhaled anesthetics. In: Barash PG, Cullen BF, Stoelting RK, et al., eds. *Clinical Anesthesia*. 6th ed. Philadelphia, PA: Lippincott Williams & Wilkins; 2009:413–443.
4. Roizen MF, et al. Anesthetic doses blocking adrenergic (stress) and cardiovascular responses to incision-MAC BAR. *Anesthesiology*. 1981;54(5):390–398.
5. Avidan MS, et al. Prevention of intraoperative awareness in a high-risk surgical population. *N Engl J Med*. 2011;365(7):591–600.

# 68.

# TRACE CONCENTRATIONS, POLLUTION, AND PERSONNEL HARZARDS

*David E. Swanson*

## INTRODUCTION

There are many occupational hazards among operating room (OR) personnel, including fire, accidents, allergic reactions, drug addiction, burnout, depression, and suicide. Of these hazards, the breathing in of trace anesthetic gases has garnered the most attention since the first report on the concern was published in 1967. Trace anesthetic gases have been associated with decreased fertility, and an increased risk of spontaneous abortions in pregnant OR personnel, as well as headaches and, theoretically, malignant hyperthermia in a person with a genetic predisposition.[1] Always using the lowest fresh gas flow needed is a good habit that will minimize the trace anesthetic gas concentration in your OR when the circle system is not a closed loop, such as during masking and intubation. This low-flow habit is also a cost-effective way to minimize volatile anesthetic expense and is better for the environment. Volatile anesthetics and nitrous oxide may be more substantial contributors to greenhouse gases than many realize. Desflurane has more than an order of magnitude worse environmental impact than sevoflurane and isoflurane. Very low-flow anesthesia with proper carbon dioxide absorbent (which minimizes formation of compound A and clinically relevant toxicity to kidneys) can further decrease the global warming potential of each anesthetic.[2] Careful filling of vaporizers to avoid spillage can decrease the trace gas concentration in the OR, and filling them at the end of each day minimizes staff exposure. The gas outlet on membrane oxygenators used for cardiopulmonary bypass can be another source of OR pollution. Finally, it is important to have routine testing and maintenance of OR ventilation systems that, when functioning properly, quickly dilute the anesthetic gases when they do escape into the room.

The infectious risk from human immunodeficiency virus and hepatitis, as well as the respiratory risk from tuberculosis (TB) have long been known and managed by use of proper personal protective equipment (PPE). The COVID-19 pandemic taught the world the importance of adequate supplies of PPE, supply chain vulnerabilities, and the challenges of an unanticipated dramatic increase in demand for PPE.

Toxic fumes in the smoke plume from the surgical field and chemicals such as methylmethacrylate have attracted attention but are not well understood regarding any long-term harm from known carcinogens in these.

There is biological plausibility of health hazards from the air we breathe in the OR, so taking steps to minimize these potential risks by understanding the sources of air pollution in the OR is important.

Radiation exposure and eye injury from lasers also warrant proper PPE.

## ANESTHETIC CONSIDERATIONS

### PREOPERATIVE

Assure that there is no significant leak of gases during the anesthesia machine check. This includes assessing the waste anesthetic gas evacuation system. Careful anesthesia technique can decrease the trace anesthesia gas concentration in the OR. In planning for airway surgery without a secure airway or surgery that is likely to involve multiple disconnections of the circuit, consider total intravenous anesthesia rather than volatile anesthetics.

Following universal precautions to avoid direct contact with blood and bodily fluid always needs to be observed, as well as preoperative testing for TB or COVID-19 when indicated and use of proper PPE when a test is positive or no result is available.

### INTRAOPERATIVE

Assuring a proper seal of the mask on our patients is important, since the anesthetics released outside the anesthesia circle system cannot be scavenged. This can be difficult during a day of quick pediatric cases with numerous mask anesthetics. Similarly, when the volatile anesthetic is on and the mask is not on the patient, this gas is not evacuated and escapes into the room. While turning the vaporizer off is helpful in that situation, less anesthetic gas enters the room if the gas flow is paused (if your machine has that function and you expect to reconnect the patient to the circuit within the time allowed by the pause) or the volatile anesthetic and the fresh gas flow are turned down or off. Assess for adequate cuff pressures in endotracheal tubes and supraglottic airways to minimize the escape of anesthetic gas into the OR during the maintenance phase. Sevoflurane concentrations in the anesthesiologist's breathing zones were found to be higher with use of supraglottic airways compared to endotracheal tubes.[2] Trace gases were also higher in turbulent flow ORs compared to ORs with laminar flow ventilation.

Use of a proper viral filter in the circuit is important for COVID-19 patients, as is avoiding circuit disconnections and minimizing the risk of aerosol-generating procedures by using a rapid sequence induction.

When fluoroscopy or plain X-rays are used, be certain to not only use a lead apron, but a thyroid shield and lead glasses as well. Staying as far away as patient safety allows from the source will minimize exposure. The source is the X-ray tube of a C-arm, so keeping away from that is a good practice. The two most important factors in reducing radiation exposure are distance and shielding. Radiation intensity from a point source is inversely proportional to the square of the distance from the source. Anesthesiologists who spend significant time in the neuro-interventional suite should wear protective eyewear.[4]

Energy-based surgical instruments can create a smoke plume and fumes from methylmethacrylate, both of which may have health implications. It seems prudent to encourage the use of smoke evacuation devices (SED), which have up to 10 times the suction flow rate as wall suction. Surveys have shown limited use. SEDs are expensive, have bulky, awkward handling, and are noisy, all of which has limited surgeon buy-in when routine use is not required in most US states. SEDs are recommended by the CDC for cases involving human papilloma virus (HPV) and TB. Also consider wearing a mask with increased filtering ability compared to an ordinary surgical mask during certain procedures to minimize exposure to carcinogens, harmful chemicals, HPV, and other possible pathogens known to be in the smoke plume.[5] The potential risk of surgical smoke was reported in 1985 and much is known about the contents of the plume, but unfortunately direct evidence of harm beyond headaches, nausea, irritation to eyes, mucous membranes, and upper respiratory tract is limited to 4 cases of HPV likely contracted from surgical smoke exposure.

## POSTOPERATIVE

Be sure to turn the vaporizer off at the end of all cases. The recovery room may have a higher trace gas concentration than ORs since there is no practical way to scavenge the anesthetics that patients are breathing out. The ventilation requirement for operating rooms is a minimum total of 15 air changes per hour, with a minimum of 3 air changes of outdoor air (fresh air) per hour. Compare this to recovery rooms' recommended minimum total of 6 air changes per hour, with a minimum of 2 air changes of outdoor air per hour.[1]

## REFERENCES

1. Heiderich S, et al. Low anaesthetic waste gas concentrations in postanaesthesia care unit: A prospective observational study. *Eur J Anaesthesiol*. 2018 Jul;35(7):534–538.
2. Feldman JM, et al. Estimating the impact of carbon dioxide absorbent performance differences on absorbent cost during low-flow anesthesia. *Anesth Analg*. 2020 Feb;130(2):374–381.
3. Herzog-Niescery J, et al. Occupational chronic sevoflurane exposure in the everyday reality of the anesthesia workplace. *Anesth Analg*. 2015 Dec;121(6):1519–1528.
4. Anastasian Z, et al. Radiation exposure of the anesthesiologist in the neurointerventional suite. *Anesthesiology*. 2011 Mar;114(3):512–520.
5. Swerdlow BN. Surgical smoke and the anesthesia provider. *J Anesth*. 2020;34:575–584.

# 69.

# COMPARATIVE PHARMACODYNAMICS
# OF INHALED ANESTHETICS

*Nicholas M. Parker*

## INTRODUCTION

The inhaled anesthetics have been discussed in detail in earlier chapters. This chapter will focus on defining the unique pharmacologic profile of each agent to best identify its role in therapy. Table 69.1 details the properties of each anesthetic, while unique features are discussed in the following.

## NITROUS OXIDE

Nitrous oxide is unique among the other inhaled anesthetics because it exists as a gas at standard temperature and pressure. It is also an oxidizer, so it can accelerate fires. This drug does not produce full anesthesia even if the patient were breathing pure nitrous oxide, so it must be combined with other anesthetics if complete sedation is required.[1] Nitrous oxide has several unique safety benefits, including neutral effects on blood pressure, no effect on ventilation, and no effect on uterine muscle.[1,2] It triggers sympathetic effects

such as increased cerebral blood flow, which can balance other anesthetics that cause the opposite effect. Prolonged use of nitrous oxide may cause megaloblastic anemia, but this is rare.[1,2]

## SEVOFLURANE

Sevoflurane features a rapid onset and low pungency; this makes it appropriate for induction of anesthesia.[1,2] The minimum alveolar concentration (MAC) is age dependent, with dose requirements falling by half for an 80-year-old patient compared to a 25-year-old. A lower concentration may also be used when combined with nitrous oxide. Sevoflurane has a context-dependent half-time due to accumulation in the tissues, with rapid recovery after less than 2 hours of use, but much longer recovery time if used for more than 2 hours.[2] Sevoflurane causes a dose-dependent vasodilatory effect, without compensation from increased cardiac output, so hypotension may ensue.[1,2]

*Table 69.1* PHARMACOLOGIC PROPERTIES OF INHALED ANESTHETICS

| INHALED ANESTHETIC | PHYSICAL PHASE | BLOOD:GAS PARTITION COEFFICIENT | BRAIN:BLOOD PARTITION COEFFICIENT | MAC (%) | PUNGENCY | CARDIAC CONTRACTILITY | HEART RATE | VASCULATURE |
|---|---|---|---|---|---|---|---|---|
| Nitrous oxide | Gas | 0.47 | 1.1 | > 100 | None | Opposing effects, overall neutral | No effect | No effect |
| Desflurane | Liquid (inhaled as vapor) | 0.42 | 1.3 | 6 to 7 | High | No effect | Increased | Vasodilation |
| Sevoflurane | | 0.69 | 1.7 | 2.0 | Low | No effect | No effect | Vasodilation |
| Isoflurane | | 1.40 | 2.6 | 1.4 | High | No effect | Increased | Vasodilation |
| Enflurane | | 1.80 | 1.4 | 1.7 | Low | Depressed | No effect | No effect |
| Halothane | | 2.30 | 2.9 | 0.75 | Low | Depressed | No effect | No effect |

MAC: minimum alveolar concentration.

*Table 69.1* CONTINUED

| INHALED ANESTHETIC | VENTILATION | UTERINE MUSCLE | INTRACRANIAL PRESSURE | EEG EFFECTS[A] | TOXICITY (PROLONGED EXPOSURE) | ONSET/ RECOVERY | OTHER FEATURES |
|---|---|---|---|---|---|---|---|
| Nitrous oxide | No effect | No effect | Increased | Fast oscillations in frontal cortex | Megaloblastic anemia | Rapid | Incomplete anesthesia |
| Desflurane | Decreased tidal volume, increased respiratory rate (greatest effect from isoflurane and enflurane) | Uterine relaxation | Decreased at 0.5 MAC; neutral effect at 1.0 MAC; increased at 1.5 MAC | Typical effects | Carbon monoxide generation | Rapid | Transient sympathetic activation; poor choice for induction |
| Sevoflurane | | | | Isolated epileptic-like patterns (1.0–2.0 MAC) | Minimal | Rapid | Suitable for induction |
| Isoflurane | | | | Electrical silence (2.0–2.5 MAC) | Minimal | Slow | Poor choice for induction |
| Enflurane | | | | Seizures possible (1.0–2.0 MAC) | Nephrotoxicity from fluoride | Slow | No longer used in United States |
| Halothane | | | | Typical effects | Hepatotoxicity | Slow | Increased catecholamine sensitivity; no longer used in United States |

EEG: electroencephalogram; MAC: minimum alveolar concentration.

[A] In addition to specific effects listed in the table, desflurane, sevoflurane, isoflurane, enflurane, and halothane initially produce increased EEG activity at low doses, followed by slowed activity at 1.0–1.5 MAC.

## ISOFLURANE

Isoflurane also causes vasodilation, but allows more compensatory tachycardia than sevoflurane.[1] The official labeling indicates isoflurane may be used for induction of anesthesia, but it is highly pungent and may cause coughing, breath-holding, or laryngospasm, as well as mildly increasing secretions. Isoflurane also has a slower onset than sevoflurane, so is not an optimal choice for induction. Given its high potency and low cost, isoflurane may be a cost-effective option for long surgeries. It also has a context-sensitive half-time, so it must be discontinued some time before the end of the surgery to allow timely recovery.[1,2]

## DESFLURANE

Desflurane has a similar hemodynamic profile to isoflurane, but has a more rapid onset and recovery. Desflurane is extremely noxious and cannot be used for induction due to intense airway irritation and transient sympathetic stimulation.[1,2] Its rapid onset does allow for quick adjustment in depth of anesthesia during particularly painful portions of the surgery.

## ENFLURANE AND HALOTHANE

Enflurane and halothane are no longer available in the United States due to the availability of newer agents.[2] These anesthetics have slower onset and recovery and cause myocardial depression. Enflurane can cause frank seizures and may cause renal toxicity from production of fluoride. Halothane can cause hepatotoxicity and increases the risk of arrhythmias due to increased sensitivity to catecholamines.[1]

## ANESTHETIC IMPLICATIONS

### PREOPERATIVE

Avoid using desflurane in patients with airway disease. Develop a plan for induction and maintenance, taking into account the length of surgery, the patient's age, and whether nitrous oxide will be used as an adjunct.

### INTRAOPERATIVE

Monitor the patient's heart rate and blood pressure. Time the discontinuation of anesthetics appropriately with respect to the anticipated end of surgery and recovery time of the anesthetic.

## POSTOPERATIVE

Monitor for and treat emergence reactions such as nausea and shivering. Desflurane in particular may cause bronchospasm and cough.

## REFERENCES

1. Eilers H, Yost S. General anesthetics. In: Katzung BG, ed. *Basic and Clinical Pharmacology*. 14th ed. New York: McGraw-Hill; 440–458. https://accessmedicine-mhmedical-com.ezproxy.libr ary.wisc.edu/content.aspx?bookid=2249&sectionid=175219294. Accessed August 30, 2020.
2. *Lexicomp*. Wolters Kluwer; 2020. http://online.lexi.com. Accessed August 30, 2020.

# 70.

# INTRAVENOUS OPIOID ANESTHETICS

*Nicholas M. Parker*

## INTRODUCTION

Opioids are highly effective analgesics with sedative and anxiolytic properties. Intravenous opioids play an important role in anesthesia induction and maintenance, in addition to treating pain postoperatively.

## MECHANISM OF ACTION

Opioid drugs act on opioid receptors found throughout the central and peripheral nervous system (CNS and PNS).[1,2] Activation of these receptors inhibits nociception by decreasing primary signal transmission, post-synaptic sensitivity to those signals, and the affective perception of pain. Opioids also activate descending pathways that further inhibit pain signaling. In addition to analgesia, opioids also have sedative, anxiolytic, and euphoric effects. They notably do *not* cause amnesia, so other agents must be used if amnesia is desired.

Three subtypes of opioid receptors exist with selective affinity for the endogenous opioids used by the body to modulate pain control and a variety of other functions. Endorphins primarily stimulate the μ-opioid receptor, enkephalins favor the ∂-opioid receptor, and dynorphins are selective for the κ-opioid receptor. Opioid drugs in general act on the μ-opioid receptor.[1]

## PHARMACOKINETICS AND PHARMACODYNAMICS

### PHARMACOKINETICS

### Absorption and Distribution

When given intravenously, absorption into the bloodstream is complete and immediate. It should be noted, however, that most opioids given orally have fairly low bioavailability; this means the intravenous dose of a given opioid will be much lower than the equivalent oral dose (Table 70.1).[1-3] Opioids readily distribute from the blood into tissues, including the CNS.[1]

### Metabolism and Excretion

In general, opioids are metabolized in the liver first by CYP3A4 or CYP2D6, then glucuronidated. This results in a hydrophilic product that is readily cleared by the kidneys. Most opioid metabolites are inactive, but morphine and hydromorphone have active metabolites that may accumulate in patients with renal dysfunction.[1,3] Remifentanil is uniquely metabolized and inactivated by plasma and tissue esterases, resulting in rapid clearance that is independent of hepatic or renal function. Note that CYP2D6 is subject to significant genetic variation, and both CYP3A4 and CYP2D6 are involved in many drug interactions.[1,3]

## Pharmacodyamics

Intravenous opioids in general are full agonists of the μ-opioid receptor, with the exceptions listed in Table 70.1. The practical difference between intravenous opioids is in onset and duration of action (Table 70.1); these parameters are a function of not only drug clearance but also receptor affinity and tolerance.

### EFFECTS ON CIRCULATION

In general, opioids have only minimal effect on circulation, if any. For this reason, opioids are a preferred sedative and anesthetic for patients with hemodynamic compromise or lability, such as in cardiac surgery or in critical illness. Opioids may cause bradycardia but this is usually not dose-limiting. One exception is meperidine, which has antimuscarinic activity which may cause tachycardia. Some opioids, especially morphine, may induce histamine release, causing vasodilation and hypotension; this is why morphine is usually not used for induction or maintenance of anesthesia.

### EFFECTS ON RESPIRATION

All opioids diminish respiratory drive, causing decreased respiratory rate.[1,2] When opioids are used for conscious sedation, the respiratory rate and blood oxygenation must be monitored closely, and the anesthesia team should be ready to manually ventilate the patient if needed. Patients with head injuries may experience cerebral vasodilation

*Table 70.1* PROPERTIES OF INTRAVENOUS OPIOIDS

| | TYPICAL INTRAVENOUS DOSE | DURATION OF ACTION | UNIQUE ATTRIBUTES | TYPICAL USES |
|---|---|---|---|---|
| Morphine | Analgesia: 1 to 4 mg | Long | Active metabolites Prototypical opioid | Acute pain, chronic pain, air hunger |
| Hydromorphone (Dilaudid®) | Analgesia: 0.2 to 0.8 mg | Long | Active metabolites | Acute pain, analgosedation |
| Methadone (Dolophine®) | Analgesia: 2.5 to 10 mg | Long | Effective in opioid-tolerant patients Unpredictable and nonlinear equivalence to other opioids | Chronic pain, maintenance in opioid use disorder, adjunct in acute pain and anesthesia |
| Fentanyl (Sublimaze®) | Analgesia: 25 to 100 mcg Induction: 0.5 to 1 mcg/kg | Medium | More potent and shorter-acting than morphine and hydromorphone | Acute pain, induction of anesthesia, analgosedation, chronic pain |
| Sufentanil (Dsuvia®) | Induction: 1 mcg/kg per hour of surgical time (given over 2 to 10 minutes) | Medium | More potent than fentanyl | Surgical anesthesia |
| Alfentanil | Induction: 130 to 245 mcg/kg Maintenance: 1 to 1.5 mcg/kg/min | Short | Less potent than fentanyl but faster onset and shorter duration | Surgical anesthesia |
| Remifentanil (Ultiva®) | Induction: 0.5 to 1 mcg/kg/min Maintenance: 0.25 to 1 mcg/kg/min | Ultra-short | Metabolized by plasma and tissue esterases (independent of hepatic or renal function) | Surgical anesthesia |
| Meperidine (Demerol®) | Shivering: 12.5 to 50 mg | Medium | Antimuscarinic effects (e.g., tachycardia) | Postoperative shivering |
| Nalbuphine (Nubain®) | Induction: 0.3 to 3 mg/kg Opioid-induced pruritus: 2.5 to 5 mg | Medium | μ-opioid receptor antagonist but κ-receptor agonist | Induction of anesthesia, opioid-related itching |

Long: 4–6 hours; Medium: 1–2 hours; Short: less than 1 hour; Ultra-short: seconds to minutes; mcg: microgram.

and increased intracranial pressure due to carbon dioxide retention when using opioids.[1] If opioids are used for induction or maintenance of surgical anesthesia, patients must be manually or mechanically ventilated. Naloxone may be administered to reverse respiratory depression caused by opioids, but will also reverse analgesic and sedative effects.

Too-rapid administration of fentanyl, sufentanil, alfentanil, or remifentanil may cause truncal rigidity and decreased thoracic compliance, making mechanical ventilation more difficult.[1,3] If this occurs, slow the infusion rate of the opioid and use a nondepolarizing paralytic (e.g., rocuronium, atracurium, etc.) if needed.

## EFFECTS ON OTHER ORGANS

Opioids reliably diminish gastrointestinal motility.[1–3] While this is not of great concern in the operating room, opioid-induced constipation can significantly hamper postoperative recovery. Unless otherwise contraindicated, patients should receive stool softeners postoperatively until they have reliable return of bowel function and no longer require opioid analgesics. Patients do not develop tolerance to opioid-induced constipation, even as other effects diminish.[2]

Opioids may also cause increased biliary and/or urinary sphincter tone, miosis, hypogonadism, leukopenia, cough suppression, hyperthermia, or hypothermia.[1–3]

## SIDE EFFECTS AND TOXICITY

The most important side effects of opioids—respiratory depression, sedation, and constipation—were discussed previously. Opioids may also cause nausea, vomiting, dysphoria, hallucinations, nightmares, and pruritus.[1–3]

Opioids also carry significant potential for dependence and addiction.[1–3] Withdrawal from opioids often presents as anxiety, tachycardia, hypertension, nausea/vomiting, and/or hyperalgesia. Opioid withdrawal is not life-threatening but is very unpleasant and may cause patients to continue using opioids even after pain has diminished. Opioid overdose, from either illicit use or unintentional overuse of prescription opioids, leads to approximately 100,000 deaths every year in the United States.[4]

## ROLE IN INDUCTION OF ANESTHESIA

During induction, intravenous opioids are typically used as an adjunct to other anesthetics like propofol. In addition to providing analgesia, opioids blunt the airway reflexes, tachycardia, and hypertension that may be triggered by intubation. Opioids also provide some sedation, which allows for a reduced dose of the primary agent, which may diminish hypotension. Due to respiratory depression at sedating doses, opioids are less ideal if mechanical ventilation is not planned.

Remifentanil, with its ultra-short duration of action, may also be used at high doses during rapid-sequence intubation in place of a neuromuscular blocking agent.

## ANESTHETIC CONSIDERATIONS

### PREOPERATIVE

Opioids are effective analgesics with useful sedative and anxiolytic properties. Assess the patient for chronic opioid use or use of opioid antagonists (naloxone, buprenorphine) that may complicate their response to opioid anesthetics.

### INTRAOPERATIVE

Choose the opioid agent and dose based on the anticipated duration of the procedure.

### POSTOPERATIVE

Ensure the patient is breathing spontaneously before extubation. Taper the patient off of opioids as soon as possible after surgery to reduce the risk of dependence, addiction, and overdose. Give stool softeners and limit opioid doses to reduce the risk of constipation and ileus. Prescribe naloxone to patients discharging with large quantities of opioids.

## REFERENCES

1. Schumacher MA, et al. Opioid agonists and antagonists. In: Katzung BG, ed. *Basic and Clinical Pharmacology*. 14th ed. New York: McGraw-Hill; 553–574. https://accessmedicine-mhmedical-com.ezproxy.library.wisc.edu/content.aspx?bookid=2249&sectionid=175220393. Accessed August 23, 2020.
2. Baumann TJ, et al. Pain management. In: DiPiro JT, Talbert RL, Yee GC, Matzke GR, Wells BG, Posey LM, eds. *Pharmacotherapy: A Pathophysiologic Approach*. 9th ed. New York: McGraw-Hill Education; 2014:925–942.
3. *Lexicomp*. Wolters Kluwer; 2020. http://online.lexi.com. Accessed August 23, 2020.
4. Ahmad FB, Rossen LM, Sutton P. Provisional drug overdose death counts. National Center for Health Statistics. 2021. https://www.cdc.gov/nchs/nvss/vsrr/drug-overdose-data.htm.

# 71.

# SUBSTANCE USE DISORDER

*Raymond C. Yu and Till Conermann*

## SUBSTANCE ABUSE

Millions of Americans suffer from substance use disorder (SUD) as characterized by the fifth edition of the *Diagnostic and Statistical Manual of Mental Disorders* (DSM-5).

### CRITERIA FOR SUBSTANCE USE DISORDER (SUD)

(1) Often taking in larger amounts or over a longer period than was intended;
(2) Unsuccessful efforts to cut down or control use;
(3) Great deal of time is spent in activities necessary to obtain, use, or recover from the substance's effects;
(4) Strong desire or urge to use the substance;
(5) Recurrent use leading to failure to fulfill major obligations at work, school, or home;
(6) Continued use despite having persistent or recurrent social or interpersonal problems caused or exacerbated by its effects;
(7) Important social, occupational, or recreational activities are given up or reduced because of use;
(8) Recurrent use in situations in which it is physically hazardous;
(9) Continued use despite knowledge of having a persistent or recurrent physical or psychological problem that is likely to have been caused or exacerbated by the substance;
(10) Tolerance;
(11) Withdrawal.

This describes a problematic pattern of use of intoxicating substance leading to clinically significant impairment or distress. The United States 2018 National Survey on Drug Use and Health on people aged 12 or older estimated that 8.1 million people had at least one illicit drug use disorder, commonly marijuana (4.4 million) and opioids (2.1 million). For surgery, they can be in an acute, intoxicated state or in withdrawal, wherein the symptoms are typically opposite of the acute or intoxicated effects. Approximately 3.7 million people per year receive medication assisted treatment (MAT) for SUD.[1]

## GENERAL MECHANISM OF SUBSTANCE USE DISORDER

Addictive and abused substances exert their reinforcing effects through the activation of the mesolimbic dopamine system due to central nervous system (CNS) increased dopaminergic signaling from and dopaminergic surge in the midbrain ventral tegmental area to the nucleus accumbens in ventral striatum (see Figure 71.1). This causes a strong reinforcing effect, leading to maladaptive behavior and sometimes compulsive consumption in individuals.[2]

## TOLERANCE, DEPENDENCE, AND ABUSE DEFINITION

Tolerance is a decreased effectiveness or response of a substance secondary to its chronic administration. Physical dependence is the emergence of negative or withdrawal signs and symptoms when drug use is discontinued. Addiction is a disease state characterized by compulsive drug seeking and use despite harmful or negative consequences.[2,3]

## ALCOHOL AND PREOPERATIVE CONSIDERATIONS

Alcohol use disorder is common and should be screened for (e.g., CAGE questionnaire). Alcohol is a small, water-soluble molecule that is metabolized in the liver through alcohol dehydrogenase via zero-order kinetics and induces the cytochrome p450 oxidases (such as CYP2E1). Acute alcohol consumption acts as a CNS depressant with synergistic depressant effects with barbiturates, benzodiazepines, opioids, and general anesthetics.[3,4]

Brain reward (dopamine) pathways

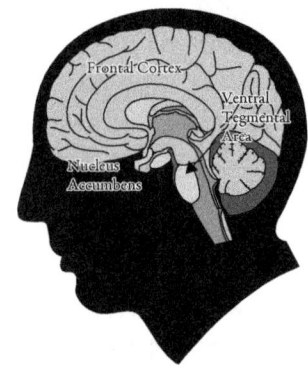

These brain circuits are important for natural
rewards such as food, music, and sex.

Drugs of abuse increase dopamine

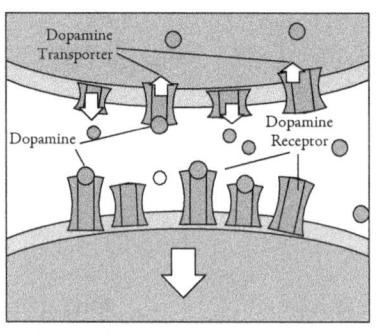

FOOD

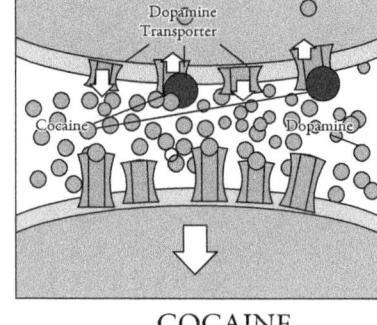

COCAINE

Typically, dopamine increases in response to natural rewards such as food.
When cocaine is taken, dopamine increases are exaggerated, and communication is altered.

Figure 71.1. Enforcing effects of addictive substances through the activation of the mesolimbic dopamine system with increased dopamine in the midbrain ventral tegmental area to the nucleus accumbens in ventral striatum.

Chronic alcohol intake leads to alterations in neuronal excitability. Alcohol withdrawal could begin as early as 6 to 24 hours after last alcohol intake. Withdrawal signs and symptoms include anxiety, nausea, headache, tachycardia, hypertension, sweating, and tremors. Treatment of withdrawal includes benzodiazepine, barbiturates, or anticonvulsants. Deliriums tremens (DT), a life-threatening condition, is characterized by severe delirium with autonomic dysfunction requiring immediate medical treatment and stabilization.[3,4]

Disulfiram is an alcohol-sensitizing medication that alters the body's response to alcohol, making it unpleasant. It inhibits aldehyde dehydrogenase, raising the blood acetaldehyde concentration, leading to disulfiram-ethanol reaction: tachycardia, palpitations, nausea, vomiting, or shortness of breath. Disulfiram has the potential for hepatotoxicity and hypotension. The recommendation is to discontinue disulfiram 10 days prior to anesthesia.[4]

## ALCOHOL USE AND INTRAOPERATIVE ANESTHETIC CONSIDERATIONS

Rapid sequence induction is advised due to delayed gastric emptying. Naso- or orogastric tube is a relative contraindication for suspected esophageal varices. Once surgery is underway, acute alcohol intoxication decreases MAC, while chronic alcohol use increases MAC. Acute alcohol intoxication can lead to serious physiologic derangements such as impaired cognition, cerebral artery vasospasm, acute hepatitis, arrhythmias, coagulopathy, and life-threatening metabolic electrolyte abnormalities.[4] Chronic alcohol abuse

can cause liver cirrhosis, dilated cardiomyopathy, oral and esophageal cancers, nutritional deficiencies, and electrolyte derangements such as metabolic acidosis and hyponatremia. Coagulopathy can be corrected by administration of fresh frozen plasma or vitamin K, and refractory cases might potentially require recombinant factor VII.[3]

## ALCOHOL USE AND POSTOPERATIVE CONSIDERATIONS

Postoperative analgesic management should consider possible physiologic derangements. Reducing opioid doses can lessen lethal interactions with benzodiazepines which are used to treat withdrawal symptoms. Close monitoring of withdrawal symptoms and DT is advised.[3]

## OPIOIDS OVERVIEW AND PREOPERATIVE CONSIDERATIONS

Opioids acutely can result in analgesia, euphoria, sedation, respiratory depression, nausea, and itching. Chronic opioid use and abuse lead to development of tolerance. For patients experiencing opioid overdose, naloxone, an opioid antagonist, is a short-acting agent used to counteract CNS and respiratory depression. Because of its short half-life, close monitoring is required since recurrence of sedation and respiratory depression can occur.[4]

Patients with opioid dependence are sometimes maintained on MAT. Naltrexone is a μ receptor competitive antagonist with no agonist properties. It blocks the activation of μ opioid receptors and helps promote opioid/alcohol abstinence; however, it antagonizes the effectiveness of opioid analgesics. It is ideal to discontinue oral naltrexone at least 3 days prior to surgery and extended-release naltrexone at least one month prior to surgery.[3,5]

Methadone is a synthetic, long-acting opioid that is primarily a μ receptor agonist and a weak NMDA receptor antagonist. In addition to MAT, it can be used in chronic pain management. Side effects of methadone include edema, hypotension, and QT prolongation, especially at higher doses of 90 to 100 mg daily, which can lead to *torsades de pointes*. Methadone should be continued for surgery.[3,5]

Buprenorphine is a semi-synthetic opiate that is a potent partial agonist of the μ opioid receptor with high affinity but with very low intrinsic activity and a κ receptor antagonist. It reduces the intensity of opioid withdrawal. Its high potency and slow dissociation rate allow it to displace other μ agonists from the receptors and overcome opioid dependence.[3,5] Buprenorphine has a ceiling effect on respiratory depression. It can be continued for surgeries with minimal anticipated postoperative pain, but for painful, elective procedures, it should be discontinued 3 to 5 days prior, with bridging to a short-acting opioid to prevent withdrawal.[5]

## OPIOID USE AND INTRAOPERATIVE ANESTHETIC CONSIDERATIONS

Opioids cause delayed gastric emptying. Acutely intoxicated individuals will require aspiration precautions and gastric decompression. Acute opioid intoxication will have lower MAC, while chronic opioid dependence can increase MAC requirements. Tolerance makes adequate analgesic doses of opioids unpredictable. Multimodal analgesia with regional anesthesia and adjuvants (NMDA-antagonists, nonsteroidal anti-inflammatory agents, alpha-2 receptor agonist, local anesthetic infiltration) is advised.[3] Patients who are on MAT often require higher doses of opioids than opioid-naïve patients due to the presence of opioid cross-tolerance and occupancy of μ receptor, but additional short-acting opioids should not be withheld for acute pain.[5]

## OPIOIDS AND POSTOPERATIVE CONSIDERATIONS

Patients should be monitored closely and provided only an adequate amount of short-acting opioids, and tapered once post-surgical pain subsides. Close follow-up is essential to the success of MAT in opioid SUD. Patients who discontinued their therapy and were placed on opioids should be made aware of the risks associated with opioid overdose and relapse.[4,5]

## CANNABINOIDS OVERVIEW AND PRE-ANESTHETIC CONSIDERATIONS

Acutely, marijuana use may result in euphoria, psychomotor impairment, sedation, dizziness, or confusion. Delta-9-tetrahydrocannabinol (THC) interacts with cannabinoid receptors, which could induce opioid and benzodiazepine receptors due to common intracellular signaling mechanisms. Chronic smoking of marijuana can lead to pulmonary pathology.[3,4]

## MARIJUANA USE AND INTRAOPERATIVE ANESTHETIC IMPLICATIONS

Anesthetic implications of marijuana use are relatively minor compared with other drugs. During anesthesia, hypotension can occur; this is usually manageable with conventional treatment. Acute intoxication from marijuana may possibly reduce MAC requirements. Some literature indicates chronic marijuana users may require increased dosages of midazolam, propofol and fentanyl. There might be higher risk of pulmonary and cardiovascular complications.[3, <3,6>]

## MARIJUANA AND POSTOPERATIVE CONSIDERATIONS

Conventional analgesics can be used. Chronic marijuana users may have higher pain scores, but the reason behind this still needs further research. Marijuana may reduce postoperative nausea and vomiting. Mild symptoms of withdrawal can occur in heavy users that suddenly stop.[3,4]

## COCAINE OVERVIEW AND PRE-ANESTHETIC CONSIDERATIONS

Cocaine has been used as a local anesthetic and vasoconstrictor. It is a CNS stimulant through inhibition of presynaptic catecholamine reuptake, leading to accumulation of extracellular dopamine in the mesolimbic system. This provides a sense of euphoria, excitement, and increased mental and physical capacity. Patients using cocaine may present with severe agitation, seizures, or delirium, which can be managed with benzodiazepines.[4]

## COCAINE USE AND INTRAOPERATIVE ANESTHETIC IMPLICATIONS

Acute use increases MAC requirements. Sympathetic stimulation during induction should be avoided, especially with the presence of abnormal cardiovascular signs. Patients are monitored closely for fever, arrhythmias, significant hypertension, and cardiac ischemia. Chronic cocaine users may have decreased MAC levels. The risk of cardiovascular compromise, such as the presence of arrhythmia and ischemia, can still occur. Indirect-acting sympathomimetic (ephedrine) agents may be less effective due to decreased sympathetic tone.[3,4]

## COCAINE USE AND POSTOPERATIVE ANESTHETIC CONSIDERATIONS

Cocaine withdrawal can be associated with agitation, tremors, and fatigue, and is usually treated symptomatically with benzodiazepines. Close monitoring is advised for patient safety and potential drug-seeking behavior.[3,4]

## OTHER SUBSTANCES: BARBITURATES, BENZODIAZEPINES, AMPHETAMINES, HALLUCINOGENICS

Benzodiazepines modulate the GABA-A receptor through specific benzodiazepine receptors. Barbiturates act directly upon the GABA-A receptor. Acute intoxication of these substances significantly reduces the doses of induction and maintenance agents required, as normal doses can cause significant hypotension. Chronic abusers develop tolerance, requiring higher MAC.[3,4]

Amphetamines are CNS stimulants as they cause presynaptic catecholamine release, leading to variable response of indirect acting sympathomimetic. Acutely intoxicated individuals present with fever, tachycardia, hypertension, and arrhythmias requiring treatment. Profound hyperthermia will require aggressive cooling intraoperatively. MAC requirements are increased. Chronic amphetamine abusers may have chronic vasculitis with aneurysm formation and infarcts. They may present with malnutrition, dehydration, and poor dentition. MAC requirements are decreased and indirect acting sympathomimetics have decreased effect.[3,4] Toxicity may

be treated with chlorpromazine, haloperidol, α blockers, and β blockers.

Hallucinogenic agents include indolamines or lysergic acid diethylamide (LSD), phenylethylamines (MDMA, ecstasy), or phencyclidine (PCP). These substances act primarily though serotonin receptor 5-HT2 subtype, with the exception of PCP which is an NMDA antagonist. PCP can block reuptake of norepinephrine and serotonin and also can inhibit pseudocholinesterase. PCP intoxication can induce dissociated state with extremely violent behavior, sweating, salivation, fever, rigidity, hyperreflexia, hypertension, tachycardia, and convulsions. Nystagmus is usually present. LSD has significant analgesic effect, anticholinesterase effects, and can cause mild hypertension, tachycardia, hyperthermia, wheezing, and salivation. General anesthesia can initiate a flashback in patients using LSD. MDMA is closely related to amphetamines, with similar anesthetic considerations. Hemodynamic instability and arrhythmias can be seen intraoperatively. For these substances, emergence can be challenging due to significant hemodynamic changes, arrhythmias, and altered mental status leading to postoperative delirium.[3,4]

## REFERENCES

1. Center for Behavioral Health Statistics and Quality. Results from the 2018 National Survey on Drug Use and Health: Detailed Tables. https://www.samhsa.gov/data/sites/default/files/cbhsq-reports/NSDUHNationalFindingsReport2018/NSDUHNationalFindingsReport2018.pdf.
2. Volkow ND. *Drugs, Brain, and Behavior: The Science of Addiction.* NIH Publication No. 20-DA-5605. Printed in April 2007, revised June 2020. https://www.drugabuse.gov/sites/default/files/soa.pdf.
3. Gutstein, HB. Management of patients with chronic alcohol or drug use. In: Evers AE, Maze M, Kharasch E, eds. *Anesthetic Pharmacology: Basic Principles and Clinical Practice.* 2nd ed. Cambridge: Cambridge University Press; 2011:1106–1116.
4. Management of intoxication and withdrawal, pharmacological interventions and other somatic therapies. In: Herron AJ, Brennan TK, eds. *The ASAM Essentials of Addiction Medicine.* 3rd ed. Philadelphia, PA: Wolters Kluwer Health/Lippincott; 2020:285–341.
5. Kampman K, Jarvis M. American Society of Addiction Medicine (ASAM) national practice guideline for the use of medications in the treatment of addiction involving opioid use. *J Addict Med.* 2015 Sept–Oct;9(5):358–367.

# 72.

# EPIDURAL AND INTRATHECAL ANESTHETICS

*Wilson Alfredo Medina II and Laura Liss Gershon*

## SPINAL, EPIDURAL, CAUDAL, COMBINED SPINAL/EPIDURAL ANESTHESIA

### INDICATIONS AND CONTRAINDICATIONS

Epidural and spinal anesthesia may be used as primary anesthetics or as adjuvants to general anesthesia for lower extremity, upper and lower abdominal, and thoracic surgical procedures. They may also be used for analgesia for obstetric indications or postoperative pain management. A combined spinal epidural (CSE) may be used to facilitate rapid onset of obstetrical analgesia.

Caudal anesthetics are most commonly utilized for surgical anesthesia, and postoperative analgesia in pediatric cases.

Absolute contraindications to neuraxial anesthesia include patient refusal, infection at the sight of injection, and underlying bleeding disorders. Relative contraindications to neuraxial block placement include hypotension, sepsis, elevated intracranial pressure, history of back surgery, neurological disease, and cardiac conditions that render patients unable to compensate for hypotension.[1]

The epidural space is a potential space in which its borders consist of the foramen magnum cranially, the sacrococcygeal ligament caudally, the posterior longitudinal ligament anteriorly, the ligamentum flavum posteriorly, and the vertebral pedicles laterally.[2] The intrathecal/subarachnoid space contains cerebral spinal fluid (CSF) and is located between the arachnoid and pia which is contiguous throughout the brain and spinal cord.[1]

Although opioids work based on their respective affinity for opioid receptors within the Rexed laminae of the substantia gelatinosa within the dorsal root ganglia, opioids administered within the neuraxial space may impact different neuraxial levels depending on their lipophilicity.[1] Lipophilic opioids are readily absorbed, impacting the dorsal root ganglia near the site of neuraxial injection. In contrast, hydrophilic opioids stay in suspension and spread rostrally within the CSF, thus attributing to their increased potential to induce a delayed respiratory depression via medullary suppression.[3]

## FACTORS INFLUENCING ONSET, DURATION, AND TERMINATION OF ACTION

### ONSET

The onset of local anesthetics is discussed in Chapters 86 and 153. The addition of bicarbonate is commonly used to speed block onset by increasing the non-ionized local anesthetic form which can freely diffuse across the cellular lipid membrane. This allows greater intracellular concentrations of the local anesthetic to bind to intracellular neuronal sodium receptors within the lipid membrane.[3]

### DURATION

The duration of action of shorter-acting agents such as 2-chloroprocaine, lidocaine, and mepivicaine can be prolonged by the addition of epinephrine in order to prevent extravasation of the anesthetic agent.[3] Vasoconstrictive agents have minimal prolonging effects when used with longer-acting local anesthetics.[3] Ropivicaine has inherent vasoconstrictive properties and is unaffected by the addition of a vasoconstricting adjuvant.[3]

### TERMINATION OF ACTION

Metabolism and excretion of local anesthetics is minimal within the neuraxial space. After the neuraxial drug reaches the plasma via passive diffusion, it follows its corresponding pharmacodynamics, which are explained in Chapters 86 and 153.

# SPINAL/SUBARACHNOID ANESTHESIA

## BLOCK HEIGHT

Major factors that have an impact on block height are drug baricity, dose, patient position, and CSF density and volume. CSF volume has an inverse relationship to block volume, also likely having the highest impact on block height. Patient weight does not impact block height.[3]

## EPIDURAL ANESTHESIA

Factors that affect epidural block level include dose, volume of drug administered, and site of injection. Pain from abdominal procedures may be blocked via low thoracic epidurals, while a laboring parturient requires a lumbar epidural for adequate sacral, lumbar, and low thoracic dermatome coverage.[1]

## PROLONGED DURATION

The use of epinephrine and alpha-adrenergic receptor agonists may be used to prolong the duration of epidural anesthesia.[3]

## SYSTEMIC TOXICITY, TEST DOSE

A test dose is administered for epidural drug administration in order to detect whether the needle or catheter has been inadvertently placed either intrathecally or intravascularly. An unrecognized intrathecal injection may result in a high or total spinal. An unrecognized intravascular injection may result in an ineffective block or, more seriously, local anesthetic systemic toxicity. Local anesthetics are responsible for intrathecal test dosing, while epinephrine commonly tests for inadvertent intravascular placement, which is indicated by marked hypertension and tachycardia.[4] It is important to remember that the absence of concerning signs after test dose administration does not completely rule out the possibility of intravascular or intrathecal placement.[4]

## COMPLICATIONS

Post-dural puncture headache (PDPH) may be a complication of either intentional (3%) or unintentional (50%) dural puncture.[5] Risk factors for PDPH are younger age, BMI under 30, history of PDPH, and history of chronic headaches.[3] PDPH typically presents between 24 and 48 hours after a dural puncture.[5] Common findings may include frontal, occipital, and retro-orbital pain that is worsened in the upright position, and relieved when supine. Treatment typically consists of symptomatic relief, as most cases of PDPH are self-limiting within 5–7 days,[3] and includes nonsteroidal anti-inflammatory drugs (NSAIDs)/acetaminophen, oral hydration, and rest in the supine position. Epidural blood patch placement has consistently been supported as the gold standard of care. Scarce data supporting the use of epidural saline infusion and/or bolus have been reported but remain controversial.

Low frequency hearing loss, although rare, may present in the elderly, although most cases are self-limiting.[3]

Initial signs of a *high spinal* include hand weakness and numbness, with progressive rostral spread resulting in poor speech and medullary respiratory effort. Risk factors include short stature, obesity, epidural after unintended dural puncture, and spinal deformity.[1] Treatment of high spinal blockade may require intubation and mechanical ventilation, with a low threshold for the use of epinephrine.[1] Increased mortality has been reported in the setting of high spinal–induced bradycardia when epinephrine administration has been delayed.[3]

Among the rarest complications is neurologic injury via direct trauma or compression from hematoma, or infection. American Society of Regional Anesthesia (ASRA) guidelines for epidural and spinal placement in anticoagulated patients are regularly updated and may be reviewed at https://www.asra.com/advisory-guidelines.2.

## PHYSIOLOGIC EFFECTS

Epidural or intrathecally administered local anesthetics may induce hypotension by decreasing systemic vascular resistance (SVR). There is little to no effect on respiratory function, although forced vital capacity (FVC) is most sensitive to inhibition.[3]

## EFFECT ON OTHER ORGANS AND SYSTEMS

Physiologic impacts may include but are not limited to profound sedation if using alpha-2 agonists, increased gastric motility and sphincter dilation, elevated gastric pH, and diffuse vasodilation which may be therapeutically used at times to prevent thrombosis.[2]

## REFERENCES

1. Chestnut DH. *Chestnut's Obstetric Anesthesia: Principles and Practice*. 6th ed. Philadelphia, PA: Mosby/Elsevier; 2019:13:274–311; 23:474–539.
2. Horlocker T, et al. *Regional Anesthesia in the Patient Receiving Antithrombotic or Thrombolytic Therapy: American Society*

*of Regional Anesthesia and Pain Medicine Evidence-Based Guidelines.* 4th ed. 2018. https://www.asra.com/advisory-guidelines/article/9/regional-anesthesia-in-the-patient-receiving-antithrombotic-or-thrombolytic-ther. Accessed September 09, 2020.

3. Barash PG, et al. *Clinical Anesthesia.* 8th ed. Philadelphia, PA: Wolters Kluwer; 2017:20:505–527; 22:564–585; 35:914–945.

4. Tanaka M, Nishikawa T. Simulation of an epidural test dose with intravenous epinephrine in sevoflurane-anesthetized children. *Anesthesia & Analgesia.* 1998;86(5):952–957.

5. Bakshi S, Gehdoo RP. Incidence and management of post-dural puncture headache following spinal anaesthesia and accidental dural puncture from a non-obstetric hospital: A retrospective analysis. *Indian J Anaesth.* 2018;62(11):881–886.

# 73.

# BARBITURATES

*Kris Ferguson and Amol Soin*

## INTRODUCTION

Thiopental is the most commonly used barbiturate for induction. Other barbiturates include thiamylal, methohexital, secobarbital, phenobarbital, and pentobarbital. Thiopental is the prototypical barbiturate in use and will be the focus of the chapter. Barbiturates have a high potency with a rapid onset and short duration of action.[1] Thiopental can be used to induce anesthesia and can be a therapeutic option for hypoxic brain injury and intracranial hypertension.[2] Thiopental can also be used to treat status epilepticus which is refractory to conventional treatment.

## PHARMACOKINETICS

Following intravenous injection, drug concentrations in the brain, heart, intestine, spleen, pancreas, and kidney quickly rise, promoting rapid onset of action.[1] Termination of action of thiopental is due to redistribution to other compartments. Barbiturates are highly albumin bound and in cases of low albumin (severe malnutrition, liver disease) or if the non-ionized fraction is increased, such as in cases of acidosis, the brain will see larger doses. Metabolism of thiopental only becomes significant when there repeat dosing or continuous infusion.[1]

## PHARMACODYNAMICS

Barbiturates act primarily at the gamma-aminobutyric acid (GABA) A receptor. Barbiturates increase the affinity of GABA to the GABA A receptor. The GABA A receptor is a chloride channel.[2] When GABA binds to the receptor, it opens the chloride channel leading to hyperpolarization of the cell.[3]

## METABOLISM AND EXCRETION

Barbiturates are metabolized in the liver and metabolites excreted in the urine. There is a context sensitive half-life such that if there is a continuous infusion of barbiturates, the duration of action is proportional to the duration of infusion. Due to thiopental's long context-sensitive half-life, it is seldom used as a continuous infusion. Women typically have a much longer elimination half-life than men. The elimination half-life is typically unaffected in renal failure.

## CIRCULATION

The impact of barbiturate on the circulatory system is modest. There is a decreased baroreceptor reflex and decreased myocardial contractility.[1] Circulatory system depression can be catastrophic if barbiturates are given to patients with severe hypovolemia, congestive heart failure, or significant beta blockade. This is caused by uncompensated peripheral pooling of blood and direct myocardial depression.

## RESPIRATORY

Laryngeal spasms and respiratory depression can occur. Barbiturates do not provide analgesia, and airway manipulation can precipitate laryngeal spasm. There is a dose-depending decrease in respiration up to and including apnea.

## CEREBRAL

The dose and speed of injection determine onset of action, with effect ranging from sedation to general anesthesia. An induction dose of 3–5 mg/kg induces anesthesia in 14–20 seconds and lasts approximately 1 minute.[1] Barbiturates reduce intracranial pressure by reducing cerebral blood flow via increased cerebrovascular resistance and blood volume. The cerebral metabolic rate also decreases, and this is beneficial in epileptics.[2] At higher doses, barbiturates can induce electrocerebral silence also known as burst suppression.

## BARBITURATE COMA

Barbiturate coma therapy is a treatment modality which can be used in severe head injuries. The barbiturate coma can lower the intracranial pressure when hyperventilation and mannitol fail. Barbiturates also lower extracellular lactate and other excitatory amino acids. Intensive monitoring is required, including electroencephalogram (EEG), arterial blood pressure, and often pulmonary artery catheter, as well as blood chemistry.[2] Treatment is initiated with a loading dose and maintained with an infusion. Using EEG monitoring, once burst suppression is achieved, a constant infusion is maintained. Blood levels of pentobarbital do not accurately reflect the physiological impact of infusion, hence EEG monitoring. Current indications for burst suppression with low levels of evidence are: refractory status epilepticus, refractory intracranial hypertension (secondary to traumatic brain injury), intraoperative neuroprotection during cerebrovascular surgery. Typically, a 1:10 burst to suppression ratio is the target. Evidence is lacking in the setting of prolonged cerebral ischemia due to cerebral aneurysm surgery, cerebral bypass surgery, or cardiac/aortic surgery with cerebral blood flow disruption. If pentobarbital or thiopental are used for burst suppression, emergence from anesthesia may take days.

## DRUG INTERACTIONS

Barbiturates are synergistic with opioids, ethanol, and antihistamines in producing central nervous system depression. Contrast media, sulfonamides, and other drugs that are highly protein bound may displace barbiturates, increasing the effects of the delivered dose.

## SIDE EFFECTS AND TOXICITY

With barbiturates there is an absence of pain on injection. There are minimal post-induction side effects, such as nausea, vomiting, delirium, or headache. Barbiturates also lower intraocular pressure. Barbiturates lack analgesic properties. Methohexital does cause epileptogenic effects in patients with psychomotor epilepsy.

## INDICATIONS AND CONTRAINDICATIONS

Contraindications include a known allergy to barbiturates. Barbiturates are contraindicated in patients with acute intermittent porphyria. Barbiturates (phenobarbital, thiopental, methohexital) enzyme induction is dependent on the duration of exposure. Acutely, barbiturates interact with cytochrome P450 enzymes and can inhibit metabolism.[1] However, chronic use of barbiturates can induce microsomal enzymes and increased drug metabolism. This enzyme induction also induces delta-aminolaevulinic acid (ALA) synthase. ALA synthase is involved in the porphyrin pathway, which is why barbiturates can precipitate an attack of acute intermittent porphyria or variegate porphyria. This would present as severe abdominal pain, nausea, vomiting, and possibly psychiatric disorders or neurologic abnormalities. Other induction agents, such as benzodiazepines, ketamine, etomidate, and propofol, are safe to use in acute intermittent porphyria.[1] Due to barbiturates' respiratory depressant effects, caution should be used in patients with myasthenia gravis.

## ANESTHETIC CONSIDERATIONS

### PREOPERATIVE

A complete history and physical exam should be done prior to induction. Elderly patients typically require dose reduction. Obesity also requires a dose reduction of dosed in mg/kg. Thiopental dose is decreased in those with liver damage, severe anemia, shock, and heart failure. No dose reduction was needed in sickle cell patients. Chronic alcoholics require a higher thiopental dose, as there is cross tolerance with alcohol. As an induction agent, it lowers the intraocular pressure and thus can be helpful in situations of elevated intraocular pressure, such as glaucoma or penetrating eye injury. Barbiturates are a safe induction agent in pregnancy.[1]

## INTRAOPERATIVE

Barbiturates are typically not used as continuous infusions due to their long half-life. For neurosurgical cases where SSEP monitoring is performed, barbiturates can decrease the amplitude and increase the latency.

## POSTOPERATIVE

There is minimal postoperative impact.

## REFERENCES

1. Russo H, Bressolle F. Pharmacodynamics and pharmacokinetics of thiopental. *Clin Pharmacokinet.* 1998 Aug;35(2):95–134.
2. Bratton SL, et al. Guidelines for the management of severe traumatic brain injury. IX. Cerebral perfusion thresholds. *J Neurotrauma.* 2007;24(suppl 1):S59–S64.
3. Brohan J, Goudra BG. The role of GABA receptor agonists in anesthesia and sedation. *CNS Drugs.* 2017 Oct;31(10):845–856.

# 74.

# PROPOFOL

*Kris Ferguson and Peter Papapetrou*

## INTRODUCTION

Propofol is a short-acting intravenous (IV) anesthetic agent that can induce and maintain anesthesia. Propofol has a quick onset and quick offset. Propofol works primarily at the gamma-aminobutyric acid (GABA) A receptor and has been shown to decrease postoperative nausea and vomiting. One formulation of propofol is an emulsion that contains egg phosphatide among other ingredients.

## PHARMACOKINETICS

Propofol is delivered via intravenous access for sedation and general anesthesia. Onset is rapid due to propofol's lipid solubility. Following injection, propofol quickly crosses the blood-brain barrier.[1] Termination of action is due to redistribution and metabolism by the liver. Propofol does have a context-sensitive half-life: the longer the propofol is infused, the longer its half-life.[2]

## PHARMACODYNAMICS

Propofol induces sedation and general anesthesia by working at the GABA A receptor to increase the affinity for GABA to the GABA A receptor.[1,2] The GABA A receptor is a chloride channel and, when activated, hyperpolarizes the cell. Propofol is not reversed by flumazenil.[2]

## METABOLISM AND EXCRETION

Metabolism is carried out in the liver by glucuronidation and the elimination half-life is between 2 and 24 hours. It has a remarkably high extraction ratio by the liver.[1] Propofol metabolism is proportional to liver blood flow. Once metabolized by the liver by glucuronidation, it is excreted in the urine.[2]

## CIRCULATION

With an induction dose, there is a decrease in sympathetic activity, a decrease in arterial blood pressure, a decrease in systemic vascular resistance, a decrease in preload, a decrease in afterload, and a decrease in cardiac contractility.[1] There is also a decrease in pulmonary arterial capillary wedge pressure. These factors lead to hypotension. The hypotension is attenuated by intubation or surgical stimulation. The hypotension is more pronounced by hypovolemia, in the elderly, and with preexisting cardiac disease.[2] Drugs such as opioids, benzodiazepines, antihypertensive medication enhance the hypotension. The hypotension leads to decreased cardiac output, cardiac index, and stroke volume.

## RESPIRATORY

An induction dose will typically cause apnea. Respiratory depression is proportional to the dose, rate of injection, and coexisting sedative medications. Propofol decreases the tidal volume, minute ventilation, and ventilatory drive. Patients with chronic obstructive pulmonary disease (COPD) are sensitive to the respiratory depressant effects. Propofol will potentiate hypoxic pulmonary vasoconstriction.[1,2] Benzodiazepines and propofol decrease the slope of the $CO_2$ response curve, whereas opioids cause a right shift in the curve. Propofol can be metabolized in the lungs, but this is not a significant contribution to total metabolism.

## CEREBRAL

Propofol causes cerebral vasoconstriction which is proportional to the dose. Propofol decreases intraocular pressure; this is noteworthy for patients with glaucoma. There is a concomitant decrease in metabolic demand and perfusion pressure. Like thiopental, propofol may be protective in cases of focal cerebral ischemia.[1]

## DRUG INTERACTIONS

### SIDE EFFECTS AND TOXICITY

The most common adverse effect of propofol is pain on injection. The cause of the pain is unknown. A lidocaine-propofol mixture or pretreatment with lidocaine, opioids, ketamine, or nonsteroidal anti-inflammatory drugs can help ameliorate the pain on injection. Smaller veins are correlated with more pain, larger veins with less pain.[1] There seems to be minimal impact by obesity, cirrhosis, or kidney failure. Long-term infusion of propofol, typically after 48 hours of infusion at rates greater than 4 mg/kg/hr has been associated with propofol infusion syndrome.[3] Propofol infusion syndrome can lead to metabolic acidosis, hyperlipidemia, rhabdomyolysis, heart failure, and kidney failure. The mechanism is thought to be propofol-induced

mitochondrial dysfunction. Risk factors for propofol infusion syndrome are critical illness, use of vasopressors, and inadequate carbohydrate intake. Laboratory workup will likely show high potassium, high triglycerides, and rarely, green urine and liver enlargement. Treatment is supportive and discontinuing the propofol infusion. The pathophysiology of propofol infusion syndrome is thought to be a mitochondrial defect or toxicity. Prolonged propofol infusion for sedation in children has also been associated impaired motor function, muscle weakness, seizures, ataxia, and hallucinations.

## INDICATIONS AND CONTRAINDICATIONS

Propofol is indicated for monitored anesthesia care, induction of general anesthesia, and sedation of intubated mechanically ventilated patients in the intensive care unit (ICU). Propofol is not recommended below the age of 3 for the induction of anesthesia.[3] It is also not recommended for maintenance of anesthesia under 2 months.[3] Propofol is contraindicated in patients with allergies to eggs, egg products, soybeans, or soy products. Anaphylaxis is immunoglobin E (IgE) mediated. Propofol contains 10% soybean oil and 1.2% egg lecithin as an emulsifying agent. It should be noted that the current literature does not support the belief that egg allergic patients are more prone to propofol anaphylaxis. Propofol is not recommended in obstetrics, including cesarian sections, as propofol crosses the placenta and can cause neonatal depression. Prior to injecting, propofol should be visually inspected for particulate matter or discoloration, as either finding contradicts injection. The propofol emulsion does support bacterial growth. Patients with an allergy to nondepolarizing muscle relaxants can have an anaphylactic reaction to propofol.

## ANESTHETIC CONSIDERATIONS

### PREOPERATIVE

Propofol is typically not used in the preoperative setting. Propofol has been used by unqualified personnel to induce sleep in non-monitored settings, leading to catastrophic outcomes. Propofol does have anticonvulsant effects and has been used to terminate status epilepticus and can be used in epileptic patients.

### INTRAOPERATIVE

Induction dose of 2–2.5 mg/kg produces rapid onset of anesthesia.[1,2,3] Induction with propofol is associated with muscle twitching and hiccupping. Valproate can increase blood levels of propofol. It should be noted that propofol does not impact depolarizing or nondepolarizing neuromuscular blocking agents. If somatosensory evoked potentials are needed for a surgical case, it should be noted that propofol decreases the amplitude and increases the latency. For elderly patients, both the induction dose and maintenance dose may have to be decreased as the hemodynamic impact may be pronounced. For electroconvulsive therapy (ECT), propofol will shorten the duration of the seizures. Propofol can cause burst suppression while allowing for a reasonable awakening time and extubating at the end of the procedure.

## POSTOPERATIVE

Propofol has been shown to decrease postoperative nausea and vomiting.[3] Even low-dose intraoperative propofol has been shown to reduce postoperative nausea and vomiting when combined with other anesthetic agents. Sub-hypnotic doses have been shown to be efficacious in preventing postoperative nausea and vomiting. Be aware that some patients and children may have emergence delirium, which is self-limited. Patients should be advised of post-anesthesia drowsiness. Patients should not operate a motor vehicle or heavy machinery, or sign legal documents.

## REFERENCES

1. Vasileiou I, et al. Propofol: A review of its non-anesthetic effects. *Eur J Pharmacol.* 2009;605:1–8.
2. Eleved DJ, et al. Pharmacokinetic-pharmacodynamic model for propofol for board application in anesthesia and sedation. *Br J Anesthes.* 2018;120(5):942–959.
3. Chidambaran V, et al. Propofol: A review of its role in pediatric anesthesia and sedation. *CNS Drugs.* 2018 Sep;32(9):873.

# 75.

# ETOMIDATE

*Kris Ferguson and Peter Papapetrou*

## INTRODUCTION

Induction of anesthesia can be performed with a variety of agents. It is a non-barbiturate anesthesia induction agent with no analgesic properties. Most of these agents have hypotension and cardiac suppression. Etomidate induces general anesthesia with minimal hemodynamic instability.

## PHARMACOKINETICS

Etomidate is typically given intravenously for induction of anesthesia.[1] It is highly lipid soluble and rapidly crosses the blood-brain barrier. Redistribution is primarily responsible for termination of action.

## PHARMACODYNAMICS

Etomidate is structurally unrelated to other induction agents. Due to its structure, it is dissolved in propylene glycol for injection. This causes pain on injection, which can be ameliorated with a pretreatment of intravenous lidocaine. Etomidate works at the gamma-aminobutyric acid (GABA) A receptor, which is a chloride channel.[2] Etomidate potentiates the binding of GABA to the GABA A receptor, which opens the chloride channel, hyperpolarizing the cell.

Etomidate disinhibits the extrapyramidal motor system, causing myoclonus with induction.

## METABOLISM AND EXCRETION

Etomidate is primarily metabolized by the liver microsomal enzymes and plasma esterases, and end products are excreted in the urine.[2] Etomidate has been safely used in patients with acute intermittent porphyria.

## CIRCULATION

When used as the sole induction agent, etomidate has minimal impact on the cardiovascular system. Of all the intravenous induction agents, etomidate has the least impact on the cardiovascular system. Pre-load, after-load, cardiac contractility, and cardiac output are negligibly impacted. There may be a mild decrease in systemic vascular resistance. There is no histamine release. However, it should be noted that as etomidate does not have analgesic properties, it does not blunt the hypertensive response to intubation. Intubation with etomidate as the sole induction agent can result in significantly increased blood pressure secondary to the sympathetic response to intubation.

## RESPIRATORY

There is less respiratory depression with etomidate than other induction agents. Etomidate typically does not induce apnea.

## CEREBRAL

With etomidate's action at the GABA A receptor, like other induction agents, etomidate decreases cerebral metabolic rate, decreases cerebral blood flow, and decreases intracranial pressure. Cerebral perfusion pressure is typically maintained for patients with traumatic brain injury; etomidate is the only agent that decreases intracranial pressure but maintains a normal arterial pressure.

## DRUG INTERACTIONS

Fentanyl increases etomidate's elimination half-life.

## SIDE EFFECTS AND TOXICITY

It is well established that etomidate inhibits cortisol and aldosterone synthesis. After an induction dose, the adrenal and aldosterone suppression typically lasts 6–8 hours,

which is likely due to blockade of 11 beta hydroxylation in the adrenal cortex.[3] If used for sedation in the intensive care unit (ICU), it can cause significant adrenal suppression. Opioids can decrease the myoclonus seen with induction. Etomidate may also cause thrombophlebitis, laryngospasm, hiccups, myoclonus, and postoperative nausea and vomiting. Exercise caution when used in patients with myotonic dystrophy as etomidate can cause myotonic reactions.

## INDICATIONS AND CONTRAINDICATIONS

Etomidate is indicated for the induction of anesthesia. It is contraindicated in patients with an allergy to etomidate. Significant caution should be exercised if considering etomidate for sedation in the setting of ICU sepsis due to etomidate's adrenal suppression.[3]

## ANESTHESTIC CONSIDERATIONS

### PREOPERATIVE

Etomidate is not typically used in the preoperative setting.

### INTRAOPERATIVE

Induction dose is 0.1–0.4 mg/kg with onset in 30–60 seconds. Maintenance is 10–20 mcg/kg/min. Consider pretreating with opioids to blunt the hypertensive response to intubation. Etomidate is associated with myoclonus with induction. There is an increase in the amplitude and increase in latency of somatosensory-evoked potential monitoring. Burst suppression occurs at higher doses.[1] Etomidate does lower intraocular pressure. Electroconvulsive therapy requires general anesthesia and paraplegia. Etomidate will increase the duration of seizure duration. There is minimal change in uterine blood flow with etomidate.

### POSTOPERATIVE

If etomidate is used and the patient has preexisting adrenal suppression, consider supplementing with corticosteroids.

## REFERENCES

1. Cohen L, et al. The effect of ketamine on intracranial and cerebral perfusion pressure and health outcomes: A systematic review. *Ann Emerg Med.* 2015 Jan (1);65:43–51.e2.
2. Warner KJ, et al. Single-dose etomidate for rapid sequence intubation may impact outcome after severe injury. *J Trauma Acute Care Surg.* 2009;Jul67(1):45–50.23.
3. Hildreth A, et al. Adrenal suppression following a single dose of etomidate for rapid sequence induction: A prospective randomized study. *Trauma.* 2008 Sep;65(3):573–579.

# 76.

# BENZODIAZEPINES

*Kris Ferguson and Peter Papapetrou*

## INTRODUCTION

Benzodiazepines are common and pervasively used as anxiolytics, sedatives, hypnotics, and anticonvulsants. Of the dozens of different types of benzodiazepines, midazolam, diazepam, and lorazepam are the most commonly used in clinical anesthesia. The reversal agent, flumazenil, is also commonly available to clinical anesthesiologists. The site of action is the gamma-aminobutyric acid (GABA) A receptor. At lower doses, benzodiazepines have anxiolytic and anticonvulsive properties. As the dose escalates, benzodiazepines facilitate sedation, amnesia, and finally general anesthesia. Benzodiazepines do not have analgesic properties.

## PHARMACOKINETICS

Benzodiazepines can be administered intramuscularly or most commonly intravenously. Intramuscular diazepam is painful and unreliable; midazolam and lorazepam are better tolerated. Benzodiazepines are lipid soluble and quickly cross the blood-brain barrier. Following an intravenous bolus, recovery is due to redistribution. Benzodiazepines could be used as an induction agent; however, propofol, thiopental, and etomidate have faster onsets of action.

## PHARMACODYNAMICS

The GABA A receptor is a GABA-activated chloride channel. Activation of the GABA receptor opens the chloride channel which hyperpolarizes the cell. The site of action of benzodiazepines is different than the other general anesthetics such as propofol. Benzodiazepines potentiate the binding of GABA to the receptor, thereby increasing the frequency of the chloride channel opening.

## METABOLISM AND EXCRETION

Metabolism of midazolam takes place primarily in the liver via hepatic microsomal oxidation by cytochrome P450 and glucuronidation. Metabolized midazolam is excreted in the urine. Midazolam is also metabolized by extrahepatic sites. Glucuronidated alpha-hydroxy midazolam, the primary midazolam metabolite, is pharmacologically active, can cross the blood-brain barrier, and can accumulate in patients with renal failure. Diazepam is extensively metabolized by the liver and metabolites excreted in the urine. Diazepam is metabolized to oxazepam and temazepam; however, as they have shorter half-lives than diazepam, they are typically not clinically impactful. Lorazepam undergoes glucuronidation in the liver without active metabolites. Lorazepam, oxazepam, and temazepam are the three benzodiazepines metabolized by glucuronidation. As midazolam and diazepam are metabolized by the cytochrome P450 microsomal oxidation pathway, they are more prone to drug-drug interaction.

## CIRCULATION

There is minimal impact on the cardiovascular system. Intravenous administration may cause a decrease in arterial blood pressure and increase in heart rate secondary to a decrease in systemic vascular resistance. There may be a blunting of the baroreceptor reflex, altering the ability to compensate for hypovolemia.

## RESPIRATORY

Typical oral doses of benzodiazepines have minimal impact on respiration.[1,2] At higher doses or with rapid intravenous dosing, there can be respiratory depression. When benzodiazepines are administered with opioids or barbiturates, the respiratory depressant effects are synergistic and apnea can quickly result. There is a dose-dependent decrease in upper airway muscular tone. Significant caution should be exercised in using benzodiazepines in patients with obstructive sleep apnea or chronic obstructive pulmonary disease (COPD) as hypercapnia may result. The ventilatory response to arterial carbon dioxide is flattened;

however, unlike opioids, the curve is not shifted to the right. There is also a decrease in tidal volume.

## CEREBRAL

GABA is the main inhibitory neurotransmitter in the brain, hence the dose-dependent sedation, amnesia, and finally general anesthesia. The thalamic and midbrain reticular formation nuclei are the cerebral sites of action. However, compared with propofol, barbiturates, and inhalational anesthetics, benzodiazepines do not cause the same degree of neural suppression. There is a ceiling effect. Benzodiazepines, unlike barbiturates, cannot cause electrical silence. Benzodiazepines reduce cerebral metabolism and cerebral blood flow, but not to the extent of barbiturates. Benzodiazepines are not well suited for maintenance of anesthesia due to the long half-life leading to prolonged sedation.

## DRUG INTERACTIONS

Cimetidine reduces the metabolism of diazepam. Erythromycin inhibits midazolam metabolism, prolonging and intensifying effect. The combination of opioids and benzodiazepines have a synergistic effect on respiratory depression, reduction of arterial blood pressure, and systemic vascular resistance. The minimum alveolar concentration (MAC) of volatile anesthetic gases is lowered approximately 30% with the addition of benzodiazepines.

## SIDE EFFECTS AND TOXICITY

There is a synergistic effect between benzodiazepines and opioids causing increased respiratory depression than either agent alone. Caution should be exercised when combining these medications, especially in patients with COPD or obstructive sleep apnea. Benzodiazepines do cross the placenta, and diazepam is particularly dangerous as neonates have difficulty excreting it.[3] Benzodiazepine withdrawal can mimic delirium tremens after prolonged infusion. Consider switching to propofol after a prolonged infusion.[4]

## INDICATIONS AND CONTRAINDICATIONS

Exercise caution in individuals with a history of alcohol, opioid, or barbiturate abuse. Benzodiazepines are either category D or X and may harm the fetus.

## ANTAGONISM

Benzodiazepine overdose is treated with flumazenil. Initial dose is 0.2 mg over 30 seconds followed by 0.3 mg every minutes as needed to reverse overdose. Total dose should not exceed 3 mg. If sedation reoccurs, an infusion can be started at 0.1–0.4 mg per hour. Flumazenil is metabolized by the liver. For the reversal of sedation caued by benzodiazepines, 0.2 mg every 20 minutes as needed. No more than 3 mg in any one hour. Dosing is individualized based on patient response.

## ANESTHETIC CONSIDERATIONS

### PREOPERATIVE

Midazolam is one of the most used pre-surgery medications, typically given intravenously. Caution should be exercised when administered to patients with myasthenia gravis, sleep apnea, COPD, or patients with a history of addiction. Ensure appropriate monitoring in preoperative area, assessing for patient level of consciousness, ventilation, and preserved ventilation, especially if given in combination with other nervous system depressants. Midazolam is ideal for short-term use. Lorazepam has a slow onset and prolonged duration of action. Diazepam has a long duration of action and can lead to prolonged sedation if given as a continuous infusion.

### INTRAOPERATIVE

Midazolam is typically not given as an intraoperative infusion due to its long context-sensitive half-life and propensity to cause delayed awakening. Benzodiazepines lower the MAC of volatile anesthetics.

### POSTOPERATIVE

Take similar precautions as in the preoperative area, specifically ensuring appropriate monitoring for level of consciousness, ventilation, and oxygenation.

## REFERENCES

1. Barash PG, et al., eds. *Clinical Anesthesia*. 6th ed. Philadelphia, PA: Lippincott, Williams and Wilkins; 2009:240.
2. Ariano RE, et al. Comparison of sedative recovery time after midazolam versus diazepam administration. *Crit Care Med*. 1994 Sep;22(9):1492–1496.
3. Stoelting R, Miller R. *Basics of Anesthesia*. 5th ed. Philadelphia, PA: Elsevier; 2007:19103–2899.
4. Saito A, et al. Sequential use of midazolam and propofol for long-term sedation in postoperative mechanically ventilated patients. *Anesth Analg*. 2003 Mar;96(3):843–848.

# 77.

# KETAMINE

*Peter Papapetrou and Kris Ferguson*

## INTRODUCTION

Initially synthesized in 1962 as a phencyclidine derivative, ketamine was intended to be less hallucinogenic than phencyclidine.[1] It acts as an antagonist on the N-methyl-D-aspartate (NMDA) receptors in the central nervous system (CNS) to produce a state of dissociative anesthesia. Ketamine was first introduced into clinical use in 1970 as a battlefield anesthetic, as well as for uncooperative children and in veterinary medicine. In recent years it has also gained popularity for its low-dose analgesic use in acute perioperative as well as chronic pain medicine. It is the only drug known to have hypnotic, analgesic, and amnestic effects.

## MECHANISM OF ACTION

Activation of transmembrane NMDA receptors in the brain and spinal cord leads to an influx of calcium ion (Ca2+), which activates the formation of prostaglandins and nitric oxide (NO). NO production leads to an increase in glutamate release, which plays a key role in nociception. By ketamine inhibiting the NMDA noncompetitively, it acts by reducing the influx of intracellular Ca2+ and thus inhibiting this nociceptive cascade. Furthermore, NMDA receptors are also involved in pain transmission and modulation. This allows ketamine to serve a purpose in preventing pain from being chronic.

## PHARMACOKINETICS AND PHARMACODYNAMICS

Ketamine is a chiral structure consisting of both the S- and R-ketamine isomers. The S(+)ketamine isomer is 3–4 times more potent than the R(-)ketamine isomer.[2] Ketamine can be administered through several routes, as shown in Table 77.1. Administration of an intravenous (IV) induction dose of ketamine produces a rapid loss of consciousness, though awakening from it is slower than most other IV anesthetics. Ketamine has a redistribution half-life of 11 to 17 minutes.[3] The loss of consciousness resembles a dissociative state rather than a sleep-like state. Patients may move or have their eyes open, but do not respond to painful stimuli, nor do they recall events during their anesthetic state. During this state, patients may experience vivid dreams or hallucinations. Cerebral metabolic rate of oxygen (CMRO$_2$), cerebral blood flow (CBF), and intracranial pressure (ICP) are all increased by ketamine, in contrast to other IV anesthetics. Light ketamine anesthesia produces increased electroencephalogram (EEG) frequency with predominant beta-wave activity. At higher depths of anesthesia, high-amplitude theta waves and intermittent delta waves can occur.

## METABOLISM AND EXCRETION

Ketamine is extensively metabolized to norketamine, which is one-fourth as potent, through N-demethylation

*Table 77.1* KETAMINE ROUTES OF ADMINISTRATION

| ROUTE OF ADMINISTRATION | DOSE |
| --- | --- |
| Intravenous | 0.25–1 mg/kg in adults (sedation) |
| | 0.25–2 mg/kg in children (sedation) |
| | 1–2 mg/kg in adults (anesthesia) |
| | 2–6 mg/kg/min in children (anesthesia) |
| Intramuscular | 4–5 mg/kg (sedation) |
| | 8–10 mg/kg (anesthesia) |
| By mouth | 3–15 mg/kg in children |
| | 500 mg maximum in adults |
| Intranasal | 0.25–4 mg/kg (sedation) |
| | 3–9 mg/kg (anesthesia) |

primarily through CYP3A4. Norketamine is then metabolized to glucuronide, which is inactive. These metabolites are excreted in the urine. A small fraction of ketamine is plasma protein bound. Ketamine has a high hepatic extraction ratio. A decrease in hepatic blood flow caused by diseases or medications will prolong ketamine's duration of action.

## EFFECT ON CIRCULATION

Ketamine has indirect effects of increasing centrally mediated catecholamines from the adrenal medulla, causes direct central sympathetic stimulation, inhibits norepinephrine reuptake, and depresses the baroreceptor reflex. This leads to an increase in heart rate, blood pressure, cardiac contractility, systemic vascular resistance, and cardiac output. It can cause increased myocardial oxygen demand greater than its increase in oxygen delivery. In the critically ill, it may cause a negative inotropic effect leading to decreased cardiac output, which reflects depletion of catecholamine stores and exhaustion of sympathetic nervous system compensating mechanisms.

## EFFECT ON RESPIRATION

Ketamine has little effect on ventilatory drive, unlike other intravenous anesthetics. Though aspiration still remains a risk, protective airway reflexes are less likely to be depressed. It produces bronchodilation, which can be useful during bronchospasm. Its bronchodilatory effects are due to its anticholinergic and adrenergic properties.[4] It may also cause copious salivation, which can be minimized with the use of an antisialagogue.

## EFFECT ON CENTRAL NERVOUS SYSTEM

Ketamine causes a dissociative anesthetic state, as patients appear dissociated from their surroundings. It increases their $CMRO_2$, CBF, and ICP, and should be used with caution in patients with intracranial lesions. Furthermore, it may cause emergence delirium in adults in doses over 2 mg/kg. Emergence delirium usually manifests early in emergency but can last for more than 24 hours in some patients.

## SIDE EFFECTS AND TOXICITY

Ketamine use can be associated with unpleasant vivid dreams or hallucinations. This can be minimized with the concomitant use of a benzodiazepine. Ketamine is also associated with an increased risk of postoperative nausea and vomiting, in addition to excessive salivation and lacrimation.

## INDICATIONS AND CONTRAINDICATIONS

Ketamine is a very good anesthetic choice in hemodynamically unstable patients as an induction agent for general anesthesia, as it preserves cardiac output. It preserves airway reflexes and respiratory drive, making it an excellent choice in monitored anesthesia care. It is short acting; consciousness returns 10–15 minutes after IV induction dose. Postoperative low-dose ketamine infusions under 1.2 mg/kg/hr can reduce postoperative pain and reduce opioid requirements with no major side effects. Due to its bronchodilator effect, it can be used during episodes of bronchospasm. Caution must be used when deciding to administer ketamine to a patient with high ICP or an intracranial mass, as ketamine can further increase ICP.

## REFERENCES

1. Peltoniemi MA, et al. Ketamine: a review of clinical pharmacokinetics and pharmacodynamics in anesthesia and pain therapy. *Clin Pharmacokinet.* 2016;55:1059–1077.
2. Gao M, et al. Ketamine use in current clinical practice. *Acta Pharmacologica Sinica.* 2016;37: 865–872.
3. Dershwitz M, Rosow C. Chapter 41. Pharmacology of Intravenous Anesthetics. In: Longnecker DE, Brown DL, Newman MF, Zapol WM, eds. *Anesthesiology, 2e.* New York, NY: McGraw-Hill; 2012:699–700.
4. Blaise GA. Chapter 74. Ketamine. In: Murray MJ, et al., eds. *Faust's Anesthesiology Review.* 4th ed. Philadelphia, PA: Elsevier Saunders; 2015:166–167.

# 78.

# DEXMEDETOMIDINE

*Kris Ferguson and R. Scott Stayner*

## INTRODUCTION

Dexmedetomidine is a versatile perioperative anesthetic. It has a rapid onset, short half-life, consistent titration parameters, preservation of airway function, minimal cardiac effects, and it decreases postoperative delirium. It also decreases the minimum alveolar concentration (MAC) of volatile anesthetics, as well as having an opioid sparing effect. It is highly efficacious as dexmedetomidine has anesthetic, analgesic, and sympatholytic properties.[1]

## PHARMACOKINETICS

Dexmedetomidine has first-order kinetics with rapid onset, usually in 5–10 minutes after an intravenous (IV) dose and rapid offset by redistribution.[2] The peak effect is typically 15–30 minutes after IV injection. The duration of action is typically 10–120 minutes with a half-life of 2–3 hours.[3] It is highly protein bound. It is metabolized in the liver by oxidation and glucuronidation and metabolized excreted in the urine. Exercise caution with use of dexmedetomidine in patients with liver failure.

## PHARMACODYNAMICS

Dexmedetomidine works via the alpha2-adrenoreceptors.[4] It has a 200:1 predilection for alpha-2 to alpha-1. Dexmedetomidine has an 8 times higher selectivity for alpha-2 adrenergic receptors than clonidine. Highly lipid soluble, dexmedetomidine is 3.5 times more lipid soluble than clonidine, allowing it to quickly cross the blood-brain barrier for rapid onset of action. It also acts at the spinal cord. Anesthesia is mediated via the pre- and post-synaptic alpha-2 adrenergic receptors in the locus coeruleus, inducing unconsciousness.[3] Unique to dexmedetomidine is that the anesthesia closely mimics natural sleep, whereby the patient is arousable and cooperative. This is particularly useful for difficult airway patients or awake craniotomies.

## METABOLISM AND EXCRETION

Dexmedetomidine has a 2-hour elimination half-life that is independent of renal function.

## CIRCULATION

Initially, there may be a small increase in blood pressure and reflex bradycardia due to activation of the alpha-2B receptors in vascular smooth muscle. As the titration increases there may be hypotension secondary to central alpha-2A receptor activation. It should be noted that severe hypotension can be caused when glycopyrrolate is used to treat dexmedetomidine-induced bradycardia.[3] Dexmedetomidine can blunt the sympathetic response (increase in epinephrine, cortisol, blood glucose) to incision, sternotomy, and cardiac bypass while decreasing postoperative delirium.

## RESPIRATORY

There is minimal respiratory depression even at higher doses. Dexmedetomidine minimized discomfort with awake fiberoptic intubations; however, it does not prevent recall.[3] Ideally, it would be supplemented with another agent such as remifentanil or midazolam. Dry mouth is a helpful side effect, especially with fiberoptic intubations.

## CEREBRAL

The combination of dexmedetomidine with or without remifentanil is ideal for awake craniotomies as cooperative anesthesia is facilitated while minimizing tachycardia and hypertension. There is also a decrease in intracranial pressure and a dose-dependent decrease in cerebral blood flow and metabolic rate. Dexmedetomidine does not impact seizure duration if used for electroconvulsive therapy.[4]

## DRUG INTERACTIONS

Dexmedetomidine enhances the sedative effects of other anesthetics such as opioids, benzodiazepines, and propofol, etc. Dexmedetomidine can enhance the hypotension caused by beta blockers.

## SIDE EFFECTS AND TOXICITY

Exercise caution in infants and neonates as dexmedetomidine blocks non-shivering thermogenesis which infants depend upon for heat generation. Significant hypothermia can develop as dexmedetomidine inhibits lipolysis by post-synaptic alpha-2 activation. Diuresis is induced by dexmedetomidine by reducing vasopressin secretion, increased renal blood flow, and increased glomerular filtration. Animal studies show it may protect against radiocontrast nephropathy. There is a tendency to impact laboratory values with prolonged infusion. Dexmedetomidine may increase serum sodium causing low urine specific gravity and increase serum osmolarity. After prolonged use there may be withdrawal symptoms such as hypertension, tachycardia, and agitation.

## INDICATIONS AND CONTRAINDICATIONS

It can be useful in pheochromocytoma as it is sympatholytic. There are no absolute contraindications to dexmedetomidine other than allergy to dexmedetomidine.

## ANESTHETIC CONSIDERATIONS

### PREOPERATIVE

It can be delivered by nasal (1–2 mcg/kg) or oral (2.5–4 mcg/kg) in children or by intravenous route with 1 mcg/kg loading dose over 5–10 min, followed by an infusion of 0.2–1.4 mcg/kg/hr.

### INTRAOPERATIVE

As spontaneous ventilation is maintained, procedures such as rigid bronchoscopy are facilitated. The patency and tone of the airway is maintained even in children and adults with obstructive sleep apnea. This facilitates sleep endoscopy and dynamic airway imaging, as sedation with dexmedetomidine mimics sleep. For spine surgery, dexmedetomidine is a useful adjunct for propofol or inhalational agents to facilitate an expedited intraoperative wake-up test.[2] Dexmedetomidine has minimal effect on motor-evoked potentials. When called for, dexmedetomidine can be used for controlled hypotension. Newer techniques of craniotomies require a period of an awake, comfortable, and cooperative patient to provide feedback. Dexmedetomidine minimizes delirium, minimizes airway obstruction, maintains respiratory drive which minimizes hypercapnia, and allows for meaningful responses to verbal instruction. Epileptiform activity is not impacted, thus localization is facilitated. Lastly, dexmedetomidine is an excellent adjunct to reginal anesthesia.

### POSTOPERATIVE

There is typically a rapid emergence from dexmedetomidine anesthesia with minimal emergence delirium. It can also be used to treat postoperative shivering.

## REFERENCES

1. Davy A, et al. Dexmedetomidine and general anesthesia: A narrative literature review of its major indications for use in adults undergoing non-cardiac surgery. *Minerva Anestesiol.* 2017 December;83(12):1294–1308.
2. Mahmoud M, Mason KP. Dexmedetomidine: Review, update, and future considerations of paediatric perioperative and periprocedural applications and limitations. *Br J Anaesth.* 2015 Aug;115(2):171–182.
3. Sottas C, Anderson B. Dexmedetomidine: The new all-in-one drug in paediatric anesthesia? *Curr Opin Anesthesiol.* 2017;30:441–451.
4. Vuyk J, et al. Basic principles of pharmacology. In: Groper MA, eds. *Miller's Anesthesia.* 9th ed. Elsevier; 2020:23, 638–679.e10.

# 79.

# THIOPENTAL

*Greta Nemergut*

## INTRODUCTION

Thiopental is a rapid-acting barbiturate that has been used as an intravenous (IV) anesthetic agent for many decades. Due to the quick onset and short action of the drug, it is generally used only for induction of anesthesia or as an adjunctive agent with other anesthesia agents. Thiopental also has use as an anticonvulsant and a treatment to help control intracranial pressure. This chapter will focus on the characteristics, pharmacology, and safety of thiopental used in the anesthesia setting. Thiopental is not FDA approved and is no longer available for use in the United States.

## DRUG CHARACTERISTICS

Thiopental is a barbiturate that is derived from barbituric acid. The drug has substitutions at the C2 and C5 positions, which make it more lipid soluble (sulfur at C2) than the original compound, as well as adding hypnotic, sedative, and anticonvulsant activity (C5 substitutions).[1,2]

Thiopental is available as a sodium salt to allow improved solubility and stability. The resultant solution is a 2.5% thiopental product and is highly alkaline (pH over 10).[2,3] Since the solution is so alkaline, it cannot be mixed with more acidic agents, like neuromuscular blockers. The mixture will form precipitates and block IV lines.[1] The nature of the solution will also cause pain and tissue injury if given into the artery or extravasated into tissue.[1]

## PHARMACOLOGY/ PHARMACOKINETICS

Thiopental is an extremely rapid-acting barbiturate that works as a sedative, hypnotic, and anticonvulsant. It does not have any analgesic effects.[2] Barbiturates are non-selective and work on many pathways and involve both an increase in inhibitory neurotransmission and a decrease in excitatory transmission. The primary action on inhibitory transmission is exerted via the gamma-aminobutyric acid (GABA)

pathway; the action on excitatory transmission is not well understood.[1] Given as a slow IV push over 10–15 seconds, the onset of action of the drug is about 30–40 seconds and the effects last 20–30 minutes after a single dose. Thiopental can be given to children and adults at similar dose for anesthesia induction (3–6 mg/kg in adults; 2–6 mg/kg in children), with a repeat dose given after 1 minute if needed for a maximum dose of 500 mg in adults and 7 mg/kg in children. The dose needs to be adjusted based on patient response. Doses should be adjusted for patients with a creatinine clearance of less than 10 ml/min and reduced in patients with hepatic impairment.[3]

Since thiopental is very lipid soluble, it passes through the blood-brain barrier quickly, resulting in the quick onset of action. It is also quickly redistributed into other areas of the body, such as the liver and fat tissue, where it is not active. The remaining amount in the plasma undergoes extensive hepatic metabolism and is excreted in the urine as inactive metabolites.[2]

## SAFETY

As is common with anesthetic agents, thiopental has effects on the cardiac and respiratory systems. Thiopental reduces arterial blood pressure, but only modest changes are seen. The reduction in blood pressure is due to vasodilation caused by decreased sympathetic nervous system function. The compensatory increases in heart rate blunt and minimize the hypotension. Dilation of peripheral vessels can also result in pooling of blood, less venous return, and reduction of cardiac output. These effects are more prominent in patients with preexisting cardiac disease and are seen with larger doses given at more rapid injection rates.[1] Thiopental causes respiratory depression and produces transient apnea during induction.[1]

As mentioned, if accidentally given intra-arterially, thiopental causes severe pain and vasoconstriction that can result in severe tissue damage.

Thiopental, like other barbiturates, induces the cytochrome P450 enzymes,[2] increasing clearance and decreasing the effects of other drugs that are extensively metabolized by this pathway. It also can enhance the effects of other blood pressure–lowering drugs and other central nervous system depressants.[3]

anesthetics.[1] Largely in practice, propofol has replaced thiopental for these uses.[1]

## USES

Due to the rapid onset and limited duration of action, thiopental is used for anesthesia induction. Often, after administered, a nondepolarizing neuromuscular blocker, such as succinylcholine, is given to aid in intubation. It can also be used to allow easier acceptance of other inhaled

## REFERENCES

1. Bokoch MP, Eilers H. Intravenous anesthetics. In: Manuel C. Pardo, Ronald D. Miller, ed. *Basics of Anesthesia*. 7th ed. Elsevier; 2018:104–122.
2. Medlock RM, Pandit JJ. Intravenous anaesthetic agents. *Anaesth Intensive Care Med*. 2016;17(3):155–162.
3. Lexicomp Online, *Lexi-Drugs Online*, UpToDate Inc.; August 17, 2020. https://online.lexi.com/lco/action/home

# 80.

# SODIUM BICARBONATE

*Greta Nemergut*

## INTRODUCTION

Sodium bicarbonate is an alkalinizing agent used to restore acid-base balance and has been used with some regional and local anesthetic agents to reduce pain on administration and to enhance the effect of the agent. The bicarbonate buffer system is one of the buffer systems in the human body. Sodium bicarbonate can be given for metabolic acidosis to replace bicarbonate and improve acid-base balance.

Increasing the pH of a local anesthetic agent is how sodium bicarbonate aids the movement into lipid membranes that can allow for an enhanced effect. It has been found that sodium bicarbonate can enhance the effect of epidural anesthetics, but data do not support this effect in peripheral nerve blocks.

Local anesthetics are acidic in order to increase their shelf life and stability.[1] Prior to injection, an alkaline solution, like sodium bicarbonate, can be added to the solution to increase the pH and increase the amount of non-ionized drug, which improves lipid solubility and can improve onset of drug activity.[2] However, the amount of alkaline product

needs to be precise so as not to cause a precipitate in the solution, rendering it unsafe and useless.

## BICARBONATE BUFFER SYSTEM

There are four main buffer systems in the human body: bicarbonate, hemoglobin, other proteins, and phosphate. The bicarbonate buffer system relies on carbon dioxide to slowly combine with water (hydration) to form carbonic acid, which then deprotonates to bicarbonate. Carbonic anhydrase rapidly changes carbon dioxide into carbonic acid and is the most important buffering system in the body when used with renal excretion of bicarbonate and pulmonary excretion of carbon dioxide. The primary management of metabolic acidosis is to correct the underlying condition causing the acidosis. Sodium bicarbonate can be given on non-gap metabolic acidosis as the issue is related to bicarbonate loss. It is used in extreme cases as a temporizing measure when the patient is hemodynamically unstable. Since administration of sodium bicarbonate makes carbon dioxide, proper ventilation is needed to eliminate the gas to avoid worsening acidosis.[3]

## SUGGESTED ALKALINIZATION CONCENTRATIONS

Sodium bicarbonate is available in a standard 8.4% solution. Lidocaine and mepivacaine are most easily combined with sodium bicarbonate. For every 10 mL of lidocaine or mepivacaine, 1 mEq of sodium bicarbonate is added.[4] Due to risk of precipitation, smaller quantities of sodium bicarbonate are used with bupivacaine (0.12 mEq per 10 mL).[4] Ropivacaine is difficult to alkalinize safely, with as little as 0.1 mEq of sodium bicarbonate in 20 mL of ropivacaine 0.2% injection creating precipitates within 10 minutes of making the mixture. The higher strengths of ropivacaine (0.75% and 1%) cannot be alkalinized with sodium bicarbonate as they easily form a precipitate.[4]

Sodium bicarbonate contains 12 mEq of sodium, so if large doses are used intravenously to correct metabolic acidosis, sodium/water retention can occur, causing edema.

## PAIN REDUCTION

Evidence supports a reduction of pain on injection when sodium bicarbonate is used to alkalinize local anesthetics. This is due to the more rapid onset of action rather than the increase in pH.[1]

A meta-analysis was completed that evaluated the efficacy of sodium bicarbonate in decreasing pain during intradermal injections of local anesthetics.[5] The analysis included randomized, controlled trials that compared buffered and unbuffered solutions. A total of 12 articles were included, which included a total of 855 patients. Lidocaine was the most commonly used anesthetic. The pooled results favored the buffered solutions, showing less pain on injection with a decrease in the visual analog score (VAS) of –1.17 (95% CI, –1.68, –0.67), $p < 0.0001$. The pH of the nonbuffered drugs ranged from 3.4 to 6.4 across studies, while the buffered groups all had pH above 7 (7.1 to 7.7).

## ENHANCED EFFECT

### EPIDURAL

Onset of action is quicker when sodium bicarbonate is added to epidural anesthetics, but not by more than several minutes.[1] Because of this, the benefit of using the alkaline agent may not warrant the time spent on making the modified solution, and a drug that is faster acting is more useful.[1] Alkalinization is not useful for spinal anesthesia because this route already provides a rapid onset. There is also no benefit seen in plexus blocks or intravenous regional anesthesia.[1]

### PERIPHERAL NERVE BLOCK

Studies have not shown consistent benefit of an improved onset of action of the local anesthetic with the addition of sodium bicarbonate.[4] One study showed that adding sodium bicarbonate to mepivacaine 1.4% and epinephrine significantly increased onset of action of the sensory and motor blocks during an interscalene brachial plexus block. This change was from 2.7 minutes down to 1 minute. Because the time to surgery after placement of the nerve block is much longer than the onset of action of the block, the clinical relevance of this change is questionable. Another study showed no effect on lumbar plexus nerve blocks when sodium bicarbonate was added to bupivacaine 0.5%. Additionally, a variable effect was seen in a larger study of axillary brachial plexus blocks, femoral nerve blocks, and sciatic nerve blocks. When sodium bicarbonate was added to mepivacaine 2%, lidocaine 2% and bupivacaine 0.5%, there was faster onset in some of the nerve blocks, but the onset of lidocaine was actually slowed in the femoral and sciatic nerve blocks. Commercial anesthetic products have varying pH levels, and it is not known what the preferred pH should be to exert the maximum effect.[2] When mixed with lidocaine, there are varying results seen, depending on the presence or absence of epinephrine that can result in a decrease in the onset of action.[2] Based on the lack of data supporting a significant clinical benefit, it currently is not recommended to use sodium bicarbonate with local anesthetics for nerve blocks.

## REFERENCES

1. Brandis K. Alkalinisation of local anesthetic solutions. *Aust Prescr.* 2011;34:173–175.
2. Prabhakar A, et al. Adjuvants in clinical regional anesthesia practice: A comprehensive review. *Best Pract Res Clin Anaesthesiol.* 2019;33:415–423.
3. Lui L. Acid-base balance and blood gas analysis. In: Manual C. Pardo, Ronald D. Miller, ed. *Basics of Anesthesia.* 7th ed. Elsevier; 2018:363–376.
4. Bailard NS, et al. Additives to local anesthetics for peripheral nerve blocks: Evidence, limitations, and recommendations. *AJHP.* 2014;71(5):373–385.
5. Hanna MN, et al. Efficacy of bicarbonate in decreasing pain on intradermal injection of local anesthetics: A meta-analysis. *Reg Anesth Pain Med.* 2009;34:122–125.

# 81.

# NITROGLYCERIN AND SODIUM NITROPRUSSIDE

*Andrew Sprowell and Archit Sharma*

## INTRODUCTION

Nitrovasodilators are a class of vasoactive medications used in clinical practice since the late 1800s, whose effect is vasorelaxation mediated by nitric oxide (NO).[1] They include the organic nitrates (nitroglycerin, isosorbide dinitrate, isosorbide mononitrate, amyl nitrite), and sodium nitroprusside. In daily anesthesia practice, nitroglycerin (aka glyceryl trinitrate, nitroglycerine) is the most commonly used, though the longer-acting nitrates isosorbide dinitrite and isosorbide mononitrate may be encountered perioperatively in patients with angina, heart failure, or esophageal spasm. Amyl nitrite is an inhaled vapor used for acute cyanide toxicity and angina, unlikely to be seen in routine anesthesia practice.

## NITROGLYCERIN

Nitroglycerin converts to nitric oxide (NO) in the body. NO then activates the enzyme guanylyl cyclase, which converts guanosine triphosphate (GTP) to guanosine 3′,5′-monophosphate (cGMP) in vascular smooth muscle and other tissues. cGMP then activates protein kinase-dependent phosphorylation, ultimately resulting in the dephosphorylation of myosin light chains within smooth muscle fibers.[2]

## PHARMACODYNAMICS

At low doses, nitroglycerin will dilate veins, then arteries, and finally resistance vessels (arterioles) at high doses. Combined venous and arterial dilation will decrease blood pressure. Pooling of circulating blood volume in the large capacitance vessels of the extremities and splanchnic circulation decreases left ventricular end-diastolic pressure (LVEDP), thus decreasing stroke volume. Reflexive increases in heart rate may serve to maintain cardiac output. Decreased preload and afterload decrease myocardial oxygen consumption. Dilation of pulmonary vessels decreases right heart afterload.

In coronary artery disease, nitroglycerin can improve myocardial oxygen supply. In addition to decreased $O_2$ demand through reduction preload and afterload, nitroglycerin improves myocardial oxygen delivery via dilation of stenotic coronary vessels. Unlike nitroprusside, nitroglycerin is not associated with coronary steal—a phenomenon whereby dilation of arteriolar resistance beds causes shunting of flow away from stenotic arteries which cannot vasodilate to decrease resistance (and thus increase flow). It is commonly prescribed to patients with poor left ventricular (LV) function in whom decreased preload and afterload reduce cardiac work, by lowering systemic vascular resistance (SVR) and favorably shifting the starling curve. Its beneficial effects appear to be greater with inferior infarctions than with anterior infarctions because the right coronary artery is more liable to spasm. Nitrates also cause smooth muscle relaxation in the esophagus, gallbladder, and uterus, all of which can be clinically useful in the appropriate context.[3]

## PHARMACOKINETICS

Nitroglycerin can be administered via intravenous (IV), intra-arterial, sublingual, transdermal, topical, and oral routes. IV administration is most common in anesthesia practice. Bolus doses range from 50 to 300 mcg IV. Sublingual dosing generally starts at 0.4 mg. Onset of effect is rapid. Nitroglycerin is short-acting with a half-life of 2.8 minutes. Isosorbide dinitrate and isosorbide mononitrate have longer duration of action but similar mechanism and desired effects.

Nitrates undergo liver metabolism with a large first-pass effect. Unlike nitroprusside, no toxic metabolites are formed from their metabolism. Nitrate, a metabolite, converts oxyhemoglobin to methemoglobin.

*Tolerance* to nitrate therapy is said to have occurred when the medication does not have the desired effect, after being on it for some time. Impaired nitroglycerin bioconversion to 1,2-glyceryl dinitrate with decreased formation of NO seems to be the projected cause.[4]

## ADVERSE EFFECTS

Adverse effects include hypotension, headache, dizziness, orthostasis, and reflex tachycardia. The risk of hypotension is increased in patients with hypertrophic cardiomyopathy, in whom nitrates can induce or increase outflow tract obstruction.

## CLINICAL APPLICATIONS

Clinical applications include angina pectoris, unstable angina, acute myocardial infarction (MI), congestive heart failure, esophageal spasm, uterine relaxation, and percutaneous coronary angioplasty, among others.

## SODIUM NITROPRUSSIDE

Sodium nitroprusside (SNP) has been used as a fast acting antihypertensive in cardiac and vascular surgery, heart failure, and other acute applications. SNP breaks down in circulation to release NO. It does this by binding to oxyhemoglobin to release cyanide, methemoglobin, and NO. NO activates guanylate cyclase in vascular smooth muscle and increases intracellular production of cGMP.

## PHARMACOKINETICS

Metabolism of nitroprusside releases cyanide (CN). Cyanide has three distinct fates: it can form cyanmethemoglobin in RBCs; it can be metabolized in the liver to form thiocyanate, which can be excreted by the kidneys (requires thiosulfate and cobalamin); or it may bind to cytochrome oxidase and inhibit oxidative phosphorylation. The latter is the feared pathway, forcing a switch to anaerobic metabolism. This can be diagnosed by checking serum cyanide levels and serum lactate. Only the combination of sodium thiosulfate and sodium nitrite is currently approved by the FDA for treatment of cyanide poisoning. SNP is typically run as an infusion starting at 0.3 mcg/kg/min and titrated to effect. In pediatrics, the highest tolerated dose may be as low as 2 mcg/kg/min.[5] Important to note that the conversion of CN to thiocyanate is inhibited by hypothermia and requires adequate vitamin $B_{12}$. Cysteine is needed to produce thiosulfate.

## PHARMACODYNAMICS

Administration of SNP causes systemic vasodilation, with a more pronounced effect on arteries than nitroglycerin, causing arterial and venous dilatation, reduced afterload, decreased ventricular filling pressures, decreased systemic blood pressure, and increased cardiac output, without significant lowering of the heart rate.

## ADVERSE EFFECTS

Nitroprusside has been shown to increase intracranial pressure (ICP) due to impaired cerebral autoregulation. NO released from nitroprusside decreases cerebral vascular resistance, and has been shown to impair brain and myocardial tissue oxygenation due to increase in arterial-venous shunting. It decreases coronary flow reserve, which is the basis for the theory that nitroprusside can cause coronary steal syndrome.

## CLINICAL APPLICATIONS

SNP is used clinically in cardiac surgery to manage perioperative hypertension, hypertensive crises, vascular surgery, and other acute hemodynamic applications. It is also used in management of heart failure as it has been shown to improve LV filling and cardiac output by decreasing the afterload.

## ANESTHETIC CONSIDERATIONS

### PREOPERATIVE

Patients on long-term nitrate therapy should not be asked to abruptly stop taking their nitrates, as it can lead to coronary spasm. Phosphodiesterase (PDE5) inhibitors, e.g., sildenafil, slow cGMP degradation via inhibition of PDE5. In combination with nitrates, which increase cGMP production, an additive effect may lead to serious consequences such as profound hypotension, tachycardia, angina, and cardiac arrest.

### INTRAOPERATIVE

SNP can cause coronary and cerebral steal by causing vasodilation in smaller resistance vessels and diverts critical pressure-dependent flow from ischemic areas.

### POSTOPERATIVE

Once the patient is stable in the postoperative phase, home dose of nitrate vasodilators should be restarted promptly, to prevent coronary vasospasm. Long-term therapy with an infusion of high-dose SNP carries the risk of cyanide toxicity. Levels should be checked promptly, and antidote administered, if needed.

## REFERENCES

1. Berlin R. Historical aspects of nitrate therapy. *Drugs.* 1987;33(4);1–4.
2. Demartini C, et al. Nitroglycerin as a comparative experimental model of migraine pain: From animal to human and back. *Prog. Neurobiol.* 2019 Jun;177:15–32.
3. Abrams J. Nitroglycerin and long-acting nitrates in clinical practice. *Am J Med.* 1983;74(6):85–94.
4. Chen Z, et al. Identification of the enzymatic mechanism of nitroglycerin bioactivation. *Proc Natl Acad Sci.* 2002;99(12):8306–8311.
5. Hottinger DG, et al (2014). Sodium nitroprusside in 2014: A clinical concepts review. *J Anaesthesiol. Clin Pharmacol.* 2014;30(4):462.

# 82.

# NICARDIPINE AND OTHER ANTIHYPERTENSIVE MEDICATIONS

*Anureet Walia and Archit Sharma*

## INTRODUCTION

A hypertensive emergency refers to presence of severe hypertension along with signs and symptoms of acute end organ damage. Examples include hypertensive encephalopathy, acute pulmonary edema, and aortic dissection. Immediate but careful reduction in blood pressure is often indicated in these settings. Various agents are used to treat hypertensive emergencies in different situations.

## NICARDIPINE

Nicardipine is a dihydropyridine calcium channel blocker that is primarily used in intravenous form, although oral forms are available. Nicardipine has a better safety profile and a similar antihypertensive effect when compared with nitroprusside.[1] The major limitations are a longer onset of action, which precludes rapid titration, and a longer serum elimination half-life (three to six hours).

## DOSAGE

Continuous IV infusion can be initiated at 5 mg/hour; may increase by 2.5 mg/hour every 5 minutes (for rapid titration) to every 15 minutes (for gradual titration) up to a maximum of 15 mg/hour.

## CLINICAL USES

Nicardipine is used frequently for treatment of angina and managing blood pressure in acute hypertensive episodes and emergencies. The strategy employed in a hypertensive emergency involves using nicardipine to reduce mean arterial BP ~10%–20% over the first hour, then 5%–15% over the next 23 hours, unless there is a compelling indication (e.g., acute aortic dissection, severe preeclampsia, eclampsia) for more rapid BP and heart rate control. Off-label use is also carried out for managing blood pressure

in cases of subarachnoid hemorrhage and intracerebral hemorrhage.

## METABOLISM

Nicardipine metabolism occurs mainly in the liver, primarily by cytochrome P450 enzyme isoforms. Excretion occurs in approximately equal proportions in the urine (49%) and feces (43%), with no unchanged drug excreted.

## ADVERSE REACTIONS

Nicardipine can cause headache, lightheadedness, dizziness, flushing, muscle cramps, and abdominal pain.

## CONCERNS

Nicardipine should be used with caution in the following clinical situations:

(1) *Aortic stenosis*: In patients with aortic stenosis, nicardipine may reduce coronary perfusion resulting in ischemia, and hence its use requires very careful monitoring.
(2) *Heart failure*: Patients with heart failure (HF) or severe left ventricular dysfunction may experience worsened symptoms of HF due to mild negative inotropic effects of nicardipine.[2]
(3) *Hypertrophic cardiomyopathy (HCM) with outflow tract obstruction*: Use with caution in patients with HCM and outflow tract obstruction since reduction in afterload may worsen symptoms associated with this condition.[3]
(4) *Pregnancy*: Nicardipine has been shown to decrease maternal blood pressure without significant changes on placental perfusion or fetal hemodynamics.[4] Although effective for the treatment of hypertension in pregnancy, nicardipine may have an increased risk of

adverse maternal events (e.g., headache, nausea, tachycardia) in comparison to other agents.

## OTHER HYPERTENSIVE MEDICATIONS

### CLEVIDIPINE

Clevidipine is an ultra-short-acting dihydropyridine calcium channel blocker that is is hydrolyzed by serum esterases and has a serum elimination half-life of 5–15 minutes. It reduces blood pressure without affecting cardiac filling pressures but can cause reflex tachycardia. The initial dose is 1 mg/hour, which can be increased as necessary to a maximum of 21 mg/hour.

### NITRATES

Nitrovasodilators such as nitroprusside and nitroglycerin provide nitric oxide that induces vasodilation via generation of cyclic GMP, which then activates calcium-sensitive potassium channels in the cell membrane

### FENOLDOPAM

Fenoldopam is a peripheral dopamine-1 receptor agonist which maintains or increases renal perfusion while it lowers blood pressure.[5] Fenoldopam may be particularly beneficial in patients with renal impairment and may increase glomerular filtration rate, urine output, and sodium excretion. After starting at 0.1 mcg/kg per minute, the dose can be titrated to 1.6 mcg/kg per minute, depending upon the blood pressure response.

### LABETALOL

Labetalol is a combined beta-adrenergic and alpha-adrenergic blocker. Its rapid onset of action (5 minutes or less) makes it a useful intravenous medication for the treatment of hypertensive emergencies. However, labetalol should be avoided in patients with asthma, chronic obstructive lung disease, heart failure, or heart block. The infusion rate is 0.5 to 2 mg/min.

### ESMOLOL

Esmolol, a relatively cardio selective beta blocker, is rapidly metabolized by blood esterases. Its effects begin almost immediately, and it has both a short half-life (approximately 9 minutes) and a short total duration of action (approximately 30 minutes), permitting rapid titration.

### HYDRALAZINE

Hydralazine is a direct arteriolar vasodilator with little or no effect on the venous circulation. The initial dose is 10 mg, with the maximum dose being 20 mg. The fall in blood pressure can be sudden and begins within 10–30 minutes and lasts 2–4 hours.

### ENALAPRILAT

Enalaprilat is the intravenously active, des-ethyl ester of the angiotensin-converting enzyme (ACE) inhibitor, enalapril. The hypotensive response to enalaprilat is unpredictable and depends upon the plasma volume and plasma renin activity in individual patients with a hypertensive emergency. The usual initial dose is 1.25 mg.

## REFERENCES

1. Neutel JM, et al. A comparison of intravenous nicardipine and sodium nitroprusside in the immediate treatment of severe hypertension. *Am J Hypertens.* 1994 Jul;7(7 Pt 1):623–628.
2. Yancy CW, et al. 2013 ACCF/AHA guideline for the management of heart failure: Executive summary: A report of the American College of Cardiology Foundation/American Heart Association Task Force on Practice Guidelines. *Circulation.* 2013;128(16):1810–1852.
3. Gersh BJ, et al. 2011 ACCF/AHA guideline for the diagnosis and treatment of hypertrophic cardiomyopathy: A report of the American College of Cardiology Foundation/American Heart Association Task Force on Practice Guidelines. *Circulation.* 2011;124(24):e783–e831.
4. Cornette J, et al. Hemodynamic effects of intravenous nicardipine in severely pre-eclamptic women with a hypertensive crisis. *Ultrasound Obstet Gynecol.* 2016 Jan;47(1):89–95.
5. Murphy MB, et al. Fenoldopam: A selective peripheral dopamine-receptor agonist for the treatment of severe hypertension. *N Engl J Med.* 2001 Nov 22;345(21):1548–1557.

# 83.

# CALCIUM CHANNEL BLOCKERS

*Andrew Sprowell and Archit Sharma*

## INTRODUCTION

First introduced in 1967, calcium channel blockers (CCBs) are an important class of medications used in the pharmacotherapy of cardiovascular disorders including hypertension, angina pectoris, and supraventricular arrhythmias.[1] CCBs inhibit calcium influx through L-type calcium channels, leading to predictable effects in various cell types: cardiac myocytes (negative inotropy), smooth muscle cells (vasodilation), and cardiac sinoatrial (SA) and atrioventricular (AV) nodal cells (negative chronotropy and dromotropy, respectively). Non-dihydropyridine (non-DHP) CCBs are negative chronotropes and inotropes (verapamil, diltiazem), whereas dihydropyridine (DHP) CCBs cause vasodilation (e.g., amlodipine, nicardipine).

## MECHANISM OF ACTION

All CCBs inhibit inward current of calcium ($Ca^{2+}$) through calcium-specific membrane spanning L-type ion channels. These channels are found in vascular smooth muscle, sinoatrial and atrioventricular nodal cells, and cardiac myocytes. The impulse for cardiac contraction is initiated by autonomous pacemaker cells in the sinoatrial node which depolarize via slow inward currents from L and T calcium channels, and the funny current (a mixed sodium/potassium channel). This slow-response action potential is characterized by a gradual upstroke and a short peak with no plateau phase. Depolarization propagates across the atria, through the AV node, and into the His-Purkinje system via the fast-response action potential. The fast-response action potential is characterized by a fast upstroke, sustained plateau phase, and rapid termination.

The wave of depolarization traveling through the cardiac conduction system translates into myocardial contraction through "excitation-contraction coupling." Calcium ($Ca^{2+}$) is the key mediator in this event. In response to depolarization, voltage-gated L-type channels on cardiac myocytes open, allowing a small influx of $Ca^{2+}$ from the extracellular space into the cytoplasm. This triggers massive release of $Ca^{2+}$ stores from the sarcoplasmic reticulum into the cytoplasm through the ryanodine receptor (RyR). Calcium allows binding of the actin/myosin complex and muscle contraction. Relaxation is facilitated by the reuptake of $Ca^{2+}$ into the sarcoplasmic reticulum through the sarcoplasmic/endoplasmic reticulum calcium ATPase (SERCA), as well as extrusion of $Ca^{2+}$ across the plasma membrane by the sodium/calcium exchanger. CCBs prevent $Ca^{2+}$ from entering the cell by inhibiting the slow voltage-dependent calcium channels, thereby leading to reduced electrical conduction within the heart, decreased force of contraction (work) of the muscle cells, and arteriodilation.

## CLASSIFICATION

Calcium channel blockers are divided into three major categories: dihydropyridines, phenylalkylamine, and benzothiazepine.

Dihydropyridines (DHPs) include nifedipine, nicardipine, israpedine, amlodipine, felodipine, nisoldipine, clevidipine, and nimodipine. These are further divided into first (nifedipine), second (felodipine), and third (amlodipine) generation. DHPs bind the "N" binding site on the L-type calcium channel. Their pharmacologic effect is systemic arterial vasodilation leading to decreased blood pressure, and coronary arterial dilation leading to increased coronary perfusion. Since they do not suppress SA nodal firing, hypotension and reflex tachycardia may be seen. All the DHPs except for nimodipine are FDA approved for treatment of hypertension. Nimodipine, available as an oral formulation, is approved only for the treatment of subarachnoid hemorrhage. Nifidipine (and verapamil) can be used for treating esophageal spasms. By far the most commonly used DHP in general medical practice is amlodipine. It has a half-life of 44 hours, and doses of 2.5–10 mg daily are prescribed. In anesthesia practice, intravenous nicardipine is frequently used for perioperative management of hypertension and in critically ill patients in whom blood pressure control is paramount (e.g., intracranial hemorrhage). With a fast onset time of 1–2 minutes, and a half-life of around 40 minutes, nicardipine is run as a titratable infusion at doses up to 15 mg/hr. Nicardipine is roughly twice as selective for vascular smooth muscle over cardiac muscle, when compared to non-DHP CCBs or first-generation CCBs such as nifedipine, making it ideal for decreasing blood pressure while increasing cardiac output. Nicardipine increases cerebral blood flow and relieves cerebral arterial vasospasm in subarachnoid hemorrhage.[2] In patients with intact intracranial autoregulatory mechanisms, nicardipine does not increase intracranial pressure (ICP), and it did not increase ICP in rats with induced cerebral ischemia, though it will decrease cerebral perfusion pressure (CPP) due to a predictable lowering of mean arterial pressure (MAP).[3,4]

Non-dihydropyridines (non-DHPs) further include *phenylalkylamine* CCBs (verapamil) and *benzothiazepine* CCBs (diltiazem). The non-DHPs bind the "V" binding site of the L-type calcium channel.[5] Both verapamil and diltiazem will reduce arterial pressure without reflex tachycardia, due to their negative chronotropic, dromotropic, and inotropic effects. Of the two, verapamil causes less vasodilatory effect and less reflex tachycardia. Verapamil has good local anesthetic potency. The non-DHP CCBs are used in management of supraventricular tachyarrhythmias. However, they are contraindicated in patients with hypotension, those with sick sinus syndrome, and second- or third-degree heart block. They should not be used for treatment of atrial fibrillation or atrial flutter in patients with an accessory bypass tract (e.g., Wolff-Parkinson-White syndrome) as they may favor conduction through the accessory tract by atrioventricular (AV) nodal slowing. Verapamil is contraindicated in severe left ventricular (LV) disfunction, and diltiazem is contraindicated in acute myocardial infarction with pulmonary congestion. Both are avoided or used with extreme caution in patients taking a beta blocker. Non-DHP CCBs significantly increase blood levels of digoxin and cyclosporine.

## ANESTHETIC CONSIDERATIONS

### PREOPERATIVE

Calcium channel blockers should be continued on the day of surgery in patients on a stable dosing regimen. Patients taking digoxin or cyclosporine may need to have dosing adjustments if diltiazem or verapamil are started perioperatively to avoid drug toxicity.

### INTRAOPERATIVE

Calcium channel blockers may prolong neuromuscular blockade caused by nondepolarizing muscle relaxants, by causing allosteric inhibition of calcium channels, meaning more channels are in the desensitized state. Calcium channel blockers should not be used in the treatment of malignant hyperthermia (MHAUS). Recall that when treating postoperative supraventricular tachyarrhythmias in patients with reduced ejection fraction and hypotension (i.e., in a patient with atrial fibrillation with rapid ventricular response), diltiazem and verapamil should be used with caution. They can also inhibit platelet aggregation.

### POSTOPERATIVE

An infusion of intravenous nicardipine may be used safely for postoperative hypertension. Diltiazem can be used for treatment of atrial fibrillation that is not hemodynamically unstable.

### REFERENCES

1. Murphy CE, Wechsler AS. Calcium channel blockers and cardiac surgery. *J Card Surg*. 1987;2(2):299–325.
2. Tobias JD. Nicardipine: Applications in anesthesia practice. *J Clin Anesth*. 1995;7(6):525–533.
3. Pepine CJ. Intravenous nicardipine: Cardiovascular effects and clinical relevance. *Clin Ther*. 1988;10(3):316–325.
4. Matsuzaki T, et al. Intravenous infusion of calcium antagonist, nicardipine, does not increase intracranial pressure: Evaluation in a rat model of transient cerebral ischemia and reperfusion. *Neurol Res*. 2008;30(5):531–535.
5. Pascual I, et al. Beta-blockers and calcium channel blockers: First line agents. *Cardiovasc Drugs Ther*. 2016;30(4):357–365

# 84.

# MONOAMINE OXIDASE INHIBITORS

*Christopher Yates and Archit Sharma*

## INTRODUCTION

Monoamine oxidase inhibitors (MAOIs) are an older, less frequently utilized class of antidepressants that are typically used in patients with illness that is refractory to other classes of medications. MAOIs have fallen out of favor due to significant adverse effects, severe interactions with anesthetic drugs, and dietary limitations.

## MECHANISM

MAOIs are responsible for blocking the monoamine oxidase (MAO) enzyme. The monoamine oxidase enzyme breaks down different types of neurotransmitters from the brain: norepinephrine, serotonin, and dopamine, as well as tyramine. MAOIs inhibit the breakdown of these neurotransmitters, thus increasing their levels and allowing them to continue to influence the cells that have been affected by depression.

MAOs are divided into two subtypes: MAO-A and MAO-B. The MOA-A are mostly distributed in the placenta, gut, and liver, but MOA-B is present in the brain, liver, and platelets. MAO-A substrates are clinically relevant to anesthesia, which include dopamine, epinephrine, norepinephrine, serotonin, and tyramine.[1] Tyramine is found in foods such as cheese, avocado, fava beans, and wine. MAO-B subtypes primarily include dopamine and phenylethylamine.[2] MAO-A antagonism is primarily responsible for the antidepressant effects of MAOIs.

There are irreversible MAOIs (phenelzine, tranylcypromine, and isocarboxazide) that are non-selective and inhibit both type A and B MAO receptors. There is also a reversible MAOI (moclobemide), which is specific for MAO-A inhibition only. Selegiline, used for the treatment of the early stages of Parkinson disease, is a selective MAO-B inhibitor at low doses, and non-selective at larger doses. The reversible MAOI have a significantly shorter duration of action than the irreversible MAOIs. The irreversible MAOIs have a duration of action up to weeks and are

associated with a period of withdrawal before starting an alternative antidepressant medication.

## CLINICAL IMPLICATIONS

Consideration must be taken in patients undergoing surgery who are taking MAOIs. The most significant consideration relates to a profound pressor effect that may be seen after administration of either indirect or direct sympathomimetics and cause an excessive sympathetic activity. MAOIs inhibit the metabolism of indirect sympathomimetics, such as ephedrine and pseudoephedrine, which will result in potentiation of their action, resulting in hypertensive crisis and tachycardia. Use of MAOIs will increase presynaptic stores of neurotransmitters, leading to post-synaptic downregulation. Direct sympathomimetics are partially metabolized by catechol-O-methyl-transferase (COMT) and as a result are less dependent on MAO for metabolism. Other signs of symptoms of excessive sympathetic activity may include mydriasis, hyperthermia, seizures, and potentially coma or death. Regardless, caution should be taken with both direct and indirect sympathomimetics and doses reduced when necessary. Likewise, vasoconstrictors in local anesthetics should be used with extreme care and close monitoring of hemodynamics.

In addition to their primary mechanism of action, MAOIs have anticholinergic properties that affect their use in the perioperative period. Sexual dysfunction, weight gain, and orthostatic hypotension are common complications. There is evidence that suggests St. John's wort, which is an herbal supplement that can be used to treat depression, has an alkaloid component that is an MAOI. As a result, it has potential to have synergistic effects of elevating neurotransmitters like norepinephrine to a dangerous level and causing a hypertensive crisis. As a result of potential adverse effects, it is recommended that St. John's wort be discontinued prior to surgery.

Due to the drug interactions and concern for unstable hemodynamic response, the need for perioperative discontinuation of MAOIs has been controversial. Typically, a tapered decrease in irreversible MAOIs over 2–3 weeks has previously been recommended. Reversible MAOIs may be discontinued on the day of surgery. However, discontinuation should only be considered after consultation with the patient's primary psychiatrist due to concern for relapse of the patient's psychiatric symptoms. If discontinued, MAOIs can be reinitiated immediately postoperatively.

Phenylpiperidine opioids (meperidine, tramadol, methadone) need to be used in caution with MAO-A inhibitors because of the risk of excessive stimulation of the 5-HT1A receptor, resulting in serotonin syndrome (confusion, fever, diaphoresis, shivering, ataxia, myoclonus, hyperreflexia, and death).[1-3] MAOIs inhibit the breakdown of norepinephrine and serotonin, and also inhibit hepatic microsomal enzymes. Hence, they can exhibit a central nervous system (CNS) "type I" reaction which manifests as a high risk of serotonin syndrome under certain conditions, resulting in agitation, headache, fever, seizures, coma, and death.[4] They can also exhibit a CNS "type II" reaction due to decreased hepatic opioid metabolism and thus opioid buildup, causing sedation, respiratory depression, and cardiovascular collapse.

Patients on MAOIs can have an increased minimum alveolar concentration (MAC) requirement due to increased levels of CNS norepinephrine. They can exhibit an exaggerated hypotension with neuraxial techniques and have a prolonged succinylcholine effect. Since they can potentiate the effect of indirectly acting sympathomimetics such as ephedrine leading to a hypertensive crisis, we should try to use direct acting vasopressors (phenylephrine) only and consider using lower doses.[5]

## ANESTHETIC CONCERNS

### PREOPERATIVE

Since MAOIs can have multiple reactions with different medications, a psychiatry consultation should be sought to see if the patient can be slowly tapered off of the MAOIs starting 2 weeks before elective surgery. If that cannot be safely done, care should be taken regarding consuming tyramine containing food items and other medications that can interact with MAOIs

### INTRAOPERATIVE

MAOIs can interact with medications like ketamine and indirectly acting sympathomimetics such as ephedrine, potentiating their response and leading to a hypertensive crisis. Avoiding these medications and keeping the anesthetic deep is key to managing these patients intraoperatively.

### POSTOPERATIVE

MAOIs can lead to serotonin syndrome and hence one must avoid use of anticholinergics and meperidine during emergence or in the recovery area to avoid these side effects. If discontinued, MAOIs can be reinitiated immediately postoperatively.

During all phases, watch for complications such as orthostatic hypotension caused by octopamine, tyramine-induced hypertension, aggravation of the action of catecholamines, interaction with opioids which can lead to central serotonergic activity, interaction with meperidine (can be fatal), inhibition of hepatic enzymes, and hepatotoxicity.

## REFERENCES

1. Saraghi M, et al. Anesthetic considerations for patients on antidepressant therapy: Part I. *Anesth Prog.* 2017;64(4):253–261.
2. Rapaport MH. Dietary restrictions and drug interactions with monoamine oxidase inhibitors: The state of the art. *J Clin Psychiatry.* 2007;68 Suppl 8:42–46.
3. Thomas SJ, et al. Combination therapy with monoamine oxidase inhibitors and other antidepressants or stimulants: Strategies for the management of treatment-resistant depression. *Pharmacotherapy.* 2015;35(4):433–449.
4. Thorp M et al. Monoamine oxidase inhibitor overdose. *West J Med.* 1997;166(4):275–277.
5. Saraghi M et al. Anesthetic considerations for patients on antidepressant therapy: Part II. *Anesth Prog.* 2018;65(1):60–65.

# 85.

# ANTICONVULSANTS

*Anish Sethi and Gaurav Trehan*

## INTRODUCTION

Anticonvulsants, also known as antiepileptic drugs, refer to a group of medications that are utilized for the management of epileptic seizures. These medications have various other indications, including for the treatment of various pain syndromes and psychiatric disorders.[1]

Based on the patient's clinical presentation, certain anticonvulsants are selected over others due to their pharmacologic properties. Broadly, anticonvulsants can be categorized based on their indication or their principal cellular target; however, anticonvulsants often act on multiple channels, or their precise mechanism of action may not be fully understood.[2]

## USE IN PAIN MANAGEMENT

Anticonvulsants are often utilized in the management of various neuropathic pain syndromes, fibromyalgia, and certain headache disorders.[3] Commonly treated peripheral neuropathic pain syndromes include peripheral neuropathy, post-herpetic neuralgia, trigeminal neuralgia, complex regional pain syndrome (CRPS), and direct neuronal trauma. Central neuropathic pain syndromes include post-stroke pain, spinal cord injury–related pain, and multiple sclerosis–related pain.

Anticonvulsant treatment for neuropathic pain includes the use of gabapentin and pregabalin as first-line agents. First-line anticonvulsant treatments for trigeminal neuralgia include carbamazepine and oxcarbazepine.[3] Topiramate has demonstrated efficacy as preventative therapy for migraine headache.[3] Pregabalin has been FDA-approved in the treatment of painful diabetic neuropathy, post-herpetic neuralgia, central pain syndrome, and fibromyalgia.[3]

Treatment of pain with multiple classes of drugs with varying mechanisms of action (multimodal analgesia) has been shown to achieve superior pain control

over monotherapy; as a result, anticonvulsants are typically coadministered with other pharmacological agents (Table 85.1).

## PHENYTOIN

### INDICATIONS

Phenytoin is used for the prevention of focal and generalized tonic-clonic seizures and can be used as a second-line agent for mixed seizures.[1]

### MECHANISM OF ACTION AND METABOLISM

Phenytoin exerts its effects by blocking voltage-gated neuronal sodium channels. The primary site of action is the motor cortex, where seizure activity is inhibited. The threshold against hyperexcitability is stabilized by promoting the sodium efflux from neurons.[1]

Phenytoin undergoes hepatic degradation to inactive forms; these inactive forms are renally excreted. Patients with impaired liver function may show early signs of toxicity. Phenytoin is an inducer of the cytochrome P450 enzymes, which contributes to its significant numerous drug-drug interactions.[1]

*Table 85.1* MECHANISMS OF COMMON ANTICONVULSANTS

| CALCIUM CHANNEL | SODIUM CHANNEL | INHIBITORY CHANNELS |
|---|---|---|
| Gabapentin | Carbamazepine | Benzodiazepines |
| Pregabalin | Oxcarbazepine | Barbiturates |
| Ethosuximide | Lamotrigine | Valproic acid |
| | Lacosamide | Cannabidiol |
| | Phenytoin | |

## SIDE EFFECTS

Common side effects include abdominal discomfort, nausea, decreased appetite, gingival hyperplasia, ataxia, and hirsutism.[1] More serious side effects include bone marrow suppression, toxic epidermal necrolysis, and suicidal ideation.[1] Rapid intravenous administration of phenytoin may result in serious cardiac arrhythmias and hypotension.

# CARBAMAZEPINE

## INDICATIONS

Carbamazepine is indicated for the treatment of epilepsy, trigeminal neuralgia, and bipolar disorder.[2] It may also be utilized for the treatment of painful diabetic neuropathy and central post-stroke pain syndrome.

## MECHANISM OF ACTION AND METABOLISM

Carbamazepine functions by the blockade of presynaptic voltage-gated sodium channels, thereby decreasing the availability of sodium channels, resulting in a net decrease in the firing of ectopic action potentials.[2] Carbamazepine is metabolized extensively in the liver by the cytochrome P450 system.

## SIDE EFFECTS

Common side effects of carbamazepine include diplopia, nystagmus, rash, visual changes, ataxia, sedation, dizziness, and hypernatremia.

As an inducer of the cytochrome P450 system, carbamazepine affects the metabolism of multiple other medications, including other anticonvulsants, antivirals, warfarin, and oral contraceptives. Use of carbamazepine in pregnancy should be avoided due to the risk of teratogenic effects.[2]

Serious dermatologic reactions, including Stevens-Johnson syndrome and toxic epidermal necrolysis, may occur with the use of carbamazepine. In rare cases, agranulocytosis and aplastic anemia may occur with long-term use.

# GABAPENTIN

## INDICATIONS

Gabapentin is utilized for the treatment of neuropathic pain syndromes, including painful diabetic neuropathy, mixed neuropathic pain, post-herpetic neuralgia, HIV neuropathy, phantom limb pain, direct nerve injury, radicular nerve pain, and spinal cord injury. It is additionally utilized as an adjunctive treatment for the management of focal epilepsy and restless leg syndrome.

## MECHANISM OF ACTION AND METABOLISM

Gabapentin's structure is similar to the neurotransmitter gamma-aminobutyric acid (GABA); however, it has not been shown to interact with GABA receptors. Instead, gabapentin has been shown to bind to the $\alpha2\delta$-1 subunit of the presynaptic L-type calcium channel. This causes a modulation of calcium influx, resulting in a reduction in excitatory neurotransmitter release with a subsequent decrease in pain signaling.[2]

Gabapentin is minimally metabolized in humans, and is eliminated renally as unchanged drug. Patients with renal dysfunction exhibit decreased plasma clearance, and thus require dose adjustment.[3]

## SIDE EFFECTS

Gabapentin overall has a favorable side-effect profile. Side effects may include sedation, encephalopathy, weight gain, peripheral edema, or confusion.[3]

Dosing of gabapentin involves a gradual period of uptitration to the desired clinical effect, while monitoring for adverse effects.

## ANESTHETIC CONSIDERATIONS

Patients should be continued on their anticonvulsants through the perioperative period; if they were receiving oral anticonvulsants and are made NPO (nothing by mouth), alternative intravenous formulations should be considered. Once patients are able to tolerate oral medications, they should be transitioned back to their usual oral anticonvulsant regimen. Serum drug concentrations should be monitored with dose adjustments or if there is concern for adverse effects. Caution should be exercised while administering perioperative medications to patients on anticonvulsants, due to the multiple potential drug-drug interactions.

Perioperative administration of gabapentin has often been utilized in an attempt to modulate postoperative pain. Recent studies on perioperative gabapentin use have demonstrated no effect on postoperative pain resolution; however, a modest effect on promoting opioid cessation and prevention of chronic opioid use was noted.[4]

Patients with a history of epilepsy should be closely monitored for the occurrence of perioperative seizures; seizures may be controlled with intravenous benzodiazepines and anticonvulsants.

## REFERENCES

1. Jensen TS. Anticonvulsants in neuropathic pain: Rationale and clinical evidence. *Eur J Pain*. 2002;6(Suppl A):61–68.
2. Beal BR, Wallace MS. An overview of pharmacologic management of chronic pain. *Med Clin North Am*. 2016;100(1):65–79.
3. Li CT, Watson JC. Anticonvulsants in the treatment of pain. In: Deer T, Pope J, Lamer T, Provenzano D, eds. *Deer's Treatment of Pain*. Springer, Cham; 2019:149–161.
4. Hah J et al. Effect of perioperative gabapentin on postoperative pain resolution and opioid cessation in a mixed surgical cohort: A randomized clinical trial. *JAMA Surg*. 2018;153(4):303–311.

# 86.

# LOCAL ANESTHETICS

*Peter Papapetrou and Kris Ferguson*

## INTRODUCTION

Local anesthetics have been widely used in perioperative anesthesia as well as chronic pain management. The delivery of local anesthetics to the skin, subcutaneous tissues, peripheral nerves, epidural, and intrathecal spaces has been extremely useful in the preoperative, intraoperative, and postoperative setting to control acute pain.

## MECHANISM OF ACTION

Local anesthetics directly bind to voltage-gated sodium channels, preventing nerve depolarization. This inhibits the generation or propagation of action potentials in peripheral nerves.[1] The most susceptible nerves are non-myelinated C fibers, whereas the least susceptible to local anesthetic blockade are small myelinated, A-delta fibers. Potency of local anesthetics is related to lipid solubility; duration of action is related to protein binding and speed of onset is related to pKa.

## BIOTRANSFORMATION AND EXCRETION

Local anesthetics are categorized as either amino ester or amides, as shown in Table 86.1 with their respective maximum doses. Amino ester local anesthetics such as

chlorprocaine are hydrolyzed by cholinesterase enzymes in plasma. Amino amide local anesthetics such as lidocaine are primarily biotransformed in the liver. Enzyme activity and hepatic blood flow account for the elimination of amide local anesthetics. Excretion of amide local anesthetics occurs via the kidneys, with less than 5% of unchanged

*Table 86.1* ESTER AND AMIDE LOCAL ANESTHETICS

| DRUG | MAXIMUM DOSE (MG/KG) |
| --- | --- |
| **Esters** | |
| Chlorprocaine | 12 |
| Procaine | 12 |
| Cocaine | 3 |
| Tetracaine | 3 |
| **Amides** | |
| Lidocaine | 5* |
| Mepivacaine | 4.5 |
| Prilocaine | 8 |
| Bupivacaine | 3 |
| Ropivacaine | 3 |

*5 mg/kg maximum dose without epinephrine; 7 mg/kg maximum dose with epinephrine

drug being found in the urine, and the remaining amount in the urine being metabolites.[2] Both congestive heart failure (CHF) and liver disease decrease the elimination of local anesthetics.

## LOCAL ANESTHETIC COMPOSITION

Local anesthetic molecules are composed of an aromatic ring, an intermediate chain, and a terminal amine.[3] The aromatic ring determines its lipid solubility, which is related to the local anesthetic's potency. The intermediate chain gives classification of the local anesthetic as either amino ester or amide, which are biotransformed differently. Amide local anesthetics are biotransformed in the liver and are therefore longer lasting, and carry decreased risk of allergic reactions than ester local anesthetics. Time of onset of local anesthetic is predicted by its pKa, which affects how rapidly the drug is ionized. The non-ionized form is lipid soluble and crosses the axonal membrane, which then becomes ionized, the form which is responsible for neural blockade.

## PROLONGATION OF ACTION

Addition of epinephrine (5 mcg/mL) to local anesthetic solutions allows more local anesthetic molecules to reach nerve membrane due to reduced vascular absorption. Clinically, this results in a greater duration of action of local anesthetics. Site of injection also determines vascular uptake of local anesthetics, as shown in Table 86.2.

## CENTRAL NERVOUS SYSTEM SIDE EFFECTS

The potency of local anesthetics impacts the degree of central nervous system (CNS) toxicity they can cause. CNS

*Table 86.2* RATE OF ABSORPTION OF LOCAL ANESTHETICS BASED ON ADMINISTRATION ROUTE

| ROUTE OF ADMINISTRATION | ABSORPTION RATE |
|---|---|
| Intravenous | Fastest |
| Intercostal | |
| Caudal epidural | |
| Lumbar epidural | |
| Brachial plexus | |
| Subcutaneous | Slowest |

toxicity can be manifested as tinnitus, dizziness, blurred vision, circumoral numbness, restlessness, agitation, and tonic-clonic seizures. Hypercarbia lowers the seizure threshold by increasing cerebral blood flow (CBF) and the acidotic state decreasing protein binding, which increases free drug availability.[4] Another devastating result of local anesthetic toxicity is cauda equina syndrome, described as prolonged neurologic injury manifested by pain, motor deficits, and sensory changes, which occurs in spinal anesthesia. The etiology of cauda equina syndrome is thought to be due to neural toxicity caused by high concentrations and doses of certain local anesthetics, which are primarily chlorprocaine and lidocaine. Patients can also experience transient neurologic symptoms (TNS), which are most often manifested as severe pain radiating down both legs. Lidocaine is the most frequently implicated local anesthetic in TNS, but other risk factors include obesity, early ambulation, and lithotomy position.

## CARDIAC SIDE EFFECTS

The degree of myocardial depression caused by a local anesthetic is proportional to its potency. In addition, high doses of local anesthetics can cause vasodilation. Bupivacaine is particularly cardiotoxic as it more strongly binds to inactivated sodium channels and dissociates more slowly than other local anesthetics in myocardial tissue.

## ALLERGIC REACTIONS

Allergic reactions to ester local anesthetics are much more common than to amide local anesthetics. Ester local anesthetics are metabolized to para-aminobenzoic acid (PABA), which is known to cause allergic reactions.

## PRESERVATIVES

Sulfites are commonly added to local anesthetic solutions to stabilize vasoconstricting agents such as epinephrine. Anaphylactoid reactions can be the result of exposure to sulfites, which can manifest as bronchospasm, angioedema, seizures, circulatory collapse, and death. Sodium bisulfite has been implicated in the development of arachnoiditis, and is the preservative used in 2-chlorprocaine. To replace sodium bisulfite, disodium ethylenediaminetetraacetate (EDTA) was used to prolong shelf life. However, large volumes of epidurally injected EDTA has been the cause of severe pain at injection sites. Methylparaben is a bacteriostatic agent used as a preservative in local anesthetics. Its chemical structure is similar to PABA, and can cause anaphylactoid reactions in certain patients.

## METHEMOGLOBINEMIA

O-toluidine is responsible for oxidizing hemoglobin to methemoglobin, which is a metabolic product of prilocaine. Methemoglobinemia makes pulse oximeter readings inaccurate, though oxygen saturation readings do not decrease below 84% despite true oxygenation. Methemoglobinemia is treated with 1 mg/kg methylene blue intravenously.

## LOCAL ANESTHETIC SYSTEMIC TOXICITY

Despite preventative measures such as using safe dose and concentration of local anesthetic, as well as use of a test dose to monitor for intravascular injection, local anesthetic systemic toxicity (LAST) still can occur. Diagnosis is made by monitoring CNS changes. Treatment is focused on maintaining an adequate airway, breathing, and circulation. Hypoxia and hypercarbia should be avoided, and 100% $O_2$ should be administered. If convulsions occur, they should be treated with a benzodiazepine. Twenty percent lipid emulsion should also be administered with a dose of 1.5–4 mL/kg initially, followed by a continuous infusion of 0.25–0.5 mL/kg/min for 10–60 minutes to ensure rapid recovery from local anesthetic toxicity.

## REFERENCES

1. Local Anesthetics. Yanagidate F, Strichartz GR. *HEP*. 2006;177: 95–127.
2. Heavner JE. Chapter 45: Pharmacology of local anesthetics. In: Longnecker et al., eds. *Anesthesiology*. 2nd edition. New York, NY: McGraw-Hill; 2012:767–782.
3. Wadlund DL. Local anesthetic systemic toxicity. AORN. 2017;106:367–374.
4. Murray MJ, et al. *Faust's Anesthesiology Review*. 4th ed. Philadelphia, PA: Elsevier Saunders; 2015.

# 87.

# MUSCLE RELAXANTS

*Peter Papapetrou and Kris Ferguson*

## INTRODUCTION

Muscle relaxants, otherwise known as neuromuscular blocking agents (NMBAs), are useful during tracheal intubation and allow for less volatile anesthetic while optimizing muscle relaxation during surgery. They are classified as either depolarizing or nondepolarizing muscle relaxants based on their mechanism of action. Succinylcholine is the only depolarizing muscle relaxant currently being used, whereas the nondepolarizing muscle relaxants primarily include rocuronium, vecuronium, pancuronium, atracurium, and cisatracurium. Each NMBA carries unique properties, side effects, and differences in metabolism. Table 87.1 lists all the commonly used neuromuscular blocking agents, as well as intubating doses, onset of action, and duration of action.

*Table 87.1* COMMONLY USED NEUROMUSCULAR BLOCKING AGENTS

| DRUG | INTUBATING DOSE (MG/KG) | ONSET | DURATION OF ACTION |
|---|---|---|---|
| Succinylcholine | 1.5 | 30–90 s | Very short |
| Rocuronium | 0.9–1.2 | 60–90 s | Intermediate |
| Vecuronium | 0.08–0.12 | 2–3 min | Intermediate |
| Atracurium | 0.5 | 3–5 min | Intermediate |
| Cisatracurium | 0.15–0.2 | 2.7 min | Intermediate |
| Pancuronium | 0.08–0.12 | 3–5 min | Long |

## SUCCINYLCHOLINE

Succinylcholine is the only current depolarizing muscle relaxant used. It produces rapid skeletal muscle relaxation by binding to nicotinic receptors at the postjunctional neuromuscular membrane. Its duration of action is relatively brief, as the vast majority of molecules are metabolized in the blood by plasma cholinesterases before reaching the muscle endplate, and the termination of muscle relaxation is due to diffusion of succinylcholine molecules away from the neuromuscular junction.[1] Peripartum patients and patients with severe liver disease have decreased plasma cholinesterases, causing prolonged responses to succinylcholine. In addition, prolongation can occur with inhibition of plasma cholinesterases with anticholinesterases, echothiophate, organophosphates, phenelzine, and cytotoxic agents.

## SUCCINYLCHOLINE SIDE EFFECTS

Though useful for rapid muscle relaxation during tracheal intubation, succinylcholine use carries certain limitations. Succinylcholine depolarization at the postjunctional membrane causes leakage of potassium into the serum with an approximate increase of 0.5–1 mEq/L. Patients who have a recent history of trauma or muscle denervation may be susceptible to a massive hyperkalemic response, which may lead to ventricular fibrillation and cardiac arrest. Patients who are susceptible to this response have a history of stroke, closed head injury, encephalitis, brain tumor, immobility, and third–degree burns.[2] Succinylcholine is a known culprit of malignant hyperthermia, and should be avoided in susceptible patients or those with a strong family history of malignant hyperthermia. Caution should be used when administering succinylcholine to children as undiagnosed myopathies may manifest as massive hyperkalemia and cardiac arrest. Furthermore, children are predisposed to bradycardia after succinylcholine administration, as they are more sensitive to muscarinic stimulation.[3] A transient though small increase in intraocular pressure can occur with succinylcholine, and caution must be used in patients with penetrating eye injuries. Intracranial pressure may increase from succinylcholine administration through various theories of mechanisms, though this has yet to be confirmed. Furthermore, though succinylcholine increases intragastric pressure, it also increases lower esophageal sphincter tone and does not increase aspiration risk.

## PSEUDOCHOLINESTERASE ABNORMALITIES

Succinylcholine is hydrolyzed by butyrylcholinesterase (BChE), resulting in 5%–10% of the drug reaching the neuromuscular junction. Its clinical effects are terminated when succinylcholine diffuses away from the neuromuscular junction. Patients with genetic variants of BChE can have a significantly prolonged duration of succinylcholine neuromuscular blockade. This can be confirmed with a dibucaine number, which represents the qualitative percentage of BChE's ability to metabolize succinylcholine. A dibucaine number of 80 represents a normal ability to metabolize succinylcholine. A dibucaine number of 50–60 represents the heterozygous enzyme variant, with prolongation of a standard succinylcholine dose by 30%,[4] whereas a dibucaine number of 20–30 represents the homozygous atypical enzyme variant and a duration of neuromuscular blockade of succinylcholine of 2–3 hours.

## PHASE 1 AND 2 BLOCKADE

Phase 1 blockade after administration of succinylcholine is the standard and expected response to the drug, which is characterized by muscle fasciculations, neuromuscular blockade, absence of post-tetanic facilitation, augmentation of muscle blockade with anticholinesterase, decreased amplitude but sustained response to continuous stimulation, train-of-four (TOF) ration >70%, and absence of fade to tetanic or TOF stimulation. With infusions or repeated doses of the drug, a Phase 2 blockade can be observed, resulting in prolonged action of succinylcholine. Phase 2 blockade is thought to be due to a distortion of the normal electrolyte balance caused by repeated channel opening, resulting in inappropriate receptor response to succinylcholine and prolonged response. Phase 2 is characterized by tetanic fade, decreased contraction to a single twitch, post-tetanic facilitation, TOF ration <30%, and reversal with anticholinesterases. Tachyphylaxis is also associated with Phase 2 blockade, which is not observed with Phase 1.

## NONDEPOLARIZING NEUROMUSCULAR BLOCKING AGENTS

Given the unwanted side effects of succinylcholine, newer muscle relaxants have been developed. Nondepolarizing muscle relaxants competitively inhibit nicotinic receptors, causing muscle relaxation. They are all highly ionized in water due to presence of a quaternary ammonium cation and thus have very little lipid solubility. The potency of these agents and degree of muscle relaxation is enhanced by inhalational anesthetics, aminoglycosides, magnesium lithium, local anesthetics, acidosis, hypokalemia, and hypothermia.

## ROCURONIUM

Duration of action and rate of recovery of rocuronium is very similar to vecuronium, but its onset is much faster when given at twice the $ED_{95}$. Typically, it can allow for excellent intubating conditions at this dose within 60 seconds in 90% of patients,[5] and can be used as an alternative to succinylcholine when expedient airway securement is necessary. Thirty percent of rocuronium is eliminated by the kidneys, and the remainder is through the biliary system. There are no metabolites of rocuronium.

## VECURONIUM

Vecuronium is stored in powdered form because it is unstable when mixed in a solution. Its onset of action is 3–5 minutes and has duration and recovery times similar to rocuronium. It is metabolized by the liver and cleared by the kidneys, with some clearance by the biliary system.

## ATRACURIUM

Atracurium has similar onset and duration as vecuronium. One-third of atracurium is metabolized via Hofmann elimination, which is the spontaneous nonenzymatic degradation of this compound, and therefore does not rely on liver and kidney elimination. The other two-thirds are metabolized by nonspecific plasma esterases. One of atracurium's metabolites is laudanosine, which is not clinically relevant in humans but can cause CNS excitation in animals. Caution should be used when administering atracurium in asthmatics, as it can cause histamine release.

## CISATRACURIUM

Cisatracurium is four times more potent than atracurium, though it does not cause histamine release. It is metabolized purely through Hofmann elimination.

## PANCURONIUM

Pancuronium is a long-acting NMBA with a duration of action between 60 and 90 minutes. Some of the drug is metabolized in the liver, but the majority is excreted unchanged in the urine. Patients with renal failure may experience a prolongation of its effects. Pancuronium is vagolytic, causing an increased heart rate, blood pressure, and cardiac output.

## ALLERGIC REACTIONS

NMBAs have been implicated as the most common cause of allergic reactions to anesthetic agents. The reactions are immunoglobin E (IgE)-mediated, and there exists significant cross-reactivity among the different nondepolarizing NMBAs.

## SIDE EFFECTS OF NONDEPOLARIZING NMBAS

Nondepolarizing muscle relaxants may cause unwanted autonomic side effects due to their interaction with receptors in autonomic ganglia of the sympathetic and parasympathetic nervous systems. An older NMBA, d-tubocurarine, can cause hypotension due to autonomic ganglia blockade at doses slightly higher than doses required for neuromuscular blockade. Pancuronium can cause vagolysis through muscarinic receptor blockade of nodal cells in the heart, resulting in increased heart rate. It also decreased norepinephrine reuptake. Histamine release is another rare side effect. The benzylisoquinolinium subgroup of nondepolarizing NMBAs causes histamine release from mast cells. This may result in peripheral vasodilation that can manifest as erythema of the torso, neck, and face. Bronchospasm is a very rare though serious manifestation of histamine release caused by NMBAs. Rapid administration of mivacurium and atracurium at high doses can cause histamine-induced hypotension.

## REFERENCES

1. Pino RM, Ali HH. Chapter 34: Monitoring and managing neuromuscular blockade. In: Longnecker et al., eds. Anesthesiology. 2nd ed. New York, NY: McGraw-Hill; 2012:492–507.
2. Mancuso, AJ. Chapter 80: Succinylcholine side effects. In: Murray MJ, et al., eds. *Faust's Anesthesiology Review.* 4th ed. Philadelphia, PA: Elsevier Saunders; 2015:177–179.
3. Hager HH, Burns B. Succinylcholine chloride. [Updated June 22, 2020]. In: *StatPearls* [Internet]. Treasure Island, FL: StatPearls; 2020 Jan–. https://www.ncbi.nlm.nih.gov/books/NBK499984/.
4. Trujillo R, West WP. Pseudocholinesterase deficiency. [2020 July 15, 2020]. In: *StatPearls* [Internet]. Treasure Island, FL: StatPearls; 2020 Jan–. https://www.ncbi.nlm.nih.gov/books/NBK541032/.
5. Buzello W, et al. Muscle Relaxants: A clinical update. *Acta Anaesthesiol Scand Suppl.* 1996;(109):165–167.

# 88.

# MEDICATION-ASSISTED OPIOID WITHDRAWAL

*Huanhuan Peng and Till Conermann*

## INTRODUCTION

According to the fifth edition of the *Diagnostic and Statistical Manual of Mental Disorders* (DSM-5), opioid use disorder is defined as a problematic pattern of opioid use during a 12-month period leading to clinically significant impairment or distress, and is manifested by at least 2 of several criteria, such as taking opioids in larger amounts than intended, craving opioids, recurrent use in dangerous situations, difficulties cutting down or controlling opioid use, continued opioid use despite harm or adverse consequences, tolerance, withdrawal, reduced social or occupational activities because of opioid use, and difficulties with fulfilling obligations at home or at work.

Withdrawal symptoms of anxiety, tachycardia, diaphoresis, gastrointestinal distress, and drug craving can occur if opioids are stopped abruptly in a patient who is opioid tolerant. Tolerance is defined by the FDA as taking at least 60 mg of morphine a day or its equivalent (60 MME) for at least one week. While opioid withdrawal is not life-threatening, the symptoms can be severe, and patients often relapse to reduce their suffering.[1]

Naltrexone can be used for full detoxification as it is a full antagonist. Methadone and buprenorphine, on the other hand, typically result in a state of continued physiological dependence since these medications rely on full and partial opioid agonism, respectively. These medications, by not creating an intense euphoria and by being prescribed as part of a monitored treatment program, are safer, with fewer side effects and risks, than the continued use of commonly abused opioids.[1]

Alpha-2 adrenergic agonists such as clonidine and lofexidine can also be used to mitigate the severity of withdrawal symptoms. The efficacy of buprenorphine and methadone are comparable to each other, but both are superior to clonidine and lofexidine in supervised withdrawal.[1]

## BUPRENORPHINE

Buprenorphine is a mixed agonist-antagonist opioid receptor modulator that is a partial agonist at the μ opioid receptor and antagonist at the kappa opioid receptor. Due to its partial agonism, buprenorphine has a ceiling effect for respiratory depression as well as for the euphoric response, which provides larger safety margins. It can be used in several forms such as a daily, trans-mucosal form (sublingual or buccal), an extended-release injected subcutaneous form, as well as a long-acting implant. The sublingual form is provided either as a tablet or as a buccal soluble film strip and is the most commonly used form for the treatment of an opioid use disorder. Buprenorphine is usually formulated with naloxone in the oral form of ratio 4:1 to prevent it from being abused intravenously by crushing and dissolving. Naloxone has minimal bioavailability when administered sublingually with buprenorphine, but when being abused parenterally, it will precipitate withdrawal symptoms. Although buprenorphine is relatively safe, it is not without potential side effects. Sedation, insomnia, constipation, headache, and nausea are some of the more commonly reported side effects. Buprenorphine can lead to fatal respiratory depression when administered with other respiratory depressants such as benzodiazepines and alcohol. The buprenorphine-naloxone combination should not be used in patients with severe liver impairment because first-pass metabolism is impaired, increasing naloxone bioavailability and neutralizing the opioid agonist effects. Buprenorphine is safe to use during pregnancy and provides the benefit of reduced duration and severity of neonatal abstinence syndrome compared to methadone.[2] It is important to note that buprenorphine initiation (induction) should occur only when a patient is in at least moderate opioid withdrawal (on the clinical opiate withdrawal scale; COWS) since buprenorphine as a partial agonist with a very high affinity for the μ receptor will displace full agonist opioids and precipitate more severe opioid withdrawal symptoms. Induction with buprenorphine is usually done under direct prescriber observation at the office or at home, with a second dose available to the patient if withdrawal symptoms are not well controlled with the first dose. The typical trans-mucosal buprenorphine starting dose is 4 mg, followed by an additional 2–4 mg if withdrawal symptoms persist after a 2-hour observation period. On the next day, a single dose of total dose received on the previous day will be given, followed by an increase in up to 4-mg increments if residual withdrawal symptoms are observed. The half-life of buprenorphine is 24–42 hours depending on the patient. It takes 5 half-lives for buprenorphine to reach its pharmacological steady-state, and it is not recommended to increase the total daily dose above 16 mg/day in most patients. It is very rare for a patient to require 24 mg/day or more. The most common maintenance dose is between 8 and 16 mg/day.[3] When buprenorphine needs to be tapered and discontinued, it should be tapered gradually, with 2-mg dose reductions every 1 to 2 weeks. For a more rapid taper, the dose can be reduced by 2 mg every 1 to 3 days.[1,4] The long-lasting buprenorphine implant (lasting 6 months) is intended for a stabilized patient with a daily dose of 8 mg or less, but requires a minor surgical procedure to be placed. The injectable form is administered monthly, with 300 mg as an initiating dose and 100 mg monthly as a maintenance dose. As part of buprenorphine treatment, to make sure the patient is not using other illicit drugs and is not diverting prescribed medication, a multi-panel test that specifically tests for buprenorphine and other common substances such as amphetamines and barbiturates will be administered prior to and during therapy.

## METHADONE

When used for medication-assisted withdrawal, methadone needs to be provided through a federally designated treatment program or inpatient hospital setting due to overdose risk and life-threatening adverse effects. Methadone can prolong the QT interval at high doses and can cause *torsades de pointes*. Patients should not receive methadone if their QT is over 500 milliseconds and should be monitored closely if their QT interval is between 450 to 500 milliseconds. Other factors that can worsen QT prolongation include concurrent use of other QT elongation medications, such as ondansetron, amiodarone, and macrolides; bradycardia; hypomagnesemia; hypokalemia; or hypocalcemia. Respiratory depression caused by a methadone overdose can be treated with naloxone. Repeat naloxone doses are often needed as it has a shorter half-life than methadone. Other common side effects of methadone are constipation, sweating, drowsiness, peripheral edema, hyperalgesia, and erectile dysfunction. Methadone is usually given as a diluted and artificially colored liquid to help prevent it from being abused intravenously. The first dose of methadone should be given at the time that mild to moderate withdrawal symptoms are observed in order to observe the efficacy of the starting dose. The first dose should be under 30 mg, and the total first-day dose should not exceed 40 mg. The typical initial dose is 10–20 mg, followed by an incremental dose of 10 mg 2 hours later if needed, based on withdrawal measured by the clinical opioid withdrawal score (COWS; see Appendix 1). Due to methadone's long half-life of 8 to 59 hours and significant interindividual variability in its pharmacokinetics, each

incremental dose should be given with close monitoring of patient response. The dose on day 2 is based on the total dose received on day 1, and if withdrawal symptoms persist and cannot be controlled, the total dose can be increased up to 40 mg and adjunctive treatment initiated (see later discussion). Maintenance therapy can be considered once withdrawal symptoms resolve. Methadone doses can be tapered gradually with slight dose decreases by 5–10 mg/week every several weeks or monthly to cease therapy.[1,4]

## ALPHA-2 ADRENERGIC AGONISTS

The alpha-2 adrenergic agonists clonidine and lofexidine are also used to help mitigate opioid withdrawal symptoms. Although they are minimally effective in reducing cravings and are no longer used as primary medications in opioid withdrawal treatment, an alpha-2 adrenergic agonist can effectively mitigate many of the autonomic withdrawal symptoms such as sweating, irritability, anxiety, intestinal cramps, nausea, and diarrhea by decreasing locus coeruleus hyperactivity and noradrenaline levels. Alpha-2 agonists should not be used if a patient is already hypotensive, has moderate or severe renal insufficiency, has cardiac instability, is pregnant, or is psychotic.[1,2]

## NALTREXONE

Naltrexone, an opioid antagonist, can be used to help prevent relapse after completion of medically supervised withdrawal from opioids. The initiation of naltrexone should be medically supervised as it can precipitate withdrawal symptoms. Side effects include headache, dizziness, fatigue, and nausea. The severe side effect of liver damage can occur with supertherapeutic doses and usually resolves once naltrexone is discontinued. If the patient is prescribed therapeutic opioids after discontinuation of antagonist therapy, extra care should be taken. Patients may lose their tolerance to opioids over time, and thus need to be started on the same doses as opioid-naïve patients to avoid the risks of overdose and death.[1,5]

## REFERENCES

1. Diaper AM, et al. Pharmacological strategies for detoxification. *Br J Clin Pharmacol*. 2014 Feb;77(2):302–314.
2. Bell J, et al. Detoxification from opiate drugs during pregnancy. *Am J Obstet Gynecol*. 2016 Sep;215(3):374.e1–6.
3. Gowing L, et al. Buprenorphine for managing opioid withdrawal. *Cochrane Database Syst Rev*. 2017 Feb 21;2:CD002025.
4. Berna C, et al. Tapering long-term opioid therapy in chronic noncancer pain: Evidence and recommendations for everyday practice. *Mayo Clin Proc*. 2015 Jun;90(6):828–842.
5. Tanum L, et al. Effectiveness of injectable extended-release naltrexone vs daily buprenorphine-naloxone for opioid dependence: A randomized clinical noninferiority trial. *JAMA Psychiatry*. 2017 Dec 1;74(12):1197–1205.

# APPENDIX 1

Clinical Opiate Withdrawal Scale (COWS)

For each item, circle the number that best describes the patient's signs or symptom. Rate on just the apparent relationship to opiate withdrawal. For example, if heart rate is increased because the patient was jogging just prior to assessment, the increase pulse rate would not add to the score.

Patient's Name: _____     Date and Time ____/____/____:_____

Reason for this assessment:_____

Restina Pulse Rate:_____beats/minute

*Measured after patient is sitting or lying for one minute*

0  pulse rate 80 or below

1  pulse rate 81-100

2  pulse rate 101-120

4  pulse rate greater than 120

Sweating: *over past ½ hour not accounted for by room temperature or patient activity.*

0  no report of chills or flushing

1  subjective report of chills or flushing

2  flushed or observable moistness on face

3  beads of sweat on brow or face

4  sweat streaming off face

Restlessness *Observation during assessment*

0  able to sit still

1  reports difficulty sitting still, but is able to do so

3  frequent shifting or extraneous movements of legs/arms

5  Unable to sit still for more than a few seconds

Pupil size

0  pupils pinned or normal size for room light

1  pupils possibly larger than normal for room light

2  pupils moderately dilated

5  pupils so dilated that only the rim of the iris is visible

Bone or Joint aches *If patient was having pain previously, only the additional component attributed to opiates withdrawal is scored*

0  not present

1  mild diffuse discomfort

2  patient reports severe diffuse aching of joints/ muscles

4  patient is rubbing joints or muscles and is unable to sit still because of discomfort

Runny nose or tearing *Not accounted for by cold symptoms or allergies*

0  not present

1  nasal stuffiness or unusually moist eyes

2  nose running or tearing

4  nose constantly running or tears streaming down cheeks

GI Upset: *over last ½ hour*

0  no GI symptoms

1  stomach cramps

2  nausea or loose stool

3  vomiting or diarrhea

5  Multiple episodes of diarrhea or vomiting

Tremor *observation of outstretched hands*

0  No tremor

1  tremor can be felt, but not observed

2  slight tremor observable

4  gross tremor or muscle twitching

Yawning *Observation during assessment*

0  no yawning

1  yawning once or twice during assessment

2  yawning three or more times during assessment

4  yawning several times/minute

Anxiety or Irritability

0  none

1  patient reports increasing irritability or anxiousness

2  patient obviously irritable anxious

4  patient so irritable or anxious that participation in the assessment is difficult

Gooseflesh skin

0  skin is smooth

3  piloerrection of skin can be felt or hairs standing up on arms

5  prominent piloerrection

Total Score _____

The total score is the sum of all 11 items

Initials of person

completing Assessment: _____

Score: 5-12 = mild; 13-24 = moderate; 25-36 = moderately severe; more than 36 = severe withdrawal

Reproduced with permission from Wesson DR, Ling W. The Clinical Opiate Withdrawal Scale (COWS). *J Psychoactive Drugs*. 2003 Apr-Jun;35(2):253-9. doi: 10.1080/02791072.2003.10400007.

# 89.

# AGENTS AND TECHNIQUES IN PEDIATRIC ANESTHESIOLOGY

*F. Cole Dooley and Charlotte Streetzel*

## INDUCTION TECHNIQUES

The two main induction methods used for children are inhalational and intravenous. Dosing schedules and minimum alveolar concentration (MAC) of induction agents vary between ages and are summarized in Table 89.1.

## INHALATIONAL INDUCTION

Compared to adults, children have greater minute ventilation-to-FRC (functional residual capacity) ratios and increased cerebral blood flow, which allows for relatively quicker inhalational induction times.[1]

Sevoflurane has a low blood solubility, allowing for rapid onset and rapid recovery, minimal odor allowing for less airway irritability, and less myocardial depression. Thus, sevoflurane is the preferred inhaled anesthetic in pediatric patients.[1,2]

Desflurane and isoflurane are avoided for pediatric inhalational induction due to their strong odor and risk of triggering airway reflexes, but may be used for maintenance. Desflurane has the lowest blood solubility, which allows for rapid recovery, while isoflurane has a higher blood solubility, resulting in a slower onset and offset.

When compared to sevoflurane, halothane has a slower onset and recovery time, a very high risk of triggering airway reflexes on single breath induction, and a greater incidence of bradycardia, hypotension, and arrhythmias.[2]

*Table 89.1* INHALATION AND INTRAVENOUS AGENTS USED IN PEDIATRICS

PEDIATRIC INDUCTION AGENTS

| INDUCTION METHOD | AGENT | KEY FACTS | PATIENT AGE | MAC/INDUCTION DOSE |
|---|---|---|---|---|
| Inhalational Volatiles | Sevoflurane | No odor | Neonates<br>Children 6mo–10y | 3.20 %<br>2.40 % |
| | Desflurane | Strong odor<br>Quick onset/offset | Children without concurrent use of nitrous | 7–9% |
| | Isoflurane | Strong odor<br>Slower onset/offset | Children | 1.50% |
| | Halothane | Cardiac instability | Children | 1.0% |
| Intravenous | Propofol | Blunting of airway reflexes | Neonates, infants and children | 2–3 mg/kg |
| | Etomidate | Adrenal suppression | Children | 0.2–0.3 mg/kg |
| | Ketamine | Catecholamine release | Neonates and children | 1–3 mg/kg |
| | Methohexital | Skeletal muscle, hyperactivity, hiccups, myoclonus | Infants, children, and adolescents | 1–2.5mg/ kg |
| | Thiopental | Not available for use in US | Neonates<br>Children | 3–4 mg/kg<br>5–6 mg/kg |

## INTRAVENOUS INDUCTION

Intravenous (IV) induction usually involves the administration of propofol, followed by a nondepolarizing muscle relaxant, and/or narcotics like fentanyl.[1] If succinylcholine is used, atropine should be administered to avoid bradycardia.[1] EMLA (eutectic mixture of local anesthetics) cream and/or the use of nitrous oxide provides adequate sedation and analgesia for IV catheter placement.[1,2]

Propofol is a short-acting hypnotic with rapid onset and offset. It depresses airway and oropharyngeal muscle tone, which aids with instrumentation and decreases risk of laryngospasm. Propofol is also associated with a smooth recovery because it protects from and treats emergence agitation. Infants and children have larger volumes of distribution compared to adults, so require larger doses for induction.

Etomidate is a hypnotic agent that is widely known for its hemodynamic stability, especially in the face of hypovolemia and cardiovascular disease.[2] Pain, myoclonus, and laryngospasm occur commonly after injection. Adrenal suppression may occur, even after one dose.

Thiopental was the most commonly used IV induction agent before propofol. Neonates and children may experience excessively prolonged effects due to increased beta-elimination compared to adults.[2]

Ketamine may be used for intravenous induction in children. Neonates and infants require slightly higher doses than adults; however, the pharmacokinetics are equivalent. It is useful for patients with hemodynamic instability because it causes catecholamine release.

Methohexital is a very short-acting agent that has a more rapid recovery compared to thiopental and may cause muscular hyperactivity, hiccups, and myoclonus.

## ANESTHETICS: ACTIONS DIFFERENT FROM ADULTS

### DRUG TOXICITIES PREFERENTIALLY OCCURRING IN CHILDREN

Premature babies and infants are at increased risk of drug toxicity because they have decreased glomerular filtration rates, decreased hepatic blood flow, immature hepatic enzyme systems, and disproportionately lower fat and muscle content. The result is a prolonged duration of action, especially in lipid-soluble drugs like fentanyl and propofol.[1]

Propofol infusion syndrome (PRIS) occurs in children who receive infusions of propofol at greater than 4 mg/kg/hr for 48 hours. PRIS impairs mitochondrial function and is associated with acute refractory bradycardia, severe metabolic acidosis, and other metabolic derangements.

Neonates, infants, and young children are at an increased risk of accidental overdose with inhalational induction due to a greater minute ventilation-to-FRC ratio, increased blood flow to the brain, and reduced blood/gas coefficients of the volatile anesthetics.[1]

## OPIOIDS

Opioids are more potent in neonates and infants than they are in adults due to decreased hepatic conjugation, hepatic blood flow, and renal clearance. Metabolism and elimination of opioids increases with maturation of cytochrome P450 pathways and increased hepatic blood flow.

Morphine is given to children at a dose of 0.05–0.1 mg/kg. Neonates are sensitive to the ventilatory depressive effects and may experience delayed blood concentration rises, as well as sporadic, transient increases due to enterohepatic recirculation.

Fentanyl is a short-acting and potent opioid analgesic given to neonates and infants at doses of 1.0–1.5 mcg/kg.[1] Its metabolism and clearance increase with increasing age and increasing hepatic blood flow. Infants and children can all experience fentanyl-induced chest wall rigidity.[3]

Remifentanil is an ultra short-acting synthetic opioid whose action is not affected by liver or renal function. It is the only opioid with a shorter half-life in neonates and infants when compared to adults. A standard pediatric induction dose is 1–2 mcg/kg.

Sufentanil has a slower clearance in infants younger than 1 month old. It can be given in larger doses in infants undergoing cardiac surgery with minimal ventricular function depression.

Alfentanil is given in 35 mcg/ml boluses with 10 mcg/kg doses every 15 minutes. It is pharmokinetically similar to adults, but clearance is slower and more variable in premature and young infants.

Meperidine is only given as a one-time dose to children in the post-anesthesia care unit (PACU) to treat shivering. Repeated use leads to the accumulation of normeperidine, which can cause seizures, especially in children with decreased renal function.[3]

Codeine undergoes O-demethylation into morphine via the CYP2D6 pathway in the liver. Neonates and young children are less sensitive to codeine compared with adults because of less CYP2D6 enzyme activity.[2,3]

## NEUROMUSCULAR BLOCKING AGENTS

The neuromuscular junction of an infant has less reserve than that of an adult; therefore, fade occurs at high rates of stimulation. Infants have a myasthenic response and are sensitive to nondepolarizing agents. Due to a larger volume of distribution, infants have similar dosing as adults, but with shorter circulation time, infants experience faster onset.

Congenital diseases that alter any step in neuromuscular transmission put the patient at high risk if a neuromuscular blocking (NMB) agent is used. Succinylcholine should be avoided in the congenital neuromuscular disease population due to the risk of potentially fatal hyperkalemia and rhabdomyolysis. Succinylcholine use in a patient with myotonia can cause severe muscle spasm that can prevent intubation and ventilation. In contrast, succinylcholine can be given to patients with myasthenia gravis, and due to relative resistance, they will require higher doses. The use of nondepolarizing muscle blockers should be avoided in patients with neuromuscular disorders due to the respiratory weakness, difficulty weaning, and the dysphagia that ensues. If they must be used, careful monitoring should be employed, potentially with dose reductions.

Complications of succinylcholine use in children include myoglobinemia, myoglobinuria, masseter spasm, malignant hyperthermia, and diffuse muscle pains postoperatively.[1] A previously undiagnosed myopathy increases their risk of rhabdomyolysis and hyperkalemic cardiac arrest. Significant bradycardia and sinus arrest can occur following the first dose of succinylcholine; therefore, pretreatment with atropine may be administered beforehand.[1]

## REGIONAL ANESTHESIA

Surgical procedures in most pediatric patients is performed under general anesthesia.[1]

Local anesthetics have different pharmacokinetics in children when compared to adults because of more rapid absorption, greater cardiac output and regional tissue blood flow, and certain anatomical spaces that contain less fat tissue. With greater volumes of distribution in neonates, half-life is prolonged compared to adults. Protein binding is decreased in neonates, reducing their metabolism and leading to a greater risk of central nervous system (CNS) toxicity since a greater proportion of the drug is unbound.[3,4] Neonates and infants have reduced plasma cholinesterase activity, which results in slower metabolism of ester anesthetics. Amide anesthetics are metabolized via hepatic conjugation, and since hepatic enzymes are immature and hepatic blood flow is decreased in neonates, these agents also have reduced metabolism.[3]

## REFERENCES

1. Pediatric anesthesia. In: Butterworth IV JF, Mackey DC, Wasnick JD, eds. *Morgan & Mikhail's Clinical Anesthesiology*. 6th ed. New York, NY: McGraw-Hill; 897–927. http://accessmedicine.mhmedical.com/content.aspx?bookid=2444&sectionid=193563052. Accessed May 28, 2020.
2. Ghazal EA, Vadi M, Mason LJ, Coté CJ. Preoperative evaluation, premedication, and induction of anesthesia. In: Charles J. Cote, Jerrold Lerman, Brian J. Anderson, eds. *A Practice of Anesthesia for Infants and Children*. Philadelphia, PA: Elsevier; 2018:35–67. https://doi.org/10.1016/B978-0-323-42974-0.00004-5.
3. Lerman J, Steward D, Coté, CJ. Clinical pharmacology. In: *Manual of Pediatric Anesthesia*. New York, NY: Churchill Livingstone; 2009:43–75.
4. Suresh S, Wheeler M. Practical pediatric regional anesthesia. *Anesthesiol Clin North Am*. 2002;20(1):83–113. doi:10.1016/s0889-8537(03)00056-7.

# Part VI

# CLINICAL SCIENCES ANESTHESIA PROCEDURES, METHODS, AND TECHNIQUES

# 90.

# AMERICAN SOCIETY OF ANESTHESIOLOGISTS (ASA) PREOPERATIVE TESTING GUIDELINES

*Timothy F. Flanagan and Karim Fikry*

## INTRODUCTION

### PREOPERATIVE CATEGORIZATION

Testing guidelines for preoperative assessment of surgical patients can largely be divided between preoperative assessment for noncardiac surgery and preoperative assessment for cardiac surgery. The noncardiac guidelines are largely defined by the American Heart Association (AHA) Guidelines on Perioperative Cardiovascular Evaluation and Management of Patients Undergoing Noncardiac Surgery; the most recent edition was published in August 2014. Preoperative assessment for cardiac surgery is beyond the scope of this chapter.

## URGENCY AND RISK

The American College of Cardiology (ACC)/AHA guidelines categorize urgency into four categories: emergent, urgent, time-sensitive, and elective. Emergency surgeries are defined by a patient's whose life, limb, or organ is threatened if surgery is not initiated within 6 hours. Urgent surgery is defined by threat to life, limb, or organ if surgical intervention is not begun within 6–24 hours. Time-sensitive procedures are defined by a negatively affected outcome if delayed by 1–6 weeks. Elective procedures are anything that could be delayed up to 1 year.

If the risk of a major adverse cardiac event (MACE) is suspected to be less than 1%, the surgery is deemed low risk. Risk above 1% is considered elevated risk. Commonly cited examples of low-risk surgery are cataracts and most cosmetic plastic surgeries.

## CALCULATING RISK

The original cardiac risk index was published in 1977; 1001 patients over the age of 40 were studied to determine the risk of fatal and life-threatening postoperative cardiac issues. The Revised Cardiac Risk Index was published in 1999; 4315 patients whose ages were greater than or equal to 50 years old were studied, and the risks of major cardiac complications were 0.5%, 1.3%, 3.6%, and 9.1% for a given number of risk factors; 0,1,2,3 and greater than 3, respectively.[1] Only patients with zero factors would be in the low risk (<1%) category. The risk factors are ischemic heart disease, congestive heart failure, cerebrovascular disease, diabetes mellitus (treated with insulin), creatinine >2 mg/dl, high-risk surgery. High-risk surgery is defined as vascular surgery or any surgery that is in the intraperitoneal, intrathoracic, or suprainguinal areas.[1]

## ACC/AHA GUIDELINES

For a healthy patient undergoing a low-risk procedure, no laboratory testing is needed and no electrocardiogram (ECG) is needed. The ACC/AHA guidelines recommend further testing for patients with risk factors for coronary artery disease based on the urgency of the surgery.

### ACC/AHA GUIDELINES: EMERGENCY SURGERY

Emergency surgery testing guidelines suggest stratifying risk, optimizing monitoring, and proceeding with surgery.

### ACC/AHA GUIDELINES: LOW RISK VS. ELEVATED RISK

For a non-emergency procedure without acute coronary syndrome (ACS) suspected, the evaluation should include an estimation of the risk of a major adverse cardiac event using the revised cardiac risk index. If the risk is <1%, no further testing is indicated. If the risk ≥1%, the patient's functional capacity guides the next steps.

Patients who can perform greater than or equal to 4 metabolic equivalents (METs) require no further testing; 4

METs is equivalent to climbing one flight of stairs, running a short distance, or walking up a hill. If a patient cannot perform 4 METs, any additional testing must only be performed if it will change the care the patient receives. If a patient cannot perform a physiologic stress test, a pharmacologic stress test may be employed and coronary revascularization may be considered if the test is abnormal.[2]

In 2012 the ASA released a Practice Advisory for Preanesthesia Evaluation which provided guidance on specific laboratory testing and the supporting evidence. Per their conclusions, preoperative tests should not be ordered routinely, and there is not enough evidence to support specific decision rules regarding testing. The considerations for testing are as follows:

- Chest X-ray: cardiac disease, upper respiratory infection, chronic obstructive pulmonary disease (COPD), smoking;
- ECG: may be indicated in patients with known risk factors, such as known cardiovascular disease, significant arrhythmia, or structural heart disease. Age alone is not an indication;
- Hemoglobin/hematocrit: indicated in invasive procedures, patients with liver disease, extremes of age, anemia history, hematologic disorders, or prior to surgeries where excessive blood loss is anticipated;
- Coagulation studies: bleeding disorders, liver and renal dysfunction, invasive procedures;
- Basic metabolic profile and liver function tests: patients with endocrine disorders, liver and renal dysfunction, and on certain medications;

- Pregnancy testing: recommendations updated in 2016, testing may be offered to patients of childbearing age and for whom the result would alter the patient's management. Informed consent should include information about the false positives and negatives rates of pregnancy testing and that the current literature is unable to determine whether anesthesia may cause unknown harmful effects during early pregnancy.[4]

## REFERENCES

1. Fleisher LA, et al. ACC/AHA Guidelines on perioperative cardiovascular evaluation and management of patients undergoing noncardiac surgery. *Circulation.* 2014;130:e278–e333
2. Eagle KA, et al. ACC/AHA Guideline update for perioperative cardiovascular evaluation for noncardiac surgery—executive summary: a report of the American College of Cardiology/American Heart Association Task Force on Practice Guidelines. J Am Coll Cardiol. 2002;39(3):542.
3. Lee TH, et al. Derivation and prospective validation of a simple index for prediction of cardiac risk of major noncardiac surgery. *Circulation.* 1999;100:1043–1049.
4. American Society of Anesthesiologists. *Pregnancy Testing Prior to Anesthesia and Surgery Committee of Origin: Quality Management and Departmental Administration* (Approved by the ASA House of Delegates on October 26, 2016). https://www.asahq.org/standards-and-guidelines/pregnancy-testing-prior-to-anesthesia-and-surgery. Accessed August 1, 2020.
5. American Society of Anesthesiologists. *ASA/APSF Statement on Perioperative Testing for the COVID-19 Virus.* https://www.asahq.org/about-asa/newsroom/news-releases/2020/04/asa-and-apsf-joint-statement-on-perioperative-testing-for-the-covid-19-virus. Accessed August 1, 2020.

# 91.

# GUIDELINES FOR PERIOPERATIVE CARDIOVASCULAR EVALUATION

*Rewais B. Hanna and Alaa Abd-Elsayed*

## INTRODUCTION

Over 8 million Americans who undergo surgery yearly have coronary artery disease or risk factors for cardiovascular disease. The risk of perioperative cardiac complications is increased in this population, with many suffering from major adverse cardiac events (MACEs), defined as death or myocardial infarction.[1] Over the next decade, this number is likely to rise due to the aging nature of our population. It is estimated that around 40% of Americans undergoing surgery yearly will have either coronary artery disease or a risk factor for cardiovascular disease.[2–5] Among hospitalizations for major noncardiac surgery, perioperative MACEs occurred in 3.0% of patients.[2] To aid in decreasing these adverse events, the American College of Cardiology/American Heart Association (ACC/AHA) Task Force conducted a literature review to provide guidelines for perioperative cardiovascular assessments using randomized controlled trials (RCTs), registries, nonrandomized comparative and descriptive studies, case series, cohort studies, systematic reviews, and expert opinion. This chapter will review class I recommendations made by the ACC/AHA task force where procedure/treatment should be performed or administered because the benefit greatly outweighs the risk (Figure 91.1).[3]

## CLINICAL RISK FACTORS

### VALVULAR HEART DISEASE

Valvular heart disease significantly increases cardiac risk for patients undergoing noncardiac surgery. Class I evidence suggests that patients with clinically suspected moderate or greater degrees of valvular stenosis or regurgitation should undergo preoperative echocardiography if there has been either no prior echocardiography within 1 year or a significant change in clinical status or physical examination since the last evaluation. For adults who meet standard indications for valvular intervention (replacement and repair) on the basis of symptoms and severity of stenosis or regurgitation, valvular intervention should occur before elective noncardiac surgery to effectively reduce perioperative risk.[3]

## CARDIOVASCULAR IMPLANTABLE ELECTRONIC DEVICES

Cardiovascular implantable electronic devices (CIEDs) pose a risk to those undergoing surgery in a number of ways. Primarily, patients with CIEDs always have underlying cardiac disease that may involve arrhythmias, structural heart disease, or other pathologic clinical conditions. Therefore, as clinicians, both the hardware, programming, and underlying condition of the patient must be considered prior to surgery. Before elective surgery in a patient with a CIED, the surgical/procedure team and clinician following the CIED should communicate in advance to plan perioperative management of the CIED.[3]

## PULMONARY VASCULAR DISEASE

It is paramount that patients optimize their pulmonary hypertension and RV status preoperatively to decrease morbidity and mortality. Studies show mortality rates of 4%–26% and morbidity rates, most notably cardiac and/or respiratory failure, of 6%–42% due to perioperative complications of pulmonary hypertension. Therefore, it is recommended that patients receive the necessary perioperative management of their pulmonary hypertension. Chronic pulmonary vascular targeted therapy (i.e., phosphodiesterase type 5 inhibitors, soluble guanylate cyclase stimulators, endothelin receptor antagonists, and

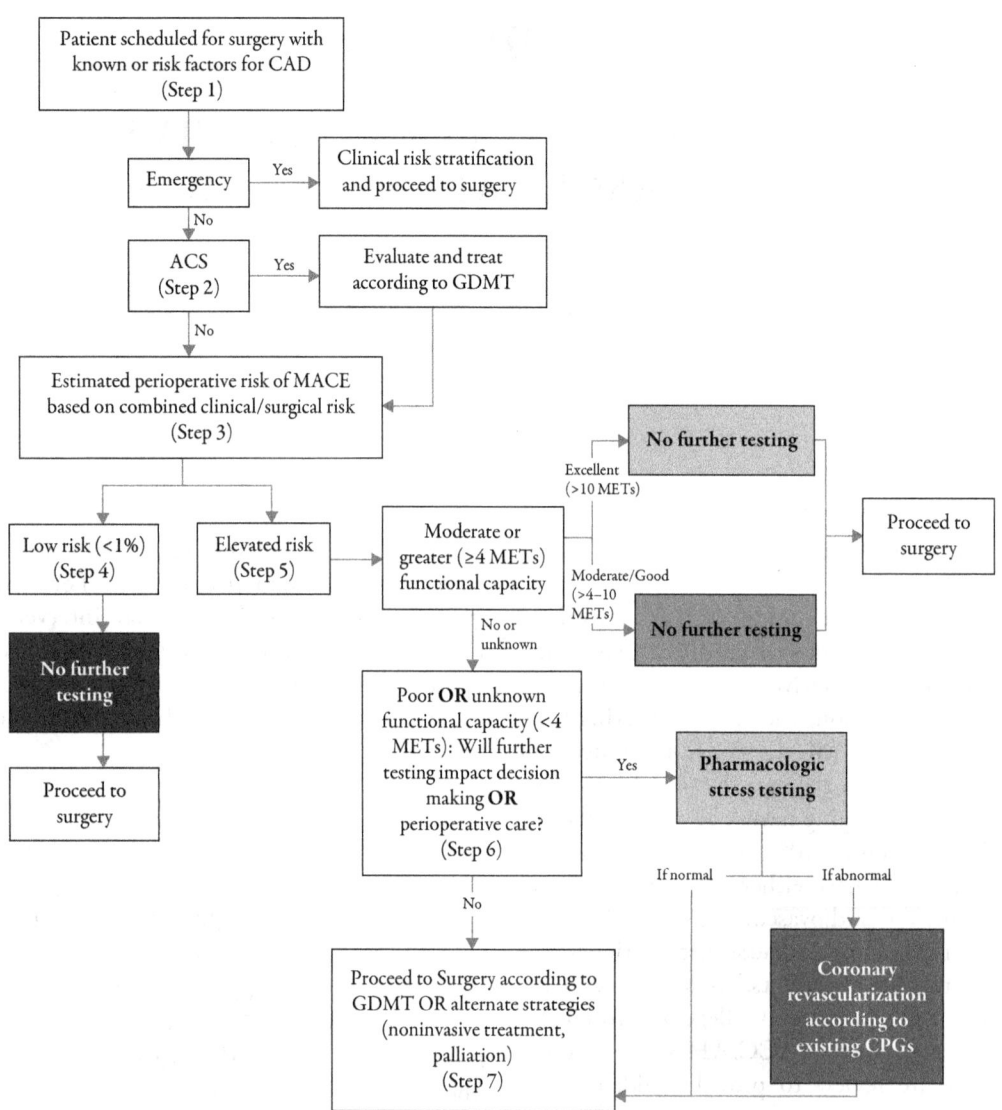

**Figure 91.1.** A stepwise approach to perioperative cardiac assessment for patients with CAD. Abbreviations in figure: CAD: coronary artery disease; ACS: acute coronary syndrome; GDMT: guideline-directed medical therapy; MACE: major adverse cardiac event; METs: metabolic equivalents; CPGs: clinical practice guidelines.

prostanoids) should be continued unless contraindicated or not tolerated in patients with pulmonary hypertension who are undergoing noncardiac surgery.[3]

## CORONARY ARTERY DISEASE

### Coronary Revascularization before Noncardiac Surgery

If a patient is undergoing noncardiac surgery, the cumulative mortality and morbidity risks of the coronary revascularization procedure should be weighed with consideration toward the individual patient's overall health, functional status, and prognosis. Revascularization before noncardiac surgery is recommended in circumstances in which revascularization is indicated according to existing clinical practice guidelines.[3]

### Timing of Elective Noncardiac Surgery in Patients with Previous PCI

An important factor in elective surgery is the timing following previous percutaneous coronary intervention (PCI). The ACC/AAHA has provided guidelines recommending elective noncardiac surgery should be delayed 14 days after balloon angioplasty and 30 days after bare-metal stent implantation. Moreover, elective noncardiac surgery should optimally be delayed 365 days after drug-eluting stent (DES) implantation.[3]

### Perioperative Beta-Blocker Therapy

Beta blockers are one of the most prescribed medications commonly used to treat ischemic heart diseases, hypertension, and cardiac arrhythmias for over a half century. Beta blockers should be continued in patients undergoing surgery who have been on beta blockers chronically.[3]

## Perioperative Statin Therapy

Similarly, lipid-lowering statin agents have been long used to decrease cardiovascular risk in a sizable portion of the United States. They have been found to significantly decrease the incidence of MACEs in patients using statins.[4] Statins should be continued in patients currently taking statins and scheduled for noncardiac surgery.[3]

## Antiplatelet Agents

Antiplatelet agents are used to decrease the formation of fibrin clots and thus vastly decrease the risk of MACEs. In patients undergoing urgent noncardiac surgery during the first 4–6 weeks after bare-metal stent or drug-eluting stent implantation, dual anti-platelet therapy should be continued unless the relative risk of bleeding outweighs the benefit of the prevention of stent thrombosis. Furthermore, in patients who have received coronary stents and must undergo surgical procedures that mandate the discontinuation of P2Y12 platelet receptor–inhibitor therapy, it is recommended that aspirin be continued if possible and the P2Y12 platelet receptor–inhibitor be restarted as soon as possible after surgery.[3]

## Perioperative Management of Patients with CIEDs

Patients with ICDs who have preoperative reprogramming to inactivate tachytherapy should be on cardiac monitoring continuously during the entire period of inactivation, and external defibrillation equipment should be readily available. Systems should be in place to ensure that ICDs are reprogrammed to active therapy before discontinuation of cardiac monitoring and discharge from the facility.[3]

## REFERENCES

1. Mangano DT, Goldman L. Preoperative assessment of patients with known or suspected coronary disease. *N Engl J Med*. 1995 Dec 28;333(26):1750–1756.
2. Smilowitz NR, Gupta N, Ramakrishna H, Guo Y, Berger JS, Bangalore S. Perioperative major adverse cardiovascular and cerebrovascular events associated with noncardiac surgery. *JAMA Cardiol*. 2017;2(2):181.
3. Fleisher LA, et al. 2014 ACC/AHA guideline on perioperative cardiovascular evaluation and management of patients undergoing noncardiac surgery: Executive summary: A report of the American College of Cardiology/American Heart Association Task Force on Practice Guidelines. *Circulation*. 2014 Dec 9;130(24):2215–2245.
4. Durazzo AES, et al. Reduction in cardiovascular events after vascular surgery with atorvastatin: A randomized trial. *J Vasc Surg*. 2004;39:967–975.
5. Mangano DT. Perioperative cardiac morbidity. *Anesthesiology*. 1990;72: 153–184.

# 92.

# ASA CLASSIFICATION

## *Sheetal Patel and Alaa Abd-Elsayed*

## INTRODUCTION

The American Society of Anesthesiologists (ASA) Physical Status classification was originally developed in 1941 by Meyer Saklad for facilitating comparison of anesthetic data.[1,2]

It went through multiple revisions since its conception. The classification underwent revision in 1963 with the number of classes reduced from seven to five. There have been also modifications to definitions and additions to the organ donor class, ASA 6.[2]

As ASA classification did not includes examples, there was a question of inter-rater reliability and reproducibility. So in October 2014, ASA included examples in the ASA physical status classification.[3]

The system is often regarded as an overall health assessment and degree of patient's comorbidities.[4] It is now used in allocation of resources, anesthetic service reimbursement, communications, and to create a uniform system for statistical analysis.

## ADVANTAGE

- Simple assessment without need for laboratory values or clinical resources.

## DISADVANTAGES

- Moderate inter-rater reliability.
- Inability of the system to account for specific factor such as gender, age.
- It cannot reliably be used alone to describe a patient's physical status. especially in pediatric patients. Certain aspects of patient histories in children may underestimate the risks.

Table 92.1 provides the ASA classification with ASA-approved examples.[1]

The classification system is also used for non-anesthesia purposes:[2]

(1) Government agencies: Justification for hospital inpatient admission of surgical patients. Site of service determination (office- or facility-based) (ASA 1, 2, 3 can be performed in office; ASA 4 and 5 cannot be performed in office).
(2) Non-anesthesia providers: Determination of administration of moderate versus deep sedation.
(3) Medical device manufacturers: Determination of eligibility for patient-controlled sedation.
(4) Pediatric surgical services: Determination of the appropriate facility and resources for specialty care.
(5) Veterinary services: Small animal anesthesia services.

Ambulatory surgeries are assumed to have expeditious recovery. Assessment of the patient's ASA physical status with history and physical examination are crucial in the screening of patients selected for ambulatory or office-based surgery. Usually, ASA 4 and 5 patients would not

*Table 92.1* ASA CLASSIFICATION

| ASA PS CLASSIFICATION | DEFINITION | ADULT EXAMPLES, INCLUDING, BUT NOT LIMITED TO: |
|---|---|---|
| ASA I | A normal healthy patient | Healthy, non-smoking, no or minimal alcohol use |
| ASA II | A patient with mild systemic disease | Mild diseases only without substantive functional limitations. Examples include (but not limited to): current smoker, social alcohol drinker, pregnancy, obesity (30< BMI <40), well-controlled DM/HTN, mild lung disease |
| ASA III | A patient with severe systemic disease | Substantive functional limitations; one or more moderate to severe diseases. Examples include (but not limited to): poorly controlled DM or HTN, COPD, morbid obesity (BMI ≥40), active hepatitis, alcohol dependence or abuse, implanted pacemaker, moderate reduction of ejection fraction, ESRD undergoing regularly scheduled dialysis, premature infant PCA <60 weeks, history (>3 months) of MI, CVA, TIA, or CAD/stents. |
| ASA IV | A patient with severe systemic disease that is a constant threat to life | Examples include (but not limited to): recent ( <3 months) MI, CVA, TIA, or CAD/stents, ongoing cardiac ischemia or severe valve dysfunction, severe reduction of ejection fraction, sepsis, DIC, ARD or ESRD not undergoing regularly scheduled dialysis. |
| ASA V | A moribund patient who is not expected to survive without the operation | Examples include (but not limited to): ruptured abdominal/thoracic aneurysm, massive trauma, intracranial bleed with mass effect, ischemic bowel in the face of significant cardiac pathology or multiple organ/system dysfunction. |
| ASA VI | A declared brain-dead patient whose organs are being removed for donor purposes | |

* The addition of "E" denotes emergency surgery (an emergency is defined as existing when delay in treatment of the patient would lead to a significant increase in the threat to life or body part). Reproduced with permission from the American Society of Anesthesiologists. *ASA Physical Status Classification System.* ASA website. https://www.asahq.org/standards-and-practice-parameters/statement-on-asa-physical-status-classification-system.

be candidates for ambulatory surgery, whereas ASA 1 and 2 patients would be prime candidates for such surgery.[5] ASA 3 patients with diabetes, hypertension, and stable coronary artery disease would not be precluded from an ambulatory procedure, provided their diseases are well controlled. Ultimately, the surgeon and anesthesiologist must identify patients for whom an ambulatory or office-based setting is likely to provide benefits (e.g., convenience, reduced costs, and charges) that outweigh risks (e.g., the lack of immediate availability of all hospital services, such as a cardiac catheterization laboratory, emergency cardiovascular stents, assistance with airway rescue, and rapid consultation).[5]

## REFERENCES

1. American Society of Anesthesiologists. *ASA Physical Status Classification System.* ASA website. http://www.asahq.org/resources/clinical-information/asa-physical-status-classification-system. Approved October 15, 2014. Accessed February 22, 2015.
2. Abouleish AE, et al. ASA provides examples to each ASA physical status class. *ASA Monitor* 2015;79:38–39. http://monitor.pubs.asahq.org/article.aspx?articleid=2434536.
3. Hurwitz EE, et al. Adding examples to the ASA-Physical Status Classification improves correct assignment to patients. *Anesthesiology.* 2017 Apr;126(4):614–622.
4. Doyle DJ, et al. *American Society of Anesthesiologists Classification (ASA Class).* 2020 Jan.
5. Ansell GL, Montgomery JE. Outcome of ASA III patients undergoing day case surgery. *Br J Anaesth.* 2004 Jan;92(1):71–74.

# 93.

# PREPARATION FOR ANESTHESIA/PREMEDICATION

*Caylynn Yao and Elisha Peterson*

## ANXIOLYTICS

Perioperative stress and high levels of anxiety commonly arise in patients presenting for surgery. Quelling such anxiety with premedication not only calms the patient, but also may in turn improve patient satisfaction, operating conditions, recovery time, cognitive impairment at discharge, and ease parental anxiety in the case of children who present for surgery. In addition to patient comfort, addressing anxiety preoperatively can influence stress hormone production, gastric secretions, initial anesthetic requirements, and the difficulty of preoperative procedure, including intravenous placement.[1]

The most widely used class of premedication is benzodiazepines, specifically midazolam; lorazepam and diazepam have also been administered in the preoperative setting. Benzodiazepines can be administered via oral, intravascular, intranasal, rectal, and intramuscular routes. In the pediatric population, midazolam is commonly used, and ketamine has been used in selected patients.

In adult patients, midazolam 1–2mg IV (intravenous) is sufficient for premedication. Its advantage over other benzodiazepines is its shorter half-life, twofold increase in potency, and decreased potential for cardiorespiratory depression. It has an onset of anxiolysis and sedation occurring in as little as 1–2 minutes in IV form. Similar to other benzodiazepines, midazolam causes anterograde amnesia with variable duration[2] with the onset of the amnestic effect concurrent with its onset of somnolence.[2] Midazolam decreases cerebral metabolic rate of oxygen (CMRO) in a dose-dependent fashion.[2] It can cause respiratory and myocardial depression, but at doses used for premedication, this is unlikely.[2] Midazolam accumulates in fatty tissue and extensively binds to plasma. Its half-life elimination is 1 to 4 hours, depending upon release of the drug from adipose tissue and protein-binding sites. The tablet form of benzodiazepine, namely oral diazepam, also has a long history of use in adults. If patients are particularly anxious, an oral benzodiazepine prescription the night before or morning of surgery has been effective.

In pediatric patients, premedication is not recommended prior to 6 months as separation anxiety has not yet formed.[3] Anxiety with parental separation most commonly culminates at 2 years of age.[3] Oral midazolam reaches peak concentrations in 30 minutes at a dose of 0.5 mg/kg without issues of aspiration.[4] Ketamine, an NMDA receptor antagonist, is a premedication commonly reserved for children who are agitated or cognitively delayed who will not cooperate[4] with an oral medication. It is most commonly administered intramuscularly at 2–4 mg/kg to produce sedation, amnesia, and analgesia.[4] It can be administered orally, nasally, rectally, or intramuscularly. Ketamine is often administered with an anti-sialogogue such as atropine or glycopyrrolate, as ketamine is associated with excessive salivation.[4]

## ANALGESICS

Opioids are considered as premedication if the patient requires analgesia or is on a preexisting opioid regimen. In these circumstances, fentanyl or one of its analogs may be given. Patients should be closely monitored with continuous pulse oximetry due to opioid side effects such as respiratory depression, sedation, and nausea/vomiting.[4] Fentanyl has significant advantages over other opioid agents in its favorable pharmacologic properties, including rapid serum clearance, high potency, and minimal release of histamine. In patients who have an opioid dependency, maintenance of their baseline opioid requirements is encouraged to avoid the physiologic and psychological effects of withdrawal during the anesthetic induction. Other preoperative analgesics includes nonsteroidal anti-inflammatory drugs (NSAIDs), namely celecoxib 400

mg PO in adults, without increasing the risk of surgical bleeding.[1]

## ANTIEMETICS

Antiemetics are typically given intraoperatively to prevent postoperative nausea and vomiting (PONV), one of the most common causes of patient dissatisfaction after anesthesia, with reported incidences up to 80% in all post-surgical patients.[5] These medications include ondansetron, dexamethasone, and droperidol. However, antiemetic agents with long duration of action or delayed onset of action can appropriately be given as premedication. Transdermal scopolamine, with a peak plasma time around 24 hours, has been shown to be as efficacious as ondansetron and droperidol for the prevention of postoperative emesis. PONV risk factors comprise of patient, anesthetic, perioperative, and surgical factors, as seen in Table 93.1.

## ASPIRATION PROPHYLAXIS

Anesthesia-related aspiration prophylaxis can prevent a range of pulmonary syndromes, from hypoxia and pneumonia to complete respiratory failure and acute respiratory distress syndrome. Risk for an anesthesia-related aspiration event increase with medications and predisposing conditions that affect the lower esophageal sphincter, level of consciousness, and loss of protective reflexes. However, administration of agents to reduce the risk of pulmonary aspiration is not routinely warranted. Non-fasted patients, patients with gastrointestinal obstruction, hiatal hernia, obesity, autonomic neuropathy, advanced pregnancy, gastroesophageal reflux disease, and scleroderma should be considered for the administration of aspiration prophylaxis. These agents decrease both gastric pH and residual

*Table 93.1* FACTORS CONTRIBUTING TO PONV

| PATIENT | ANESTHETIC | SURGICAL | POSTOPERATIVE |
|---|---|---|---|
| Non-smoker | Use of volatile agents | Duration of surgery | Ambulation |
| Female gender | Use of opioids | Type of surgery | Pain |
| Adolescents | Use of nitrous oxide | *Head:* eye muscle, tonsillectomy, inner ear | Early food ingestion |
| History of motion sickness | | *Genitourinary:* orchiopexy, inguinal hernia, penile procedures | |
| History of PONV | | *Abdominal procedures* | |
| Recent food ingestion | | *Laparoscopic procedures* | |

gastric volumes. H2-receptor blockers are effective in reducing gastric pH if given 2–3 hours prior to anesthetic induction.[1] Gastric stimulants, including metoclopramide and proton pump inhibitors, can also be helpful but have not shown additional benefit to H2-receptor antagonists.[1] Nonparticulate antacids such as sodium citrate can also be considered, as they quickly increase gastric pH and can be considered in patients at risk for aspiration.

## BETA BLOCKADE

Perioperative beta blockade is only recommended for specific preoperative populations, generally high-risk cardiac patients undergoing high-risk vascular surgery. The POISE trial indicated a higher rate of mortality and stroke with widely used metoprolol in surgical patients. If applicable, beta blockade should be started at least a week prior and titrated to a heart rate of less than 60 if there is no concomitant hypotension which has been found to reduce cardiac morbidity. Beta blockade can also decrease analgesic requirements and the control of hypertensive responses during surgery as an added benefit.[1]

## STEROIDS

Supplementation of glucocorticoid therapy should be considered in patients who are taking more than the equivalent of 20 mg of prednisone daily for more than a 3-week period prior to their scheduled surgery. These patients are at high risk for suppression of the hypothalamic-pituitary-adrenal axis and thus adrenal crisis due to secondary adrenal insufficiency. Generally, hydrocortisone or an equivalent is the steroid premedication of choice and is dosed depending on the type of surgery. For example, a dose of hydrocortisone 50 mg IV with continuation for 1–2 days postoperatively is often appropriate for most surgeries. But high-risk surgeries with a mortality of greater than 5% may require 100 mg IV doses with continuation for 2–3 days. Minimally invasive procedures, however, do not require any such supplementation.[1]

## ANTIBIOTICS

Preoperative antibiotics are warranted if there is high risk of infection or high risk of deleterious outcomes should an infection develop at the surgical site. Selecting an antibiotic, dosing, and timing it based on the patient's risk factors, the operative procedure, and wound classification can have significant impact on outcomes. The American Heart Association 2017 guidelines recommend that the highest-risk patients receive antibiotic prophylaxis to prevent infective endocarditis from dental procedures. These highest-risk patients include those with prosthetic cardiac valves, previous infective endocarditis, congenital heart disease, and in a cardiac transplant with valve regurgitation due to a structurally abnormal valve.

## REFERENCES

1. Freeman BS, Berger JS, eds. *Anesthesiology Core Review: Part One Basic Exam*. McGraw-Hill; 2014.
2. Reves JG, et al. Midazolam: Pharmacology and uses. *Anesthesiology*. 1985;62:310–324.
3. Rosenbaum A, et al. The place of premedication in pediatric practice. *Paediatr Anaesth*. 2009;19(9):817–828.
4. Coté CJ, et al. *Coté and Lerman's a Practice of Anesthesia for Infants and Children*. 6th ed. Elsevier; 2018.
5. Choi JB, et al. Incidence and risk factors of postoperative nausea and vomiting in patients with fentanyl-based intravenous patient-controlled analgesia and single antiemetic prophylaxis. *Yonsei Med J*. 2014;55(5):1430–1435.

# 94.

# INTERACTION WITH CHRONIC DRUG THERAPY

*Vincent Pinkert and Sydney E. Rose*

## INTRODUCTION

Medication management prior to surgery is one of the most important components of perioperative care. Many patients are on complicated regimens of prescription and nonprescription medications, and most patients are unaware that any medication, prescribed or not, has the potential to interact with anesthesia. Cessation of medications can result in disease progression, patient decompensation, or withdrawal. However, continuing certain medications through the perioperative period can cause changes in drug metabolism and result in drug-related complications (DRCs) such as bleeding, infection, acute renal failure, hemodynamic instability, poor wound healing, or even death.[1] The overarching goal of preoperative care is to optimize patients for surgery by reducing modifiable risks. This includes the complex task of evaluating the risks and the benefits of continuing versus stopping each individual medication in a patient's regimen.[2] In order to optimize a patient for surgery, anesthesiologists and clinicians performing preoperative assessments must have a comprehensive knowledge of pharmacology, potential drug interactions, and DRCs. This knowledge is applied within the context of an individual patient's disease processes and weighed against the potential dangers of exacerbating specific diseases.[2] The focus of this chapter is to highlight popular medications taken for common diseases, and discuss those with known or theoretical interactions with anesthetics, or that have perioperative effects.

## CLINICAL ASSESSMENT

A relevant, focused medical history of a patient should always be performed, prior to making any adjustments to a patient's chronic medication regimen prior to surgery. In addition to discussion of pertinent medical problems, the clinical assessment should include a thorough medication history that covers all prescription medications, and nonprescription pharmacotherapeutics such as over-the-counter medications, herbal and nonherbal supplements,

and vitamins. Illicit drug use and its frequency should also be discussed, as many of these have a propensity for DRCs. Understanding a patient's comorbidities and severity enables a clinician to make an educated perioperative decompensation risk assessment, and balance the risks and benefits of continuing versus holding medications in the perioperative period.[2]

## GENERAL CONSIDERATIONS

There is a paucity of literature to guide decisions when it comes to perioperative medication management. This is due to constant turnover of pharmacotherapeutics, and lack of large randomized controlled trials. For the most part, perioperative medication management strategies are derived from clinical experience, theoretical interactions, and expert opinion.[1] The medical decision-making that goes into perioperative medication management is complex and unique to each patient; however, a few general principles apply. The clinician making these decisions should:

- Have an understanding of medications associated with DRCs when combined with anesthesia.
- Consider holding medications associated with DRC's in the perioperative period.
- Continue medications associated with acute withdrawal unless continuation poses a significant DRC risk.
- Make arrangements for appropriate tapering of any medications accociated with acute withdrawal when the risk of DRC outweighs the risk of withdrawal.[2]
- Hold any non-essential medications that substantially increase a patient's risk of surgical complications.
- Consider the impact of disease flare or progression to a patient prior to stopping a given medication.
- Be aware that pharmacokinetics of medications and metabolites may be altered and absorption of oral medications may be decreased.[1]
- Be aware that most medications can be re-started post surgery once the patient is tolerating PO.

## MEDICATION CLASSES

### CARDIOVASCULAR

Most patients with cardiovascular disease take daily medications to keep their disease from advancing. These drugs have implications from both a surgical and cardiovascular morbidity standpoint. Understanding the risk and benefits of continuing these drugs is essential to any anesthetic practice.

### Beta Blockers (βbs)

Bradycardia and hypotension are serious DRCs that may occur when βbs are continued perioperatively.[2] Alternatively, abruptly stopping βb therapy puts patients at elevated risk for myocardial ischemia, tachycardia, and hypertension. The potential sequelae of either continuing or stopping βbs can be associated with severe morbidity, and even death.[3] For patients with cardiac disease, the risks associated with stopping long-term βb therapy outweigh the DRCs associated with continuing them. Therefore, chronic βb therapy should be continued perioperatively, and meticulous efforts intraoperatively, to avoid hypotension and bradycardia. Surgical patients without significant cardiovascular disease should NOT be initiated on βbs day of surgery, as there is strong evidence showing this to be associated with an increased risk of stroke and all-cause 30-day mortality.

### Statins

There is compelling evidence for continuing statin therapy perioperatively, even initiating it, in patients undergoing high-risk noncardiac surgery or vascular surgery. Perioperative statin therapy is associated with a decrease in nonfatal cardiac events, cardiac mortality, and noncardiac all-cause mortality.[3]

### Non βb Antihypertensives

Over 25% of noncardiac surgery patients have hypertension, and many of these patients are on one or more antihypertensive medications.[4] Most antihypertensive medications, taken as part of a long-term regimen, should be continued perioperatively to avoid withdrawal and increases in cardiovascular complications. These include βbs (discussed previously), alpha2-adrenergic agonists, calcium-channel antagonists, nitrates, and most diuretics.[2]

Certain antihypertensive medications are associated with significant DRCs that outweigh the benefits of continuing the medication through the perioperative period. Angiotensin converting enzyme inhibitors (ACEIs) and angiotensin II receptor blockers (ARBs) are antihypertensive medications known to be associated with significant refractory intraoperative hypotension when continued perioperatively. There is controversy over the outcome benefit in terms of continuing vs. holding these medications;[3] however, most anesthesiologists agree that ACEIs and ARBs should be held 24 hours prior to surgery,[4] as the body may rely more heavily on the renin-angiotensin system to maintain blood pressure when other mechanisms, such as vascular tone, are negated by the sympathetic blunting effects of general anesthesia. Loop diuretics can cause volume depletion and electrolyte abnormalities, and have been shown to cause more strokes in surgical patients who only take them for blood pressure control. Alternatively, patients on long-term loop diuretic therapy for heart failure often need to continue their therapy to avoid volume overload. Perioperative loop diuretic management depends on what the medication is being used to treat.[4]

### Antiplatelet Therapy (Aspirin, P2Y12 Inhibitors, NSAIDs)

In general, primary prevention antiplatelet therapy should be held 7–10 days prior to noncardiac surgery due to the increased risk of bleeding.[1] Alternatively, for secondary prevention antiplatelet therapy, at least one antiplatelet medication (typically aspirin) should be continued. Exceptions include intracranial, intraspinal, or other noncardiac surgeries in which the risk of bleeding outweighs the potential for a major cardiac event.[2]

### PULMONARY

Patients with moderate to severe pulmonary disease (asthma, COPD, sarcoid) are often taking disease-maintenance medications such as inhaled β -agonists, steroids, and anticholinergic agents.[2] Given the increased risk of respiratory compromise these patients present with, it is best to continue pulmonary disease-maintenance medications perioperatively. Albuterol, in particular, is an inhaled β -agonist used liberally during the perioperative period when bronchodilation is needed.

### ENDOCRINE/DIABETES MELLITUS

Patients on chronic medication therapy for endocrine dysfunctions are usually continued on their normal regimens perioperatively.[1] Glucocorticoids should not be stopped prior to surgery, as even a short, remote course can induce significant adrenal insufficiency. Abruptly stopping glucocorticoids puts patients at risk for hypotensive shock.[2] In fact, stress dose steroids should be readily available to administer intraoperatively for any patient on glucocorticoid therapy within the past 6 months.

### Oral Hypoglycemics/Insulin

Diabetes mellitus is the most common endocrine disorder in patients presenting for surgery. Oral hypoglycemics (sulfonylureas, meglitinides, DPP-4 inhibitors, etc) should be held the day of surgery, given the inability to quickly titrate these medications, and the potential for prolonged periods of fasting. Metformin should be held 24–48 hours prior to surgery due to the rare, but serious, risk of lactic acidosis.[1,2] For insulin-dependent patients, short-acting insulin can be continued up until the point of fasting (usually 8 hours prior to surgery); intermediate and longer-acting insulin should be taken at one-half the regular prescribed dose the night before surgery.[1] All diabetes patients should have a preoperative blood glucose check, and then have blood glucose checked at regular intervals every 1–2 hours. Regular insulin +/- glucose can be bolused or infused to maintain normoglycemia, until the patient returns to taking a normal oral diet.

## PSYCHIATRIC/NEUROLOGIC MEDICATIONS

Antidepressants, antipsychotics, antiseizure, and dementia medications should be continued in the perioperative period.[2,5] Evidence suggests that selective serotonin reuptake inhibitors (SSRIs) increase surgical bleeding risk; however, associated transfusion, reoperation, and mortality risks remain debated.[2] Monoamine oxidase A inhibitors (MAO-A inhibitors) are an exception, and should be discontinued at least 2 weeks prior to a procedure involving anesthesia, as these older class psychiatric medications can potentially interact with anesthetic medications, causing severe morbidity, including serotonin syndrome, and possibly death.[5]

Parkinson's disease medications should be continued without missing doses. Abrupt cessation of Parkinson's disease medications can lead to neuroleptic malignant syndrome, or an acute progression of disease, and can cause significant morbidity.[2] Carbidopa/levodopa, especially, should be continued with a dose administered as close to anesthesia induction as safely possible. MAO-B inhibitors, such as selegiline and rasagiline, do not affect the metabolism of serotonin at therapeutic doses, and therefore should also be continued perioperatively.[5]

## SUMMARY

Over 131 million American adults use medications regularly to maintain or improve their health. Perioperative medication management is an essential component of caring for surgical patients. Understanding a patient's medication regimen, the disease(s) being treated with individual medications, and how a particular drug may interact with anesthetics is a crucial component of anesthetic care and essential to maintaining patient safely perioperatively.

## REFERENCES

1. Pass SE, Simpson RW. Discontinuation and reinstitution of medications during the perioperative period. *Am J Health Syst Pharm.* 2004;61(9):899–914.
2. Zafirova Z, et al. Preoperative management of medications. *Anesthesiol Clin.* 2018;36(4):663–675.
3. Devereaux PJ, et al. How strong is the evidence for the use of perioperative β blockers in non-cardiac surgery? Systematic review and meta-analysis of randomised controlled trials. *BMJ.* 2005;331:313–321.
4. Hazzi R, Mayock R. Perioperative management of hypertension. *J Xiangya Med.* 2018;3(25).
5. Huyse FJ, et al. Psychotropic drugs and the perioperative period: A proposal for a guideline in elective surgery. *Psychosomatics.* 2006;47(1):8–22.

# 95.

# ADVERSE REACTIONS TO PREMEDICATION

*Caylynn Yao and Elisha Peterson*

## COGNITIVE ADVERSE EVENTS

Postoperative delirium and cognitive dysfunction (POCD) are concerning complications following surgery. Delirium is an observational diagnosis that refers to behavioral manifestations of fluctuating confusion.[1] POCD is a transient state that does not lead to dementia, requiring formal testing to identify such decline in neuropsychiatric function.[1] Delirium is associated with POCD as well as dementia. Therefore the development of delirium postoperatively could be temporary if associated with POCD or, instead, could be more serious. The relationship between delirium and dementia has yet to be elucidated; it is unclear if the manifestation of delirium occurs in patients who already have subclinical dementia or if delirium heralds a patient's vulnerability to develop dementia.[1] Medications used in the preoperative period that are implicated to increase risk of delirium are listed in Table 95.1. In general, medications that increase dopamine and/or norepinephrine, decrease acetylcholine, or alter serotonin and gamma-aminobutyric acid (GABA) can cause delirium.[2] Beta-blockers as a whole class were found to increase risk of postoperative delirium and are implicated in altering serotonin centrally.[2] Patient risk factors for developing delirium are outlined in Box 95.1. Taking more than 3 medications preoperatively was found to be an independent risk factor for postoperative delirium.[2]

## CARDIAC AND RESPIRATORY DISTURBANCES

### QT PROLONGATION

Patients who have congenital or acquired prolonged QT who present for surgery are at risk for a ventricular tachyarrhythmia perioperatively known as *torsades de pointes*; many drugs and anesthetics prolong the QT interval. A selection of QT-prolongating preoperative medications is presented in Table 95.2. In addition to continuous electrocardiogram (EKG) monitoring and avoidance of concomitant medications known to prolong QT, ensuring normal electrolytes—specifically, serum calcium, potassium, and magnesium[3] and decreasing perioperative stress[3] will mitigate the risk of ventricular arrhythmia.

### RESPIRATORY DEPRESSION

Opioids have a known risk of respiratory depression due to their action on the μ receptor. When given in conjunction with benzodiazepines, the risk of respiratory depression further increases.[4] Patients with obstructive sleep apnea (OSA) have a magnified vulnerability to developing respiratory depression with opioids and other sedative medication[3,4] that can be life-threatening. OSA results in brief repetitive hypoxic insults to the brain from airway collapse, most commonly due to obesity from redundant soft tissue around

*Table 95.1* PREOPERATIVE DRUGS IMPLICATED IN POSTOPERATIVE DELIRIUM

| DRUG CLASS | PREOPERATIVE DRUG |
|---|---|
| Anticholinergics | Scopolamine patch, glycopyrrolate |
| Antihistamines | Diphenhydramine, ranitidine, promethazine |
| Benzodiazepines | Midazolam, diazepam |
| Beta blockers | Propranolol, metoprolol, atenolol |
| Opioids | Morphine, meperidine |
| Prokinetics | Metoclopramide |

*Box 95.1* PREOPERATIVE PATIENT RISK FACTORS FOR DELIRIUM

Elderly
Smoking
Alcohol use
Baseline cognitive impairment
Preoperative polypharmacy
Baseline sleep difficulties
Liver failure
Renal failure

**Table 95.2 COMMON PREOPERATIVE MEDICATIONS THAT PROLONG QT INTERVAL**

| DRUG CLASS | PREOPERATIVE DRUG |
|---|---|
| Antihistamine | Diphenhydramine, famotidine |
| Antiemetic | Ondanestron, granisetron, dolasetron, droperidol |
| Bronchodilator | Albuterol |
| Opioid | Methadone |

---

the neck or enlarged tonsils and adenoids. These hypoxic insults can result in a decrease in hypoxia-driven arousal mechanism[3] and sleep fragmentation.[4] Opioid doses should be decreased in patients with OSA by half[3] and carefully titrated.

Use of codeine is contraindicated in children with OSA undergoing tonsillectomy. Codeine relies on the patient's cytochrome p450 (CYP) enzyme, CYP 2D6, to convert into morphine in order to have any analgesic effect. Due to the variability in this enzyme's activity, the patient could receive no analgesia (little 2D6 activity) or overdose (high 2D6 activity). Middle Eastern and African populations were found to have high 2D6 enzyme activity.[3] Given the already present increased vulnerability to respiratory depressant effects of opioids in patients with OSA, there are recent reports of African American children who have died in the recovery room from a standard dose of codeine.[3]

## PARADOXICAL REACTIONS

Benzodiazepines are frequently used for anxiolysis,[3,4] but in rare instances (less than 1% in adults[5] but can be up to 15% in children[3]) they can result in an acute increase in agitation such as anger and excitement; this is known as a paradoxical or disinhibitory reaction.[5] Box 95.2 lists the suggested patient risk factors for a paradoxical reaction. Given that paradoxical reactions to benzodiazepines are rare, the underlying mechanism is not well defined. Treatment includes supportive care[5] with flumazenil, a benzodiazepine receptor antagonist that can be used in severe cases.

## EXTRAPYRAMIDAL SYMPTOMS

Extrapyramidal symptoms (EPS) are characterized by abnormal muscle tone and movements that can occur with the administration of dopamine receptor antagonists such as metoclopramide. Metoclopramide is a prokinetic agent used in the prevention of PONV that can result in EPS.[4] Treatment is administration of an anticholinergic agent.

## REFERENCES

1. Silverstein JH, Deiner SG. Perioperative delirium and its relationship to dementia. *Prog Neuropsychopharmacol Biol Psychiatry.* 2013;43:108–115.
2. Kassie GM, et al. Preoperative medication use and postoperative delirium: A systematic review. *BMC Geriatr.* 2017;17(1):298.
3. Cote CJ, et al. *Cote and Lerman's a Practice of Anesthesia for Infants and Children*. 6th ed. Elsevier; 2018.
4. Barash PG. *Clinical Anesthesia.* 8th ed. Wolters Kluwer; 2017.
5. Paton C. Benzodiazepines and disinhibition: A review. *Psychiatr Bull.* 2002;26(12):460–462.

# 96.

# DRUG ABUSE

*Sabrina S. Sam and Maria Torres*

## INTRODUCTION

Drug abuse, also referred to as substance use disorder (SUD), affects approximately 9.2% of individuals in the United States, according to the 2012 National Survey on Drug Use and Health.[1] The most commonly used drugs are marijuana, cocaine, heroin, prescription opioids, methamphetamines, and hallucinogens.[2] Approximately 21%–29% of patients misuse prescription opioids and 8%–12% of those develop an opioid use disorder.[3] SUD is increasing and requires anesthesia providers to be familiar with the perioperative care of patients with recent substance use, those who are in withdrawal, and those in treatment or recovery. Multimodal analgesia with opioid-sparing techniques and responsible prescribing of opioids on discharge are also important. Enhanced recovery after surgery (ERAS) protocols should be used in these patients in order to accomplish our goals.

## CLINICAL FEATURES

SUD is the continued use of a substance that results in negative outcomes such as legal consequences, health issues, or social problems. Drug abuse can lead to disruption of the reward circuit leading to poor judgment, decision-making, and memory impairment.[2] Some individuals may develop tolerance to drugs or withdrawal when cessation is attempted. SUD comprises three stages that occur in a cycle: intoxication, withdrawal, and preoccupation. Intoxication is where the individual experiences positive reinforcement from using substances. Withdrawal results in adverse effects when the drug use is discontinued. Preoccupation includes cravings leading to habitual substance use and restarting the cycle. Signs and symptoms of acute intoxication and withdrawal vary with the specific substances used (Table 96.1). SUD occurs more commonly in individuals with coexisting psychiatric diseases, such as schizophrenia, depression, and bipolar disorder.[3]

*Table 96.1* COMMONLY ABUSED DRUGS IN THE PERIOPERATIVE PATIENT

| SUBSTANCE | SIGNS/SYMPTOMS OF INTOXICATION | SIGNS/SYMPTOM OF WITHDRAWAL | ANESTHETIC CONSIDERATIONS |
|---|---|---|---|
| Opioids | Inadequate analgesia, respiratory depression, coagulopathy, liver disease, hypotension | Restlessness, abdominal pain, sweating, nausea, vomiting, hypertension, tachycardia, tremors | Difficult vascular access; consider use of multimodal analgesia, naloxone for overdose |
| Cocaine | Agitation, alertness, anxiety, euphoria, paranoia, hallucinations, tachycardia, hypertension, increased temperature, pulmonary edema | Unpleasant dreams, insomnia/ somnolence, anger, increased appetite, agitation, depression, anxiety, slowing of movements and thinking | Blood pressure control, avoid beta blockers and medications that increase heart rate, elective surgery postponed until cocaine-free for one week |
| Amphetamines | Poor dentition, euphoria, hemodynamic instability, arrhythmias | Fatigue, hyperphagia, depression | Treat hypotension aggressively, increased MAC in chronic users |
| Hallucinogens | Aggression, dissociation, tachycardia, hypertension, increased temperature | Confusion, depression, memory loss, seizures, muscle rigidity | Avoid light anesthesia and exogenous catecholamines |
| Marijuana | Airway irritability, rhythm abnormalities, myocardial sensitization | Restlessness, irritability, nausea, vomiting, diarrhea | Watch for airway edema, may require increased induction medications |

# TREATMENT

Various forms of behavioral and pharmacological treatment are often combined. Behavioral therapy includes cognitive therapy, motivational interviewing, and contingency management. Medication-assisted treatment (MAT) is specific to the substances being used. Medications can be used to reproduce the effects of the drugs and then taper, as in methadone or buprenorphine for opioid use disorder. MAT can also be used to diminish the euphoria from the drugs, such as with naltrexone for opioid use disorder. Both inpatient and outpatient treatment programs are available.

Treatment goals are immediate and long-term abstinence and recovery. Individuals may require aid during abstinence if undergoing withdrawal. Relapse is threatened by a multitude of factors, such as the stigma of treatment, lack of social support, psychiatric comorbidities, and underlying pain. Success of recovery can be increased by participation in a 12-step program, group therapy, treating comorbid psychiatric illness or underlying pain, social support, and MAT.

# ANESTHETIC CONSIDERATIONS

Patients may require anesthesia while acutely intoxicated, in withdrawal, on MAT, or in recovery. Providers must recognize signs and symptoms in all stages of SUD and anesthetic considerations for these substances (Table 96.1). It is important not only to provide adequate depths of anesthesia and analgesia, but also to consider the risk of relapse in patients re-exposed to these medications.

## PREOPERATIVE

A detailed preoperative history and physical, focusing on past and present substance use, current prescribed medications as well as adherence, nonprescription drugs taken and last use, and MAT with dosing. As many individuals are reluctant to relay information on substance abuse, it is imperative to establish trust between provider and patient in a nonjudgmental manner by explaining risks with anesthetic delivery.

In acutely intoxicated patients who are unable to provide an accurate history, a urine drug screen should be obtained and surgery should be delayed if possible. The most commonly tested substances are marijuana, amphetamines, barbiturates, benzodiazepines, phencyclidine, cocaine, and opioids. In chronic users, anesthetic management should be weighed against the risks of each particular substance.

Buprenorphine, a partial opioid-agonist, should be discontinued 3–5 days prior to the procedure, and pure opioid agonists can be used to manage withdrawal symptoms if necessary. MAT prescribers should be consulted postoperatively to determine when to restart buprenorphine. In emergency cases or minor procedures, buprenorphine is continued perioperatively while utilizing multimodal techniques. Methadone, a full μ-receptor agonist and N-methyl-d-aspartate (NMDA) receptor antagonist, should be continued at the patient's regular dosing or divided into 3 doses administered every 8 hours. Methadone will decrease the requirements for other anesthetics. Naltrexone, a kappa-receptor opioid antagonist, should be discontinued at least 72 hours prior to surgery, or 30 days if extended-release naltrexone is being used. Continuing or discontinuing buprenorphine necessitates a discussion with the patient and all members of the care team. It can be stopped and restarted, or there may be no need to stop it and pain will be controlled using regional anesthesia or other non-opioid modalities.

## INTRAOPERATIVE

Important intraoperative considerations include management of patients in withdrawal and providing adequate anesthesia and analgesia. This can be achieved by utilizing multimodal analgesic techniques in order to minimize opioid use (ERAS protocols), including regional anesthesia, nonpharmacological techniques, and non-opioid medications, which decrease not only opioid consumption but also length of hospitalization, and result in improved patient satisfaction.[4]

Adjuvants frequently utilized include nonsteroidal anti-inflammatory drugs (NSAIDs), acetaminophen, ketamine, gabapentin/pregabalin, antispasmodics, anticonvulsants, and celecoxib. NSAIDs include ketorolac, diclofenac, naproxen, and ibuprofen. Acetaminophen can be administered parenterally or orally with reduction in pain scores and incidence of postoperative nausea and vomiting (Siu). Ketamine, an NMDA receptor antagonist, is generally administered via intermittent boluses intravenously or via an infusion. Gabapentin/pregabalin, which works by inhibiting voltage-gated calcium channels via binding to alpha-2-delta subunits, can decrease hyperalgesia and central sensitization. Regional anesthesia can include single-shot or catheter-inserted peripheral nerve blocks, truncal blocks, or neuraxial anesthesia. Nonpharmacologic methods of analgesia include acupuncture, hypnosis, and neurostimulation.

## POSTOPERATIVE

In the postoperative period, it is important to ensure adequate analgesia and prevention of withdrawal. Patients who have been using drugs recently develop tolerance and may require higher doses than normal to provide analgesia. If prescribing outpatient narcotics, it is imperative to discuss with the surgeon and MAT prescriber.

## REFERENCES

1. Moran S, et al. Perioperative management in the patient with substance abuse. *Surg Clin N Am*. 2016;95:417–428.
2. Beaulieu P. Anesthetic implications of recreational drug use. *Can J Anesth*. 2017;64(12):1236–1264.
3. *Analgesia and Anesthesia for the Substance Use Disorder Patient*. AANA. https://www.aana.com/docs/default-source/practice-aana-com-web-documents-(all)/analgesia-and-anesthesia-for-the-substance-use-disorder-patient.pdf?sfvrsn=3e6b7548_2. Published 2019. Accessed June 22, 2020.
4. Siu E, Moon T. Opioid-free and opioid-sparing anesthesia. *Int Anesthesiol Clin*. 2020;58(2):34–41.

# 97.

# INTRAOCULAR PRESSURE

*Camila Teixeira and Steven Minear*

## INTRODUCTION

The rapid intraocular pressure (IOP) change during surgery plays a significant role in the pathogenesis of perioperative ocular morbidity, especially in patients with preexisting eye disease like glaucoma. Perioperative visual loss (POVL) is an uncommon but catastrophic event, which exhibits a multifactorial etiology. Among all causes addressed to POVL, the ischemic optic neuropathy (ION) is the most frequently described.[1] During the preoperative assessment of patients with glaucoma, it is imperative to evaluate the predisposing elements that contribute to the IOP elevation, and therefore to POVL occurrence.

## PHYSIOPATHOLOGY

The intraocular perfusion pressure (IOPP) is defined as the difference between the mean arterial pressure (MAP) and the intraocular pressure (IOP). The balance between the aqueous humor production and outflow rates is one of the main predictors of IOP. Resistance to the aqueous humor outflow, present in some glaucomatous patients, can rapidly increase the IOP and decrease the retinal perfusion.

## ANESTHETIC CONSIDERATIONS

### PREOPERATIVE

Patient and surgical features that corroborate either to decrease the MAP or to elevate the IOP can induce an ocular perfusion imbalance and, consequently, contribute to the occurrence of ION. Other predisposition characteristics, besides glaucoma, should also be addressed during the preoperative patient evaluation and preparation. Society members of the American Society of Anesthesiologists Task Force on Perioperative Visual Loss have agreed that vascular risk factors, preoperative anemia, prolonged procedures, and substantial intraoperative blood loss all increase the risk of POVL.[2] Several non-ocular surgical procedures have been associated with POVL, although cardiac and spinal surgeries are the most commonly reported. Cardiac surgeries can be associated with reduced ocular perfusion due to hypotension, cardiopulmonary bypass, anemia, and the hyperviscosity during induced hypothermia.[3] Prone spinal surgeries and laparoscopic procedures can reduce the venous drainage, resulting in optic nerve edema. During laparoscopic surgery, IOP elevation can be a result of the venous congestion from Trendelenburg position, exacerbated by the partial pressure of carbon dioxide ($PaCO_2$) elevation from the pneumoperitoneum.[4]

## INTRAOPERATIVE

Anesthetic management significantly influences the pressure changes in the eye, and consequently, the risk of morbidity for glaucomatous patients. Vigilance in controlling IOP and safeguarding IOPP must be a central concern when planning the anesthesia management. The overall effect of general anesthesia results in IOP reduction, except during active laryngoscopic retraction. McGrath video laryngoscopes, when compared to Macintosh blade laryngoscopes, have shown advantages in regard to the effect on IOP elevation.[5] Verification of proper muscle relaxation before proceeding with tracheal intubation is key. Succinylcholine administration is associated with IOP elevation, though clinically relevant adverse events from this remain unproven. Hypercarbia, hemodilution, exacerbated periods in hypotension, and external eye compression should be avoided in patients with glaucoma disease undergoing surgery. It is recommended, when possible, to plan for staging procedures when prolonged surgical times are expected.[2] Constant checks for pressure on the globes or signs of congestion on patients in prone position can prevent POVL. Leveling the patient at regular intervals during surgeries in the Trendelenburg position can also be a helpful strategy.

## REFERENCES

1. Lee LA, et al. The American Society of Anesthesiologists postoperative visual loss registry: Analysis of 93 spine surgery cases with postoperative visual loss. *Anesthesiology.* 2006;105:652–659.
2. American Society of Anesthesiologists Task Force on Perioperative Visual Loss. Practice advisory for perioperative visual loss associated with spine surgery: An updated report by the American Society of Anesthesiologists Task Force on Visual Loss. *Anesthesiology.* 2012;116:274–285.
3. Kelly DJ, Farrell SM. Physiology and role of intraocular pressure in contemporary anesthesia. *Anesth Analg.* 2018;126(5):1551–1562.
4. Awad H, et al. The effects of steep trendelenburg positioning on intraocular pressure during robotic radical prostatectomy. *Anesth Analg.* 2009;109(2):473–478.
5. Karaman T, et al. Intraocular pressure changes: The McGrath video laryngoscope vs the Macintosh laryngoscope: A randomized trial. *J Clin Anesth.* 2016;34:358–364.

# 98.

# UREMIA

*Anureet Walia and Archit Sharma*

## INTRODUCTION

Uremia refers to high plasma levels of urea, which occur secondary to renal failure. The kidneys are responsible for maintaining the fluid and electrolyte balance, so renal dysfunction not only leads to accumulation of toxic products such as urea and creatinine, but also leads to fluid retention and edema.[1] This can occur due to both acute or chronic renal failure. There are more than 80 different compounds that build up in renal failure and lead to the uremic syndrome (urea, creatinine, cyanates, polyols, phenols, ß2 microglobulin, etc.).

Acute renal failure is defined as an increase in creatinine of 0.5 mg/dL if baseline <2.5 mg/dL, a 20% increase if baseline >2.5 mg/dL, or a 50% decrease in glomerular filtration rate (GFR). Once creatinine clearance falls below 25 mL/min, patients are at risk for significant pharmacokinetic abnormalities. When indexed GFR falls below 15 mL/min/1.73m², uremic symptoms begin to appear. Blood urea nitrogen (BUN) is a misleading marker of renal function, as it is dependent on volume status, and can be affected by gastrointestinal (GI) bleeding, a high protein diet, and steroids.

## SIGNS AND SYMPTOMS

Uremic syndrome consists of constitutional symptoms such as weakness, tiredness, fatigue, loss of appetite, and organ-specific symptoms, which have been tabulated (see Table 98.1). If left untreated, these symptoms progress to stupor, coma, and death.

A classical manifestation of uremia is uremic fetor uremic breath, which is an ammoniacal odor in the patient's breath, due to high concentrations of urea secreted in the saliva. Similarly, a patient might have uremic frost, which is a white powdery crusty appearance of the entire skin due to excretion of urea crystals in the sweat. Pallor occurs due to anemia of renal disease, and patients can have thrombosis and petechiae due to platelet dysfunction. Enamel hypoplasia and caries are very common in the early age groups due to the alkaline saliva.

## ETIOLOGY

Causes of uremia also fall under the same classification as causes for renal failure.

### PRERENAL

There is decreased blood flow through the kidneys. Examples include hypotension, dehydration, congestive heart failure, bleeding, etc.

### RENAL

Intrinsic disease processes involve renal parenchyma. Examples include glomerulonephritis, tubular necrosis, and other renal diseases.

*Table 98.1* VARIOUS ORGAN SPECIFIC MANIFESTATIONS OF UREMIA

| SYSTEM | MANIFESTATION |
| --- | --- |
| Central nervous system | Headache, fatigue, seizures, coma, encephalopathy, confusion |
| Cardiovascular | Hypertension, pericarditis, pulmonary edema |
| Gastrointestinal | Anorexia, nausea, vomiting, gastroparesis, ulcers |
| Hematological | Platelet dysfunction, anemia, bleeding problems |
| Integumentary | Itching, dryness, uremic frost |
| Skeletal | Osteomalacia, bone weakness |
| Endocrinological | Impotence, infertility, sterility |

### POSTRENAL

There is obstruction to the flow of urine, causing decreased excretion. Examples include kidney stones, tumors, ureteral strictures, and prostatic hypertrophy.

## DIAGNOSIS

In clinical assessment, looking for organ-specific signs helps to diagnose uremia, but certain laboratory tests aid in confirmation of the diagnosis. The principal diagnosis is a very low GFR (<30 ml/min). Although the most trusted test for determining GFR is iothalamate clearance, laboratories generally calculate the GFR with the Cockcroft-Gault formula.

Other tests include a basic metabolic panel (BMP) to look at the electrolytes such as serum sodium, potassium, and BUN and serum creatinine values. At the same time, assessment of serum calcium and phosphate level should also be done to assess bone health. Uremia leads to elevation of both blood urea and creatinine, elevated potassium, high phosphate, and normal or slightly high sodium, as well as likely depressed calcium levels.

## TREATMENT

Treatment of uremia is centered around treating the primary cause of renal dysfunction. Hence, if the cause is prerenal azotemia, then it is best treated by restoring perfusion to the kidneys by fluid resuscitation. If the cause is postrenal, relieving the obstructive cause will lead to improvement of renal status and slow improvement of uremia as well.

If all these measures have failed, and the patient is worsening, or in severe electrolyte disturbance and acidosis, hemodialysis is an option to remove uremic metabolites from the body.[2] During dialysis, removal of wastes, extra fluids, and toxins from the bloodstream is handled artificially by a machine, instead of by the kidneys. Patients on dialysis can acquire what is called *residual syndrome*. Residual syndrome is a non-life-threatening disease, which is displayed as toxic effects, with similar symptomatology to uremia.[3] This is likely due to the accumulation of large molecular weight solutes that are poorly dialyzed, and dialyzable solutes that are incompletely removed.

## ANESTHETIC CONSIDERATIONS

Patients with renal failure and uremia undergoing surgery are at a substantial risk for increased morbidity and mortality. There are various effects on homeostasis that are not only restricted to water and electrolyte abnormalities, but also affect multiple organ systems, making intraoperative management of these patients especially challenging.[4]

## PREOPERATIVE

Patients with chronic renal failure undergoing elective surgery should receive dialysis treatment the day before planned surgery to optimize their electrolyte, metabolic, and volume status. It is important to check their electrolytes such as a BMP, calcium, and phosphate level on the day of surgery.[5] These patients can have anemia and thrombocytopenia, and a complete blood count (CBC) should be checked to evaluate that as well.

## INTRAOPERATIVE

Neurologic sequelae, including confusion, sedation, or obtundation, can result from uremic encephalopathy, making it difficult to manage these patients' sedation, necessitating securing the airway with an intubation. Volume overload can lead to hypoxemia, and renal failure can lead to acidosis

## POSTOPERATIVE

A prompt neurologic exam should be performed in the recovery area, with special attention to degree of consciousness and ability to protect the airway.

## REFERENCES

1. Burtis CA, et al. *Tietz Textbook of Clinical Chemistry and Molecular Diagnostics*. e-book. Elsevier Health Sciences; 2012.
2. Meyer TW, Hotstetter T. Uremia. *N Engl J Med*. 2007;357: 1316–1325.
3. Depner TA. Uremic toxicity: Urea and beyond. *Semin Dialysis*. 2001 Jul;14(4):246–251.
4. Wagener G, Brentjens TE. Anesthetic concerns in patients presenting with renal failure. *Anesthesiol Clin*. 2010;28(1): 39–54.
5. Sladen RN. Anesthetic considerations for the patient with renal failure. *Anesthesiol Clin North Am*. 2000;18(4):863–882.

# 99.

# INCREASED CEREBROSPINAL FLUID PRESSURE

*Ling Tian and Christina T. Nguyen*

## INTRODUCTION

Intracranial pressure (ICP) is determined by the three compartments inside the skull: brain parenchyma, blood volume, and the cerebrospinal fluid (CSF). Changes in the volume of one compartment can lead to changes to ICP, affecting the function of the other compartments. Measurement of CSF pressure is therefore commonly used as a surrogate to assess ICP and is critical for the anesthesiologist to understand in order to preserve brain oxygen delivery and protection of neural tissue.

## CSF FORMATION AND ABSORPTION

CSF is constantly produced and reabsorbed. The average adult has around 150 ml CSF and produces 500 ml/day. CSF is actively secreted by epithelial cells in the choroid plexus by energy-requiring mechanisms involving Na/K-ATPase. Equal amounts of CSF are absorbed across the arachnoid granulations by a valve-like mechanism to maintain the stable CSF volume and therefore pressure. Normal CSF pressure is 10–15 mmHg in adults and 3–4 mmHg in infants (Figure 99.1).[1]

The skull and spinal tract are closed volume-static spaces; therefore any change to one of the three compartments (parenchyma, blood, and CSF volume) directly affects the others. In addition, cerebral venous pressure contributes more to CSF pressure than arterial pressure through two mechanisms: venous engorgement and decreased CSF reabsorption. Therefore, heart failure with associated increase of venous pressure can lead to increased CSF pressure. Another cause of decreased CSF reabsorption are the chronic changes after subarachnoid hemorrhage, namely fibrosis of the arachnoid villi, which causes the common

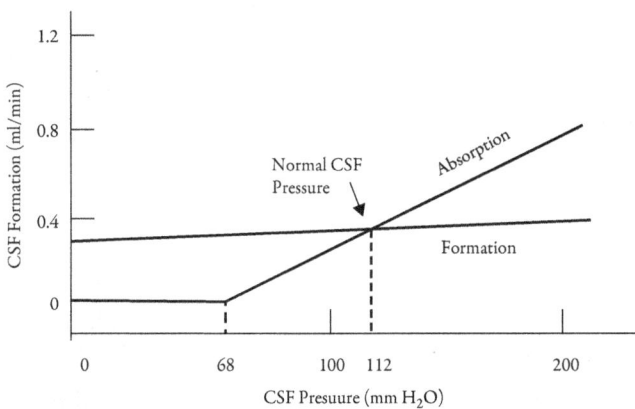

**Figure 99.1.** CSF formation and absorption as a function of outflow pressure. At 112 mm, $H_2O$ formation and absorption are equal. At 68 mm $H_2O$, absorption is zero. Reproduced from Cutler RW, et al. Formation and absorption of cerebrospinal fluid in man. Brain. 1968;91(4):707–720 by permission of Oxford University Press.

sequelae of hydrocephalus (see Table 99.1). Pseudotumor cerebri is also thought to be caused mainly by impaired CSF reabsorption.[2]

## CONSEQUENCE OF INCREASED CSF PRESSURE

Increased CSF pressure can translate to pressure on the brain parenchyma itself, resulting in neuronal damage and atrophy. Hydrocephalus is the condition in which increased CSF pressure causes enlargement of the ventricles within the brain. In cases where the increased CSF pressure is not uniform (obstructive hydrocephalus), it can lead to shifting of the brain parenchyma and brainstem, leading to devastating herniation.

*Table 99.1* CAUSES OF INCREASED CSF PRESSURE

| SPACE-OCCUPYING LESIONS | BLOOD VOLUME | CSF VOLUME |
|---|---|---|
| Tumor | Decreased venous outflow | Increased CSF production |
| Abscess | | |
| Hematoma | Intracranial hypertension | Decreased CSF absorption (pseudotumor cerebri, elevated venous pressure, sequelae of subarachnoid hemorrhage) |
| Arteriovenous malformation | Subarachnoid hemorrhage | |
| Focal or diffuse edema (trauma, ischemia, toxins) | | |
| | | Obstruction to CSF flow |
| | | Bacterial meningitis |
| | | Imbalance of proteins and electrolytes |

For the anesthesiologist, increased CSF pressure is essential to understand because it affects cerebral blood flow (CBF), which is critical to maintain adequate oxygenation and delivery of nutrients and glucose to the neuronal tissue. CBF is autoregulated by adjustments to cerebral vascular resistance in response to cerebral perfusion pressure (CPP). CPP is calculated by mean arterial pressure (MAP) – ICP. In normotensive adults, autoregulation can maintain CBF in a CPP range of 50–150 mmHg.[2] In practice, since measurement of ICP is not easily attained, MAP is used as a surrogate for CPP. Thus, if ICP is elevated, the actual CPP will be lower than the MAP would suggest and the patient will be at risk of low CBF and ensuing ischemia, decreased neuronal functioning. Therefore, for patient at risk of increased ICP, the anesthesiologist should consider continuous monitoring of ICP so that adequate MAP goals can be maintained.

## CSF PRESSURE MEASUREMENT AND CSF DRAINAGE

CSF pressure and therefore ICP can be measured by numerous methods. Continuous monitoring is usually achieved intracranially, including intraventricular, intraparenchymal, subarachnoid, and even epidural monitors. Lumbar puncture is usually used for a one-time measurement of CSF pressure; however, catheters can be left intrathecally for continuous monitoring as well as for continuous drainage for CSF. For lumbar puncture, ideally pressure is measured with the patient in the lateral recumbent position at the moment a needle is placed in the lumbar sac, prior to removal of fluid.

CSF drainage can acutely treat increased ICP in some instances. In communicating hydrocephalus, CSF drainage from lumbar puncture is generally safe. However, if the increased ICP is caused by obstructive hydrocephalus, CSF must be drained from the intracranial ventricular system; otherwise, the pressure difference created by lumbar drainage can cause cerebellar herniation.

## OTHER METHODS TO REDUCE ICP

Based on multiple large studies, the Brain Trauma Foundation recommended lowering ICP at thresholds of 22 mmHg, as it is associated with increased mortality in severe traumatic brain injury.[3] In addition to CSF drainage, other methods have been studied to decrease ICP. These methods affect the parenchyma and blood compartments of the central nervous system, thus having a downstream effect of lowering CSF.

The simplest method and most noninvasive is elevation of the head of the bed to prevent venous outflow obstruction. Mannitol boluses of 0.25–1g/kg reduce ICP in

20–30 min by causing an osmotic reduction of cerebral parenchymal cell water and decreasing the overall brain volume. Hyperventilation lowers ICP by decreasing $PaCO_2$ (partial pressure of carbon dioxide) and subsequently reducing CBF. However, since CBF may drop by as much as 50% following traumatic brain injury (TBI), the use of hyperventilation for treatment of TBI is controversial; in fact, the Brain Trauma Foundation recommends against chronic hyperventilation. Barbiturates and propofol lower ICP by causing dose-dependent reductions in cerebral metabolism and subsequently cerebral blood flow. However, they can also cause hypotension, which could decrease CPP, so care must be taken to maintain adequate arterial blood pressure. The target CPP is between 60 and 70 mmHg for survival and favorable outcomes.[3] Hypothermia lowers ICP in patients with TBI, also through a reduction in cerebral metabolism and blood flow. However, the benefit of hypothermia on functional outcome is unclear.[5] Hypo-osmolar glucose-containing fluids have the ability to aggravate cerebral edema, increase ICP, and induce hyperglycemia, which can aggravate ischemic neurologic injuries. All intravenous anesthetics except ketamine cause reduction in cerebral blood flow, metabolism, and ICP.

## REFERENCES

1. Rosenberg G. Cerebrospinal fluid: Formation, absorption, markers, and relationship to blood–brain barrier. In: *Primer on Cerebrovascular Diseases*. 2nd ed. London: Academic Press; 2017:25–31.
2. Cottrell JE, et al. Cerebrospinal fluid. In: *Cottrell and Patel's Neuroanesthesia*. 6th ed. Edinburgh: Elsevier; 2017:59–73.
3. Carney N, et al. Guidelines for the management of severe traumatic brain injury, fourth edition. *Neurosurgery*. 2017;80(1):6–15.
4. Cutler RW, et al. Formation and absorption of cerebrospinal fluid in man. *Brain*. 1968;91(4):707–720.
5. Andrews PJ, et al. Hypothermia for intracranial hypertension after traumatic brain injury. *N Engl J Med*. 2015;373(25):2403–2412.

# 100.

# CHRONIC STEROID INGESTION

*Hewenfei Li and Christina T. Nguyen*

## INTRODUCTION

Cortisone was first introduced in the mid-twentieth century for the treatment of primary adrenal insufficiency and has quickly become the fundamental treatment for many common conditions. Since the discovery of secondary adrenal insufficiency due to withdrawal from chronic glucocorticoid therapy, perioperative glucocorticoid coverage has become a standard of care. However, stress steroid administration during a perioperative period remains controversial and has been recently been challenged given the fact that true perioperative adrenal insufficiency is a rare event and excess perioperative steroid replacement therapy may be unnecessary and potentially damaging.[1]

## HYPOTHALAMIC-PITUITARY-ADRENAL AXIS (HPAA) SUPPRESSION

In immunocompetent patients, acute stress directly activates the hypothalamic-pituitary-adrenal axis and the adrenal cortex produces cortisol. Under normal conditions, adrenal glands produce a total of 10–30 mg of cortisol per day. During minor surgery or illness, cortisol secretion rate can increase up to 50–100 mg per day and may increase up to 200–500 mg per day for major surgery or trauma.[2]

Chronic steroid ingestion is well known to suppress the HPAA and cause the adrenal glands to produce inadequate amounts of cortisol. The risk of adrenal insufficiency may last up to 6–12 months after discontinuation of steroid use before the adrenal gland can recover.[3] However, it is difficult to predict the perioperative HPAA response due to interpersonal variations.

## ADVERSE EFFECTS OF CHRONIC STEROID INGESTION

Giving patients an unnecessary high steroid dosage is not without risk, especially when a true perioperative adrenal crisis is rare, occurring anywhere from 1% to 2% of major surgical procedures.[4] Patients on chronic steroid therapy are already at risk of osteoporosis, thinning of skin, hypertension, fatty liver, muscle weakness, weight gain, and Cushing syndrome. Additional high steroid dosage increases the risks of perioperative complications, including but not limited to infection, psychosis, impaired wound healing, and hyperglycemia.

## CLINICAL SYMPTOMS AND SIGNS

In an awake patient, clinical manifestation of an adrenal crisis may include altered mental status, abdominal pain, nausea, vomiting, weakness, hypotension, hyponatremia, or hypokalemia. However, in a patient under general anesthesia, severe and persistent hypotension that is refractory to fluids and vasopressors may be the only sign of adrenal insufficiency.

## ANESTHETIC CONSIDERATIONS

### PREOPERATIVE

All patients should have a complete preoperative history and physical, including a history of recent steroid use, the duration and dosage of steroid use, and any prior incidents of adrenal insufficiency or crisis. Patients should have recent labs to assess electrolyte and glucose level. Anesthesiologists should assess the anticipated surgical stress to determine the appropriate perioperative stress dose (Table 100.1).

In patients with possible HPA suppression, the presence of unexplained symptoms and signs should prompt testing a random cortisol and may require empiric corticosteroids therapy.[2]

*Table 100.1* RECOMMENDED STEROID DOSING FOR SURGERY TYPE

| SURGERY TYPE | ENDOGENOUS CORTISOL SECRETION RATE | EXAMPLES | RECOMMENDED STEROID DOSING |
|---|---|---|---|
| Superficial | 8–10 mg per day (baseline) | Dental surgery<br>Biopsy | Usual daily dose |
| Minor | 50 mg per day | Inguinal hernia repair<br>Colonoscopy<br>Uterine curettage<br>Hand surgery | Usual daily dose<br>*plus*<br>Hydrocortisone 50 mg IV before incision<br>Hydrocortisone 25 mg IV every 8 h × 24 h, then usual daily dose |
| Moderate | 75–150 mg per day | Lower extremity revascularization<br>Total joint replacement<br>Cholecystectomy<br>Colon resection<br>Abdominal hysterectomy | Usual daily dose<br>*plus*<br>Hydrocortisone 50 mg IV before incision<br>Hydrocortisone 25 mg IV every 8 h × 24 h, then usual daily dose |
| Major | 75–150 mg per day | Esophagectomy<br>Total proctocolectomy<br>Major cardiac/vascular<br>Hepaticojejunostomy<br>Delivery<br>Trauma | Usual daily dose<br>*plus*<br>Hydrocortisone 100 mg IV before incision, followed by continuous IV infusion of 200 mg hydrocortisone more than 24 h<br>*or*<br>Hydrocortisone 50 mg IV every 8 h × 24 h<br>Taper dose by half per day until usual daily dose reached<br>*plus*<br>Continuous IV fluids with 5% dextrose and 0.2–0.45% NaCi (based on degree of hypoglycemia) |

Reproduced with permission from Liu MM, Reidy AB, Saatee S, Collard CD. Perioperative steroid management: Approaches based on current evidence. *Anesthesiology* 2017;127(1):166–172. doi: https://doi.org/10.1097/ALN.0000000000001659. Copyright 2020 by Wolters Kluwer Health, Inc.

IV = intravenous.

## Low Risk for HPAA Suppression

Patients who are at low risk of adrenal insufficiency, including patients who have been treated with any dose of glucocorticoid for less than 3 weeks, morning doses of prednisone less than 5 mg/day or its equivalence for any length of time, or prednisone less than 10 mg/day or its equivalent every other day, should continue their home glucocorticoids regimen without perioperative stress steroids coverage (Grade 2C).[2]

If preoperative evaluation is clinically warranted, a standard 250 mcg ACTH (adrenocorticotropic hormone) stimulation test should be used to assess the integrity of HPAA.[1] In patients with normal response (serum cortisol >18 mcg/dL) to administration of cosyntropin (a synthetic analog of ACTH), no further evaluation and perioperative steroid are needed. For patients receiving morning cortisol test, if cortisol is <5 mcg/dL, stress dose steroids should be administered perioperatively (Grade 2C). If morning cortisol >10 mcg/dL, current glucocorticoid regimen may be continued and no additional coverage needed (Grade 2C). If morning cortisol level is between 5 and 10 mcg/dL, consider evaluating with a standard ACTH stimulation test or start empiric stress glucocorticoid therapy (Grade 2C).[2] Patients who have a diagnosis of secondary adrenal insufficiency should receive perioperative stress-dose steroids.

## High Risk for HPAA Suppression

Patients who are at risk for adrenal insufficiency, including patients who have been treated with steroid in doses equivalent to more than 20 mg per day of prednisone for more than 3 weeks or have a clinical diagnosis of Cushing's syndrome should receive perioperative glucocorticoids coverage (Grade 2C).[2]

## Intermediate Risk for HPAA Suppression

Patients currently taking 5–20 mg of prednisone for more than 3 weeks have considerable variability in HPAA suppression. Patients in this category may consider an endocrinology consult or preoperative testing to assess their HPAA function. In addition, patients who have been using high-dose inhaled glucocorticoids such as equivalent to 750 mcg per day of fluticasone for more than 3 weeks, or equivalent to 2 g per day of high potency topical corticosteroids (Class I–III) for more than 3 weeks should have their adrenal function evaluated.[2] If unable to obtain preoperative testing, anesthesiologists should exercise their best clinical judgment regarding perioperative steroid replacement therapy based on the patient's clinical picture.

## INTRAOPERATIVE

Acute hemodynamic instability should first be thoroughly assessed for common etiologies. Once common causes are ruled out, acute adrenal insufficiency is considered and hydrocortisone is the drug of choice for stress and rescue steroid therapy. Vasopressors may be necessary to support a patient's hemodynamic. The clinical impact of adrenal suppression of one-time etomidate bolus is not well defined; one should generally avoid etomidate induction in critically ill patients.[2]

Patients may have significant volume deficits during the intraoperative period, and intravenous fluid therapy should be initiated. Intraoperative electrolyte and glucose should be monitored and corrected according to institution-specific protocol. Patients may receive perioperative glucocorticoid coverage, including intravenous hydrocortisone, dexamethasone, or methylprednisolone (Table 100.2).

## POSTOPERATIVE

Blood glucose level, electrolyte, and volume status should be reassessed in the postoperative period. Patients with intraoperative hemodynamic instability due to adrenal insufficiency should be managed in the intensive care unit. All patients with suspected adrenal insufficiency should be tested for serum cortisol and ACTH stimulation test. Physicians should remain vigilant and use glucocorticoid rescue therapy in the event of unexplained perioperative hypotension.[1]

*Table 100.2* STEROID EQUIVALENT DOSES

| STEROID | GLUCOCORTICOID ACTIVITY | MINERALOCORTICOID ACTIVITY | EQUIVALENT DOSE (IV/PO) | HALF-LIFE, H |
|---|---|---|---|---|
| Dexamethasone | 30–40 | 0 | 0.5–0.75 | 36–54 |

IV = intravenous; PO = per os.

Reproduced with permission from Liu MM, Reidy AB, Saatee S, Collard CD. Perioperative steroid management: Approaches based on current evidence. *Anesthesiology* 2017; 127(1):166–172. doi: https://doi.org/10.1097/ALN.0000000000001659. Copyright 2020 by Wolters Kluwer Health, Inc.

## REFERENCES

1. Liu MM, et al. Perioperative steroid management: Approaches based on current evidence. *Anesthesiology* 2017;127(1):166–172.
2. Hamrahian A, et al. UpToDate. The management of surgical patient taking glucocorticoids.
3. Miller RD, Pardo M, eds. *Basics of Anesthesia.* 7th ed. Philadelphia, PA: Elsevier/Saunders; 2018:208–209.
4. Kehlet H, Binder C. Adrenocortical function and clinical course during and after surgery in unsupplemented glucocorticoid-treated patients. *Br J Anaesth.* 1973;45:1043–1048.
5. Zaghiyan K, et al. A prospective, randomized, noninferiority trial of steroid dosing after major colorectal surgery. *Ann Surg.* 2014;259(1):32–37.

# 101.

# OBSTRUCTIVE SLEEP APNEA

## Shivani Varshney and Adam Yu Yuan

## INTRODUCTION

Obstructive sleep apnea (OSA) is characterized by recurrent episodes of partial (hypopnea) or complete obstruction (apnea) of the pharyngeal airway during sleep. Apnea is defined as complete cessation of airflow for greater than 10 seconds, while hypopnea is defined as greater than 30% reduction in airflow for duration more than 10 seconds and associated with greater than 3% oxygen desaturation. Micro arousals from sleep are required to open the pharynx and re-establish the airway.

## PATHOPHYSIOLOGY

Multiple factors have been implicated in causation, which include obesity, facial malformations, tonsillar hypertrophy, variations in pharyngeal anatomy, impaired pharyngeal dilator muscle function, and altered respiratory arousal thresholds. Airway obstruction occurs as the negative airway pressure that develops during inspiration is greater than the distending pressure of the pharyngeal musculature. Periods of transient arterial oxygen desaturations, along with hypercapnia, trigger sympathetic activation and hemodynamic disturbances. Long-term consequences of these catecholamine surges include systemic hypertension, pulmonary arterial hypertension, and cardiac dysfunction.[1] Frequent sleep disruptions lead to fragmented sleep, daytime sleepiness, and fatigue.

## EVALUATION AND DIAGNOSIS OF OSA

It is estimated that up to 80% of patients with OSA in the general population are undiagnosed. The objective of preoperative assessment is to identify patients at high risk for OSA to allow targeted perioperative interventions. Preoperative evaluation should include a focused history taking and comprehensive airway assessment.[1,4] Patients should be questioned about symptoms of daytime sleepiness, fatigue, snoring, and morning headaches. Comprehensive airway examination should include assessment of nasopharyngeal structures, neck circumference, tonsil size, and tongue volume.

The STOP-Bang questionnaire (Table 101.1) is a simple and easy screening tool to identify patients at risk of OSA. The questionnaire requires "yes" or "no" responses to 8 questions about snoring, tiredness, observed apneas, blood pressure, BMI >35 kg/m², age >50 years, neck circumference >40 cm, and male gender (assigned one point each). Patients with 0 to 2 positive responses are considered "low risk"; those with 3 or 4 are at "intermediate risk"; and those with ≥5 positive responses are at "high risk" of having OSA.[5]

The gold standard for the diagnosis of OSA is an overnight sleep study (polysomnography). It is recommended for patients who screen at risk of moderate to severe OSA and in patients who have significant comorbid cardiopulmonary disease. Polysomnography provides classification of severity of patients with OSA based on the Apnea-Hypopnea Index

*Table 101.1* STOP-BANG QUESTIONNAIRE

| | YES | NO |
|---|---|---|
| 1. **Snoring:** Do you snore loudly (louder than talking or loud enough to be heard through closed doors)? | ☐ | ☐ |
| 2. **Tiredness/fatigue:** Do you often feel tired, fatigued, or sleepy during the daytime, even after a "good" night's sleep? | ☐ | ☐ |
| 3. **Observed apnea:** Has anyone ever observed you stop breathing during your sleep? | ☐ | ☐ |
| 4. **Pressure:** Do you have or are you being treated for high blood pressure? | ☐ | ☐ |
| 5. **Body mass index:** Do you weigh more for your height than shown in the *Height/Weight* table below? | ☐ | ☐ |
| 6. **Age:** Are you older than 50 years? | ☐ | ☐ |
| 7. **Neck size:** Does your neck measure more than 15¾ inches (40 cm) around? | ☐ | ☐ |
| 8. **Gender:** Are you male? | ☐ | ☐ |
| | SCORE | # OF YES |

**Scoring Criteria**

**For General Population**

**Low risk of OSA:** Yes to 0–2 questions

**Intermediate risk of OSA:** Yes to 3–4 questions

**High risk of OSA:** Yes to 5–8 questions

Or Yes to 2 or more of 4 STOP questions + male gender

Or Yes to 2 or more of 4 STOP questions + BMI > 35 kg/m2

Or Yes to 2 or more of 4 STOP questions + neck circumference

17"/43cm in male, 16"/41cm in female

Reproduced with permission from Chung F et al. STOP questionnaire. *Anesthesiology* 2008;108(5):812–821.

(AHI). The AHI is the sum of the number of apneas and hypopneas that occur, on average, each hour during the period of sleep.[4] It is expressed as number of events per hour of sleep. Mild sleep apnea is defined as an AHI between 5 and 15, whereas severe OSA occurs when the AHI exceeds 30.

## ANESTHETIC CONSIDERATIONS

### PREOPERATIVE

Patients with mild OSA may benefit from mandibular advancement devices.[3] Continuous positive airway pressure (CPAP) therapy should be initiated preoperatively in moderate to severe cases.[1] Time should be given to accustom the patient to the CPAP device. Patients who are already on CPAP therapy for OSA should continue treatment up to the day of surgery and should preferably bring their CPAP device with them on the day of surgery. Ideally, all sedative premedication should be avoided or used cautiously. Even minimal sedation can cause airway obstruction and ventilatory arrest.

### INTRAOPERATIVE

Patients with OSA have increased susceptibility to the depressant effects of opioids and inhaled anesthetics.[3] Thus, opioid-sparing techniques should be used whenever possible.

Regional or local anesthesia should be considered whenever possible.

For patients requiring moderate sedation, ventilation should be continuously monitored using capnography. In patients using CPAP preoperatively, use of CPAP during moderate sedation may be beneficial. Agents that are less likely to induce respiratory depression, like dexmedetomidine and ketamine, may be useful for sedation.

For general anesthesia, equipment necessary to manage a difficult airway should be readily available prior to induction, and attention to preoxygenation is very important. Awake fiber-optic intubation should be considered in high-risk cases. Short-acting anesthetic agents that facilitate rapid emergence from anesthesia with minimal residual sedation (e.g., propofol, desflurane, remifentanil) should be used instead of long-acting drugs.

Invasive arterial blood pressure (BP) monitoring may be used if noninvasive BP monitoring is impossible because of associated morbid obesity. Regional blocks and infiltrating the surgical site with local anesthetics are acceptable options to decrease the need for postoperative opioid use.

Extubation should be considered only after patients are fully conscious, purposefully responding to commands, and have no residual neuromuscular blockade.

### POSTOPERATIVE

Patients should be cared in a semi-upright (30° head-up) position. Vigilance and monitoring of oxygenation should be continued in the postoperative period. Supplemental oxygen may be beneficial for most patients; however, it should be administered with caution as it may reduce hypoxic respiratory drive and increase the incidence and duration of apneic episodes. CPAP along with oxygen, rather than oxygen alone, would be helpful in recurrent hypoxia. Patients who use CPAP preoperatively should continue use of their devices as soon as feasible in the immediate postoperative period.[2] Postoperative opioid therapy should be minimized and titrated with extreme caution. If patient-controlled systemic opioids are used, continuous background infusions should be avoided. Nonsteroidal anti-inflammatory drugs (NSAIDs), ketamine, and dexmedetomidine may be useful adjuncts.[2]

Discharge from the post-anesthesia care unit (PACU) should occur only after the patient's oxygen saturation on room air returns to baseline and hypoxemia or airway obstruction does not occur when the patient is left undisturbed.

## REFERENCES

1. American Society of Anesthesiologists Task Force on Perioperative Management of patients with obstructive sleep apnea. Practice guidelines for the perioperative management of patients with obstructive sleep apnea: An updated report by the American Society of Anesthesiologists Task Force on Perioperative Management of patients with obstructive sleep apnea. Anesthesiology. 2014; 120(2):268–286.
2. Barash PG, et al., eds. *Clinical Anesthesia*. 8th ed. Philadelphia, PA: Lippincott Williams & Wilkins; 2017.
3. Stoelting RK, et al. *Stoelting's Anesthesia and Co-Existing Disease*. 7th ed. Philadelphia PA: Elsevier; 2017.
4. Chung F, et al. Society of Anesthesia and Sleep Medicine guidelines on preoperative screening and assessment of adult patients with obstructive sleep apnea. *Anesth Analg*. 2016;123(2):452-473.
5. Chung F, et al. STOP questionnaire: A tool to screen patients for obstructive sleep apnea. *Anesthesiology*. 2008;108:812–821.

# 102.

# DEPRESSION

*Ruben Schwartz and Omar Viswanath*

## INTRODUCTION

The depression medication pharmacology discussed in this chapter includes selective serotonin reuptake inhibitors (SSRIs), serotonin-norepinephrine reuptake inhibitors (SNRIs), tricyclic antidepressants (TCAs), and monoamine oxidase inhibitors (MAOIs). These comprise the most commonly used antidepressant medications.[1] The 2013 National Ambulatory Care Survey showed that the antidepressant class of medications is the third most frequently prescribed throughout the outpatient setting.[2] These medications must be taken for an extended period of time, and often no clinical improvement in symptomatology is seen for 2–4 weeks.

## PATHOPHYSIOLOGY OF DEPRESSION

Depression has been a highly researched topic due to its increased prevalence throughout the patient population. Many postulate that depression is caused by a "chemical imbalance." Disruption in neurochemical substrates like serotonin, dopamine, epinephrine, and others have all been implicated as decreased in depressed individuals.

This is the principal reason that medications like SSRIs, SNRIs, TCAs, and MAOIs have grown in popularity. Their mechanisms of actions increase the overall concentrations of these neurotransmitters. In patients with depression, 5-hydroxyindoleacetic acid (5-HIAA), the major metabolite of serotonin, has been shown to be reduced in cerebrospinal fluid (CSF) samples. Post-mortem brain tissue samples in patients who died due to suicide demonstrated decreased serotonergic levels as well.[3] Structural imbalances within the brain have been noted in rat models of subjects submitted to an environment with increased stressors. Repeated stress has demonstrated atrophy of CA3 pyramidal neurons in the hippocampus, with a decrease in number and length of apical dendrites.[3] Alterations in the cerebral cortex have also been noted in patients with depression and bipolar disorder.

## SEROTONIN-NOREPINEPHRINE REUPTAKE INHIBITORS

SNRIs provide their effects via a similar mechanism as SSRIs with the inhibition of serotonin as well as norepinephrine within the synaptic cleft. Some of the common SNRIs include desvenlafaxine, duloxetine, levomilnacipran,

milnacipran, and venlafaxine. Side effects from SNRIs include sedation, nausea, insomnia, tachycardia, sexual dysfunction, and anticholinergic symptomatology, including xerostomia and constipation.[5] The inhibition of norepinephrine contributes to the tachycardia and elevated blood pressure with the use of SNRIs. Overall, SNRIs have been noted to cause more norepinephrine reuptake inhibition than serotonin.[4] Venlafaxine and duloxetine have both been demonstrated as weak to moderate inhibitors of the CYP 2D6 enzyme, causing a variable response to prodrugs reliant on this enzyme, as mentioned previously. SNRIs have been utilized in other disease processes besides depression, including chronic neuropathic pain, painful diabetic neuropathy, posteherpetic neuralgia, and generalized anxiety disorder.[4]

## MONOAMINE OXIDASE INHIBITORS

MAOIs work on similar principles as the other antidepressants, effectively increasing the amount of various neurotransmitters within the synaptic cleft. MAOIs inhibit presynaptic monoamine oxidase enzymes, increasing cytoplasmic concentrations of serotonin, norepinephrine, and dopamine.[1] MAOIs are utilized for refractory depression in patients not responding to other classes of medications. MAOIs are broken down into two classes, MAOI-A and MAOI-B. The substrates of MAO-A include dopamine, epinephrine, norepinephrine, serotonin, and tyramine. It is important to note that tyramine can also be found in some foods, like cheese, avocado, and fava beans, causing a potentially fatal hypertensive crisis if combined with patients on MAOIs.[1] Orthostatic hypotension is a common side effect seen with MAOIs. Indirect sympathomimetic agents should be avoided perioperatively due to the increased norepinephrine stores in these patients.[4] Meperidine is contraindicated in these patients as it can cause serotonin syndrome.[4]

## SEROTONIN SYNDROME

In the perioperative setting, one of the most feared complications with the use of serotonergic drugs is serotonin syndrome. Normally, serotonergic activity is terminated in the presynaptic neuron with the use of monoamine oxidase. Agents capable of promoting increased serotonin levels and therefore serotonin syndrome include the aforementioned antidepressants, alone or in combination with proserotonergic medications, including phenylpiperidine opioids (meperidine especially, but also potentially fentanyl), tramadol, dextromethorphan, ondansetron, metoclopramide, methylene blue, erythromycin, metronidazole, "triptan" migraine medications, second generation anti-psychotics, and St. John's wort. Serotonin syndrome manifests as a triad of autonomic instability, neuromuscular abnormalities (hyperreflexia), and changes in mental state. Patients under general anesthesia may exhibit hemodynamic collapse.[4] In the perioperative setting alpha agonists can be utilized to maintain hemodynamic stability. Propranolol should be avoided as it can cause bradycardia and hypotension resulting in cardiovascular instability. Cyproheptadine can also mitigate some of the effects of the excessive serotonin activity.

## REFERENCES

1. Saraghi M, et al. Anesthetic considerations for patients on antidepressant therapy: Part I. *Anesth Prog.* 2017;64(4):253–261.
2. National Center for Health Statistics, Centers for Disease Control and Prevention. Therapeutic drug use. 2021. Available at: https://www.cdc.gov/nchs/fastats/drug-use-therapeutic.htm.
3. Duman RS. Pathophysiology of depression: The concept of synaptic plasticity. *Eur Psychiat.* 2002;17(Suppl. 3):306–310. https://doi.org/10.1016/S0924-9338(02)00654-5
4. Saraghi M, et al. Anesthetic considerations for patients on antidepressant therapy: Part II. *Anesthesia progress*, 2018;65(1):60–65.
5. Catalani B, et al. Psychiatric agents and implications for perioperative analgesia. *Best Pract Res Clin Anaesthesiol.* 2014;28:167–181.

# 103.

# CHRONIC OBSTRUCTIVE PULMONARY DISEASE

*Shahrose Hussain and Karim Fikry*

## INTRODUCTION

Chronic obstructive pulmonary disease (COPD) is chronic, irreversible airflow limitation due to airway and/or alveolar abnormalities caused by noxious particles and/or developmental abnormalities associated with significant morbidity and mortality.[1,2] It is the fourth leading cause of death in the world, commonly seen in the elderly and smokers. While tobacco smoking is the main risk factor for COPD, nonsmokers may develop COPD as well, due to environmental exposures (i.e., biomass fuel or air pollution) or genetic factors (i.e., alpha 1 antitrypsin deficiency).[1,3] COPD usually consists of a variable level of overlapping between emphysema and chronic bronchitis.[2,3] Emphysema is a hyperinflation of the lungs, resulting in air trapping due to parenchymal destruction of the alveoli.[3] Chronic bronchitis is a chronic cough with sputum production that obstructs the airway occurring for greater than 3 months in at least 2 consecutive years, associated with increased rates of COPD exacerbations. *COPD exacerbation* is defined as an acute worsening in respiratory symptoms from baseline, necessitating additional therapy.[3]

## CLINICAL FEATURES

COPD commonly presents with dyspnea and a chronic, productive cough.[1,3] Worsening dyspnea, cough, or sputum production from baseline or signs of respiratory distress can be indicative of an acute exacerbation. Signs and symptoms related to right heart failure, such as lower extremity edema, jugular venous distension, and/or ascites, can result due to cor pulmonale from COPD. Signs of increased work of breathing, including accessory muscle use, fatigue, and weight loss, may not be apparent until progression of COPD.[3]

## DIAGNOSIS

COPD should be considered in symptomatic patients with exposure to risk factors. Spirometry establishes a diagnosis

of COPD using the post-bronchodilator forced expiratory volume in the first second divided (FEV1) by the forced vital capacity (FVC) (Figure 103.1). A value less than 0.70 confirms a diagnosis of COPD. An acute exacerbation of COPD is diagnosed clinically based on symptoms, and spirometry should not be performed in these situations. General screening for asymptomatic patients is not recommended, since it has not shown benefit.[1,3] Complete pulmonary function testing is not necessary for diagnosis but may be performed to assess the impact of the disease.[3] Other tests may be performed in the workup of a patient presenting with COPD but are not diagnostic. For example, imaging, such as a chest radiograph, may show signs of lung hyperinflation, and an arterial blood gas may show respiratory acidosis.[1]

## TREATMENT

Smoking cessation has been shown to have the greatest impact in reducing morbidity and mortality related to COPD.[1-3] Influenza and pneumococcal vaccination are

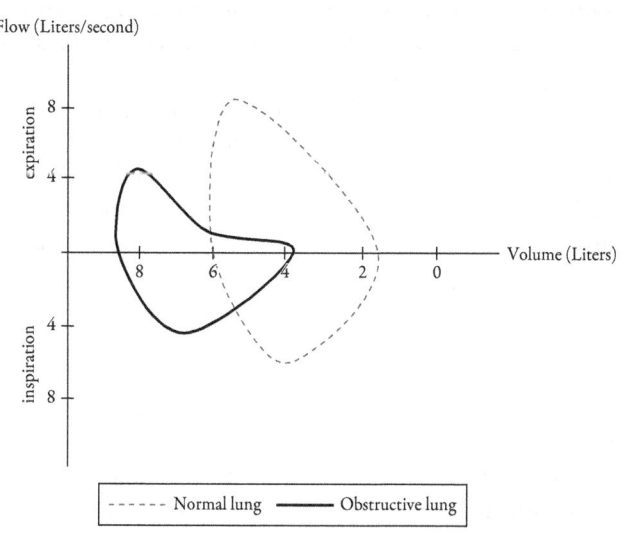

Figure 103.1 Flow volume loop.

recommended for patients with COPD to decrease the incidence of lower respiratory tract infections. Pulmonary rehabilitation has been shown to improve functional capacity. Long-term oxygen therapy is recommended only in patients with severe resting hypoxemia (pO2 <55 mmHg).[1,2] Pharmacologic treatment for stable COPD should be individualized, based on severity of the disease, and aimed at improving symptoms and preventing exacerbations. For acute symptom relief, short-acting bronchodilators are recommended.[1-3] Long-acting bronchodilators are added for maintenance therapy, and inhaled corticosteroids can be considered to improve lung function and reduce exacerbations.[1,3] In an acute exacerbation, oxygen supplementation, short-acting bronchodilators, and corticosteroids are the cornerstone of therapy.[1-3] Antibiotics may be added if there is increased sputum production or purulent sputum.[1,3]

## ANESTHETIC CONSIDERATIONS

### PREOPERATIVE

A proper pre-anesthetic evaluation allows the anesthesiologist to assess COPD disease severity, optimize the patient's condition, and develop an appropriate anesthetic plan that minimizes risks for the patient. A thorough history and physical will illustrate the presence and severity of signs and symptoms that can help predict the risk of postoperative pulmonary complications. For example, the presence of wheezing preoperatively increases the risk of postoperative pulmonary complications; therefore it is recommended to delay elective procedures in the setting of an exacerbation to allow for aggressive treatment with bronchodilators or chest physiotherapy. Smoking cessation should be recommended to patients preoperatively, with cessation 4 to 8 weeks prior to surgery showing decrease in postoperative pulmonary complications. Preoperative imaging of the chest is not routinely recommended, unless a new finding is anticipated (i.e., active infection) which may alter perioperative management. Arterial line placement may be considered in select patients based on disease severity (i.e., significant hypercapnia), comorbidity (i.e., right heart failure), or procedure (i.e., pneumonectomy) in order to obtain baseline gas analysis, to have beat-to-beat blood pressure monitoring, and/or for frequent blood gas analysis to guide management for hypercapnia.[4]

### INTRAOPERATIVE

While the anesthetic technique will be dictated primarily by the procedure, and surgeon and patient preference, regional anesthesia may be preferred as it is associated with less postoperative complications than general endotracheal anesthesia in patients with COPD. When compared with general anesthesia, regional anesthesia is associated with a lower incidence of composite morbidity and postoperative pulmonary complications, such as pneumonia, prolonged ventilator dependence, and unplanned postoperative intubation.

However, the surgical procedure or patient may necessitate general anesthesia. Due to the limited expiratory flow rate of COPD patients, positive pressure ventilation may lead to dynamic hyperinflation, which can result in hypercapnia, barotrauma, and volume trauma to the lungs, and impaired venous return to the heart with subsequent hypotension. To limit this risk, it is recommended to decrease the respiratory rate and inspiratory to expiratory ratio. However, the resultant lower minute ventilation may become a concern, and if so, it may be preferable to increase the inspiratory flow rate and tolerate slightly higher peak airway pressures. Application of external positive end-expiratory pressure in COPD patients may reduce end-inspiratory plateau pressure, leading to less dynamic hyperinflation.

During general anesthesia in a COPD patient, it is important to utilize techniques that minimize the risk of bronchoconstriction and to optimize air flow. Inhaled volatile anesthetics are useful in COPD patients, since they cause bronchodilation and can be used to treat bronchoconstriction which can commonly occur during airway instrumentation. However, desflurane is not preferred since it causes irritation with increased airway resistance, secretions, and coughing; therefore, less pungent volatiles like sevoflurane are preferred, especially during induction or emergence. Emergence from inhalational agents in COPD patients may be prolonged due to air trapping which also traps inhalational anesthetics. Intravenous anesthetics, such as propofol, and short-acting opioids can be used to blunt airway reflexes and prevent bronchoconstriction as well. It is also critical to ensure optimizing these patients' condition for extubation and ensuring adequate neuromuscular blockade reversal. Peri-extubation bronchodilator therapy and extubation to noninvasive ventilation may be considered, especially in high-risk patients, in an effort to decrease the work of breathing and air trapping.[5]

### POSTOPERATIVE

Close and careful monitoring of COPD patients is necessary in the postoperative period to prevent and provide intervention for postoperative pulmonary complications. Respiratory failure resulting in reintubation is associated with significant morbidity and mortality in COPD patients. In addition to regional anesthesia techniques, non-narcotic and nonsteroidal analgesia should be considered since these options can reduce the risk of respiratory failure secondary to over-sedation from systemic opioids.[5]

## REFERENCES

1. Global Initiative for Chronic Obstructive Lung Disease (GOLD). *Global Strategy for the Diagnosis, Management and Prevention of Chronic Obstructive Pulmonary Disease: 2020 Report.* www.goldcopd.org.
2. Rabe KF, Watz H. Chronic obstructive pulmonary disease. *Lancet.* 2017;389:1931–1940.
3. Duffy SP, Criner GJ. Chronic obstructive pulmonary disease: Evaluation and management. *Med Clin North Am.* 2019;103:453–461.
4. Edrich T, Sadovnikoff N. Anesthesia for patients with severe chronic obstructive pulmonary disease. *Curr Opin Anaesthesiol.* 2010;23:18–24.
5. Hausman MS Jr, et al. Regional versus general anesthesia in surgical patients with chronic obstructive pulmonary disease: Does avoiding general anesthesia reduce the risk of postoperative complications? *Anesth Analg.* 2015;120(6):1405–1412.

# 104.

# HYPERTENSION

*Talia H. Dagher and Lauren Beck*

## INTRODUCTION

Hypertension is one of the most prevalent medical problems in the United States today, affecting almost half of the population and inevitably influencing perioperative care. It is categorized into two stages by the American College of Cardiology/American Heart Association (ACC/AHA): stage 1 is defined as a systolic blood pressure of 130–139 or a diastolic blood pressure of 80–89; and stage 2 is defined as a systolic blood pressure ≥140 or a diastolic blood pressure ≥90.[1] A diagnosis of chronic hypertension is not made on the day of surgery, but rather by primary care providers over multiple visits. It can lead to a sequela of complications including cardiac, renal, cerebral, and vascular disease; therefore early recognition and treatment are warranted. Treatment may range from lifestyle modifications, such as dietary salt restriction, to pharmacologic therapy; however, the degree of blood pressure reduction, not the choice of antihypertensive agent, is the ultimate determinant of reduction in cardiovascular risk.[2] The presence of chronic hypertension increases the risk of perioperative blood pressure lability, myocardial ischemia, ventricular dysrhythmias, and surgical bleeding; thus careful perioperative management is crucial to prevent adverse outcomes.[3]

## ANESTHETIC CONSIDERATIONS

### PREOPERATIVE

Although ideally all patients would present for surgery with optimally controlled blood pressures, most hypertensive patients present with some degree of hypertension. A common preoperative question that many anesthesiologists face is whether there is significant benefit to delaying surgery to allow for optimization of antihypertensive therapy. It is worthwhile to note that systolic blood pressures below 180 mmHg and diastolic blood pressures below 110 mmHg have not been associated with increased perioperative risks.[4] However, while the incidence of adverse cardiac events may not differ between patients who proceed with surgery and patients who are delayed for better blood pressure control, patients with preoperative hypertension have increased likelihood of developing intraoperative hypotension, myocardial ischemia, and arrhythmias.[4] Because of this increased propensity to develop intraoperative hypotension, guidelines regarding the continuation of antihypertensives preoperatively have been created by the ACC/AHA.[1]

In general, most antihypertensives should be continued up to the time of surgery. This is especially important for beta blockers and alpha agonists since holding these medications can lead to withdrawal symptoms. Many clinicians advocate for withholding angiotensin converting enzyme inhibitors (ACE-i) and angiotensin II receptor blockers (ARB) for 24 hours prior to surgery due to the associated intraoperative hypotension; however, continuing ACE-i/ARB therapy has not been shown to increase the incidence of clinically important outcomes (stroke, myocardial infarction, kidney failure, or death). The ACC/AHA guidelines therefore state that the continuation of ACE-i or ARBs perioperatively is reasonable, and that if held, these medications should be restarted as soon as clinically feasible postoperatively.[1] Diuretics, including loop and thiazide diuretics, can be associated with potassium disturbances and fluid shifts intraoperatively. If the patient is on a diuretic for heart failure, the decision to hold or continue this medication should be based on volume status preoperatively. In addition to preoperative medication management, it is reasonable to assess for signs of end organ damage. An electrocardiogram (EKG) is often normal, but in patients with long-standing hypertension it may show signs of left ventricular hypertrophy. An echocardiogram, although not routinely recommended, may be useful to measure the effects on systolic and diastolic function. Kidney function is reflected in serum creatinine levels, and serum potassium may be prudent to obtain in patients on diuretics.[4]

## INTRAOPERATIVE

The anesthetic for patients with chronic hypertension should aim to maintain an appropriately stable blood pressure range, as these patients may experience large hemodynamic swings in the operating room. This goal range is typically defined as within 20% of the patient's preoperative blood pressure.[5] This becomes particularly important in patients with long-standing or poorly controlled hypertension, as they often have altered autoregulation of cerebral blood flow and may require higher mean arterial pressures to maintain adequate cerebral perfusion.[4]

A diagnosis of hypertension alone does not necessitate invasive intra-arterial monitoring. The decision to proceed with invasive monitoring will depend on the patient's comorbidities and surgical considerations. EKG monitoring should be employed to detect any arrhythmias or ischemia. If renal insufficiency is present, careful monitoring of urine output and fluid status is prudent.[4]

Induction of anesthesia in hypertensive patients is commonly associated with an exaggerated hypotensive response, whereas the endotracheal intubation that follows is associated with an exaggerated hypertensive response. These responses may be attenuated with a combination of vasopressors, vasodilators, opioids, and other medications. No single induction agent has been proven to be superior to others. Similarly, maintenance with either volatile or intravenous anesthetic agents is acceptable, and most produce vasodilation that will counteract elevated blood pressures.[4]

If intraoperative hypertension occurs, all possible etiologies should be considered prior to attributing the cause to the patient's chronic hypertension. This differential includes sympathetic stimulation (e.g., direct laryngoscopy, surgical stimulation), pain, inadequate depth of anesthesia, hypoxia, hypercarbia, hypervolemia, bladder distension, or increased intracranial pressure. Less common causes include alcohol withdrawal, drug abuse, thyroid storm, malignant hyperthermia, and pheochromocytoma. If due to chronic hypertension, short-acting antihypertensives are most commonly used and are summarized in Table 104.1.

If intraoperative hypotension occurs, it can be treated by decreasing anesthetic depth and administering fluids and/or vasopressors. The choice of treatment depends on the type of anesthetic, patient comorbidities, volume status of the patient, and the surgical procedure. Short-acting vasoactive medications that are commonly used to treat hypotension include phenylephrine and ephedrine.

## POSTOPERATIVE

Hypertension may continue in the postoperative period and is a common problem in the post-anesthesia care unit (PACU). This is often due to pain at the surgical site, nausea

*Table 104.1* COMMON INTRAOPERATIVE ANTIHYPERTENSIVE MEDICATIONS (IV BOLUS DOSING)

| MEDICATION | STARTING DOSE | ONSET | DURATION OF ACTION |
|---|---|---|---|
| Esmolol | 10–50 mg | 1–2 min | 10–20 min |
| Hydralazine | 5–10 mg | 5–20 min | 4–8 hours |
| Labetalol | 5–20 mg | 2–5 min | 4–8 hours |
| Metoprolol | 1–5 mg | 1–5 min | 5–8 hours |
| Nicardipine | 100–500 mcg | 1–5 min | 3–4 hours |
| Nitroglycerin | 10–100 mcg | 1–2 min | 3–5 min |

and vomiting, and shivering, but it may also be caused by respiratory abnormalities, bladder distension, or an exacerbation of chronic hypertension. Postoperative hypertension should be treated promptly, as elevated blood pressures may lead to postoperative bleeding or disruption of suture lines.[4] Underlying causes should be treated and antihypertensives may be used to achieve normotension. The most commonly used antihypertensives in this setting include labetalol and hydralazine. Labetalol is given if hypertension occurs in conjunction with tachycardia, and hydralazine is given if hypertension occurs in conjunction with bradycardia. Finally, a patient's home antihypertensive regimen should be restarted as soon as oral intake is resumed.

## REFERENCES

1. Fleisher LA, et al. 2014 ACC/AHA guideline on perioperative cardiovascular evaluation and management of patients undergoing noncardiac surgery. *Circulation*. 2014;130(24):278–333.
2. Turnbull F, et al. Effects of different regimens to lower blood pressure on major cardiovascular events in older and younger adults: Meta-analysis of randomised trials. *BMJ*. 2008;336(7653):1121–1123.
3. Barash PG, et al., eds. *Clinical Anesthesia*. Philadelphia, PA: Wolters Kluwer; 2017.
4. Morgan GE, et al. *Clinical Anesthesiology*. New York, NY: Lange Medical Books/McGraw Hill Medical; 2006.
5. Salmasi V, et al. Relationship between intraoperative hypotension, defined by either reduction from baseline or absolute thresholds, and acute kidney and myocardial injury after noncardiac surgery. *Anesthesiology*. 2017;126(1):47–65.

# 105.

# MALIGNANCY

*Vicko Gluncic*

## INTRODUCTION

Cancer is the second leading cause of death globally; in the developed world, it has already started to outpace cardiovascular disease as the leading cause. While primary excision or reduction combined with chemotherapy and/or radiotherapy and/or immunotherapy may be curative, regional recurrence and metastases remain a major source of morbidity and mortality. This chapter reviews the current state of literature regarding the anesthetic considerations and potential effects of perioperative anesthetic interventions on clinical outcomes in cancer patients.[1,2]

## CHEMOTHERAPY, RADIATION, AND IMMUNOTHERAPY

Chemotherapy, immunotherapy, radiation, and surgery are techniques for cancer treatment with different side effects. The knowledge and understanding of long-term and acute side effects caused by these modalities of treatment are critical for adequate anesthetic and perioperative management.1–3

Chemotherapy can be neoadjuvant, given before surgery to reduce the tumor size; adjuvant, given during or after surgery; and palliative, given to improve the quality of life. While most of chemotherapy drugs are antiproliferative agents specifically targeting rapidly dividing cancer cells, non-malignant dividing cells are also affected. This is the main toxicity mechanism of these drugs that leads to acute and long-term effects. Awareness of the possible effects of commonly used anticancer drugs is critical for perioperative planning. The most common toxicities include pulmonary, cardiac, renal, hepatic, and gastrointestinal systems, bone marrow, and neurological damage (Table 105.1).[1]

Radiotherapy is frequently used in combination with chemotherapy, which can achieve a complete remission for esophageal, pulmonary, cervical, head and neck, rectal, and urinary bladder cancers. Radiotherapy causes tissue damage through the production of oxygen free radicals that subsequently can cause induration of the skin, extensive adhesions, vascular stenosis, myocarditis, pneumonitis,

*Table 105.1* PERIOPERATIVE CONCERNS OF COMMON CHEMOTHERAPY AND
IMMUNOTHERAPY AGENTS

| ORGAN SYSTEM | PERIOPERATIVE CONCERN | CHEMOTHERAPY DRUGS |
|---|---|---|
| Respiratory | Pulmonary oedema | Methotrexate |
| | Pulmonary fibrosis | Bleomycin, carmustine, ifosfamide, panitumumab |
| Cardiovascular | Tachycardia | Procarbazine, cladribine, alemtuzumab, trastuzumab, muromonab-CD3 |
| | Cardiac arrhythmia | Pentostatin, fludarabine, palivizumab, interferon alfa2b, erlotinib |
| | Bradycardia | Docetaxel, lenalidomide |
| | Hypotension | Pentostatin, vincristine, alemtuzumab, daclizumab, muromonab-CD3, denileukin diftitox |
| | Hypertension | Pentostatin, vinblastine, vincristine, alemtuzumab, bevacizumab, trastuzumab, daclizumab, muromonab-CD3, sorafenib, sunitinib, nilotinib |
| | Cardiomyopathy | Doxorubicin, trastuzumab, sunitinib, dasatinib, lapatinib |
| Hepatic | Coagulopathy | Asparaginase |
| Renal | Proximal tubular dysfunction | Ifosfamide |
| | Hypomagnesemia | Cisplatin, carboplatin |
| Nervous | Peripheral neuropathy | Vinblastine, vincristine, cisplatin |
| Bone marrow | Myelosuppression and anemia | Most of the agents |
| Gastrointestinal | Nausea, mucositis, and diarrhea | Most of the agents |

pulmonary fibrosis, and delayed wound healing with frequent postoperative infections. Anesthetic management of patients with head and neck cancers can be particularly challenging. While airway management of these patients may be difficult due to the site and size of the tumor, previous radiotherapy could also lead to a limited neck extension and rigidity of the oropharyngeal tissues. This can potentially make ventilation with a face mask and laryngoscopy difficult. Furthermore, mucositis as a consequence of radiotherapy can be further exacerbated by tracheal intubation while friable oropharyngeal tissue—damaged by radiation—can cause serious bleeding if injured during laryngoscopy. In addition, radiotherapy for the head and neck can lead to a difficult central venous access. This is particularly pertinent in the cases of a long-term treatment with radiotherapy and/or chemotherapy when central or peripherally inserted central venous catheter is frequently needed.[1]

Recent discoveries in cancer immunotherapy have shifted the focus of treatment from treating the disease site to treating the specific tumor's biologic characteristics and its interaction with the immunological ability of the patient to combat malignant cells. These new therapies have already dramatically changed survival and quality of life for cancer patients. Despite the rapid advances made in

the field, immuno-oncology is still in its relative beginning, with numerous challenges and hurdles yet to be overcome, including the fact that not all cancers are equal and that very few predictors of response and toxicity currently exist (Table 105.1). The hope for the immunotherapy of cancers is that it will allow moving away from the current broad "shotgun" approaches toward treatments tailored to the factors that make each cancer and host a unique pairing.[3]

## PARANEOPLASTIC SYNDROMES

Substances secreted by the tumor or antibodies directed against tumors that cross-react with other tissue cause paraneoplastic syndromes. Up to 20% of cancer patients experience paraneoplastic syndromes, but often these syndromes are unrecognized. Symptoms may occur in any organ or physiologic system. These include fever and weight loss, hematologic abnormalities, neuromuscular abnormalities, ectopic hormone production, hypercalcemia, tumor lysis syndrome, adrenal insufficiency, renal dysfunction, and acute respiratory and cardiac complications.[1]

In fact, some of these pathophysiologic disturbances, such as superior vena cava obstruction, increased intracranial pressure, pericardial tamponade, renal failure, and hypercalcemia, may present as life-threatening medical emergencies.[1]

## ANESTHETICS IMPACT ON CANCER RECURRENCE

The immune system has developed to protect us not only from infection, but also from cancerous cells. In vitro and clinical studies have indicated that surgical stress and general anesthesia can alter the patient's immune response by suppressing the cell-mediated immune defense. In fact, data suggest that anesthetics may contribute significantly to the liberation of cancer cells into the circulation and enable survival and growth of circulating tumor cells, leading to regional recurrences and metastases, and affecting long-term outcomes after cancer surgery.[2,3]

This has raised the question whether specific anesthetic techniques might improve the ability of the body to eliminate cancer cells and improve patient survival. While it is challenging to separate anesthesia effects from adverse reactions induced by the primary disease, chemo- and radiotherapy, and surgical stress, there is some evidence that local and regional anesthesia may be beneficial in reducing the risks of cancer metastases and recurrence.[2-5]

Nevertheless, studies have definitely shown that pain-related stress reaction mediated via β-adrenergic activation promotes neoplastic propagation and metastasis, and subsequently decreases survival rates.[2,4,5]

## REFERENCES

1. Arain MR, Buggy DJ. Anesthesiology for cancer patients. *Curr Opin Anesthesiol.* 2007;20:247–253.
2. Cata JP, et al. Anesthesia options and the recurrence of cancer: What we know so far? *Local Reg Anesth.* 2020;13:57–72.
3. Esfahani K, et al. A review of cancer immunotherapy: From the past, to the present, to the future. *Curr Oncol.* 2020;27(Suppl 2):S87–S97.
4. Kim R. Anesthetic technique and cancer recurrence in oncologic surgery: Unraveling the puzzle. *Cancer Metastasis Rev.* 2017;36:159–177.
5. Perry NJS, et al. Can anesthesia influence cancer outcomes after surgery? *JAMA Surg.* 2019 Apr 1;154:279–280.

# 106.

# PEDIATRIC AND GERIATRIC DOSES

*Leah Bess and Surendrasingh Chhabada*

## INTRODUCTION

Clinical pharmacology focuses on the safe and effective use of drugs and requires understanding of age-related changes in pharmacokinetics and pharmacodynamics to determine optimal dosing in different patient populations. *Pharmacokinetics* describes how drugs are handled within the body and involves the principles of absorption, distribution, metabolism, and elimination. Changes in any of these parameters alters the amount of free drug in the circulation and subsequent delivery of the drug to the target site. *Pharmacodynamics* is often described as the effects of the drug on the body, which also varies with physiological process of ageing.

## PHARMACOKINETIC DIFFERENCES IN PEDIATRICS

The Food and Drug Administration (FDA) Guidance (1998) divided the pediatric population into groups based on age, as shown in Table 106.1.

These groups differ in pharmacokinetics and pharmacodynamics due to alterations in body composition, increased

**Table 106.1** AGE RANGES OF PEDIATRIC SUBPOPULATION

| Premature Neonate | Born before 38 Weeks Gestational Age |
|---|---|
| Neonate | 0–4 weeks postnatal age |
| Infants | 1 month–1 years of age |
| Children | 2–12 years of age |
| Adolescents | 12–16 years of age |

volume of distribution, decreased body fat and muscle mass as a portion of body weight, decreased protein binding, and immature renal hepatic function.

Pharmacokinetic differences in these groups can be realized by understanding the differences of drug absorption, distribution, metabolism, and elimination in them.

## ABSORPTION

Several age-related anatomical and physiological changes of the gastrointestinal (GI) tract affect oral drug absorption. Gastric pH is neutral at birth but falls to pH 1–3 within 24 to 48 hours after birth. The pH then gradually returns to neutral again by day 8 and subsequently declines very slowly, reaching adult values only after 2 years of age.[1] Reduced gastric acid secretion increases bioavailability of acid-labile drugs (e.g., penicillin) and decreases bioavailability of weakly acidic drugs (e.g., acetaminophen, phenytoin, and phenobarbital). Similarly, neonates have reduced bile salt formation, decreasing bioavailability of lipophilic drugs (e.g., diazepam).[2] Gastric emptying and intestinal motility are also reduced; therefore it takes longer for enteral drugs to reach therapeutic concentration. Drug-metabolizing enzymes and reduced microbial flora in young infants can also decrease drug absorption.

## DISTRIBUTION

Children have increased total body water, which results in increased volume of distribution for water-soluble drugs and therefore requires a higher loading dose. Reduced levels of total protein, albumin, and α1-acid glycoprotein results in increased free fraction of medications and can increase risk of local anesthetic toxicity.

## METABOLISM AND ELIMINATION

Immature hepatic and renal systems result in decreased metabolism of drugs and prolonged duration of action. Creatinine clearance is calculated to estimate glomerular filtration rate (GFR), and if it is reduced then reduction in drug dosage is recommended. Medications are thus typically administered in smaller and more frequent doses and are dosed according to body weight (mg/kg) as described in Table 106.2 or body surface area (BSA, kg/m²), resulting in more precise dosing despite significant heterogeneity in the pediatric population.

Drug administration in children typically occurs via the oral route except in hospital settings or emergencies where parenteral administration is preferred. Other routes used in pediatrics include rectal, cutaneous, nasal, and inhalation. Transdermal absorption of drugs may be enhanced in neonates and young infants as they have increased permeability of their skin and also have a higher body surface area to weight ratio. Intramuscular injections are generally avoided in children because of pain and the possibility of tissue damage. Water-soluble drugs are thus preferred as they do not precipitate at the injection site.

## PHARMACOKINETIC DIFFERENCES IN GERIATRICS

Aging is an irreversible and progressive physiological process that is characterized by degenerative changes in the structure and function of many organs and tissues. The nervous system experiences cognitive decline and loss of volume, which increases sensitivity to sedatives and anesthetics and also puts older patients at risk for delirium. Diminished cardiac reserve with comorbidities and polypharmacy puts them further at risk for side effects. Delayed gastric emptying, increased gastric pH, slowed intestinal transit time, and reduced splanchnic blood flow in older adults can affect drug absorption.[3] Elderly patients are thus at increased risk for aspiration during perioperative period. Changes in body composition include decreased total body water and muscle mass and increased percentage of body fat. This results in a significantly increased volume of distribution, extended clearance, and prolonged half-life for lipid-soluble medications (e.g., benzodiazepines). For water-soluble drugs (e.g., digoxin, lithium) the volume of distribution is decreased and so smaller doses are required to avoid toxicity. The elderly also have a lower plasma concentration of albumin leading to decreased drug binding and increased free fraction of drugs that are highly protein bound (e.g., phenytoin, warfarin) and require measurement of their levels. Decreased liver size and reduced hepatic blood flow result in reduced drug metabolism and decreased clearance of high extraction ratio drugs. Reduced renal mass, renal blood flow, GFR, tubular secretion, and filtration result in impaired renal clearance and decreased elimination of renally excreted drugs. Transdermal absorption of drugs in elderly patients is also extremely variable and slow (see Table 106.3).

Table 106.2 COMMONLY USED PHARMACOLOGIC AGENTS IN PEDIATRIC ANESTHESIA

| | DRUG | ROUTE | DOSE | UNIT | |
|---|---|---|---|---|---|
| **PREMEDICATION** | | | | | |
| Midazolam | | PO | 0.5–0.75 | mg/kg | (Max 10–15 mg) |
| | | Intranasal | 0.1–0.2 | mg/kg | |
| | | Sublingual | 0.2 | mg/kg | |
| | | IV | 0.05–0.15 | mg/kg | |
| Dexmedetomidine | | Nasal | 1–2 | mcg/kg | |
| | | IV | 0.5–1 | mcg/kg | |
| Ketamine | | PO | 6–10 | mg/kg | |
| | | IM | | mg/kg | |
| Glycopyrrolate | | IV | 10 | mcg/kg | |
| Atropine | | IV | 10–20 | mcg/kg | |
| | | IM | 20 | mcg/kg | |
| **IV ANESTHETICS** | | | | | |
| Propofol | Induction | IV Bolus | 2–3 | mg/kg | |
| | Maintenance | IV Infusion | 50–300 | mcg/kg/min | |
| Ketamine | Sedation | IV Bolus | 0.5–1 | mg/kg | |
| | Induction | IV Bolus | 1–2 | mg/kg | |
| | Maintenance | IV Infusion | 25–75 | mcg/kg/min | |
| Etomidate | Induction | IV | 0.2–0.3 | mg/kg | |
| Methohexital | Induction | IV | 1–2 | mg/kg | |
| | | PR | 25 | mg/kg | |
| **OPIOIDS** | | | | | |
| Fentanyl | | IV Bolus | 0.5–2 | mcg/kg | |
| | | IV Infusion | 1–2 | mcg/kg/hr | |
| | | IM | 1–2 | mcg/kg | |
| Morphine | | IV Bolus | 0.05–0.1 | mg/kg | (Max 2 mg/dose) |
| | | IV Infusion | 10–60 | mg/kg/hr | |
| Hydromorphone | | IV | 10–15 | mcg/kg | |
| Oxycodone | | PO | 0.05–0.15 | mg/kg | |
| Remifentanil | | IV Bolus | 0.5–1 | mcg/kg | |
| | | IV Infusion | 0.1–0.5 | mcg/kg/min | |
| **NSAIDs** | | | | | |
| Acetaminophen | Preterm | PO | 10–15 q6h | mg/kg mg/kg mg/kg | (Max single dose 1 g |
| | Term Neonates | PR | 20 q6h | mg/kg | (Max 90 mg/kg/day) |
| | Children <50 kg | IV | 10 q8h | mg/kg | (Max 22.5–40 mg/kg/day) |
| | Children >50kg | IV | 10 q6h | mg/kg | (Max 60 mg/kg/day) |
| | | IV | 15 q6h | | (Max 3750 mg/day |
| | | IV | 15 q6h | | (Max 4 g/day) |
| Ketorolac | | IV/IM | 0.5 q6h | mg/kg | (Max 30 mg/dose, 120 mg/day) |
| Ibuprofen | >6mo | PO/IV | 10 q6h | mg/kg | |

(continued)

*Table 106.2* CONTINUED

| DRUG | | ROUTE | DOSE | UNIT | |
|------|---|-------|------|------|---|
| **NEUROMUSCULAR BLOCKERS** | | | | | |
| Succinylcholine | | IV | 2–3 | mg/kg | *Consider anticholinergic to |
| | | IM* | 4–6 | mg/kg | prevent bradycardia |
| Rocuronium | | IV | 0.6–1.2 | mg/kg | |
| | | IM | 1.2 | mg/kg | |
| Cisatracurium | | IV | 0.1–0.2 | mg/kg | |
| Vecuronium | | IV | 0.1 | mg/kg | |
| Pancuronium | | IV | 0.1 | mg/kg | |
| Atracurium | | IV | 0.5 | mg/kg | |
| **REVERSAL AGENTS** | | | | | |
| Neostigmine | | IV | 35–70 | mcg/kg | (Max 5 mg) |
| Plus glycopyrrolate | | IV | 7–14 | mcg/kg | |
| Sugammadex | Moderate block | IV | 2–4 | mg/kg | |
| | Deep block | IV | 8–16 | mg/kg | |
| Flumazenil | | IV | 10 q1min | mcg/kg | (Max 1 mg, 0.2 mg/dose) |
| Naloxone | | IV | 10–100 | mcg/kg | (Duration 20 min) |
| | | ET | 0.1 | mg/kg | (Max 2 mg) |
| **ANTIEMETICS** | | | | | |
| Dexamethasone | AW edema | IM, IV | 0.5 | mg/kg | (Max 10 mg) |
| | PONV | IV | 0.15 | mg/kg | (Max 4 mg) |
| Ondansetron | >6 mo | IV | 0.1–0.15 | mg/kg | (Max 4 mg) |
| **VASOACTIVES** | | | | | |
| Dobutamine | | IV | 2.5–10 | mcg/kg/min | |
| Dopamine | | IV | 2.5–10 | mcg/kg/min | |
| Milrinone | Load | IV Bolus | 50–100 | mcg/kg | |
| | Infusion | IV | 0.25–0.75 | mcg/kg/min | |
| Epinephrine | Racemic (2.25%) | IV Bolus | 10 | mcg/kg | (Dilute w/ 3 ml 0.9% NaCl) |
| | | IV Infusion | 0.05–0.3 | mcg/kg/min | |
| | | ET | 100 | mcg/kg | |
| | | Nebulized | 0.05 | ml/kg | |
| Vasopressin | | IV | 0.02–0.05 | units/kg/hr | |
| Norepinephrine | | IV | 0.1–1 | mcg/kg/min | |
| Phenylephrine | | IV Bolus | 1–10 | mcg/kg | |
| | | IV Infusion | 0.1–1 | mcg/kg/min | |
| Ephedrine | | IV | 0.2–0.3 | mg/kg | (Max 30 mg/dose) |
| | | IM | 0.5 | mg/kg | |
| **EMERGENCY/RESUSCITATION** | | | | | |
| Adenosine | Rapid flush | IV | 0.1 | mg/kg | (Max 12 mg) |
| | Subsequent dose | IV | 0.2 | mg/kg | |
| Amiodarone | Load (30–60 min) | IV | 5 | mg/kg | (Max 300 mg) |
| | Infusion | IV | 5–10 | mcg/kg/min | |
| Lidocaine | Load | IV Bolus | 1 | mg/kg | |
| | Infusion | IV | 20–50 | mcg/kg/min | |

*Table 106.2* CONTINUED

| | DRUG | ROUTE | DOSE | UNIT | |
|---|---|---|---|---|---|
| Magnesium sulfate (torsades) | | IV | 25–50 | mg/kg | (Max 2 g) |
| Calcium | Chloride | IV | 5–10 | mg/kg | |
| | Gluconate | IV | 10–30 | mg/kg | |
| Sodium bicarbonate | | IV | 1 | mEq/kg | |
| Dantrolene | Load | IV | 2.5(q5min) | mg/kg | (Max 30 mg/kg) |
| | Maintenance | IV | 1.2 | mg/kg/hr | |
| Intralipid (20%) | Bolus | IV | 1.5 | ml/kg | (Over 1 min, max 10 ml/kg) |
| | Infusion | IV | 0.25–0.5 | ml/kg/min | |
| Defibrillation | Asynchronous | | 2 | J/kg | (Then 4 J/kg x2) |
| Cardioversion | Synchronous | | 0.5–1 | J/kg | (Then double) |

STEROIDS

| | DRUG | ROUTE | DOSE | UNIT | |
|---|---|---|---|---|---|
| Dexamethasone | | IV | 0.1–0.5 | mg/kg | (Max 10 mg/dose) |
| Hydrocortisone | | IV | 1–2 | mg/kg | |
| Methylprednisolone | | IV | 2–4 | mg/kg | |

ANTIHISTAMINES

| | DRUG | ROUTE | DOSE | UNIT | |
|---|---|---|---|---|---|
| Diphenhydramine | | IV, IM PO | 1–1.25 | mg/kg | (Max 25–50 mg) |
| Ranitidine | | IV | 0.25–1 | mg/kg | |
| Famotidine | | | 0.15 | mg/kg | |
| Hydrocortisone | | IV | 1–2 | mg/kg | |
| Methylprednisolone | | IV | 2–4 | mg/kg | |

LOCAL ANESTHETICS

| | DRUG | ROUTE | DOSE | UNIT | |
|---|---|---|---|---|---|
| Lidocaine | w/o | | 3–5 | mg/kg | |
| | w/ epi 1:200,000 | | 5–7 | mg/kg | |
| Bupivacaine | | | 2–2.5 | mg/kg | |
| Ropivacaine | | | 2.5 | mg/kg | |

IV = intravenous; IM = intramuscular; PO = per oral; ET = endotracheal; PR = per rectum; SL = sublingual.

*Table 106.3* DRUG DOSING IN GERIATRIC PATIENTS

| DRUG | | CHANGE IN DOSE | CLINICAL EFFECTS |
|---|---|---|---|
| SEDATIVES/HYPNOTICS | | | |
| Propofol | Induction | 50% reduction | Based on lean body mass |
| | Infusion | 50% reduction | |
| Etomidate | Induction | 25–50% reduction | |
| Midazolam | Preop/Intraop | 50–75% reduction | Increased risk of postoperative delirium |
| OPIOIDS | | | |
| Morphine | IV | 50% reduction | Morphone-6-glucuronide accumulation prolongs duration and increases risk of seizures |
| Fentanyl | IV | 50% reduction | |
| Remifentanil | Bolus | 50% reduction | Increase incidence of bradycardia w/ bolus dosing |
| | Infusion | 50% reduction | |

## REFERENCES

1. Fernandez E, et al. Factors and mechanisms for pharmacokinetic differences between pediatric population and adults. *Pharmaceutics.* 2011;3(1):53–72.
2. Anderson G. Children versus adults: Pharmacokinetic and adverse-effect differences. *Epilepsia.* 2002;43: 53–59.
3. Hämmerlein A, et al. Pharmacokinetic and pharmacodynamic changes in the elderly: Clinical implications. *Clin Pharmacokinet.* 1998;35(1):49–64.
4. Hutchison LC, O'Brien CE. Changes in pharmacokinetics and pharmacodynamics in the elderly patient. *J Pharm Pract.* 2007; 20(1), 4–12.

# 107.

# ANESTHETIC MANAGEMENT OF PATIENTS WITH ALLERGIES

*Brook Girma and Alan D. Kaye*

## INTRODUCTION

The strongest preventive measure of adverse allergy reactions in patients is performing a detailed preoperative evaluation and obtaining a thorough history of prior allergies and types of reactions to these allergens. Prior to surgery, it is important for the anesthesiologist to gather any clinical or past medical history, especially those involving medications and latex. It is also important to gather patient history of allergies to food or any other specific allergen which may suggest cross reactivity and may require a change in anesthetic management. Intraoperative drug anaphylaxis contributes to 4.3% of deaths occurring during general anesthesia, making adverse drug reactions one of the most common causes of morbidity and mortality in anesthesia. Penicillin allergy is the most reported drug allergy, with up to 10% of all patients reporting some degree of penicillin allergy.

## TYPES OF DRUG ALLERGY

Drug allergy is an immunological reaction elicited by medications. It is commonly divided into four different categories based on the cellular and molecular mechanisms of pathogenesis: (1) type 1 allergy is an immediate reaction generally mediated by immunoglobin E (IgE) activation on mast cells and basophils; (2) type 2 allergy is a delayed reaction generally related to IgG-mediated cell destruction; (3) type 3 reaction is generally mediated by the IgG-drug complex and the activation of complement systems; and (4) type 4 reaction generally has a delayed onset caused by T cell activation. Type 4 reaction has been considered the most common type of reaction.

## PREMEDICATION PROPHYLAXIS

Prophylactic treatments with corticosteroids alone or in combination with H1 antagonist have provided some benefit in clinical practice but remain a matter of debate. Premedication should be used with caution, as it does not prevent a hypersensitivity reaction but rather attenuates the response. Ultimately, there is no evidence that pretreatment can effectively prevent the onset or reduce the severity and could possibly delay the reaction, making it more difficult to recognize early signs of anaphylaxis.[1]

## PERIOPERATIVE APPROACH TO ALLERGIES

Common causes of pertinent perioperative culprits of allergic reactions include but are not limited to opioids, neuromuscular blocking agents (NMBAs), antibiotics, latex, radiographic contrast material, IgA deficiency, chlorhexadine or iodine. Patients involving allergies to NMBAs or opioids may require modification of the anesthetic plan. NMBAs are one of the most common causes of perioperative anaphylaxis, responsible for 50%–70% of perioperative hypersensitivity reactions. Local anesthetics, regional anesthesia, or inhaled anesthetics are effective alternatives. When it is mandatory to administer an NMBA or opioid in a patient with a previous allergy to a drug in this class, an incremental challenge with an NMBA or opioid different from that, which elicited the reaction, should be used.[1] If a patient has a history of allergies to penicillins, the best choice is to find an alternative antibiotic without penicillin like characteristics or molecular structure. It would also be useful to separate the administration of prophylactic antibiotic therapy and anesthetic induction in order to identify and treat the reaction as early as possible.[2] It should be noted that propofol allergic reaction occurs at an incidence of 1:60,000 exposures. Factors of concern include multiple surgical procedures, history of asthma or atopy, and advanced age.[4] Female gender and frequent prescription of antibiotics for short-term use are additional well-documented risk factors for perioperative hypersensitivity.[3]

Be aware that subsequent exposure to a known culprit agent may cause a greater response, potentially a life-threatening reaction. It is also important to appropriately time the administration of medications or antibiotics to allow time to detect possible anaphylaxis.[4]

## REFERENCES

1. Caffarellii C, et al. Prevention of allergic reactions in anesthetized patients. vol. 24. 2011.
2. Laguna JJ, et al. Practical guidelines for perioperative hypersensitivity reactions. *J Investig Allergol Clin Immunol*. 2018;28:216–232.
3. Patil SS, et al. Multiple drug allergies: Recommendations for perioperative management. *Best Pract Res Clin Anaesthesiol*. 2020.
4. Osman BM, et al. Case report: Management of differential diagnosis and treatment of severe anaphylaxis in the setting of spinal anesthesia. *J Clin Anesth*. 2016;35:145–149.

# 108.

# NPO STATUS AND FULL STOMACH

*Mallory Nebergall and Mazin T. Albert*

## INTRODUCTION

Aspiration of gastric contents during the perioperative period is a rare but serious event with significant morbidity and mortality. Aspiration increases the risk of prolonged intubation, pneumonitis, acute respiratory distress syndrome (ARDS), hypoxia from obstruction, infection, or even death. The incidence of pulmonary aspiration during the perioperative period ranges from 0.7 to 4.7 per 10,000 nonpregnant adults, 5.3 per 10,000 pregnant patients, and 3.8 to 10.2 per 10,000 children. Identification of patients during the perioperative period with elevated risk for aspiration allows for the implementation of risk-reduction strategies imperative for the safe delivery of anesthesia.[1–3]

## FASTING RECOMMENDATIONS

Fasting guidelines apply to healthy, nonlaboring individuals of all ages undergoing elective surgery with general or regional anesthesia, or procedural sedation to allow for sufficient gastric emptying, thereby reducing the risk of aspiration or complications related to aspiration should it occur (Table 108.1). Compliance with these recommendations should be verified at the time of procedure and if not followed, risks and benefits of proceeding

*Table 108.1* 2011 EVIDENCE-BASED ASA GUIDELINES FOR FASTING TIMES[1]

| INGESTED MATERIAL | MINIMUM FASTING TIME |
| --- | --- |
| Clear liquids | 2 hours |
| Breast milk | 4 hours |
| Infant formula | 6 hours |
| Nonhuman milk | 6 hours |
| Light meal | 6 hours |
| Full meal | 8 hours |

with surgery should be discussed with the surgical team and patient.

## CLEAR LIQUIDS

Clear liquids, including those used with enhanced recovery protocols, water, carbonated beverages, fruit juices without pulp, clear tea, and black coffee, may be consumed up to 2 hours prior to surgery. This excludes protein-containing carbohydrate drinks (no consumption within 3 hours before surgery) and alcoholic beverages. After 90 minutes, the stomach is empty of clear liquids with no change in gastric pH regardless of the type of overnight fasting, and this is why clear liquids are allowed up until 2 hours prior to surgery.[4]

## OTHER LIQUIDS

Non-clear liquids should be avoided 6 hours prior to elective procedures, as they empty the stomach more slowly and may leave residual particulate matter (for example, milk may curdle in the stomach and behave as a solid).[4]

## BREAST MILK

Breast milk can be ingested at least 4 hours before an elective procedure.

## INFANT FORMULA

Infant formula can be ingested at least 6 hours before an elective procedure.

## SOLIDS

A light meal, such as dry toast or cereal with clear liquids, can be consumed 6 hours prior to elective surgery, or a full meal 8 hours before elective surgery.[4]

## ENTERAL TUBE FEEDS

Enteral formulas often contain carbohydrates, protein, and fat, and are thus considered a fatty meal and are stopped 8 hours prior to anesthesia. Patients with a surgically placed post-pyloric feeding tube may continue feeds until the time of non-abdominal surgery.[4]

## GUM

Chewing gum generates saliva and stimulates gastric secretion, and for this reason is considered equivalent to clear liquids and should be stopped 2 hours prior to anesthesia. In the event a patient chews gum up until time of surgery, surgery should not be delayed given the lack of studies showing effects on gastric acid volume or pH under this circumstance. However, if the patient swallows his/her gum, this should now be treated as a solid intake and therefore a delay of procedure for 6 hours.

## MEDICATIONS

Medications taken the morning of surgery should be with a sip of water or clear liquid, ideally several hours prior to surgery. If a solid, such as applesauce, is required to take medication, this is treated as a solid and should be taken 6 hours prior to surgery.

## FULL STOMACH

The term *full stomach* refers to the presence of residual solid or liquid food in the stomach at time of induction of anesthesia, a condition that places the patient at risk for regurgitation and aspiration. A full stomach is assumed for all emergency cases, patients with gastric motility disorders, and those with diabetes. For emergency cases, surgery cannot be delayed to allow for full gastric emptying; therefore, attention should be directed at optimizing the anesthetic plan to decrease the risk of aspiration as well as the risk of morbidity and mortality in the event aspiration occurs.

## ANESTHETIC CONSIDERATIONS

### PREOPERATIVE

Identifying those at increased risk for aspiration during the perioperative period is important for optimization of the delivery of safe anesthesia. *Nil per os* (NPO) status and patient-specific risk factors (Box 108.1) need to be considered.

Interventions such as gastric decompression using a nasogastric tube or even reducing the acidity of gastric contents with medications such as H2 blockers or proton

**Box 108.1** RISK FACTORS FOR ASPIRATION

Oropharyngeal dysfunction (due to stroke)
Esophageal/gastric dysmotility disorders (diabetes, autonomic neuropathy)
Advanced age
Bowel obstruction
Obesity
Pregnancy
Emergency surgery
Trauma
Decreased level of consciousness
Patient positioning (lithotomy, Trendelenburg)
General anesthesia

pump inhibitors can also be used in an attempt to decrease the risk of aspiration.

## INTRAOPERATIVE

Rapid sequence intubation, application of cricoid pressure during intubation, and placement of an endotracheal tube are all intraoperative strategies to help reduce the chance of aspiration. Attention should also be given to patient positioning, such as torso elevation prior to induction and minimizing positions that would increase the risk for aspiration.[2]

## POSTOPERATIVE

In the event aspiration occurs, treatment strategies are broad, including supportive care, suctioning gastric contents, or even antibiotic administration. Steroids have not shown to be of benefit in the event of aspiration of gastric contents.

## REFERENCES

1. American Society of Anesthesiologists Committee on Standards and Practice Parameters. Practice guidelines for preoperative fasting and the use of pharmacologic agents to reduce the risk of pulmonary aspiration: Application to healthy patients undergoing elective procedures. *Anesthesiology*. 2011;114:495–511.
2. Apfelbaum JL, et al. Practice guidelines for preoperative fasting and the use of pharmacologic agents to reduce the risk of pulmonary aspiration: Application to healthy patients undergoing elective procedures. *Anesthesiology*. 2011;114(3):495–511.
3. Englehardt T, Webster NR. Pulmonary aspiration of gastric contents in anaesthesia. *Brit J Anaes* 1999;83(3):453–460.
4. Practice guidelines for preoperative fasting and the use of pharmacologic agents to reduce the risk of pulmonary aspiration: Application to healthy patients undergoing elective procedures: An updated report by the American Society of Anesthesiologists Task Force on Preoperative Fasting and the Use of Pharmacologic Agents to Reduce the Risk of Pulmonary Aspiration. *Anesthesiology* 2017; 126:376.

# 109.

# ALTERATION OF GASTRIC FLUID VOLUME, PH, AND SPHINCTER TONE

*Sean Beplate and Kenneth Toth*

## INTRODUCTION

Practicing anesthesia safely must always include an evaluation of a patient's aspiration risk, regardless of the surgical procedure to be performed. Pulmonary aspiration with clinical findings has an occurrence of roughly one in every 2,100–3,500 elective surgical cases and a much higher incidence in emergency cases, roughly one in every 600 to 800 cases. The mortality rate associated with such events is one in every 45,000 to 70,000 events.[1] In order to minimize the chance and severity of aspiration events, efforts should be taken to maximize gastric emptying, minimize gastric volume, and increase gastric pH when indicated.

Prior to planned surgery, patients are asked to restrict oral intake with the intent of minimizing gastric fluid volume to reduce the risk of aspiration. The goal is for a gastric volume of less than 25–30 mL preoperatively.[1] In cases of aspiration, gastric volumes of 0.4 mL/kg and greater are associated with poorer outcomes.[2] When considering gastric volume status, it is vital to be aware that patients presenting with ileus or bowel obstruction are at risk of increased gastric volumes. Additionally, any predisposition to delayed gastric emptying will also increase the risk of larger gastric volumes. Conditions and comorbidities of abdominal trauma, altered consciousness, pregnancy, renal failure, and gastroparesis resulting from diabetic autonomic neuropathy can all interfere with gastric emptying. Finally, multiple medications routinely administered by anesthesia providers, such as opioids and antimuscarinics, can also prolong gastric emptying times.[1]

The lower esophageal sphincter (LES) typically prevents both reflux and regurgitation of gastric fluid. Thus regurgitation risk is increased with any condition that decreases LES tone, such as gastroesophageal reflux disease (GERD), hiatal hernia, and pregnancy. Regurgitation risk also increases any time that intra-abdominal pressure can increase to levels greater than the pressure generated by the LES; this can be seen with laparoscopic surgeries and with abdominal compartment syndrome. Lastly, opioids and antimuscarinics also decrease LES tone.[1]

The dopamine antagonist metoclopramide increases LES tone, promotes relaxation of both the pylorus and duodenum, and increases gastrointestinal motility; 10 mg of metoclopramide should be given orally 30–60 minutes prior to induction, or 10 mg intravenously administered over 3–5 minutes given 15 to 30 minutes prior to induction.[1,2] A sub-therapeutic dose of oral erythromycin (200 mg) can also be given 1 hour prior to induction to increase gastric emptying, with the effect mediated by erythromycin binding to gut motilin receptors.[1,3]

Gastric content pH is the factor with the most influence on injury severity in cases of aspiration, with radiologic evidence of injury being seen within a few hours. Worse outcomes following aspiration correlate with gastric content pH less than 2.5. Acidity of gastric contents can be altered preoperatively using medications with various mechanisms of action. First, histamine-2 (H2) receptor antagonists decrease gastric acid secretion, thus increasing gastric fluid pH while decreasing gastric fluid volume.[1,2] Famotidine has been found to be effective when given hours before surgery, whereas ranitidine has been shown to be effective when given 30–45 minutes before surgery.[2,4] Proton-pump inhibitors also prevent gastric acid secretion, and have been found to be most effective when two repeated doses are given the night before and then again the morning of surgery. In emergent situations, the nonparticulate antacid sodium citrate can be given within an hour of proceeding to surgery and is capable of providing a rapid increase in gastric pH above 2.5.[1,2]

## REFERENCES

1. Barash P. *Clinical Anesthesia Fundamentals*. Philadelphia, PA: Wolters Kluwer Medical; 2019:534–546.
2. Freeman B, Berger J. *Anesthesiology Core Review Part One: Basic Exam*. Washington, DC: McGraw Hill Education;2014:188–189.
3. Lee A, Kim C. The effect of erythromycin on gastrointestinal motility in subtotal gastrectomized patients. *J Korean Surg Soc*. 2012;82(3):149.
4. Rout C, et al. Intravenous ranitidine reduces the risk of acid aspiration of gastric contents at emergency cesarean section. *Obstet Gynecol Surv*. 1993;48(11):734–735.

# 110.

# CONTINUATION VS. DISCONTINUATION OF CHRONIC MEDICATIONS

*Robert P. Schroell III and Ronald Harter*

## INTRODUCTION

It is imperative for the anesthesiologist to thoroughly understand the impact of preoperative medications on the perioperative setting, since both surgery and anesthesia may affect drug absorption, metabolism, and elimination.[1,2] This chapter highlights recommendations for the perioperative management of chronic medications by drug class (Table 110.1), and will aim to broadly identify the risks and benefits of their continuation or discontinuation in the perioperative setting.

## CARDIOVASCULAR

### STATINS

Statins should be always be continued perioperatively. Patients that continue their home statin therapy have a lower mortality rate.[3]

### ANTIHYPERTENSIVES, DIGOXIN, AND ANTIARRHYTHMICS

There are variations in the recommendations for the continuation of major blood pressure medications. Angiotensin converting enzyme (ACE) inhibitors and angiotensin receptor blockers (ARBs) should be held the day prior to surgery.[1,3] In contrast, beta blockers and calcium channel blockers (CCBs) should be continued including the day of surgery.[3,4] There is a theoretical risk of bronchospasm from beta-2 receptor antagonism. Nevertheless, patients with chronic use of propranolol or other non-selective beta blockers are advised to continue taking these medications on the day of surgery.

Both beta blockers and CCBs have also been found to decrease arrhythmias and diminish myocardial ischemia

in patients undergoing noncardiac surgery.[4] Importantly, however, beta-blocker therapy should not be initiated on the day of surgery, since this carries a risk for adverse outcomes. Finally, patients on long-term antiarrhythmics and/or digoxin should continue these medications on the day of surgery.

## DIURETICS

Diuretics decrease intravascular volume, which can lead to intraoperative hypovolemia, decreased preload, and hypotension, as well as electrolyte derangements. As a result of this, diuretics should be discontinued one day prior to surgery, unless the patient has diuretic-dependent heart failure.

## ANTI-ANGINALS

The decision to continue/discontinue anti-anginal medications such as nitroglycerin and nicardipine must be individualized, based on the risk of hypotension and/or hypertension.

## ANTICOAGULANTS

Most therapeutic anticoagulants, including warfarin, as well as direct oral anticoagulants, are discontinued several days prior to surgery due to the increased risk of surgical bleeding. The timing of holding therapeutic heparin and low molecular weight heparin is dependent on the indication for systemic anticoagulation, risk of surgical bleeding, and surgeon preference. Aside from certain circumstances, venous thromboembolism prophylaxis may be continued on the day of surgery. If central neuraxial or certain peripheral nerve blocks are planned, please refer to guidelines for recommendations for perioperative anticoagulant administration.[5]

*Table 110.1* QUICK REFERENCE FOR MEDICATIONS TO BE CONTINUED AND DISCONTINUED PRIOR TO SURGERY

| CONTINUE | HOLD/STOP |
|---|---|
| *Cardiac* | *Cardiac* |
| Alpha 1 blocker | ACEi/ARBs |
| Alpha 2 agonist | Diuretics |
| Beta blocker | |
| Antiarrhythmic | *Hemostasis-Affecting Agents* |
| Phosphodiesterase inhibitors (stop if used for erectile dysfunction) | Non-aspirin NSAIDs |
| | Warfarin |
| Calcium channel blockers | GII/IIIb receptor blocker |
| Digoxin | Direct thrombin inhibitors |
| Statins | TPA/alteplase |
| *Hemostasis-Affecting Agents* | *Pulmonary* |
| COX-2 inhibitors | Theophylline |
| Aspirin | |
| P2Y12 receptor blockers (depends on surgery) | *Endocrine* |
| | Short-acting insulin |
| *Pulmonary* | Oral diabetic meds and SGLT2-inhibitors |
| Short-acting beta agonists | Hormonal therapy |
| Long-acting beta agonists | Selective estrogen receptor modulators |
| Leukotriene inhibitors | |
| Corticosteroids (inhaled and oral) | *Psychiatric* |
| | Stimulants |
| *Endocrine* | *Herbal* |
| Thyroid medications | All |
| Oral corticosteroids | |
| *Gastrointestinal* | |
| Proton pump inhibitors | |
| H2 blockers | |
| Aminosalicylates | |
| *Neurological* | |
| Antiepileptic | |
| Anticholinesterase inhibitors | |
| Acetaminophen | |
| Gabapentin | |
| Parkinson's medications | |
| Chronic opioids | |
| Baclofen | |
| *Psychiatric* | |
| Selective serotonin reuptake inhibitors | |
| Serotonin norepinephrine reuptake inhibitors | |
| Antianxiety medications | |
| Benzodiazepines | |
| Antipsychotics | |

## ANTIPLATELETS

For most surgical procedures, low-dose aspirin may be continued perioperatively to reduce the risk of vascular, thromboembolic, and cardiac events. Other medications that impair platelet function are generally discontinued 3–5 days prior to surgery. The decision to hold these medications should be made in conjunction with the surgeon and cardiologist, again in keeping with recognized guidelines if a regional block is planned.[1,5]

## PHOSPHODIESTERASE INHIBITORS

If taken for erectile dysfunction, phosphodiesterase inhibitors should be held perioperatively. However, if prescribed for pulmonary hypertension, a discussion with the patient's primary care team should be initiated to determine its continuation or discontinuation.

# PULMONARY

## BETA-AGONISTS, ANTICHOLINERGICS, LEUKOTRIENES, STEROIDS, AND THEOPHYLLINE

Medications used to control asthma and chronic obstructive pulmonary disease can decrease the risk of postoperative pulmonary complications and should be continued the day of surgery.[3] Special consideration should be made for theophylline due to its narrow therapeutic window and increased risk of cardiac and neurotoxicity; this medication should typically be stopped the night before surgery.

# ENDOCRINE

## THYROID MEDICATIONS

Long-term thyroid supplementation and anti-thyroid medications should be continued the day of surgery to decrease risk of myxedema coma and thyroid storm, respectively.[3]

## STEROIDS

Patients taking long-term chronic steroids should continue to take their prescribed dose the morning of surgery, and the anesthesiologist should be aware of the need for possible stress-dose steroids intraoperatively.

## ANTIDIABETICS AND ANTIHYPERGLYCEMICS

All oral antihyperglycemic medications should be continued until the day prior to surgery except Sodium-glucose transporter 2 (SGLT2) inhibitors, which should be discontinued 2–4 days preoperatively, depending on the agent.[3] All short-acting insulins should typically be held the day of surgery, while the recommended dose of long-acting insulin the night before is dependent on whether the patient is a type 1 or type 2 diabetic. Type 1 diabetic patients should take one-third to one-half of their normal long-acting insulin; type 2 diabetic patients can take none to one-half of their normal dose.[3]

## CONTRACEPTIVES, HORMONAL THERAPY, AND ESTROGEN MODULATORS

Due to the prothrombic effects of estrogen, it is recommended that selective estrogen receptor modulators and hormone-replacement therapy be discontinued 4 weeks prior to surgery to reduce the risk of venous thromboembolism. Special consideration should be given to women of childbearing age who take modern oral contraceptives, which generally have a low estrogen content. Risks of unintended pregnancy with the discontinuation of oral contraceptives should be discussed with all patients.

## GASTROINTESTINAL

### H2 BLOCKERS AND PROTON PUMP INHIBITORS

It is recommended that H2 blockers and proton pump inhibitors (PPIs) be continued on the day of surgery.[3] These agents decrease the gastric volume and acidity of gastric contents, thereby reducing the risk of aspiration, chemical pneumonitis, and stress ulcers.

## PSYCHIATRIC

### SSRIS/SNRIS, TCAS, MAO-INHIBITORS, ANTIPSYCHOTICS, MOOD STABILIZERS, AND STIMULANTS

Many psychotropic medications should be continued during the perioperative period due to risk of withdrawal.[1,3] Ephedrine and meperidine should be avoided perioperatively due to the risk of hypertensive crisis and toxic metabolite accumulation. Stimulants such as amphetamines and methylphenidate should also be held the day prior to surgery.

## CHRONIC PAIN

### NSAIDS, OPIOIDS, GABAPENTIN, INTRATHECAL PUMPS, AND BACLOFEN PUMPS

It is recommended that nonsteroidal anti-inflammatory drugs (NSAIDs) be discontinued 24–72 hours prior to surgery due to the risk of acute kidney injury in the *nil per os* patient. It is recommended that chronic pain medications be continued preoperatively, including methadone and buprenorphine; however, opioid antagonist medications such as naltrexone should be tapered prior to surgery. Gabapentin and muscle relaxants may be continued on the day of surgery and perioperatively. Finally, it is critical to ensure that baclofen and intrathecal pumps are functioning prior to surgery, as baclofen toxicity and withdrawal may be life-threatening.

## HERBAL MEDICATIONS

It is recommended that all herbal supplements be stopped 14 days prior to surgery.[1]

## REFERENCES

1. Pass SE, Simpson RW. Discontinuation and reinstitution of medications during the perioperative period. *Am J Health-Syst Pharm.* 2004;61:899–912.
2. Kennedy JM, et al. Polypharmacy in a general surgical unit and consequences of drug withdrawal. *Br J Clin Pharmacol.* 1999;49: 353–362.
3. Preoperative evaluation. In: *Miller's Anesthesiology.* 9th ed.:918–998.
4. Fleisher LA, et al. 2014 ACC/AHA guideline on perioperative cardiovascular evaluation and management of patients undergoing noncardiac surgery. *J Am Coll Cardiol.* 2014;22:e77–137.
5. Horlocker TT, et al. Regional anesthesia in the patient receiving antithrombotic or thrombolytic therapy: American Society of Regional Anesthesia and Pain Medicine Evidence-Based Guidelines (Fourth Edition). *Reg Anesth Pain Med.* 2018;43;3: 263–309.

# 111.

# PROPHYLACTIC CARDIAC RISK REDUCTION

*Christina Gibson and Daniel S. Cormican*

## INTRODUCTION

Cardiovascular complications are a common cause of perioperative morbidity and mortality.[1] Prophylactic cardiac event risk reduction requires assessment of those patients at greatest risk for cardiac events and optimization of therapies to reduce adverse perioperative cardiac events; this chapter focuses on these topics.

## PERIOPERATIVE EVALUATION

The perioperative evaluation should start with a thorough history and physical exam, including medications, allergies, previous anesthetic reactions, and identifying patients at increased risk of cardiac events.[2] The Revised Cardiac Risk Index (RCRI) estimates cardiovascular risk and consists of 6 components: high-risk surgery; history of myocardial infarction (MI) or positive stress test; history or signs of congestive heart failure; history of stroke; preoperative treatment with insulin; and preoperative creatinine >2.0. One point is given for each.

Functional capacity is typically expressed as metabolic equivalents (METS). Perioperative cardiac risk is increased in patients capable of less than 4 METS (climbing a flight of stairs, walking uphill, or performing heavy housework) of activity.[3]

There are three risk categories for noncardiac surgeries based on 30-day cardiac event rates: low (1%); intermediate (1%–5%); and high (5%). Figure 111.1 shows a cardiac risk-assessment algorithm.

## NONINVASIVE TESTING

It is reasonable for patients at elevated risk (1% or greater) of a cardiac event who have poor or unknown functional capacity having intermediate risk surgery to undergo exercise or pharmacological stress testing if the results may change intraoperative management.[4]

Routine preoperative 12-lead electrocardiogram (ECG) is of no benefit for asymptomatic patients or for patients undergoing low-risk surgery.[3] Obtaining an ECG is reasonable for patients with considerable cardiovascular risk factors, and may be considered in those undergoing high-risk surgical procedures.[3]

Assessment of left ventricular (LV) function (e.g., echocardiogram) is indicated to evaluate patients with unknown or worsening dyspnea, sudden change in clinical status, or in a patient with stable documented heart failure.[3]

## PROPHYLACTIC REVASCULARIZATION

A large randomized control trial showed no difference in mortality or incidence of postoperative MI between patients who underwent prophylactic revascularization versus patients with optimized medical management prior to surgery.[2] There are currently no specific indications for preoperative coronary revascularization, unless the patient would have required revascularization irrespective of upcoming surgery.

### TIMING OF ELECTIVE NONCARDIAC SURGERY IN PATIENTS WITH PCI

If patients have undergone percutaneous coronary intervention (PCI) with stent placement and are on dual antiplatelet therapy (DAPT), the urgency of the noncardiac surgery and the risk of bleeding or ischemic events, including stent thrombosis, must be considered.[3] Truly elective surgeries should be delayed 14 days after balloon angioplasty, 30 days after bare metal stent (BMS) placement, and 180 days after drug-eluting stent (DES) placement.[3] If the risk of delaying surgery is greater than the risk of thrombosis, then patients with DES may undergo surgery within 3 months of stent placement.[5] Aspirin should be continued perioperatively and the $P2Y_{12}$ inhibitor restarted as soon as possible postoperatively.[3]

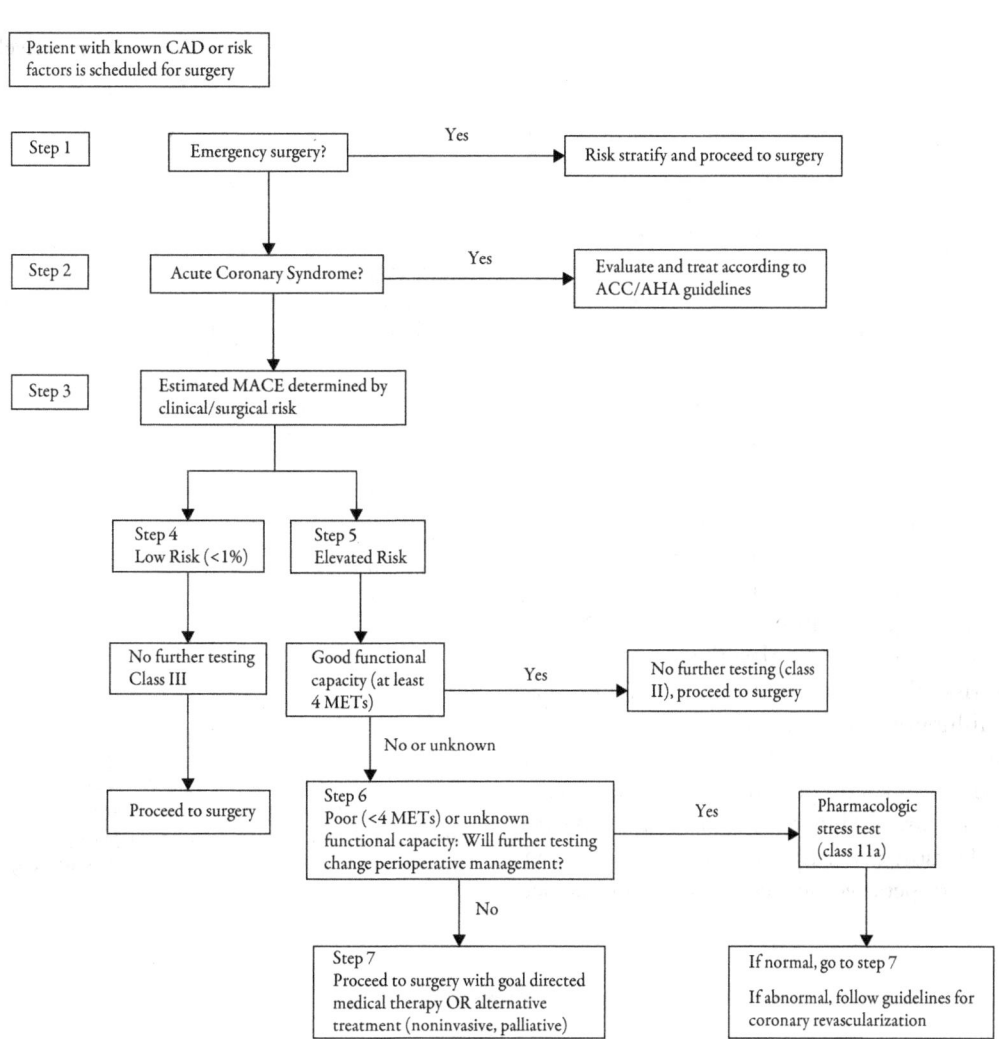

**Figure 111.1** American College of Cardiology/American Heart Association recommendations for perioperative cardiac risk assessment for noncardiac surgery.

## PERIOPERATIVE MEDICAL MANAGEMENT

Medical optimization reduces cardiac risk by facilitating favorable myocardial oxygen supply and demand, plaque stabilization, and reducing thrombus formation.[4]

### ANTIHYPERTENSIVES

#### Beta Blockers

Beta blockers are a mainstay of therapy in patients with cardiac diseases.[1] Although overall evidence suggests that beta blockers reduce the risk of MI and cardiac death, there is an overall increase in mortality and stroke.[1]

The ACC/AHA guidelines class I recommendation regarding beta blockers is that patients on chronic beta-blocker therapy should be continued perioperatively because withdrawal of therapy is associated with increased mortality.[3] A class III recommendation is that beta-blocker therapy should not be started within 24 hours of surgery due

to an increased risk of MI and cardiac death.[3] However, it is suggested that they should be initiated at least 2–4 weeks prior to surgery to allow for titration to a target heart rate of 55–65 bpm with systolic blood pressure >100 mmHg.[1] Beta blockers are typically recommended in patients undergoing vascular surgery with identified coronary heart disease, elevated cardiac risk, or 3 or more RCRI risk factors, as long as there is suitable time to assess safety and tolerability prior to surgery.[4]

#### ACE Inhibitors

Angiotensin-converting enzyme (ACE) inhibitors are often associated with hypotension in the perioperative period. However, there is no association with increased risk of perioperative cardiovascular events.[3] The ACC/AHA issued a class II recommendation that it is reasonable to continue ACE inhibitors in the perioperative period, and if they are held before surgery, it is reasonable to restart them as soon possible postoperatively.[3]

## STATINS

The ACC/AHA guidelines include a class I recommendation that statins should be continued in patients currently on statin therapy undergoing noncardiac surgery.[3] There was found to be a rebound effect of increased risk of cardiovascular events in patients who abruptly stopped statin therapy.[1] The ACC/AHA also offers a class II recommendation that statins may be started in patients undergoing vascular surgery.[3] It is recommended that statin therapy be initiated several weeks prior to surgery.[1]

## ANTIPLATELET THERAPIES

Aspirin causes the irreversible inhibition of cyclooxygenase 1 and 2 and is a mainstay of primary and secondary prevention of cardiovascular diseases.[1] The ACC/AHA guidelines include a class I recommendation that patients undergoing urgent noncardiac surgery within 4–6 weeks of BMS or DES placement continue DAPT unless the risk of bleeding outweighs the risk of stent thrombosis.[3] If discontinuation of a P2Y$_{12}$ inhibitor is necessary, it should be started as soon as possible postoperatively.[3] Discontinuing aspirin in patients who are on aspirin for prevention of cardiac events is associated with a threefold increase in the risk of adverse cardiac events.[1] In most cases, aspirin should be continued perioperatively. Perioperative management of antiplatelet therapies should be determined collaboratively by the surgeon, anesthesiologist, and cardiologist.[1]

## REFERENCES

1. Holt NF. Perioperative cardiac risk reduction. *Am Fam Physician.* 2012;85(3):239–246.
2. Miller RD, Pardo MC. *Basics of Anesthesia.* 6th ed. Philadelphia, PA: Elsevier/Saunders; 2011.
3. Fleisher LA, et al. 2014 ACC/AHA guideline on perioperative cardiovascular evaluation and management of patients undergoing noncardiac surgery: Executive summary. *Circulation.* 2014;130(24):2215–2245.
4. Poldermans D, et al Pre-operative risk assessment and risk reduction before surgery. *J Am Coll Cardiol.* 2008;51(20):1913–1924.
5. Levine GN, et al. 2016 ACC/AHA guideline focused update on duration of dual antiplatelet therapy in patients with coronary artery disease: A report of the American College of Cardiology/American Heart Association Task Force on Clinical Practice Guidelines: An update of the 2011 ACCF/AHA/SCAI guideline for percutaneous coronary intervention, 2011 ACCF/AHA guideline for coronary artery bypass graft surgery, 2012 ACC/AHA/ACP/AATS/PCNA/SCAI/STS guideline for the diagnosis and management of patients with stable ischemic heart disease, 2013 ACCF/AHA guideline for the management of ST-elevation myocardial infarction, 2014 AHA/ACC guideline for the management of patients with non-ST-elevation acute coronary syndromes, and 2014 ACC/AHA guideline on perioperative cardiovascular evaluation and management of patients undergoing noncardiac surgery. *Circulation.* 2016;134(10).

# 112.

# PROPHYLACTIC ANTIBIOTICS

*Austine Lin and Raymond Graber*

## INTRODUCTION

The ideal drug for antibiotic prophylaxis should prevent infection and the associated morbidity and costs, should be inexpensive, and should have minimal adverse effects. The drug should be active against the pathogens most likely to contaminate the surgical site. The predominant organisms causing surgical site infections (SSIs) after clean procedures are skin flora, including *Staphylococcus aureus* and coagulase-negative staphylococci such as *S. epidermidis*. Cefazolin is the drug most frequently used for prophylaxis because it has been extensively studied and has proven efficacy. It has a desirable spectrum of activity against organisms commonly encountered in surgery, has a reasonable duration of action, is relatively nontoxic to organ function, and is low cost. In clean-contaminated procedures such as colorectal procedures, the predominant organisms include gram-negative rods and enterococci in addition to skin flora, so additional coverage with metronidazole is utilized. Ciprofloxacin is the most commonly used antibiotic in genitourinary procedures that include cystoscopy. It is important to refer to guidelines published by national subspecialty organizations or your local hospital to confirm correct choice of antibiotic for specific procedures.[1,2] It is also important to consider that patients with significant beta lactam allergy will require an alternative antibiotic strategy such as vancomycin or clindamycin. In addition, patients who are colonized with methicillin-resistant *Staphylococcus aureus* (MRSA) will also need coverage with vancomycin.

## OPTIMAL TIMING

The optimal time for administration of the preoperative antibiotic is within 60 minutes before surgical incision. Some agents, such as fluoroquinolones and vancomycin, require administration over 1–2 hours; therefore, the administration of these agents should begin within 120 minutes before surgical incision and is frequently started in the preoperative holding area. The rationale for this recommendation is that successful prophylaxis requires that serum and tissue levels of antibiotics exceed the minimum inhibitory concentration (MIC) for the probable organisms associated with the procedure prior to incision. Thus, administration too early or too late may not lead to optimal drug levels. In a prospective evaluation of 1708 surgical patients receiving antimicrobial prophylaxis, the preoperative administration of antimicrobials within 2 hours prior to surgical incision decreased the risk of SSI to 0.59%, compared with 3.8% for early administration (2–24 hours before surgical incision) and 3.3% for any postoperative administration (any time after incision).[3]

## DOSING

As stated previously, adequate prophylaxis requires that serum and tissue levels of antibiotics exceed the minimum inhibitory concentration for the probable organisms. It has been shown that this did not always happen in the obese adult patient. In order to rectify this issue, weight-based dosing is frequently used. For example, cefazolin is administered as a 2 g dose for patients weighing less than 120 kg, and increased to 3 g for those weighing over 120 kg. Vancomycin is typically administered as a 15 mg/kg dose. Gentamycin is dosed at 5 mg/kg. All prophylactic antibiotics for pediatric patients are dosed based on body weight.

## REDOSING

Intraoperative antibiotic redosing is needed to ensure adequate serum and tissue concentrations of the antimicrobial if the duration of the procedure exceeds 2 half-lives of the drug or there is excessive blood loss (i.e., >1500 mL) during the procedure. For example, cefazolin (with a serum half-life of 1.8 hrs) is usually administered every 4 hours during a procedure. The caveat is that patients with significant renal dysfunction (i.e., CrCl <30 mL/min) will have delayed drug clearance, and thus a longer interval until redosing is needed.

## DURATION

The goal is to administer antibiotics for the shortest period of time so as to minimize adverse effects (such as development of antimicrobial resistance or *C. difficile* infection) and costs. For many procedures, no postoperative dosing may be necessary. The current practice is to limit postoperative dosing to less than 24 hours.

## RISKS OF ADMINISTRATION

Although antibiotics are generally safe and are tolerated well by most patients, a small percentage of patients can develop allergic reactions like rash, hives, or even anaphylaxis. A careful allergy history should be part of the preoperative evaluation. A not uncommon scenario is the patient who states they have a penicillin allergy, and the standard prophylaxis drug would be cefazolin. There are a number of things to consider. Only about 10% of patients who state they have a penicillin allergy actually test positive for a penicillin allergy. If a patient describes itch, rash, or nausea-type symptoms, it is generally safe to use a cephalosporin. If the patient describes a more dangerous reaction such as an immunoglobulin E (IgE)-mediated allergic reaction (angioedema, anaphylaxis bronchospasm, etc.), then the risk of a reaction is higher. In these patients, look for a history of prior safe administration of cefazolin—if present, it should be safe to administer it again. If there is no history of cephalosporin exposure, then it is probably better to administer a guideline-appropriate non-beta lactam agent such as vancomycin or clindamycin.

## SOME ADDITIONAL CONSIDERATIONS

Vancomycin needs to be administered over an hour or more to reduce the risk of an anaphylactoid reaction (mast cell and/or basophil release of histamine) and development of red man syndrome. Gentamycin and other aminoglycosides can enhance neuromuscular blockade by decreasing acetylcholine release at the neuromuscular junction. Antibiotic administration has the potential to lead to postoperative nausea, diarrhea, rash, and altered patient bacterial flora. However, these risks are very low if postoperative dosing is reduced or eliminated.

## REFERENCES

1. Bratzler DW, et al. American Society of Health-System Pharmacists; Infectious Disease Society of America; Surgical Infection Society; Society for Healthcare Epidemiology of America. Clinical practice guidelines for antimicrobial prophylaxis in surgery. *Am J Health Syst Pharm*. 2013 Feb 1;70(3):195–283.
2. Ban KA, Minei JP, et al. American College of Surgeons and Surgical Infection Society: surgical site infection guidelines, 2016 update. *J Am Coll Surg*. 2017 Jan;224(1):59–74.
3. Classen DC, et al. The timing of prophylactic administration of antibiotics and the risk of surgical-wound infection. *N Engl J Med*. 1992;326:281–286.

# 113.

# COMA AND HYPEROSMOLAR COMA

*Vicko Gluncic*

## COMA

Coma is a state of total absence of arousal (overall level of responsiveness, ability to experience surroundings) and awareness (ability to process self/environmental stimuli, to understand relationship to surroundings). It can be of traumatic and nontraumatic origins:[1,2]

- Neurologic disorders
  - Stroke (ischemic, hemorrhagic)
  - Nontraumatic subarachnoidal hemorrhage
  - Cerebral venous thrombosis
  - Compression of cerebral tissue by mass (tumor, bleeding, hydrocephalus), causing brainstem compression (direct or by transtentorial herniation)
  - Nonconvulsive status epilepticus
  - Central nervous infection
  - Sepsis
- Metabolic disorders
  - Dehydration
  - Hypoxia/hypercapnia
  - Hepatic failure
  - Hypoglycemia/hyperglycemia (hyperosmotic)
  - Uremia—renal failure
  - Hyponatremia/hypernatremia
  - Toxic (toxins, drugs, medications, alcohol)
  - Hypothermia
- Endocrine disorders
  - Adrenal insufficiency
  - Panhypopituitarism
  - Thyroid disorders.

## EVALUATION OF A PATIENT IN COMA

The approach to a patient with altered consciousness consists of the assessment of level of consciousness (deepness of coma), and the differentiation between structural and metabolic origins of coma.[1,2]

### Physical Examination

To assess the deepness of coma, the Glasgow coma scale (GCS) is used. Although this scale was developed for the evaluation of traumatic brain injuries, it is also used for evaluation of coma of nontraumatic origin. It evaluates eyes opening (E, maximum of 5 points), verbal communication (V, maximum of 4 points), and motor responses (M, maximum of 6 points) for the best response. The score can be expressed as a sum of all best scores (3–15), or as a point for the each section (e.g., GCS E1 + V1 + M1 = 3).

Eye opening can be spontaneous, or it can occur as a reaction to voice or pain. Although spontaneous eye opening usually indicates an aroused patient, and is accompanied by awareness, in a vegetative state patients open eyes spontaneously, but they are not aware of their surroundings.

When eye opening is assessed, usually the pupils ([an] isocoria, photoreactivity, [mid]positioning), spontaneous eye movement (nystagmus, [dis]conjugate movements), and ocular reflexes (oculocephalic, oculovestibular) are also evaluated.

Motor activity is assessed as spontaneous activity or a response to pain, if spontaneous activity is missing. Abnormal flexion upon painful stimuli indicates decortication, while abnormal extension indicates decerebration. Injuries to the lower brainstem result in flaccid extremities upon painful stimulus. Focal motor deficits, clonic movement, and spontaneous myoclonus should be noted also.

It should be noted that flaccid paralysis of all extremities accompanied with spontaneous eye opening and preserved blinking and vertical eyeball movement indicates *locked-in state*, a state characterized with complete immobility of voluntary muscles but with conserved awareness.

There are several major limitations to the GCS. The ordinary GCS for adults cannot be used in preverbal children. As an alternative, the pediatric GCS should be used. Second, in intubated patients who are unable to answer questions, the verbal response cannot be evaluated properly. In these patients, verbal response is rated as pseudoscore of 1. The third limitation is that GCS cannot be used to assess the brainstem.

If GCS ≤8, the protective reflexes in the airway are assumed to be impaired or lost, so patients should be intubated.

Alternatives to GCS are: FOUR (Full Outline of UnResponsiveness) score, AVPU (alert, voice, pain, unresponsive) scale, and Simplified Motor Score.

After assessing the deepness of coma, the full physical examination should be done with the focus on neurological functions, including the testing of brainstem functions and reflexes.

## Laboratory Evaluation

Laboratory evaluation should include complete blood count (CBC), electrolytes, renal and liver function, glycemia, assessment of acid-base balance, blood/urine cultures, lumbar puncture (after brain imaging), and endocrine function tests (if needed).[2]

## Radiographic Imaging and Electrodiagnostics

Computed tomography (CT) or/and magnetic resonance imaging (MRI) should be performed to identify structural causes of coma.[2] CT is more sensitive for compartmental shifts, intracranial hemorrhage, hydrocephalus, and edema, while MRI is more sensitive for infectious, septic, and autoimmune processes, as well as for diffuse axonal injury.

Electroencephalogram (EEG) is used to detect nonconvulsive seizures that can lead to unconsciousness.[2]

## MANAGEMENT

Management of a patient in coma consists of the protection of airways (endotracheal intubation if GCS ≤8), specific treatment of the cause, and supportive therapy.

## HYPERGLYCEMIC HYPEROSMOLAR NONKETOTIC COMA

This state is similar to diabetic ketoacidosis in pathogenesis, clinical presentation, and treatment.

### CLINICAL PRESENTATION

The major difference is that a patient in hyperosmolar nonketotic coma is typically an elderly person with several associated diseases who is severely dehydrated due to hypotonic fluid loss and present in coma (in contrast to diabetic ketoacidosis).[3-5] Also, these patients usually have type 2 diabetes mellitus, and have just enough endogenic insulin to prevent ketoacidosis.

### PATHOGENESIS

Hyperglycemia and hyperosmolarity are caused by pronounced volume depletion.[3-5] In turn, volume depletion causes reduced renal blood flow and glomerular filtration that diminish urinary elimination of glucose. In the same time, decreased peripheral utilization of glucose activates mechanisms that initiate exaggerated hepatic gluconeogenesis. All these factors combined (decreased peripheral utilization, decreased renal elimination, and hepatic gluconeogenesis) deepen hyperglycemia and hyperosmolarity further.

In these patients, different stages of altered consciousness, including coma, are probably caused by hyperosmolarity.[4,5] Mental status alters at plasma osmolarity above 320 mosm/kg $H_2O$, while coma develops when plasma osmolarity is above 530 mosm/kg $H_2O$. Both focal and generalized seizures, as well as involuntary movements, can occur.

### LABORATORY FINDINGS

Biochemical findings of a patient with hyperosmolar nonketotic coma show severe hyperglycemia (serum glucose > 600 mg/dL, but can exceed 1000 mg/dL), hyperosmolarity, and electrolyte disbalance.[3-5] Since the level of ketone bodies is not high, there is no ketoacidosis.

## TREATMENT

Treatment is similar to the treatment of diabetic ketoacidosis.[3-5] Fluid replacement is crucial to mitigate hyperosmolar state (which will reduce insulin resistance), and to prevent hypotension caused by fluid shifts that result from transport of glucose into cells. Fluid replacement should start with isotonic fluids, 1–2 L in the first hour, and fluid balance should be monitored because of the age and concomitant comorbidities of these patients. Plasma glucose should be decreased by 100 mg/dL per hour. Insulin therapy should start after the initial volume is restored, and the regimen is the same as in the treatment of diabetic ketoacidosis.

Electrolyte disbalance should be corrected also, especially hypokalemia.

## REFERENCES

1. Stevens RD, Kornbluth J. Causes and diagnosis of unconsciousness. In: Webb A, ed. *Oxford Textbook of Critical Care*. 2nd ed. Oxford, UK: Oxford University Press. 2016:1234–1239, 1083–1087.
2. Disorders of consciousness. In: *Marino's ICU Book*. 4th rev. international ed. Philadelphia, PA: Lippincott Williams & Wilkins; 2014:806–810.
3. Osmotic disorders. In: *Marino's ICU Book*. 4th rev. international ed. Philadelphia, PA: Lippincott Williams & Wilkins; 2014: 662–623.
4. Hirsch IB. Diabetic ketoacidosis and hyperosmolar hyperglycemic state in adults: Epidemiology and pathogenesis. In: Nathan DM, ed. *UpToDate*. Waltham, MA; 2020. https://www.uptodate.com/contents/diabetic-ketoacidosis-and-hyperosmolar-hyperglycemic-state-in-adults-epidemiology-and-pathogenesis. Accessed August 30, 2020.
5. Hirsch IB. Diabetic ketoacidosis and hyperosmolar hyperglycemic state in adults: Treatment. In: Nathan DM, ed. *UpToDate*. Waltham, MA, 2020. https://www.uptodate.com/contents/diabetic-ketoacidosis-and-hyperosmolar-hyperglycemic-state-in-adults-treatment. Accessed August 30, 2020.

# 114.

# MINIMALLY INVASIVE CARDIAC SURGERY

*Ellyn Gray and Archit Sharma*

## INTRODUCTION

Minimally invasive cardiac surgery (MICS) refers to a variety of operations performed through incisions that are smaller and less traumatic than the standard sternotomy.

Before patients undergo MICS, they are evaluated to ensure they are appropriate candidates for the procedure. Often, this requires adequate peripheral access, either for percutaneous techniques or for bypass. Patients with severe peripheral vascular disease may have more difficult access and be at increased risk for peripheral vascular injury. For procedures utilizing robotic or laparoscopic techniques, one-lung ventilation is used to improve visualization. If a patient has a poor pulmonary function test (PFT), this method may be contraindicated. Finally, patients with previous cardiac surgeries likely have increased scaring and

abnormal adherence of tissues that makes minimally invasive approaches more technically difficult and risky.

## CORONARY ARTERY BYPASS

Minimally invasive direct coronary artery bypass surgery (MIDVAB) was initially performed through an anterolateral thoracotomy without cardiopulmonary bypass (CPB). It is now usually performed via a left lateral thoracotomy. Performing the procedure off-pump minimizes inflammatory effects and hemodilution of CPB. Recent guidelines from the International Society for Minimally Invasive Cardiothoracic Surgery have recommended the off-pump approach, especially in high-risk patients with comorbidities that may be exacerbated by CPB (for example, severe calcification of the ascending aorta or renal insufficiency).[1] The aortic cannula is placed through the left femoral artery 2 cm distal to the aortic valve with aortic occlusion balloon, allowing anterograde perfusion of the aortic arch and descending aorta. Bilateral radial art lines detect migration of balloon.

Robots have also been employed in a variety of ways for both on- and off-pump coronary artery bypass procedures, ranging from robotically assisted, for harvesting of the left internal mammary artery (LIMA) to on- and off-pump total endoscopic coronary artery bypass (TECAB). Single lung ventilation is required for harvesting the artery with minimal left hemithorax insufflation.[2] Contraindications to this procedure include but are not limited to poor LFTs (difficult one lung ventilation), emergent coronary artery bypass grafting (CABG), diffuse left anterior descending (LAD) disease, morbid obesity, EF<30%, moderate-severe aortic or mitral valve disease, and previous thoracic surgery or radiation.

Hybrid coronary revascularization involves performing a minimally invasive LIMA to LAD bypass in conjunction with stenting of other occluded coronary arteries during the same procedure. Using a LIMA graft to the LAD is known to increase survival, more so than other coronary artery disease (CAD) therapies.[3]

## MITRAL VALVE

Minimally invasive mitral valve surgeries (MIMVS) can be performed through lower hemisternotomy, right parasternal incision, and right mini-thoracotomy. It can also be performed video-assisted or robotically assisted. The valve is visualized by exposure through the left atrium or trans-septally through the right atrium. Cardiopulmonary bypass (CBP) is typically accomplished with aortic and venous cannulas placed through the femoral artery and vein.

For the robotic approach, patients are positioned with right shoulder elevated 30 degrees while the pelvis is supine for femoral access. Single-lung ventilation is required, and complete paralysis is critical until the robot is undocked to avoid iatrogenic injury. Patients are not a candidate for robotic mitral valve surgery if they have a severely calcified mitral annulus, severe pulmonary hypertension, ischemic heart disease, will require multiple mitral valve replacements, have had a previous right hemithorax surgery, or have severe aortic/peripheral atherosclerosis.

The MitraClip™ (Abbott group) procedure is performed via a percutaneous approach through the femoral vein, and a septal puncture allows access into the left atrium. Once in the left atrium, the device is advanced, and the clip arms are extended to grab the two mitral valve leaflets. This procedure is usually performed under a general anesthetic and requires transesophageal echocardiography to verify the placement of the clip.

## AORTIC VALVE REPLACEMENT

Minimally invasive aortic valve replacement (MIAVR) can be performed via a hemi- or mini-sternotomy and right anterior thoracotomy. It is now most commonly performed using a mini-sternotomy with a J or inverted T incision, which minimizes postoperative pain and effects on thoracic cage stability. Both peripheral and central cannulation can be used for CPB. Most studies have shown minor improvement in outcomes in MIAVR over open AVR, but there is a learning curve for this procedure, although for trained surgeons, operative times are similar with MIAVR as with open AVR.[4]

Transcatheter aortic valve replacements (TAVRs) are typically performed for high-risk patients, via a retrograde approach through the femoral artery, with a catheter advanced through the stenotic valve. The device is guided into place using either fluoroscopy or transesophageal echocardiography (TEE). The most common complications of this procedure include atrioventricular block and injury to iliofemoral vessels (dissection, occlusion, or perforation). Other complications include paravalvular leak, annular rupture, aortic annular dissection, cardiac tamponade, prosthesis dislocation, renal failure, and stroke.

## ATRIAL FIBRILLATION ABLATION

Atrial fibrillation (AF) ablation accomplished by the Cox-maze procedure has evolved to enable minimally invasive approaches. The Cox-maze IV procedure utilizes cryotherapy, radiofrequency, and high-intensity ultrasound, as opposed to the cut-and-sew method of the Cox-maze III procedure.[5] Approaches for minimally invasive AF ablations include mini-thoracotomy, laparoscopic, video-assisted thoracoscopic, or robotic. Left atrial appendage exclusion can also be performed via a minimally invasive approach in conjunction with this procedure.

## ANESTHETIC CONSIDERATIONS

### PREOPERATIVE

Correct patient selection with rigorous testing is a precursor to MICS. Severe peripheral vascular disease, prior cardiac surgery, and poor LFTs can be relative contraindications.

### INTRAOPERATIVE

Various surgical procedures might require special strategies such as one lung ventilation and strict neuromuscular blockade. Adequate vascular access should be obtained prior to initiating surgery.

## POSTOPERATIVE

MICS leads to less pain, smaller incisions, and enhanced recovery.

## REFERENCES

1. Iribarne A, et al. The golden age of minimally invasive cardiothoracic surgery: Current and future perspectives. *Future Cardiol.* 2011;7(3):333–346.
2. Miller RD. *Miller's Anesthesia.* Gropper MA, et al., eds. 9th ed. Elsevier; 2020.
3. Buttar SN, et al. Long-term and short-term outcomes of using bilateral internal mammary artery grafting versus left internal mammary artery grafting: A meta-analysis. *Heart.* 2017;103(18): 1419–1426.
4. Liu J, et al. Minimally invasive aortic valve replacement (AVR) compared to standard AVR. *Eur J Cardio-Thorac Surg.* 1999;*16*(Supplement_2), S80–S83.
5. McCarthy PM, et al. The Cox-maze procedure: the Cleveland Clinic experience. *Semin Thorac Cardiovasc Surg.* 2000 Jan;12(1): 25–29.

# 115.

# ABDOMINAL AORTIC ANEURYSM

## *Ravi K. Grandhi and Claire Joseph*

## INTRODUCTION

Abdominal aortic aneurysms (AAA) occur in 3%–10% of patients older than age 50.[1] Advances in screening via the abdominal ultrasound have increased the diagnosis of asymptomatic aneurysms. The majority of aneurysms are located infra-renally. There are a number of risk factors which are associated with development of AAA—of which the primary modifiable risk factor is smoking. Other risk factors include older age, male gender, family history, genetics, coronary artery disease, high cholesterol, chronic obstructive pulmonary disease, increased height, peripheral vascular disease, and Caucasian race.[2]

AAA are caused by a compromised vascular wall strength through local elastin resorption, caused by an increased elastase activity, localized wall inflammatory changes, increased protease activity, and mural thrombus formation in the arterial wall and plasminogen activation. AAA will expand with time and eventually rupture if not repaired. The risk of rupture increases nonlinearly as the size of the aneurysm increases, and becomes clinically significant at 5 cm diameter. Elective repair is indicated if the size >5.5 cm or the rate of growth is >1.0 cm/year.[3] Mortality rates are significantly higher for emergent repairs, particularly if they require an open approach.[4] Mortality after a ruptured AAA is 75%–90% if they don't reach the operating room; however, for those who do reach the operating room the mortality rate is 40%.[4] The two types of ruptured AAA are *contained* or *confirmed rupture*. The overall mortality rate for an elective endovascular repair of AAA (EVAR) is 0.9% and 4.3% with an open repair. Risk must also take into account the 5 types of aneurysms classified by the Crawford classification system, which are as follows (Figure 115.1):

(1) Distal left subclavian to suprarenal;
(2) Distal left subclavian artery to infrarenal;
(3) Infrarenal;
(4) Aorta bifurcation;
(5) Suprarenal.

Type 2 repairs have the highest risk of complications.

## ANESTHETIC CONSIDERATIONS

### PREOPERATIVE

Patients mostly present to the hospital in two different fashions, with the majority appearing hemodynamically stable for scheduled endovascular intervention. Surgery replaces the weakened aortic segment with a synthetic graft.

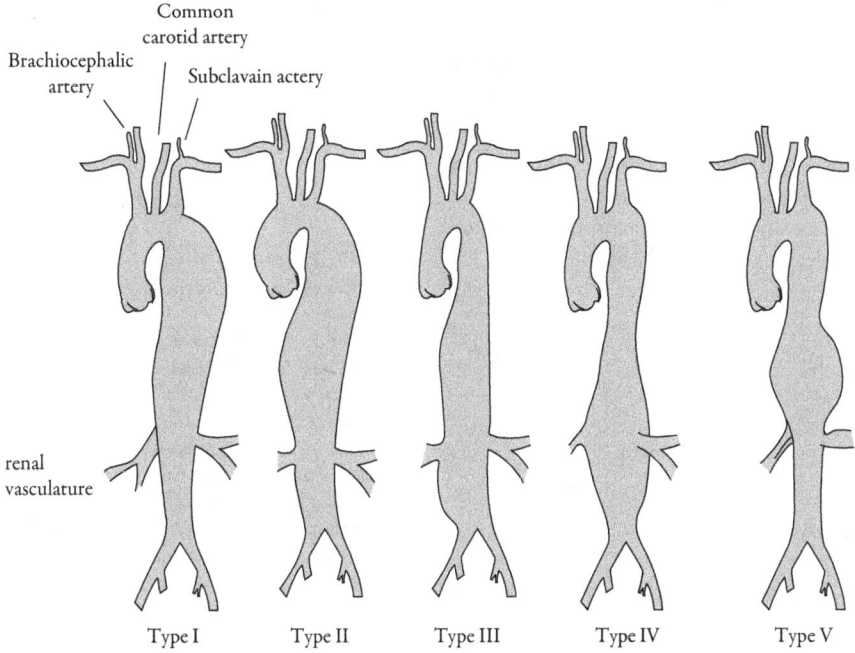

Figure 115.1 Types of Thoracoabdominal Aortic Aneurysms.

Initial therapy, if diagnosed asymptomatically, includes aggressive blood pressure control with beta blockers, antiplatelet agents, statins, and smoking cessation.

Two surgical approaches exist: EVAR or open. The approach is based on the aneurysm morphology, patient comorbidities, presentation, and age. EVAR is the preferred technique because of the lower risk of morbidity and mortality. Further, there is an increased frequency of early ambulation, decreased blood transfusion, and shorter length of stay associated with EVAR. However, with EVAR there is an increased risk of reintervention due to a proximal or distal endoleak.[4]

Of primary concern is the cardiovascular status of the patient. At a minimum a 12-lead electrocardiogram (EKG) is required; however, many require a more comprehensive cardiology evaluation including an echocardiogram or stress test. According to the Revised Cardiac Index (RCRI), there is an at least intermediate risk of preoperative cardiovascular complications. Further, if they are smokers, they may require a respiratory evaluation. If the patient is hemodynamically unstable, emergent intervention is required without comprehensive preoperative evaluation.

## INTRAOPERATIVE

Intraoperative goals vary based on the presentation and surgical approach. Despite fewer complications associated with EVAR, the anesthesiologist should be prepared for conversion to open. There are two primary anesthetic approaches: neuraxial and general anesthesia. However, neither approach has a clear advantage in terms of morbidity or mortality. Neuraxial anesthesia may have the advantage of blocking sympathetics leading to increased

coronary protection, decreased hyper-coagulability, and decreased thrombotic events postoperatively. On occasion, local anesthesia and sedation can also be used. Monitoring involves intravascular blood pressure cannulation via a radial arterial line and urine output via Foley catheter. Large bore intravenous access and maintenance of euvolemia and normotension are important. Administration of heparin and monitoring activated clotting times are vital.

Additional monitors are required in patients undergoing open repair, including a central line due to significant hemodynamic swings associated with clamping of the aorta, which increases afterload and increases blood pressure, while also decreasing cardiac output. In this setting, nitroglycerin maybe required. In addition, when the clamp is placed there is increased intracranial pressure (ICP) and as a result decreased spinal cord perfusion. Thus, patients require a lumbar drain to assist with spinal cord perfusion, with a cerebral spinal pressure goal of 8–10. Patients may also require monitoring of evoked potentials because there is decreased perfusion to the lower extremities. Further, during cross clamping, forced air warming of the lower body is contraindicated because hyperthermia can increase acidosis. Maintaining a temperature of 30°–34°C is recommended to protect the spinal cord and kidneys. Once the cross clamp is removed, there is hypotension and lactic acidosis. As a result, vasoactive agents, intravenous volume loading, electrolyte correction, Trendelenburg position, decreased anesthetic agents, and bicarbonate are needed due to the decreased preload. In addition, cerebral oximetry can be used to monitor cerebral perfusion. In some patients with extensive thoracoabdominal aneurysms, left heart bypass and transesophageal echocardiography maybe required. Epidurals are also often placed for pain management.

## POSTOPERATIVE

Postoperatively, monitoring for ischemia, acidosis, ongoing respiratory failure, and cardiac problems are important. Roughly 18% of cases have acute kidney injury and thus nonsteroidal agents (NSAIDs) should be avoided.[5] Maintaining adequate intravascular volume and limiting use of contrast die can help prevent renal injury. Complications associated with endografts are endoleaks, vascular injury during graft deployment, inadequate fixation and sealing of the graft to the wall, stent frame fractures, aneurysmal rupture, and breakdown of graft material. EVAR is associated with endothelial activation from the graft leading to fever, elevated inflammatory mediators, and leukocytosis. This is self-limited and can be treated with nonsteroidal agents if there are no renal complications. In rare cases, there is a propagation of a dissection leading to aortic regurgitation and tamponade. Even with an endovascular approach, there is still a risk of spinal cord ischemia leading to paraplegia because of exclusion of intercostal arteries. There may also be visceral or mesenteric injury with exclusion of the celiac artery. In addition to the spinal cord ischemia, those who have undergone an open repair have an increased risk of developing intra-abdominal hypertension and stroke. There is significantly greater risk of complications associated with open repair.

## REFERENCES

1. Al-Hashimi M, Thompson J. Anaesthesia for elective open abdominal aortic aneurysm repair. *Cont Educ Anaesth Crit Care Pain*. 2013 Dec;13(6):208–212.
2. Chaer R. Endovascular repair of abdominal aortic aneurysm. In Mills JL, Eidt JR, Collins KA, eds. *UpToDate*. Waltham, MA. February 2020. Accessed September 6, 2020.
3. Brewster DC, et al. Guidelines for the treatment of abdominal aortic aneurysms: Report of a subcommittee of the Joint Council of the American Association for Vascular Surgery and Society for Vascular Surgery. *J Vasc Surg*. 2003;37:1106.
4. Dalman, RA, Mell, M. Overview of abdominal aortic aneurysm. In Eidt JF, Mills JL, Creager MA, eds. *UpToDate*. Waltham, MA. March 2020. Accessed September 6, 2020.
5. Saratzis A, et al. Renal function is the main predictor of acute kidney injury after endovascular abdominal aortic aneurysm repair. *Ann Vasc Surg*. 2016;31:52–59.

# 116.

# ANESTHETIC CHOICE IN REDUCED RENAL FUNCTION

*Ling Tian and Christina T. Nguyen*

## INTRODUCTION

Perioperative acute kidney injury (AKI) is associated with elevated mortality rates. Ischemia, reperfusion injury, hypoxia, inflammation, and nephrotoxicity are major causes of perioperative AKI. The greatest concerns in determining anesthetic agents for patients with reduced renal function include prolonged action and enhanced intensity of effect.

## PATHOPHYSIOLOGY OF RENAL DISEASE

Causes of AKI can generally be divided into prerenal, intrinsic renal failure, and postrenal categories. Prerenal AKI is caused by a rapid decrease of renal blood flow (RBF) which leads to decline of glomerular filtration rate (GFR), increase of inflammation, and mismatch of metabolic demand of nephrons, leading to ischemia.

Intrinsic renal failure can be caused by nephrotoxins, myoglobinemia, nephritis, acute glomerulonephritis, and direct physical injury to the kidneys. Postrenal failure is caused by obstruction to the flow of urine. Some causes include tumors, prostatic hypertrophy, nephrolithiasis, and kinked or clotted urinary catheters.

## RISK FACTORS FOR ACUTE RENAL FAILURE

Risk factors include reoperative renal failure, congestive heart failure (CHF), advanced age, diabetes mellitus, and hypertension, as well as type of surgery, including cardiac, aortic, liver transplant, and emergent surgery.

# ANESTHETIC CHOICE IN REDUCED RENAL FUNCTION

The dosage of drugs that are cleared solely by the kidney can be reduced based on the reduction in GFR. Often this can be estimated by clearance of creatinine. However, most drugs have a combination of hepatic and renal clearance, which makes dose adjustments difficult to predict. Hepatic enzymes can be either enhanced or reduced in the setting of renal failure.

The mechanisms by which reduced renal function affects anesthetics are largely by reduced clearance of either unchanged drug or active metabolites, or by reduced protein binding caused by uremia. For drugs that rely on renal clearance, both loading dose and especially infusions or repeat doses will need to be reduced because of risk of buildup. Drugs that are usually highly protein bound will have a higher proportion of free molecules in uremic patients and therefore can exhibit exaggerated clinical effects. Consequently, loading doses in particular will need to be reduced (Table 116.1). Generally, the groups of anesthetics most affected by reduced renal function are opiates and muscle relaxants. Use of many opiates in patients with reduced renal function has the potential for over-sedation and apnea due to diminished excretion of active drug or metabolites. Prolonged neuromuscular blockade is a common concern in many of the nondepolarizing muscle relaxants. It should be noted that for neuromuscular reversal agents, no change in dose is necessary when used in patients with reduced renal function who received muscle relaxants because they also have prolonged effects.

*Table 116.1* RENAL CONSIDERATIONS FOR COMMON ANESTHETICS[2,3,4]

| MEDICATION | INTERACTIONS WITH RENAL FUNCTION |
| --- | --- |
| **INHALED ANESTHETICS** | |
| Sevoflurane | Theoretical renal toxicity from inorganic fluoride ion metabolite, and formation of "Compound A" with low fresh gas flows. In practice, sevoflurane has been safely used in CKD and dialysis patients. |
| Isoflurane | No direct effect |
| Desflurane | No direct effect |
| N2O | No direct effect |
| **INTRAVENOUS INDUCTION AGENTS** | |
| Propofol | No direct effect, may be renal protective when compared to volatile anesthetics for maintenance[2] |
| Ketamine | No direct effect |
| Etomidate | No direct effect |
| Methohexital | No direct effect |
| Thiopental | Reduced protein binding: exaggerated clinical effect, reduce dose |
| **ADJUNCT AGENTS** | |
| Dexmedetomidine | Reduced protein binding, prolonged sedation. May be renal protective[2] |
| Midazolam | Half-life of midazolam and metabolites may be prolonged if given as an infusion |
| Other benzodiazepines | Reduced protein binding, active metabolites can cause over sedation |
| **NEUROMUSCULAR BLOCKING AGENTS** | |
| Succinylcholine | Safely used if K <5.5 mEq/L |
| Rocuronium | Predominantly hepatobiliary excretions, some renal clearance. Effect may be prolonged. Sugammadex/rocuronium complex can be dialyzed. |
| Cisatracurium/atracurium | Hofmann elimination, independent of renal function |
| Vecuronium | 10%–20% renal excretion. May have prolonged effect in patients with reduced renal function. |
| Mivacurium | Lower plasma pseudocholinesterase activity in renal failure, prolonged effect |
| Pancuronium | 70%–80% renal excretion. Avoid. |

*(continued)*

*Table 116.1* CONTINUED

| MEDICATION | INTERACTIONS WITH RENAL FUNCTION |
|---|---|
| **NMB REVERSAL AGENTS** | |
| Neostigmine | Renally excreted, prolonged duration |
| Glycopyrrolate/Atropine | Renally excreted, prolonged duration |
| Sugammadex | May be used in moderate to severe renal impairment. Sugammadex-rocuronium complex can be removed by high-flux dialysis method.[6] |
| **OPIOIDS** | |
| Remifentanil | No direct effects |
| Fentanyl | No direct effects |
| Alfentanil | Reduced protein binding but clearance unchanged, therefore consider lower loading dose |
| Sufentanil | No direct effects |
| Hydromorphone | Reduced excretion of metabolite hydromorphone-3-glucuronide may cause cognitive dysfunction and myoclonus |
| Oxycodone | Reduced excretion of primary drug and metabolites |
| Buprenorphine | No direct effects |
| Methadone | Excreted mainly in feces. In anuric patients, it is exclusively excreted in feces. Safe to use. |
| Tramadol | 90% tramadol and metabolites are excreted in urine. Avoid. |
| Morphine | Reduced clearance of active 6 glucuronide metabolites. Reduced protein binding. Reduce loading dose, avoid chronic administration due to risk of oversedation and apnea. |
| Meperidine | Elevated risk of seizures and respiratory depression by metabolite normeperidine. Avoid. |
| Codeine | Prolonged narcosis. Avoid. |
| **LOCAL ANESTHETICS** | |
| | Duration of action may be diminished due to increased cardiac output and decreases in PH |

## PHARMACOLOGIC PREVENTION AND TREATMENT OF RENAL FAILURE

Preventing hypovolemia and hypotension is a proven strategy to prevent perioperative renal failure; however, caution must be taken for patients with heart failure or risk of fluid overload. Common nephrotoxic medications, including aminoglycosides, amphotericin, and radiocontrast agents, should be cautiously administered in patients at risk of having reduced renal function.

Based on randomized control trials,[5] dopamine does not prevent AKI postoperatively. Other medications, including mannitol, loop diuretics, fenoldopam, atrial natriuretic peptide, and N-acetylcysteine, have been studied and have not been shown to prevent AKI. Some studies looking at cardiac bypass patients, as well as studies on rats and porcine models, have shown some intravenous anesthetics to be renal protective. Most studies have focused on propofol and dexmedetomidine and found them to have favorable outcomes in renal protection when compared to other anesthetics, possibly due to antioxidant effects, inhibition of oxidative stress, and anti-apoptotic mechanisms.[2]

## ANESTHETIC CONSIDERATIONS

### PREOPERATIVE

Identify patients with increased risk of developing intraoperative or postoperative AKI. The greatest risk factor is a history of renal failure.

### INTRAOPERATIVE

Fluids should be administered judiciously to maintain mean arterial pressure to ensure adequate renal blood flow and oxygen delivery. Nephrotoxic medications should be avoided if possible. Choose anesthetics with consideration of their effects on blood pressure, metabolism, elimination, and protein binding associated with reduced renal function. Notably, several commonly used opiate medications have prolonged half-lives in patients with reduced renal function and therefore may have an increased risk of respiratory depression. Many muscle relaxants also have prolonged effects in patients with renal disease; therefore dose and case duration should be taken into account when choosing an agent. Carefully monitor urine output. Hemofiltration and hemodialysis may be indicated and should not be delayed.

## POSTOPERATIVE

Continue judicious fluid administration, and avoid nephrotoxic medications. Monitor patients for prolonged neuromuscular blockade or over-sedation and respiratory depression. Continue to monitor and trend renal function in order to identify postoperative AKI early.

## REFERENCES

1. Chappell D, et al. A rational approach to perioperative fluid management. *Anesthesiology*. 2008;109(4):723–740.
2. Motayagheni N, et al. A review of anesthetic effects on renal function: potential organ protection. *Am J Nephrol*. 2017;46(5): 380–389.
3. Trainor D, et al. Perioperative management of the hemodialysis patient. *Semin Dial*. 2011;24(3):314–326.
4. Stafford-Smith M, et al. The renal system and anesthesia for urologic surgery. In Barash PG, Cullen BF, Stoelting RK, Cahalan MK, Stock MC, Ortega RA, et al., eds. *Clinical Anesthesia*. Philadelphia, PA: Wolters Kluwer; 2017:1400–1415.
5. Bellomo R, et al. Low-dose dopamine in patients with early renal dysfunction: A placebo-controlled randomised trial. Australian and New Zealand Intensive Care Society (ANZICS) Clinical Trials Group. *Lancet*. 2000;356(9248):2139–2143.

# 117.

# FLUID-REPLACEMENT STRATEGIES AND CONTROVERSIES

*Jay I. Conhaim and Gretchen A. Lemmink*

## INTRODUCTION

Intravenous (IV) fluids are the most common medication used in the modern operating room, yet their administration is often haphazard and lacks a patient-centered approach. Tailoring perioperative fluid therapy to the individual patient is optimal, yet determining the correct type of fluid and appropriate amount to administer is steeped in controversy. This chapter will concisely review basic perioperative fluid-replacement strategies and highlight current evidence-based practices.

## PREOPERATIVE CONSIDERATIONS

The need, or lack thereof, for preoperative fluid replacement in elective surgery is often determined by the factors leading up to the procedure itself. Many patients are instructed to be *nil per os* (NPO) after midnight regardless of procedure

start time. Historically, a common practice was to calculate preoperative fluid losses based on NPO time and then subsequently administer a resuscitative fluid bolus in the calculated amount. This strategy is now viewed as antiquated and is not recommended. One increasingly accepted method to account for preoperative dehydration in elective surgery is to prescribe preoperative oral hydration. Carbohydrate-based oral hydration up to 2 hours prior to induction of anesthesia has demonstrated benefits with regard to patient comfort, reduction in preoperative anxiety, and reduction in intraoperative and postoperative insulin resistance.[1] Such preoperative hydration is increasingly being adopted by institutions to facilitate Enhanced Recovery After Surgery (ERAS) protocols. Patients presenting for emergency surgery (or those presenting for elective surgery who have been prescribed a mechanical bowel prep) should have a thorough evaluation of their volume status as time permits. Preoperative IV hydration should be prescribed if the evaluation indicates the patient's hemodynamics are likely to benefit from IV volume resuscitation.

## INTRAOPERATIVE CONSIDERATIONS

Modern intraoperative volume management has evolved from historical strategies of calculating volume needed for resuscitation, based on NPO time, estimated blood loss (EBL), and maintenance requirements, to a more "goal-directed" strategy. This historical "fixed volume" approach includes calculation of maintenance fluid volumes based on the patient's actual body weight and the "4 + 2 + 1 rule" (e.g., 4 mL/kg IV fluid (IVF) for the first 10 kg, 2 mL/kg IVF for the next 10 kg and 1 mL/kg IVF for every kg thereafter). In this historical model, EBL is typically replaced in a 3:1 ratio with crystalloid and in a 1:1 ratio with colloid. Such mathematical approaches to fluid management are no longer recommended.

Goal-directed volume management is based on continuous assessment of dynamic physiologic parameters and allows fluid delivery to be targeted to a patient's acute hemodynamic needs. While it is outside the scope of this chapter to delve into the different methods of goal-directed monitoring, there is a growing body of evidence that shows intraoperative utilization of objective data beyond urine output, blood pressure, heart rate, and cardiac filling pressures is beneficial to patient outcomes.

Optimal volume targets are another point of contention in the operative theater. "Liberal" and "restrictive" fluid administration strategies are vague classifications that have emerged in the past two decades to describe attempts, or lack thereof, to achieve a zero-balance intraoperative resuscitation. A restrictive, or zero-balance approach, involves only replacing the fluid that is lost during surgery (both insensible and sensible losses) in order to avoid postoperative fluid retention and its associated complications. This approach has been shown to result in several notable clinical benefits, including a decreased incidence of postoperative pulmonary edema and pneumonia, and decreased time to first flatus.[2] Conversely, a recent large trial in patients undergoing major abdominal surgery comparing liberal vs. restrictive intraoperative fluid goals found patients in the restrictive group had a higher risk of acute kidney injury (AKI) when compared to their liberal counterparts.[3] Overall, there is a growing body of evidence suggesting a liberal resuscitative strategy (or one that results in postoperative edema and excessive weight gain) is harmful; however, the precise approach to a restrictive strategy remains elusive. In major surgery, where large fluid shifts are anticipated, utilization of dynamic, goal-directed resuscitation parameters can guide the clinician around the pitfalls of being too restrictive in their intraoperative resuscitation (Figure 117.1).

Finally, the type of fluid utilized for replacement must also be considered when determining a perioperative resuscitative plan. The main categories of fluid types encountered in the perioperative period are crystalloids, colloids, and blood

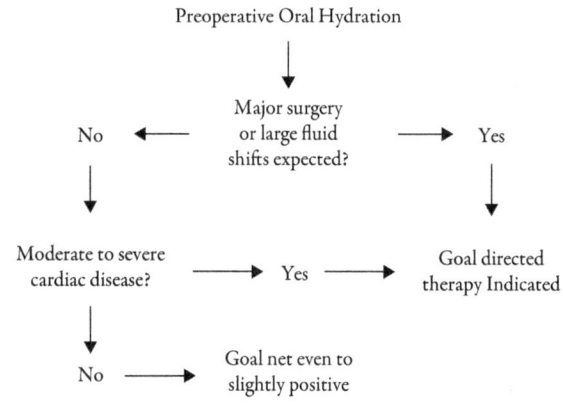

Figure 117.1 Suggested algorithm for development of a perioperative fluid management strategy.

products. Literature indicates that a balanced crystalloid solution with an acid-base and electrolyte composition similar to a patient's own plasma (e.g., Hartmann's solution, Plasma-Lyte A, Normosol, or even Lactated Ringer's) is the optimal fluid to use for maintenance therapy in the perioperative period. Evidence increasingly indicates that 0.9% saline is associated with increased risk for metabolic acidosis and AKI.[4]

The appropriate fluid to use for bolus IV resuscitation remains difficult to ascertain, and the use of colloids (e.g., albumin, hetastarches) vs. balanced crystalloids remains hotly debated. Albumin is the most commonly used colloid, and its use over crystalloids may have some benefit in certain clinical scenarios (e.g., patients with cirrhosis, especially those with ascites or patients undergoing cardiac surgery). The use of hetastarch (HES) in critically ill patients is known to increase mortality and morbidity; however, outcomes related to elective surgery are less definitive. Perioperative literature has shown a clinical correlation with increased intraoperative bleeding when HES use is compared to crystalloid and albumin; thus its routine use in the perioperative setting is not recommend.[5] Finally, patients with active major hemorrhage should be resuscitated with blood product transfusion.

## POSTOPERATIVE CONSIDERATIONS

An in-depth discussion of postoperative volume management is outside the scope of this chapter; however, early enteral intake and discontinuation of IV fluids should be attempted when clinically appropriate. This should be evaluated on a case-by-case basis, and close attention should be paid to patients who fail to meet their oral intake needs.

In summary, when developing a perioperative fluid management strategy, the clinician must consider the volume, type, and timing of perioperative fluid administration, but above all should seek to maintain euvolemia. In larger surgeries this requires continuous reassessment of the patient's volume status. The modern technique of goal-directed resuscitation, coupled with the use of balanced crystalloids for maintenance therapy, should be the backbone of any perioperative fluid-management strategy.

## REFERENCES

1. Bilku DK, et al. Role of preoperative carbohydrate loading: A systematic review. *Ann R Coll Surg Engl*. 2014;96(1):15–22.
2. Schol PB, et al. Liberal or restrictive fluid management during elective surgery: A systematic review and meta-analysis. *J Clin Anesth*. 2016;35:26–39.
3. Myles PS, et al. Restrictive versus liberal fluid therapy for major abdominal surgery. *N Engl J Med*. 2018;378(24):2263–2274.
4. Self WH, et al. Balanced crystalloids versus saline in noncritically ill adults. *N Engl J Med*. 2018;378(9):819–828. doi:10.1056/NEJMoa1711586
5. Rasmussen KC, et al. Effect of perioperative crystalloid or colloid fluid therapy on hemorrhage, coagulation competence, and outcome: A systematic review and stratified meta-analysis. *Medicine (Baltimore)*. 2016;95(31):e4498.

# 118.

# PROBLEMS OF TERM AND DELIVERY

*Mohamed Fayed and Joshua Younger*

## INTRODUCTION

Every pregnancy-related death is devastating. About 700 women die each year from complications of pregnancy. About 36% of deaths happened at delivery or in the week after. Heart disease and stroke caused more than 1 in 3 deaths (34%). Other leading causes of death included infections and severe bleeding.[1] This chapter will summarize several important labor and delivery topics. This chapter will serve as an overview for topics that will be covered in detail later. The purpose of this chapter is to provide an overview of issues that arise; in-depth discussion will follow in later chapters.

## PREECLAMPSIA AND ECLAMPSIA

### DEFINITIONS

*Preeclampsia*: New hypertension after 20 weeks gestation with significant proteinuria.

*Preeclampsia with severe features*: blood pressure (BP) >160/110 mmHg, +/– symptoms, +/– hematological or biochemical complications, +/– previous eclamptic fit.

*Eclampsia*: convulsive disorder associated with pre-eclampsia.

*HELLP syndrome*: Hemolysis, elevated liver enzymes, and low platelets.

### PRINCIPLES OF MANAGEMENT

1. Early delivery
2. Control BP: aim SBP < 160 mmHg, DBP < 110 mmHg.
3. Seizure prevention and treatment with magnesium sulfate.[2]

## SUPINE HYPOTENSIVE SYNDROME

Supine hypotensive syndrome is compression of the abdominal aorta and inferior vena cava by the gravid uterus when a pregnant woman lies on her back.

*Characterized by*: pallor, nausea, tachycardia, hypotension and dizziness.

*Management*: turning the patient to the left recumbent position, left uterine displacement, and administrating IV fluids.

## ASPIRATION OF GASTRIC CONTENTS

Aspiration may induce chemical pneumonitis, airway obstruction, or acute bronchospasm.

### MANAGEMENT

Place patient in Trendelenburg position, securing the airway with endotracheal tube, suction pharynx and trachea, positive-pressure ventilation. Bronchoscopy, pulmonary lavage, and broad-spectrum antibiotics are not indicated except possibly when particulate aspiration has occurred. Corticosteroids are generally not recommended.

## EMBOLIC DISORDERS (AMNIOTIC FLUID EMBOLISM)

### RISK FACTORS

Advanced maternal age, grand multiparty, instrumental delivery, precipitous labor, medical induction, placenta previa, placental abruption, fetal distress, eclampsia.

### CLINICAL APPROACH

This disorder may present as peripartum cardiac arrest. Conscious patients may complain of chest pain, dyspnea. Cardiogenic shock with RV (right ventricular) strain on echocardiography hypoxia DIC (disseminated intravascular coagulopathy).

### MANAGEMENT

There is no specific treatment; management is supportive, especially respiratory failure with positive pressure ventilation, cardiogenic shock, especially RV dysfunction, for example, using inotropes and pulmonary vasodilators such as dobutamine infusion, and consideration of mechanical circulatory support such as VA ECMO (extracoporeal membrane oxygenator) and treatment of coagulopathy.

## ANTEPARTUM HEMORRHAGE

### PLACENTAL ABRUPTION

*Placental abruption* is separation of the placenta from the uterus.

> *Features*: Severe abdominal pain, vaginal bleeding, fetal compromise/death.

> *Management*: Resuscitation and delivery.

## PLACENTA PREVIA

*Placenta previa* is insertion of the placenta into the lower uterine segment.

> *Features*: Typically presents with painless vaginal bleeding after 20 weeks gestation.

> *Management*: Resuscitation, ultrasound evaluation of placental position, and surgical delivery.

## POSTPARTUM HEMORRHAGE (PH)

PH is the consequence of:

> Tone (and tissue): Uterine atony (most common) associated with retained products of conception, prolonged labor, multiparity, macrosomia.

> Trauma: Tears to uterus, cervix, or vagina.

> Thrombus (inability to form thrombus): Coagulopathy or thrombocytopenia.

### MANAGEMENT

> Hemorrhage control: Urgent delivery of retained products, fundal massage, bimanual uterine compression, and examination under anesthesia.

> Uterotonic therapy: e.g., oxytocin, prostaglandin F2 alpha, e.g., carboprost.

> Extended therapies: Uterine balloon tamponade, e.g., Bakri balloon, external aortic compression, uterine arterial angioembolization, or hysterectomy.[3]

## CORD PROLAPSE

### PRESENTATION

Severe, prolonged fetal bradycardia or moderate to severe variable decelerations.

### MANAGEMENT

Prompt cesarean delivery to avoid fetal compromise. Intrauterine resuscitation, e.g., elevation of the presenting part manually, placing the patient in Trendelenburg or knee-chest position, and administering a tocolytic.

## RETAINED PLACENTA

### DEFINITION

Lack of placental expulsion within 30 minutes of delivery of an infant.

## ETIOLOGIES

The placenta may be trapped behind a partially closed cervix (incarcerated placenta); adherent to the uterine wall, but easily separated manually (placenta adherens); or pathologically invading the myometrium (placenta accreta).

## MANAGEMENT

Gentle cord traction is the initial maneuver. If unsuccessful and the lower uterus/cervix is constricted, nitroglycerin can be used to release the constriction. If the uterus is atonic, oxytocin infusion is used to promote uterine contraction.

# MATERNAL CARDIOPULMONARY RESUSCITATION

## PERIPARTUM RESUSCITATION

Key principles are advanced life-support algorithms, early intubation, manual displacement of the uterus to the left;[4] hand placement for chest compressions may need to be slightly higher. Consider bilateral (bi-axillary) defibrillator pads placement. Early call for obstetric and pediatric help. Consider perimortem Caesarean delivery.

## PERIMORTEM CAESAREAN DELIVERY

Should be commenced at 4 minutes into the cardiac arrest[5] for pregnancies over 20 weeks. There is no requirement for transfer to an operating theater, obstetric/surgical expertise.

# FEVER AND INFECTION

## SOURCES OF SEPSIS

Antepartum: e.g., Pyelonephritis, chorioamnionitis, septic abortion.

Postpartum: e.g., Caesarean wound infections, episiotomy infections, mastitis.

## MANAGEMENT

Sepsis should be managed in the standard fashion, including suitable microbiological samples, early antibiotics, appropriate hemodynamic resuscitation, and source control.

# PRETERM LABOR

*Preterm labor* is defined as the onset of labor before 37 weeks gestation.

## RISK FACTORS

Risk factors include multiple gestation, premature rupture of membrane, infection, placenta previa, abruption placenta, smoking, and substance abuse.

## TREATMENT

At <34 weeks gestation: expectant management, hospitalization, tocolytic therapy (magnesium sulfate, terbutaline, nifedipine) for 48 hours. Glucocorticoids for fetal lung maturity. Empiric antibiotics for group B Streptococcus if delivery is imminent or if there is evidence of active infection. At >34 weeks gestation: glucocorticoids for fetal lung maturity. Expectant management if lung maturity is proven, empiric antibiotic if delivery is imminent.

## REFERENCES

1. Suresh MS, et al. Cardiopulmonary resuscitation and the parturient. *Best Pract Res Clin Obstet Gynaecol.* 2010;24(3):383–400.
2. Espinoza J, et al. Gestational hypertension and preeclampsia: ACOG practice bulletin, number 222. *Obstet Gynecol.* 2020;135(6):e237–e260.
3. Apfelbaum J,L et al. Practice guidelines for obstetric anesthesia: An updated report by the American Society of Anesthesiologists Task Force on Obstetric Anesthesia and the Society for Obstetric Anesthesia and Perinatology. *Anesthesiology.* 2016;124(2):270–300.
4. Ueland K, et al. Maternal cardiovascular dynamics. IV. The influence of gestational age on the maternal cardiovascular response to posture and exercise—PubMed. 1969. Accessed July 18, 2020. https://pubmed.ncbi.nlm.nih.gov/4893386//
5. Jeejeebhoy FM, et al. Cardiac arrest in pregnancy: A scientific statement from the American Heart Association. *Circulation.* 2015;132(18):1747 1773.

# 119.

# NONOBSTETRIC SURGERY DURING PREGNANCY

*Piotr Al Jindi*

## INTRODUCTION

Approximately 1%–2% of pregnant women will need surgery during their pregnancy. These procedures, in general, have a favorable outcome for the mother and the fetus. A multidisciplinary approach is needed for these cases for optimal patient and fetal outcomes. Early during pregnancy, there is a concern about teratogenicity. Later, the problem shifts toward fetal hypoxemia and preterm labor.

## ANESTHETIC CONSIDERATIONS

### PREOPERATIVE

Current evidence does not show that there is an association between surgery or anesthesia and fetal death. Still, there is a significantly increased risk of spontaneous abortion in the first and second trimester and preterm delivery.[1-3] It is not clear if the risk of preterm labor is due to surgery or anesthesia or the mother's condition that required surgery.

### Timing of Surgery

The opinion statement of the American Society of Anesthesiology and the American College of Obstetricians and Gynecologist (ASA/ACOG) states that elective surgeries should not be performed, but if the surgery is necessary, then the pregnant patient cannot be denied surgery because of trimester consideration. The second trimester is the preferred period to perform surgeries due to the lowest risk of abortion and preterm labor during this period.[1]

Risks of maternal surgery include the teratogenicity of anesthetic agents or other drugs administered, decreased uteroplacental perfusion and/or fetal oxygenation, and subsequent preterm delivery or fetal demise.

## FETAL CONSIDERATIONS

### Teratogenicity

No currently used anesthetic agents have been shown to have any teratogenic effects in humans when using standard concentrations at any age.[1] It seems important to avoid nitrous oxide in the first trimester.[2] Opioids, neuromuscular blocking agents, barbiturates, and propofol seem to be safe.

### Fetal Brain Development

There is no current evidence that in utero human exposure to anesthetic agents has any effect on the developing fetal brain. Additionally, there is no animal data to support such an impact with limited exposure less than 3 hours in duration.[1]

Prophylactic corticosteroids should be given 48 hours before surgery between 24–34 weeks of gestation, to help with lung maturation if preterm birth is precipitated by the surgery.

Pregnant patients are at increased risk of aspiration due to lower esophageal sphincter tone and intraabdominal pressure, so aspiration prophylaxis is needed.

There is no proven benefit of prophylactic tocolytics,[3] and due to the hypercoagulable state during pregnancy, thromboprophylaxis is required.

### Fetal Heart Rate Monitoring during Surgery

Per ACOG/ASA opinion statement, if a fetus is pre-viable, then fetal heart rate (FHR) monitoring is sufficient prior to the surgery and post-surgery. Per the statement, the FHR monitoring "may be appropriate when all of the following apply: (1) the fetus is viable; (2) it is physically possible to perform intraoperative monitoring; (3) a healthcare provider with obstetric surgery privileges is available and willing to intervene during the surgical procedure for fetal indications; (4) when possible, the woman has given informed consent to emergency cesarean delivery; and (5) the nature of the planned surgery will allow the safe interruption or alteration of the procedure to provide access to perform emergency delivery."[1]

## INTRAOPERATIVE

Regional anesthesia should be the preferred modality in these cases, to minimize fetal drug exposure, and to limit the risk of hypoxemia and aspiration,[3] although no studies have shown a beneficial outcome on pregnancy when compared to general anesthesia.[3]

Loss of airway control is the most common cause of anesthesia-related maternal mortality. All pregnant patients are considered to have difficult intubation and a full stomach and are at increased risk of aspiration.

Preoxygenation is prudent due to rapid desaturation from decreased functional residual capacity (FRC) and increased oxygen consumption. It is essential to maintain normocarbia, normothermia, and avoid hypoxemia and hypotension.[3] So, hypotension should be treated aggressively.

Aortocaval compression is a major concern after the 20th week and might require a bed tilt; 15–30 degrees is advised if possible. FHR monitoring might help with the optimal positioning of the patient.

The MAC of volatile anesthetics is decreased 30%–40% during pregnancy, related to higher progesterone levels. Inhaled agents cause muscle relaxation, and they have a depressant effect on uterine contractility, which is beneficial in the setting of maternal surgery.

Since opioids and induction agents cross the placenta, if there is a need for immediate fetus delivery, fetal respiratory depression can be seen.

Anticholinesterase drugs given rapidly could stimulate the release of acetylcholine, which can precipitate uterine contraction. Thus, it is recommended to administer them after providing an anticholinergic agent and to administer them slowly. Glycopyrrolate crosses the placenta less readily than atropine, so atropine is preferred in this setting. Sugammadex per the recommendation of the Society of Obstetrics Anesthesia and Perinatology should be avoided in early pregnancy and used with caution or avoided at term or near-term pregnancy, as its effects on lactation are unknown.[4]

Cardiac surgeries and bypass carry the highest risk for the fetus. If they are necessary, then it is recommended to utilize FHR monitoring, maintain high flows on bypass, and maintain perfusion pressure >70 mmHg.[3] A normothermic bypass has shown to be advantageous over a hypothermic one. Also, normal $PaO_2$, $PaCo_2$, and acid-base balance are crucial.

For neurosurgery cases with high intracranial pressure (ICP), if induced hypotension is required, FHR monitoring is essential. Also, nitroprusside should be used with caution, as it is metabolized to cyanide, which crosses the placenta and can cause fetal death. Extreme hyperventilation to $PaCo_2$ below 32 should be avoided. Mannitol in small doses of 0.25–0.5 mg/kg seems to be safe.

Laparoscopic surgeries can be safely performed. Maintain normocarbia to avoid fetal acidosis, and low peritoneal pressure or gasless technique should be used.

## POSTOPERATIVE

No guidelines specify for how long the patient should be monitored postsurgically;[5] however, in the immediate postoperative period the patient should be monitored for uterine contractions and for FHR. Studies show that if preterm labor is not precipitated within a week after surgery, then the risk of preterm labor is the same as in the general population.[2] Since postoperative pain can precipitate uterine contraction, pain control is essential to prevent preterm labor. Nonsteriodal anti-inflammatory drugs (NSAIDs) should be avoided after 32 weeks of pregnancy, due to concern of premature closure of the fetal ductus arteriosus (if given for a longer period than 48 h).[2]

## REFERENCES

1. ACOG Committee Opinion No. 775: Nonobstetric surgery during pregnancy. *Obstet Gynecol.* 2019;133(4):e285–e286.
2. Upadya M, Nayak M. Anaesthesia for nonobstetric surgery during pregnancy. *Update Anaesth.* 2019; 34:91–96.
3. E. Reitman, P. Flood, Anaesthetic considerations for non-obstetric surgery during pregnancy. *Br J Anaesthes.* 2011;107: i72–i78.
4. Butwick W, et al.; Society for Obstetric Anesthesia and Perinatology. Statement on sugammadex during pregnancy and lactation. Ad Hoc task force, SOPA website. April 2019. https://www.soap.org/assets/docs/SOAP_Statement_Sugammadex_During_Pregnancy_Lactation_APPROVED.pdf. Accessed August 1, 2020
5. Gupta A, et al. Postoperative monitoring in pregnant patients undergoing surgery for advanced malignancy in last trimester: How long is enough? *J Anaesthesiol Clin Pharmacol.* 2014;30(2):284–286.

# Part VII

# REGIONAL ANESTHESIA

# 120.

# SPINAL, EPIDURAL, CAUDAL, AND COMBINED SPINAL/EPIDURAL ANESTHESIA

*Christopher O. Fadumiye and Brian J. Cacioppo*

## INTRODUCTION

Spinal, epidural, and caudal anesthesia are alternatives in operative management of patients that provide surgical analgesia without the need for general anesthesia.

## SPINAL ANESTHESIA

### INDICATIONS

Spinal anesthesia is indicated for patients who require anesthesia for procedures involving the lower extremities, perineum, pelvic girdle, or lower abdomen. It is especially useful in procedures where patients wish to remain conscious, or for patients who have comorbidities that put them at life-threatening risk with general anesthesia, i.e., patients whose medical history includes severe respiratory or cardiac disease, or patients with a history of difficult airway.

### CONTRAINDICATIONS

Absolute contraindications for spinal anesthesia include patient refusal of the procedure, localized infection at the desired needle entry site, and allergies to the medications (i.e., local anesthetic) that will be administered. Additionally, the inability of a patient to cooperate with instructions for placement, secondary to either comorbidities or physical limitation, classifies as an absolute contraindication.

There are numerous relative contraindications that either make accurate placement of the spinal difficult or put the patient at increased risk. These relative contraindications include:

1. *Previous spinal surgery*: Prior spinal surgery may make it challenging or impossible to access the intrathecal space, which can result in unpredictable spread of local anesthetic.
2. *Multiple sclerosis*: Patients with a diagnosis of MS may be more sensitive to local anesthetics and have prolonged sensory and motor blockade.
3. *Aortic stenosis*: Neuraxial blockade can result in marked reductions in systemic vascular resistance, putting these patients at risk of coronary hypoperfusion.
4. *Patients receiving thromboprophylaxis*: Patients receiving these medications are at increased risk of spinal/epidural hematoma formation, which can result in paralysis. See Table 120.1 for ASRA guidelines regarding discontinuation timing (guidelines change over time, so make sure you read the most recently published guidelines before the exam).
5. *Patients with inherited coagulopathy*: These patients are also at risk of hematoma formation.
6. *Systemic infection*: There is theoretical risk of seeding infection in the intrathecal space in patients with untreated or unresponsive-to-treatment systemic infections.[1,2]

### SITE OF ACTION

The desired binding sites for local anesthetic are the spinal cord, spinal nerve roots in the subarachnoid and epidural spaces, and the dorsal root ganglia. There are also various desired dermatome levels that are required for specific surgical procedures. For example, Cesarean sections require T4, hip surgery T10, and foot procedures L2. Factors that affect block distribution include dose and baricity of the medication used, cerebrospinal fluid (CSF) volume,

**Table 120.1** ASRA EVIDENCE-BASED GUIDELINES FOR NEURAXIAL ANESTHESIA IN THE PATIENT RECEIVING THROMBOPROPHYLAXIS[3]

| DRUG | NEURAXIAL NEEDLE/CATHETER PLACEMENT | | | NEURAXIAL CATHETER REMOVAL | | COMMENTS |
|---|---|---|---|---|---|---|
| | DISCONTINUE | RESTART | CATHETER | DISCONTINUE | RESTART | |
| **ANTIPLATELET AGENTS** | | | | | | |
| Aspirin | Safe for all categories | | | | | |
| NSAIDs | Safe for all categories but caution with concomitant drugs that may affect coagulation | | | | | |
| Clopidogrel | 5–7 d | Immediately If loading dose: 6 h | Catheters may be maintained for 1–2 days after restarting Clopidogrel or Ticlodipine | | Immediately. If loading dose: 6 h | |
| Ticlodipine | 10 d | | | | | |
| | | | | | | |
| Prasugrel | 7–10 d | | Avoid catheters | | | |
| Ticagrelor | 5–7 d | | | | | |
| Dipyridamole | 24 h | 6 h | Avoid catheters | | 6 h | |
| GP IIa/IIIb inhibitors | | These drugs are generally contraindicated for 4 weeks postsurgery | | | | |
| **UNFRACTIONATED HEPARIN** | | | | | | |
| Intravenous | 4–6 h and confirm normal coagulation | 1 h | Safe | 4–6 h and confirm normal coagulation | 1 h | Check platelet count before needle placement or catheter removal if duration of LMWH >4 d |
| **SUBCUTANEOUS** | | | | | | |
| Low-dose prophylaxis | 4–6 h or confirm normal coagulation | 1 h | Safe | 4–6 h and confirm normal coagulation | 1 h | 5,000 U SC bid or tid |
| Higher-dose prophylaxis | 12 h and confirm normal coagulation | | Safety of catheters not established | | | 7500–10 000 U SC bid or ≤20 000 U/d |
| Therapeutic | 24 h and confirm normal coagulation | | Avoid catheters | | | >10 000 U SC/dose or >20 000 U/d |
| **LOW MOLECULAR WEIGHT HEPARIN** | | | | | | |
| Once daily prophylaxis | 12 h | 12 h | Safe | 12 h | 4 h | Check platelet count before needle placement or catheter removal if duration of LMWH >4 d |
| Twice daily prophylaxis | | | Avoid catheters | | | |
| | | | | | | |
| Therapeutic dose | 24 h | 24–72 h | Avoid catheters | | | |
| **ORAL ANTICOAGULANTS** | | | | | | |
| Coumarins | Ideally 5 d and INR <1.5 | No delay | Monitor INR daily and check sensory/ motor function routinely | INR <1.5 | No delay | |

*Table 120.1* CONTINUED

| DRUG | NEURAXIAL NEEDLE/CATHETER PLACEMENT | | | NEURAXIAL CATHETER REMOVAL | | COMMENTS |
|---|---|---|---|---|---|---|
| | DISCONTINUE | RESTART | CATHETER | DISCONTINUE | RESTART | |
| Apixaban | 72 h | 6 h | Avoid catheters | | 6 h | Refer to ASRA guidelines if unanticipated indwelling catheter |
| | | | | | | |
| Rivaroxaban | | 6 h | | | | |

pregnancy, advanced age, and patient position during/immediately following block placement.

## ONSET

Onset for spinal anesthesia varies from 3 to 8 minutes and is dependent on the local anesthetic used. Chloroprocaine has the fastest onset time and bupivacaine the slowest.

## DURATION

Duration of blockade is dependent on the particular local anesthetic used and if any additives were used. Chloroprocaine has a duration ranging from 40 to 90 minutes, while bupivacaine can last anywhere from 130 to 230 minutes. Additives which prolong duration include opioids, steroids, vasoconstrictors, alpha-2-agonists, neostigmine, and sodium bicarbonate.

## TERMINATION OF ACTION

Termination of blockade occurs when the concentration of local anesthetic in the CSF decreases. This is due to an uptake by non-neural tissue. Of note, the time it takes for block regression is inversely correlated to CSF volume.[2] The rate of drug elimination is dependent on medication distribution (larger spread, shorter duration) and the lipid solubility, as lipid-soluble medications can bind to epidural fat and slow vascular absorption. No drug metabolism occurs in the CSF.

## SYSTEMIC TOXICITY

Local anesthetic medications at toxic systemic levels primarily affect the central nervous system (CNS), followed by the cardiovascular system. The classic sequence of events starts with minor CNS symptoms of perioral tingling, tinnitus, and/or a metallic taste in the mouth. This is quickly followed by seizures and eventual cardiovascular collapse. Treatment involves the use of a bolus dose of intralipid followed by an infusion. Propofol should never be used as a substitute for intralipid. When performing ACLS, it is important to remember that patients require a decreased dose of epinephrine.[2]

## TEST DOSE

Small volume of 1.5% lidocaine (or similar concentration) with 10–15 mcg of epinephrine are typically used as a test dose with the following endpoints to determine intravascular injection: increase in systolic blood pressure more than 15 mmHg, or an increase in heart rate more than 10 beats per minute.

## COMPLICATIONS

### NEUROLOGIC

Serious neurologic complications are quite rare. These potential catastrophic complications include paraplegia (secondary to direct needle trauma, contaminated medications, or preservative-containing medications), profound hypoperfusion/ischemia causing irreversible damage, and epidural hematomas (bleeding in the epidural space causing ischemic compression of the spinal cord).

Transient neurologic symptom (TNS) is bilateral or unilateral pain in the buttocks that radiates to the legs, occurring within 24 hours of spinal resolutions and lasting for approximately one week. TNS was traditionally associated with lidocaine administration but has been described with any local anesthetic.[1] Other potential neurologic complications include nerve injury, arachnoiditis, and post-dural puncture headache (see section on Epidural Anesthesia).

### CARDIOVASCULAR

Cardiovascular complications include hypotension, bradycardia, and, more rarely, sudden cardiac arrest.

## RESPIRATORY

There is a dose-dependent risk of respiratory depression when neuraxial opioids are used.

## INFECTIOUS

Bacterial meningitis and epidural abscess are rare but nonetheless potential and life-threatening complications.

## OTHER COMPLICATIONS
### Backache

Risk factors for backache include preexisting back pain, surgery greater than 2.5 hours, lithotomy position, body mass index (BMI) greater than 32, and multiple block attempts.

### Nausea and Vomiting

Possible causes of nausea and vomiting following neuraxial anesthesia include use of opioids in the block (morphine greater risk than fentanyl), addition of phenylephrine or epinephrine, history of motion sickness, use of procaine, and hypotension during spinal.

### Pruritus

Commonly occurs with addition of opioids. Mechanism is likely secondary to central opioid receptor activation and not histamine release. Nalbuphine can be used for treatment.

### Shivering

Shivering is related more to epidural than spinal. It can be prevented with prewarming patients, avoiding administration of cold medications/fluids, and the addition of opioids.

### Wrong Route of Administration

There is the risk of infusion of medication in the wrong compartment or intravascular injection.

## PHYSIOLOGIC EFFECTS
### Gastrointestinal

Blockade of T6 to L1 interferes with splanchnic sympathetic innervation, resulting in hyperperistalsis. This increase in gut motility causes nausea and vomiting in as much as 20% of patients. However, the primary causes of nausea and vomiting have been mentioned earlier.

### Pulmonary

Paralysis of the abdominal muscles leads to a decrease in expiratory reserve volume and vital capacity. This is typically compensated by the use of other accessory respiratory muscles. The diaphragm is unaffected given that its innervation comes from C3–C5. Respiratory arrest in the setting of neuraxial anesthesia is usually secondary to hypoperfusion of the respiratory centers of the brainstem and not phrenic nerve dysfunction.[2]

### Cardiac

Blockade of the peripheral and cardiac sympathetic fibers (T1–L2 and T1–T4) causes decreased stroke volume and heart rate. There is also a decrease in arterial blood pressure during spinals, more so than epidurals. Decreases in afterload and heart rate can also lead to a decrease in myocardial oxygen demand.

### Renal

Neuraxial blockade causes a decrease in renal blood flow; however, it is of little physiologic importance. There is a common misconception that spinal and epidural anesthesia cause urinary retention. However, studies have shown that the incidence of urinary retention was no more frequent with neuraxial anesthesia than with general anesthesia and opioids.[1]

## EPIDURAL ANESTHESIA

Epidural anesthesia is indicated for surgeries involving the same dermatomal distribution as spinal anesthesia and can be utilized in procedures even further up the thorax. They can also be administered via intermittent or continuous catheter delivery, thus extending its duration of action and allowing for longer procedures. Additionally, epidurals can be helpful in providing postoperative neuraxial analgesia.

## POST-DURAL PUNCTURE HEADACHE (PDPH)

Though a potential complication following any method of neuraxial anesthesia, PDPH is more common following unintentional dural puncture during epidural placement. This is because of the larger bore needle required for passing an epidural catheter, as well as the type of needle that is used. PDPH is characterized by frontal or occipital headache pain that worsens when in the upright or seated position and improves with lying supine.[2] It can be associated with nausea, vomiting, neck pain, dizziness, tinnitus, and diplopia. PDPH is thought to be secondary to loss of CSF, causing traction on intracranial structures and initiating compensatory intracranial vasodilation. However, these causes are theoretical and not yet proven.

Risk factors for PDPH include younger age, female gender, larger sized needle, pregnancy, and multiple punctures. Conservative management includes supine positioning, hydration, caffeine, abdominal binder, and oral analgesics. An epidural blood patch may also be used, which has up to 90% initial improvement in rate of symptoms.

## CAUDAL ANESTHESIA

Caudal anesthesia is a popular technique used in pediatric anesthesia, but it can also be performed in adults. Indications in adults are essentially the same as the indications for lumbar epidural anesthesia, and it is particularly useful when sacral spread is desired. It is also useful in patients who have a prior spinal surgery scar. This technique is commonly utilized in chronic pain and cancer pain management.

## COMBINED SPINAL/EPIDURAL

Combined spinal and epidural (CSE) anesthesia allows for the faster onset of a spinal with the extended duration of an epidural. This allows for longer duration procedures to be performed without general anesthesia. Additionally, with this technique, a smaller amount of medication can be used in the spinal with extension of the block, if necessary, using the epidural, providing improved hemodynamic stability.

## GENERAL INFORMATION

Spinal, epidural, and caudal blocks result in sympathetic, sensory, and or motor blockade depending on dose, concentration, and volume of local anesthetic administered.

The spinal cord originates at the distal end of the brainstem and terminates as the conus medullaris, which is separated into the filum terminale and the cauda equina. Termination occurs at approximately L3 in infants and L1 in adults. Surrounding the spinal cords are three membranes: the pia mater, the arachnoid mater, and the dura mater. CSF resides in the space between the pia mater and the arachnoid mater (intrathecal space).

## REFERENCES

1. Butterworth JF, et al. Spinal, epidural, & caudal blocks. In: *Morgan & Mikhail's Clinical Anesthesiology*. New York, NY: McGraw-Hill Education; 2018:937–973.
2. Gropper MA, Miller RD. Spinal, epidural, and caudal anesthesia. In: *Miller's Anesthesia*. Philadelphia, PA: Elsevier; 2020: 1413–1445.
3. Horlocker TT, et al. Regional anesthesia in the patient receiving antithrombotic or thrombolytic therapy. *Reg Anesth Pain Med*. 2018;43(3):263–309.

# 121.

# INTRAVENOUS REGIONAL ANESTHESIA

*Elizabeth Scholzen and Lisa Klesius*

## BACKGROUND

Many nerve blocks can be used as a primary anesthetic for upper or lower extremity surgeries. However, unlike peripheral nerve blocks that target a specific nerve or nerve plexus, intravenous regional anesthesia (IVRA), also known as a Bier block, provides anesthesia of the entire extremity through intravenous local anesthetic injection while a tourniquet retains the medication in the desired area, resulting in nerve blockade via diffusion into the surrounding tissues. Benefits of the IVRA technique over peripheral nerve blocks include faster onset/offset of nerve blockade, reliability of technique, and ease of performance without need for special equipment.

## TECHNIQUE

There are two similar techniques that can be used for IVRA. First is the traditional approach that involves anesthetizing the entire arm with a tourniquet placed high on the upper arm. This technique has largely fallen out of favor due to the high volume of local anesthetic required and the potential for associated local anesthetic toxicity. In addition, a minimum tourniquet time of 20–30 minutes makes the block less practical for short procedures.[1] The second approach is a newer technique that involves anesthetizing only the distal forearm, wrist, and hand, with a tourniquet placed on the forearm. This technique uses a lower volume of local anesthetic and can be used for procedures less than 30 minutes. Both techniques are described in the following.

### TRADITIONAL TECHNIQUE

1. Place an additional IV in the operative forearm (the patient should already have an IV in a non-operative extremity).

2. Place a double pneumatic tourniquet high on the upper arm.
3. Raise the arm for 1–2 minutes to allow for passive exsanguination and then actively exsanguinate the arm using an Esmarch bandage wrapped from fingers to axilla.
4. Inflate the distal tourniquet followed by the proximal tourniquet to 100 mmHg above systolic blood pressure. Release the distal tourniquet and remove the Esmarch bandage.
5. Inject an intermediate-acting local anesthetic (approximately 50–60 mL of 0.5% lidocaine) and then remove the IV in the operative arm.
6. Only one of the tourniquets is inflated at a time. If tourniquet pain develops (typically occurs after 20–30 minutes of inflation) the alternate (distal) tourniquet is inflated, checked for functionality, and then the proximal tourniquet is deflated.
7. The tourniquet must be inflated for at least 30 minutes after local anesthetic injection to avoid local anesthetic toxicity after deflation. If the tourniquet must be deflated before this time, a gradual, sequential deflation/reinflation technique may be used.

### FOREARM TECHNIQUE

1. Place an additional IV in the operative forearm.
2. Place a single tourniquet on the proximal forearm and exsanguinate the arm using the same process as the traditional technique.
3. Inflate the tourniquet to 100 mmHg above systolic blood pressure and remove the Esmarch bandage.
4. Inject 20–30 mL of an intermediate-acting local anesthetic (0.5% lidocaine) and remove the IV in operative arm.
5. Generally, there does not need to be a sequential release of the tourniquet, even after short procedures,

due to the low dose of local anesthetic involved in the block.

## CONTRAINDICATIONS

The only true absolute contraindication to IVRA is patient refusal. All other contraindications are relative, and the benefits and risks of IVRA need to be carefully weighed against other anesthetic techniques. Contraindications are outlined in Box 121.1.

---

**Box 121.1** CONTRAINDICATIONS TO IRVA

**Relative Contraindications[2]**

Cellulitis over the surgical area
Crush injury or compound fracture of the extremity
Patients with vascular injury to the extremity (i.e., Raynaud's, scleroderma)
Sickle cell disease
Allergy to local anesthetics
Surgeries anticipated to last longer than 1 hour

---

## COMPLICATIONS

The most concerning complication with IVRA is the potential for local anesthetic systemic toxicity (LAST). Thankfully, LAST is a rare complication. According to the ASA Closed Claims Project of 1980–1999, there have only been 3 cases reported of death or brain damage resulting from LAST related to IVRA.[3] The most common adverse reaction from an IVRA is tourniquet pain, which can be improved with inflation of the distal tourniquet over the anesthetized arm in the setting of a traditional IVRA, or with additional systemic sedatives and analgesics. Other rare complications from IVRA include nerve damage or compartment syndrome.

## REFERENCES

1. Arslanian B, et al. Forearm Bier block: A new regional anesthetic technique for upper extremity surgery. *Ann Plast Surg.* 2014;73(2):156–157.
2. Candido K, et al. Intravenous regional block for upper and lower extremity surgery. NYSORA. 2021. https://www.nysora.com/techniques/intravenous-regional-anesthesia/intravenous-regional-block-upper-lower-extremity-surgery/.
3. Kraus GP, et al. Bier block. [Updated July 24, 2020]. In: *StatPearls* [Internet]. Treasure Island, FL: StatPearls; 2020 Jan–. Available from: https://www.ncbi.nlm.nih.gov/books/NBK430760/.

# 122.

# NEUROAXIAL ANESTHESIA IN OBSTETRICS

*John Penner*

## LABOR EPIDURAL

Providing labor analgesia using an epidural consists of the epidural block initiation and maintenance phases. Table 122.1 summarizes the medications and concentrations of drugs used for labor analgesia.

## EPIDURAL INITIATION PHASE

Block initiation is the process during which the epidural block is established at a level that provides adequate pain relief. This is accomplished by bolus dosing of the catheter. The preferred bolus medication is a dilute local anesthetic solution, with or without narcotic. The advantages of using a dilute local anesthetic include allowing a greater volume (and thus greater spread), decreased risk of local anesthetic toxicity, and less likelihood of prolonging the second stage of labor. On occasion a higher concentration solution may be used. The total bolus dose is usually 10–20 ml of dilute local anesthetic, with or without narcotic, injected in 5 ml increments every 5–10 minutes. Adding 50–100 mcg of fentanyl into the epidural during initiation of the epidural can increase patient comfort and supplement the effect of

**Table 122.1** DRUGS USED TO INITIATE AND MAINTAIN EPIDURAL ANALGESIA

| LOCAL ANESTHETIC* (BOLUS AND INFUSION CONCENTRATIONS) | NARCOTIC (BOLUS DOSES) | NARCOTIC (INFUSION CONCENTRATIONS) |
|---|---|---|
| Bupivicaine 0.05%–0.125% | Fentanyl 50–100 mcg | Fentanyl 1.5–3 mcg/ml |
| Ropivicaine 0.08%–0.2% | Sufentanil 5–15 mcg | Sufentanil 0.2 mcg/ml |

*1% lidocaine and 2% 2-chloroprocaine may also be used to initiate an epidural. But their short duration of action limits their effectiveness in labor.

the local anesthetic but comes with the risk of pruritis and nausea.

## MAINTENANCE PHASE

The goal of the maintenance phase is to maintain the level achieved during block initiation. There are three maintenance techniques used: a continuous epidural infusion (CEI); a continuous infusion with patient-controlled bolus dosing (PCEA); and, a programmed intermittent mandatory bolus dosing with or without PCEA (PIEB).

## CONTINUOUS EPIDURAL INFUSION (CEI)

CEIs use a pump to deliver a steady infusion of dilute local anesthetic, with or without narcotic. The rate of infusion depends on several variables, including patient height, use of intrathecal medications (CSE, see later discussion), and the patient's response to the initial bolus doses. The rate is often set between 8 and 15 ml/hour. If the patient's level decreases, manual boluses are provided by the anesthesia provider. A CEI has the advantage of decreasing physician workload while maintaining a steady level. It also improves patient satisfaction. It does not eliminate the need for the provider to intermittently "top up" the epidural. The addition of fentanyl or sufentanil to the infused mix can enhance the block with minimal side effects on the mother or fetus.

## PATIENT-CONTROLLED EPIDURAL ANALGESIA (PCEA)

PCEA starts with a CEI and adds self-administered bolus doses controlled by the patient. A lock-out interval between bolus doses is set to avoid overdosing. PCEA gives the parturient a feeling of control over her pain management and can decrease provider-given top-ups. The pump is programmed with a basal rate of local anesthetic infusion, a volume for the bolus dose, and a lock-out interval during which no

bolus dose may be given. The medications used in this technique are the same as those used for CEI. The ideal settings to use for this technique remain controversial. According to Wong,[1] a reasonable approach is a background infusion of 5–8 ml/hr with a bolus dose of 5–10 ml and a lock-out interval of 10–20 minutes.

## PROGRAMMED INTERMITTENT EPIDURAL BOLUS (PIEB)

PIEB takes advantage of the observation that epidural local anesthetic spread is greater when bolus doses are given, rather than infusions. The greater spread results in a better sensory block. The idea of PIEB is to deliver a similar volume of local anesthetic as a CEI over a given time period, but to do it with intermittent boluses rather than an infusion (i.e., rather than an infusion of 10 ml/hr, the patient is given 5-ml boluses every 30 minutes). PIEB can be used alone or with PCEA, depending on the pump used. Studies have demonstrated several advantages to PIEB, including decreased local anesthetic consumption, less motor block, and improved maternal satisfaction scores.[2] The ideal dosing regimen for PIEB has not yet been established (3). A reasonable protocol is to start the PIEB 30 minutes after the initiation of the epidural or CSE with a programmed bolus dose of 5–10 ml every 30–60 minutes. The longer the duration between the programmed bolus, the larger the volume the bolus can be. It is important to monitor the patient's sensory level to ensure that the patient's level does not get too high. Some pumps allow for patient-delivered boluses (PCEA) in addition to the mandatory boluses.

## COMBINED SPINAL EPIDURAL (CSE) FOR LABOR ANALGESIA

CSE uses a dose of intrathecal medication to get a patient comfortable quickly. An epidural catheter is then used to maintain pain control. Commonly used medications and doses are summarized in Table 122.2. The primary risk of a CSE is that a nonfunctioning epidural catheter may not

**Table 122.2** INTRATHECAL AGENTS FOR CSE INJECTION

| LOCAL ANESTHETICS | OPIOIDS |
|---|---|
| Bupivicaine 1.25–2.5 mg | Fentanyl 15–25 mcg |
| Ropivicaine 2.5–4.5 mg | Sufentanil 1.5–5 mcg |

be discovered until an hour or more after it is placed. Thus, for patients at higher risk for an operative delivery, or those with an unfavorable airway exam, a CSE may not be the technique of choice. Choices for intrathecal medications include an opioid, a local anesthetic, or combination thereof. Since fentanyl and bupivacaine are synergistic, they are commonly used together for the spinal medications. Compared to fentanyl, sufentanil is both more potent and longer lasting. However, the formulation of sufentanil available in the US (50 mcg/ml) makes accurate dosing challenging. The use of intrathecal opioid is more likely to cause pruritis than epidural opioid.

Once the spinal dose is given and the epidural catheter placed, one can either initiate the catheter right away or wait 30–60 minutes. Due to the potential for intrathecal spread of a test dose given through the epidural catheter, intrathecal medications used in the CSE are often reduced if the test dose is given immediately after threading the catheter. Once the epidural catheter is initiated, its dosing is based upon the protocol chosen (CEI, PCEA, PIEB).

## NEURAXIAL ANESTHESIA FOR CESAREAN SECTIONS

The neuraxial anesthetic choice for cesarean section (c-section) depends on several variables, including the presence and functionality of an in situ epidural catheter, the urgency of the situation, the anticipated duration of the c-section, and patient comorbidities. Any neuraxial technique chosen for c-section should provide a T4 level due to the manipulation of the viscera during the operation.

## SPINAL ANESTHETIC FOR C-SECTION

Spinal anesthesia is the first choice for c-sections if no epidural is in place. It provides a rapid, reliable, and safe anesthetic with a minimum of medication. It also avoids airway manipulation and allows the parturient to be awake for the delivery. The choices of local anesthetic for c-section include bupivacaine, lidocaine, chloroprocaine, and ropivacaine (summarized in Table 122.3). However, practically, only bupivacaine and ropivacaine are used. Additives to the local anesthetic may also be used (see below) and are summarized in Table 122.4.

Hyperbaric bupivacaine (0.75% bupivacaine in 8.25% dextrose) is frequently the drug of choice for c-section due to its reliable onset and suitable duration of action. The hyperbaric solution allows the level of block to be manipulated by adjusting the bed position. Ropivacaine is less potent than bupivacaine and has a slightly shorter duration of action but offers the advantage of having faster return of motor function. Results of studies using ropivacaine for c-section suggests its use is improved when combined with an opioid. Chloroprocaine and lidocaine are rarely used in spinal anesthesia for c-section due to their shorter duration of action and the increased risk of transient neurologic symptoms with lidocaine.

Additives to the local anesthetic chosen used include opioids, epinephrine, and clonidine (see Table 122.4). The lipophilic opioids fentanyl and sufentanil improve the density of intraoperative spinal block and help manage the visceral pain that occurs with uterine manipulation. The addition of the lipophobic opioids morphine and hydromorphone to the spinal can assist in the management of postoperative pain for 12–36 hours, though their onset is too slow to reduce intraoperative pain. The addition of lipophobic opioids comes with the potential side effects of nausea, vomiting, pruritis, and delayed respiratory depression.

Epinephrine, clonidine, and neostigmine have all been found to prolong spinal anesthetics. Epinephrine (100–200 mcg) will extend surgical anesthesia and analgesia. Clonidine (50–75 mcg), when added to hyperbaric

**Table 122.3** LOCAL ANESTHETICS USED FOR SPINAL C-SECTION

| LOCAL ANESTHETIC | BARICITY | CONCENTRATION (%) | DOSE (MG) | DURATION (IN MINUTES) |
|---|---|---|---|---|
| 2-Chloroprocaine | Isobaric | 3 | 20–60 | 30–50 |
| Lidocaine | Hyperbaric | 5 | 75–100 | 60–70 |
| Ropivacaine | Isobaric | 0.75, 1.0 | 15–20 | 75–120 |
| Bupivacaine | Hyperbaric | 0.75 | 6–12 | 90–110 |
| Bupivacaine | Isobaric | 0.5 | 8–15 | 90–100 |

*Table 122.4* ADDITIVES TO SPINAL ANESTHETICS

| DRUG | DOSE (MCG) | EFFECT | ONSET (MINUTES) | DURATION (HOUR) |
|---|---|---|---|---|
| Fentanyl | 10–25 | Intraoperative analgesia | <10 | 2–4 hours |
| Sufentanil | 2.5–10 | Intraoperative analgesia | <10 | 4 |
| Morphine | 50–150 | Postoperative analgesia | 30–60 | 12–36 hours |
| Hydromorphone | 50–100 | Postoperative analgesia | 30–60 | 6–24 hours |
| Epinephrine | 100–200 | Increased spinal duration | | |
| Clonidine | 50–75 | Increased spinal duration and post-op analgesia | | |

bupivacaine, can increase the time to first analgesic request by patients. However, when compared to bupivacaine and fentanyl, it doesn't offer any advantage in 24-hour analgesic requirements.[4] Neostigmine has shown to lead to unacceptable levels of nausea and vomiting in the obstetric population.

## EPIDURAL ANESTHETIC FOR C-SECTION

Epidurals are used for c-section when already in place from labor, or in select patients based upon their airway exam, comorbidities, or expected duration of surgery. Whether the catheter is in situ or newly placed, it is dosed with a high-concentration local anesthetic to establish a surgical level (T4). Larger doses of local anesthetic may be needed if the catheter new. The choices for local anesthetic for c-section using an epidural are summarized in Table 122.5.

The preferred choice for dosing epidural catheters for c-section is 2% lidocaine with epinephrine. It has a rapid onset, reasonable duration, and carries a low risk of systemic toxicity. Epinephrine prolongs and intensifies the block. If a more rapid onset is desired, sodium bicarbonate may be added. Two-chloroprocaine (3%) is useful for urgent c-sections due to its very rapid onset and low toxicity profile. It will, however, likely need to be re-dosed prior to the end of surgery. Bupivacaine (0.5%) is usually avoided due to the

*Table 122.5* LOCAL ANESTHETICS FOR EPIDURAL C-SECTION

| DRUG | ONSET | TWO DERMATOMAL REGRESSION |
|---|---|---|
| 2% lidocaine | 10–20 minutes* | 60–120 minutes |
| 3% 2-chloroprocaine | 5–15 minutes* | 30–90 minutes |
| 0.5% bupivacaine | 15–20 minutes | 160–220 minutes |

* May be enhanced by addition of sodium bicarbonate.

potential for cardiac toxicity and its slow onset. Regardless of local anesthetic chosen, the epidural is usually dosed with 5 ml boluses until a level of T4 is achieved (usually 15–25 ml total). If the surgical procedure extends beyond the duration of the local anesthetic, additional bolus doses are given to "top up" the level back to the T4 level.

## CSE ANESTHETIC FOR C-SECTION

CSEs are used for c-sections when the duration of the operation is uncertain. The spinal dose establishes a dense and reliable block which can be extended by dosing the epidural catheter. Often a full spinal dose of local anesthetic is given, and the catheter threaded and taped in place. If the spinal begins to regress prior to the operation being complete, the epidural test dose is given. Note that a test dose in this situation will only detect an intravascular catheter; a motor block from the original spinal block will still be present. If the test dose is negative, the catheter is bolus dosed as needed with local anesthetic.

## COMPLICATIONS OF OBSTETRIC NEURAXIAL ANESTHESIA

Complications of neuraxial anesthesia are discussed elsewhere in this book. The following is a summary of complications with special relevance to obstetric anesthesia.

### HYPOTENSION

Neuraxial techniques cause a sympathectomy, which in turn reduces systemic vascular resistance, venous return, and blood pressure. Placental blood flow does not autoregulate; thus a drop in blood pressure decreases perfusion to the fetus and may cause fetal distress. The drop is greater for c-section anesthetics than labor analgesia due to the higher level obtained and denser block required. The drop in pressure can be attenuated with a fluid bolus (500–1000 ml crystalloid) prior to, or concurrent with, block placement, and pressors. For c-sections anesthetics, a prophylactic phenylephrine infusion can be started and titrated to maintain the patient's blood pressure. Labor epidurals result in less hypotension than those used for surgery. These blood pressure changes are usually managed with bolus doses of ephedrine or phenylephrine. Historically, the patient is positioned with left uterine displacement after epidural placement to improve venous return. Recent studies suggest this may not be as effective as once thought, yet it is a low-risk maneuver.

## EPIDURAL-RELATED MATERNAL FEVER (ERMF)

The use of neuraxial anesthesia in labor and delivery is associated with an increase in maternal temperature over time. The mechanism of maternal fever related to epidural analgesia is complex but seems to be primarily related to inflammation. Data supporting inflammation includes a lack of effect with prophylactic antibiotics (not infectious), little improvement with acetaminophen (anti-pyretic with little anti-inflammatory action), and successful treatment with higher dose steroids (potent anti-inflammatory). Local anesthetics used in labor epidurals have been implicated as a source of inflammation, both due to their immunomodulatory effects as well as potentially having a direct pre-inflammatory effect at the cellular level.[5]

## EFFECTS ON LABOR

The timing of neuraxial anesthesia appears to have no effect on c-section rate, operative delivery, or fetal outcome. The duration of the first stage of labor may decrease with neuraxial analgesia, while the effect on the second stage is less clear. A recent meta-analysis looking at the effect of just low-concentration labor epidurals on the second stage of labor found a statistically insignificant lengthening of the second stage of just 5.7 minutes. Based on these findings, it seems reasonable to offer neuraxial analgesia independent of the stage of dilation or delivery.

## REFERENCES

1. Wong CA. Advances in labor analgesia. *Int J Womens Health*. 2009;1:139–154.
2. Wong CA, et al. A randomized comparison of programmed intermittent epidural bolus with continuous epidural infusion for labor analgesia. *Anesth Analg*. 2006; 102: 904–909.
3. Carvalho B, et al. Implementation of programmed intermittent epidural bolus for the maintenance of labor analgesia. *Anesth Analg*. 2016;123:965–671.
4. Khezri MB, et al. Comparison of postoperative analgesic effect of intrathecal clonidine and fentanyl added to bupivacaine in patients undergoing cesarean section: A prospective randomized double-blind study. *Pain Res Treat*. 2014; 2014:513628.
5. Sultan P, et al. Inflammation and epidural-related fever: proposed mechanisms. *Anesth Analg*. 2016:122:1546–1553.

# Part VIII
# GENERAL ANESTHESIA

# 123.

# STAGES AND SIGNS OF ANESTHESIA

*Daniel Gotlib and Melinda M. Lawrence*

## INTRODUCTION

The administration of anesthesia causes a variety of physiological changes to the human body. For centuries, anesthetists have tried to explain these changes through observed object findings. However, due to numerous confounding factors, including patient physiology, anesthetic agents, administration technique, and preliminary medications, categorizing a consistent set of observable findings has proven challenging. During World War I, Guedel devised a set of four stages of anesthesia to further facilitate and standardize the administration of diethyl ether anesthetic while in the battlefield. These stages focused on anesthetic depth to changes in respiratory response, pupillary response, and eye movement. In 1943, Gillespie further categorized these stages to other physiological changes, including pharyngeal reflexes, laryngeal reflexes, and lacrimation (see Table 123.1).

## STAGE I: ANALGESIA

The stage of analgesia begins at anesthesia administration and ends at loss of consciousness. The patient continues to have normal baseline functions, including regular breathing, voluntary ocular motor movements, and normal muscle tone. All reflexes are still intact.

## STAGE II: EXCITEMENT

The stage of excitement begins with loss of consciousness and ends with regular respiration. In practice, the eyelash reflex is lost, yet the eyelid reflex remains intact during stage II. The pupils are dilated, yet still responsive to light. Respirations become irregular. Patient has high muscle tone and the ability to move if stimulated. The anesthetic depth should be increased prior to surgical stimulation to avoid patient movement. The pharyngeal and laryngeal reflexes

begin to diminish resulting in first a decrease in swallowing, and then a decrease in retching.[2] However, the glottis is still able to spasm during this stage. The anesthetic depth should be decreased prior to extubation to avoid laryngospasm and glottic closure.

## STAGE III: SURGICAL ANESTHESIA

The stage of surgical anesthesia begins at regular respiration and ends at cessation of spontaneous breathing. This stage is further divided into 4 planes.

### PLANE 1

Plane 1 begins with regular respiration. The eyelid reflex, vomiting reflex, and lacrimation are abolished, while the pupils constrict again.

### PLANE 2

Plane 2 begins with the loss of ocular movements. Spontaneous respiratory rate begins to increase, and tidal volumes decrease, resulting in minimal to no change in the minute ventilation. Pupils begin to dilate. Glottic reflex is abolished, minimizing the chance for laryngospasm during deep extubation. Muscle tone and movement to stimulus begin to diminish.

### PLANE 3

Plane 3 begins with a decrease in intercostal muscle movement. Pupils continue to dilate and the pupillary light reflex begins to diminish.

### PLANE 4

Plane 4 begins with the paralysis of intercostal muscles. Pupils continue to dilate, and pupillary light reflex is further

*Table 123.1* STAGES OF ANESTHESIA

| | RESPIRATION | OCULAR MOVEMENTS | PUPIL RESPONSE | EYE REFLEXES | LACRIMATION | PHARYNX LARYNX REFLEX | MUSCLE TONE |
|---|---|---|---|---|---|---|---|
| Stage I | Regular breathing | Voluntary control | ⬤ Light reflex intact | Intact | Intact | Intact | Normal |
| Stage II | Irregular breathing | | ⬤ Light reflex intact | Eyelid tone high, eyelash reflex absent | | Swallow reflex diminishes, retching reflex diminishes | Muscle tone high, movement to surgical stimulation |
| Stage III Plane 1 | Regular breathing | | ⬤ Light reflex intact | Eyelid reflex absent | Lacrimation decreases | Vomiting reflex diminishes | |
| Plane 2 | RR increases, TV decreases | Ocular movement abolished | ⬤ Light reflex intact | | | Glottic reflex diminishes | Muscle tone decreases |
| Plane 3 | Decreased intercostal movement | | ⬤ Light reflex diminishes | | | | |
| Plane 4 | Paralysis of intercostal muscles | | ⬤ | | | Carinal reflex diminishes | Muscle tone minimal |
| Stage IV | Respiratory failure | | ⬤ Light reflex absent | | | | |

Modified from Guedel.

diminished. Carinal reflexes are abolished, resulting in no coughing when the carina is stimulated. This reflex is typically triggered by deep placement of the endotracheal tube.

## STAGE IV: MEDULLARY DEPRESSION

The stage begins at cessation of respiration to cardiovascular failure. This stage indicates a dangerous anesthetic concentration and plans to decrease the anesthetic should be implemented immediately. Pupils are fixed, dilated, and unresponsive to light stimulus. Most reflexes are absent.

## LEVELS OF SEDATION

The American Society of Anesthesiologists (ASA) guidelines define a varying degree of sedation for clinical services which require lower levels of sedation (Table 123.2). Minimal sedation is defined as normal responses to verbal stimulation, with unaffected airway, ventilation, cardiovascular function. Moderate sedation involves purposeful response to verbal or tactile stimulation, with unaffected airway, ventilation, or cardiovascular function. Deep sedation is defined as purposeful response to repeated or painful stimulation. The

*Table 123.2* SEDATION LEVELS

SEDATION LEVELS

|  | RESPONSE LEVEL | AIRWAY | SPONTANEOUS BREATHING | CARDIOVASCULAR FUNCTION (CV) |
|---|---|---|---|---|
| Minimal Sedation | Normal response to verbal stimuli | Maintained airway | Maintained spontaneous breathing | Maintained CV function |
| Moderate Sedation | Purposeful response to verbal or tactile stimuli | No intervention required | Adequate | Usually maintained CV function |
| Deep Sedation | Purposeful response to repeated or painful stimuli | May need intervention | May need intervention | |
| General Anesthesia | Unarousable even with painful stimuli | Often need intervention | Often need intervention | May be impaired |

Adapted from the American Society of Anesthesiologists, *Definitions of General Anesthesia and Levels of Sedation/Analgesia.*

patient may have compromised airway and ventilation at this sedation level, which may require intervention. General anesthesia involves no response to stimulation. Patients under general anesthesia often have a high probability of airway and respiratory compromise, requiring further intervention. Cardiovascular function may also be impaired at this level, requiring additional intervention.[3]

## REFERENCES

1. The signs of anaesthesia. Gillespie N. A. D.M.(Oxon.) D.A. (Eng.) APA, Current Researches in Anesthesia & Analgesia: September-October 1943: 275–282.
2. Dripps, et al. Introduction. In: *Anesthesia Principles of Safe Practice. Chapter 16: Evaluation of the Response to Anesthetics: The Signs and Stages.* 5th ed., W. B. Saunders, 1977.
3. Barash P. *Clinical Anesthesia.* 8th ed. Philidelphia, PA: Wolters Kluwer

# 124.

# TECHNIQUES OF GENERAL ANESTHESIA

*Vicko Gluncic*

## TOTAL INTRAVENOUS ANESTHESIA

In total intravenous anesthesia (TIVA), general anesthesia is both achieved and maintained by intravenously given hypnotics in the form of boluses or continuous infusion.[1-3] It is the preferred choice for adult patients, because it avoids the unpleasant smell of inhalation anesthetics. TIVA offers smooth and fast induction with minimal excitatory phase (stage 2), as well as the fast emergence because of short context-sensitive time. Also, it is an elegant and safe choice for patients with impaired ventilation and lung perfusion, while the uptake of anesthetics is independent of ventilation. It is often chosen for surgical procedures requiring neuromonitoring (e.g., brain, spinal, and some ENT surgeries) because of little effects on evoked potentials. Other advantages of TIVA are:[2,3]

- Better accepted by patients
- Better hemodynamic stability in general
- Reduction of postoperative nausea and vomiting (propofol)
- Reduction of intracranial pressure (propofol)
- Some level of analgesia (ketamine)
- No risk of malignant hyperthermia
- No generation of fluoride compounds and compound A (potential nephrotoxicity)
- Less environmental pollution.

On the other hand, the disadvantages are hemodynamic instability at induction (which can be avoided by careful dose titration), and awareness due to harder control of the depth of anesthesia and unknown drug concentration (because of the variable dose requirements among the patients due to different pharmacodynamics), which can be avoided by the use of several technologies for anesthesia depth monitoring (e.g., bispectral index [BIS] monitoring).[2,3]

Except for general anesthesia, TIVA is used for procedural sedation and for deep sedation in ambulatory surgery.

## TOTAL INHALATION ANESTHESIA

Total inhalation anesthesia, or volatile induction and maintenance anesthesia (VIMA), is a general anesthesia technique in which the induction and maintenance are achieved by inhalation of potent volatile anesthetics.[4] Although the "dose" of volatile anesthetic is usually guided by end-tidal alveolar concentration (EtAC) and minimal alveolar concentration (MAC), the assessment of the phases of VIMA and its depth is based on the movements of eyeballs, changes in breathing, and signs of sympathetic stimulation (rise of the blood pressure and heart rate, sweating, mydriasis), and the titration is made according to the blood pressure, heart rate, minute ventilation, and movements.[4]

Sevoflurane, isoflurane, desflurane are volatile anesthetics delivered as vaporized gases via anesthesia machine. Nitrous oxide, a pressurized gas, is delivered via flowmeter (as oxygen and air).

Induction and emergence in VIMA are fast, but they vary for different agents. Factors that speed up induction are: low blood solubility (low blood:gas partition coefficient) and low brain solubility (low brain:blood partition coefficient) of anesthetics, high minute ventilation, and low cardiac output (increases alveolar concentration of the volatile anesthetic).[4] Induction may be even faster if the concentration of anesthetic agent is increased, if the nitrous oxide is added in the gas mixture (second gas effect), or if

the breathing circuit is primed with the combination of sevoflurane in high concentration (e.g., 8%) and nitrous oxide.[4,5]

There are three techniques of the anesthesia induction with volatile anesthetics:[4]

1. Gradual increase of volatile anesthetic concentration by 0.5–1% (slower induction, increased incidence of excitation)
2. Respiratory volume technique—normal spontaneous breathing of volatile anesthetic concentration (sevoflurane) of 7%–8% (anesthesia achieved in one minute)
3. Vital capacity technique (inhalation bolus technique)—after priming the breathing circuit with high sevoflurane concentration (8%), patient inhales a vital capacity breath and holds the breath. This achieves 2% alveolar sevoflurane concentration, which is required to tolerate the surgical stimulus.

VIMA is usually used in children (difficult placement of intravenous line) and in procedures with minimal painful stimuli.[4] Since the uptake of volatile anesthetics occurs via lungs, VIMA is not suitable in patients with impaired ventilation and lung perfusion.[4] On the other hand, due to the preservation of spontaneous breathing, VIMA is suitable for patients with difficult airway, and due to its bronchodilatory properties, it is suitable for patients with chronic obstructive pulmonary disease (COPD).[4]

The advantages of VIMA include:[4,5]

- Reduced incidence of apnea
- Cardioprotection (sevoflurane)
- Certain level of muscular relaxation
- Analgesic properties (sevoflurane, nitrous oxide)
- Increased cerebral blood flow (CBF)
- Decreased cerebral metabolic rate (CMR)
- Modern volatile anesthetics (sevoflurane, isoflurane, desflurane) and nitrous oxide undergo negligible metabolism and biotransformation.
- VIMA is (usually) less expensive than TIVA.

Disadvantages of VIMA include:[4,5]

- Risk of malignant hypertension
- Depression of respiratory and cardiovascular system (dose-dependent)
- Postoperative nausea and vomiting
- Postoperative delirium
- Generation of fluoride compounds and compound A (potential nephrotoxicity)
- Pollution of the environment in the operating theater.

VIMA is contraindicated in patients with the risk of aspiration.

## BALANCED ANESTHESIA

Balanced anesthesia is the most widespread technique of anesthesia. While the use of a single anesthetic agent does not provide all components of good anesthesia (amnesia, hypnosis, analgesia, muscle relaxation), or the agent should be given in high doses that lead to cardiovascular instability, the simultaneous use of multiple anesthetic agents of different groups provides all components of anesthesia, but with fewer side effects.[2,3] Since the agents act via different receptors, lower dose of an individual agent is needed to achieve deep anesthesia. The usual sequence of anesthetics is opioid administration, followed by an intravenous hypnotic. After reaching the third stage of anesthesia, muscle relaxant could be administered for comfortable intubation and immobility during surgery. From this point on, the anesthesia could be continued by intravenous anesthetics (in boluses or as continuous infusion) or maintained by volatile anesthetics (often combined with nitrous oxide to lower the dose of volatile agent).

Adding opioids in the anesthesia mixture provides good intraoperative and immediate postoperative analgesia, and blunts the sympathetic response to intubation and surgical stimuli.[2,3] Also, opioids lower the need of intravenous hypnotics and volatile agents (the effect is reflected in lowering BIS value, but not in the increase of MAC number, since MAC does not reflect electrophysiologic state of the brain), which contributes to hemodynamic stability.

## NEUROLEPTANESTHESIA

Another concept of anesthesia is neuroleptanesthesia. In this concept, an opioid (analgesic component) is combined with a neuroleptic agent to produce sedation and analgesia, tranquility, immobility, and amnesia (the latter achieved only in some patients).[3] Cardiovascular stability is maintained, and autonomic reflexes are suppressed. Neurolepic drugs used in neuroleptanesthesia are butyrophenones (droperidol, haloperidol) and phenothiazines (chlorpromazine). Phenothiazines are used less commonly because of more frequent hypotension.[3]

Neuroleptanesthesia is used for procedural sedation, endoscopic examinations, neurodiagnostic procedures, some ophthalmic surgeries, and awake craniotomies.[3] It is contraindicated in patients with Parkinson's disease (butyrophenones interrupt dopamine balance), patients receiving monoamine oxidase inhibitors, and patients with alcohol and drug abuse.[3]

## REFERENCES

1. Falk SA, Fleisher LA. Overview of anesthesia. In: Jones SB, ed., *UpToDate*, Waltham, MA, 2020. Retrieved August 30, 2020, from https://www.uptodate.com/contents/overview-of-anesthesia.
2. Khorsand SM. Maintenance of general anesthesia: Overview. In: Joshi GP, ed., *UpToDate*, Waltham, MA, 2020. Retrieved August 30, 2020, from https://www.uptodate.com/contents/maintenance-of-general-anesthesia-overview.
3. Fukunda K. Opioid analgesics. In: Miller RD, ed. *Miller's Anesthesia*. 8th ed. Philadelphia, PA: Churchill Livingstone/Elsevier, 2015.
4. Hays SR. Inhalation anesthetic agents: Properties and delivery. In: Joshi GP, ed., *UpToDate*, Waltham, MA, 2019. Retrieved August 30, 2020, from https://www.uptodate.com/contents/inhalation-anesthetic-agents-properties-and-delivery.
5. Forman S, Ishizawa Y. Inhaled anesthetic pharmacokinetics: Uptake, distribution, metabolism, and toxicity. In: Miller RD, ed. *Miller's Anesthesia*. 8th ed. Philadelphia, PA: Churchill Livingstone/Elsevier, 2015:6389–6369.

# 125.

# ASSESSMENT/IDENTIFICATION OF DIFFICULT AIRWAY

*Katya H. Chiong*

## ANATOMIC CORRELATES

The evaluation of the airway is a very important component in the overall evaluation of the patient and can be performed immediately preoperatively or at a formal preoperative visit. The airway evaluation should include any history of a difficult airway either by direct communication with the patient or by obtaining previous anesthetic records, or pertinent data, which may include a "difficult airway" letter that the patient may have been given at a previous encounter. The airway evaluation should include any gross abnormalities, deformities visualized (particularly in the head and neck), and overall habitus particularly noting anything in the exam that may bring difficulty in securing the airway. The evaluation of the nasal cavity should be obtained, particularly noting any deformities, trauma, or other abnormalities (e.g., septal deviation, narrowing, obstruction). The overall evaluation should also include a history of any congenital or acquired syndromes, as some anomalies may increase the difficulty of securing the airway.[1-4]

Particular components of the airway exam may indicate a difficulty in securing the airway or maintaining adequate mask ventilation. Mask ventilation requires a good seal between the patient's face and the mask in order to overcome upper airway obstruction. Independent predictors of moderate to severe difficulty with mask ventilation include the presence of a beard, obesity (BMI >26 kg/m$^{-2}$), lack of teeth, age greater than 55 years, and history of snoring.[1] Important components of the airway exam include:

- A mouth opening of 4 cm or less, measured as the distance between incisors, has been proposed as an indicator of a possible difficult intubation.[3,4]
- The overall condition of dentition, whether it is intact, normal, or abnormal (e.g., edentulous, chipped, cracked, missing, or whether dentures, caps, crowns, veneers, implants, bridges, etc., are present) is also important to note. Caries, periodontitis, loose teeth, and overall poor dentition carry an increased risk of dental damage during airway manipulation.[3,4]

- The length of incisors and the relationship of the maxillary and mandibular incisors to each other, on the other hand, may impede a proper view of the airway. The ability to prognath, or protrude, the mandibular incisors in front of the maxillary incisors is a critical part of the airway exam; in fact, the mere inability of bringing the mandibular incisors in line with the maxillary incisors is associated with a difficult intubation.[4]
- A similar evaluation of mandibular mobility, the upper lip bite test (ULBT), has been found to be more specific and has shown to have less interobserver variability than the Mallampati classification. The ULBT is divided into three classes describing the reach and ability of the lower incisors to bite the upper lip above the vermillion border; the inability of the lower incisors to bit the upper lip has been associated with a difficult laryngoscopy.[4]
- An inter-incisor distance (or inter-gum distance if edentulous) of less than 3 cm is considered a risk for a difficult laryngoscopy.[1]
- Tongue size and the presence and location of any lesions (e.g., the base of the tongue) are important to note; they may contribute to difficulty with mask ventilation and manipulation of the airway.[3,4]
- Facial hair, whether present or excessive, may also impede adequate mask ventilation.[3,4]
- A thyromental distance (with the head maximally extended and mouth closed, and measuring from the mandible to thyroid notch) of less than 6–7 cm correlates with a poor laryngoscopic view.[2] A short thyromental distance may reflect a decrease in neck mobility and degree of retrognathia which can signify difficulty in displacing the tongue. The distance is often estimated in fingerbreadths, which is typically at least 3 fingerbreadths.[3,4]
- Good compliance of the mandible is also necessary to facilitate the displacement of the tongue, which is needed for glottic visualization.[3,4] Mandible compliance may be negatively impacted by changes from scarring, radiation, localized infections, etc.

## MALLAMPATI CLASSIFICATION

The oral cavity can be formally assessed using a modification of the Mallampati classification (which assigns four gradations instead of three, Table 125.1 and Figure 125.1). However, while it is important to note that the Mallampati assessment on its own is of limited value in detecting a difficulty airway, it remains a useful and important method to indirectly assess the difficulty of endotracheal intubation.[3] The assessment is made by having the patient sit up straight (as ability allows), and asking them to open their mouth while protruding their tongue out as much as possible (without phonation), specifically noting the visibility of the uvula, tonsillar pillars, soft palate, hard palate, tongue. Patient cooperation, effort in opening mouth, and the ability to protrude the tongue may limit proper evaluation.[3]

## RANGE OF MOTION

Range of motion in the neck should be evaluated for full flexion and extension. Limited range of motion can impair direct laryngoscopy, as proper alignment of the neck in relation to the airway cannot be optimally obtained. The atlanto-occipital joint is also an important predictor. Normally, 35 degrees of atlanto-occipital joint extension is possible. A greater than two-thirds decrease of atlanto-occipital joint extension from a normal 35 degrees is associated with a technically difficult or impossible laryngoscopic view.[2] Additionally, head and neck mobility can be quantitated by measuring the sternomental distance between the sternal notch and the point on the chin with the head in full extension and mouth closed; a distance of less than 12.5 cm is associated with difficulty intubating.[4] Caution should be taken in the evaluation of trauma patients and other patients who may have cervical spine instability, such as those with rheumatoid arthritis and Down's syndrome. Extension of the head at the atlanto-occipital

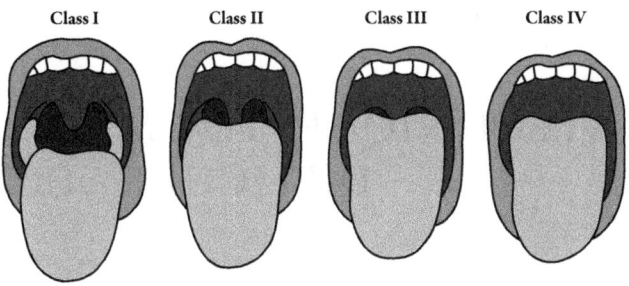

**Figure 125.1.** Mallampati Classification: Class I, soft plate fauces, entire uvula, pillars; Class II, soft palate, fauces, portion of uvula; Class III, soft palate, base of uvula; Class IV, hard palate only. Reproduced with permission from Bair AE, Caravelli R, Tyler K, et al: Feasibility of the preoperative Mallampati airway assessment in emergency departments patients, *J Emerg Med* 38:677–680, 2010.

joint aligns the oral and pharyngeal axes, while flexing the head toward the chest by elevating the head approximately 10 cm will align the laryngeal and pharyngeal axes. Implementing these maneuvers simultaneously places the patient in a "sniffing" position and aligns all three axes for an optimal laryngoscopic view. An assessment of the overall range of motion of the neck can be performed by measuring the angle created by the forehead when the neck is fully flexed and then fully extended. An angle measurement of less than 80 degrees is predictive of a difficult intubation.[2,4] A neck circumference (or thickness) of greater than 43 cm and a short neck length are both additional, non-reassuring findings that may be an indication of a difficult laryngoscopic view.[3,4] It is important to note that a large neck circumference is more predictive of a difficult intubation than a high body mass index (BMI).[4]

Causes of difficult airways are multifactorial. There is no single test that can completely predict the difficult airway; rather, the collective data from both the patient examination and their medical history can better prepare us and unmask any possible difficulty in securing and/or maintaining the airway.

*Table 125.1* MALLAMPATI CLASSIFICATION

| MALLAMPATI CLASSIFICATION (MODIFIED) | DEGREE OF DIFFICULTY[1,3] |
|---|---|
| **Class I:** Soft palate, fauces, entire uvula, and pillars are visualized | Easy |
| **Class II:** Soft palate, fauces, portion of the uvula are visualized | |
| **Class III:** Soft palate and base of the uvula are visualized | |
| **Class IV:** Only the hard palate is visualized | Potentially very difficult |

## REFERENCES

1. Rosenblatt WH, et al. Airway management. In: Barash PG, ed., *Clinical Anesthesia.* 8th ed. Philadelphia, PA: Wolters Kluwer; 2017:771–773.
2. Klinger K, Infosino A. Airway management. In: Miller RD, Pardo MC Jr, eds., *Basics of Anesthesia.* 7th ed. Philadelphia, PA: Churchill Livingstone; 2010:239–272.
3. Wijeysundera DM, Finlayson E. Preoperative evaluation. In: Gropper MA, Miller RD et al., eds., *Miller's Anesthesia.* 9th ed. Philadelphia, PA: Churchill Livingstone; 2020:918–920.
4. Artime CA, Hagberg CA. Airway management in the adult. In: Gropper MA, Miller RD et al., eds., *Miller's Anesthesia.* 9th ed. Philadelphia, PA: Churchill Livingstone; 2020:1373–1412.

# 126.

# TECHNIQUES FOR MANAGING AIRWAY (INCLUDING DIFFICULT AIRWAY ALGORITHM)

*Sahil Sharma and Archit Sharma*

## INTRODUCTION

The human airway in adults is divided into upper (above cricoid cartilage) and lower airways. The adult airway is the narrowest at the glottis, as compared to the pediatric airway, which is narrowest at the subglottis. Children younger than 12 years have a smaller cricothyroid membrane, their larynx is more compliant, funnel-shaped, and rostral in position, and laryngoscopy is challenging due to larger occiput and short neck.

## AIRWAY MANAGEMENT TECHNIQUES

### AIRWAY POSITIONING

Upper airway obstruction can be relieved by head tilt, chin lift, or jaw thrust. In infants and children, a simple suctioning of the airway will help with the clearance.

### ADJUVENTS TO UPPER AIRWAY OBSTRUCTION

An oropharyngeal airway can be used to prevent the tongue from obstructing the airway in a sedated patient. They are measured and sized from the lip to the angle of the jaw. Nasopharyngeal airway can be used in a patient with trismus or oral trauma, where the oral cavity should not be instrumented.[1]

### BAG AND MASK VENTILATION

The patient is placed in the Sniff position (neck flexion and upper cervical extension), the mask is applied with a good seal with pincer grasp. If mask ventilation is difficult, the head should be repositioned; two-hand mask ventilation or two-person bag mask ventilation should be employed.

Advanced airways include supraglottic device (laryngeal mask airway, esophago tracheal tube) and an endotracheal tube.

## SUPRAGLOTTIC AIRWAY (SGA)

An SGA is any airway device that sits outside the larynx and forms a seal around it, permitting increased ventilation and reducing the chance of gastric distention that can be encountered during face-mask ventilation. Although intubation continues as the gold standard for airway management and protection from aspiration, correct SGA use requires less expertise and training than endotracheal intubation.

### LARYNGEAL MASK AIRWAYS (LMAS)

LMAs are the most commonly used supraglottic devices, and are available in different designs such as LMA Supreme, i-gel, etc. There is no need for laryngoscopy for LMA insertion, making them an excellent rescue device in case of failed bag-mask ventilation or intubation.[2] However, when ventilation pressure exceeds 20 cm $H_2O$, it pressurizes the stomach, leading to the possibility of aspiration.

### KING LARYNGO-TRACHEAL AIRWAY (LTA)

The King (Ambu) LTA is a true SGA device that does not provide a direct seal over the glottis. It is a double-lumen, silicone tube with a large oropharyngeal blocking cuff and smaller esophageal blocking cuff that lies in the esophagus below the glottis. The ventilation port is situated between these cuffs. It has become very popular for first responders and EMTs because of its ease of insertion.[3]

## ENDOTRACHEAL INTUBATION

Endotracheal intubation involves placement of an endotracheal tube past the vocal cords with the cuff inflated, preventing aspiration of gastric contents and obtaining control of the airway. For emergencies, if the patient is not empty stomach or has a higher aspiration risk, then rapid sequence induction (RSI) using rapid-acting medications (succinylcholine or high-dose rocuronium) is the preferred strategy to obtain quick control of the airway, avoid bag masking, and decrease aspiration risk.

The patient is pre-oxygenated with 100% oxygen (if possible), to increase oxygenation reserve and prevent desaturations. After the patient has been induced, *direct laryngoscopy* can be performed with a Macintosh or Miller blade with a handheld laryngoscope. The endotracheal tube is advanced after visualization of the glottis, followed by visualization of the vocal cords. A *video laryngoscope* can be used as well, which has a camera attached to the laryngoscope blade that is placed near the vallecular space, allowing you to visualize the vocal cords and place the endotracheal tube under indirect vision. A "Sellick maneuver" or "cricoid pressure" can be applied to aid in visualization of the glottis, if needed. Some physicians consider the Bougie, which is a long, semi-rigid plastic device (a plastic stylet), as an adjunct or rescue device in difficult intubations

Other than direct visualization, correct placement of the endotracheal tube should be confirmed by auscultation of bilateral breath sounds, bilateral chest rise, end-tidal carbon dioxide measurement, chest X-ray, ultrasound, fiberoptic examination, or a combination of these strategies.

## SURGICAL AIRWAY

If all other means of ventilating and oxygenating a patient's airway have failed, then a surgical approach (tracheostomy or cricothyrotomy) is used to gain access to the airway. Use of LMA as a rescue device in failed intubations has decreased the use of a surgical airway strategy. Complications include hemorrhage, subcutaneous emphysema, pneumomediastinum, and pneumothorax.

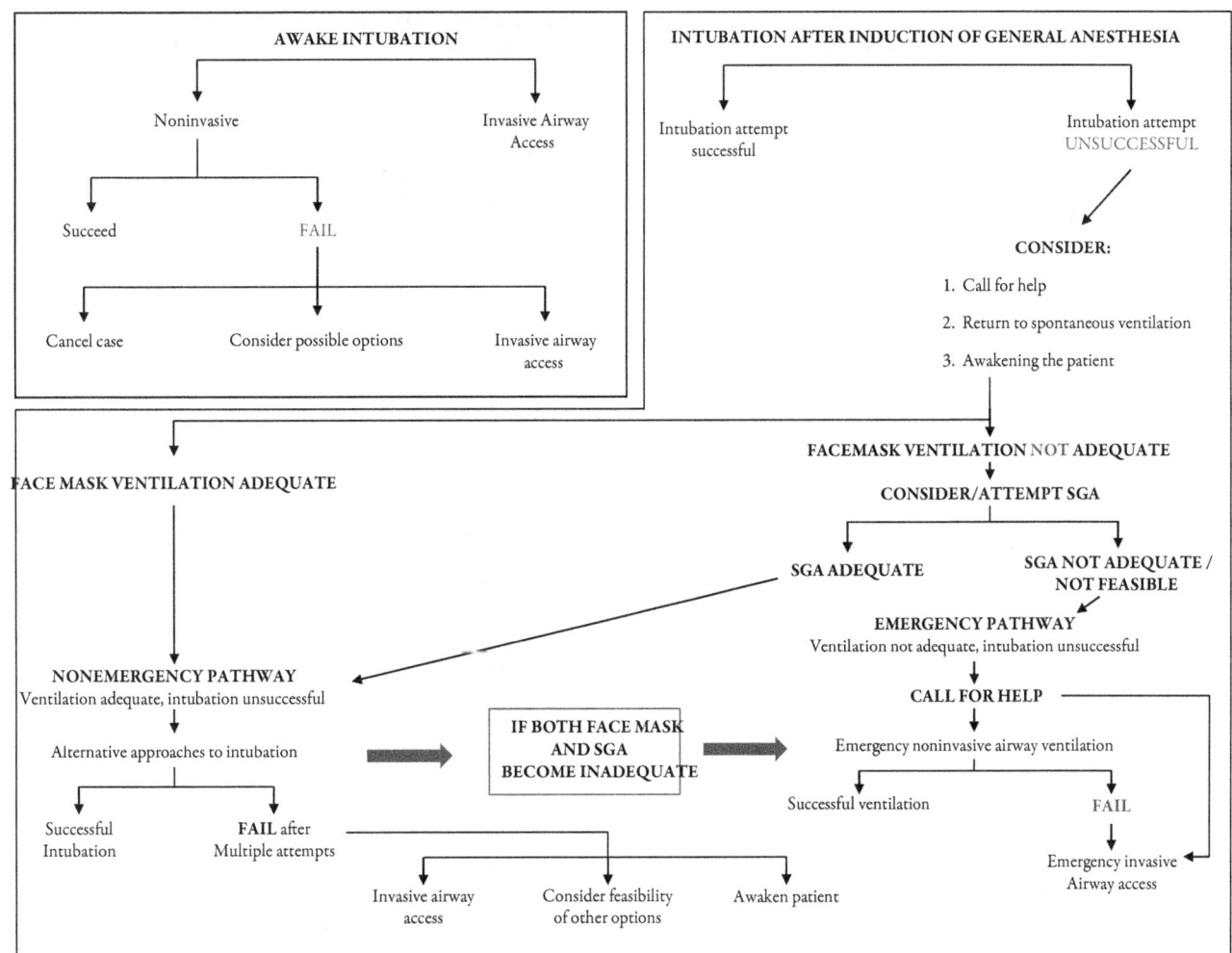

**Figure 126.1.** Difficult airway management algorithm.

## MANAGEMENT OF A DIFFICULT AIRWAY

Evaluation of the airway for signs of potential difficulty should be performed as soon as possible on any patient in respiratory distress. Using a three-tier classification, Mallampati et al. reported difficult direct laryngoscopy in the majority of patients with a poor view of the pharyngeal structures and divided them in 3 classes, with an increasing class corresponding to a higher grade of visualization on intubation and a higher difficulty level in visualization of the glottis:[4]

Class 1: Faucial pillars, soft palate, and uvula could be visualized.

Class 2: Faucial pillars and soft palate could be visualized, but uvula was masked by the base of the tongue.

Class 3: Only soft palate could be visualized.

Other predictors of difficult airway would be reduced mouth opening (less than 3 cm), decreased thyromental distance (<4 cm), limited neck mobility, presence of facial hair or beard that would limit sealing of a mask and examination of structures, large tongue, presence of masses or lymph nodes, or bleeding in the airway. The four Ds (distortion, disproportion, dysmobility, dentition) may make direct laryngoscopy with standard equipment very challenging.

The American Society of Anesthesiologists (ASA) Difficult Airway Management Algorithm, a part of the ASA Practice Guidelines, has become the gold standard in addressing the urgent response to the inability to oxygenate and ventilate, and we have provided an adaptation in Figure 126.1.[5] The guidelines are dynamic and have changed over the years to recognize newer concepts with the introduction of newer airway devices. This management algorithm stresses the early identification of patients with difficult airway and considers the use of awake fiberoptic intubation in patients that are higher risk. If the patient has been induced, if there is inability to ventilate with a bag-mask strategy, it emphasizes the use of a supraglottic airway, calling for help, using fiberoptic scope through a LMA after establishing ventilation, and even trying to wake the patient up, if safely possible. If all else fails, a surgical airway should be obtained in the essence of patient safety.

## REFERENCES

1. Avva U, et al. Airway management. In *StatPearls [Internet]*. StatPearls; 2020.
2. Benumof JL. Laryngeal mask airway and the ASA difficult airway algorithm. *Anesthesiology.* 1996;84(3):686–699.
3. Guyette FX, et al. King airway use by air medical providers. *Prehosp Emerg Care.* 2007;11(4):473–476.
4. Mallampati SR, et al. A clinical sign to predict difficult tracheal intubation: A prospective study. *Can J Anaesth Soc J.* 1985;32(4:429–434.
5. Apfelbaum JL, et al. Practice guidelines for management of the difficult airway: An updated report by the American Society of Anesthesiologists task force on management of the difficult airway. *Anesthesiology* 2013;118(2):251–270.

# 127.

# AIRWAY DEVICES

*Ben Schmitt and Jai Jani*

## INTRODUCTION

Intubation devices are used to facilitate the placement of an endotracheal tube in a timely manner. These devices use a variety of modalities including direct visualization, indirect (camera or fiberoptic based), and transillumination. This chapter will explore the unique properties of each of these devices.

## DIRECT LARYNGOSCOPE (DL) BLADES

A laryngoscope is a device inserted into the oropharynx designed to improve visualization of the glottis. Trans-oral visualization of the glottis requires alignment of the oral, pharyngeal, and laryngeal/tracheal axis, and is facilitated by displacement of the tongue and epiglottis.[1] Under anesthesia, patients have decreased muscle tone, resulting in upper airway collapse due to gravity. In the supine position this means the tongue will move posteriorly into the pharyngeal axis, and the epiglottis will fall into the laryngeal axis, blocking a trans-oral view of the vocal cords. Laryngoscope blades displace the tongue and lift the epiglottis anteriorly.

Straight Miller blades are designed to have the blade advanced to the epiglottis, where anterior motion will directly lift the epiglottis. In patients with a flaccid epiglottis, these blades can provide better epiglottis tip displacement improving glottic visualization.[1]

Curved Macintosh blades more easily follow the natural curvature of the tongue, simplifying insertion past the teeth (Table 127.1).[1] Once at the base of the tongue, the blade should be placed into the vallecula abutting the hypoepiglottic ligament. Anterior-inferior motion will tense the ligament, indirectly pulling the epiglottis anteriorly, away from the glottis. This motion requires adequate ligament rigidity and an epiglottis that is not "floppy."

In most adults, a Miller 2 or Macintosh 3 blade is an appropriate size.[1] Larger blades can be used for individuals with larger thyromental distances. In the pediatric population, blade sizing can be estimated by comparing the blade to the distance from the patient's lips to angle of the mandible (Table 127.2).

## VIDEO LARYNGOSCOPES

Video laryngoscopes use a small camera mounted on a laryngoscope connected to a viewing monitor. To prevent fogging on the camera lens, most devices are heated or use anti-fog coating to prevent water condensation.[1,2] Because the viewing point is inside the patient, the need to align

### Table 127.1  MILLER VS. MACINTOSH BLADE

|  | MILLER (STRAIGHT) BLADE | MACINTOSH (CURVED) BLADE |
| --- | --- | --- |
| Tip placement | On epiglottis | Vallecula |
| Epiglottis movement | Direct | Indirect via suspensory ligament |

*Source:* data from Gropper MA, et al. Airway management in the Adult. In: *Miller's Anesthesia.* 9th ed. Philadelphia, PA: Elsevier; 2020:1373–1412.

### Table 127.2  PEDIATRIC SIZING OF MILLER BLADES

| AGE | MILLER SIZE | MAC |
| --- | --- | --- |
| Premature | 0 | |
| Neonate | 0–1 | |
| 1 month–2 year | 1 | |
| 2–6 years old | 1–2 | 2 |
| 6–12 years old | 2 | 2–3 |
| 12+ years old | 2–3 | 3 |

*Source:* data from Salyer SW, Pediatric emergencies: A. Emergencies and resuscitations. In: Salyer SW, *Essential Emergency Medicine: For the Healthcare Practitioner.* Philadelphia, PA: Saunders/Elsevier; 2007:652–813.

the oral, pharyngeal, and laryngeal axes is eliminated. This enables the use of hyperangulated blades, prevents teeth and the tongue from obstructing the view, and may reduce cervical spine motion.[2]

Compared to direct laryngoscopy, video laryngoscopy provides improved visualization of glottis with decreased force, increased success of intubation, and decreased sympathetic response to intubation.[2] The external display enables people not preforming laryngoscopy to also examine the airway.

Issues with videolaryngoscopy include cost, need for power to video display, increased time to intubation, increased rates of desaturation in trauma population, and need for a stylet to match the curvature of the blade used (50%–70% of video intubations require stylet use).[1,2] Structures proximal to the camera may not be seen. Blind introduction of an endotracheal tube may result in damage to structures not seen.[2] Without alignment of oral-laryngeal axis, the glottis may be seen, but the anesthetist may be unable to pass an endotracheal tube. Blood, gastric contents, secretions, or oral debris may also coat the camera and impair visualization.

## FIBEROPTIC DEVICES

Fiberoptic devices use total internal reflection to propagate light through a core approximately 10–20 μm in diameter.[3] To ensure total internal reflection, the core is surrounded by a material with a lower refractive index, preventing light from escaping the core. Each of these optical fibers will then conduct color and brightness of the light it carries. If the arrangement of the fibers is identical at both ends, an image is formed, with each optical fiber behaving like a pixel in a TV. Smaller diameter of fibers will therefore result in a higher resolution. The image generated can be seen directly through a viewing lens or can be transformed into a digital image, displayed on a screen. Illumination of the distal end is provided by a second bundle of fiberoptic cables connected to an emitting light source.

Optical fibers can be housed in a rigid or flexible protective casing, enabling manipulation of the cables. Flexible fiberoptic scopes can be advanced nasally or orally into the trachea, and have an endotracheal tube advanced over them. Most have a hollow working channel for suction, irrigation, insufflation, or deployment of materials.[3] Bronchoscopes are small enough to pass into bronchi, and frequently used to examine segmental bronchi. They require very little movement of tissues as the scope moves around structures, reducing cervical motion with intubation, and can be tolerated by awake patients.[3] They come in various sizes depending upon brand, but most have adult (~5.5 cm external diameter) and pediatric sizes (~3.7 cm external diameter); the endotracheal tube should be slightly larger than the external diameter of the scope. An awake fiberoptic intubation should be considered for any difficult airway.

## TRANSILLUMINATION

Transillumination of the trachea produces visible glowing of overlying skin, which can be used to guide placement of an endotracheal tube. Light may be produced from a bulb at the distal tip of the stylet or carried via fiberoptic filaments from an external source. There is a theoretical concern for thermal injury to tissues when using a bulb-based stylet for prolonged periods of time, but no histological differences have been shown when compared to control tissue in cats.[4] Contraindications to transillumination include masses or objects in upper airway and suspected laryngeal injury where visualization is needed. Compared to direct laryngoscopy, transillumination results in decreased time to intubation, decreased airway trauma, reduced severity of sore throat, decreased cervical spine motion, and decreased hoarseness the next day.[4] Surprisingly, transillumination-based intubation without laryngoscopy has not been found to significantly reduce heart rate or blood pressure changes with intubation. Traditional devices have relied upon light being emitted from inside the trachea and visualized on the patient's neck. A newer iteration of this concept is looking at shining an external light onto the trachea to decrease larynx recognition time when performing video laryngoscopy.

## REFERENCES

1. Gropper MA, et al. Airway management in the adult. In: Artime CA, Hagberg CA, eds, *Miller's Anesthesia*. 9th ed. Philadelphia, PA: Elsevier; 2020:1373–1412.
2. Berkow LC, et al. The technology of video laryngoscopy. *Anesth Analg.* 2018;126(5):1527–1534.
3. Collins SR, Blank RS. Fiberoptic intubation: An overview and update. *Respir Care.* 2014;59(6):865–880. doi:10.4187/respcare.03012
4. Davis L, et al. Lighted stylet tracheal intubation: A review. *Anesth Analg.* 2000;90(3):745–756.
5. Salyer SW. Pediatric emergencies: A. Emergencies and resuscitations. In: Salyer SW, *Essential Emergency Medicine: For the Healthcare Practitioner*. Philadelphia, PA: Saunders/Elsevier; 2007:652–813.

# 128.

# THE SURGICAL AIRWAY

*Julia Kendrick and Alan D. Kaye*

## INTRODUCTION

Surgical airway management is defined as the creation of an opening in the trachea by invasive means to provide oxygenation and ventilation.[1] The need for a surgical airway is uncommon. However, clinicians responsible for airway management must be familiar with techniques to establish emergency front of neck access (FONA) in "Can't Intubate, Can't Ventilate" scenarios.[2] These procedures may also be used to establish an airway in situations that have a high likelihood of failing. Options for FONA include cricothyrotomy, tracheostomy, and transtracheal jet ventilation (TTJV). For the anesthesiologist, cricothyrotomy and transtracheal jet ventilation are most applicable. These procedures should not be performed when there is massive trauma to the trachea, larynx, or cricoid cartilage. Nasotracheal and orotracheal intubations should always be considered before a surgical airway is performed. When surgical airway management fails or is too hazardous, cardiopulmonary bypass is the ultimate solution.

## ETIOLOGY

A surgical airway may be required in both the operating room (OR) and out of the OR setting. The rate of failed emergency department intubations and need for surgical airway is under 0.6%.[1] In the emergency department (ED) it is estimated that a surgical airway is required for 1%–2.8% of all intubation events in patients with trauma. While there is little data regarding emergency surgical airway practices at different institutions, one study reported that 0.008% of all emergent airways required surgical access.[3]

## CRICOTHYROTOMY AND TRACHEOSTOMY

Cricothyrotomy is the creation of an opening through the cricothyroid membrane with the placement of a cuffed tracheostomy or endotracheal tube into the trachea. Tracheostomy requires a greater level of skill, is preferred for long-term management, and is usually performed by a surgeon in a controlled setting. In emergency situations, cricothyrotomy should be performed.[1]

There are two common techniques for performing a cricothyrotomy: surgical and percutaneous. The percutaneous technique has traditionally been the method of choice for anesthesiologist due to the familiarity of using the Seldinger technique for other procedures. However, surgical cricothyrotomy has recently become the technique of choice due to its faster speed and higher reliability.[4]

### SURGICAL CRICOTHYROTOMY

A number of approaches exist; however the Difficult Airway Society guidelines for management of the difficult airway describe the scalpel-bougie technique as the preferred method.[4] In emergency situations, cricothyrotomy should be performed even without informed consent. Necessary equipment includes a number 10 blade scalpel, a bougie with angled (coudé) tip, and cuffed endotracheal tube with a 6-mm internal diameter. A tracheostomy tube with an internal diameter of 6 mm is preferred, but is not always available in an emergency situation. Tracheostomy tubes are easier to secure and shorter, decreasing the likelihood of mainstem intubation and increasing ease of suction.[1]

Place the patient in the supine position. There is usually not time to drape the patient. Apply chlorhexidine or povidine iodine if time permits. If the patient is awake, anesthetize the skin with local anesthesia. Steps are provided for the right-handed provider. Side-specific designations made be reversed for left-handed operators. Stand on the patient's left side. Stabilize the larynx using the left hand. Identify the cricothyroid membrane (CTM) with the left index finger. The space between the thyroid and cricoid cartilages is the cricothyroid membrane. Make a 2.5-cm vertical incision (caudal to cranial on the patient) through the skin and subcutaneous tissue. If the CTM is not palpable, make an 8–10 cm vertical incision in the midline. Blunt dissection can be performed using a curved snap or with the index fingers of both hands until the CTM is located. Once the CTM is encountered, make a horizontal incision (patient left to patient right) through the membrane. Once the trachea is entered, the blade stays within the incision to ensure that communication to the airway is not lost. Without removing the blade from the incision, hold the scalpel in your left hand. Take the bougie in your right hand and pass it through the incision into the trachea. Remove the scalpel and pass a lubricated 6.0 mm endotracheal tube (ETT) over the bougie. Remove the bougie, inflate the cuff, and confirm ventilation with capnography.

### PERCUTANEOUS

A number of kits are commercially available that employ the percutaneous dilatational technique. The basis for this technique is the insertion of an airway catheter over a dilator that has been passed through the skin. Ultrasound guidance may be used if landmarks are difficult to locate. Make a small vertical incision through the skin over the CTM. Attach an 18-gauge catheter to a fluid-filled syringe and pass it through the incision at a 45-degree angle directed caudally. Puncture should be made in the lower one-third of the membrane due to the proximity of the CTM to the vocal cords and cricothyroid artery. Aspiration of air indicates passage into the trachea. Advance the catheter over the needle into the trachea. Remove the needle and leave the catheter in place. Insert a guidewire through the catheter to a depth of 2–3 cm. Next, the catheter is removed and a curved dilator with the airway cannula is advanced through the CTM over the wire. The dilator and guidewire are removed together, leaving the cannula in place. Inflate the cuff and start ventilation. Confirm placement with capnography and secure the airway.

## NEEDLE CRICOTHYROTOMY

In needle cricothyrotomy a catheter is placed over a needle that penetrates the membrane, allowing ventilation by a pressurized stream of $O_2$. The technique is similar to percutaneous cricothyrotomy, but a catheter is left in place and used for ventilation instead of a tracheostomy or endotracheal tube. The catheter is smaller in diameter and it is less effective in providing adequate ventilation and therefore should only be used as a temporizing measure while preparations are made for a surgical cricothyrotomy or tracheostomy. In the pediatric population (children under the age of 10), needle cricothyrotomy with transtracheal jet ventilation (TTJV) is the preferred method until tracheostomy is performed. In children, the cricoid cartilage is the narrowest part of the airway and the isthmus of the thyroid reaches the level of the CTM. The pediatric larynx is more susceptible to damage and postoperative airway complications by surgical cricothyrotomy due to its small size and structural immaturity.[5]

## COMPLICATIONS

Major complications associated with this placement of a surgical airway include esophageal perforation, recurrent laryngeal nerve damage, excessive bleeding or hemorrhage. These complications occur due to the close proximity of vital structures (esophagus, recurrent laryngeal nerves, major vessels) to the CTM.

## TRANSTRACHEAL JET VENTILATION

The ASA DAA lists TTJV as an emergent invasive technique to be used in patients who cannot be ventilated or intubated using conventional means.[4] Percutaneous TTJV is regarded as a lifesaving procedure that can provide temporary oxygenation and ventilation with less training and complications that a surgical airway. Pressurized oxygen is insufflated through a cannula placed by needle cricothyrotomy to achieve inspiration. Expiration is passive and is a result of the elastic recoil of the lungs and chest wall. To avoid breath stacking and barotrauma, sufficient time for passive exhalation is needed. Since expiration occurs through the glottis, the upper airway must not be obstructed, otherwise barotrauma and pneumothorax may occur. Bubbles resulting from the egress of air through the glottis from TTJV can also facilitate placement of an ETT. TTJV should not be performed in patients who have evidence of direct damage to the cricoid cartilage or larynx, or in patients with complete upper airway obstruction.

To perform TTJV, a 12- to 16-gauge, kink-resistant catheter is used. Several commercial devices exist, such as a 6 French, coil-reinforced, Teflon-coated catheter which prevents kinking and facilitates passage into the trachea. One must confirm proper placement in the trachea before initiating jet ventilation. The minimum pressure required to drive a jet ventilator is 15 psi. In the OR the jet ventilator can be connected straight to the pipeline supply in most cases. The pipeline pressure for oxygen in hospitals in the United States is about 55 psi. Jet ventilators contain pressure regulators to lower pipeline pressure to provide successful ventilation while avoiding barotrauma.

## COMPLICATIONS

Complications of TTJV include barotrauma, pneumothorax, subcutaneous or mediastinal emphysema, hemorrhage, aspiration, and perforation of the trachea or esophagus. It is essential to verify proper placement, allow enough time for passive expiration, and to ensure that a path for air egress exists to avoid complications.[2]

## REFERENCES

1. Hsiao J, Pacheco-Fowler V. Cricothyroidotomy. *N Eng J Med.* 2008;358(22):e25.
2. Artime CA, Hagberg CA. *44—Airway Management in the Adult*; 2020.
3. Dillon JK, et al. The emergent surgical airway: Cricothyrotomy vs tracheotomy. *Int J Oral Maxillofac Surg.* 2013;42(2):204–208.
4. Frerk C, et al. Difficult Airway Society 2015 guidelines for management of unanticipated difficult intubation in adults. *Br J Anaesth.* 2015;115(6):827–848.
5. Coté CJ, Hartnick CJ. Pediatric transtracheal and cricothyrotomy airway devices for emergency use: Which are appropriate for infants and children? *Pediatric Anesthesia.* 2009;19(Suppl. 1):66–76.

# 129.

# ENDOBRONCHIAL INTUBATION

*Hisham Kassem and Omar Viswanath*

## INTRODUCTION

Endobronchial intubation (EI) is defined as the placement of the endotracheal tube, either inadvertently or intentionally, in the right or left mainstem bronchus.[1] Unintentional EI, typically in emergency situations, occurs more commonly in the right mainstem bronchus due to the straighter trajectory and can lead to signs of hypoxemia and difficult ventilation.[1] However, specialized endotracheal tubes can be placed in certain scenarios to provide effective methods of lung isolation (Boxes 129.1 and 129.2).[1]

## INDICATIONS

EI to achieve one-lung ventilation has both absolute and relative indications, although the relative indications are more commonly seen. Lung isolation during video-assisted thorascopic surgeries (VATS) is becoming the most commonly seen utilization requiring EI as more minimally invasive surgical techniques are being employed.[1] EI may also be used to prevent spillage of massive bleeding or infection from one lung from a lung abscess or pulmonary hemorrhage, respectively.[1] Moreover, bronchopleural/bronchocutaneous fistulas often need lung isolation to maintain adequate ventilation. Relative indications for EI center around providing adequate surgical exposure during procedures such as lobectomy/pneumonectomy, thoracic/cardiac surgery, and esophagectomy.[1]

## METHODS OF ENDOBRONCHIAL INTUBATION

Endobronchial intubation and one-lung ventilation are typically achieved through the use of a double-lumen tracheal tube, a bronchial blocker, or advancing a single-lumen endotracheal tube (ETT) into the right or left bronchus.[1] The most commonly used device to achieve endobronchial intubation is a double-lumen tube.[1] These tubes consist of two single lumens that are blended together, with the longer lumen reaching the respective bronchus, and the shorter lumen sitting in the trachea, each with their own individual inflatable cuffs.[1] They are primarily made of polyvinyl chloride and have color-coded cuffs with respective pilot balloons.[2] The bronchial cuff is typically blue, while the tracheal cuff is clear.[2] Double-lumen tubes are D-shaped and have both right- and left-sided variations; sizes range from 28 to 42 French (F) for adults.[2] The particular size of tube is usually based on gender (35–37 F for females and 39–41 F for males) and height, but age can also be factored in, especially in the pediatric population. The internal diameter for each lumen is approximately 6.5, 6, 5.5, 5, and 4.5 mm for double-lumen tubes sizes 41, 39, 37, 35 and 28 F, respectively.

The placement of double-lumen tubes requires direct laryngoscopy with visualization of the vocal cords as it is introduced into the trachea, then rotated 90 degrees to the right or left side, and advanced until resistance is met.[1] While auscultation after inflation is needed to assess proper placement, confirmation is done with a fiberoptic scope to ensure no cuff herniation.[1] On the other hand, a bronchial blocker can be placed in the mainstem bronchus needed and

---

**Box 129.1** ADVANTAGES OF DOUBLE-LUMEN TUBES

- **Relatively easy to place**
- **Ability to rapidly convert from one-lung to conventional ventilation**
- **Suctioning from both lungs**
- **Possibility to provide CPAP to non-ventilated lung**

---

**Box 129.2** ADVANTAGES OF BRONCHIAL BLOCKER

- **Technically simple placement**
- **Isolation of individual lung segments possible**
- **No need to change ETT if need postoperative ventilation**
- **Useful in smaller/pediatric airways**

---

the cuff inflated. The bronchial blocker is available in 3 sizes (5 F, 7F, and 9F) with the 9 F recommended for ETT of 7.5 mm and above. Proper placement is also confirmed with a fiberoptic scope, and the cuff is inflated to ensure proper lung isolation.[1] Bronchial blocker may have more issues with dislodgement and cuff herniation into the trachea.[1] In rare cases of abnormal or distorted airway anatomy that require a nasal intubation, a bronchial blocker can be placed through the ETT lumen to provide one lung ventilation.[3]

## ANESTHETIC CONSIDERATIONS

### PREOPERATIVE

In anticipation of patients needing endobronchial intubation during a surgical procedure, it is important for the anesthesiologist to assess which device is most suitable for securing one-lung ventilation. This entails having a comprehensive discussion with the surgeon and reviewing all pertinent available radiological studies to assess necessary exposure, evaluate for any anatomical airway compromise, and identify the location of lung pathology. Furthermore, patients with preexisting lung disease (abnormal pulmonary function testing) or significant comorbidities (i.e., obesity) may be less likely to tolerate lung isolation.[1]

### INTRAOPERATIVE

There are multiple anesthetic considerations when managing endobronchial intubation intraoperatively. Of most importance is the need to understand the physiology of one-lung ventilation and the management of hypoxia.

As most surgeries with lung isolation are done in the lateral decubitus position, this creates an inherent mismatch between the over-ventilated nondependent lung and the increased perfusion of the dependent lung. The compensatory hypoxic pulmonary vasoconstriction (HPV) allows redistribution of blood to better ventilate the non-surgical lung.[1] At times, certain anesthetic agents may inhibit this HPV, which can lead to the hypoxia and oxygen desaturation seen.[1] The goals of oxygenation and ventilation during EI are based on maintaining a safe environment for the patient. Patients are often kept on higher inspired oxygen concentrations and allowed to have higher $CO_2$ levels (permissive hypercapnia).[1]

### POSTOPERATIVE

The postoperative considerations for EI include assessing the need for prolonged mechanical ventilation. The use of a double-lumen tube will make it more difficult as the patient will need a tube exchange for a traditional ETT. Also, with double-lumen tubes there is a higher incidence of tracheal or bronchial trauma during the initial "blind" placement.[1]

## REFERENCES

1. Morgan GE, et al. *Clinical Anesthesiology*. New York, NY: Lange Medical Books/McGraw Hill; 2006.
2. Bora V, Kritzmire SM, Arthur ME. Double lumen endobronchial tubes. In: *StatPearls*. Treasure Island, FL: StatPearls; June 5, 2020. https://www.ncbi.nlm.nih.gov/books/NBK535366/
3. Kaza SR, et al. One lung ventilation in a patient with an upper and lower airway abnormality. *Indian J Anaesth*. 2012;56(6):567–569.

# 130.

# TYPES OF ENDOTRACHEAL TUBES

*Aparna Jindal and Archit Sharma*

## INTRODUCTION

Endotracheal tubes (ETT) are an essential and part of anesthesiology practice. They help to maintain airway patency, permit oxygenation and ventilation, allow for suctioning of secretions, prevent aspiration of gastric contents or oropharyngeal secretions, and facilitate the use of volatile anesthetics.

## DESIGN

The most common standard ETT is cuffed and is made up of polyvinyl chloride (PVC). Uncuffed ETT are still available and are used in pediatric population including neonates.[1] Endotracheal tubes have an inner diameter and an outer diameter. The "size" of an ETT refers to its internal diameter. Therefore if you ask for a "size 7" ETT, you are asking for one with an internal diameter of 7 mm. Narrower tubes increase the resistance to gas flow, which is especially relevant in the spontaneously breathing patient who will have to work harder to overcome the increased resistance.

The shape of the ETT is curved, corresponding the shape of oropharynx. The distal end is beveled to aid in visualization, as the ETT enters the vocal cords, and to facilitate smooth passage. Opposite to the bevel is a side hole, known as a Murphy eye, that can act as an alternate port for ventilation if tip of the tube gets obstructed. Tubes without a Murphy eye are called Magill-type tubes and can have a higher risk of tube occlusion if the tip impinges against the tracheal or bronchial wall. The cuff is an inflatable balloon present near the distal end of an ETT, surrounding its entire circumference. It is a high-volume low-pressure cuff, which provides a tight seal against the tracheal wall but avoids trauma to the airway at the same time. Lateral wall cuff pressure higher than 25–35 mmHg can cause mucosal ischemia, leading to sloughing and tracheal denudation.[2] Figure 130.1 shows a standard single-lumen tube with its various components.

The cuff is attached to a pilot balloon via a pilot line through which the cuff is filled. Numbers along the length

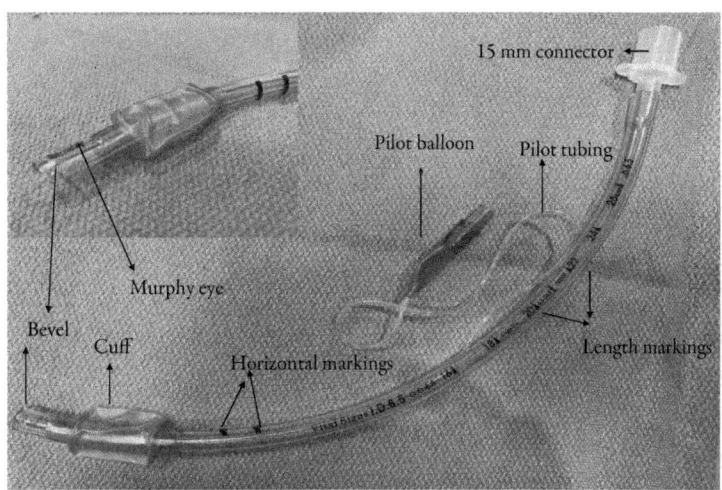

**Figure 130.1.** A standard single-lumen tube with its various components.

of ETT denote the distance in cm from the distal end. A radio-opaque line through the length can be detected on chest X-rays. A 15-mm connector is attached to the proximal end for attachment to breathing circuits.

## SPECIALTY TUBES

### DOUBLE-LUMEN TUBE (DLT)

DLTs are used in thoracic surgeries to provide one-lung ventilation, while isolating the operative lung. As the name suggests, these tubes have two different lumens, each with independent cuff and pilot balloon.[3] These can be left-sided or right-sided, corresponding to the longer endobronchial lumen.[2] The bronchial cuff and balloon are blue, whereas the tracheal is clear, for visual identification. Though either sided tube can be used to isolate lung, left-sided DLT is more commonly used due to the longer length of the left main bronchus. Right-sided DLT has an additional hole to ventilate the right upper bronchus, which requires precise positioning over the takeoff of the right upper lobe bronchus. Flexible bronchoscope is used to confirm correct placement, as mispositioning is very common. Figure 130.2 shows a left-sided DLT, with its sperate tracheal and bronchial lumens.

Another method to achieve one-lung ventilation is to use bronchial blockers, which are hollow catheters with inflatable balloons. These can be inserted through a regular ETT, under guidance with a fiberoptic scope, obviating the need to change a DLT to a regular ETT for maintenance of mechanical ventilation. Another advantage is that they can isolate a particular lobe rather than entire lung, if needed. Several types of bronchial blockers are available that differ in the techniques of inserting to left vs. right main bronchus.

### LOW-PROFILE PREFORMED TUBES

These are especially used in head and neck surgery, and are designed to stay out of the operative field. Ring-Adair-Elwyn (RAE Mallinckrodt Inc., Pleasanton, California) is one of the most common type of preformed ETT, used to provide a clear surgical field, minimizing risk of kinking.[3] Two subtypes are available—oral and nasal. Oral RAE has one curve that can be turned to either side with respect to the head. Nasal RAE has two curvatures: one is the pharyngeal curve, and the other one is to fix the tube over the forehead. Both these RAE have fixed length from curvature depending on the size (internal diameter) of the tube. This can pose a challenge where either a smaller size tube is needed, or if the patient is taller. It is to be noted that they reduce the risk of kinking but do not eliminate the risk, RAE tubes can still be kinked. Figure 130.3 shows both oral and nasal RAE tubes that are used for these specialty surgeries.

### REINFORCED TUBES

These tubes are made up of soft material with steel wire rings embedded through the entire length of the tube. These are mostly used in head and neck surgery to prevent kinking of the tube. Once kinked or bent, they cannot regain their original shape and need to be changed. Because of the soft nature of the tube, a stylet must be used for placement. There is a small length between the connector and the beginning of the steel rings where the tube is not reinforced, and it is prone to getting bent in this area.

### MICROLARYNGEAL TUBES

These are used for the surgery of the larynx. The outer diameter of these tubes is narrow to aid surgery around them. Mechanical ventilation can become challenging owing to the small diameter of these tubes.

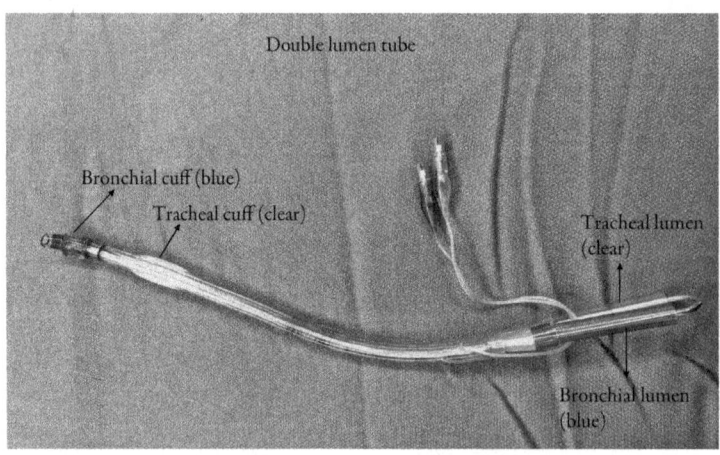

**Figure 130.2.** A left-sided double-lumen tube, with its separate trachael and bronchial lumens.

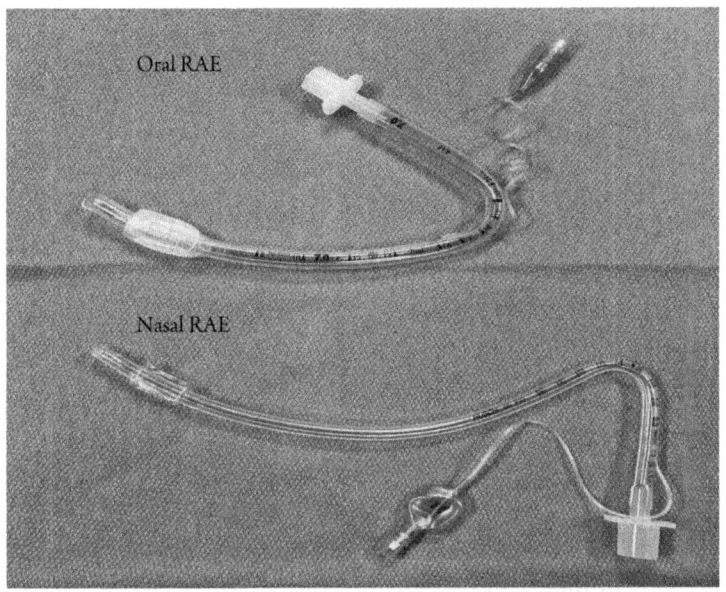

**Figure 130.3.** Oral and nasal RAE tubes that are used for these specialty surgeries.

### ETT FOR NEUROMONITORING

These are used for thyroid and other neck surgeries where the integrity of recurrent laryngeal or vagus nerve can be compromised. These special tubes have a sensor, which in properly placed tubes comes in contact with vocal cords where the recurrent laryngeal nerve runs, and can monitor the activity intraoperatively. Neural Integrity Monitor (NIM™) is one such commonly used ETT. The blue marking present on the tube helps in correct placement at the level of the vocal cords.[4]

### LASER-RESISTANT ETT

Laser beam produces extreme focused energy, which in the presence of oxygen and nitrous oxide can lead to burn injuries to the airway and other surrounding tissues, especially in conventional ETT made up of PVC. Thus, for these surgeries, special tubes are utilized that are made of either stainless steel or silicone tubes wrapped with copper or aluminum. One type of such tubes has double cuffs, to protect the airway in the event of puncture through the one. The cuff is filled with saline dyed with methylene blue, to detect any leakage. Figure 130.4 shows a laser-resistant ETT with a reinforced core.

### OTHER ETT VARIATIONS

#### Subglottic ETT

One of the variations that we commonly see is an extra channel below the cuff to allow suctioning of the pooled secretions.

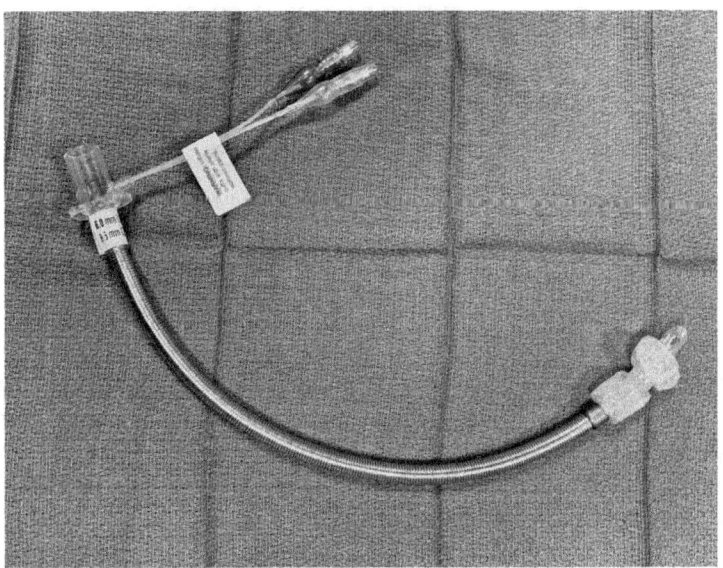

**Figure 130.4.** A laser-resistant ETT with a reinforced core.

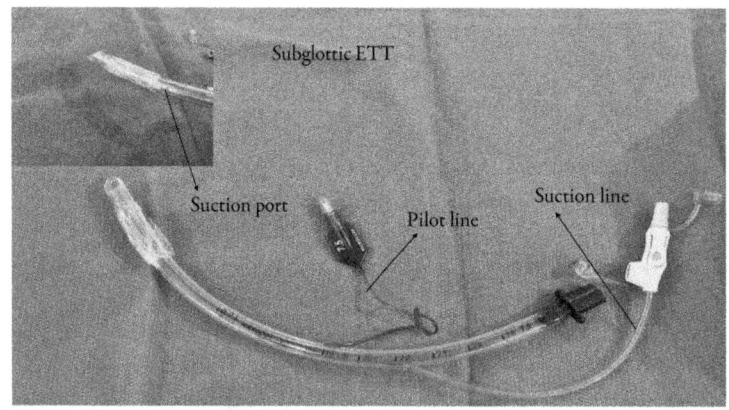

**Figure 130.5.** A subglottic tube with subglottic suctioning port.

This is to prevent micro-aspiration of the secretions through the microchannels that get created in these cuffs.[5] Figure 130.5 shows a subglottic tube with subglottic suctioning port.

## REFERENCES

1. Khine H, et al. Comparison of cuffed and uncuffed endotracheal tubes in young children during general anesthesia. *Anesthesiology.* 1997;86:627–631

2. Haas, CF, Blank, R. Endotracheal tubes: Old and new—discussion. *Respiratory care* 2014;59(6):933–955.
3. Sandberg W, Urman R, Ehrenfeld J. (2010). *The MGH Textbook of Anesthetic Equipment E-Book.* Elsevier Health Sciences; 2010:111–126.
4. Tsai CJ, et al. Electromyographic endotracheal tube placement during thyroid surgery in neuromonitoring of recurrent laryngeal nerve. *Kaohsiung J Med Sci.* 2011;27(3):96–101.
5. Hamilton A, Grap M. The role of the endotracheal tube cuff in microaspiration. *Heart & Lung,* 2012;41(2):167–172.

# 131.

# SUPRAGLOTTIC SECRETION SUCTIONING AND LASER SAFETY PROTOCOLS

*Matthew T. Connolly*

## INTRODUCTION

Supraglottic secretion management is an important component of the intraoperative course, which has implications for extubation and airway protection postoperatively. Although suctioning may seem straightforward, oropharyngeal trauma can occur if performed in a cavalier manner. LASER use by various surgical specialties has become more commonplace and comes with many important intraoperative considerations, of which the anesthesia provider must be aware for the safety of themselves and the patient.

## SUPRAGLOTTIC SECRETION SUCTIONING

### EQUIPMENT

Assessing for adequate functioning suction is an essential component of the preoperative anesthesia checklist. Inadequate suctioning or lack of proper equipment can have deleterious consequences, particularly at the time of extubation, including aspiration of sections, whether it be from salivary, gastric, or another source. Additionally, secretions have the potential to cause laryngospasm if they contact the vocal cords following extubation. The primary supraglottic suctioning modalities for general anesthesia are the Yankhauer, pediatric suction catheter, and flexible suction catheter. These devices come in various sizes and should be tailored to the clinical context based on situation and patient anatomy.

### TECHNIQUES AND ANESTHESIA CONSIDERATIONS

Supraglottic suctioning should be administered prior to extubation while the patient has an adequate general anesthetic. The provider must be cautious to avoid suctioning during Stage 2 in order to prevent agitation of the patient that could potentially lead to increased blood pressure, heart rate, laryngospasm, and premature extubation through coughing. Suctioning should also be performed after the patient is extubated and able to open their mouth to command.[1] In the event of any of the preceding responses, one should quickly deepen the anesthetic, usually with a bolus of propofol, which could assist in preventing further sympathetic response and blunt the cough and laryngospasm reflexes. Supraglottic suctioning can be performed at any time intraoperatively if secretions are a concern, as well as postoperatively following extubation. Care should be taken

with opening the mouth and navigating the hard plastic of the Yankhauer around the teeth and soft tissues to minimize oropharyngeal trauma, especially in coagulopathic patients. Flexible suction catheters help minimize and prevent trauma, particularly in patients with small mouth opening, and are also useful for suctioning the nares.

## ANESTHETIC CONSIDERATIONS WITH LASERS

### LASER USES AND TYPES

LASERs are used for ear, nose, and throat (ENT) surgeries such as microlaryngoscopy, urological procedures, and ophthalmologic procedures. As indicated in Table 131.1, there are various types of LASERs for various procedures.[2]

### GENERAL RISKS AND ANESTHESIA CONSIDERATIONS

Although LASERs used in surgery are non-ionizing, they are still deemed unsafe due to their intensity and the matter that can be produced from the surrounding tissues. Moreover, LASERs have a propensity to ignite fires, with $N_2O$ and oxygen supporting combustion. As such, $FiO_2$ should be minimized to the lowest level possible (typically less than 30%) and the level communicated to the surgery team to mitigate risk.[1,2] Anesthesia can be administered with or without an endotracheal tube (ETT), with the risk and benefits of general anesthesia versus moderate sedation being discussed with the surgery team. Microlaryngoscopy is one of several surgeries that have seen success with the use of TIVA and without the need of an ETT.[3] The key component to allowing sedation techniques is maintaining patient immobility.

*Table 131.1* COMMON LASERS USED IN SURGERY

| LASER | GAS/SOLID | COLOR | WAVELENGTH (NM) | ADDITIONAL NOTES |
|---|---|---|---|---|
| $CO_2$ | Gas | Invisible (far infrared) | 10,600 nm | Most common LASER used Limited penetration (0.01 nm); damage limited to cornea |
| Nd/YAG | Solid | Invisible (near infrared) | 1064 nm | Poorly absorbed by water Penetrates tissues more deeply |
| Argon | Gas | Blue-green | 500 nm | |
| Helium/Neon | Gas | Red | 633 nm | |
| KTP | Solid | Green | 532 nm | |
| Ruby | Solid | Red | 695 nm | |

KTP: Potassium titanyl phosphate; Nd: YAG: neodymium:yttrium-aluminum-garnet.

*Source:* data from Miller, R. *Miller's Anesthesia.* 6th ed. Chapter 70. Philadelphia, PA: Elsevier. Churchill Livingstone; 2005.

Misdirection of LASER beams can damage tissue, especially the eyes of the patient and anyone in the operating room. Eye injuries are noted to be the greatest risk with those exposed to LASERs.[2] Everyone in the operating room, including the patient, should wear eye protection with goggles appropriate for the particular wavelength. Wet gauze can also be applied on the patient's eyes as it absorbs the LASER radiation. Additionally, LASERs can cause plumes of smoke and matter from the tissue which is particularly concerning if the lesion is viral, such as with a human papilloma virus, as well as carcinogens, toxins, and bacteria.[2] These scenarios warrant personal protective equipment to prevent inhalation of the virus. Proper signage should be placed outside the procedure room for anyone entering when the LASER is in use.[1,2]

## LASER-SAFE ETTS

Standard polyvinyl chloride ETTs have the potential to ignite fires when LASERs are in use under a general anesthetic. As previously mentioned, moderate sedation techniques are being employed in which this is not an issue. However, LASER-safe ETTs are available and have traditionally consisted of wire-wrapped tubes, as well as various new designs specific for use with LASERs. Of note, ETT cuffs should be inflated with sterile saline with methylene blue added to use as an indicator of cuff rupture by a misdirected beam.[1] Some ETTs have an additional cuff for redundancy to prevent loss of cuff seal.

## REFERENCES

1. Barash, P. *Clinical Anesthesia*. 7th ed. Philadelphia, PA: Lippincott Williams & Wilkens; 2015.
2. Miller, R. *Miller's Anesthesia*. 6th ed. Philadelphia, PA: Elsevier Churchill Livingstone; 2005.
3. Yoo MJ, et al. Tubeless total intravenous anesthesia spontaneous ventilation for adult suspension microlaryngoscopy. *Ann Otol Rhino Laryngol*. 2018 Jan;127(1):39–45.

# 132.

# INTRAVENOUS FLUID THERAPY DURING ANESTHESIA

*David Guz and Connor McNamara*

## INTRODUCTION

The first recognized use of intravenous fluid was in 1831 by Dr. Thomas Latta, who described the use of a saline solution for the treatment of severely dehydrated patients suffering from cholera. Since then, various electrolyte- and carbohydrate-containing solutions have been an essential component of modern medicine, where they are used to replace fluid and electrolyte deficits for patients in whom oral intake may be unfeasible or inadequate. Intravenous fluid solutions have been listed as essential drugs by the World Health Organization and, like any other drug, improper use can be associated with adverse patient outcomes, including volume overload, acid/base disturbances, and surgical morbidity.[1]

As part of the American Board of Anesthesiology (ABA) BASIC exam curriculum, trainees are expected to have familiarity with the physiology of free water and electrolyte balance, the various classes and types of solutions commonly available, and commonly used paradigms for fluid administration.

## WATER, ELECTROLYTE, AND GLUCOSE REQUIREMENTS AND COMMON IV FLUID FORMULATIONS (CRYSTALLOID VS. COLLOID)

In adult males ~60% of body mass is composed of water (compared to ~50% in females), which is divided into

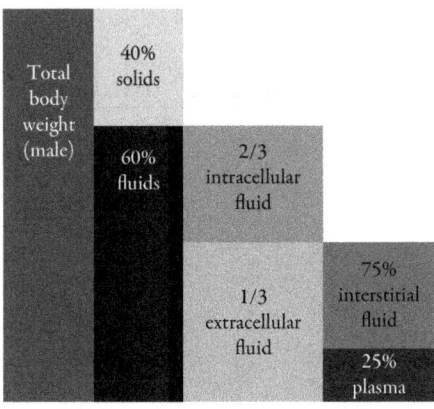

**Figure 132.1.** Body fluid composition.

intra- and extracellular compartments (Figure 132.1). The separation of these compartments is maintained by semipermeable cell membranes which utilize active and passive mechanisms to create electrolyte gradients; these gradients comprise ions, proteins, urea, and sugars, of which ionic sodium (Na+) is the primary determinant of extracellular osmolality. A total body free water deficit can thus be estimated by comparing a patient's plasma Na concentration to an established baseline, as demonstrated in the equation:

Free water deficit = % Total body water * weight in kg
(current Na/ideal Na) – 1).

Ion gradients create regions of varying tonicity and serve to facilitate osmotic transport of free water to and from the intracellular and extracellular compartments and thus maintain cellular integrity. Derangements in this system are responsible for a variety of pathologic conditions, including hemolysis and cerebral edema.[2] Normal extracellular (serum) osmolality is commonly cited as 275–295 mmol/kg and can be estimated by the formula:

Serum osm ≈ 2(Na) + (glucose)/18 + (BUN)/2.8 + 9.

Significant differences between this calculation and a directly measured serum osm (an osmolar gap) can be seen in pathologic processes involving the presence of osmotically active compounds not included in most basic metabolic panels such as ketoacids, ethylene glycol, and methanol.

While sterile distilled water is the base for all commonly used IV fluids, its use in clinical practice is limited to use via the enteric route, as irrigation, and as a solvent. Infusion of water "free" of electrolytes can catastrophically dilute the plasma, leading to expansion of the intracellular space and cell lysis. To avoid this problem, sterile water must be combined with solutes to create solutions of varying effective tonicity prior to being infused. This is accomplished with the addition of osmotically active compounds. IV fluids are commonly divided into two broad categories of crystalloid and colloid solutions; crystalloids are composed of water-soluble mineral salts, ions, and simple sugars, while colloids typically contain both soluble and larger, insoluble substances such as albumin, starches, hemoglobin, and gelatin (Table 132.1). Choice of fluid used in clinical practice can be tailored to each patient's individual situation based on intravascular volume status, solute balance, and energy requirements.

Anecdotally, colloid solutions are regarded as superior expanders of intravascular volume when compared to crystalloid solutions as they theoretically do not cross the endothelial barrier and increase plasma oncotic pressure, thus preferentially remaining in the intravascular space. For this reason, some providers prefer to use colloid solutions to resuscitate patients deemed to have total body volume overload with intravascular depletion; however, no evidence has definitively proven a mortality benefit in the setting of hypovolemic shock. Hetastarch in particular has been associated with acute kidney injury and coagulopathy.

The addition of a simple carbohydrate (typically dextrose) to IV fluids serves to provide an energy source and prevent catabolism for patients in whom PO intake is difficult or contraindicated. Dextrose is the R-isomer of the glucose molecule and is the primary substrate for glycolysis. Each gram of dextrose will provide 3.4 kcal of energy; thus, in a 5% dextrose solution (containing 50mg/ml) each ml should deliver 0.17 kcal of energy. The optimal choice of dextrose-containing solution and rate of administration will depend on individual patient needs (based on basal metabolic rate) and solute balance. In typical perioperative clinical practice, it is reasonable to provide 500 kcal of energy to the average 70kg patient to avoid muscle breakdown. Solutions like 5% dextrose in water can also be used as a parenteral free water equivalent that is isotonic when administered, unlike sterile water, and will not cause hemolysis. Dextrose may be supplemented alone or in addition to fats and proteins as a component of parenteral nutrition.

## FLUID DEFICIT CALCULATIONS, REPLACEMENT STRATEGIES, AND ERAS CONSIDERATIONS

In clinical practice, IV fluids are used to correct existing and ongoing fluid deficits, maintain solute balance, and provide substrate for metabolism. Perioperative fluid management has traditionally relied heavily upon the use of standardized formulas and "static" clinical markers of tissue perfusion such as heart rate, urine output, and central venous pressure to estimate existing volume deficits and needs for maintenance fluid. Static clinical markers may indicate true hypovolemia; however, the surgical stress response often mimics these changes and may lead to inappropriate administration of fluids.[3] Traditional guidelines for fluid administration continue to appear on tests and in situations where use of novel markers of volume status is unavailable

*Table 132.1* DIFFERENT TYPES OF FLUIDS

| SOLUTION | OSMOLARITY | PH | NA+ | CL⁻ | K+ | CA2+ | GLUCOSE | OTHER |
|---|---|---|---|---|---|---|---|---|
| 0.9% "Normal" Saline | 308 | 6.0 | 154 | 154 | — | — | — | — |
| 0.5% NS | 154 | 6.0 | 77 | 77 | — | — | — | — |
| 3% NS | 1026 | 5.0 | 513 | 513 | — | – | – | – |
| Lactated Ringer | 273 | 6.5 | 130 | 109 | 4 | 3 | – | Lactate 28 |
| Plasmalyte | 294 | 7.4 | 140 | 98 | 5 | 3 | – | Acetate 27, gluconate 23 |
| 5% Dextrose in Water | 253 | 4.5 | – | – | – | – | 50 | – |
| D5W in 0.5% Saline | 432 | 4.0 | 77 | 77 | – | – | 50 | – |
| D5W LR | 525 | 5.0 | 109 | 109 | 4 | 3 | 50 | Lactate 28 |
| 7.5% NaHCO3 | 1786 | 8.0 | – | – | – | – | – | HCO3 893 |
| Albumin 5% | 330 | 7.4 | – | – | <2 | – | – | Albumin 50 |
| Albumin 25% | 330 | 7.4 | – | – | <2 | – | – | Albumin 250 |
| 10% Dextran in NS | 308 | 4.0 | 154 | 154 | – | – | – | Dextran 100 |
| Hetastarch 6% in NS | 308 | 5.9 | 154 | 154 | – | – | – | Hetastarch 60 |

or unfeasible. These guidelines derive estimates of fluid requirements based on a multitude of factors, including patient weight, duration of time NPO, use of bowel prep, extent of surgical exposure, and strict tabulation of gross fluid losses. Classically the "4/2/1" rule was commonly utilized as a standard of care to estimate a set hourly fluid requirement based on weight; initially created for pediatric use, it gradually made its way into general adult practice for lack of alternative options. The protocol called for 4 cc/kg for the first 10 kg of total body weight, 2cc/kg for the next 10 kg, and 1 cc/kg for every kg above 20. For an average 70kg adult, this would equate to a minimum of 110 cc/hr IV fluid, which would be added onto other intraoperative fluid losses for a total hourly rate. Sources for intraoperative fluid loss include blood loss, outputs from various drains (including urinary catheters, chest tubes, and gastric tubes), as well as more difficult to quantify "third-spaced" and insensible losses, also typically derived arbitrarily based on patient weight and extent of surgical exposure.

These conventional modes for estimation and replacement of initial and ongoing fluid deficits have been criticized in recent years for a propensity toward over-resuscitation, which has been shown to be directly linked with increased surgical and intensive care unit (ICU) morbidity (including anastomotic failure, ileus, increased length of stay, and increased duration of mechanical ventilation).[4] In alignment with modern Enhanced Recovery After Surgery (ERAS) protocols, this has given way to a more restrictive strategy of resuscitation, emphasizing a "zero-balance" approach when feasible, alongside the use of dynamic markers of volume status, which may serve to better approximate losses attributable to third-spaced and insensible losses when compared to the formula-based method. These dynamic markers include predictors of fluid responsiveness including straight leg raises, pulse pressure variation and pulse contour analysis, and echocardiographic visualization of cardiac filling; these are covered in more detail as part of the advanced curriculum.

## ANESTHETIC CONSIDERATIONS

### PREOPERATIVE

- Obtain excellent history and physical exam; note factors which may impact patient's "volume status," such as use of a mechanical bowel prep, prolonged NPO time, or presence of decompensated cardiac or renal failure.
- Review the difference between patient's target and current weight as a possible measure of fluid overload/deficit.
- Review labs, assess for derangements which may favor use of a particular solution over others.

## INTRAOPERATIVE

- Patient may require small fluid bolus around time of induction to offset sympathectomy.
- Consider use of TEE or cardiac output monitoring per ERAS guidelines to dynamically manage patient's fluid requirements in real time.
- Try to monitor and chart ongoing fluid losses and administration to best of ability.

## POSTOPERATIVE

- Consider continued use of ultrasound and/or cardiac output monitors to optimize fluid administration.
- Monitor I/Os (input/output).

## REFERENCES

1. Shin CH, et al. Effects of intraoperative fluid management on postoperative outcomes: A hospital registry study. *Ann Surg.* 2018; 267:1084.
2. Shah MM, Mandiga P. Physiology, plasma osmolality and oncotic pressure. [Updated October 9, 2021]. In: *StatPearls* [Internet]. Treasure Island (FL): StatPearls Publishing; 2021.
3. Siparsky N. Overview of postoperative fluid therapy in adults. In: Cochran A, Sterns RH, Collins KA, eds., *UpToDate*, Waltham, MA, 2020. Accessed December 29, 2021.
4. Holte K, et al. Pathophysiology and clinical implications of perioperative fluid excess. *Br J Anaesth.* 2002;89:622.

# 133.

# COLLOIDS

*Stacey Watt and Anthony D'Auria*

## INTRODUCTION

It has been frequently described that under normal conditions approximately two-thirds of total water in the human body is confined to the intracellular space, and one-third in the extracellular space, which includes the plasma, interstitial space, and a small portion relegated to the glycocalyx layer. An important role of the anesthesiologist is to maintain this physiologic fluid balance, which often involves administration of intravenous fluids (IVF) in the perioperative period. Given the assortment of options, choosing an appropriate solution may seem daunting; however, like any other intervention or administered drug, IVFs have risks and benefits that should be carefully examined before selection.

The first branch point in choosing an IVF is selecting crystalloid vs. colloid solutions. Crystalloids (e.g., 0.9% normal saline or balanced salt solutions such as lactated ringers) are often the first choice as they are low-priced and readily available solutions that have demonstrated efficacy in restoring total body fluid. These solutions will be discussed separately in this text, and the focus of this chapter is on the use of colloid solutions, whose unique characteristics allow for rapid intravascular volume expansion.

Colloids are large molecules (typically greater than 70 kDa) of homogenous, non-crystalline substances dissolved in saline or other balanced crystalloids. The relatively large size of the dissolved molecules renders colloids unable to pass through the glycocalyx layer on the inner lumen of vasculature endothelium, and unlike crystalloids, colloids will therefore remain in the plasma. In other words, the entire initial volume of distribution of colloids is restricted to the plasma. This further allows for intravascular volume expansion as the solutions increase colloid osmotic pressure (COP) and pull free water into the intravascular space via oncotic drag.[1] While this results in results in hemodilution and reduction of hematocrit, it has benefit of reducing plasma viscosity and improvement of blood flow.[2]

Colloids are large (typically larger than 70 kDa) and often homogenous. Generally speaking, colloids are more expensive, are less readily available, and their overall utilization is significantly less than crystalloids. They offer no oxygen-carrying capabilities, and examples include human plasma derivatives (e.g., 5% albumin, 20% albumin), hydroxyethyl starches (e.g., hetastarches, pentastarches), dextrans, and gelatins (though not approved by the US Food and Drug Administration).

## ALBUMIN

Hypoalbuminemia has long been associated with poor outcomes in critical disease states, as endogenous albumin is responsible for approximately 80% of oncotic pressure in the plasma. Despite the intuition to simply replete albumin, it has been shown that administration of exogenous albumin does not improve outcomes in situations of hypoalbuminemia, though it should be clearly stated that the majority of research regarding albumin administration is in the critical care setting, and not the operative setting. Additionally, varying evidence on outcome demonstrated in meta-analyses further confuses the subject. Despite these complexities, the role of exogenous albumin administration continues to play a role in plasma expansion, with the major evidence-based indications being in the critically ill when crystalloids are not effective or contraindicated, in patients with advanced cirrhosis, and after large volume paracentesis. Additionally, a reduction in mortality has also been shown in burn patients who received albumin.[3] In 2004, the SAFE trial showed patients with traumatic brain injury had worse outcomes with exogenous albumin, and its use should be avoided in this patient population.[4]

Exogenous albumin is available in 5%, 20%, and 25% formulations and is prepared from human venous plasma, thus technically a blood product (consider Jehovah's Witnesses). The 5% formulation has a COP of 20 mmHg, very close to physiological levels, whereas the 20% and 25% formulations are hyperosmotic and can cause an intravascular volume expansion of 200%–400% within 30 minutes. The half-life of blood-derived exogenous albumin is approximately 12–16 hours.

Albumin is typically mixed with normal saline, and monitoring for hypernatremia should be considered as the sodium concentration 145 ± mEq/L. Sodium concentration can be decreased by mixing with D5W instead of normal saline.

## HYDROXYETHYL STARCHES: HETASTARCH AND PENTASTARCH

Hydroxyethyl starches (HESs) are a group of colloid solutions derived from corn or potato with hydroxyethyl radicals attached to the glucose molecule and have long been used as a volume expander. In 2008 the FDA approved HESs for acute blood loss. In addition, HESs have endothelium-protective properties by reducing the number of circulating adhesion molecules. The ratio of hydroxyethyl substitutions to the total number of glucose molecules, termed the molar substitution (MS) ratio, is a common method of stratifying HESs. An MS of 0.7 are hetastarches, and an MS of 0.5 are pentastarches. Most commonly, hetastarch is formulated in 6% solutions, and pentastarch in 10% formulations, and lower molecular weight solutions exist as well (3%). From a cost perspective, HESs are a more attractive option than albumin, and was at one time a favored option for intravascular volume expansion; however, HESs have fallen out of favor as there are documented deleterious effects on coagulation, platelet function, and renal dysfunction that are of considerable concern.

The effects on coagulation are partially a result of dilution, but there is also an apparent molecular weight–dependent factor VIII decrease, with higher molecular weight starches resulting in more marked reductions. Platelet function, in particular adhesion, is also affected due to the same molecular weight–dependent reduction in von Willebrand factor and glycoproteins IIb/IIIa. Impact can be as high as 80%, even when used below the recommended daily limit of 25–50 ml/kg. Increased PT and APTT were reported.

Renal dysfunction noted with HESs appears to also demonstrate the same molecular weight dependence, as shown previously. Oliguria, increased creatinine, and AKI in critically ill patients with preexisting renal dysfunction have been shown with administration of HESs. The CHEST trial demonstrated an increased risk of renal replacement therapy with HESs.[5]

## ANESTHESIOLOGY CONSIDERATIONS

### PREOPERATIVE

- An assessment of the patient's volume status, comorbid conditions (particularly cardiac, renal, and hepatic dysfunction), electrolyte disturbances, and blood loss are important considerations in fluid selection.
- Recall that the majority of major studies of colloid solutions have been done in the critical care setting, and information in the operative and perioperative period is limited.

## INTRAOPERATIVE

- Colloid solutions have the advantage of rapid intravascular expansion.
- Both crystalloid and colloid solutions offer no oxygen-carrying capability.
- Albumin is FDA approved for acute blood loss, but avoid in patients with traumatic brain injury (TBI).
- HESs have significant effects on coagulation and renal function.

## POSTOPERATIVE

- If HESs are used, consider an assessment of the patient's renal function.

## REFERENCES

1. Rehm M, et al. Endothelial glycocalyx as an additional barrier determining extravasation of 6% hydroxyethyl starch or 5% albumin solutions in the coronary vascular bed. *Anesthesiology.* 2004;100:1211–1223.
2. Grocott MPW, et al. Perioperative increase in global blood flow to explicit defined goals and outcomes after surgery: A Cochrane Systematic Review. *Br J Anaesth.* 2013;111:535–548.
3. Liumbruno GM, et al. Recommendations for the use of albumin and immunoglobulins. *Blood Transfus.* 2009;7:216–234.
4. Finfer S, et al. A comparison of albumin and saline for fluid resuscitation in the intensive care unit. *N Engl J Med.* 2004;350(22):2247–2256.
5. Myburgh, JA et al. Hydroxyethyl starch or saline for fluid resuscitation in intensive care [published correction appears in *N Engl J Med.* 2016 Mar 31;374(13):1298]. *N Engl J Med.* 2012;367(20):1901–1911.

# 134.

# ENHANCED RECOVERY AFTER SURGERY PROTOCOL FOR FLUID THERAPY

*Hisham Kassem and Ivan Urits*

## INTRODUCTION

Enhanced recovery after surgery (ERAS) pathways have emerged during the past decade to guide care for patients undergoing major surgery. These pathways have aimed to provide improved patient outcomes by setting recommendations to follow throughout the entire perioperative period. An essential component of a successful ERAS protocol and one to be integrated with the other pillars is fluid management.[1] We will discuss the anesthetic considerations for ERAS patients when managing fluids during the preoperative, intraoperative, and postoperative phases.

## PREOPERATIVE CONSIDERATIONS

The management of fluids for patients integrating an ERAS protocol begins before he/she arrives for the scheduled surgery. Traditionally, surgical patients have been told to fast for 8 hours or sometimes more.[2] This long period of fasting has been shown to lead to increased metabolic stress and insulin resistance while adding to hypovolemia.[1] ERAS protocols encourage patients to drink clear liquids for up to 2 hours before the surgery, and studies show no increased risk of aspiration or perioperative morbidity.[3] Furthermore, oral liquid carbohydrate loading is encouraged because of reported potential added beneficial effects. These benefits are predominantly a reduction in insulin resistance, as well as decreasing patient-reported weakness in the first 24 hours postoperatively.[1] The metabolic benefits are centered on creating an anabolic state before surgery that can reduce incidence of postoperative hyperglycemia, ultimately a risk factor for infection.[2]

## INTRAOPERATIVE CONSIDERATIONS

The main goal of intraoperative fluid management is based on maintaining a euvolemic state while providing adequate perfusion to vital organs. The term "goal-directed fluid therapy" (GDFT) is commonly used to describe optimization of patient fluid status based on a continuous and individualized basis.[2] Various types of fluids have been studied in the context of ERAS protocol, with most of the results inconclusive. A general rule is to provide a balanced isotonic crystalloid solution (i.e., lactated Ringer's, PlasmaLyte, Normosol) as maintenance fluids and utilize colloids (i.e., albumin) when fluid boluses are needed due to their ability to stay in the intravascular space for longer periods of time.[1] The use of 0.9% normal saline has decreased in the past few years because of the associated electrolyte abnormalities such as hypercholremia and metabolic acidosis.[3] In some instances, patients are often started on low-dose vasopressor support during the surgery to restrict the amount of fluids needed. Fluid management, as stated before, needs to be managed in a continuous manner and should be guided by parameters that can indicate proper end-organ perfusion. The most accurate monitor that can be used is a pulmonary artery catheter (PAC), but this is not often used given the invasive nature of the procedure. More frequently, volume status of a patient can be guided by factors such as heart rate, blood pressure, end-tidal $CO_2$, and urine output. Urine output is often seen as a reliable measure of volume status, with a goal of at least 0.5 ml/kg/hr.[4]

## POSTOPERATIVE CONSIDERATIONS

While anesthetic management of patients undergoing ERAS protocol for major surgery usually ends in the postanesthesia care unit (PACU), there are certain principles of fluid management that are important to know. Patients are encouraged to begin early enteral/oral fluid intake as to stimulate quicker return of bowel function, which in turn can lead to decreased hospital length of stay. While most urinary catheters are removed early after surgery, careful monitoring of fluid balance should be continued in the postoperative period by restricting intravenous fluid maintenance once adequate oral intake has been achieved.[1]

## REFERENCES

1. Zhu AC, et al. Perioperative fluid management in the enhanced recovery after surgery (ERAS) pathway. *Clin Colon Rectal Surg.* 2019;32(2):114–120.
2. Kendrick JB, et al. Goal-directed fluid therapy in the perioperative setting. *J Anaesthesiol Clin Pharmacol.* 2019;35(Suppl 1):S29–S34.
3. Miller TM, Myles PS. Perioperative fluid therapy for major surgery. *Anesthesiology.* 2019;130(5):825–832.
4. Gustafsson UO, et al. Guidelines for perioperative care in elective colonic surgery: Enhanced Recovery After Surgery (ERAS®) Society recommendations. *Clin Nutr.* 2012;31(6):783–800.

# 135.

# ACUTE POSTOPERATIVE AND POSTTRAUMATIC PAIN

*Savion D. Johnson and Brian M. Starr*

## INTRODUCTION

As the number of surgeries in the United States increases yearly, the management of acute postoperative pain is important not only for acute hospital admissions, but also to mitigate the long-term consequences of ineffective pain management. Despite the use of various pathways to manage postoperative pain, adequate pain control is still elusive for many patients, with less than half of postoperative patients reporting adequate pain relief.[1] Management of postoperative pain starts in the preoperative period with proper planning and expectation setting with patients, and pain management should be seen as a continuum of interventions from the preoperative to postoperative period.

## PREOPERATIVE MANAGEMENT

### MULTIMODAL ANALGESIA AND ADJUNCTS

The treatment of acute postoperative and trauma-related pain starts preoperatively with the use of multimodal analgesia, which is the use of drugs from different classes and different analgesic techniques to target different mechanisms of pain. This has synergistic effects and can maximize pain relief with lower doses and fewer adverse effects. Three treatments that are often used preoperatively as part of a multimodal analgesia approach include gabapentinoids, nonsteroidal anti-inflammatory drugs (NSAIDs), and acetaminophen.

Gabapentin has historically been used as an adjunct for chronic neuropathic pain, but recently has been used more in the preoperative setting. Gabapentin and pregabalin are inhibitors of the alpha-2-delta subunit of the high voltage activated calcium channel. These drugs are eliminated unchanged in the urine. The most common side effects are dizziness, fatigue, drowsiness, weight gain, and peripheral edema. Regimens for gabapentin usually range from 300 mg to 900 mg, either as a one-time dose preoperatively or as a three times a day regimen in the postoperative period, with reduced dosing in renal insufficiency, and in the elderly due to sedation.[2]

NSAIDs are used in treating mild to moderate pain. They inhibit cyclooxygenase (COX) in the arachidonic acid pathway, limiting the formation of prostaglandin and thromboxane. These drugs act via inhibition of COX-1 or COX-2, and this variance changes not only the analgesic effects, but also the side effect profile of these medications. NSAIDs that block COX-1 have greater gastrointestinal adverse effects, while those that block COX-2 have increased cardiovascular thrombotic risk due to platelet aggregation (Table 135.1).[3]

*Table 135.1* COMMONLY USED NSAIDS IN THE PREOPERATIVE SETTING

| DRUG | COX INHIBITION | ADULT DOSAGE |
|---|---|---|
| Acetaminophen (Tylenol/Ofirmev) | Yet to be fully determined | 650–975 mg q4, q6h oral 1000 mg q6h IV |
| Celecoxib (Celebrex) | COX-2 | 100–200 mg BID oral |
| Ibuprofen (Motrin) | Non-selective | 400–800 mg q6-8h oral |
| Ketorolac (Toradol) | COX-1 | 10–50 mg q6-q8h oral 15–30 mg q8h oral |
| Meloxicam (Mobic) | COX-2 | 7.5–15 mg qd oral |
| Naproxen (Aleve) | COX-1 | 250–500 mg q8–12h oral |

## INTRAOPERATIVE MANAGEMENT

### EPIDURAL ANALGESIA AND NEURAXIAL OPIOIDS

Epidural analgesia has many indications, which include abdominal surgery, thoracic surgery, lower limb surgery, and lower body vascular procedures. Epidural analgesia has been shown to have superior analgesic benefit, opioid sparing, and improved surgical outcomes.[4] Epidural placement is contraindicated in patients who refuse, are coagulopathic, are on current antiplatelet or anticoagulant therapy, or those with infection at desired insertion site. Drugs of choice for epidural analgesia include local anesthetics and neuraxial opioids. These can be administered alone, but commonly are administered together, where they act synergistically for improved pain control. See Tables 135.2 and 135.3 for commonly used solutions and settings. Clonidine can be used, in addition to local anesthetics and opioids, to provide improved analgesia and greater duration of action. In addition to their use via the epidural space, opioids can be used in the intrathecal space to reduce the need for systemic opioids. Commonly used intrathecal opioids include morphine, fentanyl, and hydromorphone.

### PERIPHERAL NERVE BLOCKS

Peripheral nerve blocks are a critical component in managing both intraoperative and postoperative pain. There are a number of upper- and lower-extremity blocks that can be utilized to provide both surgical anesthesia and pain control.[5] See Tables 135.4 and 135.5 for review of common blocks.

One medication that has changed the decision of single shot versus catheter placement for peripheral nerve blocks is the approval of Exparel (bupivacaine liposome injectable suspension). The appeal of Exparel is that it allows a single-shot procedure to produce post-surgical analgesia for up to

*Table 135.2* COMMONLY USED LOCAL ANESTHETICS FOR CONTINUOUS EPIDURAL ANALGESIA

| LOCAL ANESTHETIC | DOSE | |
|---|---|---|
| Bupivacaine | 0.0625%–0.125% at 4–8 ml/hr | Most commonly used |
| Ropivacaine | 0.08%–0.2% at 4–8 ml/hr | Better safety profile in higher concentrations |
| Levobupivacaine | 0.0625%–0.125% at 4–8 ml/hr | Not available in the United States |
| Lidocaine | 0.75%–1.0% at 4–8 ml/hr | |

*Table 135.3* COMMONLY USED OPIOIDS FOR
CONTINUOUS EPIDURAL ANALGESIA

| OPIOID | DOSE |
|---|---|
| Fentanyl | 50–100 mcg/ml starting at 6 ml/hr |
| Sufentanil | 5–10 mcg/ml at 4–8 ml/hr |
| Hydromorphone | 3–25 mcg/ml starting at 6 ml/hr |

72 hours. The maximum dose is 266 mg per patient, and the common practice at our institution is for patients who received Exparel to wear wristbands to alert providers to be cautious of administering any additional local anesthetic.

## POSTOPERATIVE MANAGEMENT

### PATIENT-CONTROLLED ANALGESIA

Patient-controlled analgesia (PCA) is routinely used in the immediate postoperative period and allows patients to control their analgesia without the need for nurse interventions. These devices have built-in safety features to limit the risk of adverse outcomes. See Tables 135.6 and 135.7 for common PCA settings for opioid naïve and tolerant patients, respectively.

### INFUSION THERAPY

In the intraoperative and postoperative period, ketamine and lidocaine infusions are often used for pain relief. Ketamine acts via NMDA antagonism and also decreases pain excitability. Normal infusions are 0.5 mg/kg bolus followed by 0.25 mg/kg/hr infusions. Contraindications include those with elevated intracranial pressure (ICP), active psychiatric disorders, uncontrolled hypertension, and ischemic heart disease.

Lidocaine works by blocking voltage gated sodium channels, resulting in inhibition of nerve conduction. Typical infusions are 1–1.5 mg/kg/hr and serum lidocaine levels should be monitored to reduce the likelihood of developing local systemic toxicity symptoms.

*Table 135.4* COMMON UPPER EXTREMITY PERIPHERAL NERVE BLOCKS

| NERVE BLOCK | ANATOMY | CONSIDERATIONS |
|---|---|---|
| Cervical plexus block | Originates from C2, C3, and C4 anterior rami<br>Coverage for carotid endarterectomy and superior shoulder procedures in combination with interscalene block | Avoid bilateral plexus blocks due to blockade of phrenic nerve.<br>Near vertebral artery, intrathecal space, and spinal cord |
| Interscalene block | Blocks C5, C6, and C7 at level of interscalene groove<br>Adequate block for upper arm procedures proximal to elbow | Avoid medial approach due to risk of puncture to carotid artery and internal jugular vein.<br>Spares ulnar distribution so not appropriate for surgeries distal to the elbow<br>Transient ipsilateral paralysis, so avoid in patients where loss of diaphragm would cause respiratory distress. |
| Supraclavicular block | Provides complete anesthesia distal to the elbow as well as upper arm to tourniquet site<br>Works at supraclavicular fossa, transition between trunks and divisions in brachial plexus | Risk of pneumothorax and phrenic nerve paralysis |
| Infraclavicular block | Works at the level of the brachial plexus where it becomes three distinct cords<br>For procedures distal to the elbow | Good block for catheter placement for procedures distal to the elbow |
| Axillary block | At the level where the radial, median, and ulnar nerves surround the axillary artery with the musculocutaneous nerve between the biceps and coracobrachialis muscles<br>Good for surgery distal to the elbow, especially forearm and hand | Avoids the risk of pneumothorax and phrenic nerve paralysis but drawback of musculocutaneous nerve being spared and need for multiple needle passes<br>With increased use of ultrasound, supraclavicular more popular |

*Table 135.5* COMMON LOWER EXTREMITY PERIPHERAL NERVE BLOCKS

| NERVE BLOCK | ANATOMY | CONSIDERATIONS |
|---|---|---|
| Lumbar plexus block | Indicated for surgeries of the hip, anterior thigh, or knee and can provide anesthesia to entire lower extremity when combined with sciatic nerve block <br> Derived from anterior rami of L1 to L4 nerve roots | Increased risk of local anesthetic toxicity due to proximity to vascular structures and use of large volumes of local anesthetic |
| Femoral block | For analgesia to the lower extremity and postop pain control for mid-shaft femoral fractures or surgeries above the knee <br> Arises from posterior branches of L2, L3, and L4 of lumbar plexus | Risk factor for falls <br> Good for catheter placement for hip fractures |
| Adductor canal block | Motor sparing peripheral nerve block for total knee arthroplasty | Less weakness of quadriceps compared to femoral blocks, with similar pain relief |
| Saphenous nerve block | Supplement to sciatic nerve block for lower extremity surgery of the medial portion of foot or leg | Largest sensory component of femoral nerve and only component that innervates below the knee |
| Lateral femoral cutaneous nerve block | Used in combination with other lower extremity blocks for complete lower extremity analgesia <br> Direct branch from lumbar plexus L2 and L3 <br> Innervation to anterolateral thigh and small portion of thigh from hip to knee | |
| Obturator nerve block | Sensory innervation for surface of the knee, used for total knee arthroplasty and ACL repairs <br> Formed from anterior division of L2, L3, and L4 | Risk of intravascular injections and hematoma |
| Sciatic nerve block | Largest of lower extremity nerves and can be used as complete anesthetic for foot and ankle surgeries when lower leg tourniquet needed <br> Used in conjunction with saphenous nerve if medial portion of ankle or leg coverage needed <br> Formed from ventral rami from L4 to S3 | |
| Ankle blocks | Sensory innervation of the foot provided by deep peroneal, superficial peroneal, tibial, sural, and saphenous nerve | Can be uncomfortable and require multiple injection sites <br> Must monitor local anesthetic values |

*Table 135.6* COMMON PCA SETTINGS FOR OPIOID-NAÏVE PATIENTS

| OPIOID | CONCENTRATION | DOSE SETTING |
|---|---|---|
| Morphine | 5 mg/ml | 0.8–1.2 mg demand dose q10 minutes with 1 hour limit of 4–6 mg |
| Fentanyl | 50 mcg/ml | 8–12 mcg q6 or q10 minutes with 1 hour limit of 64–96 mcg |
| Hydromorphone | 1 mg/ml | 0.1–0.3 mg q10 minutes with 1 hour limit of 0.5 to 1.5 mg |

*Table 135.7* COMMON PCA SETTINGS FOR OPIOID-TOLERANT PATIENTS (SICKLE CELL, CHRONIC PAIN, ONCOLOGY)

| OPIOID | CONCENTRATION | DOSE SETTING |
|---|---|---|
| Morphine | 5 mg/ml | 2–2.5 mg q10 minutes with 1 hour limit 10–12.5 mg |
| Fentanyl | 50 mcg/ml | 15–20 mcg q6 or q10 minutes with 1 hour limit of 120–150 mcg |
| Hydromorphone | 1 mg/ml | 0.3–0.4 mg q10 minutes with 1 hour limit of 1.5–2.0 mg |

## REFERENCES

1. Sharrock NE, et al. Changes in mortality after total hip and knee arthroplasty over a ten-year period. *Anesth Analg.* 1995;80:242–248.
2. Schmidt PC, et al. Perioperative gabapentinoids: Choice of agent, dose, timing, and effects on chronic post-surgical pain. *Anesthesiology.* 2013;119:1215.
3. McGettigan P, Henry D. Cardiovascular risk and inhibition of cyclooxygenase: A systematic review of the observational studies of selective and nonselective inhibitors of cyclooxygenase 2. *JAMA.* 2006;296(13):1633. Epub 2006 Sep 12.
4. Wu CL, et al. Effect of postoperative epidural analgesia on morbidity and mortality following surgery in medicare patients. *Reg Anesth Pain Med.* 2004;29(6):525.
5. Ray N et al. Management of acute postoperative pain. In: Longnecker DE, Mackey SC, Newman MF, Sandberg WS, Zapol WM, eds. *Anesthesiology.* 3rd ed. McGraw-Hill; 2017.

# 136.

# INDICATIONS AND CONTRAINDICATIONS

*Elizabeth Kremen and Sahel Keshavarzi*

## INTRODUCTION

In a move to increase cost effectiveness and efficiency, there is a tendency to have more pediatric procedures performed in ambulatory surgical centers.[1] Patients qualifying for outpatient surgeries have the advantage of potentially lessening the disruption to families in terms of cost and time commitment, compared with surgeries requiring a full inpatient admission. However, the appropriateness of treatment in an ambulatory center may be assessed in three main categories: patient factors, surgical factors, and location factors (Figure 136.1).[2]

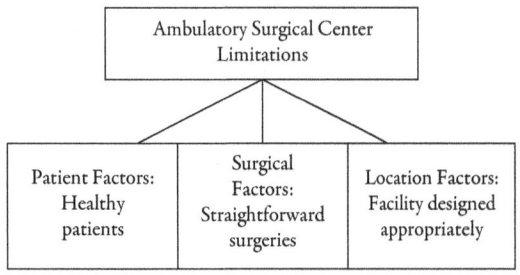

**Figure 136.1.** General requisites for effective ambulatory surgical cases.

## PATIENT FACTORS

- Patient should have no risk factors for, or history of, a difficult airway.
- Patient and patient's family members should not have a history of adverse reactions to anesthesia, or history of a muscular dystrophy.
- Patients should be healthy overall, or have well-managed, stable chronic conditions, namely are ASA class 1 or 2.
- Patients with complex cardiac conditions or congenital dysrhythmias are generally poor candidates for outpatient surgery in a free-standing ambulatory surgical center.
- If the patient has a history of prematurity, their current age must be greater than 60 weeks post-conceptual age (PCA).
- If the patient is a healthy, full-term infant, their current age must be greater than 4 to 6 weeks old.
- The patient is unlikely to need invasive monitoring for the procedure.
- The patient's home caregiver should be available, reliable, and willing to provide care at home before (including enforcing *nil per os* rules) and after the surgery.
- Patients should not be acutely sick or unstable.

## SURGICAL FACTORS

- The surgical procedure is expected to be of short duration.
- The surgical procedure is unlikely to require overnight admission.
- The procedure is unlikely to have significant anesthetic or surgical complications.
- The procedure is unlikely to require specialized equipment unavailable at an outpatient center and can be performed safely at the outpatient facility.
- The procedure has a low likelihood of requiring blood products or transfusions.
- Post-discharge home care instructions should be straightforward and easy to follow.
- Postoperative pain is expected to be well-controlled without intravenous medication. On the day of surgery, postoperative pain should be controlled with regional blocks or with oral medications.

## LOCATION FACTORS

- The ambulatory surgical center should maintain supplies and have staff trained to adequately manage malignant hyperthermia acutely.
- The center should have a plan in place for patient care if an inpatient transfer or admission becomes necessary.
- Ancillary services should be easily accessible, if not in house, such as laboratory, respiratory care, or radiology imaging services.
- Staff are trained to handle preoperative and postoperative services, give instructions, and follow up with patients in the 24-hour perioperative window.
- Staff should be able to handle patient care in a high-patient-turnover setting.
- Standard anesthesia equipment, including ASA monitors, should be available and should be used.[3]
- Emergency airway equipment available and in good working order, with staff trained for use, for managing surprise difficult airways.

Overall, ambulatory surgical center cases are best equipped to handle healthy children for short, straightforward procedures. If patients are sicker or more fragile, and do not meet the preceding guidelines, there should be consideration either to delay surgery or to undergo the surgery at a facility with more resources and ability to admit to the inpatient setting. Similarly, if a complex procedure is planned, or one with significant fluid shifts expected, or high risk of complications, or with complicated postoperative care instructions, it should be undertaken at a facility equipped to provide a higher level of care.[2]

## SPECIAL CONSIDERATIONS

### UPPER RESPIRATORY TRACT INFECTIONS (URTI)

There is not a clear consensus on how long it is appropriate to wait after a child clears an URTI for surgery to proceed. Some suggest waiting 2 weeks, others as long as 7 weeks. Considering that children often get common otolaryngology interventions such as myringotomy tube placement, tonsillectomy, or adenoidectomy procedures for having frequent recurrent infections or being unable to clear infections, the decision to delay surgery in order to wait for a clear, healthy window may be difficult. Longer waits may be impractical or impossible with young children contracting new URTIs within that timeframe. Some studies suggest that the use of a supraglottic device instead of endotracheal intubation, if possible, may result in fewer airway complications by avoiding triggering bronchial hyperreactivity. There is conflicting data around the benefits of pretreating pulmonary symptoms with inhalers.[2,4]

### CONSIDER RESCHEDULING IF

- The patient appears acutely unwell, with systemic symptoms.
- The patient is newly sick or has recently developed symptoms, including a decreased appetite, lethargy, malaise, or the patient appears significantly dehydrated.
- The patient has purulent nasal discharge, or a cough.
- The patient has persistent pulmonary signs, including rales that do not clear, or wheezing.
- The patient is febrile with a temperature greater than 38.5°C.
- A major operation is planned, or extensive airway instrumentation is required.
- The patient has significant underlying medical conditions likely exacerbated by acute illness, or a history of prematurity.

### USE BEST CLINICAL JUDGMENT IF

- The patient has minimal symptoms, appears active and playful, or if caregivers report that the patient is at their baseline.
- The caregiver reports improvement or resolution of symptoms.
- The patient is afebrile.
- The child is older.
- There are significant social factors affecting the patient and family, such as large distance traveled, the limited ability to take time away from work, or the family is nearing the end of insurance coverage.

# OBSTRUCTIVE SLEEP APNEA

## ADDITIONAL RELATIVE CONTRAINDICATIONS

- Obesity: Obese patients have a higher risk of postoperative airway obstruction and apnea, thus will likely require further monitoring to prevent adverse outcomes.[2,4]
- If a patient has a high apnea hypopnea index, they will similarly be at higher risk of complication, including hypoxemia or hypercarbia.
- If a patient has an ASA class greater than II, including syndromic patients, the patient should be preferentially scheduled for intervention in a location with more resources than an ambulatory surgical center.

## REFERENCES

1. Fabricant PD. et al. Cost savings from utilization of a pediatric ambulatory surgery center for orthopaedic day surgery. *Pediatrics*. Jan 2018;141:616.
2. Politis G. Pediatric ambulatory anesthesia. In: Gregory GA, Andropoulos DB, eds. *Anesthesia Care of Pediatric Patients in Developing Countries*. Global HELP;2015:487–522.
3. American Association for Accreditation of Ambulatory Surgery Facilities. *Procedural Standards and Checklist for Accreditation of Ambulatory Surgery Facilities*, Version 4.3. February 2019.
4. Ghazal EA, et al. Preoperative evaluation, premedication, and induction of anesthesia. In Coté CJ, Lerman J, eds. *A Practice of Anesthesia for Infants and Children*. 6th ed. Elsevier; 2019.

# Part IX

# COMMON COMPLICATIONS

# 137.

# TRAUMA

*Mallory Nebergall and Mazin T. Albert*

## INTRODUCTION

Traumatic injuries sustained while under the care of an anesthetist are often multifactorial, but iatrogenic causes account for a large portion. It is the duty of the anesthetist to minimize the risk of physical injury to the patient through high standards of clinical practice.

## TRAUMA TO UPPER AIRWAY: EPISTAXIS

Epistaxis is a common complication of nasal airway manipulation. Insertion of nasal trumpets and endotracheal tubes can cause trauma to the nasal mucosa overlying Kisselbach's plexus in the anterior nasal septum resulting in epistaxis. Risk factors and common causes are listed in Box 137.1.

If bleeding occurs during nasal intubation, intubation should be completed to tamponade the bleeding and protect the airway. Mild epistaxis usually resolves spontaneously or with external pressure to affected nares for 10–60 seconds. If moderate or persistent nasal bleeding, apply a topical vasoconstrictor (epinephrine, phenylephrine, cocaine, or oxymetazoline solution). If local therapy fails, nasal packing can be used to achieve tamponade. Rarely, surgical ligation or embolization is needed.[1,2]

---

*Box 137.1* RISK FACTORS AND COMMON CAUSES OF EPISTAXIS

- Inexperienced clinician, repeated attempts, poor technique (using oversized tube, excessive force)
- Inadequate vasoconstriction
- Avulsion of nasal polyps, adenoids, tonsils, or damage to posterior pharyngeal wall
- Anatomic deformities, nasopharyngeal tumors
- Inflammatory/granulomatous diseases (allergic rhinitis, nasal polyposis, Wegner's granulomatosis)
- Use of anticoagulation

---

## TRAUMA TO LARYNX, TRACHEA, AND ESOPHAGUS

Airway injury during general anesthesia is a well-recognized complication of anesthesia, with most frequent sites of injury being the larynx, pharynx, and esophagus. Esophageal and tracheal injuries are associated with difficult intubations, while injury to the larynx is associated with nondifficult intubations.

### LARYNX

Laryngeal injury can occur from mucosal abrasion from movement of the endotracheal tube, but is more commonly secondary to pressure necrosis from the tube itself.

### TRACHEA

Most tracheal injuries occur from surgical tracheostomy during emergency airway management with difficult intubations. Tracheal perforation is a rare, but severe injury occurring with routine tracheal intubation. Sign of tracheal injury include development of subcutaneous emphysema or pneumothorax, postoperative chest pain, or nonspecific respiratory complaints.

### ESOPHAGUS

Perforation of the esophagus is a serious, life-threatening injury associated with poor outcomes. Risk factors include difficult or emergency intubation and intubation by inexperienced personnel. In nondifficult airways, causes include instrumentation of the esophagus by esophageal intubation, placement of an orogastric or nasogastric tube, esophageal dilator, esophageal stethoscope, or transesophageal echocardiography. Early symptoms of perforation are nonspecific and include sore throat, deep cervical pain, chest pain, and cough. Later symptoms include fever, dysphagia, and dyspnea, and could result in infectious sequelae (deep cervical abscess, mediastinitis or mediastinal abscess, retropharyngeal abscess, or pneumonia). Despite improved survival with early diagnosis and treatment within 24 hours, overall mortality remains high (25%).[3]

# TRAUMA TO THE EYES: CORNEAL ABRASIONS, BLINDNESS, POSTOPERATIVE VISUAL LOSS

Eye injuries are well-known complications of surgery and anesthesia, ranging from corneal abrasions to more rare devastating complications such as blindness or postoperative visual loss (POVL). POVL is a catastrophic multifactorial event with incidence from 0.002%–0.2% for higher risk surgeries, namely cardiac and spine, and should be considered in any patient complaining of visual loss during the first week after surgery. The most frequent cause of POVL is ischemic optic neuropathy (ION), with other less common causes including central retinal artery occlusion, hemorrhagic retinopathy, retinal ischemia, cortical blindness, ophthalmic vein obstruction, and acute glaucoma.[3]

## CORNEAL ABRASION

Corneal abrasion is the most common ocular complication of general anesthesia. Symptoms include foreign body sensation, pain, tearing, decreased visual acuity, and photophobia. The pain is exacerbated by blinking and ocular movement. Iatrogenic mechanisms of injury include oxygen masks, surgical drapes, IV tubing, stethoscopes, ID cards, watch bands, or chemical injury from antiseptic solutions. Ocular injury may also occur due to the loss of pain sensation, decreased tear production, or patient rubbing eyes during emergence. Immediate ophthalmologist consultation should be obtained. Treatment consists of artificial tears, prophylactic topical antibiotic ointment, and patching the injured eye shut. Healing usually occurs within 24 hours, although permanent injury is possible.[3]

## HEMORRHAGIC RETINOPATHY

Retinal hemorrhages are often asymptomatic and can be a complication from turbulent emergence from anesthesia, protracted vomiting, or even after injection of local anesthetics, steroids, or saline into the lumber epidural space (usually rapid administration of volumes - 40 mL into the epidural space). These venous hemorrhages are usually self-limiting and resolve completely within days to months.[3]

## ISCHEMIC OPTIC NEUROPATHY (ION)

The optic nerve can be divided into anterior and posterior segments, depending on blood supply. The central retinal artery and small branches of the ciliary artery supply

---

> **Box 137.2** RISK FACTORS FOR ISCHEMIC OPTIC NEUROPATHY
>
> - Increased venous congestion in optic canal reducing optic nerve perfusion (obesity, prone positioning, use of Wilson frame for spinal surgeries, increased EBL, capillary leak, interstitial edema)
> - Reduced venous return/cardiac output (blood pressure >40% below baseline for - 30 minutes, blood loss >1 liter)
> - Male sex
> - Increased crystalloid administration
> - Long anesthetic durations (–6 hours)
> - Preexisting comorbidities (older age, hypertension, atherosclerosis, smoking, diabetes, vascular disease)
>
> *EBL: estimated blood loss.*

the anterior portion of the optic nerve, while the small branches of the ophthalmic and central retinal arteries supply the posterior portion of the optic nerve.

Due to the different blood supplies, the underlying causes and presentations differ between anterior and posterior segments. Causes are multifactorial, but hypoperfusion or decreased oxygen delivery to the optic nerve has been shown to be largely associated with the development of ION. Anterior ischemic optic neuropathy (AION) is often associated with cardiac surgery (underlying comorbid conditions), and posterior ischemic optic neuropathy (PION) with spinal fusion surgery (optic nerve edema).

Clinical findings of ION include painless visual loss and impaired color vision. Fundoscopic exam findings will show optic disc edema in AION, but not for PION due to its location. Risk factors for ION are listed in Box 137.2.[3]

Preventive strategies include avoiding external pressure to eyes, minimizing time in prone position, positioning head level with or higher than heart, maintaining head in neutral forward position with avoidance of neck flexion, extension, lateral flexion or rotation, and maintaining blood pressure as close to baseline as possible. Staged spine procedures should be considered in high-risk patients to avoid excessive periods of prone position.

There is no treatment, but various therapies may be used, including IV acetazolamide, furosemide, mannitol, and steroids.

## RETINAL ISCHEMIA OR INFARCTION

Retinal ischemia/infarction results from decreased perfusion pressure or increased ocular venous pressure. It is very important for careful positioning of the patient to avoid pressure to the orbit, as well as decreasing factors leading to increased venous pressure around the orbital nerve.

## CENTRAL RETINAL ARTERY OCCLUSION AND BRANCH RETINAL ARTERY OCCLUSION

Central retinal arterial occlusion and branch retinal arterial occlusion are important and often preventable causes of postoperative visual loss. Most cases follow spinal, nasal, sinus, neck, or coronary artery bypass graft surgery. Causes include external pressure to the eye, as well as emboli from carotid plaques, vasospasm, thrombosis, hypotension, and intranasal injection of alpha-adrenergic agonists. Presentation includes painless, monocular blindness, limited visual field deficit, or blurred vision. Visual field defects can be severe initially but improve with time, unlike ION. Pathognomonic findings on funduscopic examination reveal a pale, edematous retinal and a cherry-red spot. Prevention is more successful than treatment. It may be possible to apply ocular massage to dislodge an embolus to more peripheral sites. IV acetazolamide and 5% carbon dioxide inhalation have been used to increase retinal blood flow. Prognosis is poor, and about 50% of patients with central retinal arterial occlusion eventually have optic atrophy.

Unlike ION, central retinal artery occlusion may be caused by emboli from an ulcerated atherosclerotic plaque of the ipsilateral carotid artery, vasospasm, or thrombosis. It can also occur following intranasal injection of alpha-adrenergic agonists. Stellate ganglion block usually improves vision in these patients.[3]

## CORTICAL BLINDNESS

Cortical blindness has been observed after profound hypotension or circulatory arrest resulting from hypoperfusion and infarction of watershed areas in the parietal or occipital lobes of the brain. Cortical blindness has been observed following surgical procedures such as cardiac surgery, craniotomy, laryngectomy, and cesarean section. It may also result from air or particulate emboli during cardiopulmonary bypass. Cortical blindness is characterized by loss of vision, but retention of pupillary reactions to light. Funduscopic examination is usually normal. Patients may not be aware of focal vision loss, which usually improves with time. Computed tomography (CT) or magnetic resonance imaging (MRI) abnormalities in the parietal or occipital lobes confirm the diagnosis. Preventive strategies include maintenance of adequate systemic perfusion pressure, and in cardiac surgery, minimizing manipulation of the aorta, meticulous removal of air and particulate matter during valvular procedures, and the use of an arterial line filter in selected patients during bypass.[3]

## OPHTHALMIC VENOUS OBSTRUCTION

Obstruction of venous drainage from the eyes may occur intraoperatively as a result of external pressure on the orbits during patient positioning. Ophthalmoscopic examination reveals engorgement of the veins and edema of the macula.

## REFERENCES

1. Fatakia A, et al. Epistaxis: A common problem. *Ochsner J.* 2010;10:176–178.
2. Jeffrey L, et al. Reducing epistaxis during nasotracheal intubation. *Anesth Analg.* 2008 Jun;106(6):1923–1924.
3. Domino K, et al. Airway injury during anesthesia: A closed claims analysis. *Anesthesiology.* 1999;91:1703.

# 138.

# VASCULAR INJURIES

*Yasser M. A. Youssef and Nawal E. Ragheb-Mueller*

## PERIPHERAL CATHETER-RELATED INJURIES

### PERIPHERAL VENOUS CATHETERS

The most common complications related to intravenous (IV) catheters are skin slough, or necrosis, followed by swelling, inflammation, infection, nerve damage, fasciotomy scars from compartment syndrome, and air embolism. Miscellaneous complications involve rashes from tape, sheared-off catheters, ecchymosis, and accidental placement in a radial artery. Vasculitis leading to hand ischemia after administration of cold blood also has been reported.

### Extravasation

Approximately half of peripheral IV complications are related to the extravasation of drugs or fluids. The most commonly implicated medications causing skin slough are calcium chloride, thiopental, and vasopressors (e.g., dopamine, dobutamine, epinephrine).[1] Extravasation may lead to compartment syndrome and result in nerve damage. Anesthesia providers should recognize any early signs of infiltration, such as an IV drip that slows for no apparent reason, and should visually check the site of IVs, particularly in arms-tucked positions. If it is necessary to administer vasopressors into a peripheral vein urgently, the infusion pump should be set to detect small changes in infusion pressure to detect extravasation promptly.

### PERIPHERAL ARTERIAL CATHETERS

Invasive arterial monitoring is associated with risks of bleeding, hematoma, pseudo-aneurysm, infection, nerve damage, and distal limb ischemia. The most common cannulation sites are the radial, femoral, and axillary arteries. The radial artery is preferred given its consistent anatomic accessibility, ease of cannulation, and low complication rate.[2]

### Distal Ischemia

Indwelling artery catheters may induce intimal damage that can promote thrombus formation and lead to stenosis or even occlusion. Thrombotic occlusion has been described as early as 2 hours after placement, or as late as a week after catheter removal. The incidence of permanent hand ischemic damage is 0.09%.[2] Use of modified Allen's Test to assess adequacy of collateral blood flow to the hand before radial artery cannulation is controversial due to lack of evidence that it can predict ischemia after radial artery cannulation. Absent pulse, dampened waveform, blanched or mottled skin, delayed capillary refill, and painful cold hand with motor weakness are the initial presentations. Blistering and skin ulceration are late findings. Arterial color flow Doppler ultrasound, angiography, or even magnetic resonance imaging (MRI) can be used to evaluate arterial blood flow. Immediate vascular surgery consultation is imperative. The catheter should be removed to ensure it is not contributing to flow obstruction if intra-arterial drug administration or arteriography is not under consideration. Treatment is aimed at the underlying mechanism of injury (e.g., thrombus, vasospasm, or digital embolization). Aspiration of thrombus at the catheter tip has been reported to restore arterial pulsation in 60% of patients with suspected thrombosis.[2] Intra-arterial verapamil, prilocaine, and phentolamine have been successfully used to reverse ischemic symptoms. Other proposed treatments include low-molecular-weight dextran and low-dose heparin. Hot compresses may resolve vasospasm (but may aggravate the ischemia if applied to the hand). Sympathetic nerve block should be considered for suspected arterial vasospasm. Surgical exploration may be necessary if blood flow is absent and severe ischemia results.

### Inadvertent Intra-Arterial Injection

Accidental arterial injections of anesthetic medications like benzodiazepines or barbiturates, for example, can lead to cyanosis or gangrene of the limb and possible extremity loss.[3] Obese and darkly pigmented skin are at increased risk of injury. Bright red or pulsatile movement of blood in the IV tubing or within the catheter, as well as signs of ischemia distal to it, suggests unintentional arterial catheterization. Symptoms suggestive of arterial injection include pain after injection of medication that is worse than expected. Additional signs include skin pallor; hyperemia; cyanosis; hyperesthesia; profound edema; muscle weakness, paralysis, and/or gangrene with tissue necrosis proximal and distal to the injection site. The intra-arterial catheter should be left in place. This allows confirmation of arterial injection either through transduction or blood gas analysis, as well as direct treatment to the site of injury. Starting a slow infusion of isotonic fluid to maintain catheter patency is recommended. Anticoagulation with heparin is the accepted first step in treatment if the situation allows. Elevation of the extremity may decrease the local edema and provide symptomatic relief to the affected area. Administration of local anesthetic and/or Stellate ganglion block may prevent reflex vasospasm. Papaverine, an opium alkaloid that causes smooth muscle relaxation, has been injected with varying success. Selective intra-arterial injection of calcium channel blockers, thrombolytics, hyperbaric oxygen therapy, and corticosteroids have all been used with varying benefit.

## CENTRAL VENOUS CATHETER-RELATED INJURIES

Vascular injuries from central venous catheterization range from minor complications such as local hematoma to serious consequences, including perforation into the pleural space or mediastinum, and result in hydrothorax, hemothorax, and/or chylothorax.

### ARTERIAL PUNCTURE

Unintended arterial puncture is the most common acute mechanical complication with an incidence of 1.9% to 15%.[4] Most of these injuries result in localized hematoma formation but may lead to arterial thromboembolism. Under normal circumstances, arterial puncture is usually easy to identify by the pulsatile flow into the syringe and the bright-red color of the blood. If there is any doubt, a small gauge single-lumen catheter can be connected to a pressure transducer to confirm the presence of venous waveforms and venous pressure. If the arterial puncture occurs via a small gauge needle, it should be removed, and external pressure applied for several minutes to prevent hematoma formation. Large-bore needles or dilator-induced punctures require a vascular surgery consult and the needle and/or dilator should remain in place until evaluation. If the needle or dilator is immediately removed, hemothorax, an arterio-venous fistula, or pseudo-aneurysm may develop.

## CARDIAC PERFORATION

The most catastrophic complication is cardiac tamponade resulting from perforation of the intra-pericardial superior vena cava, right atrium, or right ventricle. These injuries can cause hemopericardium or unintentional pericardial instillation of intravenous fluid, leading to cardiac compression. The delayed presentation (1–5 days) indicates that this complication is related to catheter maintenance rather than the vascular access procedure itself. The most important preventive measure is to confirm the catheter tip position radio-graphically for early recognition of a tip abutting the superior vena cava wall at a steep angle. Cardiac arrhythmias may provide an early clue for an intra-cardiac location of the catheter tip.[4]

### AIR EMBOLISM

A spontaneously breathing patient generates negative intrathoracic pressure during inspiration. If a catheter is open to room air, this negative intrathoracic pressure can draw air into the vein, resulting in air embolism. Even small amounts of air can be fatal, especially if transmitted to the systemic circulation through an atrial or ventricular septal defect. To prevent this, catheter hubs should always be occluded and the patient placed in Trendelenburg position during the procedure. If air embolism occurs, the patient should be placed in Trendelenburg with a left lateral decubitus tilt to prevent movement of air into the right ventricular outflow tract. Administration of 100% oxygen is recommended to speed the resorption of the air. If a catheter is located in the heart, aspiration of the air should be attempted.

## PULMONARY ARTERY CATHETER-RELATED INJURIES

### PULMONARY ARTERY RUPTURE

Pulmonary artery (PA) rupture occurs in 0.02%–0.2% of catheterized patients and leads to mortality in 50%. Risk factors include pulmonary hypertension, hypothermia, anticoagulation, and advanced age.[5] Suggested mechanisms of injury include forceful inflation of the balloon, chronic erosion by the catheter tip abutting the vessel wall, unnecessary catheter manipulation, excessive insertion depth, prolonged balloon inflation, or improper balloon inflation with liquid rather than air. The hallmark of catheter-induced pulmonary artery rupture is hemoptysis, which may signal life-threatening exsanguination or hypoxemia. Chest radiograph aids diagnosis by revealing hemothorax or new infiltrate near the tip of a distally positioned catheter. Diagnosis may be confirmed by performing wedge angiogram, in which radiopaque dye injected through the wedged pulmonary artery catheter (PAC) will extravasate into the pulmonary parenchyma to identify the site of arterial disruption. Treatment focuses on resuscitation and immediate control of hemorrhage. The first priority is to ensure adequate oxygenation and this may require endobronchial intubation with a single- or double-lumen endotracheal tube to selectively ventilate and protect the unaffected lung. Positive end-expiratory pressure applied to the affected lung may help control hemorrhage. Any anticoagulation should be reversed unless the patient must remain on cardiopulmonary bypass. Bronchoscopy can be performed to localize and control the site of bleeding. Despite all these measures, many patients may require definitive surgical therapy, such as over-sewing the involved PA or resecting the involved segment, lobe, or lung.

## REFERENCES

1. Bhananker SM, et al. Liability related to peripheral venous and arterial catheterization: A closed claims analysis. *Anesth Analg.* 2009;109(1):124–129.
2. Brzezinski M, et al. Radial artery cannulation: A comprehensive review of recent anatomic and physiologic investigations. *Anesth Analg.* 2009;109(6):1763–1781.
3. Sen S, et al. Complications after unintentional intra-arterial injection of drugs: Risks, outcomes, and management strategies. *Mayo Clin Proc.* 2005 Jun;80(6):783–795).
4. McGee DC, Gould MK. Preventing complications of central venous catheterization. *N Engl J Med.* 2003;348(12):1123–1133.
5. Miller RD, et al. *Miller's Anesthesia E-Book.* Elsevier Health Sciences; 2014.

# 139.

# NEUROLOGICAL COMPLICATIONS

*Yasser M. A. Youssef and Nawal E. Ragheb-Mueller*

## INTRODUCTION

Although perioperative peripheral nerve injury is a rare complication with a reported incidence as low as 0.03%, it is a significant morbidity that can affect the patient's quality of life and subject the anesthesiologist to professional liability.[1] It comprises the second leading cause of claims in the American Society of Anesthesiologists (ASA) Closed Claims project data (22% of reported cases).[2] In general anesthesia, malposition is the main etiology, with the mechanism of injury resulting from prolonged stretch, lengthy compression, or ischemia of the nerves. It is important to note that despite appropriate padding and precautions during positioning, nerve injuries may still occur; this suggests that there may be other poorly understood factors leading to these injuries.[2] In regional anesthesia practice, direct trauma by the block needle and intra-neural injection of the local anesthetic with subsequent chemical injury are the main proposed mechanisms of injuries.[3]

## PERIPHERAL NERVE INJURIES

Peripheral neuropathies related to general anesthesia encompass the majority of the ASA Closed Claims associated with nerve injury. The most commonly reported injuries involve the brachial plexus (27%), followed by, specifically, ulnar neuropathy (22%) and those associated with the spinal cord (19%).[2] Many of these injuries are related to malpositioning during general anesthesia. As a rule of thumb, the patient should tolerate the anticipated position when s/he is awake. A high index of suspicion is required so the anesthetist can anticipate potential nerve injuries and look for risk factors during the preoperative evaluation. All weight-bearing surfaces of the extremities should be well padded, all body curvatures should be supported, the head should remain in a neutral position, and the eyes should be closed with no external pressure. Long duration surgeries require more attention and frequent rechecking of pressure points. Extreme surgical positions require limiting the duration of surgeries. A safety strap is crucial to prevent a fall from the operating table. The following is a summary of the ASA Task Force recommendations for perioperative management of such cases.[4]

## PREOPERATIVE MANAGEMENT

A prudent anesthesia provider anticipates the risk of perioperative peripheral neuropathy by looking for preexisting risk factors and clinically assessing whether the patient will be able to tolerate the proposed position, especially in surgeries that require extreme positioning. Potential risk factors include the following: diabetes mellitus, preexisting neuropathy, peripheral vascular disease, alcohol dependence, smoking, arthritis, extremes of body weight, male gender (more prone to ulnar neuropathy).

## INTRAOPERATIVE MANAGEMENT

A periodic intraoperative assessment is required to maintain the desired position. The following recommendations should be followed during intraoperative positioning. For a summary of specific recommendations, see Table 139.1.

- Limit arm abduction to less than 90 degrees.
- Avoid excessive lateral rotation of the head.
- Avoid direct pressure on the axillae.

*Table 139.1* SUMMARY OF PREVENTIVE MEASURES FOR SPECIFIC PERIOPERATIVE NEUROPATHY

| SITE | AT-RISK POSITION | PREVENTION |
|---|---|---|
| **Brachial plexus** | Greater in lateral and prone position | • Avoid stretch or compression at the axillae<br>• Avoid shoulder braces in Trendelenburg position<br>• Avoid excessive rotation of the head<br>• Arm abduction <90 degrees |
| **Ulnar nerve** | Any position | • Padding of the elbow<br>• Forearm in neutral or supine position |
| **Radial nerve** | Any position | • Avoid compression at the lateral humerus |
| **Common peroneal nerve** | Greater in lithotomy and lateral positions | • Padding of the fibular head |
| **Sciatic nerve** | Greater in lithotomy position | • Simultaneous movement of both legs during positioning<br>• Avoid excessive hip flexion and knee extension |

- Arms should remain in either supine or neutral position.
- Avoid prolonged pressure on the spiral groove of the humerus to protect the radial nerve.
- Avoid excessive flexion/extension of the elbow above the comfortable range to protect the median and ulnar nerves.
- Avoid excessive hip flexion and knee extension to protect the sciatic nerve.
- Avoid prolonged pressure on the fibular head to protect the peroneal nerve.
- Pad arm boards and provide padding at the elbows.
- Pad the fibular head (padding which is too tight may increase the risk of neuropathy).
- A non-sliding mattress is recommended over shoulder braces in Trendelenburg position to avoid excessive pressure on the brachial plexus.

## POSTOPERATIVE MANAGEMENT

Perioperative neuropathy usually manifests between 48 and 72 hours postoperatively, with a median of 3 days in most injuries (especially ulnar neuropathy). Lower extremity neuropathies are symptomatic immediately after the analgesic effects of anesthetics dissipate. Lower extremity neuropathies are usually related to intraoperative causes, but ulnar neuropathy is usually related to causes in the postoperative period. Although the clinical picture differs according to the nerve injured, most manifest with pain as an initial symptom, followed by paresthesias in the areas supplied by the injured nerve. Paresis or paralysis may follow, and joint stiffening and bone demineralization are late sequelae. A careful clinical exam of the extremity involved should be conducted. When suspected, a full neurological examination is required to rule out any central causes. Once confirmed, full disclosure to the patient must take place with appropriate referral to neurology consultation. Imaging such as plain X-rays can be helpful to rule out any local fractures or dislocations that can lead to compression injuries. Magnetic resonance imaging (MRI) may be required to visualize the nerve plexus or routes for any abnormal signals. Nerve conduction studies (NCS) and electromyography (EMG) are the gold standard of investigation for diagnosis and prognosis as well. These studies help to localize the lesions and differentiate the mechanism of injury, whether it is due to axonal degeneration or demyelination. Serial examinations can help in prognostication. Although it is recommended that the EMG/NCS be done 3 weeks following the injury to allow for the full degeneration process to be complete, some practitioners recommend a baseline study prior to 3 weeks to help recognize any potential preexisting injury. Prognosis depends on the type of nerve injury. Neuropraxia carries the best prognosis, with recovery of function occurring within weeks to months. Axonotmesis with loss of axonal continuity, but intact nerve sheaths, has a variable prognosis ranging from prolonged recovery to permanent injury. Some cases may require surgical intervention when there is axonal discontinuity, provided the epineurium remains intact.

## PERIPHERAL NERVE INJURIES IN REGIONAL ANESTHESIA

Peripheral nerve injury is a recognized complication that can follow peripheral nerve blocks, although most reported cases have other contributing factors, such as a tightly applied cast, surgical dressings, or malposition-related injuries.[5] In regional anesthesia, the most common claims result from injuries to lumbosacral roots (39%), followed by those to the spinal cord (29%).[2] Mechanisms of injury include neural ischemia, traumatic injury to the nerves during needle or catheter placement, infection, and local anesthetic neurotoxicity.[5] Anesthesia providers should adhere to the following recommendations to prevent nerve injury during regional anesthesia.

• Preoperatively identify patients at risk and avoid using potent local anesthetics. Reduce the concentration and doses to the extent possible and avoid or limit vasoconstrictive additives for these patients. Patients at particular risk are those with any preexisting nerve diseases, diabetics, individuals with severe peripheral vascular disease, and those receiving chemotherapy.

• During the procedure, if any pain or paresthesias occur during injection, the operator should immediately stop and reposition the needle to avoid possible intra-neural injection.
• High injection pressures should be avoided as they can lead to intra-fascicular injury. The effectiveness of injection pressure-monitoring devices is still a subject of research.
• Direct visualization of local anesthetic deposition under ultrasound is the optimal technique for a successful regional block without increasing the risk of direct nerve injuries.

## REFERENCES

1. Welch MB, et al. Perioperative peripheral nerve injuries: A retrospective study of 380,680 cases during a 10-year period at a single institution. *Anesthesiology*. 2009;111(3):490–497.
2. Cheney FW, et al. Nerve injury associated with anesthesia: A closed claims analysis. *Surv Anesthesiol*. 2000;44(1):59.
3. Lee LA, et al. Complications associated with peripheral nerve blocks: Lessons from the ASA Closed Claims Project. *Int Anesthesiol Clin*. 2011;49(3):56–67.
4. American Society of Anesthesiologists Task Force on Prevention of Perioperative Peripheral Neuropathies. Practice advisory for the prevention of perioperative peripheral neuropathies: An updated report by the American Society of Anesthesiologists Task Force on Prevention of Perioperative Peripheral Neuropathies. *Anesthesiology*. 2011;114(4):741.
5. Neal JM, et al. ASRA practice advisory on neurologic complications in regional anesthesia and pain medicine. *Reg Anesth Pain Med*. 2008;33(5):404–415.

# 140.

# BURNS

*Sohail K. Mahboobi and Ramaiza Sohail*

## INTRODUCTION

Burns are life-threatening injuries. The mortality increases with advancing age, burn size, and the presence of inhalational injury. Perioperative anesthetic management of burn is complicated by the physiological systemic changes and altered response to anesthetic agents.

## PATHOPHYSIOLOGY

Burns involves all systems of the body and are classified in four types (Table 140.1). Within a short time after burn injury, the initial shock phase, tissues release inflammatory and vasoactive mediators, including histamine, prostaglandins, kinins, and nitric oxide, that result in increased capillary

*Table 140.1* CLASSIFICATION OF BURNS

| TYPES OF BURNS | DEFINITION |
| --- | --- |
| First-degree | Also called superficial burn. It involves the outer layer of the skin (i.e., epidermis) with redness, pain, and no blisters. |
| Second-degree | Also called partial thickness burn. It involves epidermis and deeper skin layers (i.e., dermis). Blisters occur with pain and redness. |
| Third-degree | Also called full thickness burn. It involves epidermis and all the dermis and may extend to the subcutaneous tissues. The burn site may be blackened and charred. |
| Fourth-degree | In this the burn involves all the skin layers, subcutaneous tissues, muscles, and can even extend to bones. There is no pain as nerve endings are destroyed. |

permeability and localized edema. This further causes significant fluid leak and electrolytes from the intravascular space into the interstitial space. Replacement of intravascular volume is critical in burn patients. Hypermetabolic phase develops in a few weeks, with a surge in catecholamines and steroids. Persistent tachycardia, hypertension, muscle degradation, insulin resistance, and liver dysfunction can occur. Cardiac output and heart rate remain elevated, and immune system is impaired for a significant time after the injury. Burn patients develop a hypercoagulable state due to the activation of clotting factors and increased risk for venous thrombosis, pulmonary embolism, and disseminated intravascular coagulation.

Carbon monoxide (CO) and cyanide are two toxic components of smoke. CO poisoning is diagnosed by elevated carboxyhemoglobin (COHb) levels.[1] Signs and symptoms include headache, mental status changes, dyspnea, nausea, weakness, and tachycardia. Patients with CO poisoning have a normal $PaO_2$ and oxygen saturation by routine pulse oximetry and are not cyanotic. Co-oximetry is helpful for diagnosis. CO binds to hemoglobin and cytochromes with an affinity 200 times stronger than that of oxygen. The treatment includes administration of 100% oxygen, which will reduce carboxyhemoglobin half-life from 4 hours with room air to 1 hour. Hyperbaric oxygen treatment is required in severe cases.

Burning of certain plastic products can result in cyanide inhalation. Cyanide impairs the ability of cells to utilize oxygen. Signs and symptoms include headache, mental status changes, nausea, lethargy, and weakness. Treatment begins with high inspired oxygen concentration and methemoglobin generators such as the nitrates (amyl nitrite inhalation or sodium nitrite). Methemoglobin competes with cytochrome oxidase for cyanide but itself can be toxic in higher concentration.

## ANESTHETIC CONSIDERATIONS

The anesthetic management is challenging. With adequate initial resuscitation, early surgery is tolerated well as later patients develop reduced immunity and a hypermetabolic state.

### PREOPERATIVE

Assessment of airway, pulmonary status, and the distribution of the burn wounds is important. The patient's current physiologic status should be assessed regarding hemodynamic status, vasopressor requirements, ventilator settings, pulmonary compliance, adequacy of resuscitation, and laboratory values, particularly acid-base disturbances.

The possibility of laryngeal edema that can cause airway obstruction should be noted and requires early intubation. Signs of an inhalation injury can be delayed, but history of entrapment in a closed space, facial burns, symptoms of respiratory distress, and the presence of carbonaceous sputum should increase the suspicion. Chemical injury from incomplete products of combustion causes damage to the tracheal and lung parenchyma that can lead to partial or complete airway obstruction, decreased pulmonary compliance, and atelectasis.[2] Fiberoptic bronchoscopy is helpful for diagnosis and evaluation of inhalational injury. Chest radiographs underestimate lung damage immediately after injury.

In order to assess the extent of burn injury, various methods are used, e.g., rule-of-nine for adults and the Lund-Browder age/growth-adjusted chart for children. Fluid resuscitation is guided by formulas that estimate initial fluid requirements based on burn severity and body weight and provide an initial starting point for resuscitation. For the first 24 hours after burn injury, resuscitation is usually performed using the Parkland formula. Patients receive lactated Ringer's solution, 4 mL/kg per percentage of burned surface area, within the first 24 hours. Half of the calculated volume is administered within the first 8 hours, followed by the rest in the next 16 hours. This is accompanied with continuous clinical assessment in the form of hemodynamics and urine output to ensure adequate resuscitation.[3]

### INTRAOPERATIVE

Intraoperative management is challenging due to airway edema and narrowing. The patient may have facial injury with contractures causing limitations in mouth opening and neck extension. Burn patients are at risk for perioperative hypothermia and should be monitored. Warming the operating room, forced-air warmers, and warm intravenous fluids are useful in preventing hypothermia.[4]

Uses of perioperative anesthetic medications undergo a biphasic pharmacokinetic response. In the acute phase, lower doses are usually required due to decreased circulating volume and decreased renal and hepatic clearance. In the hypermetabolic phase, the duration of action is decreased, requiring frequent re-dosing due to high blood flow to the liver and kidneys and decreased binding plasma proteins.[5] Propofol is safe to use; etomidate carries a theoretical risk of adrenal suppression in already immunocompromised patients. Ketamine can be used as an alternative induction due to its hemodynamic stability and analgesia.

There is a proliferation of extrajunctional acetylcholine receptors that results in increased resistance to nondepolarizing muscle relaxants (e.g., vecuronium), and increased sensitivity to depolarizing muscle relaxants (e.g., succinylcholine).[5] Administration of succinylcholine after 24 hours of burn can result in a hyperkalemic response which is proportional to the dose, burned surface area, and time since the injury. This response can persist for up to 18 months after the burn. Resistance to nondepolarizing muscle relaxants may develop within a week of burn injury and persist for up to a year, and twitch monitoring is recommended to avoid overdosing.

Lung protective ventilation strategy should be used with low tidal volume (6 ml/kg predicted body weight), higher ventilator rate, and positive end expiratory pressure (PEEP). Burn patients develop acute lung injury and acute respiratory distress syndrome (ARDS) due to circulating inflammatory mediators, increase in lung vascular permeability, and pulmonary vascular resistance.

## POSTOPERATIVE

Extubation decision should be made after assessment of clinical extubation criteria, need for multiple operating room visits, and pulmonary rehabilitation. Adequate analgesia is required to avoid adverse physiological and psychological outcomes. Multimodal analgesia should be used for the treatment of pain and anxiety. Pain management ranges from utilization of opioids in the acute phase to the use of ketamine and regional nerve blocks if warranted.

## REFERENCES

1. Varon J, et al. Carbon monoxide poisoning: A review for clinicians. *J Emerg Med*. 1999;17:87–93.
2. Rehberg S, et al. Pathophysiology, management and treatment of smoke inhalation injury. *Expert Rev Respir Med*. 2009;3:283–297.
3. Tricklebank S. Modern trends in fluid therapy for burns. *Burns*. 2009;35:757–767.
4. MacLennon N, et al. Anesthesia for major thermal injury. *Anesthesiology*. 1998;89:749–770.
5. Blanchet B, et al. Influence of burns on pharmacokinetics and pharmacodynamics of drugs used in the care of burn patients. *Clin Pharmacokinet*. 2008;47:635–654.

# 141.

# CHRONIC ENVIRONMENTAL EXPOSURE

*Sarah C. Smith*

## INTRODUCTION

Anesthesia providers and other workers in the perioperative environment are at risk for chronic occupational exposure to waste anesthetic gases (WAGs). Although there is conflicting evidence regarding whether typical occupational exposure to WAGs results in serious adverse health outcomes, regulatory agencies and professional societies agree that this exposure should be kept to an absolute minimum. To achieve this goal, there are a number of engineering controls and clinical practice modifications that can minimize the presence of WAGs in the perioperative environment.[1]

## POTENTIAL ADVERSE EFFECTS OF OCCUPATIONAL EXPOSURE TO WAGS

Acute exposure to large amounts of WAGs, such as occurs after an accidental spill, is associated with transient neurological manifestations, including sedation, confusion, and headaches. More relevant to the anesthesia practitioner and other workers in the perioperative environment are the cumulative effects of relatively low levels of exposure over the course of months to years. Animal and human studies have shown that chronic exposure to WAGs can result in cellular oxidative damage[2] and genotoxicity,[3] potentially resulting in carcinogenesis or other forms of end-organ damage, including hepato- and renal toxicity. These effects appear to be both dose- and time-dependent, while occupational exposure to multiple inhalational anesthetic agents appears to have additive adverse effects.[1,3] Nitrous oxide additionally inactivates vitamin $B_{12}$, and long-term deficiency has been linked to cardiovascular and cerebrovascular disease. However, the results of studies examining the negative health effects of WAG exposure in anesthesia providers and other operating room (OR) personnel have been conflicting, so a causal link cannot be firmly established.[1]

Epidemiologic studies conducted in the 1970s of workers chronically exposed to WAGs also indicated a number of adverse reproductive outcomes, including reduced fertility, an increased risk of spontaneous abortion and stillbirth, prematurity, low birth weight, and congenital malformations. However, these studies suffered from methodological problems and do not reflect subsequent changes to improve the safety of anesthesia workspaces, such as scavenging systems, improved ventilation, and newer anesthetics. Interestingly, more recent studies do show a predominance of female offspring in workers exposed to WAG, suggesting an adverse effect specifically to the Y chromosome.[4]

## SOURCES OF WAG EXPOSURE IN THE PERIOPERATIVE ENVIRONMENT

Faulty equipment, such as cracked vaporizers or improperly functioning scavenging systems, may result in unacceptably high levels of WAGs in the OR or other anesthetizing location. Leakage of WAGs from around poorly fitting airway devices can also be a source of occupational exposure that is most pronounced in personnel located close to the patient's airway. This is particularly relevant in the practice of pediatric anesthesia due to the difficulty in consistently matching the size of airway devices to patient anatomy. Not surprisingly, multiple studies have shown that pediatric anesthesiologists are exposed to higher levels of WAGs than those caring for adult patients.[5] After removal of the airway device, patients continue to exhale inhalational agents into the environment for varying periods of time during the recovery phase, so post-anesthesia recovery units may also be significant areas of exposure.[1]

## PRECAUTIONS TO MINIMIZE EXPOSURE TO WAGS

While the nature and magnitude of negative adverse health outcomes resulting from WAG exposure in the modern anesthesia workspace remain unknown, minimizing exposure through certain clinical practices and engineering controls is essential (Table 141.1). The National Institute for Occupational Safety and Health (NIOSH), therefore, sets limits on the concentration of anesthetic gases to which workers may be exposed. The NIOSH limit for nitrous oxide exposure is 25 ppm as a time-weighted average over the course of the anesthetic, while the limit for halogenated agents must be below 2 ppm for a time period not to exceed 1 hour. However, there is evidence that these limits are exceeded in anesthetizing and anesthesia recovery locations with a fair degree of frequency.

Utilization of scavenging systems and adequate ventilation are the most important safety measures that can be implemented to minimize occupational exposure to WAGs. Scavenging systems may be attached directly to the anesthesia circuit or near the patient's airway to directly remove WAGs and prevent them from entering the environment. Even in well-ventilated areas, the use of scavenging systems can decrease the level of WAGs in the air by a factor of 20, compared to when these systems are absent. Utilization of a closed-loop anesthesia circuit and low-flow anesthesia (fresh gas flows less than 1–2 L/min) can also help minimize the release of WAGs.

When halogenated agents are used, detectable anesthetic odor by the anesthesia practitioner or someone else

*Table 141.1* METHODS TO MINIMIZE OCCUPATIONAL WAG EXPOSURE

| | |
|---|---|
| Engineering modifications | • Utilize scavenging systems<br>• Ensure adequate ventilation in anesthetizing and recovery locations<br>• Maintain anesthesia equipment to prevent leaks<br>• Consider closed-loop anesthesia circuits |
| Anesthetic management | • Ensure proper fitting of airway devices to prevent leaks<br>• Avoid inhalation inductions when possible<br>• Utilize low-flow anesthesia technique |
| Safe practices | • Investigate the source of halogenated anesthetic odors<br>• Maximize personnel distancing from patient's airway<br>• Practice safe storage of inhalational anesthetic agents<br>  • Securely cap bottles<br>  • Store in locked cabinets |

in the operating room (OR) should prompt an investigation to identify the source. This may indicate compromise of the circle-system, a problem with a vaporizer, unrecognized spill, or a malfunctioning scavenging system. If the source of the odor is a poorly fitting airway device, the device should be repositioned and replacement considered. Maximizing the positioning of personnel from the patient's airway can also minimize exposure in this circumstance.[1] As inhalation inductions of anesthesia result in far greater escape of WAGs into the environment compared to intravenous inductions, this technique should be limited to instances of clinical necessity.[5]

## REFERENCES

1. Deng HB, et al. Waste anesthetic gas exposure and strategies for solution. *J Anesth.* 2018;32(2):269–282.
2. Turkan H, et al. Effect of volatile anesthetics on oxidative stress due to occupational exposure. *World J Surg.* 2005;29(4):540–542.
3. Yilmaz S, Calbayram NC. Exposure to anesthetic gases among operating room personnel and risk of genotoxicity: A systematic review of the human biomonitoring studies. *J Clin Anesth.* 2016;35:326–331.
4. Gupta D, et al. Does exposure to inhalation anesthesia gases change the ratio of X-bearing sperms and Y-bearing Sperms? A worth exploring project into an uncharted domain. *Med Hypotheses.* 2016;94:68–73.
5. Raj N, et al. Evaluation of personal, environmental and biological exposure of paediatric anaesthetists to nitrous oxide and sevoflurane. *Anaesthesia.* 2003;58(7):630–636.

# 142.

# HYPOTHERMIA

*Syena Sarrafpour*

## INTRODUCTION

Hypothermia is defined as a core temperature of less than 35°C (Table 142.1).[1] It is a very common occurrence under anesthesia due to four main types of heat loss: radiation, evaporation, conduction, and convection. The majority of heat loss (approximately 60%) is a result of radiation due to loss of heat to the environment. Evaporation accounts for ~25% of heat loss as energy in the form of heat is lost during water vaporization. Conduction describes the loss of kinetic energy from tissue to the surrounding environment. Convection describes warmed air moving away from the skin by currents. Approximately 15% of heat loss is in the form of conduction and convection.[1]

## ETIOLOGY

Thermoregulation is the body's ability to sense and have a response for deviations from normothermia. Afference sensing is executed by A-delta and C fibers integrating sensory information within the hypothalamus. The hypothalamus is the central control, since it is the primary center for thermoregulation. Lastly, the efferent response ranges from thermogenesis, altering subcutaneous blood flow, sweating, skeletal muscle tone, and metabolic activity.[1]

## PREVENTION AND TREATMENT

In order to both prevent and treat hypothermia, temperature must be monitored. Preferred sites of monitoring core temperature include the nasopharynx, distal esophagus, tympanic membrane, and rectum. Monitoring skin

*Table 142.1* CLASSIFICATION OF HYPOTHERMIA

| Normothermia | 36°–38°C |
| --- | --- |
| Mild hypothermia | 32.2°–35°C |
| Moderate hypothermia | 28°–32.2°C |
| Severe hypothermia | <28°C |

temperature is inaccurate as there are large amounts of fluctuations.[2,3]

Prewarming a patient perioperatively is the most effective way to prevent heat loss from the largest source, redistribution, which can lead to radiative loss. Forced air systems help to minimize the drop in core temperature if placed on the patient for at least 30 minutes and help require less heat to warm patients once redistribution occurs.[2,3]

Room conditions are also helpful in preventing and treating hypothermia as they decrease radiation and convective heat loss from the skin and tissue.[2] Ideally, the room will be warmed to 24°C during induction, and once the patient is prepped and draped, the room temperature can be lowered. Forced air systems placed over patients are the most effective way to decrease heat loss and increase cutaneous warming and increasing insulation.[2,3] They preserve body heat and maintain normothermia. Warm blankets and intravenous fluid warming can also help hypothermia; however, they are less effective than forced air systems.[2]

## ANESTHETIC CONSIDERATIONS

There are primarily three phases of hypothermia under general anesthesia. The first phase results in the greatest decline within the first 30 minutes, due to redistribution as the core temperature is 2°–4°C higher. Vasodilation, along with a depressed hypothalamic response, results in redistribution and causes heat loss through radiation. Phase two describes heat loss after 1 hour in which core temperature decreases at a slow linear rate. Phase three describes heat loss between 3 and 5 hours in which an equilibrium state is reached, as heat production is matched to heat loss.[1] Under general anesthesia, there are many ways in which hypothermia is accelerated. Refer to Table 142.2.

Regional anesthesia can also induce hypothermia, especially neuraxial blocks. The blockade of afferent fibers blocks colder input to the hypothalamus, resulting in the hypothalamus believing the temperature is, in fact, increased.[1] The thermoregulation incorrectly believes the temperature in the regional anesthetized location to be increased.[1] There is a drop in core temperature; however, patients experience more warmth because of the misinterpretation of the skin temperature.[1]

## COMPLICATIONS AND PROGNOSIS

Hypothermia can result in an efferent response of shivering during the postoperative period, which can be quite uncomfortable for patients. Shivering can occur with even small decreases of temperature. Shivering can result in physiologic stress and can result in tachycardia, hypertension, increased catecholamines, and increased oxygen consumption.[1] This can even lead to myocardial events. In fact, even mild hypothermia triples the incidence of postoperative adverse myocardial events.[1,2] Treatment of hypothermia in the postoperative stage includes warm blankets, forced air systems, and even pharmacologic treatments, including meperidine to reduce the threshold for shivering.[2,3]

Hypothermia also results in increased wound infection from impairment of the immune system and can delay duration of hospitalization.[1] Coagulopathy also occurs due to

*Table 142.2* PERIOPERATIVE ANESTHETIC CONSIDERATION ASSOCIATED WITH HYPOTHERMIA

| | COMPLICATIONS | PREVENTION/TREATMENT |
|---|---|---|
| Preoperative | | • Pre-warm via forced air systems (>30 minutes) to increase temperature and reduce redistribution and radiation losses.[2,3] |
| Intraoperative | • Decreased MAC[1,2]<br>• Volatile anesthetics and propofol promote heat loss via redistribution/vasodilation, impairing hypothalamic thermoregulation in a dose-dependent fashion[1]<br>• Opioids depress sympathetic outflow[1]<br>• Nitrous oxide depresses thermoregulation[1]<br>• Regional anesthesia also results in hypothermia[1] | • Warm room to 24°C during induction until the patient is prepped and draped.[2,3]<br>• Utilize forced air systems to decrease heat loss (the most effective way to warm the patient).[2,3]<br>• Warm blankets[2]<br>• Warm intravenous fluids[2] |
| Postoperative | • Shivering increases physiologic stress through increased catecholamines and oxygen consumption[1,2]<br>• Increase in adverse myocardial events<br>• Impaired wound healing[1,2]<br>• Coagulopathy due to interruption with platelet dysfunction and coagulation enzymes[2]<br>• Increased blood loss and transfusion requirements<br>• Delayed PACU recovery[2]<br>• Increased costs[2] | • Optimize with warm blankets, forced air systems[2]<br>• Pharmacologic interventions, such as meperidine[2] |

decreased platelet function and coagulation cascade enzymes which can result in increased blood loss and increased transfusion requirements. It can also interfere with drug metabolism and delay awakening due to prolongation of both inhaled and IV anesthetics, neuromuscular drugs.[1,2] There are associated increased costs and delayed post-anesthesia care unit (PACU) recovery time with hypothermia.[2]

## REFERENCES

1. Díaz M, Becker DE. Thermoregulation: Physiological and clinical considerations during sedation and general anesthesia. *Anesth Prog.* 2010;57(1):25–34.
2. Reynolds L, et al. Perioperative complications of hypothermia. *Best Pract Res Clin Anaesthesiol.* 2008;22(4):645–657.
3. Sessler, DI. Complications and treatment of mild hypothermia. *Anesthesiology.* 2001;95(2):531–543.

# 143.

# NON-MALIGNANT HYPERTHERMIA

*Kyle Ferguson and Angela Johnson*

## INTRODUCTION

Hyperthermia is an elevation in body temperature secondary to failure of the hypothalamic thermoregulatory systems; that is, there is no change in the thermoregulatory set point in the hypothalamus. Many causes of hyperthermia are secondary to pharmacologic interventions or pathologic states that overwhelm the body's ability to regulate body temperature. Medications that affect the serotonergic, dopaminergic, adrenergic, and cholinergic systems can alter the thermoregulatory actions of the hypothalamus, resulting in systemic temperature dysregulation. In addition, endocrine disorders can alter the normal hypothalamic-pituitary axis, leading to hormonal and temperature abnormalities. Due to the significant morbidity associated with severe hyperthermia, quick recognition and treatment are paramount. This chapter will review some of the major causes and treatment of non-malignant hyperthermia, including neuroleptic malignant syndrome, serotonin syndrome, and anticholinergic toxicity (Table 143.1).

## NEUROLEPTIC MALIGNANT SYNDROME

### ETIOLOGY

Neuroleptic malignant syndrome (NMS) results from dopamine receptor blockade in the basal ganglia, specifically D2

receptor antagonism. D2 dopamine receptor blockade within the nigrostriatal, hypothalamic, and mesolimbic pathways in the basal ganglia can lead to dysregulation of the thermoregulatory systems and parkinsonian-type symptoms. NMS is typically seen in patients taking antipsychotic medications. High-potency first-generation antipsychotics such as haloperidol are most likely to induce NMS; however, all antipsychotic medications carry this risk, including the second-generation atypical antipsychotic medications.[1] Anti-emetics with antidopaminergic activity, such as metoclopramide and promethazine, have also been known to increase the development of NMS. In addition, cases have been reported after abrupt withdrawal or reduction in Levo-Dopa doses.[1]

### SYMPTOMS

Symptoms include hyperthermia, mental status changes, muscular rigidity, tremor, and autonomic instability.[1] NMS typically develops over days to weeks. Patients often experience profuse diaphoresis and very high body temperatures. Severe cases can lead to rhabdomyolysis, precipitating acute renal failure.[1,5] Patients typically have very elevated creatine kinase (CK) levels and significant leukocytosis.

### TREATMENT

Treatment includes the cessation of causative agents. Cooling blankets, ice water lavage, and ice packs are used to control hyperthermia. Patients with significantly elevated CK levels and rhabdomyolysis need liberal fluid resuscitation in an effort to prevent renal failure. Management is ultimately supportive therapy; however, some advocate the use of dantrolene, bromocriptine (a dopamine agonist), or amantadine (an anticholinergic medication with dopaminergic activity) for severe symptoms. Benzodiazepines are used for neuropsychiatric symptoms.[1,5]

## ANESTHETIC CONSIDERATIONS

Review the medications a patient is taking in an effort to prevent drug interactions. In patients taking any antidopaminergic medications, such as antipsychotics, it may be best to avoid precipitating agents such as the anti-emetics metoclopramide and promethazine. Intraoperatively, closely monitor temperature and hemodynamics, as well as monitoring for muscular rigidity and diaphoresis. If any signs concerning for NMS occur, cooling blankets, cool saline, and ice packs can be used to lower body temperature. Liberal fluid resuscitation is appropriate in this setting. Obtaining a CK level may be warranted if there is concern for rhabdomyolysis. Finally, dantrolene, bromocriptine, or amantadine can be used for pharmacologic management. Patients should be closely monitored postoperatively in an intensive care unit (ICU) with further supportive care and administration of bromocriptine or amantadine if necessary.

## SEROTONIN SYNDROME

### ETIOLOGY

Serotonin syndrome occurs due to an overstimulation of 5-HT2A receptors in the central nervous system (CNS).

The most common cause includes the SSRI (selective serotonin reuptake inhibitor) and SNRI (serotonin-norepinephrine reuptake inhibitor) classes of medications. Other medications that affect serotonin activity which are frequently used in the perioperative setting include anti-emetics such as ondansetron; opiates such as fentanyl, meperidine, and tramadol; as well as trazodone, bupropion, and other antidepressant medications.[2]

### SYMPTOMS

Symptoms include hyperthermia, diaphoresis, autonomic hyperactivity, altered mental status, hyperreflexia, clonus, and tremors.[2,5] The hyperreflexia associated with serotonin syndrome is classically more exaggerated in the lower extremities.[2,4] Other symptoms include mydriasis, nausea, vomiting, and diarrhea. Onset typically occurs within hours to days. The diagnosis is clinical and based on symptoms and medication history.[5] Elevated CK, leukocytosis, and metabolic acidosis, albeit rare, may be present in severe cases.

### TREATMENT

Treatment consists of cessation of causative agents but is otherwise largely supportive. Cyproheptadine, an antihistamine with 5-HT antagonistic properties, has been used as a treatment modality, as well as benzodiazepines to assuage agitation and mental status changes.[4]

### ANESTHETIC CONSIDERATIONS

Preoperatively it is important to recognize medications that alter serotonin activity to minimize pharmacologic

*Table 143.1* CAUSES OF PERIOPERATIVE HYPERTHERMIA

|  | NMS | SEROTONIN SYNDROME | ANTICHOLINERGIC TOXICITY | THYROID STORM | MH |
|---|---|---|---|---|---|
| Neuromuscular/ Psychiatric Sx | Rigidity Hyporeflexia | Hyperreflexia Tremors Myoclonus | Hyperactive delirium Confusion | — | Rigidity Hyporeflexia |
| Temperature |  |  |  |  |  |
| Blood pressure | Elevated | Mild elevation | Mild elevation | Elevated | Elevated |
| Heart rate |  |  |  | Arrhythmias |  |
| Skin | Diaphoretic | Diaphoretic | Anhidrotic Red, hot |  | Diaphoretic |
| Eyes | — | Mydriasis Ocular clonus | Mydriasis Blurry vison | — | — |
| Bowel symptoms | — | Increased bowel sounds N/V/diarrhea | Decreased bowel sounds |  | Decreased |
| Onset | Days to weeks | Hours to days | Hours to days | Rapid | Variable: Typically minutes–hours |

interactions associated with elevated serotonin. Intraoperatively, monitor temperature and hemodynamics while being cognizant of other symptoms such as ocular clonus. Autonomic instability is best treated with short-acting vasoactive agents. Severe cases should be admitted to the ICU postoperatively for further monitoring and supportive care.

## ANTICHOLINERGIC TOXICITY

### ETIOLOGY

Symptoms occur due to competitive inhibition of acetylcholine at the muscarinic acetylcholine (ACh) receptors, thereby blocking parasympathetic stimulation. Many drugs can affect these receptors, including antihistamines such as diphenhydramine and doxylamine, tricyclic antidepressants, scopolamine, and antidiarrheals. The condition can also be caused by some plants that are known to contain atropine, scopolamine, and antimuscarinic alkaloids, such as Datura stramonium (Jimson weed), Mandragora officinarum (mandrake), Hyoscyamus niger (henbane), and Atropa belladonna (deadly nightshade).

### SYMPTOMS

Anticholinergic toxicity can be remembered by the well-known mnemonic of clinical features; "Red as a beet, dry as a bone, hot as a hare, blind as a bat, and mad as a hatter."[4] Cutaneous vasodilation caused by an anticholinergic state results in flushing of the skin. Sweat glands are innervated by muscarinic acetylcholine receptors, so anticholinergic toxicity produces an anhidrotic hyperthermia secondary to lack of heat dissipation via diaphoresis.[3] Anhidrosis distinguishes anticholinergic toxicity from other hyperthermic states. Patients also experience dry mouth, urinary retention, blurred vision, and nonreactive mydriasis, secondary to pupillary dilation and ineffective visual accommodation. In contrast to the increased bowel sounds, nausea, and vomiting seen with serotonin syndrome, patients experience decreased or absent gastrointestinal activity. Lastly, patients frequently develop neuropsychiatric symptoms, including hyperactive delirium and hallucinations. Diagnosis is typically clinical; however, a trial of physostigmine can be both diagnostic and therapeutic, as it will improve symptoms. Organic causes of delirium must be ruled out; however, delirium in anticholinergic toxicity is typically more abrupt in onset than that of an organic etiology such as sepsis or uremic encephalopathy.

### TREATMENT

Treatment is gastric lavage, and the treatment of choice is physostigmine. Physostigmine, a tertiary amine that is able to cross the blood-brain barrier, is an acetylcholinesterase inhibitor that binds and reversibly inhibits acetylcholinesterase in both the peripheral and central nervous systems leading to an increase of ACh at the muscarinic receptors. This local increase of ACh overcomes the anticholinergic blockade, leading to improvement in symptoms.[3,5] Physostigmine should be used with caution in patients with asthma or cardiac conduction abnormalities, such AV block or bradyarrthymias. Physostigmine can cause hypotension, asystole, and bronchospasm. Benzodiazepines may be necessary for the treatment of neuropsychiatric symptoms.

### ANESTHETIC MANAGEMENT

Due to the large number of prescribed and over-the-counter medications with anticholinergic activity, preoperative review to minimize drug interactions is paramount. Intraoperative monitoring of hemodynamics and temperature remains pivotal. If a patient experiences symptoms of anticholinergic toxicity in the perioperative period, the source medication should be discontinued, physostigmine should be given to treat the symptoms of toxicity, and temperature regulated with supportive measures. Postoperatively the patient should be transferred to the ICU for further monitoring and management.

### REFERENCES

1. Berman BD. Neuroleptic malignant syndrome: A review for neurohospitalists. *Neurohospitalist*. 2011;1(1):41–47.
2. Iqbal MM, et al. Overview of serotonin syndrome. *Ann Clin Psychiatry*. 2012;24(4):310–318.
3. Eyer, F, Zilker, T. Bench-to-bedside review: Mechanisms and management of hyperthermia due to toxicity. *Crit Care*. 2007;11:236.
4. Walter E, Carraretto M. Drug-induced hyperthermia in critical care. *J Intensive Care Soc*. 2015;16(4):306–311.
5. Jamshidi N, Dawson A. The hot patient: Acute drug-induced hyperthermia. *Aust Prescr*. 2019;42(1):24–28.

# 144.

# ACETYLCHOLINESTERASE-INHIBITOR TOXICITY

*David Guz and Angela Johnson*

## INTRODUCTION

The use of acetylcholinesterase-inhibiting agents (AChI) is widespread, spanning applications in the realms of medicine, industry, and armed conflict. These agents have been of particular importance since the 1930s, when research on carbamate and organophosphate compounds culminated in the development of physostigmine, which quickly found use as a remedy for myasthenia gravis and as an antidote for anticholinergic toxicity. The events leading up to the development of physostigmine for therapeutic purposes was fraught with reports of cholinergic toxicity, which is the mechanism behind many commonly used pesticides and chemical nerve agents.[1] Organophosphates are used also as commercial insecticides and in chemical warfare; they can be rapidly absorbed through the skin and mucous membranes. They are also used for medical purposes, such as echothiophate which is used to treat glaucoma. This chapter will review acetylcholinesterase inhibitors, cholinergic toxicity, and its treatment.

## PHYSIOLOGY

Acetylcholinesterase-inhibiting (AChI) medications work indirectly by preventing the breakdown of the endogenous neurotransmitter acetylcholine (ACh) via inactivation of the enzyme acetylcholinesterase, which resides primarily at the synaptic basal lamina and functions to cleave ACh into choline and acetic acid, which do not participate in neurotransmission.[2] This increased concentration of acetylcholine at the nerve synapse results in agonism of both nicotinic and muscarinic receptors, which clinically mediate the motor end-plate and end-organ parasympathetic drive.[2] AChI medications also inactivate to a lesser extent the enzyme butyrylcholinesterase, a nonspecific cholinesterase found in plasma, synthesized in the liver, which can be used as a marker of liver synthetic function. Clinically, butyrylcholinesterase is notable for succinylcholine metabolism; as such, the use of succinylcholine in patients with acute AChI toxicity may lead to prolonged neuromuscular

blockade. Most clinically used agents like physostigmine and donepezil bind acetylcholinesterase reversibly, resulting in a shortened duration of action and greater titratability, while pesticides and nerve agents irreversibly inactivate the enzyme (see Table 144.1).[2]

## SIGNS AND SYMPTOMS

Cholinergic toxicity/cholinergic crisis is diagnosed by history and clinical signs. While laboratory measurements of red blood cell (RBC) acetylcholinesterase activity exist, their utility in the acute setting is minimal. Symptoms of anticholinergic toxicity range from mild to life-threatening, and may mimic other conditions. The most common signs include bradycardia, hypersalivation, and generalized weakness. The classic muscarinic manifestations can be remembered with the SLUDGE/BBB mnemonic device (see Box 144.1). Severe manifestations include hemodynamically significant bradyarrhythmias and weakness leading to respiratory compromise. Organophosphate compounds commonly seen in pesticides and nerve agents may also cause a delayed cholinergic neurologic syndrome, leading to sensory and cognitive deficits weeks after exposure. Rapid diagnosis and treatment are critical to minimize adverse outcomes.[3]

## TREATMENT

Initial treatment focuses on termination of exposure (e.g., removing soiled clothing) resuscitation, and supportive

*Table 144.1* ACETYLCHOLINESTERASE INHIBITORS

| ACETYLCHOLINESTERASE INHIBITORS | |
|---|---|
| PHARMACOLOGIC | INDUSTRIAL/MILITARY |
| -stigmine medications | Parathion |
| Donepezil | Carbofuran |
| Edrophonium | Malathion |
| Echothiophate | Nerve agents (Sarin/VX) |

care. Patients may be in need of respiratory support and emergent intubation. In the setting of AChI toxicity, succinylcholine may have decreased efficacy; a rapid sequence induction (RSI) dose of a nondepolarizing agent such as rocuronium may be needed to achieve adequate blockade. Early administration of the centrally acting anticholinergic drug atropine may be diagnostic and therapeutic, illustrating absence of typical anticholinergic symptoms and resolution of cholinergic symptoms (specifically salivation and bronchoconstriction) serving as markers of toxicity and effective treatment.[4] As atropine binds specifically to muscarinic receptors sparing nicotinic receptors at the motor end-plate, coadministration of the acetylcholinesterase-reactivating drug pralidoxime may be required to reverse the somatic effect of toxicity and prevent irreversible binding of organophosphate compounds to the enzyme.[4] This is especially relevant in the setting of toxicity caused by pesticide or nerve agent exposures, which may build up in adipose tissue and have effects ranging up to several weeks following exposure.[4]

## ANESTHETIC CONSIDERATIONS

### PREOPERATIVE

The perioperative physician should take precautions in patients with risk factors for adverse reactions to cholinergic medications, including the elderly, those with polypharmacy, existing neuromuscular or pulmonary insufficiency, and those with renal or hepatic dysfunction. Patients may also be taking medications with pro-cholinergic activity that are continued into the perioperative period.

### INTRAOPERATIVE

A patient may receive several different cholinergic medications for various indications in the course of a single anesthetic, contributing to the possibility for toxicity (Table 144.1). Monitor for signs and symptoms of toxicity, which may be nonspecific while under anesthesia. Care must be taken to ensure the AChI used for reversal is paired with an anticholinergic drug with similar duration of action (neostigmine/glycopyrrolate or edrophonium/atropine), otherwise unopposed action from either agent may be observed.[5] Patients with myasthenia gravis requiring the use of high-dose pyridostigmine are at particular risk for the development of cholinergic toxicity, with further AChI use possibly overshooting the therapeutic index and leading to worsened weakness. For these patients, sugammadex should be strongly considered as the reversal agent of choice in the absence of other contraindications.

### POSTOPERATIVE

Monitor for toxicity, obtain appropriate studies and labs. Consider consultation with hospital pharmacist or poison control (1-800-222-1222 in the US) if cholinergic toxicity is suspected. Manage symptoms accordingly and consider use of atropine and/or pralidoxime with low threshold for intensive care unit (ICU) admission for monitoring and treatment.

## REFERENCES

1. Scheindlin S. Episodes in the story of physostigmine. *Mol Interv*. 2010;10(1):4–10.
2. Tafuri J, Roberts J. Organophosphate poisoning. *Ann Emerg Med*. 1987;16(2):193–202.
3. Indira M, et al. Incidence, predictors, and outcome of intermediate syndrome in cholinergic insecticide poisoning: a prospective observational cohort study. *Clin Toxicol (Phila)*. 2013;51(9):838–845.
4. Eddleston M, et al. Management of severe organophosphorus pesticide poisoning. *Crit Care*. 2002;6(3):259.
5. Azar I, Pham, A. The heart rate following edrophonium-atropine and edrophonium-glycopyrrolate mixtures. *Anesthesiology*. 1983;59:139–141.

# 145.

# BRONCHOSPASM

*Jeffery James Eapen and Jason Bang*

## INTRODUCTION

Bronchospasm is a respiratory condition in which the smooth muscle surrounding the bronchioles constrict, resulting in airflow obstruction primarily in the expiratory phase of the respiratory cycle. Reactive airway disease such as asthma, chronic obstructive pulmonary disease (COPD), anaphylaxis, or intervention by an anesthesiologist increases the risk of bronchospasm. Bronchospasm occurs 0.2% of the time during general anesthesia, but the incidence increases to 6% in patients who have reactive airway disease.[1]

Risk factors for bronchospasm include asthma, upper respiratory tract infection, smoking history, and carcinoid syndrome. Noxious stimuli such as allergens, dust, cold air, endotracheal intubation, secretions, desflurane, beta-blockers, nonsteroidal anti-inflammatory drugs (NSAIDs), cholinesterase inhibitors, and histamine-releasing drugs such as morphine can result in stimulation of afferent sensory fibers that eventually stimulate the nucleus tractus solitarius, which in turn stimulates efferent fibers of the vagus nerve to result in bronchial smooth muscle contraction.[1]

Release of inflammatory mediators is another cause of bronchospasm. These inflammatory mediators can be a result of allergic reactions or anaphylactic shock in which bronchospasm is either mediated by anaphylactoid or immunoglobin E (IgE)-mediated anaphylaxis. Bronchospasm is also a complication seen in carcinoid syndrome and occurs in 15%–19% of patients.[2]

## CLINICAL FEATURES

Perioperative bronchospasm can occur following noxious stimulus such as endotracheal intubation. Observed signs and symptoms during bronchospasm are dependent on if the patient is being mechanically ventilated. If the patient is not being mechanically ventilated, respiratory distress is noted with physical examination findings of decreased breath sounds and expiratory wheezing. While mechanically ventilated, a rapid rise in peak airway pressures from baseline are observed. Capnography will show delayed rise

in end tidal carbon dioxide, and decreased exhaled tidal volumes are noted.[3] If bronchospasm persists, the patient will begin to desaturate and hypotension is often experienced due to decreased preload from air trapping, resulting in increased intrathoracic pressure.

## MANAGEMENT

If bronchospasm is suspected, quick action should be taken to prevent further complications from arising. Management should aim to increase delivered oxygen content to the patient, improve ventilation, relax bronchial smooth muscle, and stop stimulation such as surgery.[3] Increasing inspired oxygen concentration to 100%, increasing inspired concentration of non-noxious volatile anesthetics for their bronchodilating properties, and positive pressure ventilation can facilitate relaxation of bronchial smooth muscle. B2 agonists such as albuterol via MDI or nebulized forms should be immediately introduced into the endotracheal tube (ETT) to relax bronchial smooth muscle that is causing bronchospasm.[1] Ingtravenous (IV) agents such as propofol and ketamine are often employed in scenarios of continued bronchospasm. Ketamine in particular is a known bronchodilator. Initiate manual ventilation, as it can serve as a diagnostic tool for ruling out mechanical complications and assessment of pulmonary compliance during the bronchospasm. If the bronchospasm is refractory to various techniques employed to terminate the bronchospasm, epinephrine should be used, usually starting with 10 mcg per dose, IV.[3]

## ANESTHETIC CONSIDERATIONS

### PREOPERATIVE

Identification and appropriate planning of the management in patients who are at increased risk of bronchospasm can impact the incidence and outcomes of bronchospasm. Physical examination by auscultation and taking history from the patient are vital on the day of the surgery to assess if further action is necessary to optimize the patient's respiratory status prior to proceeding with the anesthetic plan. Patients should be counseled about smoking cessation 6–8 weeks prior to surgery as this reduces the risk of respiratory complications, including bronchospasm.[4] Respiratory infections should have resolved with absence of symptoms for 2 weeks to decrease the chance of bronchospasm.[5] In patients with reactive airways such as asthma, pretreatment with beta agonist nebulized agents 30 minutes prior to the procedure has been associated with decreased incidence of bronchospasm.[3]

## INTRAOPERATIVE

On induction, appropriate depth of anesthesia should be a goal prior to proceeding with laryngoscopy and intubation, as this can promote the development of bronchospasm. Emergency medications, such as epinephrine, should be prepared in anticipation of refractory bronchospasm. During the maintenance of general anesthesia, avoid histamine-releasing drugs and maintain an adequate depth of anesthesia. At the end of the procedure, consider a deep extubation, as this can decrease the stimulatory effects of extubation on the smooth muscle of the bronchioles.

## POSTOPERATIVE

During recovery the patient should be assessed for continued airway reactivity; this can necessitate continued use of bronchodilator therapy, corticosteroids, and chest physiotherapy.

A chest radiograph should be obtained to evaluate for pulmonary edema or pneumothorax. If anaphylaxis was a suspected cause, ordering a tryptase level is warranted.[3]

## REFERENCES

1. Freeman B. *Anesthesiology Core Review*. McGraw Hill; 2014:390–392
2. Ferrari AC, Glasberg J, Riechelmann RP. Carcinoid syndrome: Update on the pathophysiology and treatment. *Clinics*. 2018;73(Suppl 1):e490s.
3. Looseley A. (n.d.). *Update in Anaesthesia*. Retrieved August 30, 2020, from https://www.wfsahq.org/components/com_virtual_library/media/3fe4887e14541ff43fc8b0d7c6c477f8-Bronchospasm-During-Anaesthesia--Update-27-2011-.pdf
4. Dudzińska K, Mayzner-Zawadzka E. Tobacco smoking and the perioperative period. *Anestezjol Intens Ter*. 2008;40:108–113.
5. Nandwani N, Raphael JH, Langton JA. Effects of an upper respiratory tract infection on upper airway reactivity. *Br J Anaesth*. 1997;78:352.

# 146.

# LATEX ALLERGY

*Kelsey E. Lacourrege and Alan D. Kaye*

## INTRODUCTION

Allergy to natural rubber latex (NRL) presents a potential source of perioperative anaphylaxis. Though the general population has a small risk of developing latex allergy, most cases are associated with certain high-risk populations. Awareness of the populations most at risk for this allergy, knowledge of potential sources of latex in the clinical environment, and prompt recognition of anaphylaxis and other allergic reactions are essential skills for clinicians in the perioperative environment.[1]

## ETIOLOGY

The overwhelming cause of latex allergy development is exposure to NRL allergens through healthcare equipment, especially gloves. Beginning in the 1980s, the introduction of universal precautions spurred an epidemic of latex allergy development among healthcare workers, patients with certain chronic conditions, and individuals in other industries such as food service. Among those with chronic illness, individuals with spina bifida, those with urologic conditions, those with indwelling catheters, and those who have undergone multiple surgeries are at highest risk.[1]

Exposure to latex allergens through skin contact, such as gloves, has been shown to lead to localized allergic reactions consisting of erythema and urticaria. However, the use of powdered latex gloves and associated aerosolization of latex allergens can also trigger allergic asthma, rhinitis, ocular symptoms, and anaphylaxis, especially in healthcare workers. For reasons not entirely understood, patients with spina bifida also have heightened susceptibility to latex allergy. Type IV cell-mediated and type I immunoglobulin E (IgE)-mediated immune responses were reported. At the height of the epidemic in 1991, 1 of every 8 patients with spina bifida would experience anaphylaxis perioperatively. Overall in the 1990s, allergy rates soared to as high as 17% among healthcare workers and 70% among spina bifida patients. Today the rate of allergy development has declined to 1% for the entire population.[1]

# DIAGNOSIS

Skin testing for latex allergy is associated with high rates of anaphylaxis and thus is not performed in the United States. Serologic testing provides an alternative option and has excellent specificity but low sensitivity. Therefore patients with a clinical history consistent with latex allergy should be considered high risk even in the absence of serologic confirmation.[1]

Of additional clinical relevance is the latex-fruit syndrome. Due to cross-reactivity between allergens in latex and those in many varieties of fruit, individuals with allergies to particular fruits—especially tropical fruits like banana, avocado, kiwi, pineapple, and papaya—may be more likely to have or develop a latex allergy.[1,2]

For a patient with new-onset latex allergy intraoperatively, diagnosis is made by correctly identifying the presence of an allergic reaction and investigating the source. Clinical features of anaphylaxis include cardiovascular instability (tachycardia, bradycardia, hypotension, arrest) and bronchospasm. Cutaneous reactions such as urticaria and angioedema may be seen in both anaphylaxis and in milder reactions. Measurement of plasma histamine and tryptase concentrations can also help support the diagnosis of an allergic reaction. The next step, identifying the source of the reaction, requires consideration of all possible allergens. The most common culprits of perioperative anaphylaxis are neuromuscular blocking agents, antibiotics, and latex. If other potential allergens have been excluded and latex is the primary suspect, serologic testing as described earlier can be used to support the diagnosis.[2]

# ANESTHETIC MANAGEMENT

Due to recognition of the cause of the latex allergy epidemic and appropriate policy responses, the use of latex-containing products in healthcare has dwindled significantly in the United States. This has led to a decline in the incidence of new latex allergies. Nevertheless, prevalence of latex allergy may still be relatively high in some patient populations. Clinicians should be especially cautious with any individual with spina bifida, with anyone who frequently uses latex gloves or catheters, and with atopic patients.[1] Over 40,000 everyday items and some medical supplies, such as indwelling urinary catheters and red rubber catheters, still contain latex.[3] Patients who use these pieces of equipment may be particularly high risk, as mucosal exposure may be associated with more severe reactions compared to cutaneous exposure.[4]

For any patient with known latex allergy or for those considered to be high risk, key preventive measures should be taken to eliminate intraoperative exposure risk. This requires that operating room (OR) personnel be aware of the patient's allergy or high-risk status and be knowledgeable about which supplies in the OR contain latex. Thorough history taking, comprehensive documentation of previous exposures and reactions, and use of a surgical checklist can all ensure awareness of at-risk patients.[4] All OR staff should also be attentive to labeling of supplies and be able to recognize which items are and are not latex-free.[3] Those cases can be scheduled as first case in the morning. Airborne particles containing latex can be suspended in air for up to 5 hours.

If a patient develops anaphylaxis secondary to latex exposure in the OR, prompt recognition and management are key. Anaphylaxis can occur immediately upon exposure but may take up to 60 minutes to present. Immediate resuscitation with intravenous epinephrine and intravascular fluid should be initiated. Additionally, if the source of latex exposure is still present, such as a catheter, it should immediately be removed and replaced with a latex-free alternative.[2]

# REFERENCES

1. Kelly KJ, et al. Clinical commentary review latex allergy: Where are we now and how did we get there? *J Allergy Clin Immunol Pr* [Internet]. 2017;5:1212–1218. Available from: http://dx.doi.org/10.1016/j.jaip.2017.05.029.
2. Dewachter P, et al. Anaphylaxis and anesthesia: Controversies and new insights [Internet]. *Anesthesiology*. 2009;111:1141–1150. Available from: www.anesthesiology.org.
3. Liberatore K, et al. Latex allergy risks live on. *J Allergy Clin Immunol Pract* [Internet]. 2018;6(6):1877–1878. Available from: https://doi.org/10.1016/j.jaip.2018.08.007.
4. Minami CA, et al. Management of a patient with a latex allergy. *JAMA*. 2017;317:309–310.

# 147.

# LARYNGOSPASM

*David S. Beebe and Kumar G. Belani*

## INTRODUCTION

Laryngospasm is the forceful contraction of the vocal cords and muscles of the upper airway, usually in response to irritation or stimulation, which halts ventilation. Although laryngospasm can occur in people of all ages, most commonly it is seen in infants or children undergoing induction or emergence from general anesthesia. Laryngospasm may be partial where some ventilation still occurs, or complete. If the laryngospasm is complete and ventilation not restored, it can result in hypoxia, bradycardia, and even mortality.[1]

## PATHOPHYSIOLOGY

The pathophysiology of laryngospasm was described by Bernard Fink in 1956.[2] Laryngeal reflexes are elicited by stimulation of the afferent fibers contained in the internal branch of the superior laryngeal nerve. These reflexes control the laryngeal muscle contractions which protect the airway during swallowing. A stimulus can cause forceful adduction of the vocal cords, probably as a protective mechanism, but is unopposed by the abductors in the anesthetized state. Adduction of the false vocal cords can have consequences. This may result in a ball-valve effect, which will obstruct air flow through the vocal cords even if positive pressure is applied from above.[2] Restoration of ventilation often requires deepening the depth of anesthesia or other measures to relax the adductor muscles.[1]

## ANESTHETIC CONSIDERATIONS

### PREOPERATIVE

Although any patient receiving anesthesia may develop laryngospasm, certain patients are more susceptible. Infants and children are more susceptible than older children or adults. Patients who have an upper airway infection, either acute or chronic, are also more at risk. Obese patients are also more susceptible. Laryngospasm is often associated with and/or precipitated by aspiration. Patients with chronic reflux may therefore be at particular risk. Finally, surgery on the throat or upper airway such as a tonsillectomy is associated with a greater risk of laryngospasm.[1]

### INTRAOPERATIVE

There is no specific anesthetic technique that will guarantee that laryngospasm will not occur sometime during the case in a patient who is susceptible. Laryngospasm may occur with either inhaled or intravenous induction of anesthesia. However, adequate depth of anesthesia prior to airway instrumentation or tracheal intubation is necessary to depress the laryngeal reflexes that may stimulate laryngospasm. Tracheal intubation will prevent laryngospasm as long as the patient remains intubated but may occur when the tracheal tube is removed. Indeed, that is when laryngospasm is most likely to occur.[1]

The best technique for tracheal extubation (deep or awake) of patients susceptible to laryngospasm is unclear. Removing the tracheal tube while the child is still anesthetized theoretically would not stimulate the larynx and trigger laryngospasm. However, the tissue has been irritated from the presence of the tracheal tube and perhaps the surgery and laryngospasm may occur as the patient emerges from anesthesia. Proponents of extubating patients when awake feel that laryngospasm is less likely to occur if consciousness and vocal cord function have been regained. This technique also reduces the risk of aspiration. There are little data supporting either technique.[1] A recent study of pediatric events requiring rapid response during anesthesia showed that 44% of the events were due to laryngospasm. Of these, 28% were following deep extubation, most (60%) of which occurred in the recovery room.[3] This study suggests that deep extubation did not prevent laryngospasm and may have only delayed it until the recovery room.

However, one technique that has been shown to be beneficial in preventing laryngospasm is the administration of lidocaine. It has been shown to be beneficial in a recent meta-analysis whether administered intravenously (1–2 mg/kg) or topically to the vocal cords (4 mg/kg) at the time of tracheal intubation.[4]

If laryngospasm does occur upon induction of general anesthesia, a jaw thrust maneuver and positive pressure ventilation with 100% oxygen should be applied, as well as insertion of an oral airway. If an intravenous catheter is present, anesthesia may be deepened with an intravenous agent such as propofol. A rapid-acting, skeletal muscle relaxant such as succinylcholine or rocuronium may need to be administered if that is not successful, and the trachea intubated, or, if ventilation becomes adequate, managed with a laryngeal mask airway. The situation becomes much more difficult if an intravenous catheter is not yet placed and laryngospasm causing complete airway obstruction develops. If an intravenous catheter can rapidly be established, 0.5–1 mg/kg of succinylcholine can be administered to break the laryngospasm. If one cannot be established, intramuscular succinylcholine (4 mg/kg) can be administered. Although its onset can be slow using this technique compared to the intravenous route, and since complete laryngeal relaxation is usually not needed to break laryngospasm, it usually proves adequate. Alternatively, succinylcholine may be administered via the femoral vein, sublingually, or via an intraosseous needle.[1,5]

Laryngospasm occurring upon emergence from anesthesia is managed in the same manner. If ventilation cannot be established by standard airway maneuvers, either intravenous propofol or succinylcholine may need to be administered. Often only a small dose (0.1–0.2 mg/kg) of succinylcholine needs to be administered to stop the laryngospasm. The patient can then be ventilated until the relaxant wears off.[1]

## POSTOPERATIVE

Laryngospasm may result in significant morbidity and mortality, including cardiac arrest (0.5%), post-obstructive negative pressure pulmonary edema (4%), pulmonary aspiration (3%), bradycardia (6%), and oxygen desaturation (61%).[1] As such, patients should be observed for several hours in the recovery room to be sure the patients are fully recovered from anesthesia with normal oxygenation, clear lung fields, and no evidence of laryngeal irritability or recurrent laryngospasm.

## REFERENCES

1. Alalami A, et al. Laryngospasm: Review of different prevention and treatment modalities. *Pediatr Anesth*. 2008;18:281–288.
2. Fink B. The etiology and treatment of laryngeal spasm. *Anesthesiology*. 1956;17:569–577.
3. Schleelein L, et al. Pediatric perioperative adverse events requiring rapid response: a retrospective case-control study. *Pediatr Anesth*. 2016;26:734–741.
4. Qi X, et al. The efficacy of lidocaine in laryngospasm prevention in pediatric surgery: A network meta-analysis. *Sci. Rep.* 6:32308. doi:10.1038/srep32308 (2016).
5. Mazze RI, Dunbar RW. Intralingual succinylcholine administration in children: An alternative to intravenous and intramuscular routes? *Anesth Analg*. 1968;47:605–615.

# 148.

# POSTOBSTRUCTIVE PULMONARY EDEMA

*Benjamin Kloesel and Balazs Horvath*

## INTRODUCTION

Postobstructive pulmonary edema (POPE) describes a unique form of gas-exchange impairment that can be encountered in the perioperative period. It is triggered by vigorous respiratory efforts against an obstructed airway, which lead to a chain of events that facilitate trans-vascular fluid filtration. The resulting pulmonary edema causes impairment of gas exchange, which manifests as hypoxemia, dyspnea, tachypnea, and expectoration of pink, frothy sputum. Airway obstruction can have many different etiologies, but in anesthetic practice, the most frequent situations that lead to POPE include laryngospasm and occlusion of the endotracheal tube caused by the patient biting down when no protective bite block is in place.

## PATHOPHYSIOLOGY

The main pathophysiological factor for the development of POPE remains the generation of negative pleural pressures significantly below the physiological level during the attempt to spontaneously inhale against an obstructed airway (modified Mueller maneuver).[1] During physiologic breathing via an unobstructed upper airway, the diaphragm generates negative inspiratory pressures of −2 to −8 cm $H_2O$, while forceful inspiration against an obstructed airway can result in negative inspiratory pressures of up to −140 cm $H_2O$ (Figure 148.1).[2] Some sources categorize POPE into two different types: type I occurs after relief of an acute upper airway obstruction, while type II is characterized by occurrence after relief of a chronic upper airway

obstruction, for example after tonsillectomy or airway tumor removal.[3]

During type I POPE, inhalation against an obstructed airway generates an increase in right ventricular preload, along with negative intrapleural pressures that are transmitted to the alveoli. Negative pleural pressure facilitates an increase in venous return and creates a large gradient between alveoli and pulmonary capillaries, resulting in fluid movement into the interstitial space. Furthermore, high pressure gradients can disrupt pulmonary epithelium and blood vessel membranes, resulting in microhemorrhage and further fluid translocation.[3] In type II POPE, patients experience long-standing, intermittent episodes of airway obstruction, resulting in wide swings in intrathoracic pressure, generation of intrinsic positive end-expiratory pressure (PEEP), hypoventilation, and hypercarbia. Sudden relief of the obstruction removes intrinsic PEEP and causes an increase in venous return and right ventricular preload. Chronic changes from the long-standing obstructive episodes, such as systemic vasoconstriction, hypoxic pulmonary vasoconstriction, increased

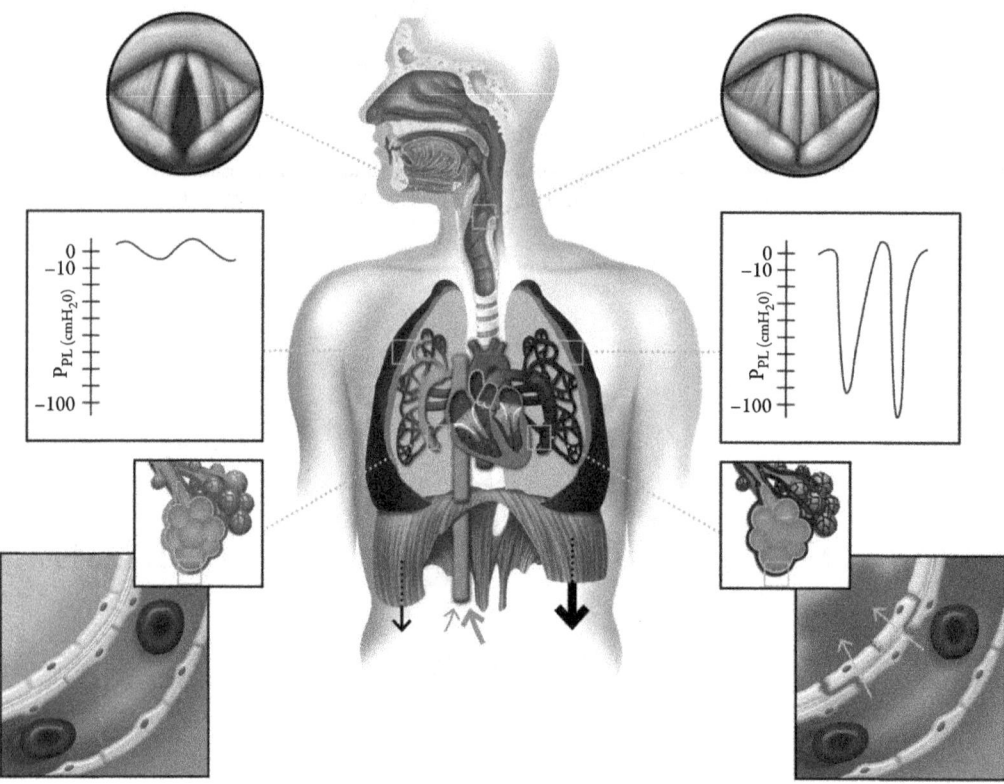

**Figure 148.1.** As shown in the *left part* of the illustration, breathing through the normally open upper airway requires minimal diaphragmatic efforts (*thin black arrow*) that generate small levels (−2 to −8 $cmH_2O$) of negative pleural pressure ($P_{PL}$) during inspiration. In normal conditions, the alveolar–capillary pressure gradient is small, and when hydrostatic pressures slightly increase in the pulmonary capillary bed, the fluid overload may be offset by increased lymphatic drainage. Conversely, inspiration against an obstructed upper airway—as represented by closed vocal cords in the *right side* of the illustration—requires forceful diaphragmatic efforts (*large black arrow*) generating high levels (−50 to −140 $cmH_2O$) of negative $P_{PL}$ that increase venous return to the right side of the heart. This may result in higher hydrostatic pressures in the pulmonary capillaries and a sudden drop of pressures in the alveolar spaces, creating a huge pressure gradient across the pulmonary capillary wall and disruption of the alveolar–capillary membrane, leading to alveolar flooding and pulmonary edema (Grey Arrows).

Reproduced with permission from Lemyze M, Mallat J. Understanding negative pressure pulmonary edema. *Intensive Care Med.* 2014;40(8):1140–1143.

pulmonary artery pressures, and myocardial dysfunction, impair the body's ability to handle the sudden fluid load imposed on the pulmonary circulation and result in development of pulmonary edema.[3]

## ETIOLOGY AND RISK FACTORS

The most common triggering factors of POPE differ within the pediatric and adult population. In children, the majority of upper airway obstruction resulting in POPE is caused by infectious croup or epiglottitis. In adults, post-extubation laryngospasm, upper airway infection, and tumors are the predominant etiologic factors. Other risk factors include difficult intubation, hanging, strangulation, goiter, expanding hematoma, obstructive sleep apnea, airway foreign body, and bilateral vocal cord paralysis. Young, healthy adults are at higher risk for development of POPE due to their ability to generate large negative intrathoracic pressures.[1,4]

## DIAGNOSIS

The first and probably most important clue for the diagnosis should be drawn from the situation in which POPE occurs and the timeframe to symptom onset. Events such as laryngospasm in the perioperative phase, the patient biting down on the endotracheal tube, or airway obstructions after medication administration should raise the index of suspicion for POPE if the patient develops otherwise unexplained hypoxemia and dyspnea. POPE is furthermore characterized by a rapid onset of symptoms (seconds to minutes after the precipitating event), although delayed presentations (30–60 minutes and even 24 hours after a precipitating event) have been reported.[5] The patient may exhibit tachycardia, tachypnea, dyspnea, tachypnea, agitation, and cough. Expectoration of pink frothy sputum or even frank hemoptysis may occur. Auscultation of the lungs may reveal rales and rhonchi. A chest X-ray can show alveolar and/or interstitial edema, typically in a bilateral distribution. Bronchoscopy is often unnecessary for diagnosis but may show bloody return consistent with alveolar hemorrhage. The differential diagnosis for POPE should include cardiogenic pulmonary edema, neurogenic pulmonary edema, aspiration pneumonia, anaphylaxis, and iatrogenic fluid overload.[4]

## ANESTHETIC CONSIDERATIONS

### PREOPERATIVE

POPE typically occurs in the postoperative period. Risk factors such as potential difficult intubation, obesity, and obstructive sleep apnea that may predispose a patient to develop POPE should be elicited.

### INTRAOPERATIVE/POSTOPERATIVE

POPE most frequently occurs after extubation or in the post-anesthesia care unit, but cases occurring during induction of anesthesia have also been reported.[2] The most important step to address POPE is relieving the precipitating airway obstruction, either by simple basic life support maneuvers (head extension, jaw thrust) or more advanced techniques (oropharyngeal/nasopharyngeal airway, supraglottic airway device, endotracheal intubation). Further treatment of POPE is supportive. A majority of cases can be managed with supplemental oxygen and patient observation.[2] If hypoxemia is refractory, noninvasive positive pressure ventilation (NIPPV) may be trialed. This allows application of oxygen to address hypoxemia, along with continuous positive airway pressure (CPAP), which supports fluid resorption from the alveoli back into the vascular space.[2,4] If noninvasive positive pressure ventilation is unsuccessful or not possible, the patient may require endotracheal intubation and mechanical ventilation. A lung-protective ventilation strategy should be targeted (e.g., tidal volume of 4–8 mL/kg predicted body weight with target plateau pressures <30 cmH$_2$0) and PEEP should be utilized to facilitate fluid resorption. Diuretics have been used but are often unnecessary; they may hasten the resolution of pulmonary edema, although care must be taken to avoid the administration in a hypovolemic patient.[2,3] Some sources recommend the use of inhaled ß$_2$-agonists, although it is important to point out that both interventions (diuretics and inhaled ß$_2$-agonists) have not been studied in POPE and are therefore not evidence-based.[3,5] Rescue therapies for severe refractory hypoxemia despite mechanical ventilation include neuromuscular blockade, prone positioning, and extracorporeal membrane oxygenation (ECMO). The majority of cases resolve within 12 to 48 hours. Sequelae are uncommon and patients usually experience a full recovery.[1]

## REFERENCES

1. Bhattacharya M, et al. Negative-pressure pulmonary edema. *Chest.* 2016;150(4):927–933.
2. Lemyze M, Mallat J. Understanding negative pressure pulmonary edema. *Intensive Care Med.* 2014;40(8):1140–1143.
3. Udeshi A, et al. Postobstructive pulmonary edema. *J Crit Care.* 2010;25(3):508 e1–5.
4. Krodel DJ, et al. Case scenario: Acute postoperative negative pressure pulmonary edema. *Anesthesiology.* 2010;113(1):200–207.
5. Liu R, et al. Negative pressure pulmonary edema after general anesthesia: A case report and literature review. *Medicine (Baltimore).* 2019;98(17):e15389.

# 149.

# ASPIRATION OF GASTRIC CONTENTS

*Mariam Sarwary and Nathan Schulman*

## INTRODUCTION

Aspiration is defined as the entry of solid or liquid contents into the trachea and lungs. It is estimated to occur between 1 and 5 times for every 10,000 anesthetics, with a mortality rate of approximately 4%.[1] The results of aspiration can vary greatly, from mild or no symptoms to respiratory failure and acute respiratory distress syndrome. In this chapter we discuss the factors increasing the risk of aspiration during anesthesia, the sequelae of aspiration, and possible treatment measures.

## FACTORS INCREASING RISK OF GASTRIC ASPIRATION

During the normal physiological state, there are mechanisms in place to prevent regurgitation or aspiration. These include the presence of the lower esophageal sphincter (LES), the upper esophageal sphincter (UES), and the laryngeal reflexes.

The LES is found at the border of the stomach and the esophagus and is responsible for protecting the esophagus from gastric reflux. Several anesthetic drugs have been shown to affect LES tone. Notably propofol, opioids, anticholinergics, and some inhaled anesthetics may cause a decrease in LES tone and hence an increased risk of aspiration (Table 149.1). Underlying gastroesophageal pathology, i.e. gastroesophageal reflux disease (GERD), may predispose patients to a baseline decrease in their LES tone and hence an increased risk of aspiration. It should be noted that LES tone alone does not predict the likelihood for regurgitation, but rather it is determined by the difference between the LES pressure and gastric pressure, known as the barrier pressure. Therefore, any state that increases retention of gastric contents, and hence an increase in gastric pressure, may also lead to aspiration.

When performing a preoperative history and physical, the anesthesiologist must be mindful of conditions that increase the risk of esophageal regurgitation and aspiration, including but not limited to gastroparesis, GERD, hiatal hernias, ileus, obesity, pregnancy, pain, previous gastric surgery, inadequate starvation, and emergency surgeries.

*Table 149.1* EFFECT OF DRUGS USED IN ANESTHESIA ON LOWER ESOPHAGEAL SPHINCTER TONE

| INCREASE | DECREASE | NO CHANGE |
|---|---|---|
| Metoclopramide | Atropine | Propranolol |
| Domperidone | Glycopyrrolate | Oxprenolol |
| Cyclizine | Sodium nitroprusside | Ranitidine |
| Edrophonium | Ganglion blockers | Atracurium |
| Succinylcholine | Thiopental | ?Nitrous oxide |
| Pancuronium | β adrenergic stimulants | |
| Metoprolol | Halothane | |
| α adrenergic stimulants | Enflurane | |
| Antacids | Opioids | |
| | ?Nitrous oxide | |
| | Propotol | |

Reprinted from British Journal of Anaestehsia, Vol. 56, B.R Cotton, G. Smith, *The Lower Esophageal Sphincter and Anasthesia*, pg. 37–46, Copyright 1984, with permission from Elsevier.

The UES is formed by the cricopharyngeal muscle, one of the two inferior constrictor muscles of the pharynx, which is continuous with the circular muscular coat of the esophagus. In the normal physiological state, it functions to prevent reflux of contents from the esophagus into the pharynx. Studies have shown that function of the UES is impaired during anesthesia and normal sleep. In addition, neuromuscular blockers can significantly decrease UES tone, therefore causing patients with inadequate reversal of neuromuscular blockers to be at increased risk of aspiration during recovery.[2]

The protective airway reflexes include expiration, coughing, panting, and laryngospasm. Protective upper airway reflexes are reduced by decreased levels of consciousness caused by most anesthetics, as well as in elderly patients.[2]

## TYPES OF PULMONARY ASPIRATION

There are several different types of matter that can be aspirated into the lungs, and depending on the type and volume, a variety of physiological reactions may be seen.

One may aspirate on clear oral secretions during induction, face mask ventilation, or emergence. Assuming low-volume aspirate, the patient may only respond with a cough or transient laryngospasm. Aspiration of blood may occur after trauma, epistaxis, or airway surgery and may lead to changes on chest X-ray. Low-volume blood causes minor airway obstruction that can be cleared by mucociliary support; however, larger volumes may lead to airway obstruction and pulmonary hemochromatosis from iron accumulation in phagocytic cells.

The most common type of aspiration feared during induction of anesthesia and prior to securing of the airway is that of acidic gastric contents. Vomiting or regurgitation may lead to aspiration of such contents, causing a chemical pneumonitis, which results in damage to the lung parenchyma and can present as diffuse bronchospasm, hypoxemia, and atelectasis. The pH of the gastric contents plays a role in the risk of developing a chemical pneumonitis, with decreased likelihood for contents with a pH greater than 2.5. Aspiration of partially digested food worsens the prognosis, as it may obstruct the airways and serve as a nidus for infection.

## TREATMENT OF GASTRIC ASPIRATION

Most cases of aspiration will likely manifest as a chemical pneumonitis rather than an infection; however, the initial steps to be taken remain the same. As soon as regurgitation is witnessed or suspected, the patient should be placed in the Trendelenburg position to allow for gastric contents to drain out of the mouth rather than into the trachea. Subsequently the pharynx and, if possible, the trachea should be thoroughly suctioned. The airway should be secured as soon as possible, and if gastric contents are noted in the oropharynx during intubation, they should immediately be suctioned before positive pressure ventilation, as this will prevent pushing gastric contents further into the lungs. Flexible bronchoscopy should be performed to further suction the aspirate, and rigid bronchoscopy may be needed if particulate matter is noted.[3] Broad spectrum antibiotics, pulmonary lavage, and corticosteroids are not recommended for routine use, but should be individualized to the patient.[3]

## ANESTHETIC CONSIDERATIONS

The following actions can be taken to minimize the morbidity related to aspiration of gastric contents.

## PREOPERATIVE

1. Perform a history and physical, noting diseases that increase the risk of aspiration, as discussed earlier.
2. Preoperative starvation: Inform patient of NPO guidelines: 2 hours for clear liquids, 4 hours for breast milk, 6 hours for infant formula, 6 hours for a light meal, and 8 hours for a large meal (fatty foods, fried foods, meat).[4]
3. Chemoprophylaxis: According to most recent ASA practice guidelines, gastrointestinal stimulants (metoclopramide), pharmacologic blockade of gastric acid secretion (histamine-2 receptor antagonists and proton pump inhibitors), and nonparticulate antacids may be administered preoperatively to patients at increased risk of aspiration. However, routine use of these agents is not recommended. In addition, anticholinergics are not recommended to reduce the risk of aspiration.[4]

## INTRAOPERATIVE

1. Airway protection with tracheal intubation, preferably inserted with rapid sequence induction.
2. Nasogastric tube (NG) placement: Evidence supporting the routine placement of NG tubes prior to induction is lacking. However, if an NG tube is in place, suctioning of the stomach should be performed.
3. Cricoid pressure: Historically, cricoid pressure has been recommended. However, in 2018, a large randomized double-blind trial failed to show cricoid pressure reduced the risk of pulmonary aspiration. In addition, it showed that cricoid pressure resulted in increased difficulty of tracheal intubation.[5]

## POSTOPERATIVE

1. Antiemetics: Administer prophylactically to prevent nausea and vomiting in patients with potentially altered airway reflexes as they recover from anesthesia. Also ensure appropriate antiemetics are available in the post-anesthesia care unit (PACU) in the event the patient experiences nausea or vomiting.
2. Extubation: This should only occur after patient is awake and meets all extubation criteria, with particular emphasis on ensuring neuromuscular blockade is fully reversed, oropharynx is suctioned, and protective airway reflexes are intact.

## REFERENCES

1. Benington S, Severn A. Preventing aspiration and regurgitation. *Anaesth Intensive Care Med*. 2007;8(9): 368–372.
2. Robinson M, et al. Aspiration under anaesthesia: Risk assessment and decision-making. *Cont Educ Anaesth Crit Care Pain*. 2014 Aug;14(4):171–175. https://doi.org/10.1093/bjaceaccp/mkt053 .

3. Nason KS. Acute intraoperative pulmonary aspiration. *Thorac Surg Clin*. 2015;25(3):301–307.
4. Practice guidelines for preoperative fasting and the use of pharmacologic agents to reduce the risk of pulmonary aspiration: Application to healthy patients undergoing elective procedures: An updated report by the American Society of Anesthesiologists Task Force on Preoperative Fasting and the Use of Pharmacologic Agents to Reduce the Risk of Pulmonary Aspiration. *Anesthesiology*. 2017;126(3):376–393.
5. Birenbaum A, et al. Effect of cricoid pressure compared with a sham procedure in the rapid sequence induction of anesthesia: The IRIS Randomized Clinical Trial. *JAMA Surg*. 2019;154(1):9–17.

# 150.

# MALIGNANT HYPERTHERMIA

*Priyanka H. Patel and David Matteson*

## INTRODUCTION

Malignant hyperthermia (MH) is a rare, life-threatening, genetic disorder triggered by volatile anesthetics and/or succinylcholine, the latter being the most common. Malignant hyperthermia is autosomal dominant, and the most common affiliated gene is the ryanodine receptor 1 (RYR1) calcium channel gene. This chapter will focus primarily on the genetics, pathophysiology, and anesthetic considerations of the disease.

## EPIDEMIOLOGY

The incidence of MH ranges from 1:10,000 to 1:250,000, though the prevalence of a genetic abnormality associated with MH susceptibility is 1 in 2000.[1] The disease affects all ethnicities, occurs more frequently in males, and has a higher documented incidence in children. Multiple anesthetic administrations may be required prior to manifestation of MH.[1] Mortality is >70% if unrecognized and untreated; proper treatment decreases mortality to <5%–10%.

## GENETICS

Malignant hyperthermia is inherited in an autosomal dominant pattern with variable penetrance and expression. The most common gene affiliated with MH is the RYR1 gene encoded on chromosome 19. A less common gene with known association to MH is the CACNA1S gene (calcium voltage-gated channel subunit alpha 1 S).[3]

## TESTING OPTIONS

The gold standard test for MH is the caffeine-halothane contracture test, which involves a muscle biopsy. The test is highly sensitive, which helps rule out the diagnosis of MH. However, the test has a 20% false-positive rate.[1] Those who have a positive contracture test are encouraged to undergo genetic testing to help determine MH susceptibility.

Genetic testing looks for mutations with known associations to MH, but there is a high false-negative rate, as not all mutations that cause MH have been identified. Regardless of the false-negative rate, patients prefer genetic testing to avoid the cost and invasive nature of the contracture test.

## PATHOPHYSIOLOGY

During normal skeletal muscle contraction, depolarization leads to a brief opening of the RYR1 channel located on the sarcoplasmic reticulum. Channel opening allows the efflux of calcium responsible for muscle contraction and propagation of depolarization, leading to further calcium release. The increase in intracellular calcium permits contraction by inhibiting the inhibitory effects of troponin.

**Table 150.1** CLINICAL SIGNS AND SYMPTOMS OF MALIGNANT HYPERTHERMIA

| | |
|---|---|
| Neurologic and neuromuscular | Hyperthermia, muscle rigidity, rhabdomyolysis, compartment syndrome |
| Cardiovascular | Tachycardia, arrhythmias, myocardial depression, myocardial ischemia |
| Respiratory | Respiratory acidosis, tachypnea, hypercarbia |
| Renal/fluids/ electrolytes | Metabolic/lactic acidosis, hyperkalemia, diaphoresis, acute kidney injury |
| Gastrointestinal and hepatobiliary | Liver injury/failure, bowel ischemia |
| Hematologic | Disseminated intravascular coagulation, general coagulopathy |

In patients with MH, the RYR1 channel defect leads to prolonged opening and, consequently, prolonged release of calcium, resulting in sustained muscle contraction. Prolonged contractions cause a global hypermetabolic state characterized by increased carbon dioxide ($CO_2$), heat production, oxygen consumption, and glucose metabolism.[3] As this cycle continues, there are many systemic sequalae that manifest. A summary of findings can be seen in Table 150.1.

### NEUROLOGIC AND NEUROMUSCULAR

Rising temperature (up to 1°–2°C every 5 minutes) is the hallmark of MH, but it can occur later in the disease process.[4] Hyperthermia increases oxygen demand and $CO_2$ production, leading to organ damage and dysfunction.

Sustained skeletal muscle contraction leads to generalized muscle rigidity, seen in 50%–80% of cases.[4] Specifically, masseter muscle rigidity is clinically significant and can make airway management difficult.[2]

Rhabdomyolysis, a late sequela of MH, occurs as cellular ATP is depleted, which causes acidosis, cellular membrane destruction, then cell death. It is recognized by monitoring for elevated creatine kinase and brown-colored urine caused by excretion of myoglobin. Compartment syndrome can be both a cause and result of rhabdomyolysis.

### CARDIOVASCULAR

The earliest sign of MH is unexplained tachycardia, especially when noticed with an increase in end-tidal $CO_2$ ($EtCO_2$).[4] Acidosis, electrolyte abnormalities, and increased metabolic demand can cause arrhythmias and myocardial depression. Myocardial infarction may occur, especially in patients with coexisting coronary artery disease.[2]

### RESPIRATORY

Hypercarbia is an early sign of MH but may be masked by increased minute ventilation. The rapid rise in $CO_2$ is attributed to the hypermetabolic state, leading to a metabolic acidosis, which in turn contributes to a respiratory acidosis (mixed metabolic and respiratory acidosis) unless minute ventilation is significantly increased.

### RENAL/FLUID/ELECTROLYTES

The hypermetabolic state of MH depletes ATP and glucose stores, leading to anaerobic metabolism, lactic acid production, and metabolic acidosis. Concurrently, destruction of muscle cells releases intracellular potassium and produces hyperkalemia, which is worsened by the metabolic acidosis.[2]

Hyperthermia can trigger diaphoresis (though this can be blunted by many anesthetic agents), which may contribute to hypovolemia and exaggerate electrolyte abnormalities.

Excessive myoglobin from rhabdomyolysis can precipitate in the renal tubules. This, coupled with increased metabolic demands, can lead to acute kidney injury.[4]

### GASTROINTESTINAL/HEPATOBILIARY

Widespread organ dysfunction and failure are notable complications of MH. This includes liver failure and bowel ischemia.

### HEMATOLOGIC

Disseminated intravascular coagulation is a late clinical sequala of MH due to hyperthermia and release of tissue thromboplastin.[5] The coagulopathy that results is due to overconsumption of coagulation factors, requiring transfusion of platelets and clotting factors.

## ANESTHETIC CONSIDERATIONS

A brief overview of the anesthetic management of patients with MH is presented here. However, a complete discussion on perioperative management of MH is not possible given the scope of this chapter. For additional details, please see the Malignant Hyperthermia Association of the United States at https://www.mhaus.org/.

### PREOPERATIVE

Patients with a personal or family history of MH should be identified prior to the day of the procedure. These patients should be the first case of the day in order to thoroughly prepare the anesthesia workstation and minimize the possibility of contamination.

The anesthesia workstation should be prepared according to manufacturer recommendations, which typically include replacing the $CO_2$ absorbent, removing vaporizers, flushing the system, and placing a new breathing circuit. Activated charcoal filters may be utilized to rapidly remove residual inhaled agents.

Succinylcholine should be removed from the room or protected from accidental use. Total intravenous anesthesia will be utilized in most situations with nondepolarizing muscle relaxants (NDMR) for paralysis. Difficult airways or the need for rapid sequence intubation should be identified and plans must be made accordingly.

Prior to starting the case, the designated MH cart (or equivalent) should be brought into or immediately outside the operating room. The cart should be regularly checked and stocked with unexpired medications, often in coordination with the hospital pharmacy.

### INTRAOPERATIVE

If you suspect MH intraoperatively:[2]

1. Call for help and notify all personnel in the room of discovery (initiate patient transfer if not at a facility capable of providing advanced care).
2. Discontinue volatile anesthetics and succinylcholine.
3. Hyperventilate and administer 100% oxygen.
4. Administer recommended dantrolene dose(s).
5. Ensure appropriate monitoring is utilized:
   a. Continuous electrocardiography, capnography, pulse oximetry, and frequent blood pressure monitoring
   b. Core temperature monitoring
   c. Urinary output
   d. Metabolic (renal/hepatic) and coagulation profile (arterial line will be required for serial blood gases)
   e. Consider additional IV access and/or central line placement.
6. Provide symptomatic and supportive care (Table 150.2).

### POSTOPERATIVE

Patients should be admitted to the intensive care unit for at least 24 hours of monitoring. There is a 25% incidence of

*Table 150.2* TREATMENT OF ACUTE MALIGNANT HYPERTHERMIA

| | |
|---|---|
| Administer dantrolene | Initial dose 2.5 mg/kg IV repeated every 5 minutes to effect or to a maximum of 10 mg/kg; limit can be exceeded if necessary. After successful treatment, it is then continued as 1mg/kg every 6 hours for 24–48 hours. |
| Maintain anesthesia if surgery must continue | Non-triggering agents only: IV anesthetics, narcotics, benzodiazepines, NDMR |
| Treat arrhythmias | Most standard antiarrhythmics are safe, but avoid calcium channel blockers (can cause myocardial depression) |
| Treat hyperkalemia | Sodium bicarbonate, insulin/glucose; refractory hyperkalemia: β-agonist, kayexalate, dialysis calcium chloride/gluconate for cardiac dysfunction/arrhythmias |
| Treat hyperthermia | Goal core temperature <38°C, cool IV fluids, ice packs on patient, lavage open body cavities, cardiopulmonary bypass or ECMO for extreme temperatures |
| Cardiac arrest | ACLS, consider ECMO |

MH recrudescence following the acute episode.[5] After recovery, patients and family members should be counseled for further workup and precautions.

### REFERENCES

1. Ellinas H, Albrecht MA. Malignant hyperthermia update. *Anesthesiol Clin.* 2020;38(1):165–181.
2. Guo GJ, Sutin KM. Neuromuscular blockers. In: Nelson LS, Howland M, Lewin NA, Smith SW, Goldfrank LR, Hoffman RS, eds. *Goldfrank's Toxicologic Emergencies*, 11th ed. New York, NY: McGraw-Hill; 2019. http://accessemergencymedicine. mhmedical.com.sladenlibrary.hfhs.org:2048/content.aspx?bookid=2569&sectionid=210274440.
3. Kaur H, et al. Malignant hyperthermia. *Mo Med.* 2019;116(2):154–159.
4. Kim D-C. Malignant hyperthermia. *Korean J Anesthesiol.* 2012;63(5):391.
5. Rosenberg H, et al. Malignant hyperthermia: A review. *Orphanet Journal of Rare Diseases.* 2015;10(1):1–19.

# 151.

# PAIN RELIEF

*Adi Cosic and Melinda M. Lawrence*

## INTRODUCTION

Pain, as described by the International Association for the Study of Pain (IASP), is "an unpleasant sensory and emotional experience associated with actual or potential tissue damage, or *described* in terms of such damage." Careful interpretation of this definition leads the reader to conclude that pain is a subjective and unique experience to each patient, and while this is true, it is also nearly a universal experience following surgery that can have unwanted lasting effects. Studies have shown that the prevalence of postoperative pain that can be as high as 35% for as long as 2 days following surgery, while others have demonstrated moderate to severe pain in as many as 13% of patients for as long as 2 weeks following surgery.[1,2] Further, the mismanagement of postoperative pain in some patients can lead to unfavorable chronic pain conditions.

## PAIN PATHWAYS

A thorough understanding of pain pathways, as well as the receptors involved in these pathways, is essential in the adequate management of postoperative pain. In a simplified explanation, surgical incisions cause injury to tissues, which leads to the release of inflammatory mediators (bradykinin, prostaglandins, etc.). These inflammatory molecules proceed to activate peripheral nociceptors, leading to transduction and transmission of information from the periphery to the central nervous system, and start the process of neurogenic inflammation via the release of substance P and calcitonin-related gene peptide, among others. The pain signals initiated by the peripheral nociceptors are generally transmitted by the primary pain nerve fibers, the A-delta and C fibers, to the dorsal horn of the spinal cord. At this point, descending modulatory input from the upper central nervous system (CNS) occurs via molecules such as serotonin, norepinephrine, enkaphalin, etc. Noxious stimuli almost always travel to the higher CNS centers, where cortical processing produces the perception of pain. Ultimately, a complex interaction between higher neurological function, such as memory and emotion, and the current ongoing pain occurs.

## EFFECTS OF PAIN ON THE BODY

Pain has multiple effects on the body in many body systems. The predominant neuroendocrine effects of pain involve the hypothalamic-pituitary-adrenocortical and sympathoadrenal effects, which include the release of catecholamines, catabolic hormones such as cortisol, and causes an overall hypermetabolic state with sympathetically dominant characteristics—a stress response. Clinically, this can be witnessed with signs such as a sudden increase in heart rate, blood pressure, sweating, and muscle tensing. Thought should be placed into the effects of the pain and the patient experiencing them. For example, in patients with comorbidities such as vascular disease, consideration should be taken into alleviating pain appropriately to decrease the sympathetic response, in an effort to decrease myocardial oxygen demand.

## CHRONIC PAIN AND SENSITIZATION

If pain is left untreated, and unremitting noxious stimulus is experienced by the peripheral nociceptors, sensitization of the receptors as well as activation of dormant receptors can occur. It is also possible to have central sensitization and hyperexcitability after strong, continuous noxious stimulus input from the periphery with correlation between sensitization and intensity of pain following surgery. Although the exact mechanism is still not fully understood, it is thought that an overload of information from the periphery causes a functional change in the dorsal horn of the spinal cord, a change in the interplay between the ascending and descending pain tracts, and new gene expression leading to sensitization in as little as 1 hour of acute pain. Currently, strong evidence points to the N-methyl-D-aspartate (NMDA) receptor as a central agent in the development of chronic pain after an acute injury.[4]

Chronic effects of postsurgical pain have also been studied. Chronic postsurgical pain (CPSP) is a condition that can rather quickly transition from acute pain after more complicated surgeries such as limb amputation, thoracotomy, and sternotomy. Predictive factors include the type of surgery, history of chronic pain, a genetic predisposition, and psychological factors. CPSP is a difficult condition to treat, and difficult to predict as well, making postoperative pain control all the more important.[5]

## TREATMENT OF PAIN

Treatment of postoperative pain relies, like many things, on a multimodal approach that targets numerous receptors involved in the pain response, as well as appropriate dosing and routing of the medication. By approaching pain control with medication, early mobilization, and enteral nutrition, attenuation of the surgical stress response can be achieved, leading to quicker recovery.

Generally, two broad classes of medications can be discussed, opioids and non-opioids. Opioids have historically been considered the cornerstone of pain management due to their theoretical absence of analgesic ceiling, limited only by their effects of respiratory depression, nausea, and constipation. In fact, save for the lack of amnesia, prolonged and painful surgeries can be performed solely under opioid analgesia. Their wide range of administration routes (epidural, oral, sublingual, transdermal, IV-PCA, etc.) also provides a flexible path to treatment. More recently there has been more interest in opioid-sparing perioperative pain treatment strategies.

Non-opioids, such as nonsteroidal anti-inflammatory drugs (NSAIDs) are a diverse group of medications that work by targeting the cyclo-oxygenase enzymes (both type 1 and 2) and block the synthesis of prostaglandins. Although the majority of these enzymes are located in the periphery, some are also located in the CNS and exhibit central effects. Pain relief achieved with NSAIDs may not always be as effective as that with opioids, but they do not have side effects like respiratory depression or death. NSAIDs are not completely devoid of negative effects; gastrointestinal upset via mucosal injury, renal dysfunction, and platelet aggregation dysfunction are common.

Regional anesthesia can also be employed as a powerful tool against pain. A diverse arsenal of techniques for limb as well axial surgery exists, and can be employed as either a single shot or catheter, with or without the aid of ultrasound guidance. The benefit of regional anesthesia is the limited side effects in comparison to opioid or non-opioid medication. Some unwanted effects do exist, however, such as local anesthetic toxicity, potential for bleeding, nerve damage, and injury to surrounding tissues.

## REFERENCES

1. Scher C, et al. Moving beyond pain as the fifth vital sign and patient satisfaction scores to improve pain care in the 21st century. *Pain Manag Nurs.* 2018;19(2):125–129.
2. Buvanendran A, et al. The incidence and severity of postoperative pain following inpatient surgery. *Pain Med.* 2015;16(12):2277–2283.
3. Mwaka G, et al. The prevalence of postoperative pain in the first 48 hours following day surgery at a tertiary hospital in Nairobi. *Afr Health Sci.* 2013;13(3):768–776.
4. Andrei P, et al. The role of N-methyl-D-aspartate (NMDA) receptors in pain: A review. *Anesth Analg.* 2003 Oct;97(4):1108–1116.
5. Bruce J, Quinlan J. Chronic post surgical pain. *Rev Pain.* 2011;5(3):23–29.

# 152.

# OPIOIDS

*Lauren McGinty*

## INTRODUCTION

Opioids have a wide variety of therapeutic uses due to their ability to relieve somatic, visceral, and neuropathic pain. These medications are commonly prescribed for cancer pain, chronic noncancer pain, end-of-life care, and for short-term use following an injury or surgery.[1] There are, however, many initiatives to decrease opioid use where appropriate, due to the opioid epidemic and risk for misuse and overdose, so these medications should be used with caution.

## MECHANISM OF ACTION

Opioids are substances that exert their actions by binding to mu (μ), kappa (κ), and/or delta (δ) opioid receptors in the central and peripheral nervous system. This can be done by endogenous opioid peptides, which consist primarily of endorphins, dynorphins, endomorphins, and enkephalins, or by exogenously administered opioid medications. Most clinically used opioids act primarily as μ receptor agonists. When agonists bind to opioid receptors, this allows for opening of potassium channels and also inhibits opening of voltage-gated calcium channels. This ultimately prevents release of pain neurotransmitters and decreases excitability of neurons.[1-3]

Most opioids have poor oral bioavailability, making it important to pay attention to dose conversions when switching between enteral and parenteral dosage forms. These medications generally have large volumes of distribution and undergo hepatic metabolism, followed by renal excretion. The duration of action for various opioids ranges dramatically, with remifentanil being ultra-short acting and agents like methadone having a variable and prolonged half-life.[1,3]

## ADVERSE EFFECTS AND PRECAUTIONS

Opioid medications carry many black box warnings in their prescribing information. Some are common among all opioids, including a warning that these agents expose users to risks of addiction, abuse, and misuse, which may lead to overdose and death. The prescribing info for these medications also includes a black box warning addressing serious, life-threatening, and potentially fatal respiratory depression, particularly following drug initiation or dose increases.[4]

Other notable side effects of opioids include sedation, dizziness, nausea/vomiting, constipation, and miosis. Patients may also experience euphoria, hypotension, pruritus, urinary retention, dysphoria, headache, biliary spasm, and cough suppression. Patients do develop tolerance to many of these adverse effects, but two notable exceptions are miosis and constipation. As a result, it is important to put patients on an adequate bowel regimen throughout the duration of their opioid use.[1,2] Fortunately, there are some situations in which opioid adverse effects can be used to benefit patients, such as giving codeine as an antitussive or tincture of opium as an antidiarrheal.

When possible, the use of concurrent opioids and benzodiazepines should be avoided due to the additive risk of central nervous system (CNS) and respiratory depression. Caution should also be used when giving opioids to patients who are elderly or have renal or hepatic dysfunction due to the higher likelihood of side effects. Morphine and meperidine, in particular, should be avoided or used in low doses in renal dysfunction, as their active metabolites are renally excreted and can accumulate and lead to significant toxicity. Patients who have impaired respiratory function from underlying diseases, such as chronic obstructive pulmonary disease, can be at higher risk for respiratory depression from opioids.[1,3,5]

Upon discontinuation or tapering of an opioid, it is important to watch for and manage withdrawal symptoms due to the potential development of physical dependence. These symptoms may include tachycardia, hypertension, anxiety, nausea, vomiting, diarrhea, sweating, lacrimation, and rhinorrhea.[1,3]

Opioids can also cause muscle rigidity, myoclonic or athetoid movements, vertical nystagmus, and biliary colic (due to spasm of sphincter of oddi through μ receptor

*Table 152.1* OPIOID CHARACTERISTICS[1-5]

| DRUG | MECHANISM OF ACTION | SYSTEMIC ROUTES OF ADMINISTRATION | SPECIAL PRECAUTIONS | OTHER |
|------|---------------------|-----------------------------------|---------------------|-------|
| Alfentanil | μ receptor agonist | IV | Risk of serotonin syndrome<br>Major substrate of CYP3A4 | Commonly used in the perioperative setting<br>Causes minimal or no histamine release |
| Buprenorphine | Partial μ receptor agonist and κ receptor antagonist | IV, IM, subQ, buccal, sublingual, transdermal, and subdermal | QTc prolongation<br>Major substrate of CYP3A4 | Can be used for pain management and opioid use disorder<br>Ceiling effect for pain relief |
| Butorphanol | μ and κ receptor agonist | IV, IM, and intranasal | Risk of serotonin syndrome | |
| Codeine | μ receptor agonist | PO | Major substrate of CYP2D6<br>Codeine (prodrug) is metabolized via CYP2D6 to morphine.<br>CYP2D6 ultra-rapid metabolizers may have excessive side effects, but CYP2D6 slow metabolizers derive little to no pain relief. | Typically used for its antitussive effect<br>Limited analgesic effect |
| Fentanyl | μ receptor agonist | IV, IM, subQ, transdermal, buccal, sublingual, intranasal, epidural, and intrathecal | Risk of serotonin syndrome<br>Major substrate of CYP3A4 | IV form commonly used in the perioperative setting<br>Causes minimal or no histamine release |
| Hydrocodone | μ receptor agonist | PO | Major substrate of CYP3A4 | |
| Hydromorphone | μ receptor agonist | PO, IV, IM, subQ, and rectal | | May be used in the perioperative setting |
| Meperidine | μ receptor agonist | PO, IV, IM, and subQ | Risk of serotonin syndrome<br>Use within 14 days of MAOIs is contraindicated.<br>Accumulation of active metabolite, normeperidine, can lead to tremors, delirium, and seizures. | Can be used for rigors and postoperative shivering<br>Use for chronic pain management has fallen out of favor due to toxicities.<br>No antitussive effect |
| Methadone | μ receptor agonist and N-methyl-D-aspartate (NMDA) antagonist | PO, IV, IM, and subQ | QTc prolongation<br>Risk of serotonin syndrome<br>Major substrate of CYP3A4 and CYP2B6<br>Prolonged and highly variable half-life: use caution when initiating and titrating dose | Can be used for pain and opioid use disorder<br>Does not cause significant euphoria |
| Morphine | μ receptor agonist | PO, IV, IM, subQ, rectal, epidural, and intrathecal | | May be used in the perioperative setting |
| Nalbuphine | κ receptor agonist and μ receptor antagonist | IV, IM, and subQ | | Can be used for pain management and to relieve opioid-induced pruritus |
| Oxycodone | μ and κ receptor agonist | PO | Major substrate of CYP3A4 | |
| Oxymorphone | μ receptor agonist | PO | | |

*Table 152.1* CONTINUED

| DRUG | MECHANISM OF ACTION | SYSTEMIC ROUTES OF ADMINISTRATION | SPECIAL PRECAUTIONS | OTHER |
|---|---|---|---|---|
| Remifentanil | μ receptor agonist | IV | Risk of serotonin syndrome | Fastest onset of action of any opioid (1–2 minutes) Commonly used in the perioperative setting Causes minimal or no histamine release |
| Sufentanil | μ receptor agonist | IV, sublingual, and epidural | Risk of serotonin syndrome Major substrate of CYP3A4 | IV form commonly used in the perioperative setting Causes minimal or no histamine release |
| Tapentadol | Weak μ receptor agonist and inhibitor of norepinephrine reuptake | PO | Risk of serotonin syndrome | |
| Tramadol | Weak μ receptor agonist and inhibitor of serotonin and norepinephrine reuptake | PO | Risk of serotonin syndrome Risk of seizures Major substrate of CYP3A4 and CYP2D6 | |

MAOIs: monoamine oxidase inhibitors;

phenomenon). Opioid-induced biliary colic can be treated with naloxone, glucagon, and nitroglycerin.

Additional information on specific opioids, mechanisms of action, routes of administration, and unique features or precautions are outlined in Table 152.1.

## REFERENCES

1. Yaksh T, Wallace M. Opioids, analgesia, and pain management. In: Brunton LL, Hilal-Dandan R, Knollmann BC, eds. *Goodman &* *Gilman's: The Pharmacological Basis of Therapeutics*. 13th ed. New York, NY: McGraw-Hill; 2018.
2. Waller DG, Sampson AP. Opioid analgesics and the management of pain. In: *Medical Pharmacology and Therapeutics*. 5th ed. Philadelphia, PA: Elsevier; 2018.
3. Lee MC, Abrahams M. Pain and analgesics. In: Brown MJ, Sharma P, Mir FA, Bennett PN, eds. *Clinical Pharmacology*. 12th ed. Philadelphia, PA: Elsevier; 2019.
4. Lexicomp Online, Lexi-Drugs, Hudson, OH: Lexi-Comp; August 1, 2020.
5. Brenner GM, Stevens CW. Opioid analgesics and antagonists. In: *Brenner and Stevens' Pharmacology*. 5th ed. Philadelphia, PA: Elsevier; 2018.

# 153.

# AGONIST-ANTAGONISTS

*Gaurav Trehan and Anish Sethi*

## INTRODUCTION

The agonist-antagonist opioid analgesics are a very interesting group of drugs with unique properties. Unlike pure opioid agonists (e.g., morphine), the agonist-antagonists either act as competitive inhibitors (exert no action on mu [μ] receptors) or partial agonists (cause limited action on the mu receptors). They may also have partial agonist activity on other receptors such as kappa and sigma. Examples include nalorphine, pentazocine, butorphanol, nalbuphine, buprenorphine, bremazocine, dezocine, and meptazinol, among others.

## KEY POINTS

- Strong enough analgesia to be used for moderate to severe pain.
- Shallow dose response curve with a ceiling effect on analgesia, but also on respiratory depression and gastrointestinal side effects such as constipation.
- Ceiling effect on analgesia, so may not be appropriate for cancer pain. In acute pain, use of pure opioid agonists is preferable.
- Low potential for diversion or abuse.
- Potential for dysphoric reactions.
- May precipitate withdrawal in patients on chronic opioid therapy.[1-3]

## MEDICATIONS

### NALBUPHINE

#### Action

Nalbuphine is a competitive antagonist at the mu receptors and a partial agonist at the kappa receptor. It exhibits strong antagonistic activity, and when administered to a patient dependent on chronic opioid therapy, it can precipitate withdrawal. At lower doses, nalbuphine is equipotent to morphine; but as with all drugs in this class, analgesia has a ceiling at higher doses. It is currently not regulated by the Controlled Substance Act (CSA).

#### Systemic Effects

Ceiling effect for respiratory depression is at 30 mg for adults.[4] Nalbuphine reduces cardiac workload and may reduce heart rate. It does not seem to affect the systemic blood pressure and pulmonary artery pressure.[2]

#### Administration

Intravenous, intramuscular, subcutaneous (IV, IM, SC): Usual adult dosages 10 mg repeated every 3–6 hours as needed for pain. 2.5–5 mg may be used for opioid-induced pruritus.

### PENTAZOCINE (TALWIN)

#### Action

Pentazocine acts as an antagonist on mu receptors and an agonist on kappa receptors. It is one-fifth as potent as morphine when given parenterally.[3] This is a schedule IV drug (CSA).

#### Systemic Effects

Ceiling to analgesia and respiratory depression may be at 30–70 mg.[2] Dysphoric effects are common with high doses (usually >60 mg). Pentazocine increases cardiac workload potentially by increasing plasma catecholamines—elevation in heart rate, left ventricle end-diastolic pressure, systemic and pulmonary artery pressure.[2] A pure mu agonist such as morphine is a better choice in patients with myocardial ischemia or infarction. Use limited by high incidence of postoperative nausea and vomiting.

## Administration

SC, IM, or IV: Usual dose is 30 mg every 3–4 hours (max. 360 mg/day). Oral: Pentazocine/naloxone (50mg/0.5 mg), 1 tablet every 3–4 hours (max 600 mg pentazocine).

### BUPRENORPHINE

### Action

Buprenorphine differs from the other agonist-antagonists. It is primarily a partial agonist at the mu receptor and an antagonist at the kappa and delta receptors. It is almost 33 times more potent than morphine. It has a high affinity and a relatively low intrinsic activity at the mu receptors. It can displace other mu agonists (e.g., morphine) from the receptor and reduces opioid binding by 80% to 95%; this may potentially precipitate withdrawal when given to patients who are dependent on chronic opioid therapy.[2] This is a schedule III drug per the CSA.

### Systemic Effects

The ceiling effect for respiratory depression is at 0.15–1.2 mg in adults.[2] The ceiling effect phenomenon has raised concern that prescribers and patients might get a false sense of security that buprenorphine is not likely to cause any adverse reactions. Some recent studies have suggested that in opioid naïve patients, especially children, the respiratory depression might occur before the ceiling is reached.[5] Buprenorphine may prolong the QT interval. It tends to reduce cardiac workload, systemic blood pressure, as well as heart rate.[2] Compared to other drugs in this class, buprenorphine is likely to cause a greater increase in intrabiliary pressure.

### Administration

Buprenorphine has very low bioavailability of <15%.[4] Multiple formulations are available (Table 153.1).

### Indications

Chronic opioid use may result in changes in the neural reward pathways. Buprenorphine, on the other hand, reduces brain responses to opioid-induced cues and thus may lessen the potential for opioid abuse. Patients on buprenorphine maintenance for OUD are at a potentially higher risk for relapsing. Every attempt should be made to avoid changes to the buprenorphine therapy in the perioperative setting. A multimodal pain management approach is the backbone for treatment plans, utilizing non-opioid adjuncts and regional/neuraxial anesthetic techniques. Active discussions between the patient and proceduralist, in consultation with the primary prescriber, are par for the course.

For minor procedures with none or low anticipated postoperative opioid requirements, the recommendation is to continue buprenorphine therapy. Similarly, those on low dose buprenorphine (≤8 mg daily sublingual equivalent) may continue their buprenorphine regardless of the magnitude of the surgery. Patients on high dose buprenorphine (>24 mg daily sublingual equivalent) may gain analgesic benefit from tapering down their doses prior to the procedure. This is not recommended for patients at high risk for OUD relapse. Complete discontinuation of buprenorphine therapy is usually not recommended.[4]

### BUTORPHANOL

### Action

Butorphanol is a kappa receptor agonist and a very weak mu antagonist or a partial agonist. It therefore produces a mild withdrawal when given to patients who are dependent on chronic opioid therapy. It is 5–8 times as potent as morphine when given parenterally. This is a schedule IV drug per the CSA.

### Systemic Effects

Ceiling effect for respiratory depression is at 30–60 mcg/kg. Butorphanol usually results in an increase in cardiac workload and pulmonary artery pressure. Systemic blood pressure and heart rate tend to be equivocal.[2] Butorphanol may cause sweating, nausea, drowsiness, and CNS stimulation. Acute biliary spasm can occur, but biliary pressure is lower that after equipotent fentanyl or morphine

### Administration

Toxicity can be reversed with naloxone. Reduce dose by 50% in hepatic and renal impairment. Intramuscular: 2 mg every 3–4 hours as needed. Intravenous: 1 mg every 3–4 hours as needed. Intranasal (indicated for migraine and postoperative pain): 1 mg (1 spray from the metered-dose device) repeated in 60–90 minutes if needed. The 2-dose sequence may then be repeated every 3–4 hours as needed.

Table 153.1 FORMULATIONS OF BUPRENORPHINE WITH APPROXIMATE EQUIVALENT DOSING[a]

| ROUTE | BRAND NAME | INCLUDES NALOXONE | FORMULATION | AVAILABLE STRENGTHS[b] | ADMIN FREQUENCY | MAXIMUM RECOMMENDED DAILY DOSE | BIOAVAILABILITY (%) | FDA INDICATIONS | EQUIVALENT DOSE TO BUPRENORPHINE 8 MG SUBLINGUAL |
|---|---|---|---|---|---|---|---|---|---|
| Buccal | Bunavail | Yes | Film | 2.1 mg/0.3 mg, 4.2 mg/0.7 mg, 6.3 mg/1 mg | Once daily | 12.6 mg/2.1 mg | 50–60c | Opioid dependence | 4.2 mg/0.7 mg |
| Buccal | BelBuca | No | Film | 75 mg, 150 mg, 300 mg, 450 mg, 600 mg, 750 mg, 900 mg | Every 12 hours | 1800 mg in divided doses | 46–65 | Pain, chronic | Maximum dose less than 8 mg SL |
| Intradermal | Probuphine | No | Implant | 80 mg | Replaced every 6 months | 320 mg | 31 | Opioid dependance | 320 mg once every 6 months is equivalent to 8 mg/day[c] |
| Injection (IV) | Buprenex | No | Injection solution | 0.3 mg/ml | Every 6 hours as needed | N/A | 100 | Pain, acute | 2.4 mg per day in divided doses[d] |
| Subcutaneous ER | Sublocade | No | SC injection | 100 mg/0.5 mL, 300 mg/1.5 ml | Monthly | 300 mg monthly | 60–80 | Moderate-to-severe opioid use disorder | 100 mg once every month is equivalent to 8–12 mg/day[c] |
| Sublingual | Generic | No | Tablet | 2 mg, 8 mg | Once daily | 24 mg | 29 ± 10 | Opioid dependance | 8 mg |
| Sublingual | Zubsolv | Yes | Tablet | 0.7 mg/0.18 mg, 1.4 mg/0.36 mg, 2.9 mg/0.71 mg, 5.7 mg/1.4 mg, 8.6 mg/2.1 mg, 11.4 mg/2.9 mg | Once daily | 17.2 mg/4.2 mg | 40–50c | Opioid dependance | 5.7 mg/1.4 mg |
| Sublingual | Suboxone, generic | Yes | Film | 2 mg/0.5 mg, 4 mg/1 mg, 8 mg/2 mg, 12 mg/3 mg | Once daily | 24 mg/6 mg | 29±10 | Opioid dependance | 8 mg/2 mg |
| Transdermal | Butrans, generic | No | Patch | 5 mg/h, 75 mg/h, 10 mg/h, 15 mg/h, 20 mg/h | Every 7 days | 20 mg/h once weekly | 15 | Pain, chronic | Maximum dose less than 8 mg SL |

[a] ER: extended release; FDA: US Food and Drug Administration; IM: intramuscularly; IV: intravenously; N/A: not available; SC: subcutaneously.

[b] Doses provided as buprenorphine/naloxone when naloxone present, otherwise presented as buprenorphine dose.

[c] EXTRAPOLATED from package insert information.

[d] Equivalent dose extrapolated from bioavailability data.

Reproduced with permission from Warner SN et al. A Practical Approach for the Management of the Mixed Opioid Agonist-Antagonist Buprenorphine During Acute Pain and Surgery. Mayo Clin Proc. 2020 Jun;95(6):1253–1267. doi: 10.1016/j.mayocp.2019.10.007.

## REFERENCES

1. Hoskin PJ, Hanks GW. Opioid agonist-antagonist drugs in acute and chronic pain states. Review article. *Drugs*. 1991;41(3):326–344.
2. Zola EM, McLeod DC. Comparative effects of analgesic efficacy of the agonist-antagonist opioids. *Drug Intell Clin Pharm*. 1983;17:411.
3. Flood P, et al. *Stoelting's Pharmacology and Physiology in Anesthetic Practice*. 5th ed. Philadelphia, PA: Lippincott Williams & Wilkins; 2015.
4. Warner NS, Warner MA, Cunningham JL, et al. A practical approach for the management of the mixed opioid agonist-antagonist buprenorphine during acute pain and surgery. *Mayo Clin Proc*. 2020;95(6):1253–1267.
5. Centers for Disease Control and Prevention (CDC). Buprenorphine prescribing practices and exposures reported to a poison center—Utah, 2002–2011. *MMWR Morb Mortal Wkly Rep*. 2012;61(49):997–1001.

# 154.

# ALPHA-2 AGONISTS

*Balazs Horvath and Benjamin Kloesel*

## INTRODUCTION

Alpha-2 adrenergic receptors are present in both the central (CNS) and the peripheral nervous system (PNS). Alpha-2 adrenergic receptor agonists were originally developed to manage hypertension by inhibiting endogenous norepinephrine release that results in vasodilation and bradycardia.

Clonidine was the first alpha-2 receptor agonist that was approved for human clinical use. It was first introduced in chronic pain management and subsequently became an integral element of perioperative balanced multimodal analgesia. However, clonidine is not selective to the alpha-2 receptor, and by blocking the binding of catecholamines to alpha-1 receptors it frequently induces hypotension, an unwanted side effect for pain management purposes. This led to the development of dexmedetomidine, which is an 8 times more selective alpha-2 receptor agonist compared to clonidine.[1,2]

The sedative effect of alpha-2 agonists is mediated by the locus coeruleus without inhibiting the respiratory center that is found in the same region. Analgesia is attributed to two mechanisms. Inhibition of the medullospinal tract via the presynaptic alpha-2 receptors–mediated modulation of norepinephrine release augments the antinociceptive effect of the descending inhibitory pathway.[1,3] Postsynaptic alpha-2 receptor stimulation in the dorsal horn of the spinal cord decreases the release of excitatory neurotransmitters, such as glutamate and substance P. Both A delta– and C fiber–mediated reflexes and central sympathetic activity are attenuated.[5] This mechanism inhibits the ascending nociceptive pathway, resulting in analgesia, sedation, and reduced anesthetic requirement. In the PNS, alpha-2 receptor stimulation also inhibits spinal substance P release and nociceptive neuron transmission at the presynaptic and postsynaptic receptors in the spinal cord. These mechanisms inhibit the propagation of a noxious signal from the periphery to the higher cerebral centers.

The rostral ventrolateral medulla is responsible for the cardiovascular effects of the alpha-2 agonists by modulating the sympathetic nervous system. The resulting decrease of the sympathetic outflow and concomitant increased parasympathetic tone are responsible for bradycardia, vasodilation, and hypotension.[1,2]

## PHARMACOKINETICS

### CLONIDINE

Clonidine is a highly lipid-soluble compound with fast redistribution in adipose tissue. Its bioavailability is 70%–95% when administered orally and transdermally; 20%–40% is bound to protein in the serum. The drug is metabolized by the liver into inactive metabolites that are primarily cleared by renal excretion. Its elimination half-life depends on age and route of administration: neonates 22–40 hours; children 8–12 hours; adults 12–16 hours; transdermal patch 20 hours (after patch removal); cerebrospinal fluid 1.3 hours.

## DEXMEDETOMIDINE

Dexmedetomidine is highly lipophilic and the majority is found in protein-bound form in the serum. It is readily redistributed to peripheral tissue compartments with a distribution half-life of about 5–7 minutes. The elimination half-life is approximately 2 hours. When administered parenterally the context-sensitive half-time is approximately 4 minutes after an initial 10-minute bolus and increases to more than 250 minutes after an 8-hour long continuous infusion. Dexmedetomidine is deactivated by hepatic metabolism via glucuronidation and by cytochrome P2A6 oxidation. The vast majority of the inactive metabolites are excreted by the kidneys, and a small fraction is eliminated in the feces.

## PHARMACODYNAMICS

### CLONIDINE

Receptor site affinity: Alpha-2 > Alpha-1 (200:1).

### DEXMEDETOMIDINE

Receptor site affinity: Alpha-2 > Alpha-1 (1,600:1).

### EFFECTS OF ALPHA-2 ADRENORECEPTOR STIMULATION ON THE ORGAN SYSTEMS

### CNS

- Decreased sympathetic outflow, decreased A delta– and C fiber–mediated somato-sympathetic reflexes, sedation, analgesia, reduction in anesthetic agent requirements, decreased cerebral blood flow, decreased cerebral metabolic rate of oxygen, decreased intracranial and intraocular pressures

### Cardiovascular

- Decreased heart rate, decreased blood pressure, decreased systemic vascular resistance, no effect on contractility and cardiac output.

### Respiratory System

- Insignificant respiratory depression when administered alone in children and adults; apnea has been described in neonates, potentiation of opioid induced respiratory depression, upper airway obstruction.

### Renovascular System

- Decreased renovascular resistance, increased diuresis, decreased serum catecholamine concentrations, decreased activity of the renin-angiotensin system.

### Endocrine

- Inhibition of insulin secretion.

### Drug Interactions

- Decreased anesthetic requirement, decreased MAC of volatile anesthetic agents, increased sensitivity to opioid induced respiratory depression, tricyclic antidepressant, phenothiazines, and butyrophenones; co-administration may result in increased unwanted side effects.
- Clonidine and dexmedetomidine are used widely in contemporary anesthesia practice.[1-4] Alpha-2 adrenoreceptor agonists can be administered *via* different routes (see Tables 154.1 and 154.2). Compared to clonidine, dexmedetomidine has 8 times higher affinity to the alpha-2 receptor, and is a more versatile drug with less significant side effects for perianesthetic and periprocedural purposes. In addition, unlike clonidine, dexmedetomidine can be given and titrated as continuous infusion with minor respiratory and cardiovascular side effects.
- The side effects of clonidine and dexmedetomidine administration are airway obstruction (continuous dexmedetomidine infusion) apnea (neonates), hypotension, bradycardia, rebound hypertension, hypertension with reflex bradycardia (high doses, via alpha-1 receptor stimulation in the peripheral vascular musculature causing vasoconstriction), drowsiness, and dry mouth. Common contraindications to alpha-2 agonists are bradycardia, prolonged P-R interval, AV-block, severe valvular stenosis with decreased cardiac output, hypovolemia, and hepatic dysfunction/failure.[1-3]

*Table 154.1* PERIOPERATIVE CLONIDINE ADMINISTRATION

| ROUTE | ADULT | PEDIATRIC |
|---|---|---|
| Oral | 0.1–0.2 mg | 2–4 mcg/kg |
| Intrathecal adjuvant | 15–150 mcg | 1 mcg/kg |
| Caudal adjuvant | — | 1 mcg/kg |
| Continuous epidural adjuvant | 0.1 mcg/kg/HR | 1–2 mcg/mL |
| Peripheral nerve block adjuvant | Unknown (30–150 mcg) | 1.5 mcg/kg |

**Table 154.2 PERIOPERATIVE DEXMEDETOMIDINE ADMINISTRATION**

| ROUTE | ADULT | PEDIATRIC |
|---|---|---|
| Oral | 2–4 mcg/kg | 4 mcg/kg |
| Nasal | 0.5–1 mcg/kg | 1–2 mcg/kg |
| Intravenous (IV) bolus | 0.5–1 mcg/kg | 0.5–1 mcg/kg |
| Continuous IV sedation | 0.5–1 mcg/kg loading: 10 min 0.2–0.7 mcg/kg/h | 0.5–1 mcg/kg loading: 10 min 0.2–0.5 mcg/kg/h |
| Intrathecal adjuvant | 5 mcg | — |
| Caudal adjuvant | — | 1–2 mcg/kg |
| Epidural adjuvant | 0.25–1 mcg/mL | Insufficient data |
| Peripheral nerve block adjuvant | 1–2 mcg/kg | 1 mcg/kg |

## PREOPERATIVE UTILIZATION

- Anxiolysis: dexmedetomidine

## INTRAOPERATIVE UTILIZATION

- Sedation for diagnostic and minor therapeutic procedures: dexmedetomidine
- Adjuvant to general anesthesia: dexmedetomidine
- Regional anesthesia: clonidine and dexmedetomidine
- Balanced multimodal anesthesia and analgesia: dexmedetomidine
- Prevention of post-anesthesia agitation: dexmedetomidine
- Decrease the incidence of postoperative nausea and vomiting (PONV): dexmedetomidine

## POSTOPERATIVE UTILIZATION

- Treatment of postoperative agitation, emergence delirium: dexmedetomidine
- Management of postoperative shivering: clonidine and dexmedetomidine
- Extended sedation in the recovery room and in intensive care unit (ICU): dexmedetomidine.

Table 154.1 and Table 154.2 summarize the route of administration and doses of clonidine and dexmedetomidine.

## REFERENCES

1. Nguyen V, et al. Alpha-2 agonists. *Anesthesiol Clin.* 2017;35(2):233.
2. Kamibayashi T, Maze M. Clinical uses of α2-adrenergic agonists *Anesthesiology.* 2000;93(5):1345–1349.
3. Giovannitti JA, et al. Alpha-2 adrenergic receptor agonists: A review of current clinical applications. *Anesth Prog.* 2015;62(1):31.
4. Prabhakar A, et al. Adjuvants in clinical regional anesthesia practice: A comprehensive review. *Best Pract Res Clin Anaesthesiol.* 2019;33(4):415–423.

# 155.

# NONSTEROIDAL ANTI-INFLAMMATORY DRUGS (NSAIDS)

*Austin Reilly and Dalia Elmofty*

## INTRODUCTION

The basis of nonsteroidal anti-inflammatory drug (NSAID) therapy began in the fourth century BC, when people were advised to chew willow bark to treat fever and musculoskeletal pains.[1] Salicin is the active ingredient in willow bark. It was isolated in 1828, and commercial production of acetylsalicylic acid, under the brand name Aspirin, began in 1874.[2] Nonselective NSAIDs (nsNSAIDs) came to market in the 1960s with the introduction of ibuprofen, followed by indomethacin, diclofenac, and naproxen.[2] In 1971, John Vane and Priscilla Piper were credited with describing the mechanism of action for NSAIDs by inhibiting prostaglandin synthesis.[1] The two isoforms of cyclooxygenase (COX) enzymes, COX-1 and COX-2, were later discovered.

## CLASSIFICATION

### NONSELECTIVE NSAIDS

Nonselective NSAIDs (nsNSAIDs) inhibit both COX-1 and COX-2 enzymes; these enzymes are expressed in numerous organs and tissue types. Prostaglandin end products are involved in a wide range of physiologic and pathologic processes. Prostaglandins from COX-1 activity regulate renal function, protect gastrointestinal mucosal, and aggregate platelets.[3] Prostaglandins from COX-2 activity increase body temperature, propagate inflammation, and sensitize perception of pain.[3]

### COX-2 SELECTIVE NSAIDS

COX-2 selective NSAIDs (sNSAIDS) have a higher affinity for the COX-2 active binding site than the binding site for COX-1.[3] COX-1 is constitutively expressed, but COX-2 activity is induced by inflammatory mediators and cytokines.[2] sNSAIDs were developed in an attempt to decrease inflammation and pain from inflammatory mediators without incurring the bleeding, renal dysfunction, blood pressure dysregulation, and gastrointestinal distress side effects of nsNSAIDs.[2]

## MECHANISM OF ACTION

### ARACHIDONIC ACID PATHWAY

Phospholipase A2 is an enzyme that increases the release of arachidonic acid (AA) from phospholipids.[3] AA is catalyzed by COX into prostaglandin G2 (PG2), which is converted into prostaglandin H2.[3] These intermediates become various forms of prostaglandins, thromboxanes, and prostacyclins via tissue specific synthases.[3]

NSAIDs inhibit AA from binding to the active site on COX. COX inhibition decreases the production of prostanoids, such as prostaglandins and prostacyclins. NSAIDs decrease the production of these molecules, resulting in symptom relief from fever, inflammation, and pain sensitization.

### ANTIPYRETIC

Body temperature is regulated by the hypothalamus. An increase in COX-2 activity and an increase in prostaglandin E2 (PGE2) production increases internal body temperature through effects at the hypothalamus.[3] NSAIDs decrease body temperature by inhibiting COX activity.

### PAIN SENSITIZATION

PGE2 induces peripheral (peripheral nerves/tissues) and central (brain/spinal cord) sensitization to pain.[3] The spinal cord contains both COX-1 and COX-2, indicating that both are involved in modulating nociception.[3] NSAIDs provide analgesia by inhibiting COX activity.

## INFLAMMATION

Inflammation and edema in tissue are increased by the production of PGE2 and prostacyclin (PGI2).[3] PGE2 and PGI2 increase vasodilation, vascular permeability, and attract leukocytes.[3] NSAIDs decrease PGE2 and PGI2 production.

## PHARMACOLOGY

### COX-2 SELECTIVITY

The IC80 is an ex vivo assay that can predict the potency and COX-2/COX-1 selectivity of NSAIDs in vivo.[3] IC50 is the concentration of an NSAID needed to achieve 50% inhibition of COX enzyme activity.[3] IC80 was used instead of IC50 because standard dosing of an NSAID achieves plasma concentrations in the range that produce 80% inhibition of COX enzymes.[3] Dividing the IC80 of the COX-2 enzyme by the IC80 of the COX-1 enzyme gives you the IC80 ratio (COX-2/COX-1), allowing for COX-2 selectivity comparison between different NSAIDs.

### ABSORPTION

NSAIDs are well absorbed following oral ingestion, conferring a high bioavailability (80%–100%).[3] Peak plasma concentrations are observed within 2–3 hours.[3] Food intake may delay absorption but rarely affects systemic availability.

### CIRCULATION

NSAIDs are highly bound to plasma proteins (90%–95%).[3] Sufficient plasma concentration is achieved by most NSAIDs to produce central analgesic effects.[2] There is variability between different NSAIDs on their distribution into inflamed tissues and subsequent ability to produce peripheral analgesia.

### CLEARANCE

NSAIDs are cleared hepatically and excreted as inactivated metabolites renally.[3] Hepatic biotransformation of NSAIDs varies and either occurs by both phase I (oxidation, hydroxylation, demethylation) and phase II (glucuronidation, conjugation) or phase II reaction.[3] Clearance of NSAIDs is reduced in elderly populations.[3]

## SIDE EFFECTS/TOXICITY

### GASTROINTESTINAL (GI)

The use of nsNSAIDs increases the risk of serious upper GI injury by 3- to 4-fold compared to no NSAID use.[2] The mechanism of GI insult is due to the inhibition of COX-1 activity, which is an important component of regulating GI mucosal integrity.

The use of sNSAIDs results in a lower risk of GI injury compared to nsNSAIDs due to their higher COX-2/COX-1 activity. Risk factors that increase the incidence of developing GI injury include high NSAID dose, elderly patient, and concomitant use of aspirin.[2]

### CARDIOVASCULAR

Vascular endothelium expresses COX-1 and COX-2, producing prostacyclin which inhibits platelet aggregation, causes vasodilation, and natriuresis.[4] Platelets express only COX-1 and produce thromboxane A2 (TXA2) which stimulates platelet aggregation, vasoconstriction, and cardiac remodeling.[4] Disrupting the balance of this physiology can increase blood pressure, retain body fluid, and increase thrombotic events.

#### Myocardial Infarction (MI)

NSAIDs are associated with an increased risk of MI and perioperative mortality. This association was prevalent in patients with preexisting coronary artery disease (CAD).[4] NSAIDs that carried the highest risk for MI and perioperative mortality were include diclofenac and ibuprofen.[4] Naproxen carried the lowest cardiovascular risk profile.[4]

#### Heart Failure

Patients with heart failure should avoid NSAIDs due to the risk of increased blood pressure and fluid retention.[4] Observational and population-based studies showed an increased risk of hospitalization for heart failure exacerbations in patients taking NSAIDs with established heart failure.[4]

### BONE HEALING

NSAIDs decrease bone healing due to its effect on PGE2, although evidence is limited.[5] In animal and in-vitro studies, osteoblast activity is increased by PGE2.[5] NSAIDs decrease bone union by inhibiting COX activity.

## ANESTHETIC CONSIDERATIONS

### PREOPERATIVE BLEEDING

TXA2 is a powerful platelet aggregator produced by platelets. NSAIDs decrease TXA2 production by inhibiting COX-1 and increase the risk of perioperative bleeding. NSAIDs should be discontinued before surgery, and special attention should be taken when regional or neuraxial anesthesia techniques are planned. NSAIDs are to be discontinued for different lengths of time prior to interventions based on their duration of action. The American Society of Regional Anesthesia (ASRA) guidelines are a helpful resource in guiding perioperative medication management. Aspirin impairs platelet function for the life of the platelet (7–10 days). Some patients may have aspirin-induced asthma; patients will typically have a history of perennial vasomotor rhinitis with development of nasal polyps.

## INTRAOPERATIVE

Ketorolac is commonly used intraoperatively. It is administered intravenously and is a powerful analgesic. Risks and benefits should be evaluated before administering when the following concerns pertain to your patient: surgical bleeding, GI bleeding, renal insufficiency, heart failure, CAD, delayed bone healing, and neuraxial anesthesia.

## POSTOPERATIVE

NSAIDs should be avoided postoperatively in elderly patients and patients who had major orthopedic surgeries such as spinal fusions due to their negative effects on bone healing. Surgeries in which cadaveric bone grafts were used are of special importance, although the recommended time of avoidance is not well established.[5]

## REFERENCES

1. Vane JR, Botting RM. Mechanism of action of nonsteroidal anti-inflammatory drugs. *Am J Med*. 1998 Mar 30;104(3A):2S–8S.
2. Conaghan PG. A turbulent decade for NSAIDs: Update on current concepts of classification, epidemiology, comparative efficacy, and toxicity. *Rheumatol Int*. 2011;32(6):1491–1502.
3. Calatayud S, Esplugues JV. Chemistry, pharmacodynamics, and pharmacokinetics of NSAIDs. In *NSAIDs and Aspirin*. Cham: Springer; 2016:3–16.
4. Schjerning A-M, et al. Cardiovascular effects and safety of (non-aspirin) NSAIDs. *Nature Rev Cardiol*. 2020;17(9):574–584.
5. Wheatley BM, Nappo KE, Christensen DL, Holman AM, Brooks DI, Potter BK. Effect of NSAIDs on bone healing rates: A meta-analysis. *JAAOS—Journal of the American Academy of Orthopaedic Surgeons*. 2019 Apr 1;27(7):e330-6.

# 156.

# N-METHYL-D-ASPARTATE (NMDA) RECEPTOR ANTAGONISTS

*Ethan R. Leonard and Maxim S. Eckmann*

## INTRODUCTION

N-methyl-D-aspartate (NMDA) receptor antagonists are a group of drugs used widely in medicine as anesthetics. NMDA receptor antagonists induce a state of dissociative anesthesia, that causes a patient to have distorted perceptions of sight and sound and produces feelings of detachment between the patient and the environment. NMDA receptor antagonists and synthetic opioids with NMDA receptor antagonistic properties are sometimes used as recreational drugs due to their euphoric and hallucinogenic effects.[1]

NMDA receptors are located at many excitatory glutamate synapses in the central nervous system. NMDA receptor dysfunction can be linked to a variety of central nervous system disorders including epilepsy, and Alzheimer's, Huntington's, and Parkinson's disease.

## NMDA ANTAGONIST PHARMACEUTICAL AGENTS

There are several NMDA receptor antagonist agents available with varied routes of administration, including intravenous, oral, and intramuscular preparations. Table 156.1 outlines the most common agents used to treat pain and gives a summary of dosing and common side effects.[2] The main side effects in adults include hallucinations, light-headedness, dizziness, fatigue, headache, out-of-body sensation, nightmares, and sensory changes. Developed from phencyclidine, which was not clinically useful due to its potency and limited therapeutic window, ketamine has the strongest affinity for the NMDA receptor among currently available NMDA active pharmaceuticals. The other agents outlined are weaker NMDA receptor blockers. Because ketamine is the strongest clinically used NMDA antagonist, it is the least tolerable of the agents and has higher incidence of hallucinations and dissociative mental state.

### KETAMINE

Currently, ketamine is the most thoroughly studied NMDA receptor antagonist and is commonly used for induction of anesthesia and rapid sequence intubation. It also acts as a sympathomimetic and can be useful for induction of hypotensive patients. Current dose recommendations are 0.5–2 mg/kg, or 0.5–1 mg/kg in patients with shock. Lower doses may be used with concurrent administration of an additional sedative (e.g., midazolam). Ketamine can also be used perioperatively in subanesthetic doses to treat pain for patients whose pain is poorly controlled with opioids alone due to tolerance, or for extremely painful surgical procedures.

### METHADONE

Methadone is a synthetic opioid that is a μ-opioid receptor agonist and NMDA receptor antagonist that is commonly used to treat opioid dependence disorder. Methadone has proven to be effective in treating patients whose chronic pain is poorly controlled or who experience dose-limiting adverse effects of other opioids.[3] Methadone has a logarithmic equianalgesic estimation based on daily dose as well, requiring vigilance with dose conversion to other opioid analgesics. QT prolongation is a known side effect of methadone.

### MEMANTINE

Memantine is typically used to treat Alzheimer's disease and is currently being studied for use in chronic pain reduction, although its benefits remain unclear.[4]

### DEXTROMETHORPHAN

Dextromethorphan is a drug commonly used as an over-the-counter (OTC) cough suppressant, and research suggests that it can be used to reduce postoperative opioid consumption.[5]

## NMDA PERIOPERATIVE ADMINISTRATION

### CONSCIOUS SEDATION OR GENERAL ANESTHESIA

Ketamine is the NMDA antagonist drug of choice for procedures that require conscious sedation of the patient or general anesthesia. Ketamine produces bronchodilation, making it among the most beneficial drugs for induction of anesthesia in patients with severe asthma or acute bronchial constriction. Ketamine has hemodynamic advantages over other traditional anesthetic drugs and is the agent of choice for patients who are hemodynamically unstable or at risk of becoming hemodynamically unstable, including patients who are in shock, hemorrhaging, or hypotensive. Ketamine is known to increase sympathetic tone, subsequently increasing blood pressure, heart rate, and cardiac output. Anesthesia induction by ketamine is also known to maintain the patient's airway reflexes and respiratory drive. Other advantages of ketamine as an induction agent include that it has a rapid onset and recovery after intravenous administration and that alternative routes of administration are available in the event that intravenous infusion is not accessible.

Ketamine should not be used in cases where sympathomimetic effects could prove detrimental, such as patients with high blood pressure, increased heart rate, ischemic heart disease, pulmonary hypertension, and right heart dysfunction. Adverse neurologic effects include hallucinations, vivid dreams, and nightmares as the effects of the drug begin to wear off. Increased cerebral blood flow and intracranial pressure (ICP) are also side effects of ketamine as an induction agent.

### ACUTE PAIN MANAGEMENT

Ketamine has been thoroughly studied in the treatment of acute postoperative pain and has been shown to be an effective analgesic with concurrent opioid use. Current evidence-based contraindications include poorly controlled cardiovascular disease, severe hepatic dysfunction, elevated intracranial or intraocular pressure, and active psychosis. The other NMDA receptor antagonists require further study to determine their efficacy in perioperative pain management.

**Table 156.1** NMDA ANTAGONISTS FOR PAIN MANAGEMENT[2]

| DRUG | ANALGESIC DOSING | SIDE EFFECTS |
|---|---|---|
| Ketamine | IM: 2–4 mg/kg<br>IV: 0.2–0.75 mg/kg<br>Continuous IV infusion: 2–7 mcg/kg/min | *CNS effects*: hallucinations, confusion, dream-like state, irrational behavior<br>*Other effects*: respiratory depression, increased CSF pressure, hypertension, tachycardia, tremor, nystagmus, myocardial depression |
| Methadone | Opioid naïve: Initial dose, 2.5–10 mg q8–12h (interval may range from 4–12h as analgesic duration is short during initial therapy, although it increases with prolonged therapy)<br>Opioid tolerant: Oral morphine to oral methadone conversion is variable | CNS depression, respiratory depression, QTc prolongation, constipation, nausea and vomiting, dizziness, disorientation |
| Memantine | PO: 10–30 mg/day | Hypertension, dizziness, drowsiness, confusion, anxiety, hallucinations, cataract |
| Dextromethorphan | PO: 45–400 mg/day | Light headedness, drowsiness, confusion. Nervousness, visual disturbances, serotonin syndrome |

## CHRONIC PAIN

Ketamine use for the treatment of chronic pain has been an area of research interest over the past couple of decades. Current data suggest that intravenous (IV) ketamine can be used to treat chronic therapy-resistant neuropathic pain, particularly complex regional pain syndrome. IV administration of ketamine in the clinical setting is well tolerated when combined with benzodiazepines to reduce the psychotropic side effects.

The other NMDA antagonists require further study to determine their role in chronic pain treatment. Methadone should not be a first choice for an extended-release or long-acting opioid to control chronic pain.

## REFERENCES

1. Luethi D, Liechti ME. Designer drugs: Mechanism of action and adverse effects. *Arch Toxicol.* 2020;94(4):1085–1133.
2. Hewitt DJ. The use of NMDA-receptor antagonists in the treatment of chronic pain. *Clin J Pain.* 2000;16(2 Suppl):S73–S79.
3. Toombs JD, Kral LA. Methadone treatment for pain states. *Am Fam Physician.* 2005;71(7):1353–1358.
4. Kurian R, Raza K, Shanthanna H. A systematic review and meta-analysis of memantine for the prevention or treatment of chronic pain. *Eur J Pain.* 2019;23(7):1234–1250.
5. King MR, et al. Perioperative dextromethorphan as an adjunct for postoperative pain: a meta-analysis of randomized controlled trials. *Anesthesiology.* 2016;124(3):696–705.

# 157.

# TRICYCLIC ANTIDEPRESSANTS

*Ronny Munoz-Acuna and Ricardo Munoz-Acuna*

## INTRODUCTION

The first tricyclic antidepressant (TCA) developed was imipramine in 1958; other cyclic antidepressants were subsequently developed, such as amitriptyline, amoxapine, clomipramine, desipramine, doxepin, nortriptyline, protriptyline, and trimipramine. Antidepressants are indicated for treating depression or anxiety disorders, which include generalized anxiety disorder, obsessive-compulsive disorder, panic disorders, phobias, and post-traumatic stress disorder. Furthermore, some antidepressants are prescribed off-label to treat chronic pain, low energy, and menstrual symptoms. Antidepressant use in chronic pain is especially promising for providing non-opioid analgesia. Therefore, many surgical patients will be taking antidepressant drugs, and the anesthesiologist must be aware of common side effects and potential interactions with anesthetic agents. Side effects result from the blocking of muscarinic M1, histamine H1, and alpha-adrenergic receptors. This results in cardiac, anticholinergic, and antihistaminic effects, decreased seizure threshold, sexual dysfunction, diaphoresis, and tremor. The following chapter reviews the considerations for patients taking tricyclic antidepressants in the perioperative period.

## PHARMACOLOGY

TCAs are absorbed rapidly from the gastrointestinal (GI) tract in the small intestine. TCAs may impair gastric emptying and delay peak serum levels up to 12 hours after ingestion. TCAs are lipophilic and highly protein-bound, resulting in a large volume of distribution (10–50 L/kg). Once absorbed, TCAs enter the portal circulation, Metabolism and elimination occur mainly in the liver. The elimination half-life for the tricyclics and related drugs averages about 24 hours.

TCAs competitively block the reuptake of noradrenaline and serotonin from the synaptic cleft, increasing their synapse concentration. They also block muscarinic, histaminergic, and alpha adrenoceptors.[1]

## CLINICAL FEATURES

Cyclic antidepressants tend to have dose-related side effects at therapeutic doses. Amitriptyline, clomipramine, doxepin, imipramine, and trimipramine generally cause more side effects than other cyclic antidepressants. Nortriptyline and desipramine tend to have the best overall tolerability. We can divide the adverse effects by system as follows:[2]

### CENTRAL NERVOUS SYSTEM EFFECTS

These include coma, seizure, myoclonic twitches/tremor, hyperreflexia, altered mental status (agitation, confusion, lethargy), and dizziness.

### CARDIAC EFFECTS

Cardiac effects include hypertension, tachycardia, orthostasis and refractory hypotension (rare), arrhythmias, and electrocardiogram (ECG) changes (prolonged QRS, QT and PR intervals).

### PULMONARY EFFECTS

Pulmonary effects include hypoventilation resulting from central nervous system (CNS) depression.

### GASTROINTESTINAL TRACT EFFECTS

These include decreased or absent bowel sounds, constipation, and emesis.

## OTHER ANTICHOLINERGIC EFFECTS

Other effects include dry mouth, flushed skin, blurred vision, urinary retention, dry mucous membranes, mydriasis (pupil dilation), and fever.

## OTHER TESTS

Besides history and physical exam and reviewing the electronic medical record to review each patient's past and current prescriptions, the single most crucial test is the 12-lead surface ECG. Common findings include the following:

- Prolongation of the QRS complex (QRS intervals longer than 100 milliseconds are at risk for seizures, and patients with QRS intervals longer than 160 milliseconds are at risk for arrhythmias)
- QT prolongation
- Heart blocks (any degree).

## ANESTHETIC CONSIDERATIONS

### PREOPERATIVE

- Assess indication for the use of TCAs.
- Consider the interaction between TCAs and concomitant medications (Table 157.1).
- Continue TCAs during the perioperative period.
- Asses for the use of other QT-prolonging medications.
- If possible, assess a baseline EKG for QRS and QT changes.[3,4]

### INTRAOPERATIVE

- Monitor as per ASA guidelines.
- Chronic TCA therapy may lead to depletion of catecholamine stores; some patients may present with refractory hypotension.
- Hypertension and arrhythmias may result from the use of sympathomimetic drugs (and indirectly acting sympathomimetics given the increased sensitivity to catecholamines).
- Other medications that should be used with caution are pancuronium and ketamine since these also increase circulating catecholamines.
- TCAs may result in an increased response to intraoperatively administered anticholinergics.

### POSTOPERATIVE

- Patients can usually resume TCAs.
- Avoid other QT-prolonging drugs
- TCA may predispose patients to urinary retention in the post-anesthesia care unit (PACU).

*Table 157.1* INTERACTION OF TCAS AND MEDICATIONS GIVEN IN THE PERIOPERATIVE PERIOD[5]

| INTERACTING DRUGS(S) | POSSIBLE EFFECT(S) |
|---|---|
| SSRIs | Increased TCA causing concentration and adverse effects Serotonin syndrome possible, especially with clomipramine |
| Alcohol | Increased CNS depression, sedation |
| Antiarrhythmic drugs, e.g., amiodarone, flecainide, quinidine | Increased risk of ventricular arrhythmias |
| CNS depressants, e.g., benzodiazepines antihistamines antipsychotics | Increased CNS depression, sedation |
| Clonidine | Antihypertensive effects of clonidine are reduced or abolished |
| Warfarin | Occasional reports of changes in INR |
| Lithium | Neurotoxic symptoms and serotonin-like syndrome occasionally reported |
| Antipsychotics | Increased sedation, additive anticholinergic effects Plasma concentrations of phenothiazines and/or the TCA may be increased |
| Selegiline | CNS excitation, serotonin syndrome |
| Ritonavir | Plasma concentrations of TCAs may be increased. |
| Tramadol | Increased risk of seizures Possibility of serotonin syndrome, especially with clomipramine |

Abbreviations: TCA: tricyclic antidepressants; INR: international normalized ratio; CNS: central nervous system; SSRIs: Selective serotonin reuptake inhibitors.

- Increased response to anticholinergic use for neuromuscular blockade reversal may cause postoperative confusion.

## REFERENCES

1. Gillman PK. Tricyclic antidepressant pharmacology and therapeutic drug interactions updated. *Br J Pharmacol.* 2007 Jul;151(6):737–748.
2. Elvir-Lazo OL, et al. Impact of chronic medications in the perioperative period: Anesthetic implications (Part II). *Postgrad Med.* 2021;133(8):920–938.
3. Saraghi M, et al. Anesthetic considerations for patients on antidepressant therapy: Part I. *Anesth Prog.* 2017;64(4):253–261.
4. Saraghi M, et al. Anesthetic considerations for patients on antidepressant therapy: Part II. *Anesth Prog.* 2018;65(1):60–65.
5. Huyse FJ, et al. Psychotropic drugs and the perioperative period: A proposal for a guideline in elective surgery. *Psychosomatics.* 2006 Jan;47(1):8–22.

# 158.

# SELECTIVE SEROTONIN REUPTAKE INHIBITORS (SSRIS)

*David Rosenblum and Hila Elias*

## INDICATIONS

Selective serotonin reuptake inhibitors (SSRIs) are commonly used medications to treat depression and anxiety. They are used to treat mild to moderate depression, obsessive-compulsive symptoms, panic disorders, post-traumatic stress disorder, and social phobias. They have also been used off-label in the treatment of chronic pain, low energy states, and menstrual symptoms. Their unique mechanisms of action that are responsible for these properties, may lead to unexpected complications and warrant careful consideration when evaluating the perioperative patient.

## MECHANISM OF ACTION

### SELECTIVE SEROTONIN REUPTAKE INHIBITORS (SSRIS)

While the exact mechanism is not always known, it is thought that SSRIs treat depression by increasing the amount of serotonin at the synapse. It usually takes 2–4 weeks until the clinical symptoms improve, and this delay may be related to the down regulation of postsynaptic central nervous system (CNS) receptors.

SSRIs include citalopram, escitalopram, fluoxetine, fluvoxamine, paroxetine, and sertraline.

Side effects may include, but are not limited to bruxism, anxiety, gastrointestinal upset, weight loss or gain, dizziness, blurred vision, dry mouth, excessive sweating, sleep disturbances, headaches, and sexual dysfunction.

Citalopram appears to be the best tolerated, followed by fluoxetine, sertraline, paroxetine, and fluvoxamine. Side effects are dose related and can be attributed to serotonergic effects.

Differences exist between different SSRIs' half-lives, clinical activity, side effects, molecular structures, and drug interactions. Among SSRIs, these differences are clinically significant, justifying each SSRI's distinct pharmacological influence. SSRIs are not addictive, although one should be aware of possible withdrawal symptoms such as nausea, headache, and flu-like symptoms that can arise once discontinued.

## SELECTIVE NOREPINEPHRINE REUPTAKE INHIBITORS (SNRIS)

Selective norepinephrine reuptake inhibitors (SNRIs), like tricyclic antidepressants (TCAs), inhibit both the reuptake of serotonin and norepinephrine. SNRIs tend to be more selective for norepinephrine reuptake inhibition than serotonin.

SNRIs include desvenlafaxine, duloxetine, levomilnacipran, milnacipran, and venlafaxine.

Side effects may include but are not limited to constipation, insomnia, dizziness, gastrointestinal upset, headache, hot flushes, nausea, drowsiness, and sexual dysfunction.

These drugs differ from TCAs in that there are minimal effects on other neurotransmitters or receptors. Venlafaxine and duloxetine have been used for treatment of chronic neuropathic pain. Duloxetine is FDA approved for painful diabetic neuropathy, postherpetic neuralgia, and chronic musculoskeletal pain. Milnacipran is FDA approved for the treatment of fibromyalgia.

## SIDE EFFECTS

After discontinuing the use of SSRIs or SNRIs, post-SSRI sexual dysfunction (PSSD) may be common. Symptoms include but are not limited to reduced sex drive, genital anesthesia, premature ejaculation, and impotence. Further studies are required for the pathophysiology of PSSD in order to cultivate effective treatment. It may be important to inquire about side effects as patients may be taking other medications to counteract them.[1]

## ANESTHETIC CONSIDERATIONS

### PREOPERATIVE

When performing a preoperative assessment of a patient with a history for depression and anxiety, a thorough history of medications use must be obtained and scrutinized. Medications such as SSRIs and SNRIs are not the only ones that may be associated with perioperative morbidity. Monoamine oxidase inhibitors (MAOIs), lithium, and TCAs each have their own risks and associated medication interactions. Patients may be on chronic benzodiazepine therapy and may have tolerance to midazolam or may require higher doses. This population may also have a higher risk of alcohol and drug abuse. Anticoagulant use should be noted and any abnormal bleeding documented. Some SSRIs can increase warfarin levels and therefore PT/INR should be reviewed prior to surgery.

Preoperative assessments should include a thorough review of systems to ensure that the patient is not displaying any symptoms of a drug-drug interaction or toxicity due to a recent change in health, antidepressant dosage, or initiation of a new medication.

The decision to hold or continue antidepressants preoperatively should be carefully considered. Mood is unlikely to be affected by cessation of an SSRI or SNRI for 1 day due to surgery and may mitigate some unwanted cardiovascular effects.[5]

### INTRAOPERATIVE

As with all patients, hemodynamic monitoring and noting blood loss is necessary. Patients who are at a higher risk due to comorbidities or where suspicion of serotonin syndrome and excessive bleeding exist may benefit from an arterial line and Foley catheter. Central venous cannulation may also be necessary to assist in fluid resuscitation or administration of vasoactive drugs.

### POSTOPERATIVE

Postoperatively, antidepressants should be reinstituted as soon as possible to avoid lack of efficacy. The drug should be held if there is suspicion of a related reaction, postoperative bleeding, or hemodynamic instability.

## SEROTONIN SYNDROME

Serotonin syndrome is one of the most feared and infamous complications when treating patients taking SSRIs. It can be life-threatening and precipitated by use of serotonergic drugs and overactivation of post-peripheral and central postsynaptic 5HT-1A and, most notably, 5HT-2A receptors. Patients present with a combination of neuromuscular hyperactivity, mental status change, and autonomic hyperactivity.

The syndrome may occur via the therapeutic use of serotonergic drugs alone, intentional overdose of serotonergic drugs, or via a complex drug interaction between two serotonergic drugs that work by different mechanisms.[2]

### DIAGNOSIS

Diagnosis by a medical toxicologist has been labeled to be the gold standard. As the diagnosis is often hard to make, the actual incidence is unknown, and can occur at any age. A history of chronic pain or psychiatric comorbidities may alert to the possibility of serotonin syndrome. Changes in medication doses, new therapy, or substance abuse may alert the clinician. Patients who are on SSRIs and hemodialysis may have a higher incidence.[3]

Laboratory abnormalities are nonspecific. Serotonin syndrome needs to be differentiated from neuroleptic malignant syndrome, malignant hyperthermia, and anticholinergic toxicity. The causative agent in question is key to guiding diagnosis.

### PRESENTATION

Symptoms begin usually within 24 hours of an increased dose of a serotonergic agent, or if another drug is added to the regimen. Patients with mild symptoms typically will have hypertension and tachycardia, mydriasis, diaphoresis, shivering, hyperreflexia, tremor, and myoclonus. Patients presenting with severe symptoms will have the preceding symptoms, dramatic swings in heart rate and blood pressure, hyperthermia greater than 41.1°C, delirium, and muscle rigidity. This can progress to seizures, rhabdomyolysis, myoglobinuria, metabolic acidosis, renal failure, acute respiratory distress syndrome, respiratory failure, diffuse intravascular clotting, coma, and death. The most well-known combination that causes serotonin syndrome is an SSRI with an MAOI.[4]

### MANAGEMENT

When the diagnosis is made or suspected, it is paramount to discontinue all serotonergic agents. Provide supportive therapy through supplemental oxygen to maintain an oxygen saturation greater than 93%. Maintain euvolemia with intravenous fluids, cardiac monitoring, and sedation with a benzodiazepine. Serotonin antagonists may be necessary in moderate cases. The condition usually resolves within 24 hours. If the case is severe and life-threatening, then sedation, paralysis, and intubation with admission to the intensive care unit should be performed. Of note, diazepam has been shown to blunt the hyperadrenergic symptoms and sedate the patient. It can correct mild hypertension, tachycardia, and reduces fever. Serotonin antagonists such as cyproheptadine and chlorpromazine in high doses can be used. Chlorpromazine can cause orthostatic hypotension and should not be used in hypotensive patients. It is important to distinguish serotonin syndrome from neuroleptic malignant syndrome, as dantrolene is not efficacious and bromocriptine may exacerbate the condition by increasing serotonin levels.

## CYTOCHROME P450 INHIBITION

SSRIs such as fluoxetine, paroxetine, and fluvoxamine are potent cytochrome P (CYP) inhibitors. The SNRI venlafaxine is an inhibitor and a substrate of CYP 2D6. Codeine and tramadol are both prodrugs that require metabolism by CYP 2D6 to their active metabolites. Inadequate analgesia will result from this combination due to less prodrug being converted to their active metabolites. Some SSRIs, SNRIs, and TCAs inhibit CYP 2D6 to varying degrees, and this should be taken into consideration.

## BLEEDING

Platelet release of serotonin may have a role in clot formation and platelet aggregation. There may be a reduction in platelet surface serotonin receptor density due to reuptake inhibition. Those treated with SSRIs have a 3-fold increase in serious upper gastrointestinal bleeds. Those on NSAIDs, especially the elderly, are at particular risk. Aspirin has been implicated and caution is advised.

SSRIs such as fluoxetine, paroxetine, and sertraline have a relatively higher degree of serotonin reuptake inhibition and are associated with a higher risk of bleeding episodes.[5]

## ADRENERGIC AGONIST INTERACTIONS

As with patients taking TCAs, those on SNRIs may have exaggerated effects on blood pressure and heart rate when administered a local anesthetic containing epinephrine due to the increased synaptic norepinephrine activity.

Additionally, SSRIs may inhibit NSAID metabolism. This may lead to higher plasma levels of NSAIDs and increase the risk of GI perforations, bleeds, and ulceration. CYP 2C9 metabolizes naproxen, diclofenac, and celecoxib. This action is inhibited by paroxetine, sertraline, and fluvoxamine.

## REFERENCES

1. WJG, et al. Post-SSRI sexual dysfunction: A literature review. *Web.* 2018 Jan;6(1):29–34.
2. Volpi-Abadie J, et al. Serotonin syndrome. *Ochsner J.* 2013;13(4):533–554.
3. Takata J, et al. Serotonin syndrome triggered by postoperative administration of serotonin noradrenaline reuptake inhibitor (SNRI). *JA Clinical Reports.* U.S. National Library of Medicine. 2019 Aug 27;5(1):55.
4. Dunkley EJ, et al. The Hunter Serotonin Toxicity Criteria: Simple and accurate diagnostic decision rules for serotonin toxicity. *QJM.* 2003 Sep;96(9):635–642.
5. Saraghi M, et al. Anesthetic considerations for patients on antidepressant therapy: Part II. *Anesth Prog.* 2018;65(1):60–65.

# 159.

# OTHER MODALITIES

*Ethan R. Leonard and Maxim S. Eckmann*

## ACETAMINOPHEN

Acetaminophen use in perioperative pain management has been extensively researched and can be administered orally, rectally, or intravenously. A meta-analysis of randomized trials found that using oral or intravenous (IV) acetaminophen in combination with morphine postoperatively resulted in a reduced use of morphine. In addition, acetaminophen used in combination with nonsteroidal anti-inflammatory drugs (NSAIDs) can improve pain control and reduce the use of morphine postoperatively. IV acetaminophen is more expensive than the oral formulation but may aid in reducing length of hospital stays.[1]

## CORTICOSTEROIDS

Corticosteroids are a class of drugs commonly used to treat inflammatory and autoimmune diseases. Dexamethasone, the most used corticosteroid, is currently being researched for its potential in relieving perioperative pain. Specific advantages for using dexamethasone for postoperative pain are inconclusive and are likely different depending on the procedure. A 2011 meta-analysis of 24 randomized trials including multiple surgical procedures showed that patients who received more than 0.1 mg/kg IV had a slight reduction in postoperative pain and opioid use. Patients who received less than 0.1 mg/kg IV had no benefits. Reduced pain and opioid consumption for specific surgical procedures, including spinal surgeries, may exist but need further study.[2]

## CALCIUM CHANNEL BLOCKERS (GABAPENTIN AND PREGABALIN)

Gabapentin and pregabalin are calcium channel blockers that specifically act on the alpha-2-delta protein in the central nervous system (CNS) to reduce specific pain conditions. It is believed that their anti-nociceptive properties come from inhibiting calcium-mediated neurotransmitter release in dorsal root ganglia and dorsal horn neurons. Historically, gabapentin has been used to treat partial seizures and post-herpetic neuralgia. The perioperative use of these agents in reducing acute pain is an area of research interest. A 2016 meta-analysis of 132 randomized controlled trials of varied surgical procedures showed that gabapentin use for postoperative pain control was inconclusive. Further research and analysis are required to determine the efficacy of gabapentin and pregabalin on reducing postoperative pain. Studies have shown that gabapentin has a moderate effect on decreasing postoperative opioid consumption.[3] Continued research on perioperative use of the gabapentinoids in reducing postoperative pain is needed to establish indications and dosing regimens.

## PRESYNAPTIC CALCIUM CHANNEL MODULATORS (LEVETIRACETAM)

Levetiracetam is a calcium channel modulator that is commonly used to treat partial and generalized tonic-clonic seizures. Antiepileptic drugs have been used to treat neuropathic pain, and the efficacy of levetiracetam in treating pain is an area of research currently. Preliminary studies show little evidence in the indication of levetiracetam for the treatment of perioperative or chronic pain.

## SODIUM CHANNEL BLOCKERS (MEXILETINE, CARBAMAZEPINE, OXCARBAZEPINE)

Intravenous and regional use of sodium channel blockers in the treatment of acute and chronic pain is a thoroughly studied field of anesthesia. Mexiletine is an oral lidocaine analog that has been used in various chronic pain conditions. It has been indicated in the treatment of neuropathic pain and fibromyalgia but is generally considered a second- or third-line treatment due to lack of efficacy and increased neurologic and gastrointestinal side effects. Carbamazepine is a sodium channel blocker that is considered a narrow spectrum anticonvulsant but also has indications in the treatment of trigeminal neuralgia.

## NALTREXONE

Naltrexone is a reversible competitive antagonist at μ-opioid and κ-opioid receptors that is typically used to treat opioid and alcohol use disorders. At lower doses, it has been found to act as a glial cell modulator with neuroprotective effects via inhibition of glial cell activation. It acts by binding to Toll-like receptor 4 as an antagonist, thus inhibiting the downstream signaling pathway that promotes inflammatory cytokine release. Activation of glial cells and inflammatory cytokine release is a proposed mechanism of initiation and maintenance of neuropathic pain. Initial studies of low dose naltrexone have shown promising results in the treatment of fibromyalgia pain. Low dose naltrexone has minimal adverse events, no drug-drug interactions, and is a relatively inexpensive therapy when compared with other treatments for chronic pain.[4]

## TRANSCUTANEOUS ELECTRICAL NERVE STIMULATION (TENS)

Transcutaneous electrical nerve stimulation (TENS) has been used since the 1970s and could be a potential adjunct therapy in the treatment of postoperative pain. TENS is performed by electrically stimulating an area of the body with electrodes and has been hypothesized to reduce pain via inhibition of nociceptive firing at the dorsal horn of the spinal cord and increasing endogenous opioid release. A review of the literature shows that use of TENS to reduce postoperative pain is controversial, and further research is needed to determine its efficacy in postoperative pain relief.

## GUIDED IMAGERY

Guided imagery is a form of psychotherapy in which a trained practitioner helps a patient to evoke certain mental images that simulate sensory perceptions of sight, sound, taste, and touch without being in the presence of true stimulus. Evidence for the efficacy of guided imagery as a form of perioperative pain relief is limited and requires further research.[5]

## RELAXATION METHODS

Relaxation therapy is another psychological intervention that aims at inducing a state of both mental and physical rest. Relaxation therapy employs the use of diaphragmatic breathing, progressive muscle relaxation, and is often used in conjunction with guided imagery techniques. Many research studies employing relaxation methods have shown promising results, but more research needs to be done to provide conclusive evidence for the efficacy of relaxation methods in perioperative pain management.

## SLOWED BREATHING EXERCISES

Slowed breathing exercises are another alternative therapy in which a patient will actively breathe slower and deeper in an effort to control or minimize pain. It has been theorized that slowing breathing activates the parasympathetic nervous system through the primitive mammalian diving reflex, which has a modest analgesic effect (36). Research on the effects of slowed breathing exercises on perioperative pain management is limited, and currently no conclusive evidence is available.

## CRYOTHERAPY

The use of adjunct cryotherapy in treating postoperative pain has been well documented in orthopedic, gynecologic, and hernia operations. Cryotherapy is an inexpensive therapy that has minimal adverse effects and should be explored as an additional therapy in postoperative pain.

## REFERENCES

1. McDaid C, et al. Paracetamol and selective and non-selective non-steroidal anti-inflammatory drugs (NSAIDs) for the reduction of morphine-related side effects after major surgery: A systematic review. *Health Technol Assess*. 2010;14(17):1–iv.
2. De Oliveira GS Jr, et al. Perioperative single dose systemic dexamethasone for postoperative pain: A meta-analysis of randomized controlled trials. *Anesthesiology*. 2011;115(3):575–588.
3. Fabritius ML, et al. Gabapentin for post-operative pain management: A systematic review with meta-analyses and trial sequential analyses [published correction appears in *Acta Anaesthesiol Scand*. 2017 Mar;61(3):357–359]. *Acta Anaesthesiol Scand*. 2016;60(9):1188–1208.
4. Trofimovitch D, Baumrucker SJ. Pharmacology update: Low-dose naltrexone as a possible nonopioid modality for some chronic, nonmalignant pain syndromes. *Am J Hosp Palliat Care*. 2019;36(10):907–912.
5. Nelson EA, et al. Systematic review of the efficacy of pre-surgical mind-body based therapies on post-operative outcome measures. *Complement Ther Med*. 2013;21(6):697–711.

# 160.

# ACUPUNCTURE AND HYPNOSIS

*Hovik Mazmanyan and Bozana Alexander*

## ACUPUNCTURE

The understanding of acupuncture comes from theories in traditional Chinese medicine (TCM), where a compilation of records over thousands of years studied specific anatomic points which restore the body's homeostatic flow. According to TCM, acupuncture regulates "qi and blood" throughout the body in channels called meridians and is likely to affect the bioavailability, absorption, distribution, metabolism, and excretion of substances taken internally. Although various theories in the Eastern mechanism explain the relationship of these acupoints and their physiological effects, the Western mechanism investigates acupuncture effects on "neuropeptides, local circulation, inflammation, and the CNS."[1,2]

The mechanism of pain modulation with electroacupuncture (EA) has been described at the peripheral, spinal, and supraspinal levels. In the periphery, EA was shown in study rats to activate the sympathetic nerve fibers, which led to an increase of endogenous opioid at inflammatory sites. The downstream effect was a migration of endogenous opioid peptides such as B-endorphin and *met*-enkephalin. In other studies, low-frequency (2 Hz) EA have been shown to activate mu- and delta-opioid receptors through the release of enkephalin, beta-endorphin, and endomorph in supraspinal CNS regions, whereas high-frequency (100 Hz) EA has been shown to enhance the actions of dynorphins on kappa opioid receptors in the spinal cord.[2] Evidence is supported by the administration of opioid antagonists, such as naloxone, which increases the sensation of pain after patients receive acupuncture. In inflammatory tissues, cannabinoid CB2 receptors are also stimulated by EA, subsequently upregulating endogenous opioids, which were shown to be attenuated by cannabinoid receptor antagonists. Substance P (SP) is another studied neuropeptide that functions as a key modulator in the transmission of pain in inflammatory conditions, which was shown to be decreased with EA. In response to noxious stimuli, SP initiates a cascade of vasodilation through nitric oxide release, inflammation via release of cytokines, and regulation of stress. For example, studies in patient with irritable bowel syndrome (IBS) have shown that EA downregulates expressions of increased colonic mucosa-associated neuropeptide SP.

Auricular acupuncture, or auriculotherapy, is a widely studied site that has shown to play a role in vagal activity modulation of autonomic function, such as regulation of heart rate, cardiac contractility, ventricular electrical stability, and baroreflex sensitivity. This ancient method of practices has been utilized for thousands of years, dating back to the Sui and Tang dynasties (581–907 AD). Approximately 20 anterior and posterior ear points were known throughout this time and have been widely used in recent decades in China and Western-medicine countries, such as France and Germany. Thanks to French physician Paul Nogier, ear acupuncture has been rediscovered, with evidence of a comprehensive auricular reflex system representing the entire body. Interestingly, the auricular branch of the Vagus nerve (ABVN) is the only peripheral branch of this nerve that distributes to the skin. "Mechanism studies suggested that afferent projections from especially the ABVN to the nucleus of the solitary tract (NTS) form the anatomical basis for the vagal regulation of auricular acupuncture."[3]

## ANESTHETIC CONSIDERATIONS

Based on systematic reviews for acupuncture from the existing literature, most notably from the Evidence Map of Acupuncture evidence-based Synthesis Program at the West Los Angeles VA Medical Center, there is great utility of acupuncture in healthcare and in anesthesiology practice. An example of intraoperative acupuncture was studied specifically in the pediatric population and was shown to be useful for controlling pain after tonsillectomies. In this example, acupuncture was quite feasible, well tolerated by the children, well accepted by their parents, and resulted in improved pain with earlier return of diet postoperatively. In addition, the anti-inflammatory benefits were shown to have organ-protective effects in myocardial, gastrointestinal, brain tissue, and other vital organs.

Postoperatively, pain control, autonomic regulation, and postoperative nausea and vomiting (PONV) have been the most observable benefits of acupuncture. Pain control and PONV are two of the most common complications and complaints after surgery. Acupuncture point Pericardium P6, "which lies between the tendons of palmaris longus and flexor carpi radialis muscle, 4cm proximal to the wrist crease," has been widely studied and was shown to be as effective as many of the pharmacological agents used in controlling PONV, with minimal side effects.[4,5]

Although an absolute clear benefit with acupuncture monotherapy over pharmaceutical agents has not been established, in China acupuncture is used in combination with herbal medicine, dietetic regimens, and psychological guidance. In the same way, we may use it as an adjunct to a broader approach to patient care. In the meantime, well-designed evidence-based randomized controlled trials (RCTs) are needed to confirm the role of acupuncture on the quality of recovery after anesthesia and surgery.

## HYPNOSIS

According to the American Psychological Association, the practice of hypnosis incorporates a set of techniques designed to enhance a patient's responsiveness to suggestion in order to change thoughts, feelings, behaviors, and/or psychological states. By heightening concentration and minimizing distractions, hypnosis can be used in a subset of patients for potential perioperative benefits. Although hypnosis is not a full treatment modality, it could potentially harness individual hypnotic susceptibilities in order to optimize perioperative recovery in areas of pain control, anxiety, and PONV.

Historically, hypnosis was studied early in the field of obstetrics and dentistry. In the early 1900s, hypnosis was commonly used in dentistry to manage patient anxiety and fears prior to painful procedures. In the 1950s, a clinical series by Dr. Ralph August was conducted in the field of obstetrics which highlighted the benefits of clinical hypnosis in decreasing exposure to hazardous anesthetics to both mother and infant.[1] In addition, the intimate nature of hypnosis was shown to enhance rapport between the patient and clinician, which ultimately led to a better overall healthcare experience in both fields. As an adjunct to standard treatments for chronic pain, such as pharmacological and physical therapy, hypnosis was shown to have additional benefits in comparison to other alternative health practices, "which included group support, biofeedback, relaxation, autogenic training, attention control and CBT."[1]

Anesthesia considerations in hypnosis are variable and can present individual complexities depending on biological, psychological, and social factors. Perioperative considerations will need to be highly individualized based on patient's beliefs, overall susceptibility to suggestions, optimal environment, and patient rapport. Although there are limitations in the current research for hypnosis and hypnoanesthesia, future research in the perioperative arena can begin to study potential target effects on heart rate variability, respiratory rate, blood pressure, stress hormone levels, and enhanced patient recovery.

## REFERENCES

1. Moss D, Willmarth E. Hypnosis, anesthesia, pain management, and preparation for medical procedures. *Ann Palliat Med.* 2019;8(4):498–503.
2. Zhang R, et al. Mechanisms of acupuncture-electroacupuncture on persistent pain. *Anesthesiology.* 2014;120(2):482–503.
3. Usichenko TI, et al. Auricular acupuncture for postoperative pain control: A systematic review of randomized clinical trials. *Anaesthesia.* Dec 2008;63(12):1343–1348.
4. Hempel S, et al. Evidence map of acupuncture. VAESP Project #05-226; 2013.
5. Lee A, Fan LT. Stimulation of the wrist acupuncture point P6 for preventing postoperative nausea and vomiting. *Cochrane Database Syst Rev.* 2009;2:CD003281.

# 161.

# RESPIRATORY CONSEQUENCES OF ANESTHESIA AND THE SURGICAL INCISION

*Behdad Jahromi and Jai Jani*

## INTRODUCTION

Anesthesia impairs pulmonary function, resulting in hypoxemia in both spontaneously breathing and mechanically ventilated patients. More than 50% of anesthesia-related claims in the United States are due to critical respiratory incidents. The primary function of the respiratory system is ventilation and gas exchange; both key functions are affected during anesthesia, in many cases extending to the postoperative period.[1,2] Upper airway patency and the patient's respiratory effort must be closely monitored. All patients who received general anesthesia (GA) should receive supplemental oxygen in postoperative care. In one study, breathing room air was the single most significant factor correlating with hypoxemia on arrival to the post-anesthesia care unit (PACU), especially in patients of advanced age (>60 years) and weight (>100 kg).[1]

## RESPIRATORY CONSEQUENCES IN THE POSTOPERATIVE PERIOD

### UPPER AIRWAY OBSTRUCTION

Acute upper airway obstruction is a medical emergency typically occurring in the immediate postoperative period. It can manifest as stridor with incomplete obstruction or aphonia with complete obstruction.

### Loss of Pharyngeal Muscle Tone

In the immediate postoperative period, the most common cause of airway obstruction is the loss of pharyngeal muscle tone in sedated or obtunded patients, likely due to the continuous effect of inhaled and intravenous anesthetics, neuromuscular blocking drugs, and opioids.[1] In the awake state, the tongue and soft palate are pulled forward, keeping the airway open during inspiration. If pharyngeal muscle tone is decreased and the airway becomes obstructed, every respiratory effort will cause a reflex compensatory increase in effort and negative inspiratory pressure, which worsens the airway obstruction. This manifests as a paradoxical breathing pattern, retracted sternal notch, and increased abdominal muscle activity. The abdomen protrudes while the chest wall collapses, resulting in a rocking motion.[3]

### Residual Neuromuscular Blockade (NMB)

Stimulation from tracheal extubation, the activity of transferring the patient, and mask airway support will help keep the airway patent. However, in the PACU, residual neuromuscular blockade (NMB) can cause difficulty in breathing and clearing secretions despite adequate pharmacological reversal and evidence of diaphragm recovery from NMB. While a 5-second sustained head lift is the routine standard clinical evaluation for pharyngeal muscle tone, the ability to strongly oppose the incisor teeth against a tongue depressor is more reliable. In addition, hypothermia, respiratory acidosis, or both are common etiologies for persistent weakness in PACU patients, which can be treated with patient warming, airway support, and correction of electrolyte abnormalities.[1]

### Laryngospasm

Sudden spasm of the vocal cords and laryngeal occlusion usually happens after extubation in patients emerging from GA in the operating room. However, it can also occur in the PACU. Jaw thrust maneuver and continuous positive airway pressure (CPAP) of up to 40 cmH$_2$O usually breaks the laryngospasm. If needed, succinylcholine can be used to achieve immediate skeletal muscle relaxation. A tracheal tube should not be forced through a closed glottis during laryngospasm.[1]

## Edema or Hematoma

Airway edema is seen in patients receiving large-volume resuscitation, undergoing prolonged procedures in the Trendelenburg or prone position, neck and airway procedures, and cervical spine surgeries. Also, direct injury from difficult intubation or airway instrumentation can cause airway edema. Patients can develop facial and scleral edema and fail the cuff leak test. To reduce edema, the patient may sit upright to ensure adequate venous drainage, and IV dexamethasone and diuretics can be administered. Following thyroid, parathyroid, or carotid surgical procedures, hematomas might develop, causing external airway compression. If patients complain of pain, pressure, respiratory distress, or dysphagia, the surgical suture or clips would need to be released to evacuate the hematoma. This is a temporizing measure, and an emergency tracheal intubation might be crucial.[1]

## Obstructive Sleep Apnea

Patients with obstructive sleep apnea (OSA) syndrome have redundant compliant pharyngeal tissue, leading to an increased risk of airway obstruction causing hypoxemia and hypercapnia. Therefore, they should be fully awake and following commands before tracheal extubation. They should be managed with upright or semi-upright positioning, goal-directed fluid administration, and CPAP machine use in the immediate postoperative period.[1]

## DIFFERENTIAL DIAGNOSIS OF POSTOPERATIVE ARTERIAL HYPOXEMIA

Alveolar hypoventilation and atelectasis are the most common causes of transient postoperative arterial hypoxemia.

### ALVEOLAR HYPOVENTILATION

All anesthetic drugs except ketamine, nitrous oxide, and ether result in a dose-dependent decrease in minute ventilation and subsequent arterial hypoxemia and hypercapnia caused by a decrease in respiratory rate (i.e., opiates), reduction in tidal volume (i.e., volatile anesthetics), or both (i.e., propofol).[4] Generalized weakness due to residual NMB, underlying neuromuscular disease, preexisting chest wall deformity, postoperative abdominal binding, or abdominal distention all contribute to inadequate ventilation.[1] Hypercapnia will manifest as tachycardia, arrhythmias, hypertension, and vasodilation and in an awake patient can cause headache, tremor, confusion, sedation, and ultimately coma due to carbon dioxide ($CO_2$) narcosis.[4] The arterial hypoxemia secondary to hypercapnia can be treated with supplemental oxygen or by decreasing hypercapnia using controlled mechanical ventilation, reversing the effect of opioids or benzodiazepines and external stimulation of patients.[1]

### DECREASED ALVEOLAR OXYGEN PRESSURE

At the end of a nitrous oxide ($N_2O$) anesthetic, $N_2O$ rapidly diffuses into the alveoli, dilutes alveolar gas, and leads to a transient decrease in the arterial partial pressure of oxygen ($PaO_2$) and carbon dioxide ($PaCO_2$), which is referred to as "diffusion hypoxia." Diffusion hypoxia can persist for 5 to 10 minutes after discontinuation of $N_2O$ anesthetic, and, in the absence of supplemental oxygen, decreased $PaO_2$ leads to arterial hypoxemia. $PaCO_2$ is the predominant factor controlling ventilation, and its reduction will decrease the respiratory drive.[1]

### VENTILATION-PERFUSION MISMATCH AND SHUNT

Hypoxic pulmonary vasoconstriction (HPV) refers to diversion of pulmonary blood flow from areas with low alveolar oxygen content or collapsed alveoli to areas with higher oxygen content to optimally match ventilation and perfusion and increase oxygenation. Residual effects of anesthetics and vasodilators such as dobutamine and nitroprusside suppress HPV and lead to hypoxemia. Immediate postoperative pulmonary shunt is caused by atelectasis, pulmonary edema, gastric content aspiration, pulmonary emboli, and pneumonia. A true pulmonary shunt does not respond to supplemental oxygen. Transitioning the patient to a sitting position, utilizing incentive spirometry, and positive airway pressure with facemask can treat atelectasis.[1]

### INCREASED VENOUS ADMIXTURE

In low cardiac output states or conditions worsening pulmonary shunt, such as pulmonary edema and atelectasis, blood returns to the heart severely desaturated. The mixing of desaturated blood with saturated arterialized blood will lead to hypoxemia.[1]

### DECREASED DIFFUSION CAPACITY

Preexisting pulmonary conditions such as interstitial lung disease, pulmonary fibrosis, emphysema, or primary pulmonary hypertension can cause decreased diffusion capacity and hypoxemia.[1]

### INADEQUATE OXYGEN DELIVERY

Arterial hypoxemia can result from an unrecognized empty tank or disconnection of the oxygen source.[1]

## PULMONARY EDEMA

### POSTOBSTRUCTIVE PULMONARY EDEMA

Laryngospasm can lead to an exaggerated negative intrathoracic pressure caused by an inspiratory force against a closed glottis, i.e., reverse Valsalva maneuver. The high intrathoracic pressure increases the hydrostatic pressure gradient across the pulmonary vascular bed and triggers a cascade of hypoxemia, catecholamine release, and systemic and pulmonary hypertension, leading to a transudative interstitial and alveolar edema.[5] This is referred to as negative pressure pulmonary edema and is usually seen in healthy young, muscular patients. Upon relief of the obstruction, patients can develop hypoxemia within 90 minutes, dyspnea, pink frothy sputum, bilateral fluffy infiltrates on chest radiograph, and, rarely, pulmonary edema with hemoptysis. Treatment is supportive with supplemental oxygen, diuresis, bronchodilators, and in severe cases, positive-pressure ventilation.[1] However, most cases resolve spontaneously in a short period without long-term sequela.[5]

### TRANSFUSION-RELATED ACUTE LUNG INJURY (TRALI) AND TRANSFUSION-ASSOCIATED CIRCULATORY OVERLOAD (TACO)

TRALI occurs within 2 to 4 hours of receiving plasma-containing blood products where recipient neutrophils can become activated and release inflammatory mediators, leading to lung injury and pulmonary edema. TACO is caused by hypervolemia from products, and patients with renal failure or heart failure are more susceptible. Treatment for both include supportive supplemental oxygen, diuresis, and, if needed, mechanical ventilation.[1]

## RESPIRATORY CONSEQUENCES OF SURGICAL INCISION

The surgical site is the single most important factor in evaluating the risk of postoperative respiratory complications. The distance of the surgical incision from the diaphragm is inversely related to the incidence of pulmonary complications. Therefore, thoracic and upper abdominal surgeries have a higher incidence of complications compared to the lower abdomen and all other procedures. This is related to the effects on diaphragmatic function and respiratory muscles. Procedures such as abdominal aortic aneurysm repair, neurosurgery, and head and neck procedures also have a higher rate of pulmonary complications.[2]

## REFERENCES

1. Berg SM, Braehler MR. The postanesthesia care unit. In: Gropper MA, ed. *Miller's Anesthesia*. 9th ed. Philadelphia, PA: Elsevier; 2020:2586–2613.
2. Karcz M, Papadakos PJ. Respiratory complications in the postanesthesia care unit: A review of pathophysiological mechanisms. *Can J Respir Ther*. 2013;49(4):21–29.
3. Benumof JL. Obstructive sleep apnea in the adult obese patient: Implications for airway management. *J Clin Anesth*. 2001;13(2):144–156.
4. Davison R, Cottle D. The effects of anaesthesia on respiratory function. *WFSA*; 2010:2. Available at: https://resources.wfsahq.org/atotw/the-effects-of-anaesthesia-on-respiratory-function/.
5. Mulkey Z, et al. Postextubation pulmonary edema: A case series and review. *Respir Med*. 2008;102(11):1659–1662.

# 162.

# CARDIOVASCULAR CONSEQUENCES OF GENERAL AND REGIONAL ANESTHESIA

*Jared Herman and Omar Viswanath*

## INTRODUCTION

A thorough understanding of cardiovascular function and physiology is essential for anesthesiologists. An in-depth understanding of cardiovascular function and rapid changes in physiology associated with the surgeries and the agents used for general and regional anesthesia is imperative. Despite the advances in our field, surgery and anesthesia are still a time of physiologic stress on the cardiovascular system, with increased sympathetic activity, inflammation, hemodynamic compromise, bleeding, and hypothermia. All of these factors can trigger cardiac complications.[1]

## CARDIOVASCULAR CONSEQUENCES OF GENERAL ANESTHESIA

The phases of general anesthesia can be broken down into induction, maintenance, and emergence, and different agents and medications can be used during these phases to facilitate the depth of anesthesia needed for a successful operation. General anesthesia may decrease psychological stress when compared to regional anesthesia or monitored anesthesia care. However, the induction of anesthesia, laryngoscopy, intubation, stimulation from surgery, extubation, and the postoperative care period are all associated with stress on the systems of the body and subsequent increased cardiac work.[2]

The induction of general anesthesia leads to a reduction in systemic vascular resistance, arterial blood pressure, and cardiac output. Maintaining tissue perfusion of the organs is essential, and mean arterial pressure must be kept within strict parameters. Failure to maintain hemodynamic stability can lead to poorly perfused organ tissues and further complications.

The effect of volatile anesthetics typically used in the maintenance of general anesthesia leads to a dose-dependent decrease in systemic blood pressure. This effect is either due to decreases in systemic vascular resistance (isoflurane, desflurane, and sevoflurane) or attenuation of cardiac contractile function (halothane and enflurane). All arcs of the baroreceptor reflex are obtunded with volatile anesthetics.[2] However, the effect of the inhaled gases is ultimately a decrease in oxygen demand for the heart since contractility, afterload, and preload are all reduced. Most of the agents are coronary vasodilators.[2]

Induction of anesthesia mainly utilizes the intravenous (IV) agents. The evidence suggests that propofol, the most common IV agent, has at least a moderate effect on reducing contractility of the heart and decreasing systemic vascular resistance (SVR). Benzodiazepines and narcotics have mild sympatholytic effects that may lead to small decreases in mean arterial pressure (MAP).

Thiopental leads to a direct negative inotropic action and increased capacitance of the venous system results in a decrease in filling of the ventricles; caution should be utilized when administering thiopental to a patient with right ventricular failure, cardiac tamponade, or hypovolemia. Etomidate and ketamine are both IV agents that maintain hemodynamic stability the most and are excellent options for patients with a low cardiac output, tamponade, or hypovolemia. Administration of ketamine results in increases in heart rate, cardiac index, SVR, pulmonary artery pressure, and systemic artery pressure.

Dexmedetomidine, an alpha-2 adrenergic agonist, reduces the need for other anesthetic agents while maintaining hemodynamic stability and providing sedation and analgesia.[2]

## CARDIOVASCULAR CONSEQUENCES OF REGIONAL ANESTHESIA

Neuraxial blocks and peripheral nerve blocks comprise regional anesthesia. Physiologic changes to the cardiovascular system due to these different techniques need to be monitored and vigilantly treated to avoid complications.

Sympathetic block can result from the spread of local anesthetic moving to dependent areas of the subarachnoid space following spinal anesthesia. If a patient is supine, the block can be extended to the upper mid-thoracic region, result in sympathetic block (blocking fibers from T1 to T4), and decrease SVR 15%–25% due to sympathectomy. Sympathectomy results in a reduction in stroke volume, heart rate, and coronary blood flow. This unintentional spread, otherwise known as a high thoracic, can be avoided with isobaric medications that will remain near the level of injection. Treatment includes ephedrine due to its mixed adrenergic effects without sole alpha-1 agonism and IV crystalloids.[3]

Less profound changes in SVR may occur with epidural anesthesia. Onset is typically slower and is a less dense block. However, both epidural and neuraxial anesthesia can result in hypotension and bradycardia, resulting in an imbalance between myocardial oxygen supply and demand which should be addressed and corrected.[3]

## PERIPHERAL NERVE BLOCKS

Overall, peripheral nerve blocks will not create a systemic inhibition of sympathetic activity when compared to neuraxial anesthesia. Paravertebral blocks, although designed to limit the effect to a single spinal nerve, run the risk for potential local anesthetic spread to the epidural space leading to previously discussed sympathectomy. Local anesthetics are often combined with epinephrine to keep local anesthetic in the desired location, thus prolonging the duration of action and allowing for easier recognition of accidental intravascular injection.[2]

## CARDIOVASCULAR MANIFESTATIONS OF LOCAL ANESTHETIC TOXICITY

Cardiovascular manifestations of local anesthetic toxicity initially include hypertension, increased heart rate, and ventricular arrhythmias as a physiologic response to the impending progressive hypotension. Signs will progress to bradycardia, heart block, asystole, or ventricular arrhythmias (*torsades de pointes*, ventricular fibrillation, ventricular tachycardia). This may occur following epidural anesthesia (increased dose required compared to spinal) or incidental intravascular injection, resulting in high concentrations of local anesthesia in the serum. Initiate advanced cardiac life support if cardiac arrest occurs due to local anesthetic toxicity followed by lipid emulsion therapy.[2]

## CARDIOVASCULAR COMPLICATIONS

Patients with preexisting cardiac disease are predisposed to several complications in the perioperative period. These complications include perioperative myocardial infarction, systolic and diastolic heart failure, pulmonary edema, stroke and thromboembolism. These combined account for 25%–50% of deaths after noncardiac surgery.[4] Certain conditions predispose patients to increased risk of cardiovascular complications, including ischemic heart disease, congestive heart failure, cerebral vascular disease, high risk surgery, diabetes mellitus, and preoperative creatinine greater than 2 mg/dL. These conditions are used as predictors of major cardiac complications in the most widely used model for assessment for preoperative risk for noncardiac surgery. This model is the Revised Cardiac Risk Index (RCRI), which provides 1 point for the presence of each of the 6 predictors. With the presence of 1, 2, or 3 or more predictors, the original study estimated cardiac complications to be 0.4%, 0.9%, 7%, and 11%, respectively. A thorough medical history will lend itself to estimating preoperative cardiac risk and allow the opportunity for intervention an optimization before "clearing" a patient for surgery.[5]

## REFERENCES

1. Devereaux PJ, Sessler DI. Cardiac complications in patients undergoing major noncardiac surgery. *N Engl J Med.* 2015;373(23): 2258–2269.
2. Kaplan JA. *Kaplan's Essentials of Cardiac Anesthesia for Noncardiac Surgery.* 1st ed. Amsterdam, Netherlands: Elsevier; 2019. https://www-clinicalkey-com.access.library.miami.edu/#!/content/book/3-s2.0-B9780323567169000126?scrollTo=%23top.
3. Gropper MA, Miller RD. *Miller's Anesthesia.* 9th ed. Philadelphia, PA: Elsevier; 2020. https://www-clinicalkey-com.access.library.miami.edu/#!/content/book/3-s2.0-B9780323596046120012.
4. Butterworth IV JF, Mackey DC, Wasnick JD. *Morgan & Mikhail's Clinical Anesthesiology.* 6th ed. Malley J, Naglieri C, eds. New York City, NY: McGraw-Hill Education; 2018. https://accessmedicine-mhmedical-com.access.library.miami.edu/content.aspx?bookid=2444&sectionid=189634642.
5. Poldermans D, et al. Pre-operative risk assessment and risk reduction before surgery. *J Am Coll Cardiol.* 2008;51(20):1913–1924.

# 163.

# POSTOPERATIVE NAUSEA AND VOMITING

*David E. Swanson*

## INTRODUCTION

One of the first recognized complications of anesthesia was postoperative nausea and vomiting (PONV). As surgeries shifted from inpatient to outpatient over the last few decades, the management of PONV not only involved compassion for our patients, but also carried financial implications for patients with prolonged recoveries, especially if an overnight admission was required. In addition to patient distress, PONV can lead to additional complications, such as hypotension, aspiration, wound dehiscence, and electrolyte disturbances. Patient satisfaction is highly correlated with the appropriate management of PONV.

## CLINICAL FEATURES

The emesis center in the medulla can be activated by pain, volatile anesthetics, and opioids. This can be countered by medications with the following mechanisms of action: serotonin receptor antagonists, anticholinergics, dopamine receptor antagonists, antihistamines, neurokinin 1 receptor antagonists, as well as steroids whose mechanism of action is unclear.

## DIAGNOSIS

Recognition of patients at high risk of PONV is critical to ensure the proper choice of anesthesia. Apfel's[1] simplified risk index has been very helpful to determine a patient's relative risk of PONV. He recognized that female gender, nonsmoking status, anticipated postoperative pain, and a history of PONV or motion sickness were the key determinants, with each factor increasing the risk of PONV by roughly 20%. For example, a nonsmoking woman with a history of motion sickness, who is coming for a surgery with expected pain requiring opioids postoperatively, would have an 80% chance of PONV with no prophylaxis given, if a standard volatile anesthetic were administered. This is compared to

a male smoker having a simple nonpainful procedure. He would have a 10% chance of PONV, even if he had the same medications.

## TREATMENT

The breakthrough study in 2004 made it clear that multimodal prophylaxis was very important in minimizing patient morbidity related to PONV.[2] Nonpharmacologic treatments can also be helpful. In combination with thoughtful risk assessment and consideration of potential medication side effects, pharmaceutical cost compared to length of stay expenses could be optimized. Multimodal opioid-sparing analgesics have become common and have improved patient outcomes further, and many protocols for enhanced recovery after surgery have been created with this as a cornerstone.

## ANESTHETIC CONSIDERATIONS

### PREOPERATIVE

Place a scopolamine patch in high-risk patients (≥3 risk factors) without contraindications such as glaucoma. Evaluate the risk/benefit of this for elderly patients, since confusion becomes common. Consider opioid-sparing oral medications like acetaminophen, celecoxib, and gabapentin. The American Pain Society recommends perioperative use of gabapentinoids. Evidenced-based medicine supporting this is weak, at best. A recent systematic review did show that the use of gabapentinoids was associated with a lower risk of postoperative nausea and vomiting, but with more dizziness and visual disturbance. The authors conclude that the analgesic effect is not clinically significant and that their results do not support the routine use of pregabalin or gabapentin for the management of postoperative pain in adult patients.[3] Nonpharmacologic therapies, such as acupressure and transcutaneous electrical stimulation, can be applied at this time.

## INTRAOPERATIVE

The choice of anesthesia is very important with consideration for regional anesthesia (RA) as the sole anesthetic or in combination with general anesthesia (GA) to minimize the need for narcotics. GA with a volatile anesthetic has a substantially higher risk of PONV than pure RA. Surgical infiltration of local anesthetics is another useful adjunct. Be aware not to allow a toxic dose of local anesthesia if RA or if intravenous (IV) lidocaine is being used.

Total intravenous anesthesia (TIVA) is another way to minimize risk, as well as avoidance of nitrous oxide ($N_2O$). As an added benefit, the greenhouse gas effects of volatile anesthetics and $N_2O$ are eliminated when using TIVA. High-dose neostigmine is another factor in PONV that can be controlled by the provider with proper timing and dosing of neuromuscular blocking medications, use of sugammadex, or choice of a supraglottic airway which needs no muscle relaxation.

Administer at least 4 mg dexamethasone IV for most nondiabetic patients, ideally prior to incision. Do not give as a bolus to awake patients to avoid an unpleasant perineal burning sensation. Caution should be used with dexamethasone in diabetic patients since it may cause hyperglycemia. Waldron found that perioperative single-dose dexamethasone was associated with small but statistically significant reductions in postoperative pain, postoperative opioid consumption, need for rescue analgesia, post-anesthesia care unit (PACU) stays, and a longer time to first analgesic dose. The effect on postoperative opioid consumption was not dose-dependent. In addition, they found no increased risk of infection or delayed wound healing, although dexamethasone was associated with slight hyperglycemia on the first postoperative day.[4] A serotonin 5-HT3 receptor antagonist, such as ondansetron, should be given in patients with PONV risk factors. Keep in mind that 5-HT3 antagonists and dopamine receptor antagonists should be avoided in patients with long QT intervals, and cases of *torsade de pointes* have been reported. Droperidol saw decreased use after a 2001 FDA black box warning for this reason. Many have questioned the clinical relevance of this warning since the doses cited were magnitudes of order higher than had been used for PONV. With pharmaceutical shortages in recent years, it is important to keep haloperidol and droperidol as options. Steroids and 5-HT3 receptor antagonists have the advantage over many alternatives of being non-sedating.

If not given preoperatively, IV acetaminophen and an IV nonsteroidal anti-inflammatory (ketorolac) can be given intraoperatively. Other opioid-sparing medications can be given, including ketamine, magnesium, dexmedetomidine, and lidocaine infusion. Intravenous ketamine is effective in reducing total opioid requirements and delaying the time to first analgesic dose for many patients with postoperative pain.[5] Fluid management is also important, and adequate hydration can also help enhance recovery.

## POSTOPERATIVE

Best practice in the recovery room is to have a medication order for first-line treatment of PONV from a different pharmaceutical class than those given prophylactically.

## REFERENCES

1. Apfel CC, et al. A simplified risk score for predicting postoperative nausea and vomiting: conclusions from cross-validations between two centers. *Anesthesiology*. 1999;91:693–700.
2. Apfel CC, et al. IMPACT Investigators: A factorial trial of six interventions for the prevention of postoperative nausea and vomiting. *N Engl J Med*. 2004;350(24):2441–2451.
3. Verret M, et al. Perioperative use of gabapentinoids for the management of postoperative acute pain: A systematic review and meta-analysis. Canadian Perioperative Anesthesia Clinical Trials (PACT) Group. *Anesthesiology*. 2020 August;133(2):265–279.
4. Waldron NH, et al. Impact of perioperative dexamethasone on postoperative analgesia and side effects: Systematic review and meta-analysis. *Br J Anaesth*. 2013;110(2):191–200.
5. Laskowski K, et al. A systematic review of intravenous ketamine for postoperative analgesia. *Can J Anaesth*. 2011 Oct;58(10):911–923.

# 164.

# NEUROMUSCULAR COMPLICATIONS OF ANESTHESIA

## Suwarna Anand and Anand Prem

## INTRODUCTION

General endotracheal anesthesia often involves the use of neuromuscular blockade (NMB) and manipulation of the airway. Recovery of airway reflexes after anesthesia and eliminating airway reactivity are key to ensuring safe and smooth postoperative course. The impact of *residual neuromuscular blockade* on postoperative pulmonary complications and *muscle soreness* account for most of the adverse *neuromuscular consequences of anesthesia*. These events can be avoided by optimizing our dosing, monitoring, and reversal practices of neuromuscular blocking agents, thus reducing the risk of residual blockade and associated postoperative complications.

## RECOVERY OF AIRWAY REFLEXES

Airway reflexes play a vital role in preservation of airway patency and protection of the airway. Airway reflexes such as coughing, sneezing, bronchoconstriction, swallowing, laryngeal closure, the expiration reflex, negative pressure, mucous secretion, and apnea are pivotal in protecting the lower airway from aspiration.[1]

These reflexes are modified by various factors such as sleep, chemical ventilatory drive, and general anesthesia. Both depression and exaggeration of upper airway reflexes can have clinical consequences. Topical anesthesia depresses the upper airway reflexes, facilitating endotracheal intubation in an awake patient, but it can increase the risk of aspiration. Neuromuscular blockade can affect the efferent neural pathway and effector organs, leading to the impairment of the upper airway reflexes and increasing the risk for aspiration. Hence the rapidity of the recovery of airway reflexes shortly after emergence is protective. Manipulation of the upper airway under light anesthesia or irritation of the airway can exacerbate upper airway reflexes, leading to laryngospasm and prolong paroxysms of cough.

General anesthesia depresses upper airway reflexes in a dose-dependent manner through its effect on the central nervous system. Differences in sensitivity of different types of reflex responses to anesthesia may be a valuable sign in the clinical assessment of the depth of anesthesia. Cough reflex is most sensitive, and apneic reflex is most resistant to the deepening of anesthesia.[1]

McKay et al. demonstrated that desflurane facilitates more rapid recovery of airway reflexes than sevoflurane.[2]

## RESIDUAL PARALYSIS

Thousands of patients postoperatively are at risk for adverse events associated with *residual neuromuscular blockade* (Box 164.1), an important safety issue when physicians fail to use quantitative neuromuscular monitoring.

RECITE-US, a prospective observational study, found that 65% of patients had a train-of-four (TOF) ratio <0.9 with residual weakness at the time of extubation.

Residual blockade was twice as high in elderly patients compared to younger patients, as they were more sensitive to the effects of muscle relaxants, metabolized these drugs less effectively, and reversal with neostigmine was less effective.

---

**Box 164.1** EFFECTS OF RESIDUAL NEUROMUSCULAR BLOCKADE

Clinical Consequences of Residual Paralysis
Respiratory failure, reintubation
Impaired pharyngeal function
Increased risk of aspiration
Airway obstruction
Hypoxemic events
Postoperative pulmonary complications
Unpleasant symptoms of muscle weakness
Prolonged stay in PACU

*PACU: post-anesthesia care unit.*

---

Residual effects of neuromuscular blockade (NMB) lead to partial impairment of muscular activity in the postoperative period, resulting in impaired contraction of ventilatory muscles causing atelectasis, inability to cough, and impaired swallowing with accumulation of airway secretions and aspiration of gastric contents. Asai and Isono found residual NMB to be a cause of postoperative aspiration leading to pneumonia.[3,4]

Residual NMB increases the incidence of oxygen desaturation, airway obstruction, and reintubation, with impairment of pulmonary function manifested as reductions in forced vital capacity and peak expiratory flow in the immediate postoperative period.[3] Mild residual NMB can impair hypoxic respiratory drive, leading to hypoxemia and culminating in early postoperative mortality.

Arbous et al., through a large retrospective study in 2005, demonstrated that the lack of intraoperative reversal of residual NMB was an independent risk factor for 24-hour anesthesia-related postoperative morbidity and mortality. Patients who did not receive a reversal agent following a neuromuscular blockade were more likely to develop postoperative complications.[3]

## STRATEGIES TO AVOID POSTOPERATIVE RESIDUAL WEAKNESS

1. Avoid long-acting neuromuscular blockers like pancuronium with active metabolites.
2. Site of intraoperative monitoring: Monitoring is typically performed by ulnar nerve stimulation and evaluation of twitches at adductor pollicis. A 5-fold higher incidence of residual paralysis was found when monitoring facial nerve stimulation.
3. When no other option exists but to monitor the eye muscle intraoperatively, always assess the adductor pollicis before administering reversal with neostigmine or sugammadex.
4. Optimal neuromuscular blockade management involves the routine administration of reversal agents unless adequate recovery is confirmed utilizing quantitative monitoring.
5. Select the correct reversal agent:
   i. Sugammadex: reverses deep levels of blockade and is fast acting.
      Rocuronium and vecuronium block of any depth can be reversed with sugammadex. 2 mg/kg when the TOF count has reached at least 2 and 4 mg/kg for deeper blocks, but the post-tetanic contraction (PTC) needs to be at least 1. A higher dose is necessary for PTC of 0.
   ii. Neostigmine: reverses shallow levels of blockade. Neostigmine is effective for reversal of minimal block, which is defined as TOF ratio of 40% to 90% if we use objective monitoring, or as four twitches without fade if we use a nerve stimulator.

## MYALGIA

Succinylcholine is the drug of choice for producing rapid onset and offset paralysis, particularly for urgent tracheal intubation but has side effects.

*Postoperative myalgia* (POM) is one of the most common side effects of this drug, with an incidence of 41%–92%. Myalgia accompanied by muscle stiffness is most prevalent following succinylcholine use in the first 24 hours of surgery. It can last several days and sometimes cause significant discomfort. Myalgias resemble the pain or muscle soreness experienced after significant physical activity.[5] There is no clear relation between succinylcholine-related fasciculation and myalgia.

Myalgias occur less frequently in children and patients over 60 years of age, less commonly in females, and during pregnancy possibly due to hormonal influences. It is common among patients undergoing outpatient surgery since ambulation increases the possibility and intensity of myalgia.

### MECHANISM OF POSTOPERATIVE MYALGIA

It is postulated that the pain occurs due to muscle damage produced by shear forces associated with the fasciculations at the onset of phase one block. While there is no correlation between the elevation of creatine phosphokinase and the development of muscle pain, the increase in serum potassium concentration was greater in patients who develop myalgia.[5]

### PRETREATMENT AND PREVENTION OF MYALGIA

Small doses of nondepolarizing muscle relaxants (10%–30% of the $ED^{95}$) prevent fasciculations and myalgia to some extent. Following pretreatment with a nondepolarizing muscle relaxant 2–3 minutes before succinylcholine, a standard dose of succinylcholine is likely to have a weaker paralyzing effect, requiring an increased dose to achieve optimal intubating conditions. It also delays the onset of succinylcholine and is not recommended in emergency situations.

Administration of 0.5 mg/kg of ketamine in conjunction with propofol for induction of anesthesia is effective in reducing the incidence of POM. Pretreatment with magnesium, sodium channel blockers (lidocaine), or nonsteroidal anti-inflammatory drugs may prevent myalgia. Opioids had no effect.

If untreated, myalgia is self-limited and of minor harm. Only some patients are affected, and none of the pretreatments is universally effective. Consequently, it is reasonable to treat myalgia in patients who complain about it, rather than trying to prevent it in all patients.[5]

## REFERENCES

1. Nishino T. Physiological and pathophysiological implications of upper airway reflexes in humans. *Jpn J Physiol*. 2000;50:3–14.
2. McKay RE, et al. Airway reflexes return more rapidly after desflurane anesthesia than after sevoflurane anesthesia. *Anesth Analg*. 2005;100(3):697–700.
3. Cammu G. Residual neuromuscular blockade and postoperative pulmonary complications: What does the recent evidence demonstrate? *Curr Anesthesiol Rep*. 2020 Mar 27:1–6.
4. Asai T, Isono S. Residual neuromuscular blockade after anesthesia: A possible cause of postoperative aspiration-induced pneumonia. *Anesthesiology*. 2014; 120:260–262.
5. Shafy S, et al. Succinylcholine-induced postoperative myalgia: Etiology and prevention. *J Med Cases, N Am*. 2018 August;9:264–266.

# 165.

# NEUROLOGIC CONSEQUENCES OF ANESTHESIA

*Dustin Latimer and Alan D. Kaye*

## INTRODUCTION

Differentiating between neurologic complications and postoperative recovery attributable to the anesthetic drug is a difficult task to accomplish. This may result in a premature neurologic consult, but there are occasionally neurologic consequences of anesthesia that require assessment by neurologists. Complications affecting the nervous system are infrequent, but the results can have devastating implications for a patient's life. This chapter examines some of the more common neurologic consequences that can occur with anesthesia and neurologic complications that are mistakenly attributed to anesthesia.

## FAILURE TO WAKE

One of the most common reasons for a neurologic evaluation after general anesthesia is a patient failing to wake up after surgery. Some of these cases can be attributable to prolonged effects of various anesthetic agents used during surgery, but it is wise to be aware that the patient may have or may be experiencing a primary neurologic dysfunction impairing the patient's ability to regain consciousness. The possible primarily neurologic explanations could include stroke, global ischemia, encephalopathy, and status epilepticus. If any of these neurologic consequences are suspected, it is paramount to collect a detailed history, perform a

neurologic exam, and consult neurology. With the patient unable to provide a history, it is crucial to review the preoperative, intraoperative, and postoperative records, consult with the anesthesiologist and surgeon working the case, and assess for any disruptions in hemodynamic stability, adequate oxygenation, and hemostasis. Assessing the level of consciousness, brainstem reflexes, muscle tone, response to pain, gaze, and presence of adventitious movements in the eyes, face, or limbs should be the focus of the neurologic exam.[1] Newly discovered asymmetry during the neurologic physical exam needs an immediate imaging of the patient's head to assess for bleeding, clotting, or swelling. Status epilepticus may manifest as subtle nystagmus or minimal twitching in the distal fingers. A thorough neurologic physical exam can provide a great deal of information that directs the plan appropriately to potentially have profound effects on the outcome for the patient.

## POSTOPERATIVE DELIRIUM

Postoperative delirium is a fairly frequent complication in certain populations (elderly, polypharmacy [specifically benzodiazepine-prescribed patients], and patients with preexisting cognitive impairment) and may affect upward of 50% of these susceptible patients. It has been shown that postoperative use of benzodiazepines is associated with higher levels of postoperative delirium and should be avoided. Patients experiencing postoperative delirium may require sedation due to agitation; dexmedetomidine is recommended for sedation, and antidopaminergic drugs are first-line choice for agitation in this group.[1] Agitation is not always present in these cases, and it is worth noting that most of the postoperative delirium cases are hypoactive. With hypoactive cases, a standardized and validated scale is necessary to screen for delirium and track its progression.

## SEROTONIN SYNDROME, NEUROLEPTIC MALIGNANT SYNDROME, MALIGNANT HYPERTHERMIA

The differential diagnosis in febrile patients experiencing rigidity include serotonin syndrome, neuroleptic malignant syndrome, and malignant hyperthermia, so it is crucial to discover the underlying cause and treat it appropriately. Patients taking multiple psychotropic medications (specifically SSRIs/SNRIs) are susceptible to experiencing serotonin syndrome. This is most commonly due to drug interactions between the patient's psychotropic medications and a variety of anesthetic agents. Serotonin syndrome is typically seen as a febrile patient with clonus, reactive mydriasis, diffuse hyperreflexia, and hyperactive bowel sounds. The most important part of this treatment plan is discontinuation of all serotonergic drugs, but cyproheptadine has been shown to accelerate recovery.[1] The distinguishing features between serotonin syndrome and neuroleptic malignant syndrome (NMS) include NMS having a less acute presentation (taking 1–3 days to develop), bradykinesia, and lead-pipe rigidity. Creatine phosphokinase levels are often elevated in NMS. If NMS is suspected, the offending agents, usually an antidopaminergic agent, should be

discontinued, and administration of a dopamine agonist can accelerate recovery. If the patient is experiencing severe rigidity, dantrolene, a muscle relaxer, is indicated. Malignant hyperthermia is not a neurologic consequence of anesthesia, but it must be considered in febrile patients with rigidity. Patients that develop malignant hyperthermia will develop neuromuscular paralysis and become febrile within minutes of anesthesia induction or anesthesia cessation. Immediate discontinuation of the anesthetic and administration of dantrolene are effective in reversing malignant hyperthermia. Inadequate measures to reverse this can result in hypercapnia, acidosis, severe rhabdomyolysis, and cardiac arrhythmias.[1]

## SEIZURES

While most anesthetic agents have antiepileptic properties, seizures can result from several reasons. Individuals at risk of seizures include individuals with epilepsy, structural brain injury, and individuals with substance use disorder. In individuals with a history of epilepsy, it is important to avoid epileptiform-inducing drugs to minimize the amount of epileptiform changes. Seizures must be differentiated from seizure-like movements that may be seen upon waking from anesthesia. If a postoperative patient experiences a seizure but does not regain consciousness after the seizure, nonconvulsive status epilepticus should be suspected and an electroencephalogram (EEG) must be ordered to monitor seizure activity.

## REFERENCE

1. Rabinstein AA. Neurologic complications of anesthesia. Continuum (Minneapolis, Minn.). 2011; 17(1):134–147. https://doi.org/10.1212/01.CON.0000394679.20738.9c.

# Part X

# CENTRAL NERVOUS SYSTEM PHYSIOLOGY

# 166.

# FUNCTIONAL ORGANIZATION OF THE CEREBRAL CORTEX

*Dustin Latimer and Alan D. Kaye*

## INTRODUCTION

The human brain is composed of billions of neurons and is categorized into three major divisions: cerebrum, cerebellum, and brainstem. The cerebrum is divided into two hemispheres, and those hemispheres are divided into the outer layer, called the cortex, and the inner layer. The cortex is composed of gray matter, and the inner layer is composed of white matter. The cortex is developed from the most anterior part of the neural tube called the forebrain region. One of the most prominent landmarks in the cerebral cortex is the central sulcus (Figure 166.1). The central sulcus separates the precentral gyrus from the postcentral gyrus. The precentral gyrus is the primary motor cortex for humans and is often best functionally described with the infamous homunculus figure (Figure 166.2). Within the cerebral cortex, there are four lobes: frontal, parietal,

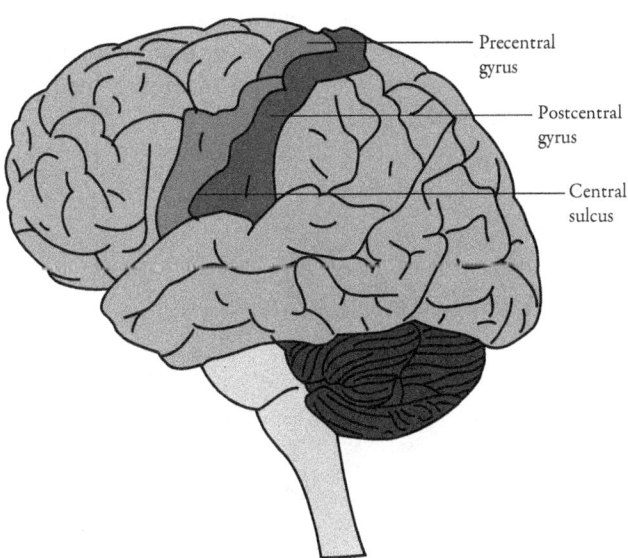

**Figure 166.1.** The central sulcus shown with the precentral gyrus (primary motor cortex) and postcentral gyrus (primary sensory cortex).

temporal, and occipital. This organizational pattern is illustrated in Figure 166.3. This chapter will examine the functional organization of the cerebral cortex.

## FRONTAL LOBE

Much of what distinguishes humans from other animals is found in the largest lobe of the brain, the frontal lobe. Comprising two-thirds of the brain, the frontal lobe is responsible for speech and language, executive function, prospective memory, personality, reasoning, learning, creativity, and movement control (Figure 166.3).[1] Broca's area, the speech production region of the brain, is located in the posterior inferior frontal gyrus.[1] Case studies involving disruption of the front lobe have shown the frontal lobe to be responsible for inhibition of inappropriate social behaviors, regulation of emotion and distress, executive decision-making and functionality, and rational judgement.[1] The frontal lobe also contains the primary motor area and the nonprimary motor area, which make up the motor cortex controlling voluntary movement.[1]

## PARIETAL LOBE

The parietal lobe is located posterior to the frontal lobe and superior to the temporal lobe (Figure 166.3). It can be broken down into two function regions: the anterior parietal lobe and posterior parietal lobe. The primary sensory cortex is housed in the anterior parietal lobe and this area is responsible for interpreting the somatosensory signals it receives from the thalamus, such as touch, pain, pressure, vibration, position, and temperature.[1]

The superior parietal lobule and inferior parietal lobule form the posterior parietal lobe. The superior parietal lobule's functions include planned movements and attention. The inferior parietal lobule contains the secondary somatosensory cortex which receives somatosensory inputs

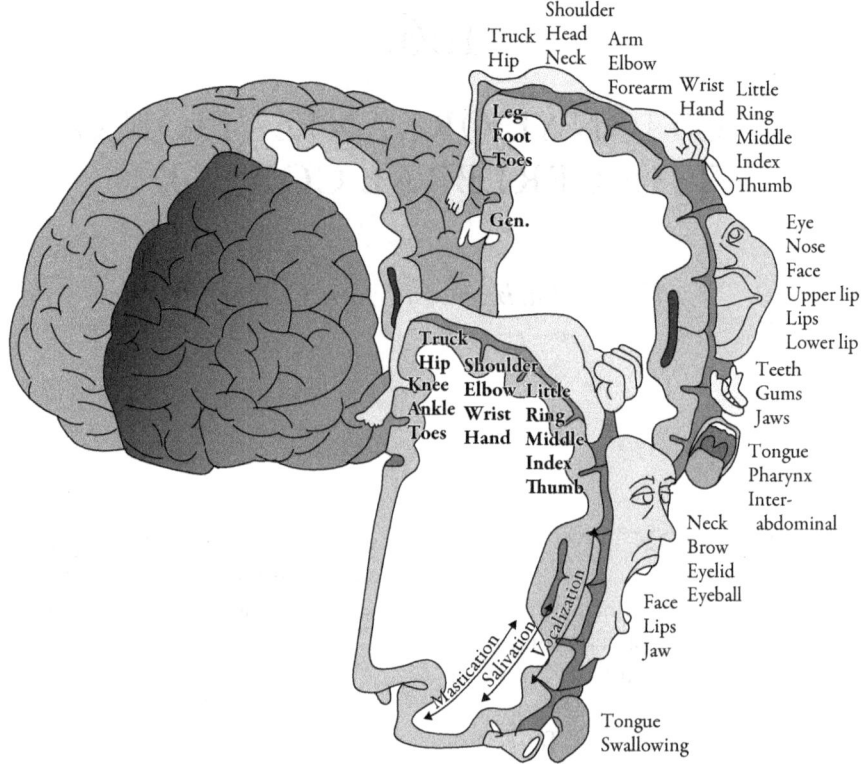

**Figure 166.2.** Drawing of the motor and sensory homunculus. Notice that the face and upper extremity are represented laterally, and the lower extremity and genitalia are represented medially.

from the thalamus and contralateral secondary somatosensory cortex. The inferior parietal lobule functions to execute sensorimotor planning, learning, language, and spatial recognition.[1]

These functions have been described in retroactive analysis of individuals who experienced damage to the regions of interest. Individuals who have lesions in the parietal lobe have been seen to experience astereognosis (inability to identify an object by touch), aphasia (inability to form or understand speech), apraxia (inability to execute skilled movements), and loss of sensation.[2]

## TEMPORAL LOBE

The temporal lobe sits posterior to the frontal lobe and inferior to the parietal lobe; it is broken down into two surfaces: the lateral surface and the medial surface (Figure 166.3).[3] The lateral surface of the temporal lobe is bound by the superior temporal sulcus and lateral temporal sulcus and within those confines are three gyri: the superior temporal gyrus, middle temporal gyrus, and inferior temporal gyrus.

The superior temporal gyrus contains Heschl's gyrus, which is the primary auditory cortex responsible for processing all sounds. Wernicke's area is housed in the superior temporal gyrus and this area has, historically, been associated with speech perception and comprehension; however,

modern evidence and research have challenged how much of speech perception is actually attributable to this region.[4] The middle temporal gyrus is bound by superior temporal gyrus dorsally and inferior temporal gyrus inferiorly and contains four subregions: anterior, middle, poster, and sulcus.

The medial surface of the temporal lobe is responsible for declarative memory because of the anatomical relationship with the hippocampus, entorhinal, perirhinal, and parahippocampal cortex. Declarative memory is long-term memory, necessary for remembering ideas and concepts, events, and learned lessons.

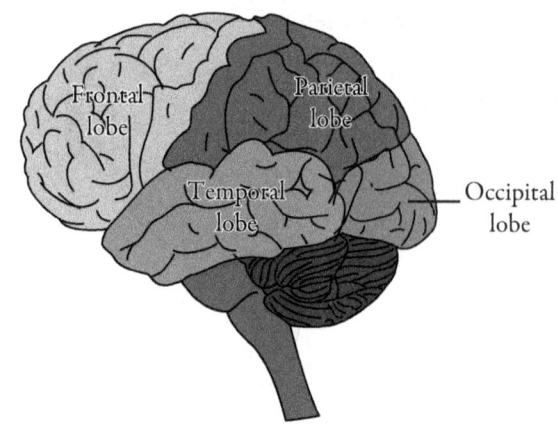

**Figure 166.3.** The anatomic lobes of the cerebral cortex.

## OCCIPITAL LOBE

The occipital lobe is the smallest, most posterior portion of the cerebral cortex. It houses the visual cortex responsible for processing and interpreting visual stimuli. The primary visual cortex receives these stimuli first from the thalamus, and this information is processed and interpreted so that it may be further analyzed by regions of the brain equipped to recognize, compare, and determine what objects are.[5]

## POSTERIOR FOSSA

Located in the most posterior and inferior portion of the cranium, the posterior fossa contains the brainstem and the cerebellum. Cranial nerves IV–XII traverse or are contained within the fossa. It also contains the following venous structures: great cerebral vein of Galen, petrosal vein, superior petrosal sinus, straight sinus, left and right transverse sinuses, lateral sinus, and occipital sinus. Major arteries within the posterior fossa include: left and right vertebral, basilar, posterior inferior cerebellar, anterior inferior cerebellar, superior cerebellar, and labyrinthine and posterior cerebral arteries. The boundaries of the posterior fossa are as follows: anteriorly—posterior surface of the petrous temporal bone; laterally—squamous and mastoid part of the temporal bone; anteriorly—occipital bone. The brainstem is comprised of the medulla oblongata, pons, and midbrain. The brainstem exits the posterior fossa though the foramen magnum. The brainstem is responsible for basic physiologic functions such as regulation of heart rate, breathing, blood pressure, and swallowing. The cerebellum plays a vital role in coordination and balance.

## REFERENCES

1. Jawabri KH, Sharma S. *Physiology, Cerebral Cortex Functions*. 2019.
2. Klingner CM, Witte OW. Somatosensory deficits. In: *Handbook of Clinical Neurology*. 2018.
3. Kiernan JA. Anatomy of the temporal lobe. *Epilepsy Res. Treat.* 2012;2012(176157). https://doi.org/10.1155/2012/176157.
4. Binder JR. The Wernicke area: Modern evidence and a reinterpretation. *Neurology.* 2015;85(24):2170–2175. doi: 10.1212/WNL.0000000000002219.
5. Huff T, Dulebohn SC. Neuroanatomy, visual cortex. In *StatPearls [Internet]*. StatPearls; 2018.

# 167.

# SUBCORTICAL AREAS

*Dustin Latimer and Alan D. Kaye*

## INTRODUCTION

The basal ganglia, hippocampus, internal capsule, cerebellum, brainstem, and reticular activating system are all considered to be a part of the subcortical region of the brain. Subcortical regions have become increasingly recognized as structures important in human cognition, affective, and social function, rather than functioning only as relay structures between the periphery and the cerebral cortex. The subcortical regions of the brain relay information to the cerebral cortex directly or via the thalamus (Figure 167.1).

In this chapter, we will discuss the function of subcortical regions of the brain.

## BASAL GANGLIA

The basal ganglia's primarily functions are motor control, but it has become apparent in recent years that the basal ganglia serve a crucial role in motor learning, executive function, and behavior and emotions as well.[1] Disruption of basal ganglia has long been understood to cause movement

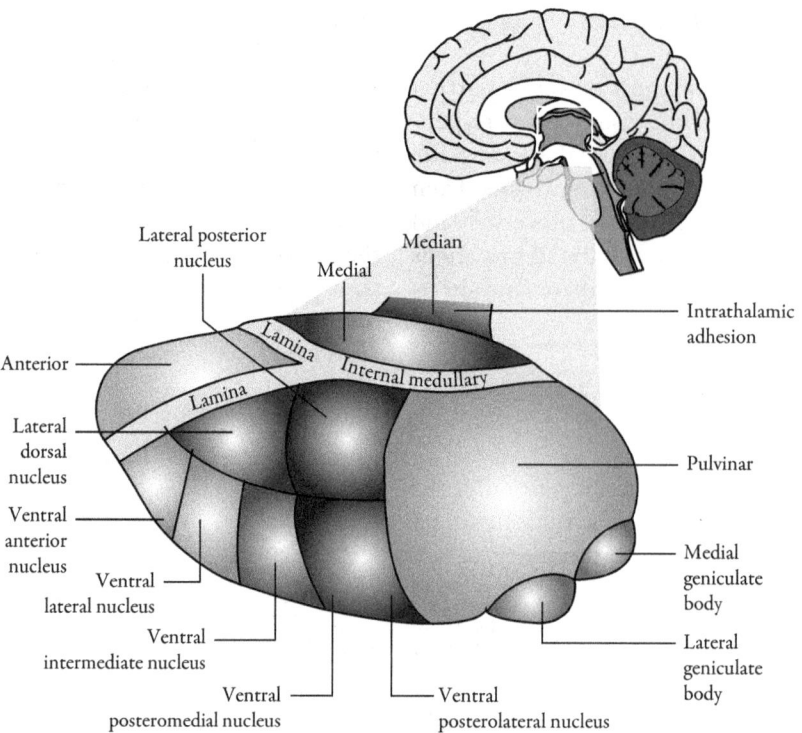

Lateral posterior
nucleus

Median

Medial

Intrathalamic
adhesion

Anterior

Lamina

Internal medullary

Lamina

Lateral
dorsal
nucleus

Pulvinar

Ventral
anterior
nucleus

Ventral
lateral nucleus

Medial
geniculate
body

Ventral
intermediate nucleus

Lateral
geniculate
body

Ventral
posteromedial nucleus

Ventral
posterolateral nucleus

**Figure 167.1** Organization of the human thalamus.

disorders.[1] The term *basal ganglia* refers to the deeply embedded nuclei in the brain hemisphere; functionally, the basal ganglia can be subdivided into the motor, associative, and limbic/emotional regions.[1] In the broader sense, the basal ganglia are categorized as having input nuclei, output nuclei, and intrinsic nuclei; this categorization allows for the visualization of the basal ganglia being viewed as multiple parallel loops and re-entering circuits.[1] A disruption of these circuits is responsible for Parkinson's disease, akathisia, muscle spasms, dystonia, Tourette's syndrome, and a list of different movement disorders and symptoms.[1] More recent research has shown a disruption of basal ganglia to be associated with psychiatric disorders such as obsessive-compulsive disorder and alterations of moods.[1]

## HIPPOCAMPUS

Embedded in the temporal lobe, the hippocampus derives its name from its Greek origin, meaning "seahorse." Due to its seahorse-like shape, it can be divided into three parts—head, body, and tail. The posterior cerebral artery supplies the hippocampus with supplemental supply from the anterior choroidal artery.[2] The hippocampus is roughly 100 times smaller in volume than the cerebral cortex.[2] The hippocampus functions primarily in learning and memory and makes up the posterior portion of the limbic system responsible for motivation, hunger, pain, pleasure, and libido.[2] Patient Henry Gustav provided ample knowledge about the

hippocampus following the removal of his hippocampus as a result of refractory epilepsy.[2] Following the removal of the hippocampus, Gustav was unable to form new episodic memories and experienced profound anterograde and partial retrograde amnesia.[2] These discoveries were consistent with the findings of individuals with Alzheimer's disease. It is common to find Alzheimer's disease patients to have atrophic hippocampus, as it is the earliest region of the brain affected, as well as the most severely affected region.[2] Pharmacologic agents to slow down the atrophy of the hippocampus in patients with Alzheimer's disease are actively being sought. Another common pathophysiologic process involving the hippocampus is epilepsy; up to 50%–70% of patients with epilepsy have sclerosis of the hippocampus at postmortem analysis.[2] It remains unclear if the sclerosis of the hippocampus is the cause of epilepsy, or if the repeated seizures throughout the patient's life cause sclerosis of the hippocampus.[2]

## INTERNAL CAPSULE

The internal capsule is a key structure functioning to transmit information to and from the cerebral cortex. Bundles of myelinated fibers course past the basal ganglia and transmit signals between the spinal cord, subcortical regions, brainstem, and cerebral hemispheres.[3] The internal capsule is a V-shaped structure located in the inferomedial portion of each cerebral hemisphere, and it separates the

*Table 167.1* LESIONS WITHIN THE INTERNAL CAPSULE

| REGION OF INTERNAL CAPSULE | FIBER TRACT | SYMPTOMS |
|---|---|---|
| Anterior limb | Frontopontine fibers Anterior thalamic radiation fibers | Confusion, impaired attention, agitation, and dysarthria |
| Genu | Corticobulbar tract fibers | Face and tongue weakness, dysarthria |
| Posterior limb | Pyramidal and extrapyramidal tract Posterior thalamic radiation fibers | Anterior half: pure motor hemiparesis contralateral to lesion location Posterior third: contralateral hemisensory deficits |

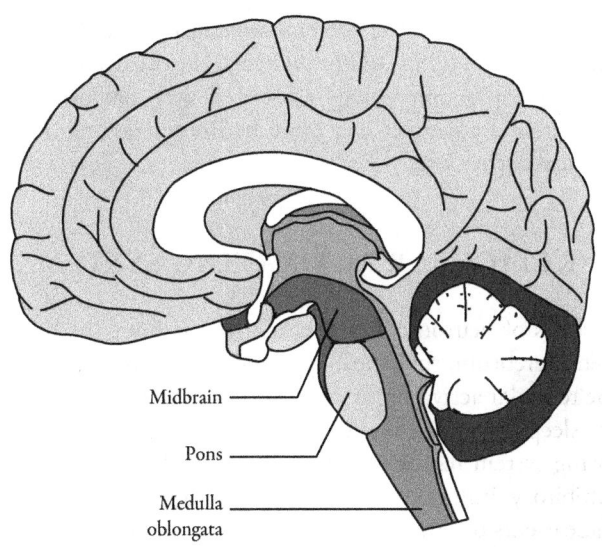

Figure 167.2. Lateral view of the brainstem (midbrain, pons, and medulla oblongata) within the neuraxis.

Midbrain

Pons

Medulla oblongata

caudate nucleus and thalamus from the lentiform nucleus.[3] The clinical significance of the internal capsule is its susceptibility to be a region of ischemia.[3] The internal capsule receives most of its blood supply from perforating arteries originating from the anterior cerebral artery, middle cerebral artery, anterior choroidal artery, and internal carotid artery.[3] There is an increased susceptibility to ischemia in these perforating arteries because they are prone to the development of lipohyalinosis.[3] Occlusion or rupture of these perforating vessels can produce lacunar strokes within the internal capsule, and depending on the location of the stroke, the symptoms can vary from seizures to pure motor symptoms to ataxic hemiparesis; the list of possible symptoms is extensive.[3] It is important to understand the blood supply to the different arms of the internal capsule to localize the stroke lesion based on the presenting symptoms. Table 167.1 lists some commonly observed symptoms with lesions within the internal capsule.[3]

## CEREBELLUM

Deriving its name from the Latin for "little brain," the cerebellum is located posterior and inferior to the cerebrum in the posterior cranial fossa. The tentorium cerebelli, a layer of dura mater, separates the cerebrum from the cerebellum; the cerebellum can be divided into two cerebellum hemispheres connected by the vermis. There are three layers of the cerebellum cortex; molecular layer, Purkinje cell layer, and the granule cell layer. The most popular function associated with the cerebellum is motor control. Individuals who experience cerebellar dysfunction have difficulty with precision, experience erratic movements, and can lack coordination.[4] A common physical exam test for cerebellar function is the "finger-to-nose" test where a patient is asked to touch the tip of their nose and then, at an arm's length

away, touch the examiner's finger; the inability to repeat this task appropriately suggests cerebellar dysfunction.[4] More recently, the cerebellum's role in cognition has become a topic of discussion in a conversation that is still ongoing; it is largely accepted that the cerebellum does play a role in cognition, but an understanding of the extent to which that role serves a purpose is in its infancy.[4]

## BRAINSTEM

The brainstem consists of 3 main parts—midbrain, pons, and medulla (Figure 167.2). The brainstem connects the spinal cord to the base of the cerebrum and is considered the most primitive part of the brain evolutionarily because it controls vital body functions such as breathing, swallowing, and vasomotor control.[5]

The medulla is the most inferior portion of the brainstem and is continuous with the spinal cord; it contains the cardiac, respiratory, vomiting, and vasomotor control centers responsible for heart rate, respiratory rate, and blood pressure maintenance.[5] The medulla connects the spinal cord to the pons, the junction connecting the medulla to the spinal cord at the foramen magnum.[5]

The pons is located between the medulla and the midbrain; it mainly functions to carry information between the cerebrum, medulla, and cerebellum.[5] Four cranial nerves (V–VIII) are present in the pons, and the pons is also the location of the pneumotaxic center. The pneumotaxic center controls the rate and pattern of breathing.

The midbrain is the most superior part of the brainstem; its associated functions relate to vision, hearing, circadian rhythm, temperature regulation, and motor control.[5] An important structure associated with the midbrain is the cerebral aqueduct. The cerebral aqueduct allows for cerebrospinal fluid (CSF) to flow between the third and fourth ventricles; pathophysiology associated with narrowing of the cerebral aqueduct can cause hydrocephalus requiring surgical correction.

## RETICULAR ACTIVATING SYSTEM

A series of neuron circuits located throughout the brainstem, cerebrum, thalamus, hypothalamus, and cerebellum, the reticular activating system is known for its control over the sleep-wake cycle and consciousness.[6] The reticular activating system regulates sleep-wake cycles by providing an inhibitory influence from external stimuli and filtering these events to slow neuronal firing.[6] For anesthetic agents, the primary site of action is the sleep-wake control system, and it has been said that anesthetic agents "hijack" the sleep-wake cycle and turn off the reticular activating system to achieve desired effects.[6]

## REFERENCES

1. Lanciego JL, Luquin N, Obeso JA. Functional neuroanatomy of the basal ganglia. *Cold Spring Harb Perspect Med*. 2012;2(12):a009621. https://doi.org/10.1101/cshperspect.a009621.
2. Anand KS, Dhikav V. Hippocampus in health and disease: An overview. *Ann Indian Acad Neurol*. 2012;15(4):239–246. https://doi.org/10.4103/0972-2327.104323.
3. Emos MC, Agarwal S. *Neuroanatomy, Internal Capsule*. In *StatPearls [Internet]*. StatPearls; 2019.
4. Koziol LF, et al. Consensus paper: The cerebellum's role in movement and cognition. *Cerebellum*. 2014; doi: 10.1007/s12311-013-0511-x.
5. Ngeles Fernández-Gil MR, et al. Anatomy of the brainstem: A gaze into the stem of life. *Semin Ultrasound, CT MRI*. 2010; doi: 10.1053/j.sult.2010.03.006.
6. Garcia-Rill E. Reticular activating system. In: *Encyclopedia of Neuroscience*. 2009.

# 168.

# CEREBRAL BLOOD FLOW

*Surangama Sharma and Lovkesh Arora*

## INTRODUCTION

The brain has a high metabolic rate (CMR), expressed in terms of oxygen consumption (CMRO$_2$) and averages 3–3.8 mL/100 g/min (50 mL/min) in adults. The average adult brain consumes 20% of total body oxygen, even though it carries only 2%–3% of the total body weight. It receives approximately 15% of the cardiac output. Sixty percent of the brain's oxygen consumption supports electrophysiologic function, and the remaining 40% helps in maintaining cellular integrity.

## CEREBRAL BLOOD FLOW

Cerebral blood flow (CBF) is approximately 50 mL/100 g/min, higher in cortical gray matter and lower in subcortical white matter. CBF below 20–25 mL/100 g/min is usually associated with cerebral impairment and slowing on the electroencephalogram (EEG). CBF rates between 15 and 20 mL/100 g/min produce a flat (isoelectric) EEG, whereas rates below 10 mL/100 g/min are usually associated with irreversible brain damage.[1]

## REGULATION OF CEREBRAL BLOOD FLOW

### AUTOREGULATION

Cerebral autoregulation is the ability of the brain to maintain relatively constant blood flow despite changes in mean arterial pressure (MAP). CBF is autoregulated between a

MAP of 70 and 150 mmHg. *Cerebral perfusion pressure* (CPP) is the difference between the MAP and the intracranial pressure (ICP): CPP = MAP – ICP or CVP, whichever is higher. Assuming a normal ICP of 5 to 10 mmHg, autoregulation can also be expressed as a function of CPP. CBF is pressure dependent, above and below these limits.[2] The cerebral autoregulation curve is shifted to the right in patients with chronic arterial hypertension, which means both higher and lower limits are right shifted. Patients can attain a near normal curve after long-term antihypertensive treatment. Proposed mechanisms for autoregulation include *myogenic mechanisms*, with intrinsic response of smooth muscle cells in cerebral arterioles to changes in MAP, and *metabolic mechanisms*, with mediators like nitric oxide and prostanoids causing changes in vascular caliber.[2]

## FACTORS AFFECTING CEREBRAL BLOOD FLOW

### CEREBRAL METABOLIC RATE

*CBF is coupled to CMR*, i.e., when cerebral metabolism (or oxygen consumption) increases, blood flow to that region increases as well. Any factor affecting CMR, such as temperature or medications, can affect CBF. All volatile and intravenous (IV) anesthetics decrease the CMR, except ketamine. Intracranial pathology may *uncouple* the relationship, and CBF and cerebral metabolism may become independent of each other.

### CEREBRAL AUTOREGULATION

Cerebral vasculature has an ability to rapidly (seconds to minutes) regulate the blood flow over a wide range of MAP or CPP. Decreases in CPP result in cerebral vasodilation, whereas elevations induce vasoconstriction. CBF can be affected in any condition that impairs the autoregulatory response. Hypercapnia can impair cerebral autoregulation by causing cerebral vasodilatation. Hemodilution and anemia can cause a decrease in vascular tone, and decrease in cerebral autoregulation capacity. Mild hypothermia impairs and mild hyperthermia enhances cerebral autoregulation. Finally, several anesthetic drugs can affect cerebral autoregulation. Propofol and remifentanil tend to maintain cerebral autoregulation, whereas inhalational anesthetics (excluding sevoflurane at clinically relevant doses) tend to impair cerebral autoregulation in a dose-dependent manner. Cerebral pathology, such as ischemia, tumor/lesion, inflammation, and trauma, can impair autoregulation.[3]

### CEREBRAL PERFUSION PRESSURE, MEAN ARTERIAL PRESSURE, AND INTRACRANIAL PRESSURE

There is a directly proportional relationship between CPP and CBF. The higher the CPP, the higher the CBF. We already know the fact that CPP = MAP – ICP or CVP, so any decrease in MAP will decrease the CPP and CBF, and any increase in ICP will decrease the CPP or CBF even if the MAP is kept constant.

### RESPIRATORY GASES

CBF is directly proportional to $PaCO_2$ between 20 and 80 mmHg. Blood flow changes 1–2 ml/100g/min per mmHg change in $PaCO_2$. In contrast, only marked changes in $PaO_2$ alter CBF; hyperoxia causes minimal decrease in CBF, while hypoxia <50 mmHg will cause significant increase in CBF.

### TEMPERATURE

Hypothermia decreases $CMRO_2$ by 6%–7%/°C, with a proportional decrease in CBF. Hypothermia can even cause complete burst suppression or an isoelectric EEG at which all activity has ceased (at about 18°–20°C). Further decrease in temperature will continue to produce a further decrease in CMR. Hyperthermia increases $CMRO_2$ and therefore CBF. However, above 42°C, a reduction in $CMRO_2$ occurs, indicating a toxic threshold likely a result of protein denaturation.

### RHEOLOGY OR VISCOSITY OF BLOOD

Hematocrit is the single most important determinant of blood viscosity. In anemia, cerebral vascular resistance is reduced and CBF increases, not only from a reduction in viscosity, but also as a compensatory response to reduced oxygen delivery. Of note, due to loss of autoregulation and maximal vasoplegia in focal ischemia zones, manipulation of viscosity in patients with acute ischemic stroke is not of benefit in reducing the extent of cerebral injury.

### MEDICATIONS

Systemic vasodilators such as sodium nitroprusside, nitroglycerin, and hydralazine cause cerebral vasodilation and increase CBF, CBV (cerebral blood volume), and ICP. α-1 agonists (phenylephrine, norepinephrine) keep CBF preserved when autoregulation is intact, despite increasing MAP, but when autoregulation is not intact, CBF increases proportionately to increase in MAP. β-receptor agonists (epinephrine, dobutamine) both increase CBF due to increase in cardiac output and MAP. β-adrenergic blockers decrease CBF secondary to changes in MAP and CPP. Calcium channel blockers (CCBs) induce vasodilation; intra-arterial nimodipine is used in treating cerebral vasospasm after subarachnoid hemorrhage while maintaining MAP, whereas nicardipine is a cerebral vasodilator but reduces systemic MAP.[4]

## Anesthetic Medications

In general, all IV anesthetics cause dose-dependent decrease in CMR and CBF, with the exception of ketamine, which increases both CMR and CBF (Table 168.1). IV anesthetics maintain cerebrovascular coupling. The change in CBF is due to similar change in CMR, with preserved autoregulation and $CO_2$ responsiveness. All opioids cause minimal to no decrease in CMR and CBF. All volatiles decrease CMR in a dose-dependent manner, but independently increase CBF. At <1 MAC, the CMR decreases and the CBF reduction predominates, whereas at a MAC >1, the vasodilatory effect predominates, increasing CBF, even though the CMR reduction is still present (flow metabolism coupling is intact, just altered).

*Table 168.1* EFFECT OF ANESTHETICS ON CEREBRAL PHYSIOLOGY

| ANESTHETICS | CMR | CBF | ICP |
|---|---|---|---|
| Volatiles (isoflurane/sevoflurane/desflurane) | ↓ | ↑ | ↑ |
| Nitrous oxide | ↓ | ↑ | ↑ |
| Barbiturates | ↓ | ↓ | ↓ |
| Propofol | ↓ | ↓ | ↓ |
| Etomidate | ↓ | ↓ | ↓ |
| Ketamine | ↑ | ↑ | ↑ |

## ANESTHETIC IMPLICATIONS

1. Identifying a target MAP for every patient is important, since cerebral perfusion depends on this range. Recognize that autoregulation is affected by chronic disease like hypertension, neuropathologic states, and volatile anesthetics.
2. Realize that with increase in ICP, cerebral perfusion will be affected if MAP is constant, so efforts at reducing ICP need to be instituted insync with efforts at increasing MAP.
3. Understand the consequences of higher MAC of volatile anesthetics, i.e., increase in CBF and ICP. Vasodilating potency in decreasing order is approximately halothane ≫ enflurane > desflurane ≈ isoflurane > sevoflurane.[5]

## REFERENCES

1. Butterworth IV JF, Mackey DC, Wasnick JD. Neurophysiology and anesthesia. In: *Morgan & Mikhail's Clinical Anesthesiology*. 6th ed. McGraw-Hill Education; 2018. Accessed December 17, 2021. https://accessmedicine.mhmedical.com/content.aspx?bookid=2444&sectionid=193560975.
2. Slupe AM, Kirsch JR. Effects of anesthesia on cerebral blood flow, metabolism, and neuroprotection. *J Cereb Blood Flow Metab*. 2018 Dec;38(12):2192–2208.
3. Dagal A, Lam AM. Cerebral autoregulation and anesthesia. *Curr Opin Anaesthesiol*. 2009 Oct;22(5):547–552.
4. Patel PM, Drummond JC, Lemkuil BP. Cerebral Physiology and the Effects of Anesthetic Drugs. In: Gropper MA, et al., eds. *Miller's Anesthesia*. 9th ed. 2 vols. Elsevier Publication; 2020:294–332.
5. Drummond JC. Baseline cerebral metabolic rate is a critical determinant of the cerebral vasodilating potency of volatile anesthetic agents. *Anesthesiology*. 2018;129(1):187–189.

# 169.

# PATHOPHYSIOLOGY OF ISCHEMIA/HYPOXIA

*Dustin Latimer and Alan D. Kaye*

## HYPOXIC-ISCHEMIC BRAIN INJURY

The brain has a high metabolic demand that is compromised in times of ischemia or hypoxemia. The extent of the injury to the brain during these times is dependent upon the degree of absent blood flow, duration of time without oxygen or adequate blood flow, and how quickly blood flow is restored.[1] In animal studies, within 10–12 minutes of ischemic onset, the brain is depleted of nearly all glucose, glycogen, adenosine triphosphate (ATP), and phosphocreatine.[1] The energy stores of tissue are the first to be depleted, followed by an accumulation of lactic acid causing acidosis, and finally, the blood-brain barrier is altered and unable to maintain ion homeostasis.[2] Consciousness is lost within 10 seconds of cerebral blood flow loss, and within 20 seconds, the human brain ceases to have spontaneous or evoked electrical activity.[2] Ischemic damage is categorized into the initial ischemic insult and manifestation of major cell damage.[1] The manifestation of major cell damage is dependent upon the duration of injury and type of cells experiencing the ischemic insult.[1]

## BIOCHEMICAL MANIFESTATIONS

The initial depletion of blood flow or oxygen to the brain causes a depolarization of neurons shifting intra- and extracellular electrolytes outside of the homeostatic location.[1] The cellular membranes are not able to maintain their electrostatic differences in intra- and extracellular fluid, and extracellular levels of sodium, chloride, and calcium decrease while the intracellular potassium leaks out of the intracellular space.[1] In an anoxic state, ATP is depleted, and the consequence of ATP depletion is an increase in lactic acid and hydrogen ions, resulting in a lowered pH.[1] Cerebral ischemia can cause initiation of apoptosis, resulting in cell shrinkage, chromatin aggregation, and attempts to preserve cell membranes.[3] Lipases, proteases, and nucleases are all activated by an increased concentration of excitotoxic neurotransmitters, glutamate, and aspartate, causing neuronal death and an increase in reactive oxygen species to further damage the neurons.[1,3]

## GLOBAL ISCHEMIA

*Global ischemia* refers to nonfocal, diminished cerebral blood flow to the point of brain damage, most commonly caused by hypoperfusion due to ventricular fibrillation or asystole.[3] Hypoperfusion lasting 5–10 minutes results in a well-documented pattern of predictable histologic changes within the neurons damaged.[3] While restoration of cerebral blood flow is necessary to sustain life, the reperfusion causes an influx of neutrophils and reactive oxygen species, as well as cerebral edema and hemorrhage, that may cause secondary damage.[3] When brain tissue experiences a lack of cerebral brain flow, the neuronal cells undergo apoptosis or cellular necrosis.[3] Apoptosis is a programmed cell death characterized by cellular shrinkage, chromatin aggregation, and preservation of the cellular membrane; necrosis is characterized by cellular swelling, membrane lysis, edema, and inflammation.[3] The clinical consequences of global ischemia are dependent on the duration and severity of ischemia, with the most susceptible regions of the brain being affected first. The most susceptible regions of the brain are the hippocampus, cortex, prefrontal cortex, thalamus, cerebellum, and putamen.[4] Humans who have experienced prolonged transient global ischemia have been observed to have new cognitive deficits that affect memory, executive function, motor function, and anxiety levels.[4] Global cerebral ischemia probability increases with age.[4]

## FOCAL ISCHEMIA

*Focal ischemia* refers to insufficient cerebral blood flow to a specific region of the brain, most commonly caused by thromboembolic event. Similar to global ischemia, the pathophysiology of focal ischemia can be broken into two phases: initial ischemia with injuries associated with anoxia, and reperfusion injuries that occur after cerebral blood flow is restored.[5] While hypoperfusion is typical in global ischemic events, focal ischemia is usually the result of a clot traveling from the periphery to restrict cerebral blood flow or hemorrhage of a cerebral vessel; both of these require markedly different approaches to minimize the amount of time the cerebral tissue is without adequate blood flow. The initial response to vascular occlusion from a thromboembolism is determining the onset of symptoms to evaluate if this patient is eligible for tPA. When a thromboembolic event occurs, the tissue immediately adjacent to the occluded vessel experiences the anoxia first and will, almost always, be the most severely affected region; this area is called the infarct core.[5] The infarct core will begin experiencing depolarization and metabolic abnormalities, and eventually will undergo the pathophysiology discussed with global cerebral ischemia.[5] Restoration of blood flow, by clot-dissolving medication or surgical extraction, is the most immediate desired treatment, but doing this will expose the infarcted region to reperfusion injuries such as an influx of reaction oxygen species and neutrophils.[5] The initial ischemia injury from a thromboembolic event will be present within 1 to 3 hours of the event; reperfusion injuries are not present until 6 to 12 hours post-thromboembolism.[5] Due to these two unique pathophysiologic models, studies have shown that tPA may do more harm if administered after 3 hours of the onset of symptoms.[5] The absolute and relative contraindications are under constant evaluation and are subject to change pending further studies. If a patient is experiencing focal ischemia due to hemorrhaging of a cerebral vessel, clot-dissolving medication, tPA, is contraindicated and immediate neurosurgical evaluation and treatment are necessary.

## GLUCOSE EFFECTS ON CEREBRAL ISCHEMIA

Glycemic control during and after focal and global ischemic events has been shown to a critical contributing factor in animal models.[3] Poor glycemic control has been associated with clinically worsened outcomes of individuals who experience traumatic brain injury, focal ischemia, or global ischemia.[3] In individuals who receive insulin treatment in critically ill conditions or who have undergone cardiac surgery, there has been a clinical correlation with positive neurologic outcomes, but further studies are necessary to observe a direct correlation between glycemic control using insulin in patients with global or focal ischemia.[3]

## BRAIN ISCHEMIA DURING SURGERY

Focal or global cerebral ischemia during surgery is one of the most severe complications of surgery that can occur. Appropriate monitoring of adequate cerebral blood flow via transcranial Doppler, electroencephalography to monitor brain activity, oxygen levels, and blood pressure monitoring are crucial for preventing this debilitating consequence because a neurologic physical exam cannot be fully performed in an anesthetized patient.[6] Anesthetics have been demonstrated to have different effects in terms of near ischemia models in which inhalational agents in general have shown improved outcomes. In this regard, research in humans utilizing brain tissue monitoring level assessment has demonstrated double brain tissue oxygen levels with standard inhalational agent delivery. It is the responsibility of the anesthesia/surgical team to reduce the risk of cerebral ischemia from occurring by assessing the patient's past medical history, current home medications, electrocardiogram (ECG), and continually assessing the patient's status during the surgery.[6] Meticulous blood pressure management to ensure adequate cerebral perfusion pressure and the use of arterial lines for beat-to-beat assessment should be considered in all applicable patients.

## REFERENCES

1. Busl KM, Greer DM. Hypoxic-ischemic brain injury: Pathophysiology, neuropathology and mechanisms. *NeuroRehabilitation*. 2010;26(1): 5–13. https://doi.org/10.3233/NRE-2010-0531.
2. Raichle ME. The pathophysiology of brain ischemia, *Ann. Neurol*. 1983 Jan;13(1):2–10. doi: 10.1002/ana.410130103.
3. Harukuni I, Bhardwaj A. Mechanisms of brain injury after global cerebral ischemia. *Neurologic Clinics*. 2006;24(1):1–21. https://doi.org/10.1016/j.ncl.2005.10.004.
4. Neumann JT, Cohan CH, Dave KR, Wright CB, Perez-Pinzon MA. Global cerebral ischemia: Synaptic and cognitive dysfunction. *Curr. Drug Targets*. 2013;14(1):20–35. https://doi.org/10.2174/138 945013804806514.
5. Hossmann KA. The two pathophysiologies of focal brain ischemia: Implications for translational stroke research. *J Cereb Blood Flow Metab*. 2012;32(7). doi: 10.1038/jcbfm.2011.186.
6. Bin Zhou Z, Meng L, Gelb AW, Lee R, Huang W-Q. Cerebral ischemia during surgery: An overview. *J Biomed Res*. 2016;30(2):83–87. doi: 10.7555/JBR.30.20150126.

# 170.

# EFFECTS OF BRAIN TRAUMA AND TUMORS

*Dustin Latimer and Alan D. Kaye*

## INTRODUCTION

Traumatic brain injury (TBI) is the leading cause of death and disability in the world.[1] Even with the prevalence being as high as it is, the prognosis for individuals with TBI remains poor. TBI injuries can be broken into two pathophysiologic categories: the primary injury accounting for the mechanical impact to the skull and the acceleration-deceleration injury sustained, and the secondary injury that is the result of the inflammatory process that follows the primary injury.[1] The primary injury is the major determining factor in the prognosis of the patient, but the secondary injury can occur over the next hours to weeks and cause further injury, most commonly by hypotension or hypoxemia.[1]

## PERIOPERATIVE PERIOD AND TBI

Given the poor prognosis of TBI, the most important actions to take are preventing primary injury from occurring, and managing secondary injury to prevent further damage. Quick resuscitation, efficient triage of the patient, rapid surgical evaluation, controlling intracranial pressure, and maintaining appropriate cerebral perfusion pressure are paramount to optimizing TBI outcomes.[1] The patient will need to undergo a computed tomography (CT) scan once resuscitated and stabilized to determine the extent of injury and to guide the treatment plan.[1] During this initial evaluation, anesthesia should be continually reassessed to ensure that airway, breathing, and circulation are adequate. The patient's neurologic status should be continually evaluated and scored with the Glasgow Coma Scale and attainable physical examination tests such as pupillary responses.[1] Most patients with TBI will require endotracheal intubation and airway management. Given the urgency of a TBI, it must be assumed that the patient is not fasted and that possible cervical spine injuries are present.[1] Nasal intubations should be avoided in patients with a high probability of base skull fractures or facial fractures.[1] The guidelines for severe TBI are listed in Table 170.1.

## BRAIN TUMORS

### INTRODUCTION

Brain tumor surgery of any kind takes significant perioperative care from the anesthetic side of surgery. It is important to access neurologic function before, during, and after surgery by physical exam and appropriate perioperative monitoring that will not be discussed in this chapter. The size of tumor mass, midline shift, cerebrospinal fluid (CSF) pressure within the ventricles, and any CSF flow obstruction are all potential complications that must be monitored.[3] Similar to TBI, a patient's cerebral perfusion pressure must be maintained, as well as appropriate oxygenation of cerebral tissue, and blood pressure must be controlled. The anesthetics used during surgery must cooperate with the desired intracranial pressure, blood pressure, and cerebral perfusion pressure; a few of these agents are discussed in Table 170.2 and Table 170.3.[3]

*Table 170.1* ANESTHETIC MANAGEMENT FOR PATIENTS WITH TPI[1,2]

| PARAMETERS | RECOMMENDATION |
| --- | --- |
| Systolic blood pressure | ≥ 100 mmHg for individuals 50–69 years old<br>≥110 mmHg for individuals 15–49 or over 70 years old |
| Cerebral perfusion pressure | Between 60–70 mmHg |
| Oxygenation | PaO₂ <60 mmHg or O₂ saturation percentage about 90% |
| Ventilation | Prophylactic hyperventilation is not recommended unless it is used as a temporary measure to decrease intracranial pressure. |
| Intracranial pressure | Monitor intracranial pressure (ICP) in patients with severe TBI and abnormal CT scan or in patients with a normal CT scan but who meet 2 or more of the qualifying criteria: >40 years old, motor posturing, or systolic blood pressure of less than 90 mmHg |

**Table 170.2** EFFECTS OF DIFFERENT INTRAVENOUS ANESTHETICS

| AGENT | EFFECT | NOTE |
|---|---|---|
| Barbiturates | Decrease cerebral blood flow, cerebral blood volume, and intracranial pressure | |
| Etomidate | Decreases cerebral blood flow, cerebral metabolic rate of oxygen, and intracranial pressure | Prolonged use may suppress adrenocortical response to stress |
| Propofol | Decreases cerebral blood flow, cerebral metabolic rate of oxygen, and intracranial pressure | Can reduce cerebral blood flow more than cerebral metabolic rate of oxygen, causing ischemia in certain conditions |
| Benzodiazepines | Minimal hemodynamic effects on cerebral circulation | |

**Table 170.3** EFFECTS OF DIFFERENT INHALATIONAL ANESTHETICS[3-5]

| AGENT | EFFECT | NOTE |
|---|---|---|
| Isoflurane | Depresses cerebral metabolism | With hyperventilation, no significant increase in intracranial pressure |
| Sevoflurane | Depresses cerebral metabolism | With hyperventilation, no significant increase in intracranial pressure; biodegraded metabolite may be toxic in high concentrations |
| Desflurane | Depresses cerebral metabolism | With hyperventilation, no significant increase in intracranial pressure |
| Nitrous oxide | Increases intracranial pressure | |

## VENTILATION AND POSITIONING

CSF flow and intracranial pressure (ICP) are affected by the levels of carbon dioxide in the blood, so ventilation plays a crucial role in maintaining the appropriate ICP. At baseline, the mechanical ventilation should maintain a $PaCO_2$ of about 35 mmHg and the $PaO^2$ of >100 mmHg, but hypo- and hyperventilation can be used to alter ICP.[3] Hypoventilation has been used to increase cerebral blood flow, but it is most common to see mild hyperventilation present during brain tumor surgeries.[3] The position of the patient is dependent on the location and approach to the tumor, but a patient undergoing surgery from an anterior approach will be positioned in a supine position with a head tilt of 15 degrees to aid in the draining of cerebral venous blood.[3]

## REFERENCES

1. Curry PD, et al. Perioperative management of traumatic brain injury. *Int. J. Crit. Illn. Inj. Sci.* 2011 Jan;1(1):27–35. doi: 10.4103/2229-5151.79279.
2. Dash HH, Chavali S. Management of traumatic brain injury patients. *Korean J Anesthesiol.* 2018;71(1):12–21. https://doi.org/10.4097/kjae.2018.71.1.12.
3. Goma H. Anesthetic considerations of brain tumor surgery. In: *Diagnostic Techniques and Surgical Management of Brain Tumors.* 2011.
4. Kaye AD, et al. The effects of desflurane vs. isoflurane in patients with intracranial masses." *Anesth and Analges.* 2004;98:1127–1132.
5. Bundgaard H, et al. Effects of sevoflurane on intracranial pressure, cerebral blood flow and cerebral metabolism: A dose-response study in patients subjected to craniotomy for cerebral tumours. *Acta Anaesthesiol Scand.* 1998 Jul;42(6):621–627.

# 171.

# CEREBROSPINAL FLUID

*Christina T. Nguyen and Nathan Schulman*

## INTRODUCTION

Cerebrospinal fluid (CSF) is critical to the central nervous system, as it bathes the entire brain and spinal cord. It provides a buoyant environment in which the brain and spinal cord are suspended, thus acting as a fluid buffer from shock. It also helps regulate brain interstitial fluid homeostasis and therefore neuronal functioning.

## PHYSIOLOGY OF CSF

The majority of CSF is produced in the lateral, third, and fourth ventricles by choroid plexuses. It then flows through the ventricles and out the foramen of Magendie and the foramina of Luschka to the subarachnoid space, where it fills the space around the brain and spinal cord between the arachnoid and pia matter. The normal adult CSF volume is about 125–150 ml with a production rate of 20 ml/hr. Therefore, over the course of a day, 400–600 ml of CSF is created and the CSF is completely renewed 3–5 times daily. The turnover rate is reduced with age due to a decrease in cerebral volume and compensatory increase in total CSF volume without increase in CSF production rate.[1]

Cells of the choroid plexus are interconnected by tight junctions, helping to create a blood-CSF barrier. This barrier helps control the environment around the brain, preventing cells, protein, and glucose from entering the CSF, while allowing an entry for small ions and nutrients. CSF is passively absorbed by the arachnoid villi, found in the dural venous sinuses and around the roots of spinal nerves.[2]

Sympathetic stimulation reduces CSF production via receptors on the choroid plexus, while parasympathetic stimulation increases CSF production. Medications can also affect production. Loop diuretics and carbonic anhydrase inhibitors can decrease production.

## CSF COMPOSITION

Chemically, CSF is similar to blood plasma and is initially passively filtered, driven by a pressure gradient. However, transport proteins also actively regulate the passage of ions. Aquaporins then transport water, following the osmotic gradient created by these pumps. Compared to plasma, CSF has lower protein, glucose, potassium, and calcium; and higher sodium, chloride, and magnesium (see Table 171.1). Due to tight junctions on the blood-brain barrier, CSF is generally acellular and low in protein. Glucose levels in CSF usually follow a ratio of 0.6 of serum glucose levels. Low CSF glucose may indicate infection; high levels may indicate hyperglycemia.

## CSF PRESSURE

The pressure of CSF is important to proper neuronal metabolism and function. The cranium and spinal cord create a volume static space comprising three compartments: parenchyma, blood, and CSF. Changes in volume to one affect the others by increasing pressure which is transmitted via CSF to the other compartments.

CSF pressure is measured with the patient supine with legs extended via a puncture into the subarachnoid space,

*Table 171.1* CSF AND PLASMA COMPOSITION

| SOLUTE | PLASMA | CSF |
|---|---|---|
| Sodium | 138 mmol $l^{-1}$ | 138 mmol $l^{-1}$ |
| Potassium | 4.5 mmol $l^{-1}$ | 2.8 mmol $l^{-1}$ |
| Calcium | 2.4 mmol $l^{-1}$ | 1.1 mmol $l^{-1}$ |
| Magnesium | 1.7 mmol $l^{-1}$ | 0.3 mmol $l^{-1}$ |
| Chloride | 102 mmol $l^{-1}$ | 119 mmol $l^{-1}$ |
| Bicarbonate | 24 mmol $l^{-1}$ | 22 mmol $l^{-1}$ |
| Glucose | 5.0 mmol $l^{-1}$ | 3.3 mmol $l^{-1}$ |
| Total protein | 70 g $l^{-1}$ | 0.3 g $l^{-1}$ |

From: May R, Reddy U. Cerebrospinal fluid and its physiology. *Anaesth Intensive Care Med.* 2019;21(1):60–61. Copyright 2019, with permission from Elsevier.

commonly at the lumbar level, but also possibly in the cranium. Normal pressure is 10–15 mmHg in adults and 3–4 mmHg in infants. Variations can occur from systolic pulse wave, respiratory cycle, abdominal pressure, jugular venous pressure, physical activity, and posture.[1]

Increased CSF pressure can be due to an imbalance of CSF production and absorption. The main determinant for rate of CSF absorption is CSF pressure and venous pressure; thus states of elevated venous pressure such as chronic heart failure and fluid overload can upset the balance of formation and absorption of CSF. Other factors that can indirectly increase CSF pressure include mass effects such as tumors, bleeding, and infections. Consequences of increased CSF pressure include hydrocephalus, shifting of brain parenchyma causing herniation, and impaired cerebral blood flow leading to ischemia. Underproduction of CSF or an increased drainage can lead to intracranial hypotension.

CSF production and reabsorption are often altered under anesthesia. Regarding CSF production, sevoflurane and halothane decrease production, and high concentrations of enflurane increase production. Anesthetics can also alter reabsorption of CSF. Sevoflurane increases resistance to reabsorption, whereas high concentrations of isoflurane decrease resistance to absorption. Halothane has a dual effect, decreasing production and increasing resistance to reabsorption, with an end result of increased intracranial pressure. Intravenous anesthetics also have varying effects on CSF production and reabsorption. For example, ketamine increases resistance to reabsorption and thus increases intracranial pressure, while propofol does not appear to alter production or reabsorption. At low doses, fentanyl decreases resistance to reabsorption, and at high doses it decreases CSF production, resulting in decreased intracranial pressure.[4]

## REFERENCES

1. Sakka L, Coll G, Chazal J. Anatomy and physiology of cerebrospinal fluid. *Eur Ann Otorhinolaryngol Head Neck Dis.* 2011;128:309–316.
2. Telano L, Baker S. Physiology, cerebral spinal fluid (CSF). In: *StatPearls* [Internet]. Treasure Island, FL: StatPearls; 2020. https://www.ncbi.nlm.nih.gov/books/NBK519007/.
3. May R, Reddy U. Cerebrospinal fluid and its physiology. *Anaesth Intensive Care Med.* 2019;21(1):60–61.
4. Cottrell J, Patel P. *Cottrell and Patel's Neuroanesthesia.* 6th ed. New York, NY: Elsevier; 2017.

# 172.

# BLOOD-BRAIN BARRIER

*Allyson L. Spence and Elyse M. Cornett*

## INTRODUCTION

The *blood-brain barrier* is a term used to describe the highly selective, semipermeable microvasculature of the central nervous system (CNS) that is crucial for CNS regulation and proper neuronal function. This dynamic, restrictive barrier protects the brain from potentially harmful substances such as toxins, pathogens, and drugs. Loss of this barrier from pathological conditions exposes the brain to these toxic, inflammatory substances. Likewise, the blood-brain barrier plays a key role in the onset and progression of such pathological conditions.[1]

## ACTIVE AND PASSIVE MOLECULAR TRANSPORT ACROSS THE BLOOD-BRAIN BARRIER

The endothelial cells of the blood-brain barrier are characterized by specialized tight junctions that contain unique proteins (e.g., claudins, occludins, and junctional adhesion molecules) that enable the highly restrictive nature of the blood-brain barrier. These tight junctions restrict the movement of small ions (e.g., $Na^+$, $K^+$, $Ca^{2+}$, and $Cl^-$), hydrophilic molecules, and most charged molecules, while allowing lipophilic and small gaseous substances to passively diffuse across the blood-brain barrier. The two primary types of transporters expressed by these endothelial cells are nutrient transporters and efflux transporters. Nutrient transporters enable the transport of nutrients from the blood into the CNS while removing waste products from the CNS into the blood. Efflux transporters, such as adenosine triphosphate-binding cassette (i.e., ABC) transporters, actively translocate a wide array of lipophilic substrates from the CNS back into the blood circulation, thus providing an extra layer of protection from molecules that would otherwise passively diffuse through the endothelial cell membrane.[1,2]

## BYPASSING THE BLOOD-BRAIN BARRIER WITH DRUGS

The aforementioned protective mechanisms provided by the blood-brain barrier also provide a barrier for delivering drugs to the brain. To overcome this barrier, researchers have identified, designed, and altered drugs to enable them to more readily cross the blood-brain barrier. Some of these alterations include increasing lipophilicity, utilizing prodrugs that can more readily pass the blood-brain barrier, and designing drugs that target endogenous receptors found at the blood-brain barrier. However, most of these pharmaceuticals may still be unable to sufficiently penetrate the CNS due to the complexity of the restrictive blood-brain barrier. For example, although small, lipophilic chemotherapeutic drugs may easily penetrate the CNS, the efflux mechanism of ABC transporters decreases intracellular drug concentrations, often contributing to the chemoresistance associated with these drugs.[3]

## BLOOD-BRAIN BARRIER DISRUPTION

Blood-brain barrier disruption has been observed in several neurological disorders (e.g., Alzheimer's disease, multiple sclerosis, epilepsy, stroke, and traumatic brain injuries). This dysfunction can lead to cerebral edema, neuroinflammation, neurotoxicity, and degeneration. Soluble factors associated with these diseases (e.g., glutamate; endothilin-1; pro-inflammatory mediators, such as tumor necrosis factor a [TNF a], bradykinin, and histamine) are responsible for the breakdown of the blood-brain barrier. It is still largely unclear whether these disease states lead to blood-brain barrier

disruption or whether the blood-brain barrier dysfunction is the primary pathogenic factor.[1,4]

## DIAGNOSIS OF BLOOD-BRAIN BARRIER DISRUPTION

Diagnostic tools are available to evaluate blood-brain barrier dysfunction. Among the highly preferred methods for evaluating blood-brain barrier intactness are the assessment of the cerebrospinal fluid/plasma albumin ratio (i.e., Qalb). Under normal, healthy conditions, albumin does not readily cross the blood-brain barrier, and thus, albumin accumulation in the cerebrospinal fluid can indicate a disruption of the blood-brain barrier. Direct measurements (i.e., lumbar puncture) can be used to assess these albumin levels, or albumin can be chemically linked to radiopaque ions to reveal albumin accumulations through a contrast-enhanced CT-MRI.[4]

## ANESTHETIC MANAGEMENT

Although more studies evaluating the effects of anesthesia on blood-brain barrier functionality are needed, numerous studies have indicated that general anesthesia agents (e.g., isoflurane, fentanyl, ketamine, and pentobarbital) can increase blood-brain barrier permeability, which may lead to neuroinflammation, postoperative cognitive impairment, and postoperative delirium. It has been shown that blood-brain barrier disruption is smaller during isoflurane anesthesia than during pentobarbitol anesthesia. Furthermore, the degree of this disruption could be decreased by adding morphine or pentobarbital during isoflurane anesthesia. Therefore, it is important to assess patients, particularly those who are vulnerable to experiencing blood-brain barrier dysfunction (e.g., the elderly and immunocompromised), for symptoms of these postoperative conditions.[5]

## REFERENCES

1. Daneman R, Prat A. The blood–brain barrier. *Cold Spring Harb Perspect Biol*. 2015; 5;7(1):a020412.
2. Barar J, et al. Blood-brain barrier transport machineries and targeted therapy of brain diseases. *BioImpacts* [Internet]. 2016;6(4):225–248.
3. Dong X. Current strategies for brain drug delivery. *Theranostics*. 2018;8(6):1481–1493.
4. Marchi N, Rasmussen P, Kapural M, Fazio V, Kight K, Mayberg MR, et al. Peripheral markers of brain damage and blood-brain barrier dysfunction. *Restor Neurol Neurosci*. 2003;21(3–4):109–121.
5. Almutairi MMA, et al. Factors controlling permeability of the blood-brain barrier. *Cell Mol Life Sci*. 2016;73(1):57–77.

# 173.

# RELATION TO BLOOD CHEMISTRY AND ACID-BASE BALANCE

*Evan DaBreo and Lynn Kohan*

## INTRODUCTION

The physiologic mechanisms of cerebrospinal fluid (CSF) buffering in relation to blood chemistry and acid-base balance are crucial in understanding the ventilatory response to metabolic derangements[1,2] and induced changes in intracranial pressure.[3,4] Hyperventilation is often used in the context of head trauma or neurosurgical procedures to reduce intracranial pressure (ICP); however, careful use of this technique is critical. The physiology of CSF is affected by blood chemistry and acid-base balance in several ways; however, the most clinically relevant relationship is its ability to buffer $CO_2$ changes in the brain. In anesthesia this concept is central to our understanding of how central chemoreceptors increase or decrease spontaneous respiration in response to hypercapnia and hypocapnia, respectively.[1,2] Additionally, this concept underpins the time-variable response of intracranial pressure/cerebral blood flow to systemic changes in $PaCO_2$.

## RESPIRATORY PATTERNS AND CSF ACID-BASE BALANCE

Chemoreceptors, which are sensitive to $CO_2$/H+ changes, exist throughout the brainstem; however, the primary chemoreceptors of the respiration system exist on the central surface of the medulla. While the chemoreceptor sites of the brainstem have variable effects on respiratory frequency and tidal volume,[1] the general trend is an increase in minute ventilation as $CO_2$ levels rise. Clinically, this can be seen in diabetic ketoacidosis as respirations go through a series of changes induced by the prolonged activation of central receptors. In Diabetic Ketoacidosis, the rate of respiration will increase initially during early acidosis. This is followed by an increase in tidal volume as the acidosis worsens. Lastly, the respiratory pattern transitions to deep and fast Kussmaul respirations in late acidosis (see Figure 173.1).[2] Animal studies suggest that the pattern of respiration change is variable depending on if the nature of the systemic acidosis is metabolic versus respiratory.[1]

## CEREBROVASCULAR BLOOD FLOW REGULATION AND CSF ACID-BASE BALANCE

Arterial $CO_2$ ($PaCO_2$) is often viewed as the major regulator of cerebrovascular smooth muscle tone, causing vasodilation and vasoconstriction as $CO_2$ levels rise and fall, respectively.[3] Because non-ionized $CO^2$ molecules, and not

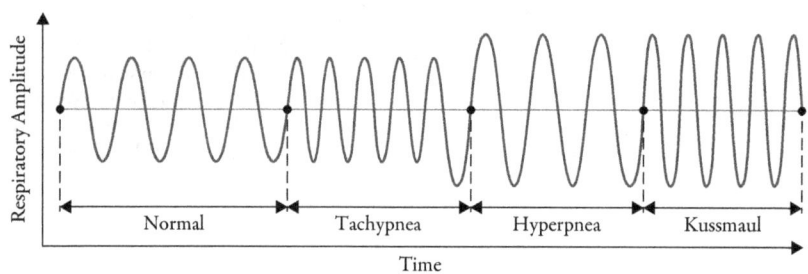

**Figure 173.1** Example of transition from normal respiratory pattern to Kussmaul respiration due to CSF acid-base disturbance in the setting of DKA.
Reproduced courtesy of Evan DaBreo, Resident, Department of Anesthesiology, University of Virginia Health, Charlottesville, VA

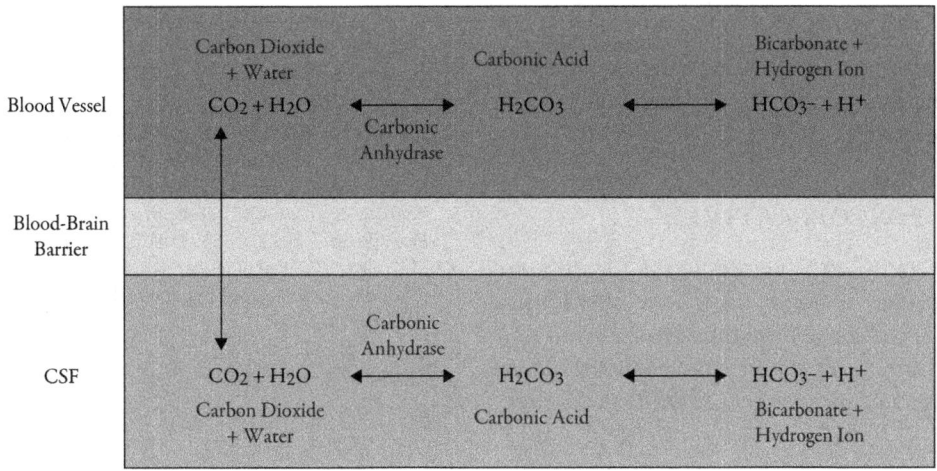

**Figure 173.2** Diagram of $CO_2$ transfer across the blood-brain barrier and conversion of $CO_2$ to H+ and $HCO_{3-}$ ion in the CSF by carbonic anhydrase.
Reproduced courtesy of Evan DaBreo, Resident, Department of Anesthesiology, University of Virginia Health, Charlottesville, VA.

ionized molecules such as H+, are able to cross the blood-brain barrier, this relationship is largely independent of systemic arterial pH.[4] Further, numerous animal studies have shown that local perivascular pH, and not dissolved $CO_2$, is the major driving factor of cerebrovascular smooth muscle tone. The implication of this finding is that while clinically we equate the rise and fall of $PaCO_2$ levels with the degree of cerebrovascular blood flow (CBF), the buffering capacity of CSF is ultimately the determinant of this phenomenon.[4] After crossing the blood-brain barrier, carbonic anhydrase breaks down $CO_2$ into $HCO_{3-}$ and H+ (see Figure 173.2).[5] The presence of increased H+ has a profound effect on perivascular pH and consequently the degree of cerebral arteriole dilation. Conversely, a reduction in H+ and concomitant increase in perivascular pH result in vasoconstriction and reduced CBF.[3,4,5]

The dilation and contraction of cerebral vasculature occurs both with variation in HCO3- with constant $CO_2$, and with variation in $CO_2$ with constant $HCO_{3-}$. This finding reaffirms the idea that changes in CSF pH are the most important factor in direct smooth muscle tone changes.[1] While dissolved $CO_2$ in CSF likely has some indirect effects on vasoconstriction via endothelium, nerves, and astrocytes,[3] the importance of CSF pH helps to explain why sustained hyperventilation is unable to maintain a depression of CBF.[4]

pH units.[3] Despite this finding, it has been observed that CBF will return to baseline as both blood and CSF pH return to normal over 6–24 hours regardless of ventilatory changes. The underlying mechanism of this return toward normal pH is due to renal compensation in the blood and a decreased bicarbonate secretion by the choroid plexus in the CSF.[4] The return to normal CSF pH despite continued hyperventilation is a cause for concern in clinical anesthesia as the brain not only loses the ability to reduce CBF with further reductions in $PaCO_2$, but also increases in reactivity. This increase in reactivity occurs due to decreased bicarbonate secretion and the CSF's diminished capacity for buffering.[4] Clinically this can manifest as a rebound increase in CBF and ICP when prolonged hyperventilation is discontinued abruptly. Alternatively, this alteration in "$CO_2$ reactivity" can result in a potentially larger increase in CBF during periods of acute $CO_2$ rise such as airway suctioning.[4]

The preceding findings support the use of hyperventilation only during periods of actual ICP increase, or during periods where contraction of the intracranial volume is needed to improve the surgical field. Prophylactic use of hyperventilation may be deleterious as the CSF loses its buffering capacity and cerebrovascular smooth muscle becomes less responsive to further reductions in $PaCO_2$.[4]

## INDUCED CHANGES IN CEREBROVASCULAR BLOOD FLOW

Alteration of mechanical ventilation to induce hypocapnia and hypercapnia has been shown to raise and decrease CSF pH, respectively, in the short phase by approximately 0.3

## ANESTHETIC CONSIDERATIONS

### PREOPERATIVE

Close communication with the neurosurgical team prior to procedure is key for planning any potential need for reduction in ICP to improve operative conditions.

## INTRAOPERATIVE

Judicious use of hyperventilation is important to allow for a predictable reduction in CBF when needed and to avoid increased "$CO_2$ reactivity."

## POSTOPERATIVE

The increased "reactivity" to acute rises in $PaCO_2$ after prolonged hyperventilation can last for many hours after surgery. This is an important consideration in the intensive care unit as the need for ventilator circuit maintenance or airway suction may cause an exaggerated increase in CBF/ICP as $CO_2$ rises.

## REFERENCES

1. Kawai A, et al. Mechanisms of $CO_2$/H+ chemoreception by respiratory rhythm generator neurons in the medulla from newborn rats in vitro. *J Physiol.* 2006;572(Pt 2):525–537.
2. Gallo de Moraes A, et al. Effects of diabetic ketoacidosis in the respiratory system. *World J Diabetes.* 2019;10(1):16–22.
3. Yoon S, et al. pCO(2) and pH regulation of cerebral blood flow. *Front Physiol.* 2012;3:365. doi:10.3389/fphys.2012.00365.
4. Muizelaar JP, et al. Pial arteriolar vessel diameter and $CO_2$ reactivity during prolonged hyperventilation in the rabbit. *J Neurosurg.* 1988;69:923–927.
5. Kazemi H, Johnson DC. Regulation of cerebrospinal fluid acid-base balance. *Physiolog Rev.* 198;66(4):970–966.

# 174.

# INCREASED INTRACRANIAL PRESSURE

*Kenan Alkhalili and Ned F. Nasr*

## PATHOPHYSIOLOGY OF ELEVATED INTRACRANIAL PRESSURE

Approximately 20 mL/hour of cerebrospinal fluid (CSF) is produced by choroid plexus (~500 mL/day) and reabsorbed via the arachnoid granulations into the venous system. The intracranial compartment is protected by the skull (fixed volume); hence, the sum of volumes of brain, CSF, and intracranial blood is constant. An increase in one should cause a decrease in one or both remaining two. Accordingly, intracranial pressure (ICP) is a function of the volume and compliance of each component of the intracranial compartment, an interrelationship known as the Monro-Kellie hypothesis. Intracranial pathologies such as mass lesions, hemorrhage, edema, increased CSF production, decreased CSF absorption, obstruction of venous outflow, and obstructive hydrocephalus may result an alternation of brain compliance, which often leads to increased ICP.

## ANESTHESIA CONSIDERATIONS

### PREOPERATIVE

#### ICP Monitoring

The purpose of monitoring ICP is to improve the clinician's ability to maintain adequate cerebral perfusion pressure (CPP) and oxygenation. Monitoring can be invasive or noninvasive. Noninvasive methods include transcranial Doppler ultrasound (TCD), which can be used to estimate ICP based on characteristic changes in waveforms. TCD, however, is a poor predictor of ICP, and is more helpful in assessment of vasospasm. Optic nerve sheath ultrasound provides a useful quick noninvasive tool for assessment of elevated ICP. Using a cut-off of 5.9 millimeters optic sheath diameter for elevated ICP has been associated with 93% sensitivity.[1] Intraventricular monitors are considered the gold standard of invasive ICP monitoring. The main advantages of this system are the accuracy, and the ability to drain CSF to treat

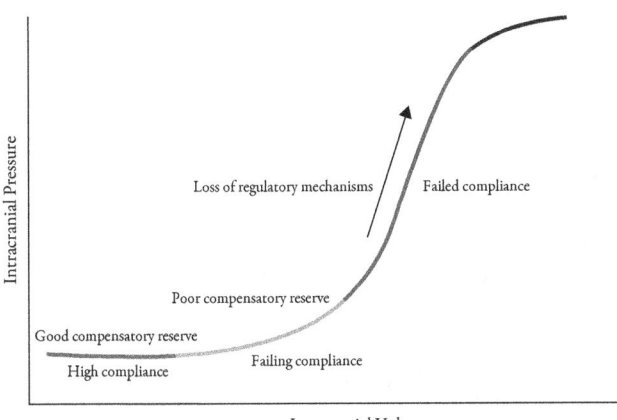

Figure 174.1 Compliance curve.

elevated ICP. However, there is an increased risk of infection in up to 20% of patients, and increased risk of bleeding particularly in coagulopathic patients.[2] Another commonly used method for ICP monitoring is the fiberoptic Camino system, which are inserted directly into the brain parenchyma. The disadvantage of this system is the lack of the ability to drain CSF in elevated ICP patients.

ICP exhibits cyclic variation based on the superimposed effects of cardiac contraction, respiration, and intracranial compliance. The P1 wave, also known as the percussion wave, correlates with the arterial pulse transmitted through the choroid plexus into the CSF. The P2 wave, also known as the tidal wave, represents cerebral compliance; it can be thought of as a "reflection" of the arterial pulse wave bouncing off the springy brain parenchyma. The P3 wave, also known as the dicrotic wave, is caused by aortic valve closure. Under normal conditions P1 > P2; however, when the brain starts losing compliance, P2 becomes > P1, and there will be rounding of waveform and appearance of plateau waves (Lundberg B and A waves) (Figures 174.1 and 174.2).

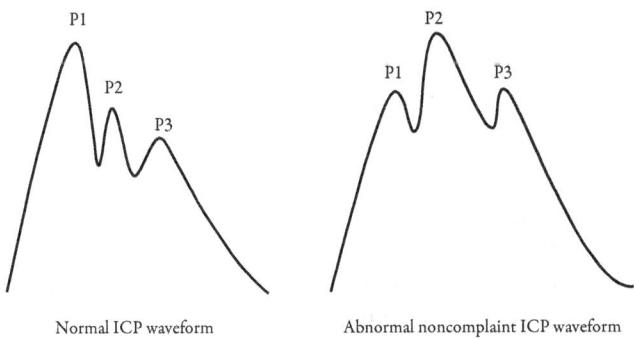

Figure 174.2 ICP wave forms: normal and noncompliant waveforms.

## INTRAOPERATIVE

### Management of Increased ICP

The first line of management of intracranial hypertension is the treatment of the cause (e.g., evacuation of blood clot, tumor resection, CSF diversion in obstructive hydrocephalus). Generally accepted levels: ICP ≤ 20–25. Interventions should be utilized only when ICP is elevated for >5–10 minutes.

General principles that should be routinely done include elevating the HOB 30 to 45 degrees and keeping the head midline to prevent obstruction of jugular veins.

CSF drainage can be highly effective, even if only a small amount is removed. Over-drainage leads to ventricular collapse over the tip of ventriculostomy catheter, resulting in its malfunction. Additionally, it could worsen already existing subdural hematoma.

Appropriate sedation can decrease ICP by reducing metabolic demand, overcoming ventilator asynchrony, alleviating venous congestion, and blunting sympathetic responses of hypertension and tachycardia. Propofol is the most commonly used sedative for ICP control. It increases the depth of sedation in a dose-dependent manner: at doses <4 mg/kg/h, CBF/CMRO$_2$ coupling, cerebrovascular reactivity, and brain oxygenation are preserved, while at higher doses (>5 mg/kg/h), propofol can induce electroencephalogram (EEG) burst suppression that can be effective to treat status epilepticus. Midazolam is more susceptible to tissue accumulation, leading to delayed ventilation weaning; however, it may be preferred over propofol in case of hemodynamic instability. Of note, both agents may alter hemodynamics and cause a reduction in CPP, though this is more frequent with propofol than with midazolam. The use of ketamine has been debatable, yet recent studies have shown that it decreases ICP while maintaining CPP.[3] There is no clear evidence of barbiturates' benefit in improving the outcome in patients with intracranial hypertension.

There is no clear evidence of superiority of either mannitol or hypertonic saline in reducing ICP. Increasing the serum osmolarity initially to a target of 300–320 mOsm/L improves osmotic gradient and alleviates brain edema. Mannitol boluses (0.25–1 g/kg, q 6 hours) are preferred over continuous infusion, as the infusion increases uptake into brain tissue. Hypertonic saline (3% or 23.4%) can be used in alternating fashion with mannitol, aiming to maintain serum sodium at high normal levels. Its principal mechanism of action is to increase plasma osmolality, resulting in water movement out of the brain along the osmotic gradient.

It is noteworthy that serum osmolality is not predictive of mannitol-induced acute renal insufficiency; thus its use as a limiting factor is unwarranted.[4] Furosemide can be used as an ICP-reduction agent, by inducing systemic diuresis and decreasing CSF production. It can be used as monotherapy (5–1 mg/kg), or in combination with mannitol at lower doses.

Hyperventilation to $PaCO_2 = 30$–35 mmHg has been shown to rapidly reduce ICP. It has been reported that for every 1 mmHg decrease in $PaCO_2$, there is a 3%–4% cerebral blood flow drop. Thus, aggressive hyperventilation $PaCo_2 < 25$ mmHg may worsen cerebral ischemia secondary to vasoconstriction.[5] It is also important to maintain proper oxygenation and glucose control.

The value of induced hypothermia has remained controversial in elevated ICP management. Hypothermia decreases cerebral metabolism and may reduce cerebral blood flow and ICP. Hypothermia can be achieved by whole-body cooling to a goal core temperature of 32° to 34°C.

In medical refractory cases, decompressive craniectomy might be considered in selected cases to increase potential volume of the intracranial contents, circumventing the Monroe-Kellie doctrine.

## POSTOPERATIVE

Patients with intracranial hypertension require close monitoring in the intensive care unit (ICU), particularly those with ventriculostomy catheter. Close $EtCO_2$ monitoring is paramount, as the ICP is sensitive to hypercarbia. Thus, extubation might be delayed to ensure adequate spontaneous ventilation and appropriate $CO_2$ levels. ICP elevation can be managed as described previously.

## REFERENCES

1. Lochner P, et al. Feasibility and usefulness of ultrasonography in idiopathic intracranial hypertension or secondary intracranial hypertension. *BMC Neurol.* 2016;16:85.
2. Mayhall CG, et al. Ventriculostomy-related infections: A prospective epidemiologic study. *N Engl J Med.* 1984;310(9):553–559.
3. Oddo M, et al. Optimizing sedation in patients with acute brain injury. *Crit Care.* 2016;20(1):128.
4. de Gondim FA, et al. Osmolality not predictive of mannitol-induced acute renal insufficiency. *J Neurosurg.* 2005;103(3):444–447.
5. Marik PE, et al. Management of head trauma. *Chest.* 2002;122(2): 699–711.

# 175.

# GENERAL ORGANIZATION OF THE SPINAL CORD

*Asli Ozcan and Till Conermann*

## INTRODUCTION

The spinal cord can be described as central nervous tissue that extends caudally from the brainstem and ends in the conus medullaris as the filum terminale and the cauda equina. It is important to note that the conus medullaris is typically located at the lower L1 level in adults, in contrast with its location at the L3 level in infants, due to developmental growth rate differences between the vertebral column and the spinal cord.

## VERTEBRAL COLUMN

The vertebral column consists of 33 vertebrae divided into 5 sections (7 cervical, 12 thoracic, 5 lumbar, 5 sacral, and 4 coccygeal). The vertebrae of the sacral and coccygeal regions are fused together, typically resulting in 24 mobile segments, though this segmentation can have congenital variations.[1] The structural organization of bony vertebrae gives rise to the cavity known as the spinal canal (also referred to as *vertebral canal*, or *vertebral cavity*) through which the spinal cord runs.

# SPINAL CORD

## GROSS ANATOMY AND SPINAL NERVES

The spinal cord is enveloped by the meninges, which are three protective membranes known as pia, arachnoid, and dura mater (listed in order of innermost to outer layering). The subarachnoid space (also called *intrathecal space*) contains the cerebrospinal fluid (CSF) and separates the pia and arachnoid membranes. The dura is surrounded by the epidural space. The epidural space is lined posteriorly by the ligamentum flavum, and anteriorly by the posterior longitudinal ligament.[2]

At each level of the spinal cord, a pair of ventral and dorsal roots emerge, combining into what is known as the mixed spinal nerve (Figure 175.1). A total of 31 pairs of spinal nerves exit the vertebral canal below their corresponding levels, with the exception of cervical spinal nerves that exit above.[3]

Transverse sectioning of the spinal cord reveals a small central canal that contains CSF, surrounded by butterfly-shaped gray matter, and an outermost layer of white matter.

## GRAY MATTER

The gray matter of the spinal cord consists of neuronal cell bodies, dendrites, axons, and glial cells. Gray matter can be primarily divided as follows. Regions in the dorsal half of the gray matter are referred to as the *dorsal horns* (posterior), the ventral half is referred to as the *ventral horns* (anterior); and the region around the central canal is called the *intermediate region*. The *intermediolateral horn* (also referred to as the *lateral gray column*) is a projection of the gray matter present in the thoracic and upper lumbar levels. Histologic analysis further divides the spinal gray matter into 10 layers based on cellular architecture, known as the laminae of Rexed.[4] These defined regions also correspond to specific functionality.

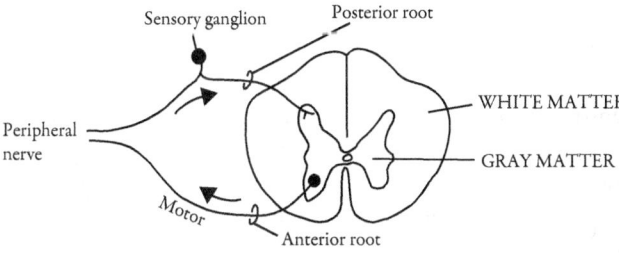

**Figure 175.1.** Cross-section of spinal cord. Digital illustration of cross-section showing posterior, anterior, and lateral columns of gray and white matter.

Reproduced with permission from Betts JG et al. *Anatomy and Physiology*. Houston, TX: OpenStax; 2013.

Here are some important structures to highlight:

- The dorsal horn contains Rexed laminae I to VI and serves as an essential sensory relay station for the transmission of sensory and noxious input from the periphery to the brain.[5]
  - In Laminae I and II, also known as substantia gelatinosa, opioid receptors are abundantly expressed, indicating an important role for this region in analgesia.
- The ventral horn contains Rexed laminae VIII to IX, which house cell bodies of motor interneurons and primary alpha, beta, and gamma neurons.
- Lateral gray column contains Rexed laminae VII and X, with lamina VII housing the intermediolateral and the intermediomedial nuclei, and Rexed lamina X surrounding the central canal.[5] The intermediolateral horn carries preganglionic sympathetic fibers. The intermediolateral cell column (IML, Rexed Lamina VII) present at T1–L2 is responsible for sympathetic outflow of the autonomic nervous system.

## WHITE MATTER

The white matter layer surrounding the gray matter is largely made of myelinated axons and glial cells. The white matter is also divided into three regions: dorsal, lateral, and ventral.[4]

- The dorsal columns consist mostly of axons of second-order sensory neurons originating in the dorsal horn of the gray matter, which make up the main pathway for skin sensation and proprioception from limbs and trunk to the central nervous system (CNS).
- The lateral and ventral columns of white matter carry numerous ascending and descending fiber groups, such as:
  - Ascending (Sensory): lateral spinothalamic tract (pain, temperature), ventral spinothalamic tract (light touch)
  - Descending (Motor): ventral corticospinal tract, lateral corticospinal tract.

## ARTERIAL SUPPLY OF THE SPINAL CORD

The spinal cord receives its arterial blood supply from one anterior spinal artery, two paired posterior spinal arteries, and segmental spinal arteries, which originate from intercostal and lumbar arteries.

- The anterior spinal artery originates from the vertebral artery and descends ventrally along the spinal cord, receiving contribution from anterior segmental medullary and radicular arteries, to supply the anterior one-half to two-thirds of the spinal cord.[3]

- The largest anterior segmental medullary artery is the artery of Adamkiewicz, which most commonly arises on the left side of the aorta and travels with the T9–12 roots, though there is significant anatomic variability between individuals. The artery of Adamkiewicz (also called the great radicular artery) is a major contributor of blood supply for lower thoracic and upper lumbar regions of the spinal cord.[2] It is crucial that the artery of Adamkiewicz is identified in its variable location prior to cross-clamping in major aortic surgery, to reduce risk of paralysis.

- Structures supplied by the anterior spinal artery and its segmental spinal arteries include the anterior and lateral corticospinal tracts, the anterolateral system, and the anterior horns. Of note, the dorsal columns are not supplied by the anterior spinal artery; hence injury to the anterior spinal can lead to paralysis, fecal/urinary incontinence, and loss of pain and temperature sensation below the level of the lesion, while sparing sensation of vibration and proprioception. This is referred to as *anterior spinal artery syndrome*.[3] The anterior, deep portion of the cord is especially prone to ischemia.[2]

- The paired posterior spinal arteries originate from the inferior cerebellar artery and supply the posterior one-third of the spinal cord, supported by contributions from posterior segmental medullary arteries. Important structures supplied by the posterior spinal arteries include the dorsal columns and dorsal horns of the spinal cord and posterior spinal nerve roots.[3]

## REFERENCES

1. Gardocki RJ. Spinal anatomy and surgical approaches. In: Azar FM, Canale ST, Beaty JH, eds. *Campbell's Operative Orthopaedics.* Philadelphia, PA: Elsevier Health Sciences; 2016:1572–1609.
2. Brull R, et al. Spinal, epidural, and caudal anesthesia. In: Gropper MA, et al., eds. *Miller's Anesthesia.* Philadelphia, PA: Elsevier Health Sciences; 2019:1413–1449.
3. Moussazadeh N, Fu KMG. Spinal anatomy. In: Winn HR, ed. *Youmans and Winn Neurological Surgery.* Philadelphia, PA: Elsevier Health Sciences; 2017:2259–2270.
4. Watson C, et al., eds. *The Spinal Cord: A Christopher and Dana Reeve Foundation Text and Atlas.* Burlington, MA: Academic Press; 2009.
5. Benzon HT, et al. Chronic pain management. In: Barash PG, et al., eds. *Clinical Anesthesia.* Philadelphia, PA: Wolters Kluwer; 2017:1607–1631.

# 176.

# SPINAL CORD REFLEXES

*Alex Woodrow and Archit Sharma*

## INTRODUCTION

In addition to transmitting sensory and motor impulses to and from the cerebral cortex and brainstem, the spinal cord also contains reflex arcs that are independent of higher cortical function to work. A *reflex* is an involuntary, stereotypical response of the effector tissue from the stimulation of receptors. A *reflex arc* is the pathway by which nerves carry sensory information from the receptor to the spinal cord, and then carry the response from the spinal cord to peripheral organs during a reflex action. The brain analyzes the signal, after the reflex action has already occurred. There are two types of reflex arcs: the *autonomic* reflex arc, affecting inner organs, and the *somatic* reflex arc, affecting muscles.[1]

Based on how many neurons are involved in one arc, the reflexes can be **monosynaptic** or **polysynaptic**.

## MONOSYNAPTIC REFLEXES

The monosynaptic reflexes consist of just two neurons. The sensory neuron is located within the spinal ganglion, which detects the stimuli from the muscle and conducts this signal to the ventral horn of the spinal cord, where the second neuron is situated. The second neuron, which is a motor neuron, sends the appropriate signal via its axon back to the same muscle. The entire arc has only one neuronal synapse that is directly between neuron I and neuron II.

The simplest reflex arc is the myotatic reflex that is known by different names, such as deep tendon reflexes (DTRs), the muscle stretch reflex, or a monosynaptic stretch reflex. The clinically utilized DTRs have been described in Table 176.1.

## POLYSYNAPTIC REFLEXES

Polysynaptic reflexes involve one or more interneurons that communicate between the afferent and efferent neurons. The afferent neuron sends signals to interneurons located in the gray matter of the spinal cord, which then direct these signals to the adequate motor neurons of their specific spinal cord segments, as well as adjacent and distant motor neurons. Because of this, one sensory stimulus transmitted can cause multiple alpha motor neurons (AMNs) to get excited or inhibited, and therefore can cause more than one muscle to contract or relax. Most common polysynaptic reflexes have been described in Table 176.2.

Spinal reflexes include the stretch reflex, the Golgi tendon reflex, the crossed extensor reflex, and the withdrawal reflex.[2]

### STRETCH REFLEX

The stretch reflex, also known as the *myotatic reflex*, is a muscle contraction in response to muscle stretch. It is a monosynaptic in nature and provides automatic regulation of skeletal muscle length.

A myotatic reflex originates from muscle spindle fibers. Spindle fibers are specialized sensory fibers that are arrayed

*Table 176.1* THE MOST COMMON CLINICALLY EVALUATED MONOSYNAPTIC REFLEXES

| MONOSYNAPTIC REFLEXES | |
| --- | --- |
| Biceps brachii | C5, C6 |
| Triceps brachii | C6, C7, C8 |
| Brachioradialis | C5, C6, C7 |
| Quadriceps femoris | L2, L3, L4 |
| Triceps surae (ankle reflex) | S1, S2 |

*Table 176.2* THE MOST COMMON CLINICALLY EVALUATED POLYSYNAPTIC REFLEXES

| POLYSYNAPTIC REFLEXES | |
| --- | --- |
| Upper abdominal | T7–T10 |
| Lower abdominal | T10–T12 |
| Cremasteric | L1 |
| Plantar | S1, S2 |
| Anal | S4, S5 |

parallel within intrafusal muscle fibers and are surrounded by extrafusal muscle fibers. Group 1a afferent neurons synapse with the spindle fiber and transmit impulses to the spinal cord when the spindle fiber is stretched. The afferent axon then travels to the spinal cord and bifurcates within the gray matter of the dorsal horn. One of the branches synapses with the corresponding AMN for the muscle that was stretched. That AMN then transmits the impulse back to the neuromuscular endplate of the stimulated muscle, resulting in contraction. The second branch of the afferent neuron synapses with an inhibitory interneuron in the dorsal horn of the spinal cord and travels to the level associated with the corresponding antagonistic muscle group. This results in the unopposed contraction of the stimulated muscle.[3] For example, a contraction of the biceps would be triggered while contraction of the triceps would be inhibited.

### GOLGI TENDON REFLEX

The Golgi tendon reflex is another monosynaptic reflex that is independent of cortical function. This reflex is initiated tension measured by the Golgi apparatus, which is located in the tendons at the insertion and origin of every muscle. Any increase in tension results in a discharge by the Golgi apparatus that is transmitted via group 1b afferent neurons to the dorsal horn of the spinal cord. There it synapses with an inhibitory interneuron, which then synapses with the AMN that corresponds with the muscle group where the signal originated. This results in a reduction in tone that is proportionate to the degree of tension sensed by the Golgi apparatus whether it is active or passive. This reflex is also referred to as the *inverse myotatic reflex*.[4]

### CROSSED EXTENSOR REFLEX

The crossed extensor reflex occurs when the flexors in the withdrawing limb contract and the extensors relax, while in the other limb, the opposite occurs. When a person steps on a nail, the leg that is stepping on the nail flexes and pulls away, while the other leg extends to bear the weight of the whole body.

## WITHDRAWAL REFLEX

The withdrawal reflex (nociceptive reflex) is intended to protect the body from painful stimuli. It is polysynaptic, and causes the stimulation of sensory, association, and motor neurons. When a person touches a hot object and withdraws his hand from it without thinking about it, the heat stimulates both the temperature and danger receptors in the skin, triggering a sensory impulse that travels to the synapses with interneurons, which further trigger motor impulses to the flexors to allow withdrawal.

## CLINICAL CORRELATION

Deep tendon reflexes are measured on a scale from 0 to 4+ with 0 representing absent tone, 2+ being normal, and 4+ representing clonus or persistent tone. DTRs that are absent are representative of a lower motor neuron lesion

(LMN) where one or more elements of the myotatic reflex are disrupted (e.g., spindle fiber, Ia afferent, alpha motor neuron). A DTR of 4+ indicates an upper motor neuron lesion that originates either in the cortex, the brainstem, or the descending pathways. The clonus observed clinically is from the loss of descending inhibitory pathways.[5]

## REFERENCES

1. Hultborn H. Spinal reflexes, mechanisms and concepts: from Eccles to Lundberg and beyond. *Prog Neurobiol.* 2006;78(3–5):215–232.
2. Floeter MK. Spinal reflexes. In: *Handbook of Clinical Neurophysiology*, Vol. 1. Elsevier; 2003:231–246.
3. Dolbow J, Bordoni B. Neuroanatomy, spinal cord myotatic reflex. In *StatPearls* [Internet]. StatPearls; 2019.
4. Stuart DG, et al. Stretch responsiveness of Golgi tendon organs. *Exper Brain Res.* 1970;10(5):463–476.
5. Walker HK. Deep tendon reflexes. In: *Clinical Methods: The History, Physical, and Laboratory Examinations.* 3rd ed. Butterworths; 1990.

# 177.

# SPINAL CORD TRACTS

*Brannon Y. Altenhofen and Nathan Schulman*

## REVIEW OF SPINAL CORD ANATOMY

The spinal cord is divided into two categories of neuronal tissue. Gray matter, composed of the cell bodies of the neurons and many synapses, is located centrally. The white matter, composed of the myelinated axons which form neuronal fiber pathways, is located peripherally.[1] These fiber pathways are organized into the spinal cord tracts, and can be further subdivided into ascending and descending pathways. Ascending pathways carry sensory information from the body to the brain. Descending pathways carry instructions from the brain to the body and include motor fibers. These major subdivisions of the spinal cord are demonstrated in Figures 177.1 and 177.2. We will discuss the specific spinal cord tracts in the following. It is important

to understand the *information* that is carried by each tract (i.e., motor vs. sensory), the *location* of each tract (i.e., anterior vs. posterior), and the relation of a lesion to the *site of crossing over* (i.e., ipsilateral vs. contralateral deficits).

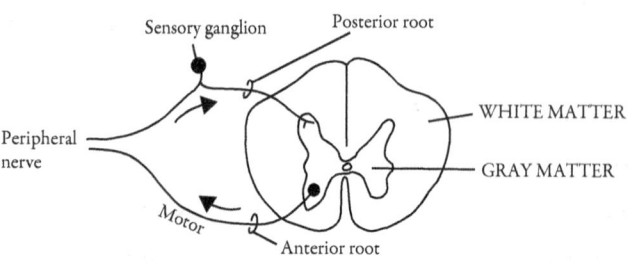

**Figure 177.1** Major subdivisions of the spinal cord.
Reproduced with permission from Goldberg S. *Clinical Neuroanatomy Made Ridiculously Simple*, Medmaster.

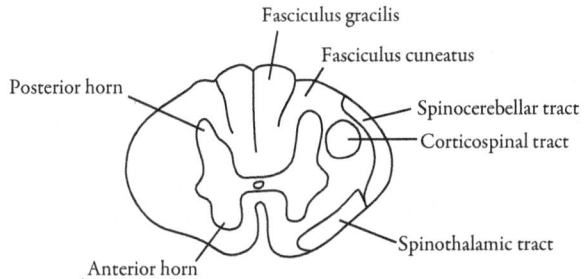

**Figure 177.2.** Major subdivisions of the spinal cord.
Reproduced with permission from Goldberg S. *Clinical Neuroanatomy Made Ridiculously Simple*, Medmaster.

## SPINAL CORD TRACTS

The ascending white matter pathways carry sensory information, receiving input from peripheral nerves with cell bodies in the sensory ganglion that enter the spinal cord via the posterior root,[1] as shown in Figure 177.1.

The *spinothalamic tract* is the pathway for pain and temperature. It is an anterior and peripheral structure, as shown in Figure 177.2. This pathway crosses over almost immediately after entering the spinal cord before ascending to the thalamus on the opposite side, as shown in Figure 177.2. Thus, a lesion of the spinothalamic tract results in a *contralateral loss* of pain and temperature sensation below the level of the lesion.[1]

The *posterior columns* (also known as the dorsal columns) are formed by a pair of ascending tracts, the medially located *fasciculus gracilis* and the more laterally located *fasciculus cuneatus*. The posterior column carries conscious proprioceptive, vibratory, and light touch information. A spinal cord lesion affecting these tracts results in *ipsilateral loss of these sensations* below the level of the lesion, as they do not cross over until reaching the brainstem, as shown in Figure 177.2.[1,2]

The *spinocerebellar tract* is a lateral structure that carries unconscious proprioceptive information from the body to the cerebellum. Unlike the other sensory pathways which immediately or eventually cross over, the spinocerebellar tract primarily remains ipsilateral.[1] This phenomenon explains why cerebral injuries tend to result in contralateral deficits, whereas cerebellar lesions result in *ipsilateral proprioceptive malfunctioning.*

The major descending white matter pathway carries motor commands from the cerebral cortex to the body via the neurons of the *corticospinal tract.*[1,2] Upper motor neurons (UMNs) descend from the brain, cross over, and continue to the appropriate spinal cord level to synapse in the gray matter of the anterior horn. After synapsing, lower motor neurons (LMNs) leave the spinal cord via the anterior nerve root, ultimately terminating at the motor end plate of a muscle fiber. The distinction between UMNs and LMNs is due to the different clinical signs that result from their lesions. Disruption of UMNs of the spinal cord results in *ipsilateral spastic paralysis*, *hyperreflexia*, and a *positive Babinski reflex*, though cortical lesions result in contralateral deficits. Disruption of the LMNs of the anterior horn or

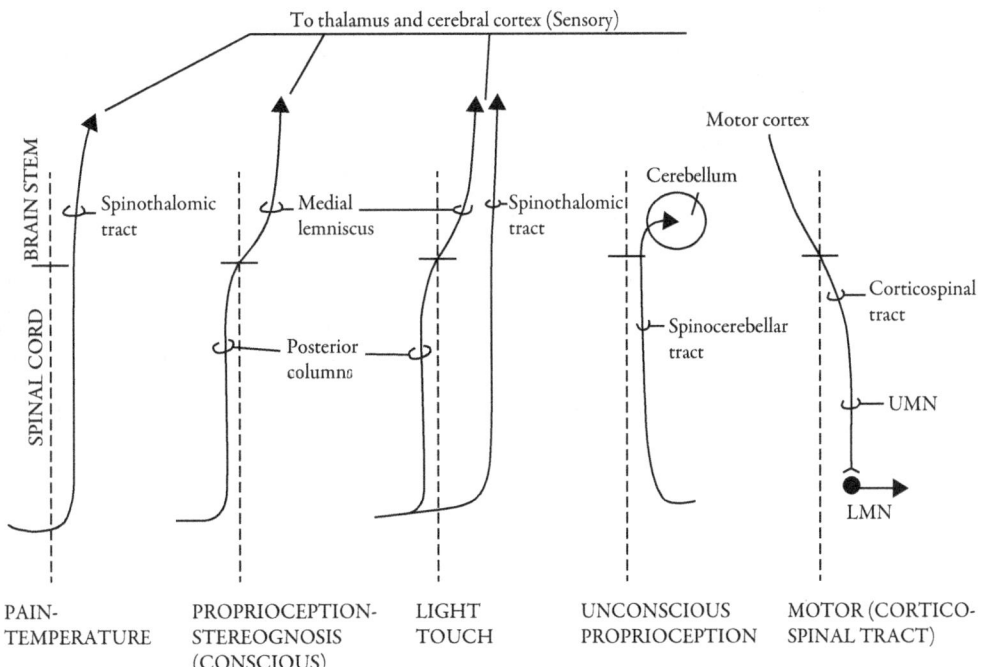

**Figure 177.3.** Schematic view of the major ascending and descending pathways. UMN, upper motor neuron; LMN, lower motor neuron.
Reproduced with permission from Goldberg S. *Clinical Neuroanatomy Made Ridiculously Simple*, Medmaster.

of the peripheral nervous system results *in ipsilateral flaccid paralysis, muscle atrophy, fasciculations or fibrillations*, and *hyporeflexia* (Figure 177.3).[1]

## SPINAL CORD SYNDROMES AND FUNCTIONAL ANATOMY

Spinal cord syndromes result from selective losses or lesions to the various spinal cord tracts. A classic example is injury to the *artery of Adamkiewicz*, the largest of the segmental arteries of the thoracolumbar region (most commonly between levels T9–T12) that critically feeds into the anterior spinal artery providing blood supply to the anterior two-thirds of the spinal cord.[3,4] Inadvertent disruption of this artery—such as during thoracoabdominal aortic aneurism surgery—can result in an *anterior spinal cord syndrome* due to injury to the spinothalamic tract (resulting in bilateral loss of pain and temperature sensation) and injury to the anterior horns (resulting in bilateral motor deficits).[3] Because the dorsal columns are supplied by the posterior spinal arteries, there is sparing of light touch, vibration, and proprioception.[2,3]

*Posterior cord syndrome* is uncommon, but causes include trauma, tabes dorsalis from syphilis, multiple sclerosis, and dorsally compressive tumors.[2] Because there is a selective lesion to the posterior columns, clinically this results in loss of vibratory, tactile, and proprioceptive sensations below the level of injury, while sparing pain, temperature, and motor function.

*Brown-Sequard syndrome* is the result of a lateral hemisection of the spinal cord.[2] At the dermatomal level of the lesion, there is ipsilateral flaccid paralysis due to disruption of the LMNs of the anterior horn, as well as an ipsilateral total loss of sensation from disruption of the posterior horn. Below the dermatomal level of the lesion, there is UMN injury from disruption of the cerebrospinal tract, resulting in ipsilateral spastic paralysis; there is ipsilateral loss of proprioception and vibration sensation from disruption of the posterior columns; and there is contralateral loss of pain and temperature sensation due to injury of the spinothalamic tract.[2]

*Conus medullaris syndrome* is due to injury of the spinal cord at the level of L1–L2, usually from direct spinal cord

trauma.[2] Clinically, it manifests as a saddle distribution of sensory deficits, and mild mixed upper and lower motor neuron deficits. In contrast, *cauda equina syndrome* is the result of injury to nerve roots below the level of where the spinal cord terminates, often from disc herniation or burst fractures. Clinically it results in prominent lower motor deficits such as flaccid paralysis.[2] Both syndromes can present with bladder and bowel dysfunction.

## NEUROMONITORING

*Intraoperative neuromonitoring* is often performed to assess the functional integrity of the nervous system during surgeries in which these structures are at risk.[5] Somatosensory evoked potentials (SSEPs) rely on the integrity of the dorsal columns and all neurons of the central nervous system (CNS) or peripheral nervous system (PNS) involved in that pathway. Motor evoked potentials (MEPs) are used to assess motor cortex and the corticospinal tracts of the anterolateral spinal cord. Electromyography (EMG) is used to monitor specific peripheral or cranial nerves or nerve roots. Brainstem auditory evoked potentials (BAEPs) assess the integrity of all structures involved in the auditory pathway and include cranial nerve VIII (vestibulocochlear nerve). Visual evoked potentials (VEPs) similarly assess the integrity of all structures in the visual pathway. When forming an anesthetic plan, one must be cognizant that neuromonitoring is often affected by the various anesthetic agents used during surgery.

## REFERENCES

1. Goldberg S. *Clinical Neuroanatomy Made Ridiculously Simple*. 3rd ed. Miami, FL: MedMaster; 2003. https://hdl.handle.net/2027/mdp.39015052698274.
2. Diaz E, Morales H. Spinal cord anatomy and clinical syndromes. *Semin Ultrasound, CT MRI*. 2016;37(5):360–371.
3. Gofur EM, Singh P. Anatomy, back, vertebral canal blood supply. *StatPearls*. 2019. http://www.ncbi.nlm.nih.gov/pubmed/31082127.
4. Butterworth JF, et al. *Morgan & Mikhails Clinical Anesthesiology*. 6th ed. New York, NY: McGraw-Hill Education; 2018.
5. Bebawy JF, Pasternak JJ. Anesthesia for neurosurgery. In: Barash PG, Cullen BF, Stoelting RK, et al., eds. *Clinical Anesthesia*. 8th ed. Philidelphia, PA: Wolters Kluwer; 2017:1003–1028.

# 178.

# SPINAL CORD MORPHOLOGY

*Alex Woodrow and Archit Sharma*

## INTRODUCTION

The spinal cord is located in the upper two-thirds of the adult spinal canal. It is continuous with the brainstem starting at the inferior portion of the medulla and exits the foramen magnum and terminates at the L1–L2 level as the conus medullaris. The spinal cord is surrounded a continuation of the dura, arachnoid, and pia mater. The dural sac extends until the termination of the spinal canal and the spinal cord and spinal nerves are surrounded by cerebrospinal fluid (CSF) between the arachnoid and pia mater. The pia mater and glial fibers form the filum terminale, which connects the conus medullaris to the distal dural sac.

The cord itself has approximately 30 segments: 8 cervical, 12 thoracic, 5 lumbar, and 5 sacral segments. Each of these segments corresponds with a pair of spinal nerves that extend from the spinal cord through the intervertebral foramen and travel to innervate somatic sensory and motor dermatomes.[1]

## CROSS-SECTIONAL ANATOMY

The spinal cord is symmetrical and can be split into two halves marked by the deep anterior median fissure and the shallower posterior (dorsal) sulcus. The lateral spinal cord consists of white matter and contains the axons of the lateral, ventral (anterior), and dorsal (posterior) columns, as well as the ascending and descending axonal tracts. Medially, gray matter forms the dorsal, lateral, and ventral horns, which contain dendrites, glial cells, and neural cell bodies.

## WHITE MATTER

White matter surrounds the gray matter and is formed by tracts that transmit information up and down the spinal cord. Table 178.1 describes the different descending pathways, their paths and roles in controlling various body functions. Similarly, Table 178.2 describes the various ascending pathways and the nerve fibers carried by them.

## GRAY MATTER

Gray matter of the spinal cord consists of the dorsal horn (posterior), which is responsible for transmitting sensory information, and the ventral horn (anterior), which

*Table 178.1* DESCENDING PATHWAYS OF THE SPINAL CORD

| | |
|---|---|
| Lateral corticospinal tract | Fine motor<br>Origin: Motor/pre-motor cortex<br>Path: Decussates from pyramidal tract (lower medulla) to lateral column. Synapses in the anterior horn. |
| Anterior corticospinal tract | Gross and postural motor<br>Origin: Motor/pre-motor cortex<br>Path: Decussates from anterior column across white commissure at the level. Synapses in anterior horn. |
| Vestibulospinal tract | Role in postural reflexes<br>Origin: The lateral and medial vestibular nuclei<br>Path: Down ventral column and synapses in anterior horn. |
| Rubrospinal tract | Minor role in motor function<br>Origin: Red nucleus<br>Path: Down lateral column and synapses in ventral horn. |
| Reticulospinal tract | Role in pain and spinal reflex modulation<br>Origin: Brainstem reticular formation<br>Path: Down anterior column and synapses with dorsal and ventral horn. |
| Descending autonomic tract | Modulates autonomic function<br>Origin: hypothalamus and brainstem nuclei<br>Path: Down lateral columns and synapses with preganglionic autonomic neurons. |
| Tectospinal tract | Reflexive head turning<br>Origin: Midbrain<br>Path: Down ventral column and synapses with ventral. |
| Medial longitudinal fasciculus | Coordinates head and eye movement<br>Origin: Vestibular nuclei<br>Path: Down ventral column and synapses in cervical gray matter. |

**Table 178.2 ASCENDING PATHWAYS OF THE SPINAL CORD**

| | |
|---|---|
| Dorsal column | Fine touch, proprioception, two point-discrimination<br>Path: 1st order synapses with 2nd order neuron in either the **gracile** (lower extremities) or **cuneate** (upper extremities) nuclei. The 2nd order neuron decussates to the contralateral medial lemniscus. |
| Spinothalamic tract | Sharp pain, temperature, crude touch<br>Path: 1st order synapses with 2nd order neuron in substantia gelatinosa of ipsilateral dorsal horn where it then synapses with 3rd order neurons. 3rd order neurons decussate at the level of entry to contralateral spinothalamic tract. |
| Dorsal/ventral Spinocerebellar tract | Movement and position sensation<br>Path: Travels within lateral column to cerebellar paleocortex via 2nd order neurons in dorsal column after synapsing with 1st order neurons in the dorsal nucleus of Clarke. |
| Spinoretricular tract | Deep somatic and chronic pain<br>Path: Along ventrolateral column to reticular formation of brainstem. |

is responsible for motor function. The gray matter is functionally delineated into 9 laminae, with the dorsal horn containing lamina I–VII and the ventral horn with lamina VIII and IX.

## SPINAL ROOTS AND NERVES

At each level, the spinal cord gives rise to four spinal roots—a dorsal (sensory) and ventral (motor) nerve root on each side. The ventral nerve root exits at the anterolateral sulcus. The dorsal and ventral roots combine after the dorsal root ganglion (DRG) and exit the spinal canal as a spinal nerve.

## VASCULAR SUPPLY

The spinal cord receives vascular supply primarily from a singular anterior spinal artery (ASA) and two posterior spinal arteries (PSA). The ASA is formed from branches of the vertebral arteries prior to the formation of the basilar artery. The PSA are formed from either the posterior inferior cerebellar artery or branches of the pre-atlantal vertebral arteries. The anterior spinal artery provides blood to the anterior two-thirds of the spinal cord, while the two posterior spinal arteries only provide blood for the posterior one-third of the spinal cord.

The ASA and PSA are supplemented by a series of segmental arteries that are branches of the aorta. The largest segmental artery is the artery of Adamkiewicz (radiculomedullary artery),

which arises from the left side of the aorta around T9 to T12 and then connects to the ASA. The artery of Adamkiewicz provides the ASA with a substantial amount of blood in the thoracolumbar region and thus is considered a watershed area. Lastly, blood supply to the lumbosacral area is provided by branches of the internal iliac arteries.[3]

## EVOKED POTENTIALS

Evoked potentials are a form of intraoperative monitoring that utilizes electrical stimuli to monitor sensory and motor pathways. The most commonly utilized are somatosensory evoked potentials (SSEP) and motor evoked potentials (MEP), but others include auditory evoked potentials and visual evoked potentials.

SSEPs are produced by stimulating distal sensory nerves. The nerves that are primarily used are the median, ulnar, and posterior tibial nerves. Stimulation of large-diameter, fast-conducting nerve fibers are recorded by a series of electrodes placed along the sensory pathway. The use of multiple recording sites is used to verify that the nervous system is activated and to identify specific locations of neural damage. SSEPs are most commonly used to reduce the risk of spinal cord injury during major spine surgery.

MEPs are utilized to monitor for motor pathway compromise. They are produced by electrical stimulation of the motor cortex through electrodes placed in the scalp. Stimulation is then transmitted through the cortical spinal tract, resulting in a compound muscle action potential (CMAP) in targeted muscle groups that are at risk during the surgery. Each CMAP elicited has a consistent onset latency and amplitude that is monitored intraoperatively. The medications used for anesthesia can also influence the obtainability and interpretation of MEPs.[5]

## BROWN-SEQUARD SYNDROME

Transection of the spinal cord can lead to ipsilateral flaccid paralysis and loss of sensation at the level of the lesion (posterior horn). Ipsilateral spastic paraparesis and loss of vibration and proprioception occur below the level of the lesion (posterior column). Lastly, contralateral loss of pain and temperature sensation occur several segments below the lesion (spinothalamic tract).

## CORD SYNDROMES

### CENTRAL

This is the most common; in elderly patients it results from cord compression from hyperextension injury with concomitant cervical spondylosis. It presents as upper extremity impairment more than lower extremity. Bladder involvement and loss of sensation below the level can be seen.

## POSTERIOR

This is the least common. It presents as loss of touch, proprioception, and vibratory sensation below the level of the lesion. Pain, temperature, and motor function are spared.

## ANTERIOR

This is the worst prognosis. Etiologies include emboli, postoperative complication, and hypotension. It presents as motor deficits and impairment of pain and temperature sensation at or below the level of the lesion.

## CAUDA EQUINA SYNDROME

This presents as flaccid paralysis with lower limb weakness, saddle paresthesia, and loss of bowel and bladder control.

## ANESTHETIC CONSIDERATIONS: SPINE SURGERY

### PREOPERATIVE

Obtain detailed history and perform a physical examination specific to preexisting neurological comorbidities such as peripheral neuropathies, myelopathies, prior cerebrovascular accident (CVA), peripheral vascular disease, and stroke risk.

## INTRAOPERATIVE

*SSEPs*: Volatile anesthetics increase signal latency and decrease amplitude. Nitrous oxide only decreases amplitude. Opiates, benzodiazepines, and barbituates have little effect on SSEP signal. Most commonly used anesthetic is a total intravenous anesthesia (TIVA) with less than 0.5 minimum alveolar concentration (MAC) of volatile.

*MEPs*: Volatile anesthetics have similar effect on MEP signal. Avoid full muscle paralysis during period of monitoring as it will eliminate the signal.

## POSTOPERATIVE

An immediate postoperative neurological exam is usually conducted to establish or rule out new deficits.

## REFERENCES

1. Ganapathy MK, Reddy V, Tadi P. Neuroanatomy, spinal cord morphology. [Updated 2021 October 30]. In: StatPearls. Treasure Island, FL: StatPearls.
2. Jameson J, Fauci AS, Kasper DL, Hauser SL, Longo DL, Loscalzo J, eds. Spinal cord diseases. *Harrison's Manual of Medicine*. 20th ed. McGraw Hill; 2020.
3. Gofur EM, Singh P. Anatomy, back, vertebral canal blood supply. In: *StatPearls*. Treasure Island, FL: StatPearls; 2020.
4. Ropper AH, Brown RH. *Adams and Victor's Principles of Neurology*. 2005:1382–1382.
5. Sloan T, et al. Evoked potentials. In: Patel P, Cottrell JE, eds. *Neuroanesthesia*. 6th ed. Elsevier; 2017:114–126.

# 179.

# NEUROMUSCULAR TRANSMISSION

*Gurpreet Mundi and Dmitry Roberman*

## MEMBRANE POTENTIAL

Neurons, like most eukaryotic cells, maintain an electric potential across their cell membranes. This potential is maintained by the sodium-potassium pump (Na+/ K+-ATPase). This pump uses ATP to actively transport 3 Na+ ions out of the cell while transporting 2 K+ ions into the cell. Chloride ions (Cl–) can passively diffuse across the cell membrane.[1–3] The net result is a resting membrane potential of –70mV (with the extra cellular space considered to be at 0).[3] This resting potential sets up conditions that allow the transmission of the action potential down the axon of the nerve cell.

## NEURONAL STRUCTURE

In brief, the components of a neuron are as follows:

- *Soma*: The cell body, contains the nucleus and DNA
- *Dendrites*: Receive the input for the neuron, either from another nerve cell or sensory tissue.
- *Axon*: Relays the information away from the neuron, either to another nerve or tissue.
- *Myelin sheath*: Produced by Schwann cells. Insulates the axon, somewhat similar to rubber insulating an electric wire. Different types of neurons are insulated to different degrees; in general, motor neurons are heavily myelinated.[2,3]

## ACTION POTENTIAL

The action potential is the means by which neurons conduct a signal across their length. Physiologically, the action potential is a sudden rise and fall of membrane potential that travels down the axon of a neuron.[1]

Voltage gated Na+ channels are at the heart of the action potential's physiology. They elicit an *all or none* response in the neuron. When a signal arrives at the proximal axon. The axon hillock, the membrane potential begins to rise in that portion of the axon. Once it has reached a threshold of –55 mEq, the voltage gated sodium channels are activated.[3] They open and sodium rushes into the axon from the extracellular space (following the concentration gradient), quickly raising the membrane potential to +20 mEq.[2] As the membrane potential rises, further voltage gated channels are triggered further down the length of the axon.

As the membrane potential approaches +20 mEq, the influx of sodium slows, and voltage gated potassium channels open, resulting in potassium rushing out of the axon (following the concentration gradient) into the extracellular space. These two occurrences, along with the baseline function of the sodium-potassium channel, quickly restore the axon to resting potential of –70 mEq.[2]

The sum of the ion exchanges discussed results in the propagation of the action potential, a quick rise and fall of membrane potential, down the axon of a neuron. Once the action potential reaches the end of the axon, chemical messengers are used to transmit a signal from the neuron, across the synapse, to the next component in the signal, which may be another neuron or another tissue such as muscle fibers. The synapse between neurons and muscle fibers is known as the *neuromuscular junction*.[2]

## THE NEUROMUSCULAR JUNCTION

The neuromuscular junction is composed of:

- *Presynaptic terminus*: the terminus of the neuronal axon. Neurotransmitters (acetylcholine in this case) are produced and released from here.
- *Motor end plate*: located on the muscle fibers, contains receptors for acetylcholine.
- *Synaptic cleft*: the space between the presynaptic junction and the motor end plate.

Acetylcholine (Ach) is the neurotransmitter used at the neuromuscular junction, and its produced by the enzyme **choline O-acetyltransferase** in the terminal axon. The Ach is stored in vesicles until it is needed.[1]

When the action potential depolarizes the terminal axon, voltage gated calcium channels allow an influx of calcium from the extracellular space into the terminal axon. This calcium binds to SNARE proteins on the Ach-containing vesicles and causes them to fuse to the axon's cell membrane, releasing the Ach into the synaptic cleft.[3]

Acetylcholine diffuses across the synaptic cleft and binds to Ach receptors on the motor endplate. This results in the opening of an associated sodium ion channel, allowing the influx of sodium ions into the muscle fiber. Each activated receptor results in a small localized rise in membrane potential, called endplate potentials, in the muscle fiber (which also has a normal resting potential of –70 mEq).[1] When there are sufficient endplate potentials to raise the membrane potential above a certain threshold, an action potential is activated in the muscle fiber, similar to the action potential in a neuron.

Acetylcholine is broken down by acetylcholinesterase in the synaptic cleft to choline and acetate. This terminates the action of Ach on the motor endplate. Since the choline molecule is difficult to produce, it is the limiting step in the production of Ach; it is actively reabsorbed by the terminal axon for reuse.[2]

## SKELETAL MUSCLE CONTRACTION

Resting membrane potential and the action potential are at the heart of muscle contraction as well. Ach stimulates the motor endplate and initiates an action potential in the muscle fibers. The action potential produces an influx of sodium through voltage gated channels. In muscle fibers, there is an exchange channel that exchanges the sodium in the cell for calcium from the extracellular space and the sarcoplasmic reticulum (a primary storage of calcium for muscle cells). The calcium initiates the contraction of muscle fibers via the muscle proteins.[1,3]

The skeletal muscle is composed of **long thin filaments of actin** that run in parallel with **thick filaments of myosin.** The filaments are connected by **cross bridges of** myosin. These cross bridges are called **myosin heads** and attach to the **tropomyosin-myosin complex** that is integrated with the actin filaments.[1,2,3]

The following are the steps involved in muscle fiber contraction.

1. Calcium binds to troponin and exposes the myosin head binding site on the actin (thin) filament.[1,3]
2. The myosin head binds to the actin filament and an ADP (depleted ATP) is released from the myosin.[1,3]
3. Actin binding and ADP release causes a conformation change in the myosin head, resulting in a "**power stroke**" which causes the thin and thick filaments to slide past each other and contracts the muscle fiber.[1,3]
4. ATP binds to the myosin and causes it to detach from the actin filament.[1,3]

5. The ATP is degraded to ADP, which causes the myosin head to return to its original conformation.[1,3]

If calcium is still present in the muscle fiber, the myosin head can again attach to the actin filament, repeating the process. If the muscle fiber is no longer being stimulated at the motor endplate, the calcium will be returned to the sarcoplasmic reticulum. [1]

## REFERENCES

1. Barash PG. *Clinical anesthesia.* 7th ed. Philadelphia, PA: Wolters Kluwer Health/Lippincott Williams & Wilkins; 2013.
2. Miller RD. *Miller's Anesthesia.* New York, NY: Elsevier/Churchill Livingstone; 2005.
3. Berg JM, et al. *Biochemistry.* New York, NY: W. H. Freeman; 2002:527–566.

# 180.

# PSYCHOLOGICAL, SOCIAL, AND VOCATIONAL INFLUENCES ON PAIN PERCEPTION

*Timothy Rushmer and Alaa Abd-Elsayed*

## PSYCHOLOGICAL INFLUENCES ON PAIN AND PAIN PERCEPTION

Studies have conclusively shown that psychological factors influence pain perception. Even in laboratory studies of pain, a variety of psychological factors have been shown to impact the level of pain reported by test subjects. Additionally, treatments aimed at addressing psychological factors have also been shown to be effective at altering patient pain and pain perception.

## EXPERIMENTAL STUDIES OF PAIN AND PSYCHOLOGICAL FACTORS

Experimental studies have confirmed what clinical providers have known for a long time: attention and

awareness affect pain perception. For example, distracting a patient while putting in an IV is an easy and effective way to reduce a patient's perception of pain. Functional magnetic resonance imaging (MRI) studies have confirmed this, showing reduced activity in somatosensory cortices in subjects distracted from painful stimuli compared to when they were not distracted. Similarly, patients' expectations regarding a painful experience play a role in pain perception. In a study illustrative of this point, test subjects with expectations that a stimulus would be more painful had higher reported pain intensity ratings than those not primed with this expectation. Less intuitively than attention and expectations about pain, beliefs about the cause of patients' pain, and their ability to control it, also affect pain perception. In one study, cancer patients who believed their pain was due to disease progression used more opioids than those who believed the cause of their pain was benign or unrelated, despite similar levels of actual disease progression.[1] In another study, patients' beliefs about the original cause of their pain, either a traumatic cause or a gradual, insidious onset, affected pain severity rankings, despite no differences in physical pathology.[2] Patients who believed a traumatic event had caused their pain reported higher pain severity. Finally, several studies have shown that a sense of personal control can lessen experimentally induced pain. Subjects exposed to the same painful stimuli rated it as less intense when they could administer it themselves, as opposed to having it administered by an experimenter.[1]

## PSYCHOTHERAPEUTIC APPROACHES

Several psychotherapeutic treatments have been shown to impact pain and pain perception. Cognitive behavioral therapy (CBT) is a type of therapist-guided, talk therapy that addresses beliefs, attitudes, and cognitive biases that underlie maladaptive emotional and behavioral responses to pain. CBT has been shown to decrease pain intensity and disability while increasing quality of life. Another psychotherapeutic treatment that has been shown to impact pain is mindfulness-based training. Mindfulness techniques encourage patients to focus on the current moment and to accept feelings, thoughts, and sensations in a neutral way, instead of with negative judgments. Mindfulness interventions have been shown to decrease reported pain intensity.[3]

## SOCIAL INFLUENCES ON PAIN PERCEPTION

Social influences on pain perception were summarized in a recent meta-analysis by Che et al. and were found to have a variety of effects. The presence of a stranger decreased pain-related arousal, while the presence of a significant other increased facial expression of pain. Verbal support, as well as the touch of a romantic partner, during a painful experience was found to decrease pain perception.[4]

## VOCATIONAL INFLUENCES ON PAIN AND PAIN PERCEPTION

Studies have investigated what role vocational factors have on the development of chronic pain. Most studies have looked at neck and back pain. Unsurprisingly, the type of work performed impacts the development of pain. Individuals with occupations involving heavy lifting, strenuous work, and repetitive movements are more likely to develop neck and back pain. Even in the occupational setting, psychological factors play a role in pain development and perception, as several studies found dissatisfaction with the workplace environment and psychological stress to be a factor predicting workplace development of pain.[5]

## REFERENCES

1. Wiech K, et al. Neurocognitive aspects of pain perception. *Trends Cogn Sci.* 2008;12(8):306–313.
2. McMahon SB, et al. *Wall and Melzack's Textbook of Pain.* 6th ed. Philadelphia, PA: Saunders Elsevier; 2013:256–272.
3. Benzon HT, et al. *Essentials of Pain Medicine.* Philadelphia, PA: Elseiver; 2018:539–544.
4. Che X, et al. Investigating the influence of social support on experimental pain and related physiological arousal: A systematic review and meta-analysis. *Neurosci Biobehav Rev.* 2018;92:437–452.
5. Jun D, et al. Physical risk factors for developing non-specific neck pain in office workers: a systematic review and meta-analysis. *Int Arch Occup Environ Health.* 2017;90(5):373–410.

# 181.

# SEX, GENDER, AND AGE DIFFERENCES IN PAIN AND PAIN PERCEPTION

*Timothy Rushmer and Alaa Abd-Elsayed*

## TERMINOLOGY

First, it is important to highlight some terminology as it has been used in prior pain research. A recent consensus report on gender and sex differences in pain, by Greenspan et al., defined *sex* as referring to biologically based differences and the term *gender* as referring to socially based phenomena. Greenspan et al. go on to say, "Although biological sex exerts a major influence on one's gender identity, sex and gender are not equivalent, and the terms are not interchangeable."[1,2] In this consensus report, the authors acknowledge that gender is not a categorical variable and instead is continuous, with a range of gender characteristics.[2] In this chapter, we will present the relative contributions of sex and gender on pain and pain perception, while acknowledging that most prior research has looked at sex as a categorical variable without the influence of gender. Implied in this acknowledgment is a call for more research to be done on gender and gender identity and their roles in pain and pain perception.

## SEX DIFFERENCES IN PAINFUL DISEASES

Research has conclusively shown that individuals of the female sex experience more pain than individuals of the male sex. The question that remains to be definitively answered is: why? Many epidemiologic studies have found that individuals of female sex have a higher prevalence of painful diseases, especially for "pain conditions involving the head and neck, of musculoskeletal or visceral origin, and of autoimmune cause." If the female sex has a higher burden of diseases or conditions that cause pain, that in itself would be a reason for the disparity. However, individuals of the female sex also experience a higher prevalence of unspecified pain syndromes, as well as more severe pain, more frequent pain, pain in more locations, and longer duration of pain, than that reported by the male sex. Some theories to try to explain these epidemiological findings include (1) the female sex-specific complications of

obstetrics and higher rates of sex-organ specific disorders, and (2) differences in sex hormones and variations across the menstrual cycle. However, these theories have only limited and often conflicting evidence to support them. Research has shown that individuals of the male sex do experience a greater prevalence of some painful conditions such as duodenal ulcers and Buerger's disease. Notably, no consistent, significant differences between the sexes have been found in studies of cancer pain.[3]

## SEX DIFFERENCES IN PAIN PERCEPTION

In addition to the differential epidemiological burden of painful diseases between the sexes, pain perception has also been shown to be different experimentally. A variety of studies have been conducted using different types of experimental pain (cold, heat, electrical, pressure, etc.) and a meta-analysis concluded that, overall, individuals of the female sex are more sensitive to painful stimulation as assessed in the laboratory. Pain sensation has been studied across the menstrual cycle, with several studies measuring hormone levels; however, results have been conflicting and no consistent effect of either could be conclusively shown.[3]

## GENDER DIFFERENCES IN PAIN PERCEPTION

Although few studies have looked at gender identity and pain perception specifically, several have used the concept of gender roles and the spectrum of masculinity and femininity, in addition to the categorical variable of sex as described earlier. A meta-analysis by O. A. Alabas et al. (2012) looked at the relationship between gender roles and experimental pain, defining gender roles as: "culturally and socially constructed meanings that describe how women and men should behave in certain situations according to feminine and masculine roles learned throughout life." They ultimately showed that individuals with high masculinity scores showed higher pain tolerance and individuals with high femininity scores showed higher pain sensitivity. Masculine gender roles are reported to endorse stoicism and contribute to increased pain tolerance and decreased chronic pain complaints in some studies, whereas female gender roles are reported as more sensitive and open to reporting pain.[4] Based on this research, it seems likely that one's perception of their own gender and gender roles has a great deal of influence on their pain perception.

## THE EFFECT OF AGE ON PAIN PERCEPTION IN THE EXPERIMENTAL SETTING

Studies investigating age differences in pain threshold and pain tolerance have reported conflicting results. Both increases and decreases in pain threshold and pain tolerance with age have been reported. But when looking at specific types of pain, slightly more consistent results have been shown; for instance, as age increases, so does pain threshold to thermal and pressure pain. While pain tolerance for thermal and pressure pain is decreased with age, sensitivity to ischemic pain seems to increase with age, while sensitivity to electrical stimulation is unchanged.[3]

## THE EFFECT OF AGE ON PAIN IN THE CLINICAL SETTING

Epidemiologically, studies have reported conflicting results about the effect age has on the prevalence of pain.[3]

However, it is known that as patients age, the prevalence of many painful conditions increase, especially cancer. Regardless of the specific prevalence, pain and painful disease states continue to affect individuals as they age and have a unique impact on elderly individuals. Elderly individuals with pain are at increased risk for falls, loss of independence, and social isolation. Older adults also have unique physiologic changes, such as altered pharmacokinetics and pharmacodynamics, changes in volume of distribution, renal impairment and decreased hepatic function, leading to changes (frequently decreases) in drug metabolism and elimination. As we age, total body fat increases and total body water decreases, leading to higher peak plasma concentrations of water-soluble drugs and decreased elimination of lipid-soluble drugs.[5] All of these physiologic changes necessitate increased caution when implementing pharmacologic treatments of pain in the elderly.

## REFERENCES

1. Raja SN, et al. The revised International Association for the Study of Pain definition of pain: concepts, challenges, and compromises [published online ahead of print, 2020 May 23]. *Pain*. 2020;10.1097/j.pain.0000000000001939.
2. Greenspan JD, et al. Studying sex and gender differences in pain and analgesia: A consensus report. *Pain*. 2007;132(Suppl 1): S26–S45.
3. McMahon SB, et al. *Wall and Melzack's Textbook of Pain*. 6th ed. Philadelphia, PA: Saunders, Elsevier; 2013:221–231, 315–319.
4. Alabas OA, et al. Gender role affects experimental pain responses: A systematic review with meta-analysis. *Eur J Pain*. 2012;16(9): 1211–1223.
5. Benzon HT, et al. *Practical Pain Management*. 5th ed. Philadelphia, PA: Mosby, Elsevier; 2014:467–473.

# Part XI

# AUTONOMIC NERVOUS SYSTEM

# 182.

# THE SYMPATHETIC NERVOUS SYSTEM

*Adi Cosic and Melinda M. Lawrence*

## INTRODUCTION

The sympathetic nervous system (SNS) is one of two divisions in the autonomic nervous system. Together with the parasympathetic nervous system (PSNS), the SNS serves to regulate a multitude of unconscious body functions, such as breathing, digestion, cardiovascular responses, reflex arcs, and the often described "fight-or-flight" reaction that the body experiences under stress. It is through the antagonistic actions of both the SNS and PSNS that the body achieves homeostasis. The enteric nervous system, previously listed as a component of the PSNS, is now thought to be an individual subdivision apart from both the SNS and PSNS given its set of separate reflex arcs.

## ANATOMY AND FUNCTION

In general, two types of neurons exist within the SNS, the preganglionic and the postganglionic. The preganglionic neurons originate in the lateral horn (within the intermediolateral cell columns) of the thoracolumbar divisions of the spine (T1 to L2 or L3). The preganglionic neuron typically synapses in a sympathetic chain or ganglia, a neurotransmitter is released, and then the postganglionic neuron is activated and a signal travels to a target site. In the SNS, three target sites exist, including the bilateral paravertebral ganglia of the sympathetic chain, the prevertebral ganglia (e.g., the celiac ganglia), and the chromaffin cells of the adrenal medulla. All of these pathways include a two-neuron transit system, with the exception of the adrenal medulla, which involves only the preganglionic neurons innervating the chromaffin cells directly. It is important to remember that the neurons of the SNS can travel superiorly, inferiorly, or innervate at the level of origin, allowing an instantaneous body-wide reaction in response to stimulus.[1]

Within the pre- and paravertebral ganglia, the synapse is an area of interest due to the exchange of neurotransmitters produced and recycled there. In all ganglionic synapses within the sympathetic nervous system, the primary messenger is acetylcholine (Ach), a neurotransmitter that is produced in the terminal end of cholinergic preganglionic neurons. Ach is synthesized by an enzyme, choline acetyltransferase (ChAT), from the substrates acetyl-CoA and choline. The neurotransmitter is then stored within vesicles near the synaptic end of the preganglionic neuron, anticipating release. Upon the arrival of an action potential to the terminal end of a preganglionic neuron, Ach is released into the synaptic cleft, binding to nicotinic ligand-gated ion channels on the postganglionic neuron, which trigger the influx of Na+. It is worth noting that there are two subtypes of the nicotinic receptor, the muscle type and the neuronal type. The neuronal type is discussed here, as it is found in the autonomic ganglia, while the muscle type is located at the neuromuscular junction (NMJ). A surge of positive ions in the postganglionic neuron causes depolarization, and it is through this chemical transmission that the signal is propagated further to the target tissue. In addition to Ach, cotransmitters such as adenosine triphosphate (ATP) and neuropeptide Y are present and serve to modulate sympathetic activity.

Acetylcholine's termination of action occurs after detachment of the molecule from the postganglionic receptor. Acetylcholinesterase, an enzyme abundantly found in the synaptic cleft, serves to degrade the molecule into the inactive metabolites choline and acetate. Choline, a substrate in the formation of acetylcholine, is reabsorbed into the cytosol of the preganglionic neuron for further use.

The postganglionic neuron receives the stimulus and carries it to the effector organ. Typically in the SNS, the neurotransmitter in postganglionic neurons is norepinephrine (NE), whose synthesis stems from tyrosine in the nerve ending. By converting L-tyrosine to L-3,4-dihydroxyphenylalanine (L-DOPA) via the enzyme tyrosine hydroxylase (the rate-limiting step in this reaction), the nerve endings can convert a simple amino acid to dopamine, NE, and epinephrine (Epi). Due to the presence of NE and Epi in these nerve fibers, they are deemed adrenergic.[2]

*Table 182.1* DRUGS WITH SYMPATHETIC ACTIVITY

| DRUG | RECEPTOR | EFFECTS | TYPICAL START DOSE | ADVERSE EFFECTS | INDICATIONS |
|---|---|---|---|---|---|
| Norepinephrine | ⇑⇑A1 > ⇑B1 | ⇑⇑ BP<br>⇑HR, SV | 0.1 mcg/kg/min | Tachyarrhythmia, peripheral ischemia, ⇑myocardial oxygen demand | First-line therapy for distributive shock |
| Epinephrine | ⇑B1<br>High doses cause ⇑A1 | ⇑⇑⇑HR, SV<br>⇑⇑⇑ BP<br>Dose dependence | 0.1 mcg/kg/min | Tachyarrhythmia, peripheral ischemia, ⇑myocardial oxygen demand | Cardiogenic shock or inotropic and chronotropic support |
| Phenylephrine | ⇑A1 | ⇑BP | 0.1 mcg/min | Peripheral and splanchnic ischemia, bradycardia | Hypotension |
| Vasopressin | ⇑V1 | ⇑⇑⇑BP | 0.01–0.03 units/min | Splanchnic ischemia | Refractory low BP, able to add to other vasopressors without pulmonary vasculature involvement |
| Dopamine | ⇑D1<br>⇑B2<br>⇑A1 | ⇑⇑HR<br>⇑⇑SV<br>⇑BP | 1–5 mcg/kg/min low dose, to increase urine output<br>5–15 mcg/kg/min, increase cardiac output/ contractility/HR | Tachyarrhythmia, myocardial splanchnic and peripheral ischemia | Bradycardia |

Much like Ach, these neurotransmitters are stored in vesicles near the terminal end of the neuron, awaiting the arrival of an action potential. When depolarized, the release of these neurotransmitters via vesicle binding causes a variety of effects based on their effector organ and the target receptors. Of note, approximately only 1% of stored NE is released with each depolarization, amounting to a large reserve of adrenergic compounds in the body. To add to this, some of the NE (as well as Ach) is recycled into the presynaptic neuron and stored again, forming a highly efficient system. Given their adrenergic nature, NE and Epi bind to α and β receptors on both the end organ and the presynaptic neuron (α-2 preganglionic receptors acting in a negative feedback loop), these g-coupled adrenergic receptors are found throughout the body, from smooth muscle to organs. For example, the effects of NE on blood vessels triggers vasoconstriction through its α-1 effects, while its β-1 effects on the heart cause an increase in heart rate.

NE is rapidly terminated once it has achieved its effect by one of three methods, all of which are utilized simultaneously. Degradation occurs via the enzymes catechol-O-methyltransferase (COMT) or monoamine oxidase (MAO), reuptake into nerve endings via the norepinephrine transporter (NET), and lastly diffusion away from binding sites occurs as well. If NE is reabsorbed into the cytosol of the presynaptic cell, it is repackaged into vesicles ready for release with the next action potential.[2]

Though the SNS typically innervates target tissues with NE and a postganglionic neuron, this is not the case for the adrenal medulla and sweat glands. The adrenal medulla's chromaffin cells are directly innervated by the preganglionic cells of the SNS, and stimulation of the cells causes release of NE into the bloodstream. Sweat glands are divided into two classes, the eccrine sweat glands and the apocrine sweat glands. Eccrine sweat glands are found throughout the body except for the lips, are used for cooling purposes, and are activated via Ach acting on muscarinic receptors. Apocrine sweat glands are activated by catecholamines acting on α-1 receptors.

In anesthesia we commonly use medications that have effects on the autonomic nervous system. Table 182.1 outlines the commonly used drugs and describes their effect on the sympathetic system.

## REFERENCES

1. Taylor P, Brown JH. Synthesis, storage and release of acetylcholine. In: Siegel GJ, Agranoff BW, Albers RW, et al., eds. *Basic Neurochemistry: Molecular, Cellular and Medical Aspects*. 6th ed. Philadelphia, PA: Lippincott-Raven; 1999. Available from: https://www.ncbi.nlm.nih.gov/books/NBK28051/
2. McCorry LK. Physiology of the autonomic nervous system. *Am J Pharm Educ*. 2007;71(4):78.

# 183.

# PARASYMPATHETIC NERVOUS SYSTEM

*Tanya Lucas*

## INTRODUCTION

The sympathetic nervous system (SNS) and the parasympathetic nervous system (PSNS) form the autonomic nervous system and are thought of as the visceral motor system. Together the SNS and PSNS modulate activity of organ systems (rather than initiate actions) to maintain homeostasis in the response to a changing environment. While the SNS is responsible for responding during stressful situations (fight or flight), the PSNS maintains function during times of energy conservation (rest and digest).[1]

## PARASYMPATHETIC NERVOUS SYSTEM ANATOMY

Like the SNS, the PSNS consists of a two-neuron chain—a preganglionic nerve and a postganglionic nerve that then synapses on the target organ. Unlike the sympathetic nervous system, the ganglia of the PSNS are found near or within the target organs, necessitating a long preganglionic nerve and a short postganglionic nerve. Because PSNS has ganglia located near or in the organs it has a more *specific, localized effect on individual organs* than the SNS. The PSNS originates in the brainstem (nuclei of CN III, CN VII, CN IX, and CN X) and at the S2–S4 level of the spinal cord. Preganglionic fibers from the CN III, CN VII, and CN IX synapse in ganglia located in the head and neck (ciliary, submandibular, and otic ganglia), from which postganglionic fibers run to organs in this region, including smooth muscles of the eye, and lacrimal and salivary glands. In contrast, preganglionic fibers from the CN X, or the vagus nerve, run directly to target organs where they synapse on postganglionic fibers at ganglia within the target organs.[2] The vagus nerve is the dominant parasympathetic output, with nearly 75% of all PSNS fibers, and it innervates the heart, lungs, and gastrointestinal (GI) tract. The caudal portion of the GI tract and the urinary bladder are innervated by parasympathetic fibers from S2–S4 that run in splanchnic nerves and synapse on postganglionic fibers near or within these organs (Table 183.1).

*Table 183.1* ANATOMY OF THE PARASYMPATHETIC NERVOUS SYSTEM

| ORIGIN | NERVE | GANGLIA | TARGET ORGANS |
| --- | --- | --- | --- |
| Midbrain<br>  Edinger Westphal<br>  nucleus | CN III<br>Oculomotor | Ciliary ganglion | Iris<br>Ciliary muscle of the eye |
| Medulla oblongata<br>  Superior salivatory<br>  nucleus | CN VII<br>Facial<br>Chorda tympani branch | Submandibular ganglion | Submandibular salivary glands<br>Sublingual salivary glands |
| Superior salivatory<br>  nucleus | Facial<br>Greater petrosal branch | Sphenopalatine ganglion | Nasal glands<br>Lacrimal glands |
| Medulla oblongata<br>  Dorsal nucleus | CN IX<br>Glossopharyngeal | Otic ganglion | Parotid gland |
| Medulla oblongata<br>  Dorsal nucleus<br>  Nucleus ambiguus | CN X<br>Vagus | Many within the target<br>  organs | Trachea, esophagus, bronchial<br>  tree, upper GI tract<br>Cardiac muscle |
| Spinal cord<br>  Lateral gray horn | S2–4 | Celiac ganglion,<br>  superior and inferior<br>  mesenteric ganglia | Lower GI tract, prostate, bladder,<br>  reproductive organs |

## PARASYMPATHETIC NEUROTRANSMITTERS AND RECEPTORS

All preganglionic PSNS nerves secrete acetylcholine (ACh), which binds to nicotinic ACh receptors (subtype N2) on the postganglionic nerve, and all postganglionic PSNS fibers secrete Ach, which binds to muscarinic ACh receptors on the target organ. Interestingly, nicotinic (subtype N1) receptors are also found at the neuromuscular junction of skeletal muscles responsible for voluntary movement, and muscarinic receptors can be found in the central nervous system (CNS), where they have a role in learning and memory. Nicotinic and muscarinic receptors are both activated by Ach, but otherwise they are unrelated. The nicotinic receptors bind 2 molecules of ACh and are ion channels, while muscarinic receptors are 7-transmembrane domain receptors coupled to G-proteins that bind 1 molecule of ACh. Therefore, muscarinic receptors are more closely related to the adrenergic receptors, as they are also 7-transmembrane domain receptors coupled to G-proteins, than they are to cholinergic, nicotinic receptors. See Table 183.2 for drugs affecting the cholinergic receptors.

## SYNTHESIS AND DEGRADATION OF ACETYLCHOLINE

Acetylcholine (ACh) is generated in the cytoplasm when the enzyme choline acetyl transferase (ChAT) transfers an acetyl group from AcetylCoA to choline. Degradation of Ach occurs when it is cleaved into choline and acetate by acetylcholinesterase (AChE), an enzyme found in the synaptic cleft. Plasma cholinesterase (also known as pseudocholinesterase or butyrylcholinesterase) is another enzyme that can degrade Ach. It is abundant in the liver and blood and hydrolyzes ACh more slowly than AChE; however, plasma cholinesterase is responsible for the metabolism of the depolarizing neuromuscular blocking agent, succinylcholine.[3]

## PARASYMPATHETIC STIMULATION EFFECTS ON TARGET ORGANS

As mentioned earlier, the PSNS, along with the SNS, helps to maintain a stable internal environment in response to changing internal and external conditions. The PSNS effects are predominant in the rest state.[3] Table 183.3 summarizes the organ responses to PSNS stimulation.

*Table 183.2* DRUGS AFFECTING THE PARASYMPATHETIC NERVOUS SYSTEM

|  | MUSCARINIC RECEPTORS | NICOTINIC N2 RECEPTORS (AUTONOMIC GANGLIA) | NICOTINIC N1 RECEPTORS (SKELETAL NM JUNCTION) |
|---|---|---|---|
| Anticholinesterase (increases Ach) |  |  |  |
| • Physostigmine | + | + | + |
| • Neostigmine | + | + | + |
| • Nerve agents (sarin) | + | + | + |
| • Organophosphates (insecticides) | + | + | + |
| Muscarinic Agonist |  |  |  |
| • Bethanechol | + |  |  |
| • Pilocarpine | + |  |  |
| Muscarinic Antagonist (Anticholinergic) |  |  |  |
| • Atropine | − |  |  |
| • Glycopyrolate | − |  |  |
| • Scopolamine | − |  |  |
| Nicotinic Agonist |  |  |  |
| • Nicotine |  | + | + |
| • Dimethylphenylpiperazinium |  | + | + |
| • Succinylcholine |  |  |  |
| Nicotinic Antagonist |  |  |  |
| • Trimetaphan |  | − |  |
| • Nondepolarizing muscle relaxants (rocuronium) |  |  | − |

**Table 183.3 PARASYMPATHETIC NERVOUS SYSTEM EFFECTS ON TARGET ORGANS**

| ORGAN | PARASYMPATHETIC STIMULATION EFFECT |
|---|---|
| Eye | Constriction of the pupil (miosis)—sphincter muscle of the iris<br>Accommodation for near vision—ciliary muscle |
| Heart | Decreased sinus rate, decreased AV nodal conduction, decreased contractility in the atria |
| Peripheral vasculature | No effect |
| Lung | Constriction of bronchial smooth muscle, increased secretions, no effect on blood vessels |
| GI tract | Increased motility, increased secretions |
| Urinary bladder | Voiding |
| Salivary glands | Increased secretions |
| Sweat glands | No effect |

## TONIC AUTONOMIC ACTIVITY

Many organs rely on the autonomic nervous system for constant baseline activity. This is known as tonic activity. Depending on the organ, tonic activity can be from the PSNS or the SNS. An example of tonic activity is the PSNS effect on heart rate. At rest, the heart rate is under PSNS control, leading to a slower heart rate than the intrinsic rate of the heart. This baseline PSNS effect on the heart is revealed if PSNS input is blocked by atropine, leading to a dramatic rise in heart rate. However, if beta blockers are given to block the SNS, there is minimal change because there is little SNS input into the heart at baseline. Thus, PSNS tone predominates in the heart at rest. If both SNS and PSNS are blocked, the intrinsic heart rate is revealed at about 100 beats/minute.[2]

## CHOLINERGIC CRISIS

Cholinergic crisis is a pathological state caused by antagonism of AChE, leading to an increase in ACh and overstimulation of the neuromuscular junctions of skeletal muscles and synapses of the PSNS. Symptoms include paralysis, leading to respiratory failure from accumulation of Ach at the neuromuscular junctions of skeletal muscles, and salivation, lacrimation, urination, defecation, GI distress, and miosis from stimulation of the PSNS. This can be caused by exposure to nerve agents (sarin) or organophosphates (insecticides) and inappropriate doses of anticholinesterases (neostigmine).[4]

## REFERENCES

1. Glick DB. The autonomic nervous system: Function. In: Gropper M, et al., eds. *Miller's Anesthesia*. 8th ed. Elsevier Health Sciences; 2015. https://www.r2library.com/Resource/Title/0702052833/ch0016s0555. Accessed August 20, 2020.
2. Koeppen B. Organization of the autonomic nervous system. In: Koeppen B, Stanton B, eds. *Berne & Levy Physiology*. 7th ed. Elsevier Health Sciences; 2018. https://www.r2library.com/Resource/Title/0323393942/ch0011s0322. Accessed August 20, 2020.
3. Taylor P. Anticholinesterase agents. In: Brunton LL, et al., eds. *Goodman & Gilman's: The Pharmacological Basis of Therapeutics*. 13th ed. McGraw-Hill; 2018. https://accessmedicine.mhmedical.com/content.aspx?bookid=2189&sectionid=167889828. Accessed August 20, 2020.
4. Baker, DJ, The role of the anesthesia provider in natural disasters. In: Gropper M, et al., eds. *Miller's Anesthesia*. 8th ed. Elsevier Health Sciences; 2018. https://www-r2library-com.umassmed.idm.oclc.org/Resource/Title/0702052833/ch0083s4196. Accessed August 20, 2020.

# 184.

# TERMINATION OF ACTION

*Robin B. Stedman*

## INTRODUCTION

The autonomic nervous system is a bipolar system comprising pre- and postganglionic fibers with interceding ganglia that are located either in paravertebral or more distal locations. The ganglia may be paired or unpaired. A detailed description of the anatomy and physiology of the autonomic nervous system may be found in the preceding chapters. Aside from one exception, the adrenal glands, the autonomic fibers produce two neurotransmitters.

These are norepinephrine and acetylcholine. The chromaffin cells of the adrenal glands also produce epinephrine.

## NOREPINEPHRINE

Norepinephrine is produced in the terminals of the adrenergic postganglionic fibers. The termination of action is by three means.[1] The most important mechanism is reuptake into presynaptic terminals and storage in vesicles, which accounts for the majority of termination of action. This energy-requiring process is very fast. It is also a stereospecific process, meaning that similar molecules can be taken up into vesicles and displace neurotransmitters. The second mechanism occurs in extraneuronal tissues that can take up norepinephrine, where it is broken down by the enzymes monoamine oxidase (MAO) and catechol-O-methyl transferase (COMT) into vanillylmandelic acid (VMA). The third mechanism is the metabolism by liver and kidney of minute amounts of norepinephrine that diffuse into the circulation.

The final metabolic product of catecholamines is VMA and is found in urine. The concentration of VMA in urine reflects the activity of the sympathetic nervous system. Measurement of urine VMA can facilitate the diagnosis of pheochromocytoma, a catecholamine-secreting tumor of the adrenal medulla.

## EPINEPHRINE

The termination of action of epinephrine is the same as that for norepinephrine.[1]

However, stimulation of the adrenal medulla, and the resultant circulating norepinephrine and epinephrine surge, produces a more prolonged adrenergic effect than the brief duration of action of norepinephrine on postganglionic effector cells in the sympathetic nerve synapse. This effect reflects the time necessary for metabolism by liver and kidneys. Likewise, exogenously administered catecholamines have a longer duration of action than norepinephrine at the local synapse.

## ACETYLCHOLINE

Acetylcholine is produced in nerve terminals of all autonomic preganglionic fibers, as well as the terminals of the cholinergic postganglionic fibers. The termination of action of acetylcholine is very different from that of the catecholamines norepinephrine and epinephrine.[2] Termination of action of acetylcholine is by acetylcholinesterase (AchE), an enzyme synthesized in nerve terminals that rapidly hydrolyzes acetylcholine to acetate and choline. Acetylcholine is not reused.

## TERMINATION OF ACTION: IMPLICATIONS FOR ANESTHESIA

Drugs that affect the enzymes involved in the termination of action of the neurotransmitters of the autonomic nervous system may have implications for anesthesia practice.

### TERMINATION OF ACTION OF ACETYLCHOLINE

In the relatively rare incidence of patients encountering irreversible inhibitors of acetylcholinesterase, as in organophosphate poisoning, the action of acetylcholine will be prolonged and will result in excessive cholinergic symptoms.[3]

Dibucaine number (DN) and fluoride number reflect reduced pseudocholinesterase activity resulting from addition of dibucaine or sodium fluoride to the assay.

Pseudocholinesterase abnormalities can lead to prolongation of action of succinylcholine (Sch):

- Homozygous typical, DN 70–80, normal response to Sch
- Heterozygous atypical, DN 50–60, lengthened by 50%–100%
- Homozygous atypical, DN 23–30, prolonged to 4–8 hours.

Pesudocholinesterase is decreased in hepatitis, cirrhosis, malnutrition, cancer, myxodema, acute infarction, and myocardial infarction.

## TERMINATION OF ACTION OF NOREPINEPHRINE

When caring for patients administered inhibitors of monoamine oxidase,[4] anesthesiologists should be wary of the potentiating action of indirect acting sympathomimetics such as ephedrine that release norepinephrine from nerve cells. Tricyclic antidepressants and cocaine inhibit reuptake of norepinephrine into presynaptic terminals, increasing the concentration of norepinephrine at receptors with exaggerated response.[1]

## REFERENCES

1. Grecu L. Autonomic nervous system: Physiology and pharmacology In Barash PG, ed. *Clinical Anesthesia*. 7th ed. Philadelphia, PA: Lippincott Williams & Wilkins; 2013:371.
2. Grecu L. Autonomic nervous system: Physiology and pharmacology In Barash PG, ed. *Clinical Anesthesia*. 7th ed. Philadelphia, PA: Lippincott Williams & Wilkins; 2013:368–369.
3. Grecu L. Autonomic nervous system: Physiology and pharmacology In Barash PG, ed. *Clinical Anesthesia*. 7th ed. Philadelphia, PA: Lippincott Williams & Wilkins, 2013:384
4. Saraghi M, et al. Anesthetic considerations for patients on antidepressant therapy: Part I. *Anesth Prog.* 2017 Winter;64(4):253–261.

# 185.

# GANGLIONIC TRANSMISSION

*Natalie H. Strand and Jillian A. Maloney*

## INTRODUCTION

The autonomic nervous system (ANS) plays a key role in homeostasis, and it is crucial that the anesthesiology trainee fully understand this system. The ANS controls involuntary functions such as heart rate, blood pressure, temperature regulation, respiratory function, and gastrointestinal responses.[1,2] The ANS is divided into the sympathetic and parasympathetic systems. The ANS reaches the end organ via two neurons: the preganglionic neuron and the postganglionic neuron. These neurons synapse in the autonomic ganglia. Autonomic ganglia are aggregations of nerve cell bodies and their dendrites where synapses are made—a connection between autonomic nerves originating in the central nervous system and the autonomic nerves that innervate the target end organs in the periphery. Preganglionic neurons release acetylcholine as the neurotransmitter, and most postganglionic neurons utilize norepinephrine. Acetylcholine is the neurotransmitter involved in ganglionic transmission for both the sympathetic and parasympathetic branches of the autonomic nervous system. When a nerve impulse reaches the end of the preganglionic neuron, it triggers the fusion of synaptic vesicles containing acetylcholine with the synaptic membrane, releasing acetylcholine into the synaptic cleft. Acetylcholine then binds to receptors on the postganglionic nerve membrane, and triggers an action potential by altering permeability to ions.

## PRESYNAPTIC VOLTAGE GATED CALCIUM CHANNELS

Action potentials in preganglionic nerves activate voltage gated calcium channels (VGCC), allowing calcium to enter the neuron and trigger neurotransmitter release via the fusion of synaptic vesicles containing acetylcholine with the cell membrane.[3] Stated another way, depolarization of the preganglionic neuron results in increased calcium permeability and triggers the release of the neurotransmitter acetylcholine into the synaptic cleft in the autonomic ganglia. Modulation of the presynaptic VGCC has a significant effect on synaptic transmission.[4]

## LIGAND GATED SODIUM CHANNELS

Nicotinic acetylcholine receptors are ligand gated sodium channels. When the receptor binds two molecules of acetylcholine, the sodium channel opens and allows sodium to enter the cell, triggering depolarization. All autonomic ganglia have nicotinic receptors on the postganglionic neurons.

## ACETYLCHOLINE

All preganglionic neurons (sympathetic and parasympathetic) in the autonomic nervous system release acetylcholine at the synapse in the ganglion. In addition, all postganglionic neurons of the parasympathetic system release acetylcholine. The cholinergic receptors are categorized as either nicotinic or muscarinic. In the synapse, termination of action of acetylcholine is by degradation by acetylcholinesterase or by reuptake into the preganglionic neuron (Table 185.1).

*Table 185.1* NEUROTRANSMITTERS

| Acetylcholine (from cholinergic fibers) | Released by all preganglionic neurons in the ANS | Released by postganglionic neurons of the parasympathetic system *and* postganglionic neurons of the sympathetic system innervating sweat glands |
|---|---|---|
| Norepinephrine (from adrenergic fibers) | Not released by preganglionic neurons in the ANS | Released by most postganglionic fibers |

## NOREPINEPHRINE

Norepineprhine (also known as noradrenaline) is released by most postganglionic neurons of the sympathetic system. In the synapse, termination of action of norepinephrine occurs by degradation by catechol-o-methyl transferase (COMT) enzyme or by reuptake into the preganglionic neuron (Table 185.1).

## ANESTHETIC CONSIDERATIONS

### PREOPERATIVE

There are several important clinical concerns in patients with known autonomic neuropathy that need to be considered in the perioperative period (Table 185.2). Preoperatively, it is important to do a thorough history and physical exam to identify any signs and symptoms of autonomic neuropathy. Asking the patient about exercise tolerance, and signs of orthostatic hypotension such as dizziness, fainting, visual changes, and lightheadedness, is important. It is also noteworthy that patients with autonomic neuropathy may have silent or asymptomatic ischemia, so history alone may miss symptoms of angina. Autonomic neuropathy in the cardiovascular system can lead to resting tachycardia up to 130 bpm, and if other causes of tachycardia are ruled out, this can be an important clue to underlying autonomic disease. Patients who are high risk for autonomic neuropathy include those with type 1 diabetes, type 2 diabetes, and/or patients with other microvascular complications such as peripheral neuropathy.[5]

### INTRAOPERATIVE

Patients with autonomic neuropathy can present with increased autonomic instability during induction and intubation. In addition, positional changes can lead to profound hypotension. As temperature dysregulation can lead to hypothermia, temperatures should be monitored and corrected swiftly to avoid prolonged hypothermia. Neuraxial blockade can also lead to profound hypotension due to the sympathetic blockade (Table 185.2).

### POSTOPERATIVE

Supplemental oxygen should be considered in the post-anesthesia care unit (PACU) given the risk of silent ischemia in patients with autonomic neuropathy. Shivering should be aggressively treated for the same reason. Patients may require hemodynamic monitoring and a higher level of postoperative care when compared to patients without autonomic neuropathy (Table 185.2).

Table 185.2 ANESTHETIC CONSIDERATIONS IN PATIENTS WITH AUTONOMIC NEUROPATHY

| AUTONOMIC NEUROPATHY | PREOPERATIVE CONCERNS | INTRAOPERATIVE CONCERNS | POSTOPERATIVE CONCERNS |
|---|---|---|---|
| Cardiovascular | Resting tachycardia, defective angina warning, painless ischemia | Hemodynamic instability, prolonged QTc can increase risk of MI, arrythmias, and sudden deth. | Increased risk of MI, painless ischemia |
| GI | Consider H2 receptor antagonists like ranitidine and prokinetics like metoclopramide as premedication | Gastroparesis—increased risk of aspiration | Nausea/vomiting |
| Sudomotor | | Hypothermia | |

MI: myocardial infarction; H2: Histamine H2-receptor antagonists.

## REFERENCES

1. McCorry LK. Physiology of the autonomic nervous system. *Am J Pharm Educ.* 2007;71(4):78.
2. Bankenahally R, Krovvidi H. Autonomic nervous system: Anatomy, physiology, and relevance in anesthesia and critical care medicine. *BJA Education.* 2016;16(11):381–387.
3. Clarke SG, et al. Neurotransmitter release can be stabilized by a mechanism that prevents voltage changes near the end of action potentials from affecting calcium currents. *J Neurosci.* 2016;36(45):11559–11572.
4. Mochida S, et al. Regulation of presynaptic Ca(V)2.1 channels by Ca2+ sensor proteins mediates short-term synaptic plasticity. *Neuron.* 2008;57(2):210–216.
5. Serhiyenko VA, Serhiyenko AA. Cardiac autonomic neuropathy: Risk factors, diagnosis and treatment. *World J Diabetes.* 2018;9(1):1–24.

# 186.

# AUTONOMIC REFLEXES

*Natalie H. Strand and Jillian A. Maloney*

## INTRODUCTION

The autonomic nervous system (ANS) regulates the cardiovascular and gastrointestinal systems as well as temperature maintenance. The ANS is divided into the parasympathetic and sympathetic nervous systems. The sympathetic nervous system increases heart rate, blood pressure, cardiac output, and causes bronchodilation.[1] The parasympathetic system's functions include reducing heart rate and increasing gastrointestinal activity.[1] The parasympathetic and sympathetic nervous systems compete to maintain homeostasis within the body via inhibitory and excitatory reflex pathways. The ANS targets smooth muscle, while the somatic system targets skeletal muscle. The ANS reflexes are involuntary. However, some reflexes may be altered consciously, such as heart rate, sexual arousal, and respiratory rate. An autonomic reflex is a response that occurs when nerve impulses pass through an autonomic reflex arc. Interneurons within the central nervous system (CNS) relay signals from sensory neurons to motor neurons. The main integrating centers are located in the hypothalamus and brainstem.

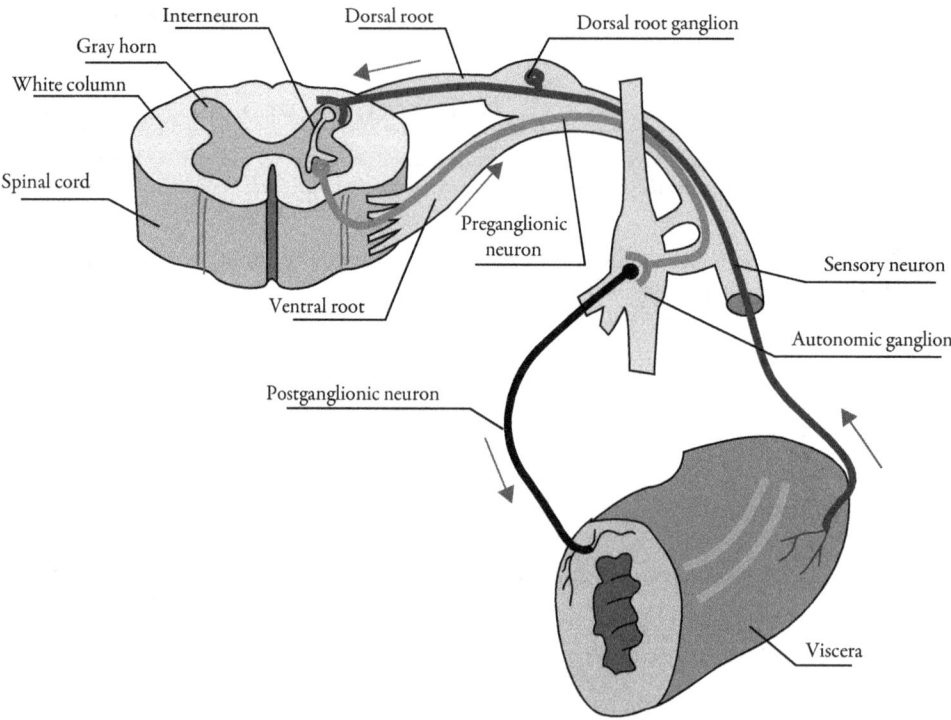

**Figure 186.1.** The autonomic reflex arc of the autonomic nervous system.
From: Stihii/Shutterstock.com.

Autonomic reflexes have two sequential neurons, as opposed to somatic reflexes which have one. Autonomic reflexes occur via spinal, cranial, and splanchnic nerves. An autonomic reflex arc has an efferent and afferent branch. The efferent branch begins with preganglionic fibers from the spinal cord or brainstem, which then synapse with a postganglionic fiber to the tissue target. The afferent branch is a sensory neuron which responds to a stimulus in the periphery and results in a change that will ultimately trigger the reflex (Figure 186.1). An example of an autonomic reflex is the baroreceptor reflex. Arterial baroreceptors are located in the carotid sinus and the aortic arch, which regulate the body's blood pressure. These baroreceptors react to stretching of the vascular walls by increased arterial pressure or blood volume, which leads to increased parasympathetic activity and decreased sympathetic activity. This will subsequently reduce the heart rate and also cause the blood pressure to decrease. Baroreceptors also respond to decrease in blood pressure. A reduction in wall tension would increase sympathetic tone and decrease parasympathetic activity, leading to increased heart rate and systemic vascular resistance to elevate the blood pressure.

The sympathetic and parasympathetic systems complement each other to maintain appropriate organ function. While organ systems have both parasympathetic and sympathetic input, there generally is a predominance of one system at the resting state, called the autonomic tone. Resting heart rate is an example of parasympathetic tone. The intrinsic rate of the sinoartial node is around 100 beats per minute.[2] At rest, parasympathetic efferents from the vagus nerves slows the resting heart rate to 55–75 beats per minute; thus resting heart rate is a parasympathetic tone.

## AUTONOMIC HYPERREFLEXIA/ DYSREFLEXIA

After traumatic spinal cord injury (usually at or above T4–7), disruption of autonomic reflex arcs can result in a potentially life-threatening syndrome called autonomic dysreflexia/hyperreflexia. Autonomic hyperreflexia is an exaggerated sympathetic response to stimuli below the level of spinal cord injury. It generally occurs 3 weeks to 9 months after the initial spinal cord injury and is most commonly seen in patients with lesions at or above the sixth thoracic spinal segment.[3] There are several hypotheses as to what causes autonomic dysreflexia; the majority suggest a hyperactive nervous system. After spinal cord injury, the regulation by higher centers on the sympathetic output from the spinal cord is lost.[4] This allows for an uninhibited exaggerated sympathetic reaction of preganglionic neurons to afferent stimuli.[4] Triggers of autonomic dysreflexia include: bladder distension, urinary tract infections, urologic procedures like cystoscopy, rectal distension, fractures, skin infections, pressure ulcers, pregnancy, and labor.[4] These stimuli can cause severe hypertension, which activates the baroreceptor reflex, resulting in profound bradycardia. The severe hypertension can cause hypertensive encephalopathy, stroke, and seizure.[5] In addition to hypertension, patients can complain of headaches, nasal congestion, sweating, and flushing of the skin above the level of the spinal cord injury.[4] Patients develop vasodilation above the level of the lesion and vasoconstriction below.

## ANESTHETIC CONSIDERATIONS

### PREOPERATIVE

It is important to ensure that the patient has proper bowel care and voids prior to surgery to reduce the risk of bladder or bowel distension intraoperatively. Spinal anesthesia has been reported as a reliable technique for prevention; epidural anesthesia, epidural meperidine, and general anesthesia also have been reported to be effective in prevention.

### INTRAOPERATIVE

If the patient develops severe hypertension intraoperatively, the patient can be treated with vasodilators like nicardipine or nitroglycerin; position the patient in an upright position to take advantage of orthostatic blood pressure drop,

administer 100% oxygen, deepen the volatile anesthetic or bolus with propofol, and most importantly, attempt to remove or reduce the noxious stimuli if possible.[5]

### POSTOPERATIVE

The most common cause of autonomic dysreflexia is bladder distension.

## REFERENCES

1. Wehrwein EA, et al. Overview of the anatomy, physiology, and phamacology of the autonomic nervous system. *Compr Physiol.* 2016 Jun 13;6(3):1239–1278.
2. Jose AD, Taylor RR. Autonomic blockade by propranolol and atropine to study intrinsic myocardial function in man. *J Clin Invest.* 1969;48(11):2019.
3. Bankenahally R, Krovvidi H. Autonomic nervous system: Anatomy, physiology, and relevance in anaesthesia and critical care medicine. *BJA Education.* 2016;16(11):381–387.
4. Bycroft J, et al. Autonomic dysreflexia: A medical emergency. *Postgrad Med J.* 2005;81(954): 232–235.
5. Eldahan KC, Rabchevsky AG. Autonomic dysreflexia after spinal cord injury: Systemic pathophysiology and methods of management. *Auton Neurosci.* 2018;209:59–70.

# 187.

# AFFERENT AND EFFERENT PATHWAYS

*Simranjit Singh and Taruna Waghray-Penmetcha*

## INTRODUCTION

The autonomic nervous system (ANS), also known as the visceral system, is responsible for control of involuntary functions. Like the somatic nervous system, the ANS can be divided into afferent and efferent pathways. While efferent pathways are divided into sympathetic and parasympathetic branches, a single afferent sensory system conducts information for the ANS. Afferent fibers are responsible for transmitting sensory information from vasculature and viscera, and initiating reflex responses. In response to the

information received, efferent fibers transmit information from the brain to the periphery in order to maintain homeostasis. Although there are exceptions, both afferent and efferent signals are transmitted by the same postganglionic nerves.

## AFFERENTS PATHWAYS

Afferent pathways relay information from periphery to the central nervous system (CNS). The impulses from the receptors located in thoracic and abdominal viscera are transmitted to the spinal cord via the dorsal root ganglion or to the brainstem via cranial nerves (CN). The afferent pathways are not as clearly defined as the efferent pathways and can be divided into 2 main sensory systems:

*Cranial afferents* enter the CNS along with cranial nerves II, V, VII, IX, and X, and transmit sensory information from face, head, tongue, palate, oropharynx, carotid body, larynx, trachea, esophagus, and thoracic and abdominal organs. These fibers terminate in the nucleus tractus solitarius (principal visceral sensory nucleus) located in medulla oblongata.[1-4]

*Spinal afferents* transmit sensations of temperature and tissue injury from the thoracic and abdominal viscera to the brainstem via afferent fibers of the vagus nerve. Sensory afferents from the pelvis enter at spinal levels S2–S4 and regulate parasympathetic outflow.

## EFFERENT PATHWAYS

The efferent limb is made up of preganglionic and postganglionic fibers and the associated autonomic ganglia. The efferent limb is further subdivided into sympathetic and parasympathetic components. The sympathetic system is responsible for "flight or fight" response, while the parasympathetic system is responsible for "rest and digest" response.[4]

### SYMPATHETIC NERVOUS SYSTEM

Preganglionic fibers originate from the cell bodies in intermediolateral columns of the thoracolumbar spinal cord from T1 to L2/L3 (thoraco-lumbar outflow). The short, myelinated fibers exit the spinal cord with the anterior roots, form white rami, and synapse with the postganglionic neurons in the sympathetic chain.[1,4] A single preganglionic neuron may synapse with multiple postganglionic neurons, which results in coordinated sympathetic stimulation to tissues throughout the body. Preganglionic neurons also synapse directly with adrenal tissue. The cells of the adrenal medulla function as postganglionic neurons and release neurotransmitter directly into the bloodstream. The long postganglionic neurons originate in the ganglia, travel along the 31 pairs of spinal nerves, and terminate on the effector tissues. The sympathetic system innervates structures of the head, thoracic, abdominal, and pelvic viscera. Vascular smooth muscle tone and sweating are also regulated by the sympathetic system. Bilateral paravertebral sympathetic chains are located anterolateral to the spinal cord. The ganglia within this chain are 3 cervical, 11 thoracic, 4 lumbar, and 4 in sacral region. Unpaired prevertebral ganglia lie ventral to the spine and receive input from the splanchnic nerves and innervate organs of the abdominal and pelvic region. These include

the celiac ganglia, superior mesenteric ganglia, and inferior mesenteric ganglia.

## PARASYMPATHETIC NERVOUS SYSTEM

Preganglionic fibers arise from the central nervous system and the sacral nerves craniosacral outflow[3]). Cranial parasympathetic fibers arise from brainstem motor nuclei of the III, VII, IX, and X cranial nerves. Sacral outflow arises from ventral rami of nerves S2–S4. The axons of the preganglionic neurons are long and synapse with short postganglionic neurons in terminal ganglia within the effector tissues. The effects of the parasympathetic system are more discrete and localized, as the terminal ganglia are located within the innervated tissue.

## ORGAN-SPECIFIC PATHWAYS

### EYE

The afferent pathway in the eye begins with changes in the amount of light on retina. This information is transmitted via neurons of optic nerve (CN II) which synapse at the mesencephalic pretectal nucleus in the midbrain. This nucleus connects to the Edinger-Westphal nucleus of the oculomotor nerve (CN III), which initiates the parasympathetic efferent pathway and ventrolateral hypothalamus, which initiates efferent sympathetic signals.[2,3] Parasympathetic fibers travel via CN III to postganglionic neurons of the ciliary ganglion, which projects to ciliary body and the sphincter pupillae muscle of the iris. Sympathetic signals are transmitted to preganglionic neurons in the lateral horn of the spinal segments T1–T3. The axons then exit with ventral roots and ascend via white rami communicans to the superior cervical ganglion, which terminates at the dilator pupillae muscle.

### LACRIMAL GLAND

Secretion is initiated with stimulation of corneal and conjunctival epithelium. This information is carried by the ophthalmic branch of the trigeminal nerve (CN V) to the trigeminal ganglion and the sensory trigeminal nucleus. The efferent parasympathetic pathway begins in the superior salivary nucleus of the facial nerve (CN VII) located in the pons. CN VII courses through the geniculate ganglion without synapsing and gives off the greater superficial petrosal nerve. This nerve joins the deep petrosal nerve to form the vidian nerve, which synapses with the postganglionic neurons of pterygopalatine ganglion that innervates the lacrimal gland.[2,3] Sympathetic efferent innervation, although insignificant, originates from T1–T4 preganglionic neurons, which synapse with superior cervical ganglion and terminate at the lacrimal gland.

## SALIVARY GLAND

Secretion begins with afferent chemoreceptors in gustatory cells or mechanoreceptors in the periodontal ligament. Information is transmitted to the solitary nucleus via fibers of the CNs V, VII, and IX. The efferent pathways originate in the superior and inferior salivatory nuclei located in the pons. The superior salivatory nucleus sends signals via the facial nerve branches, chorda tympani, and lingual nerves to postganglionic neurons of the submandibular ganglion which innervate the submandibular and sublingual salivary glands. The inferior salivatory nucleus is the initial location for efferent signals of the glossopharyngeal nerve, which branches off at the tympanic plexus to give lesser petrosal nerve. This synapses at the postganglionic otic ganglion. Axons then terminate at the parotid gland. Sympathetic innervation is less significant; preganglionic neurons are located at T1–T4, and postganglionic neurons of the superior cervical ganglion send efferents to all three glands.

## CARDIOPULMONARY SYSTEM

Afferent signals from the cardiopulmonary system are transmitted by the branches of the CN IX and X. Changes in blood pressure are sensed by stretch receptors located in aortic arch and carotid sinus, while changes in oxygen and carbon dioxide are detected by chemoreceptor cells on the carotid and aortic bodies. The carotid sinus and body are innervated by the glossopharyngeal nerve, while the aortic arch is innervated by the vagus.[2,3] These nerves transmit the signals to the nucleus of the solitary tract located in the medulla. Efferent signals are then sent to the parasympathetic vagal neurons in the nucleus ambigus and dorsal motor nucleus of the vagus or sympathetic neurons in the ventrolateral medulla. The vagus nerve is responsible for parasympathetic output, while sympathetic outflow is conducted by preganglionic neurons located in the intermediolateral columns of the spinal cord from T1–T4 levels which synapse with postganglionic neurons of the superior, middle, and inferior cervical ganglia. Sympathetic innervation of the sinoatrial and atrioventricular nodes, conduction system, myocardial muscle, and bronchioles is primarily by the inferior cervical ganglion.

## ABDOMEN AND PELVIC VISCERA

Afferent transmission begins with activation of stretch receptors in the gastric, intestinal, or bladder walls. The peripheral receptors on these organs are innervated by neurons that have cell bodies located in the dorsal root ganglion. These neurons synapse on viscero-somatic neurons in the dorsal horn. Convergence of these two signals at the dorsal horn is responsible for the phenomena of referred pain. From here, the signal is carried through the spinothalamic and spinoreticular tracts. Fibers cross midline at the level of the spinal cord and are propagated along the anterior commissure up to the solitary nucleus located in the medulla. Information is then relayed via the parabrachial nucleus to the ventroposteromedial nucleus in the thalamus, followed by the somatosensory cortex. The efferent parasympathetic signals for entire gastrointestinal tract, excluding the proximal esophagus and distal colon, are controlled by the dorsal nucleus of the vagus, located in the medulla. Sympathetic outflow is from the preganglionic neurons located at T1–L1 segments of the spinal cord, with postganglionic fibers located in the celiac and mesenteric ganglia.[3] Efferent outflow to the bladder, distal colon, and sexual organs is emitted from the sacral parasympathetic (S2–S4) neurons and lumbar sympathetic neurons (T12–L2) via the postganglionic hypogastric plexus.

## REFERENCES

1. Brunton L, Chabner B, Knollman B. *Goodman & Gilman's The Pharmacological Basis of Therapeutics.* 12th ed. New York, NY: McGraw-Hill, Health Professions Division; 2011.
2. Goetz CG. *Textbook of Clinical Neurology.* 3rd ed. Philadelphia, PA: W. B. Saunders; 2003.
3. Kandel ER. *Principles of Neuroscience.* 5th ed. New York, NY: McGraw-Hill; 2013.
4. Bankenahally R, et al. Autonomic nervous system: Anatomy, physiology, and relevance in anaesthesia and critical care medicine. *BJA Education.* 2016;16(11):381–387.
5. Furness JB. The organisation of the autonomic nervous system: Peripheral connections. *Auton Neurosci.* 2006;30(1–2):1–5.

# Part XII

# TEMPERATURE REGULATION

# 188.

# TEMPERATURE SENSING, HEAT PRODUCTION, AND CONSERVATION

*Jayakar Guruswamy and Matthew Epelman*

## THERMOREGULATION

Normal core body temperature can fluctuate by approximately 1°C and is influenced by circadian and menstrual cycles. Temperature regulation has three elements: (1) an afferent input, (2) a central control, and (3) an efferent response. The afferent component involves both heat and cold receptors, which are widely distributed in the body. Transient receptor potential proteins play the most important role in the transmission of these sensations. Among them, transient receptor potential vanilloid (TRPV) receptors 1–4 transmit heat sensation, whereas transient receptor potential melastatin (TRPM8) and transient receptor potential ankyrin (TRPA1) transmit cold stimuli. Heat and warmth receptors travel primarily through unmyelinated C fibers, whereas cold receptors travel along A-δ nerve fibers, although some overlap does occur. Ascending sensory thermal input is then transmitted to the hypothalamus, which is the primary thermoregulatory control center of mammals, via the spinothalamic tracts in the anterior spinal cord. Although most thermal information is integrated by the hypothalamus, some processing and response occurs within the spinal cord itself.[1] Central thermoregulatory control is based on thermal input from structures throughout the body; mean skin temperature contributes about 50% to thermal information,[2] with the upper chest and face contributing more than other areas. Each thermoregulatory response can be characterized by the threshold, gain, and response. The *threshold* is the temperature at which a response will occur. The *gain* represents the intensity of that response.[3] The threshold for responses to warmth (sweating and vasodilation) normally exceeds the threshold for the first response to cold (vasoconstriction) by 0.2°C to 0.4°C. Temperatures within this *interthreshold range*—the range between the threshold for response to cold and the threshold for response to warmth (0.2°–0.4°C)—do not trigger any thermoregulatory responses. However, temperatures outside the interthreshold range do trigger a response (Figure 188.1).

Efferent responses are the activation of effector mechanisms, which either increase metabolic heat production or adjust environmental heat loss and can be broadly categorized into behavioral and autonomic responses. Quantitatively, the most effective responses are behavioral ones:[4] dressing appropriately, moving voluntarily, or adjusting ambient temperature, which are not applicable to patients under general anesthesia. The major autonomic responses to heat are sweating and active cutaneous vasodilation. Sweating is mediated by postganglionic cholinergic (acetylcholine) nerves, and sweat is an ultrafiltrate of plasma. Sweating is the only mechanism by which the body

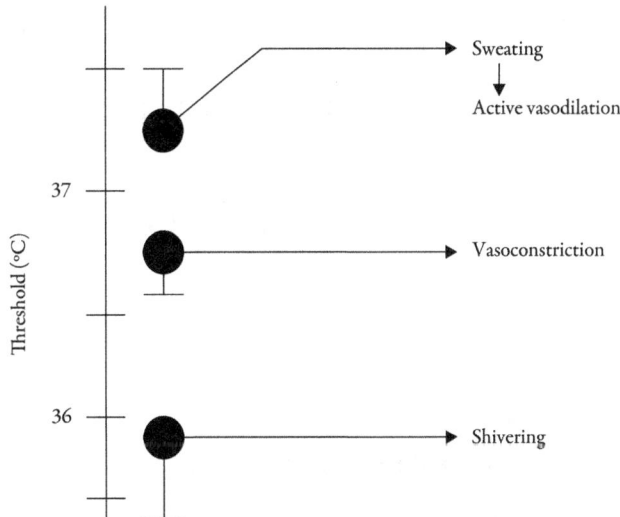

**Figure 188.1.** The major thermoregulatory thresholds in human beings. Temperatures between the sweating and vasoconstriction thresholds define the interthreshold range—a narrow margin—which do not activate thermoregulatory defenses and thus define normal core temperature. Sweating promotes heat dissipation via the skin surface into the environment. The shivering threshold is 1°C below the vasoconstriction threshold; thus, by the time a human has begun shivering, they are already hypothermic.

Reproduced with permission from Sessler DI. Perioperative thermoregulation and heat balance. *Lancet.* 2016;387:2655–2664.

can dissipate heat in an environment in which ambient temperature exceeds core temperature. Cutaneous vasodilation, a unique effector mechanism of humans mediated by the cholinergic system, diverts blood to the periphery, where heat can be dissipated more easily and ultimately can lower core temperature. Several specific vasodilators play a role in this mechanism, including nitric oxide, vasoactive intestinal peptide, histamine, substance P, and prostaglandins.[5] The primary autonomic thermoregulatory responses to cold are cutaneous arteriovenous shunt vasoconstriction, mediated by α-1 and α-2 adrenergic receptors, and shivering. Cutaneous vasoconstriction reduces the amount of blood vulnerable to heat loss from the skin surface primarily through radiation, but also by convection. Shivering, an involuntary muscular activity, significantly increases metabolic heat production by up to 100%. The response of shivering is absent in the newborn and may take several years to become fully functional. Infants therefore rely on nonshivering thermogenesis, an important thermoregulatory response that doubles heat production in infants.[5] Nonshivering thermogenesis is mediated by β-3 adrenergic receptors via activation of brown fat by an uncoupling protein, thermogenin, which allows the direct transformation of substrate into heat. The thermoneutral zone is defined as the range of ambient temperature where healthy adults can maintain normal body temperature without using energy above normal basal metabolic rate. The range is 25°–30°C (77°–86°F) for a naked adult man, standing upright, in still air.

## REFERENCES

1. Simon E. Temperature regulation: The spinal cord as a site of extrahypothalamic thermoregulatory functions. *Rev Physiol Biochem Pharmacol*. 1974;71:1–76.
2. Frank SM, et al. Relative contribution of core and cutaneous temperatures to thermal comfort and autonomic responses in humans. *J Appl Physiol. (1985)*. 1999;86:1588–1593.
3. Sessler DI. Perioperative thermoregulation and heat balance. *Lancet*. 2016;387:2655–2664.
4. Schlader ZJ, et al. The independent roles of temperature and thermal perception in the control of human thermoregulatory behavior. *Physiol Behav*. 2011;103:217–224.
5. Charkoudian N. Skin blood flow in adult human thermoregulation: How it works, when it does not, and why. *Mayo Clin Proc*. 2003;78:603–612.

# 189.

# TEMPERATURE-REGULATING CENTERS

*Karthik Dwarki and Matthew McConnell*

## INTRODUCTION

Core body temperature is a highly regulated process in order to remain within a narrow window, thus maintaining cellular function within the body. The body temperature is kept around 37°C, with small daily variations due to circadian rhythm and monthly changes in fertile women. The body's primary defenses against temperature changes include behavioral changes, e.g., dressing warmly during cold weather. Incremental changes occur based on the relative body temperature in order to once again obtain optimal temperature. It is believed that many neurotransmitters, including catecholamines and neuropeptides, determine the overall temperature threshold. A number of mechanisms can significantly alter threshold temperatures, including infection, hypo/hyperthyroidism, and anesthetics.[1]

The hypothalamic-pituitary-adrenal (HPA) axis helps to maintain homeostasis; core body temperature is specifically maintained within the preoptic area (POA) of the anterior hypothalamus. Studies have also found that the gamma-aminobutyric acid (GABA)-ergic neurons in the ventral part of the lateral preoptic nucleus (vLPO) and the glutamatergic and GABAergic neurons in the dorsomedial hypothalamus (DMD) play a major role in thermoregulation.[2]

Thermoregulation occurs in three phases, afferent thermal sensing, central regulation, and efferent response. The neural network activates once a set point is crossed, when the change in body temperature goes above or below a certain threshold. Specifically, A-δ fibers and C fibers convey cold and heat information to the spinal cord, respectively. This information travels up the spinal cord to the central nervous system, specifically integrating with the hypothalamus. Accordingly, it has been found that the skin, deep tissues including abdominal and thoracic tissues, the spinal cord, and brain including nonhypothalamic areas contribute 20% to the autonomic thermoregulatory control.[1]

Efferent responses will correlate with the body's requirement and progress based on the extent of temperature deviation. These responses include vasodilation and sweating in the setting of hyperthermia or vasoconstriction and shivering in the setting of hypothermia. In infants, nonshivering thermogenesis remains the most important method the body has to combat hypothermia, specifically with the use of brown fat. Brown fat is a specialized adipose tissue with a high mitochondrial density that is able to produce an enormous amount of heat.[1] Like the hormonal aspect of the HPA, core body temperature acts in negative feedback loop to shut down efferent responses once homeostasis is achieved.[3] Of note, thermoregulatory control remains the same between genders and intact in infants; however, it is reduced in the elderly population.[1]

## ANESTHETIC CONSIDERATIONS

As noted, hypothalamic thermoregulation is considered essential for maintaining normothermia. This axis and its response to temperature changes are downregulated secondary to anesthetic drugs. Most anesthetics, not only those used for general anesthesia and monitored anesthesia care, but also those used for regional anesthesia, will cause hypothermia through unique mechanisms of action. Volatile anesthetics and propofol, two of the most popular anesthetics, cause vasodilation, leading to increased heat loss. Interestingly, opioids not only blunt sympathetic response, but also widen the hypothalamus threshold response to temperature, with the range being anywhere from ~0.2°C to 4°C.[4] Neuraxial techniques, including both epidural and spinal, will restrict afferent fibers from communicating cold input to the hypothalamus. Interestingly, after undergoing neuraxial anesthesia, regions of skin block by the anesthetic are incorrectly assessed by the thermoregulatory center as being elevated in temperature. Thus patients will endorse subjective feelings of increased temperature even as they are clinically diagnosed with hypothermia.[4]

## REFERENCES

1. Kurz A. Physiology of thermoregulation. *Best Pract Res Clin Anaesthesiol.* 2008;22(4):627–44.
2. Correction for Zhao et al. A hypothalamic circuit that controls body temperature. *Proc Natl Acad Sci USA.* 2017;114(9):E1755.
3. Charkoudian, N. Hypothermia and hyperthermia. In: Robertson D, Biaggioni I, eds. *Primer on the Autonomic Nervous System.* Academic Press; 2012:287–289.
4. Díaz M, Becker DE. Thermoregulation: Physiological and clinical considerations during sedation and general anesthesia. *Anesth Prog.* 2010;57(1):25–32.

# 190.

# HEAT LOSS MECHANISMS

*Samuel MacCormick and Lynn Kohan*

## INTRODUCTION

Hypothermia can be defined as a core temperature of <36°C or a core to peripheral temperature gradient of 2°–4°C.[1] Hypothermia is an important physiologic mechanism to understand, as there is an association with increased perioperative mortality rates.[2] Efferent responses of thermoregulation can be behavioral or autonomic, depending on the trigger. Decreases in skin temperature can trigger a behavioral response, such as layering of clothing or seeking shelter. However, decreases in core temperature lead to autonomic responses, such as shivering and changes in vascular tone, to ensure that essential organs remain well perfused with normal core temperature blood.[3] Of note, there are also warmth-induced autonomic responses, such as vasodilation and sweating. As previously mentioned, there are risks associated with hypothermia; however, hypothermia can offer some benefits. The risks and benefits of hypothermia are outlined in Table 190.1.

As noted earlier, there are many perioperative risks associated with hypothermia. Therefore, it is imperative to know how hypothermia occurs and interventions that can be implemented to minimize these risks in a surgical setting. Undesired heat loss leading to hypothermia may occur via two mechanisms: impaired thermoregulation as a result of anesthesia and low environmental ambient temperatures.[5] Table 190.2 provides a broad overview of how anesthetics are related to thermoregulation.

*Table 190.1* RISKS AND BENEFITS OF HYPOTHERMIA

| BENEFITS OF HYPOTHERMIA | RISKS OF HYPOTHERMIA |
|---|---|
| Myocardial protection by decreasing metabolic rate[3] | Coagulopathy leading to increased bleeding times[3] |
| | Delayed wound healing with increased infection rates[2,3] |
| | Cardiac effects→negative inotropy and chronotropy, possible dysrhythmias[1] |
| CNS protection during cardiac or cerebral ischemia (iatrogenic or physiologic cause)[3] | Increased peripheral and systemic vascular resistance[1,2] |
| | Increased postop shivering and thermal discomfort[4] |
| Improved neurologic recovery in asphyxiated neonates[4] | Reduced drug metabolism (i.e., prolonged effects of muscle relaxants→impacts extubation)[3] |
| Decreases triggering and severity of malignant hyperthermia[4] | Impaired renal function[2] |

*Table 190.2* ANESTHETIC EFFECTS ON THERMOREGULATION

| TYPE OF ANESTHESIA | EFFECT ON THERMOREGULATION |
|---|---|
| General anesthesia (IV and inhaled) | Dose-dependent effects on adaptive responses[1] |
| | Minimal increase in threshold for warmth-induced responses (i.e., vasodilation and sweating)[1] |
| | Large decrease in threshold for cold-induced responses, which decreases triggering of vasoconstriction and shivering response by 2°–4°C (normal threshold triggers a response at 0.4°C)[4] |
| | Leads to 10-fold increase in interthreshold range (ITR)* which results in hypothermia via vasodilation and redistribution of core temperature)[4] |
| Neuraxial anesthesia (spinal and epidural) | Disrupts thermoregulation specifically below level of block[1] |
| | ITR changes are smaller (4-fold increase) since thermoregulation remains intact above block.[1] |
| Regional anesthesia | Alters perception of temperature of anesthetized areas in hypothalamus (reduces afferent input to hypothalamus)[2] |
| | Impairs peripheral responses such as vasoconstriction[4] |

* ITR: core temperature range between sweating and shivering responses. ITR is regulated by hypothalamic reflex.[1,2,3]

| PHASE OF HYPOTHERMIA | TIMING | CHARACTERISTICS |
|---|---|---|
| Phase 1 (most important cause of perioperative hypothermia) | 1st hour | Redistribution (No change in total body heat) <br> • Rapid drop in core temperature (1°–2°C) <br> • Anesthetic-induced vasodilation leads to heat redistribution from core to peripheral tissues.[5] |
| Phase 2 | Next 3–4 hours | Environmental losses:[5] Heat loss > heat production (in order of importance) <br> • Radiation Occurs frequently from all surfaces when object is above absolute zero <br> • Convection Layer of air over skin is disturbed; air turnover in OR plays a role. <br> • Conduction Less likely to occur since patients are usually lying on well-insulated materials <br> • Evaporation Less likely to sweat under anesthesia, less likely from airway if humidifiers and low fresh gas flow are used |
| Phase 3 | Ongoing once equilibrium is achieved | Heat production = heat loss |

## GENERAL ANESTHESIA

Given the increased perioperative mortality associated with hypothermia, understanding how hypothermia occurs is important. Table 190.3 outlines the 3 phases of hypothermia associated with general anesthesia.

## MANAGEMENT

Hypothermia occurs as a result of both anesthesia (disrupts thermoregulation) and ambulatory conditions (cold OR)[5]. Moreover, age extremes, longer procedures, and abdominal surgeries are more at risk for hypothermia. Identifying perioperative techniques and strategies to mitigate or treat hypothermia and improve mortality rates are important.

## ANESTHETIC CONSIDERATIONS

### PREOPERATIVE

Techniques such as active prewarming (i.e., warming blankets, active warming devices for 30–60 min preop) can be employed to decrease the core-peripheral temperature gradient. Therefore, when anesthesia is induced, heat redistribution will not be as prominent.[2]

### INTRAOPERATIVE

Intraoperative contributors that increase the risk of hypothermia include cold ambient room temperatures, large volume of room temperature intravenous (IV) fluids, prolonged time of exposure of large wounds, and high flows of humidified gas.[2] Both passive and active techniques can be used to prevent or slow heat loss, with a goal of maintaining normothermia (core temp >36°C). Passive techniques decrease heat loss by 30% and include covering the patient with drapes or heat reflective "space" blankets.[4] Active techniques are generally required and may include forced air warmers (1°C/hr), conductive circulating water mattresses, IV fluid warmers, airway heating, humidification, bladder irrigation with warm fluids, heating lamps, and resistive heating blankets.[4] The efficacy of airway heating and humidification as intraoperative techniques to prevent hypothermia is debated among sources.[4]

### POSTOPERATIVE

In the postoperative period, shivering can be a clue to ongoing hypothermia or iatrogenic effects (i.e., general anesthesia). Other causes of shivering that should be considered and ruled out prior to treatment include sepsis, transfusion reactions, and drug allergy.[2] Both spinal and epidural anesthetics lower shivering and vasoconstriction threshold to respond to hypothermia.[2] Shivering can increase the risk of myocardial ischemia via increase in oxygen consumption, and carbon dioxide and carbon monoxide production, resulting in a decreased arterial oxygen saturation.[2] Therefore, addressing the underlying cause of shivering such as hypothermia is important in the postoperative period. The most effective management for postoperative hypothermia is to maintain normothermia during the perioperative period.[4] If a patient is intubated or mechanically ventilated, nondepolarizing paralytics can be employed until anesthetic effects on thermoregulation have ceased and the core temperatures return to normal ranges.[2] However, if patients continue to experience hypothermia further into the postoperative phase, active heating with forced air warming devices would be most efficacious.[2] Passive techniques such as heat reflective "space" blankets can also be used, but are less effective than the active mechanisms.

## REFERENCES

1. Murray M, et al. *Faust's Anesthesiology Review.* 4th ed. Philadelphia, PA: Elsevier Health Sciences; 2014:385–386.
2. Butterworth JF, et al. *Morgan and Mikhail's Clinical Anesthesiology.* 5th ed. McGraw-Hill Education/Medical; 2013:1184–1185.
3. Sessler, DI. Mild perioperative hypothermia. *N Engl J Med.* 1997;336(24):1730–1737.
4. Fleisher LA, et al. Mild hypothermia. In: *Essence of Anesthesia Practice.* 4th ed. Philadelphia, PA: Elsevier Health Sciences Division; 2017:233.
5. Sessler, DI. Perioperative heat balance. *Anesthesiology.* 2000;92(2):578–596.

# 191.

# BODY TEMPERATURE MEASUREMENT

*Jayakar Guruswamy and Matthew Epelman*

## TRANSDUCERS AND DEVICES FOR MEASURING TEMPERATURE

### MERCURY THERMOMETERS

The mercury-in-glass thermometer is one of the oldest and simplest devices currently available for use. Mercury thermometers have largely been replaced by electronic devices.

### THERMISTORS AND THERMOCOUPLES

The two most common thermometers are thermocouples and thermistors. These electronic thermometers are inexpensive, accurate, and disposable. Thermistors are metal-oxide semiconductors that depend on electrons as charge carriers and have reliable conductivity. Thermistor thermometers operate at acceptably low impedances and are relatively immune from interference. A single battery cell is a sufficient energy source. These transducers are inexpensive and stable, and their readings are reproducible at an accuracy of 0.1°C to 0.2°C. Esophageal temperature probes are an example of a thermistor. Thermocouples are junctions of two different metals, typically copper and nickel. This combination produces a small temperature-dependent voltage most easily measured with an amplifier. Probes are less expensive and are available in very small sizes.

### LIQUID CRYSTAL THERMOMETERS

These devices use an ordered layer of optically active liquid crystals to measure skin surface temperature. The optical properties are extremely sensitive and the color changes with temperature. Unfortunately, the liquid crystals create significant discrepancy between core and skin temperatures, especially under rapidly changing physiologic conditions, and are thus not useful in the perioperative setting.[1]

### INFRARED THERMOMETER

The infrared thermometer is a noninvasive device that collects radiation emitted by a warm object. Infrared thermometers have become increasingly popular for determining temperatures in the post-anesthesia care unit because the method is quick and noninvasive. Probes are inserted into the external auditory meatus to extrapolate the tympanic membrane temperature. Newer probes have been made for use over the forehead (Figure 191.1). These infrared devices are placed in the center of the forehead and are scanned along the hairline over the temporal artery. These devices are not appropriate for intraoperative use, given their inability to provide accurate core body temperature readings.

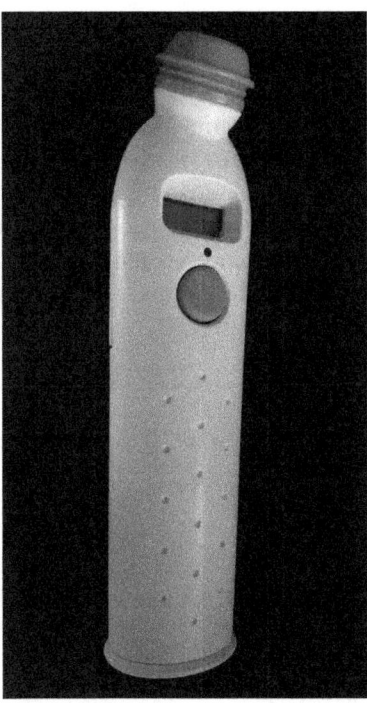

Figure 191.1. Infrared thermometer.

## ZERO-HEAT FLUX THERMOMETERS

The transcutaneous zero-heat flux thermometers measure the tissue temperature approximately 1–2 centimeter below the skin surface. Several designs are available. In comparison to standard temperature-monitoring sites, zero-heat flux thermometry has been found to correlate well with pulmonary artery temperature, while the measurement taken at the forehead and neck appears to reasonably estimate core temperature during the nonbypass portions of cardiac surgery.

## INGESTIBLE TELEMETRIC SENSOR

Ingestible core temperature monitoring devices, first described more than 50 years ago, have recently gained widespread use in the perioperative setting. The patient ingests a silicon-coated "pill" or "capsule" containing a micro-battery, quartz crystal, communication coil, and circuit board, all encapsulated in a medical-grade epoxy material. The crystal sensor vibrates at a frequency relative to the body temperature, producing a magnetic flux and transmitting the signals by radio waves to an external receiver. Multiple studies have demonstrated that intestinal temperature is a valid surrogate of core body temperature, comparable to distal esophageal temperature. These devices continue to gain widespread clinical acceptance.

## TEMPERATURE-MONITORING SITES

Various sites are available for temperature monitoring during anesthesia (Figure 191.2). Choice of site depends on the surgical procedure, type of anesthesia, and need for temperature monitoring. Pulmonary arterial blood is the gold standard for measuring core temperature. The temperature of pulmonary arterial blood correlates well with tympanic membrane temperature, distal esophageal temperature, and nasopharyngeal temperature. Even during rapid thermal fluctuations, such as cardiopulmonary bypass, these temperature-monitoring sites remain reliable. If a pulmonary arterial catheter is not placed, any of these other sites may be utilized.[2] These sites are largely interchangeable, rarely varying by more than a few tenths of a degree Celsius.

Tympanic membrane temperature approximates that at the hypothalamus; however, placement of a temperature probe near the tympanic membrane risks perforation. The external auditory canal is safer, but gives a skin temperature rather than an approximation of tympanic membrane temperature. Nasopharyngeal temperature closely reflects the brain temperature,[3] but is more prone to error from misplacement. The esophagus is a safe, easily accessible, highly resistant to artifact, and accurate site for core temperature measurement during anesthesia, especially in intubated patients. The optimal position for the sensor is the distal esophagus, approximately 45 cm from the nose in adults.[4] This site avoids cooling by respiratory gases in the trachea.

Core temperature can be estimated with reasonable accuracy using oral, axillary, rectal, and bladder temperatures, except under conditions associated with rapid temperature changes.[2,5] Rectal temperatures are in poor equilibrium with core temperatures, lagging substantially compared to the core, and are therefore inaccurate. In addition, a small risk of perforation exists with this method, and contraindications include obstetrics, gynecologic, and urologic procedures. Bladder temperature correlates well with core temperature and is easily measured with combination Foley catheter-thermistor probe devices. Bladder

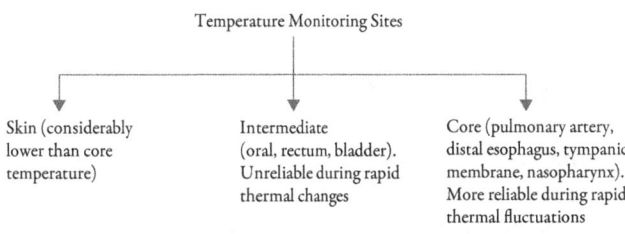

Figure 191.2. Temperature-monitoring sites.

temperatures are highly dependent on urine flow. Bladder temperature is close to core temperature when urine flow is high, but correlates poorly with core temperature when flow is low.

Axillary temperature gives a reasonable estimate of core temperature, especially if the probe is placed directly over the axillary artery and the arm is adducted. It is most reliable in infants and small children.[5] Sublingual temperature remains a good estimate of core temperature, and awake patients generally tolerate the thermometer well, although measurement is subject to error. Skin temperature reflects peripheral perfusion and is considerably lower than core temperature. With a 2°C compensation, however, skin temperature is a reasonable estimate of core temperature, except in rapidly changing conditions such as malignant hyperthermia.[1] Skin temperature is most commonly measured at the forehead because it is easily accessible and less variable than other sites. Readings can be affected by ambient temperature, skin-surface warming devices, and regional vasoconstriction.

Other sites may be of value in special situations. Myocardial temperature is readily measured with a needle probe during cardiopulmonary bypass, and skeletal muscle temperature provides the earliest indication of temperature change in malignant hyperthermia. Mostly, the measurement site, rather than the device, determines precision and accuracy. The challenge is to measure at sites that reasonably estimate core temperatures. In situations such as cardiopulmonary bypass, where there can be substantial temperature differences between core and peripheral compartments, temperature measurements at multiple sites might be needed to characterize the thermal state of the patient.

## REFERENCES

1. Larach MG, et al. Clinical presentation, treatment, and complications of malignant hyperthermia in North America from 1987 to 2006. *Anesth Analg.* 2010;110:498–507.
2. Cork RC, et al. Precision and accuracy of intraoperative temperature monitoring. *Anesth Analg.* 1983;62:211–214.
3. Siegel MN, Gravenstein N. Use of a heat and moisture exchanger partially improves the correlation between esophageal and core temperature. *Anesthesiology.* 1988;69(Suppl 3): A284.
4. Erickson RS. The continuing question of how best to measure body temperature. *Crit Care Med.* 1999;27:2307–2310.
5. Bissonnette B, et al. Intraoperative temperature monitoring sites in infants and children and the effect of inspired gas warming on esophageal temperature. *Anesth Analg.* 1989;69:192–196.

# 192.

# EFFECT OF DRUGS/ANESTHETIC TECHNIQUE ON TEMPERATURE REGULATION

*Jayakar Guruswamy and Santhalakshmi Angappan*

## TEMPERATURE REGULATION

The effect of both general anesthesia and regional anesthesia on temperature regulation is associated with impaired thermoregulatory control. The fall in temperature with general anesthesia has a characteristic pattern. It occurs in 3 phases: (1) initial rapid decrease of 0.5° to 1.5°C over the first 30 minutes, (2) slow linear reduction of about 0.3°C per hour, and (3) a plateau phase (Figure 192.1). The decrease in temperature in the first phase is from the anesthesia-induced vasodilatation, which causes increased heat loss due to redistribution of body heat from core to cooler peripheral tissues[1] (Figure 192.2).

General anesthesia decreases the metabolic rate by 20%–30%, and as a result, heat loss exceeds metabolic heat production, which causes a slower linear decrease in temperature.[2] General anesthesia also inhibits any behavioral responses to temperature fluctuations. The autonomic

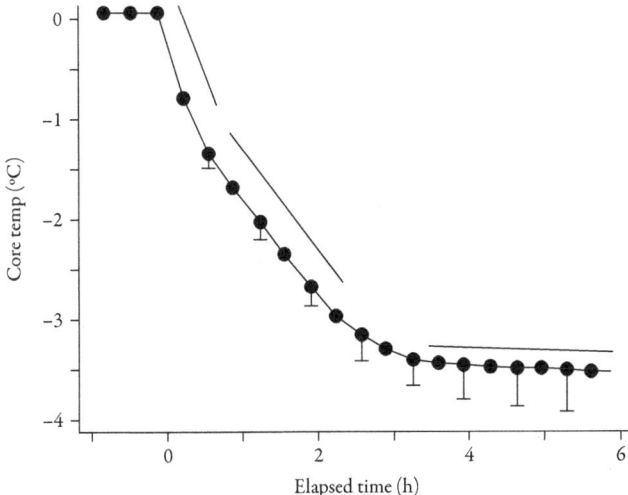

**Figure 192.1.** Hypothermia during general anesthesia develops with a characteristic pattern. An initial rapid decrease in core temperature results from a core-to-peripheral redistribution of body heat. This redistribution is followed by a slow, linear reduction in core temperature that results simply from heat loss exceeding heat production. Finally, core temperature stabilizes and subsequently remains virtually unchanged. This plateau phase may be a passive thermal steady state or may result when sufficient hypothermia triggers thermoregulatory vasoconstriction. Results are presented as mean ± standard deviation.

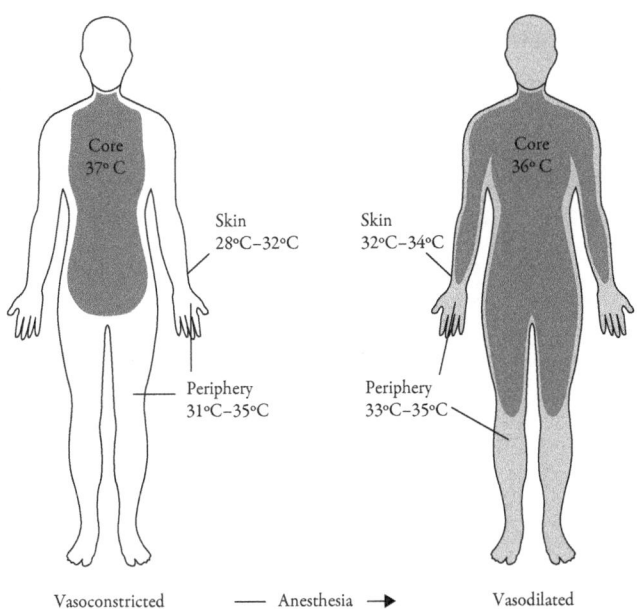

**Figure 192.2.** The periphery may be 3°C cooler than the core, but body temperature is maintained because of vasoconstriction. With general anesthesia, the vasoconstriction is reduced, leading to mixing of warm core blood with the cooler periphery. Hypothermia after induction of spinal or epidural anesthesia shows similar results, but redistribution is restricted to the legs.

responses are also markedly impaired under anesthesia. The interthreshold range increases up to 10-fold, from 0.2°–0.4°C to 2°–4°C, which makes anesthetized patients poikilothermic (cold-blooded) over a wide range of core temperatures. When the core temperature exceeds the sweating threshold or declines to below the vasoconstrictive threshold, thermoregulatory defenses are activated in anesthetized patients. Volatile anesthetics such as sevoflurane or nitrous oxide and intravenous anesthetics such as propofol and opioids impair thermoregulatory control. These agents have minimal effects on the sweating threshold, but significantly reduce the vasoconstriction and shivering thresholds. Sedatives like midazolam have minimal effects on thermoregulation. While volatile anesthetics inhibit TRPV1 receptors, their mechanism by which they impair thermoregulation is unknown.

The impairment in thermoregulation with neuraxial anesthesia occurs through 3 mechanisms. (1) Neuraxial anesthesia inhibits the central thermoregulatory control, decreasing the vasoconstriction and shivering threshold. This impairment is a linear function of the dermatomal block height and is linked to the anesthetic blocking tonic cold signals from the lower body. (2) Neuraxial anesthesia impairs autonomic thermoregulatory defenses, including active vasodilation, sweating, vasoconstriction, and shivering. (3) Hypothermia does not provoke as much thermal discomfort when under neuraxial anesthesia and hence patients do not complain of feeling cold even when they are hypothermic.[3]

Behavioral responses are impaired by neuraxial anesthesia. The initial decrease in core temperature is caused by vasodilation and a slow linear decline since heat loss exceeds heat production.[4] Unlike general anesthesia, the decrease in temperature may not plateau since the peripheral vasoconstriction is inhibited by neuraxial anesthesia and the vasoconstriction threshold is centrally altered, decreasing by 0.6°C. The effects of general anesthesia and regional anesthesia on thermoregulation are additive. Core temperature during general or neuraxial anesthesia continues to decrease throughout the surgery. In contrast, the peripheral nerve blocks have minimal effects on thermoregulation.[5]

## REFERENCES

1. Vale RJ. Cooling during vascular surgery. *Br J Anaesth.* 1972;44:1334.
2. Hynson JM, Sessler DI. Intraoperative warming therapies: A comparison of three devices. *J Clin Anesth.* 1992;4:194–199.
3. Glosten B, et al. Central temperature changes are poorly perceived during epidural anesthesia. *Anesthesiology.* 1992;77:10–16.
4. Matsukawa T, et al. Heat flow and distribution during epidural anesthesia. *Anesthesiology.* 1995;83:961–967.
5. Sessler DI. Temperature monitoring and perioperative thermoregulation. *Anesthesiology.* 2008;109:318–338.

# Part XIII

# BRAIN ANATOMY

# 193.

# CEREBRAL CORTEX

*Rutvij Shah*

## INTRODUCTION

The cerebral cortex comprises 83% of the total brain tissue. The cerebral cortex is divided into two hemispheres (left and right) and each hemisphere contains 4 lobes (frontal, parietal, temporal, and occipital). Both the hemispheres are connected to each other by a subcortical white matter band called corpus callosum. The thick folds in the cortex are called gyri, and shallow grooves are called sulci. The cerebral cortex constitutes the highest control areas for memory, attention, vision, language, motor control, and sensory perception. Microscopically, the cerebral cortex is made up of gray matter on the outer surface, with subcortical white matter tracts inside. Functionally, the cerebral cortex is divided into 47 areas called Brodmann areas (Figure 193.1).[1]

## GROSS ANATOMY OF THE CEREBRAL CORTEX

Both left and right hemispheres of the cerebral cortex are separated by a dural fold called falx cerebri. Both the hemispheres are attached to each other by a white matter tract called corpus callosum. Cortex has the highest control centers for attention, memory, vision, motor control, language, hearing, and sensory perception. Each hemisphere controls the opposite side of the body. The hemisphere that contains the areas of language is considered the dominant hemisphere. The left hemisphere is dominant in about 90% of people.[1]

The cerebral cortex is divided into 4 lobes:

- Frontal lobe:
  - The frontal lobe contains areas that control higher levels of thinking; for example, reasoning, abstract thinking, problem-solving, decision-making, emotions, impulse control, and social/sexual behavior.
  - Language area (Broca/Brodmann areas 44 and 45): This is a motor speech area located on the left frontal lobe.
  - Motor areas (Brodmann areas 4 and 6): Voluntary and planned motor controls on the opposite side of the body.[1]
  - Sensory reception and integration for taste
  - Frontal eye fields (Brodmann area 8): Responsible for conjugate saccadic gaze toward the opposite side.
- Parietal lobe:
  - Sensory reception and integration of somatic sensations (Brodmann areas 3, 1, and 2) such as pressure, pain, touch, temperature, stretch, and movement.[1]
  - Damage to the right (nondominant) parietal lobe results in visual-spatial deficits due to damage to the superior parietal lobule (Brodmann areas 5 and 7).
  - Damage to the left (dominant) parietal lobe results in characteristic Gerstmann syndrome, which causes the following deficits:[1]
    - Acalculia—inability to count fingers
    - Agraphia—word blindness
    - Finger agnosia—inability to name or identify fingers
    - Right and left confusion.
- Temporal lobe:
  - Wernicke speech area (Brodmann area 22): Situated in the anterior part of dominant temporal lobe. Damage to the area causes receptive aphasia.
  - Primary auditory cortex (Brodmann areas 41 and 42): Bilateral damage to these areas result in cortical deafness.[1]
  - Hippocampal cortex: responsible for memory formation and consolidation
  - Meyer loop: it contains the optic radiations. Damage to the Meyer loop results in contralateral superior quadrantanopia.
  - Anterior temporal lobe contains amygdala ,and damage of the amygdala results in Kluver-Bucy

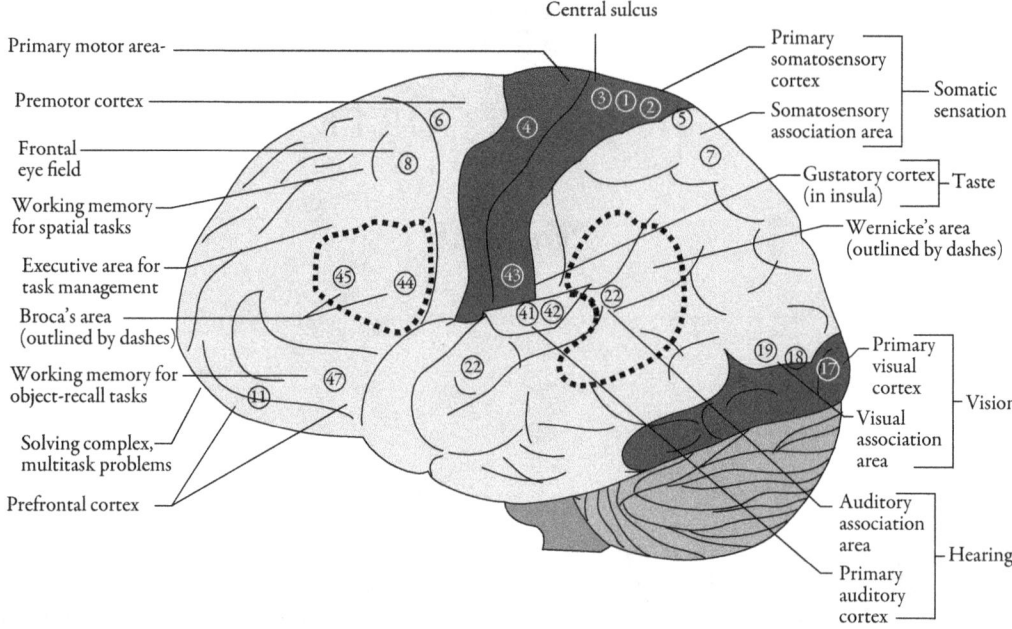

**Figure 193.1.** Cerebral cortex with the Brodmann areas and their functions.

syndrome, characterized by visual agnosia, hyperphagia, hypersexuality, and docility.[1]
- Occipital lobe:
  - It contains visual receptive cortex and calcarine cortex (Brodmann areas 17, 18, 19): Lesion to these areas result in contralateral homonymous hemianopsia or quadrantanopia.
- Insular lobe:
  - It has a role in emotion and homeostasis.

**Microscopic six layers of cortex (Layers I to VI):** Layers II and IV are mainly afferent. Layers V and VI are efferent are efferent layers. [1,2]

- Layer I: Molecular layer
- Layer II: External granular layer
- Layer III: External pyramidal layer
- Layer IV: Internal pyramidal layer
- Layer V: Internal pyramidal layer
- Layer VI: Multiform layer.

## ANESTHETIC CONSIDERATIONS

### PREOPERATIVE

Understanding the effects of anesthetic agents on the cerebral cortex is very crucial to anesthesiologists. Anesthetic agents work by interacting with ion channels to regulate synaptic transmission and membrane potentials in the specific areas of the cerebral cortex, thalamus, and spinal cord.

All the anesthetic agents have a different sensitivity to these ion channel targets.[3]

### INTRAOPERATIVE

The cerebral cortex has areas of the highest functions that include the areas of consciousness. Consciousness during general anesthesia is a dreadful condition. Unconsciousness is likely to result when several complex brain regions in the posterior parietal area are inactivated. Anesthetics cause functional disconnection in the posterior complex, while interrupting the communication and causing a loss of integration in the posterior cingulate cortex and precuneus. This leads to stereotypic responses resulting in the loss of information capacity. Midazolam and propofol produce equivalent effects, but the duration of the effects of propofol is shorter.[3,4] The thalamus also plays a key role in consciousness, as loss of consciousness is evidenced by reduced thalamic blood flow and metabolism. Gradual deterioration of consciousness can be monitored with the use of intraoperative electroencephalogram (EEG) with a gradual transition from low voltage and high frequency pattern of wakefulness, to slow wave low frequency EEG of deep non-rapid eye movement (NREM) sleep to eventually an EEG burst-suppression pattern.[3]

### POSTOPERATIVE

As mentioned earlier, the thalamus acts as a consciousness switch. Once the anesthetic agent infusion or inhalation is discontinued, the consciousness is regained by functional restoration of the thalamus and cingulate cortex.[3]

## REFERENCES

1. Gould D, et al. *High-Yield Neuroanatomy.* Philadelphia, PA: Wolters Kluwer; 2016.
2. Jacobson S, et al. *Neuroanatomy for the Neuroscientist.* 3rd ed. Springer; 2018:605–613.
3. Alkire M, et al. Consciousness and anesthesia. *Science.* 2008;322 (5903):876–880.
4. Baron Shahaf D, et al. *The Effects of Anesthetics on the Cortex: Lessons from Event-Related Potentials. Front Syst Neurosci.* 2020;14.

# 194.

# CEREBELLUM AND BASAL GANGLIA

*Alan D. Kaye and Harlee Possoit*

## INTRODUCTION

The subcortical areas of the brain are interconnecting structures that connect to the cerebral cortex as well as the periphery. They each provide higher order functions to be able to complete complex tasks, human cognition, and social functions. This chapter will describe the anatomy, functions, major nuclei, and pathways of the cerebellum and basal ganglia.

## CEREBELLUM

The cerebellum is located in the back of the brainstem within the posterior fossa. The tentorium cerebelli, a reflection of dura mater, extends over the posterior fossa, providing the separation between the cerebellum and the occipital and temporal cerebral lobes. The cerebellum is separated into three lobes: the flocculonodular lobe, posterior lobe, and anterior lobe. The cerebellum is also divided sagittally into three zones that run from medially to laterally, the midline vermis, directly lateral is the intermediate zone, and the lateral hemispheres.[1] The cerebellum has a variety of functions, the primary one being the maintenance of balance and posture through shifting the body's position in time and space, which is controlled through the vestibular receptors and proprioceptors, and coordinating voluntary movements. The centrally located vermis is responsible for the proximal muscle groups and the regulation of eye movements in response to vestibular inputs, whereas the lateral parts are primarily concerned with distal muscle groups such as gross motor movements in walking.[2] Motor learning skills can also be coordinated through the cerebellum to help with fine tuning and adaptation, such as learning to play the piano. The cerebellum is also thought to play a role in cognitive function such as language, but this role is poorly understood.[1] The input and output signals for the previously mentioned functions are relayed through subdivisions of the cerebellar cortex and deep cerebellar nuclei which travel to the cerebral cortex to perform the function or back to the cerebellar cortex (Figure 194.1).

The subdivisions of the cerebellar cortex are the cerebrocerebellum, which projects to the large dentate nuclei; spinocerebellum to the interposed nuclei; and vestibulocerebellum to the fastigial nucleus and vestibular nuclei.[3] The function of the dentate nucleus is to regulate fine-control of voluntary movements, cognition, language, and sensory functions.[4] The cerebellum, via the superior cerebellar peduncle, receives input from the lateral cerebral hemispheres and cerebellar afferent fibers. The interposed nuclei receive input from the intermediate zone of the cerebellum which connects through the superior cerebellar peduncle to the red nucleus that carries spinal, auditory, visual, and somatosensory information. The fastigial nucleus's

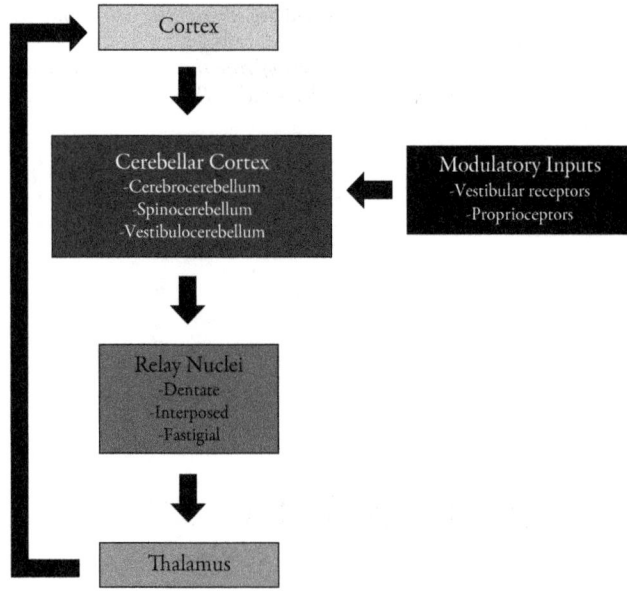

**Figure 194.1.** Basic motor organization of the cerebellar pathway.

primary function is motor control, which is executed by sending signals, via the inferior cerebellar peduncle, to the brainstem, as well as relaying information involving the somatosensory system, eye movement, and arousal. From the deep cerebellar nuclei, the afferent and efferent fibers project through three cerebellar peduncles. The superior cerebellar peduncle has efferent fibers that project to the red nucleus, upper motor neurons, and the superior colliculus before passing through the thalamus and ultimately the primary motor and premotor areas of the cerebral cortex. The middle cerebellar peduncle is primarily an afferent pathway. The cell bodies that project through this pathway form the pontine nuclei, which receive input from many areas of the cerebral cortex and superior colliculus.[2] The inferior cerebellar peduncle is a mixed afferent pathway (axons from the vestibular nuclei, spinal cord, and brainstem areas) and efferent pathway (projections to the vestibular nuclei and reticular formation). The inputs of the cerebellum are conveyed primarily through the inferior and middle cerebellar peduncles, whereas the outputs are conveyed via the superior cerebellar peduncle.[1] The cerebellar motor inputs and outputs control the ipsilateral movements of the body, separating it from the cerebral cortex which controls the lateral movements of the body.

## PATHOLOGICAL CONSIDERATIONS OF THE CEREBELLUM

Cerebellar dysfunction can present as uncoordinated smooth muscle movement, involuntary tremor exposed when moving toward a target, problems with rapid movement or dysdiadochokinesia, and defective balance and vestibuloocular reflex. Movement deficits due to

cerebellar damage will present ipsilateral to the site of the lesion. Lesions of the cerebellum can be displayed clinically through physical exam tests such as the Romberg test, which is performed by having the patient stand with their feet together, eyes closed, and arms crossed over their chest, observing for instability. Rapid alternating movements of the hands can also test several aspects of coordination. When a patient has cerebellar lesions or disease, one movement cannot be quickly followed by its opposite, resulting in movements that are slow, irregular, and clumsy.

## BASAL GANGLIA

The basal ganglia are composed of a set of nuclei located deep within the cerebral hemisphere. The structures included within the basal ganglia are the caudate-putamen (also known as the striatum), globus pallidus, subthalamic nucleus which sits at the base of the forebrain, and the substantia nigra in the midbrain. The basal ganglia are organized in parallel cortico-basal ganglia-thalamo-cortical loops which function primarily to control motor functions such as motor learning, executive functions, and behaviors and emotions. Information flows through two pathways which have opposing effects that facilitate the initiation as well as the proper execution of movement.[5] The direct pathway is responsible for increased movement, whereas the indirect pathway is responsible for decreased movement (Figure 194.2).

The nuclei within the two pathways can be divided into input nuclei (caudate nuclei, putamen, and nucleus accumbens), output nuclei (globus pallidus interna [GPi] and substantia nigra pars reticulata [SNr]), and the intrinsic nuclei (globus pallidus externa [GPe], subthalamic nucleus, and substantia nigra pars compacta [SNc]). Dopamine released onto the input nuclei from the SNc is required for proper functioning of the system, along with systematic control from the release of inhibitory (GABA) and excitatory (glutamate) neurotransmitters. The direct pathway is triggered when movement is desired. The cortex sends glutamate to the striatum, which allows for the release of GABA to the GPi and SNr. These actions decrease the amount of GABA released onto the thalamus from the GPi and SNr, allowing it to become disinhibited. The thalamus is able to send excitatory signals back to the motor cortex, resulting in muscle movement. The indirect pathway is enabled when decreased movement is desired. The cortex again sends glutamic excitatory signals to the striatum, which allows for the release of inhibitory GABA signals onto the GPe. The inhibition of the GPe allows the subthalamic nucleus to release glutamate onto the GPi, which increases its release of GABA onto the thalamus. This inhibits the release of glutamate from the thalamus, resulting in decreased excitatory signals onto the motor cortex and decreased motor movements. The proper

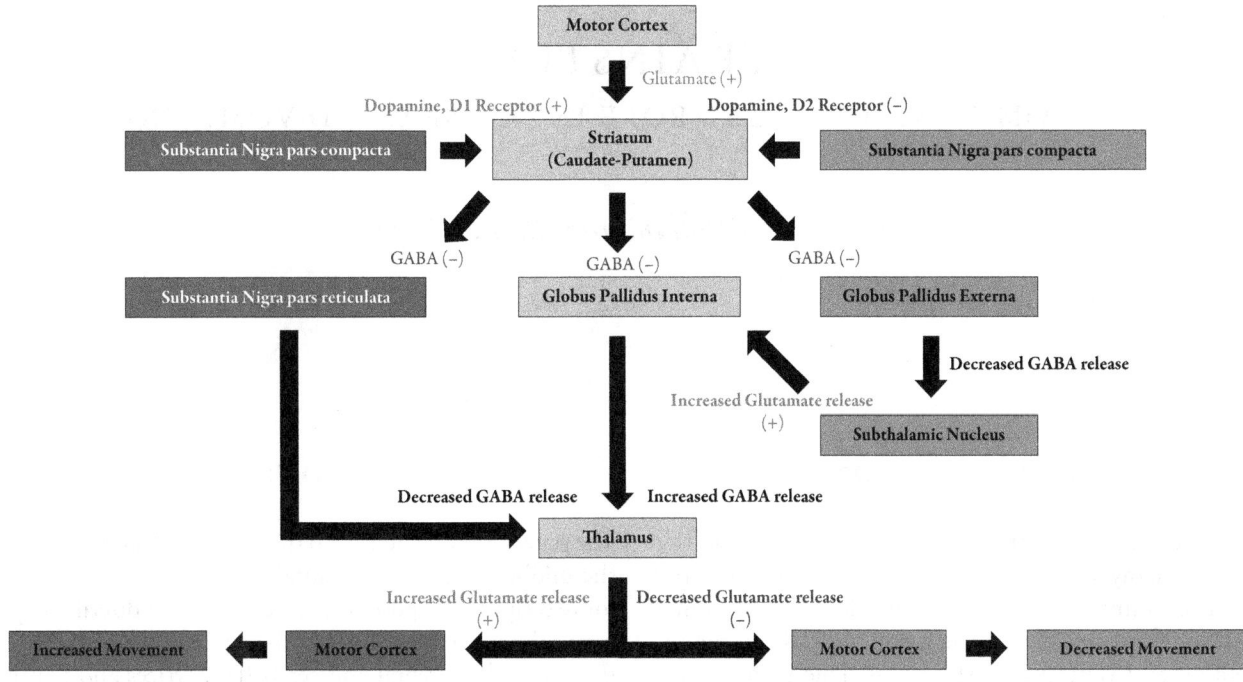

Direct Pathway                                                    Indirect Pathway

**Motor Cortex**

Glutamate (+)

Dopamine, D1 Receptor (+)                     Dopamine, D2 Receptor (−)

**Substantia Nigra pars compacta**    →    **Striatum (Caudate-Putamen)**    ←    **Substantia Nigra pars compacta**

GABA (−)          GABA (−)          GABA (−)

**Substantia Nigra pars reticulata**    **Globus Pallidus Interna**    **Globus Pallidus Externa**

Decreased GABA release

Increased Glutamate release (+)

**Subthalamic Nucleus**

Decreased GABA release          Increased GABA release

**Thalamus**

Increased Glutamate release (+)          Decreased Glutamate release (−)

**Increased Movement**    ←    **Motor Cortex**          **Motor Cortex**    →    **Decreased Movement**

Figure 194.2. Direct and indirect pathways of the basal ganglia.

balance between the direct and indirect pathways allows for adaptation of fluent body movements.

The nigrostriatal pathway is important for further modulation of the direct and indirect pathways through the use of dopamine as a neurotransmitter from the SNc. The direct pathway utilizes the D1 receptors, which allows an increase in activity and movement. The indirect pathway modulates input from the SNc via the D2 receptors, which decrease the activity of the indirect pathway and allow for movement. The delicate balance between the direct, indirect, and nigrostriatal pathways allows for appropriately executed motor functions.

## PATHOLOGICAL CONSIDERATIONS OF THE BASAL GANGLIA

Dysfunction of the basal ganglia can manifest itself in a variety of ways. Loss of dopaminergic neurons within the SNc can lead to overactivity of the indirect pathway. This results in over-inhibition and can lead to clinical manifestations such as bradykinesia, or slow movements, and akinesia, the absence of movements. On the opposing side is the hyperkinetic movement disorders, which

include manifestations such as chorea (excessive, spontaneous, snakelike writhing movements), dyskinesia (uncontrolled, involuntary movements), and dystonia (uncontrolled contracted muscles). The hallmark disease of the basal ganglia is Parkinson's disease, which usually begins with a resting tremor and can manifest as a mix of both hypokinetic and hyperkinetic movements.

## REFERENCES

1. Cerebellum (section 3, chapter 5). In: *Neuroscience Online: An Electronic Textbook for the Neurosciences | Department of Neurobiology and Anatomy*. The University of Texas Medical School at Houston. https://nba.uth.tmc.edu/neuroscience/m/s3/chapter05.html Accessed August 15, 2020.
2. Purves D, et al. Organization of the cerebellum. 2001:2–3. [Online]. https://www.ncbi.nlm.nih.gov/books/NBK11132/. Accessed August 15, 2020.
3. Purves D, et al. Projections from the cerebellum. 2004. [Online]. https://www.ncbi.nlm.nih.gov/books/NBK11100/. Accessed August 15, 2020.
4. de Leon AS, Das JM. *Neuroanatomy, Dentate Nucleus*. StatPearls; 2020.
5. Lanciego JL, Luquin N, Obeso JA. Functional neuroanatomy of the basal ganglia. *Cold Spring Harb. Perspect. Med*. 2012;2(12): .

# 195.

# BRAINSTEM
## ANATOMY AND CRITICAL ROLE IN NAUSEA AND VOMITING

*Charles deBoisblanc and Alan D. Kaye*

## INTRODUCTION

The brainstem is a primitive region of the brain that controls many basic functions required for sustaining life. The brainstem is bordered inferiorly by the spinal cord, superiorly by the diencephalon, dorsally by the cerebellum, and ventrally by the clivus. Due to its central location, the brainstem acts as a conduit for the reticular formation and multiple ascending and descending fiber tract. The brainstem is also composed of cranial nerve nuclei, and it is responsible for many primitive reflexes.[1] The brainstem is constituted by the midbrain, the pons, and the medulla.

## MIDBRAIN

The midbrain is the most superior component of the brainstem and contributes to functions such as hearing, temperature regulation, circadian cycles, arousal, and vision. The cerebral aqueduct divides the midbrain into the tectum and the cerebral peduncles. The tectum is located dorsal to the cerebral aqueduct and is formed by superior and inferior colliculi.[2] The superior colliculi are involved in vision, and the inferior colliculi function in audition.[3] The cerebral peduncles are found anterior to the cerebral aqueduct and are constituted by the tegmentum, the substantia nigra, and the crus cerebri. The tegmentum contains the reticular formation, and the substantia nigra helps to coordinate movement.[3] The crus cerebri predominantly conveys motor fibers from the cerebral hemispheres to the spinal cord and caudal brainstem.[1] The midbrain contains notable nuclei and is the source of two cranial nerves. The midbrain houses the red nucleus, which modulates muscle tone, and the oculomotor nucleus, which controls ocular smooth muscle function.[3] Cranial nerves III and IV originate from the midbrain.[3]

## PONS

The pons is found anterior to the cerebellum and inferior to the midbrain. Like the midbrain, the pons can be divided for descriptive purposes into a ventral and a dorsal component. The ventral pons is mostly formed by a fiber system that links the cerebral and cerebellar cortices and pontine nuclei with their associated fibers.[1] The aforementioned pontine nuclei include cranial nerve nuclei, as well as the trapezoid body, a collection of cochlear fibers.[3] The dorsal pons primarily functions to house the fibers of the reticular formation.[2] Multiple cranial nerves emerge from the pons. Cranial nerve V exits the brainstem bilaterally at the junction of the middle cerebral peduncle and the pons. A sulcus separates the medulla from the pons, and from this sulcus, cranial nerves VI–VIII exit the brainstem.[2]

## MEDULLA

The medulla is the most inferior portion of the brainstem and is continuous with the spinal cord. It functions to conduct signals between the brain and spinal cord and has multiple nuclei that control autonomic functions, including reflexes, swallowing, respiration, and vomiting, among others.[2] The medulla may be best understood if examined in a rostral-caudal manner. Grossly, the inferior portion of the medulla is similar in structure to the spinal cord, but the superior portion divides into dorsal and ventral limbs, with the dorsal limb contributing to form the floor of the fourth ventricle.[1] At the ventral aspect of the inferior medulla, the bulk of the pyramidal tract neurons decussate.[3] At the dorsal aspect of the inferior medulla, the dorsal horn is supplanted by the trigeminal sensory nucleus, a homologous structure.[1] At the level of the mid-medulla, the dorsal columns terminate on their respective nuclei, which then give off second-order neurons that decussate and form the medial lemniscus.1 The rostral medulla contains the inferior olivary nucleus, which aids in motor function. It also contains continuations of the raphe nucleus, fibers from the trigeminal sensory nucleus, spinothalamic fibers, and cranial nerve nuclei.[1] Cranial nerves IX–XII originate from the medulla.[2]

## ANESTHETIC CONSIDERATIONS

Postoperative nausea and vomiting (PONV) are a fairly common problem seen in patients who have undergone general anesthesia. The pathophysiology is, in part, related to the chemoreceptor trigger zone, part of the medullary area postrema.[1] The area postrema lacks the protection of the blood-brain barrier and is sensitive to emetogenic substances, related to the presence of the chemoreceptor trigger zone (CTZ). The CTZ and the nucleus tractus solitarius (NTS) of the medulla constitute the major parts of the vomiting center. Emetogenic substances activate receptors in the CTZ, and this signal is conducted to the NTS. Upon receiving the signal, the NTS then activates the vomiting reflex. The vomiting center can also be activated by signals relayed from gut chemoreceptors and mechanoreceptors.[4]

The CTZ is rich in serotonin ($5\text{-HT}_3$), dopamine ($D_2$), and opioid receptors, and the NTS has plentiful muscarinic, histaminic, and cholinergic receptors, as well as enkephalin receptors. All of these receptors, when activated, can stimulate the vomiting reflex. The greatest risk factor for PONV is the use of volatile anesthetic.[4] Additional risk factors for PONV include intraoperative or postoperative opioid use, nonsmoking, and history of PONV or motion sickness. Patients with a moderate to high risk of PONV can be treated prophylactically with transdermal scopolamine, dexamethasone, or $5\text{-HT}_3$ receptor antagonists, with a combination of these agents yielding better results.[4]

## REFERENCES

1. Crossman AR, Neary D. Brainstem. In: *Neuroantaomy: An Illustrated Colour Text*. 6th ed. 2014:89–98.
2. Gupta D. Neuroanatomy. In: *Essentials of Neuroanesthesia*. Elsevier; 2017;3–40.
3. Mancall E. Brain stem. In: *Gray's Clinical Neuroanatomy: The Anatomic Basis for Clinical Neuroscience*. Philidelphia, PA: Elsevier Saunders; 2011:157–184.
4. Pollard R. Evidence-based prevention of post-operative nausea and vomiting. In: *Case-Based Anesthesia: Clinical Learning Guides*. Philidelphia, PA: Lippincott Williams & Wilkins; 2009:127–130.

# 196.

## RESPIRATORY CENTERS

*Ricardo Murguia-Fuentes and Alan D. Kaye*

### INTRODUCTION

Respiration, specifically ventilation, is an essential function for survival that occurs involuntarily most of the time, as two separate mechanisms exist, one for voluntary control and the other for automatic control.[1] The latter is related to the capability of the nervous system to modify and to adjust the required demands for alveolar ventilation, so parameters such as the oxygen partial pressure ($PO_2$) and carbon dioxide partial pressure ($PCO_2$) are kept stable even after changes in activity or if modifications of the respiratory stress occur.

The nervous system conducts this through the respiratory center, which includes a group of neurons located in the medulla oblongata and pons. The neural mechanisms to achieve this include chemoreflexes, central drive, and neuronal feedback from muscles involved in ventilation.[2]

The respiratory center is composed of various neurons collections, which include: a dorsal respiratory group in the dorsal portion of the medulla, which has mainly inspiratory function; a ventral respiratory group in the ventrolateral portion of the medulla, which can be involved in inspiration and expiration; and finally, the pneumotaxic center, which is located in the dorsal portion of the upper part of the pons, and which regulates respiratory rate and depth of breathing.[3]

## DORSAL RESPIRATORY GROUP

Most of its neurons are in the nucleus of the solitary tract (NST) and, in less significant quantity, can be found as neurons in the adjacent reticular substance of the medulla. The NST represents a point of connection of the afferences of the vagal and glossopharyngeal nerves, which transmits the afferences from peripheral chemoreceptors, baroreceptors, and receptors located in the lungs.

The main function of the dorsal respiratory group is the generation of the basic inspiratory rhythm, through repetitive bursts of inspiratory neuronal action potentials, which continues throughout the life of an individual. The final signals sent to the diaphragm and other inspiratory muscles begin weakly and follow a ramp pattern during inspiration, which is cut abruptly after approximately 3 seconds, to allow the elastic recoil of the chest wall and pulmonary tissue, causing ventilatory expiration during this process.

## VENTRAL RESPIRATORY GROUP

Located about 5 millimeters anterior and lateral to the dorsal respiratory groups, this group of neurons is based on the nucleus ambiguous and retroambiguous.[3] The neurons that conform this group remain inactive during normal quiet ventilation, and do not appear to regulate the basic rhythmical oscillation. However, it activates with increased respiratory drive, showing activity in both inspiration and expiration.

The ventral respiratory group has three regions with specific functions. The rostral region, or Bötzinger complex, has interneurons that regulate the expiratory activity; the intermediate region contains motor neurons that innervate the pharynx, larynx, and nearby structures for increasing the caliber of the airway during inspiration, and also includes the pre-Bötzinger complex,[4] which is also involved in the respiratory rhythm generation; the caudal region has premotor neurons that innervate the accessory muscles of expiration.[5]

## PNEUMOTAXIC CENTER

The pneumotaxic center is located dorsally in the parabrachial nucleus of the upper pons. It exerts its effects

*Table 196.1* NEURAL AND CHEMICAL FACTORS THAT MODIFY THE ACTIVITY OF THE RESPIRATORY CENTER

| NERVOUS AFFERENCES | CHEMICAL FACTORS |
| --- | --- |
| Vagal nerve | Carbon dioxide |
| Pons, hypothalamus, and limbic system | Oxygen |
| Propioceptors | Hydrogen ions |
| Baroreceptors | |

through inhibiting the inspiratory ramp and controlling the duration of the filling phase, as it has neurons that become active during inspiration and other neurons that become active during expiration. When its signal is more intense, inspiration can be cut up to 0.5 seconds. Meanwhile, lower intensity signals can prolong the inspiration for 5 seconds or longer.[3]

## CHEMICAL REGULATION OF RESPIRATION

Excess $CO_2$ or excess $H^+$ in the blood exerts direct effects over the respiratory center, as it strengthens the respiratory center efferences to the inspiratory and expiratory muscles. The central medullary chemoreceptors mediate hyperventilation after increases in arterial $PCO_2$, and are separate from the dorsal and ventral groups, this is in the ventral surface of the medulla.

Oxygen, on the other hand, does not have a major and direct effect in the regulation of the respiratory center, but exerts its effects through the peripheral chemoreceptors of the carotid and aortic bodies, to achieve an indirect effect through signaling that goes from the glossopharyngeal and vagal nerve, respectively, to the dorsal respiratory area of the medulla.

A summary of the chemical and neural factors than can change the activity of the respiratory center can be seen in Table 196.1

## REFERENCES

1. Barret KE. *Ganong's Review of Medical Physiology.* 25th ed. Lange; 2016:655–667.
2. Wijdicks EFM. Noeud vital and the respiratory centers. *Neurocrit Care.* 2019;31(1):211–215.
3. Hall ME. Guyton and Hall. *Textbook of Medical Physiology.* 14th ed. Elsevier; 2021:531–540.
4. Smith J, et al. Pre-Botzinger complex: A brainstem region that may generate respiratory rhythm in mammals. *Science.* 1991;254(5032): 726–729.
5. Boron WF. *Medical Physiology.* 2nd ed. Elsevier; 2012:725–735.

# 197.

# RETICULAR ACTIVATING SYSTEM

*Rutvij Shah*

## INTRODUCTION

The reticular formation (RF) constitutes a loose group of neurons longitudinally extended through the hypothalamus, thalamus, brainstem, and upper cervical cord caudally. The RF is divided into ascending and descending pathways. The ascending pathway is also called the ascending reticular activating system (RAS), as it is responsible for arousal of a person by stimulating cortical and subcortical structures. The descending pathway is responsible for the modulation of nociception. This chapter will discuss the anatomy of the reticular activating system, with its nuclei, their connections, and functions. The chapter will also discuss the anesthetic implications of the RAS.[1]

## ANATOMY

- The RAS travels through anterior segment of the brainstem.[1]
- *Afferent connections*: RAS receives inputs from
  - Spinal cord
  - Sensory pathways (spinothalamic tract and dorsal column)
  - Thalamus
  - Cerebral cortex.
- *Efferent connections*: throughout the nervous system.
- *Components of RAS*: As depicted in Figure 197.1, several brainstem nuclei (locus coeruleus, dorsal raphe, median raphe, parabrachial raphe, and pedunculopontine nuclei), nonspecific thalamic nuclei, and hypothalamus and basal forebrain.[1] Detailed type of nuclei and their functions are mentioned in Table 197.1.
- *Blood supply*: Branches of vertebral (anterior spinal artery and posterior inferior cerebellar artery) supply the lateral aspect of the reticular formation. Medial party is supplied by the branches of basilar artery (paramedian pontine arteries and anterior inferior cerebellar artery). Posterior cerebral artery branches supply the midbrain and hypothalamic portion of RAS.[2]
- *Clinical significance*:
  - Lesion to RAS results in rapid eye movement (REM) sleep disturbances.
  - Damage to pedunculopontine neurons is associated with schizophrenia.
  - RAS stimulation results in generation of pain responses.
  - Parkinson's disease and post-traumatic stress disorder patients have shown reduced neurons in RAS.[2]

## ANESTHETIC CONSIDERATIONS

### PREOPERATIVE

Not applicable.

### INTRAOPERATIVE

The pontine and medullary reticular nuclei control the antigravity muscles. The rapid atonia during general anesthesia by a bolus dose of propofol is most likely due to the drug's effects on these reticular nuclei and gamma-aminobutyric acid (GABA)-ergic neurons of the spinal cord. Intraoperative pain management is very crucial. The synthetic opioid fentanyl controls the pain and reduces arousals by decreasing acetylcholine in the medial pontine reticular formation. Opioids reduces arousals by reducing acetylcholine in dorsolateral tegmental reticular nuclei.[3]

### POSTOPERATIVE

Postoperative pain management is very crucial. Reticular formation has the centers that modulate the bidirectional balance (enhance or decrease) of the painful stimuli. Three key RAS nuclei, the rostroventromedial (RVM), caudal ventrolateral medulla (VLM), and subnucleus reticularis dorsalis (DRt), play a prominent role in pain modulation.[4]

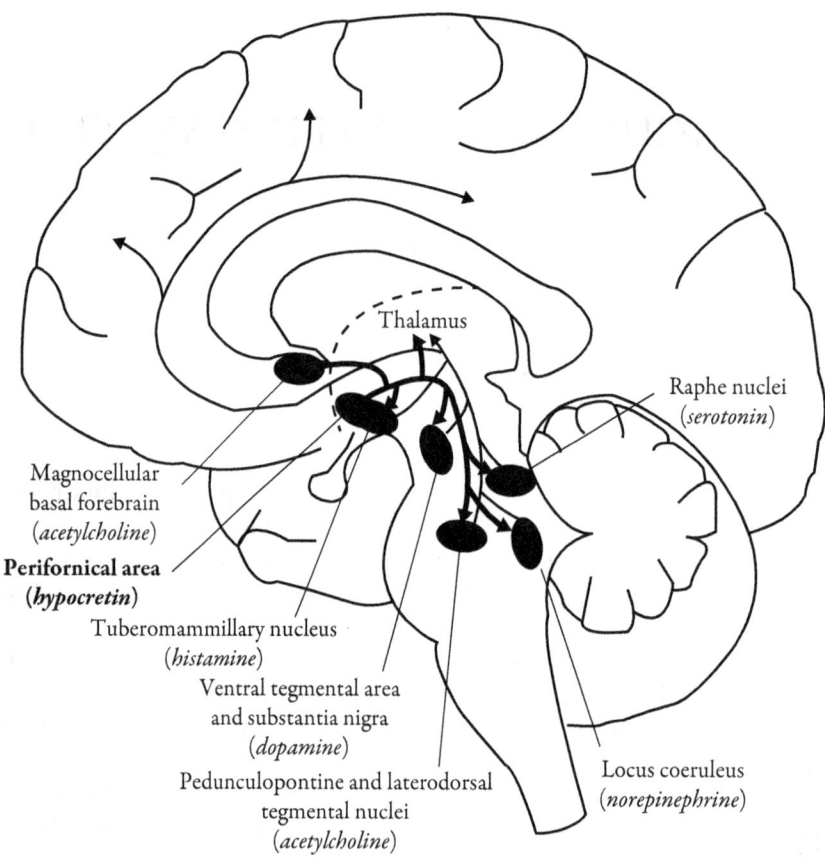

Thalamus

Raphe nuclei
(*serotonin*)

Magnocellular
basal forebrain
(*acetylcholine*)

**Perifornical area
(*hypocretin*)**

Tuberomammillary nucleus
(*histamine*)

Ventral tegmental area
and substantia nigra
(*dopamine*)

Pedunculopontine and laterodorsal
tegmental nuclei
(*acetylcholine*)

Locus coeruleus
(*norepinephrine*)

**Figure 197.1** Nuclei of the reticular activating system.

*Table 197.1* RAS NUCLEI, TYPE, AND FUNCTION[1,2]

| NUCLEI | TYPE OF NUCLEUS | FUNCTION |
|---|---|---|
| Locus coeruleus | Noradrenergic nuclei | Wakefulness and arousal |
| Dorsal and median raphe nucleus | Serotonergic nuclei | Circadian rhythms, arousal, and attention |
| Pedunculopontine nucleus | Cholinergic and glutamatergic nuclei | Switch from slow-wave sleep rhythms to high-frequency, low-amplitude wake rhythms |
| Tubulomamillary nucleus | Histaminergic nuclei | Cognition, wakefulness, and arousal |

DRt alone increases the painful responses, whereas the triad RVM-VLM-DRt reduces pain perception through emotional and cognitive modulation of pain. Opioid analgesics modulate all three RAS nuclei to control pain.[4]

## REFERENCES

1. Jacobson S, et al. *Neuroanatomy for the Neuroscientist*. 3rd ed. Springer; 2018:605—613.
2. Arguinchona J, Tadi P. *Neuroanatomy, Reticular Activating System*. [Online]. 2020. https://www.ncbi.nlm.nih.gov/books/NBK549835/
3. Brown E, et al. General anesthesia, sleep, and coma. *N Engl J Med*. 2010;363(27):2638–2650.
4. Martins I, Tavares I. Reticular formation and pain: The past and the future. *Front Neuroanat*. 2017;11:1–14.

# 198.

## CEREBRAL CIRCULATION
### CIRCLE OF WILLIS, VENOUS SINUSES, AND DRAINAGE

*Rutvij Shah*

## INTRODUCTION

The arterial supply of the brain is divided into anterior and posterior circulation. The anterior circulation is made up of the right and left internal carotid arteries, and the posterior circulation consists of right and left vertebral arteries. Branches of these two circulations connect with each other and make the circle of Willis at the base of the brain. This continuous circulation of the brain tries to provide consistent blood supply to the important brain structures. The normal blood flow of the brain is about 50 ml/100 g brain tissue/minute.[1] The cerebral veins are different than other veins of the body as they have very thin walls, no valves, and no muscular layer, which makes spread of infection from the scalp to inside the cranium possible.[2] The venous drainage follows this pathway: cerebral veins > dural venous sinuses > internal jugular veins > brachicephalic vein > left atrium of the heart.[1,2]

## CIRCLE OF WILLIS

The circle of Willis is depicted in Figure 198.1.

- Anterior circulation: Consists of 70% of the blood supply to the brain.[1,2]
  - Internal carotid artery (ICA): Intracranial branches of the ICA are:
    - Ophthalmic artery: It supplies the optic nerve (cranial nerve II) and inner aspect of retina. Occlusion of ophthalmic artery causes ipsilateral painless vision loss.[1]
    - Posterior communicating artery (PCA): It connects the middle and posterior cerebral arteries. It gives rise to small lenticulostriate branches and supplies optic chiasm and tract, anterior half of thalamus, hypothalamus, and subthalamic nuclei. It is a common site for the berry aneurysm, in which compression of the cranial nerve (CN) III results in

paralysis of extraocular muscles supplied by it and unilateral mydriasis.[1]
    - Anterior choroidal artery: It supplies the choroid plexus of the temporal horn of lateral ventricle, posterior limb of internal capsule, lateral geniculate body, optic tract, and globus pallidus.[1]
    - Anterior cerebral artery (ACA): It supplies the optic chiasm, medial frontal and parietal lobe. Occlusion of ACA causes weakness of contralateral leg, foot, and perineum. Anterior communicating artery (AComm) connects both the ACAs. The junction of ACA and AComm is the most common site for berry aneurysm.[1]
  - 95% of all aneurysms can be found near the circle of Willis at one of the following five sites:
    - ACA
    - Middle cerebral artery
    - Internal carotid artery between PCA and anterior choroidal arteries
    - Basilar bifurcation
    - Internal carotid bifurcation.
- Middle cerebral artery (MCA): It supplies the majority of lateral cerebral convexity. It supplies the cortical areas that control the motor and sensory areas of trunk, arm, and face. It also supplies language areas (Broca and Wernicke). Deep branches of MCA supply caudate nucleus, putamen, globus pallidus, and part of internal capsule.[1]
- Posterior circulation: Consists of 30% of the blood supply to the brain.[2]
  - Vertebral artery
  - Anterior spinal artery: It supplies ventral two-thirds of the cervical and midthoracic spinal cord.
  - Posterior inferior cerebral artery: It supplies the dorsolateral part of medulla, which consists of inferior cerebellar peduncle, medial and lateral vestibular nuclei, intra-axial fibers of glossopharyngeal (CN IX) and vagus (CN X) nerves, spinal trigeminal nucleus, and lateral spinothalamic tract. It also supplies the

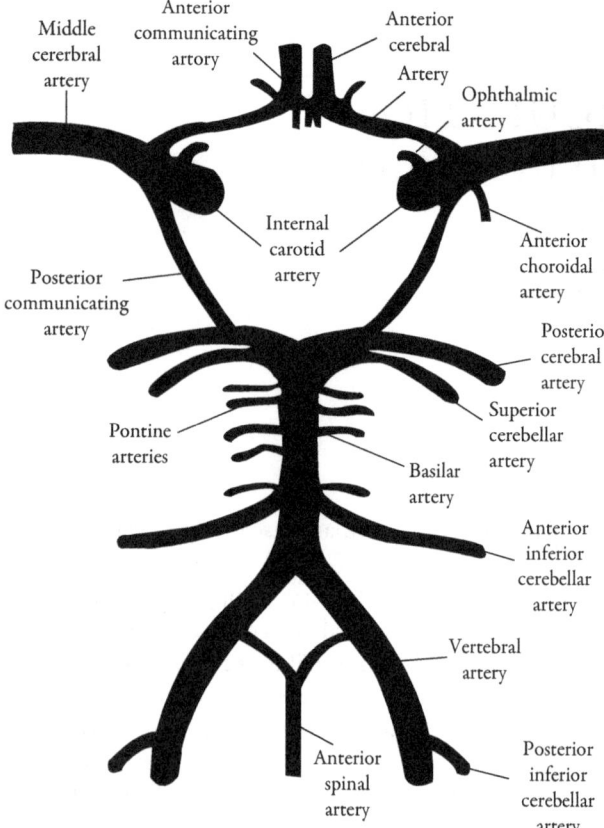

**Figure 198.1.** Circle of Willis with its contributory branches.

sympathetic fibers of the ciliospinal center of Budge, injury to which causes ipsilateral Horner's syndrome.[1]

- Basilar artery: The basilar artery is formed at around pontomedullary junction by merging of both the vertebral arteries. The following are the branches of the basilar artery.
  - Pontine arteries: They are penetrating branches to ventromedial pons. It supplies corticospinal tracts and the abducent nerve (CN VI) fibers.[1]
  - Labyrinthine artery: It supplies the inner ear.[1]
  - Anterior inferior cerebellar artery (AICA): It supplies the inferior surface of the cerebellum, facial nerve and nucleus, vestibulocochlear nerve, inferior and middle cerebellar peduncles, and spinothalamic tract.[1]
  - Superior cerebellar artery: It supplies superior surface cerebellar peduncle, lateral pons, and spinothalamic tract.[1]
  - Posterior cerebral artery (PCA): The basilar artery gives rise to two terminal branches in form of PCAs. It supplies the midbrain, occipital lobes, visual cortex, and inferior medial temporal lobe. PCAs give rise to posterior choroidal arteries that supply to the choroid plexus, posterior part of thalamus, and pineal gland.[1]

## VENOUS DRAINAGE AND VENOUS SINUSES

Figure 198.2 depicts the cerebral veins and venous sinuses.

- Superficial cerebral veins: They drain into superior sagittal sinus.
- Deep cerebral veins
  - Internal cerebral veins: There are four deep cerebral veins: the septal vein, thalamostriate vein, terminal vein, and venous angle.
  - Great cerebral vein (of Galen): Internal cerebral veins drain into great cerebral veins, which further drain into straight sinus.
- Dural venous sinuses
  - Superior sagittal sinus: It is situated at the superior edge of falx cerebri and from foramen cecum to occiput. It receives blood from superficial cerebral veins, emissary veins, and diploic veins, and terminates in the right transverse sinus.[1,2]
  - Inferior sagittal sinus: It is situated in the inderior edge of falx cerebri.[1,2]
  - Straight sinus: It is formed by joining great cerebral vein and inferior sagittal sinus.[1,2]
  - Transverse sinuses (right and left).
  - Confluence of the sinuses: Superior sagittal sinus, straight sinus, and both the transverse sinuses join to make confluence of sinuses.[1,2]
  - Sigmoid sinus: It is the continuation of the transverse sinuses. They pass through jugular foramen.[1,2]
  - Sphenoparietal sinus: It lies in the lesser wing of the sphenoid bone and drains into the cavernous sinus.[1,2]
  - Superior and inferior petrous sinuses.
  - Cavernous sinus: It receives blood from superior and inferior ophthalmic veins. It is a very important sinus as it contains very critical structures as follows:
    - Within the sinus: Internal carotid artery and CN VI.
    - Within the wall of the sinus: CNs III, IV, V1 and V2.[1,2]

## ANESTHETIC CONSIDERATIONS

### PREOPERATIVE

Poor collateral flow through circle of Willis has a higher risk of intraoperative cerebral ischemia during the carotid endarterectomy surgery. A four-vessel cerebral angiogram is needed as a preoperative workup.[3]

### INTRAOPERATIVE

Cerebral perfusion is dependent on the patency of the arterial blood supply and the venous drainage of the brain. Positioning of the head is critical during surgeries. For example, the head is to be turned up and opposite to the side

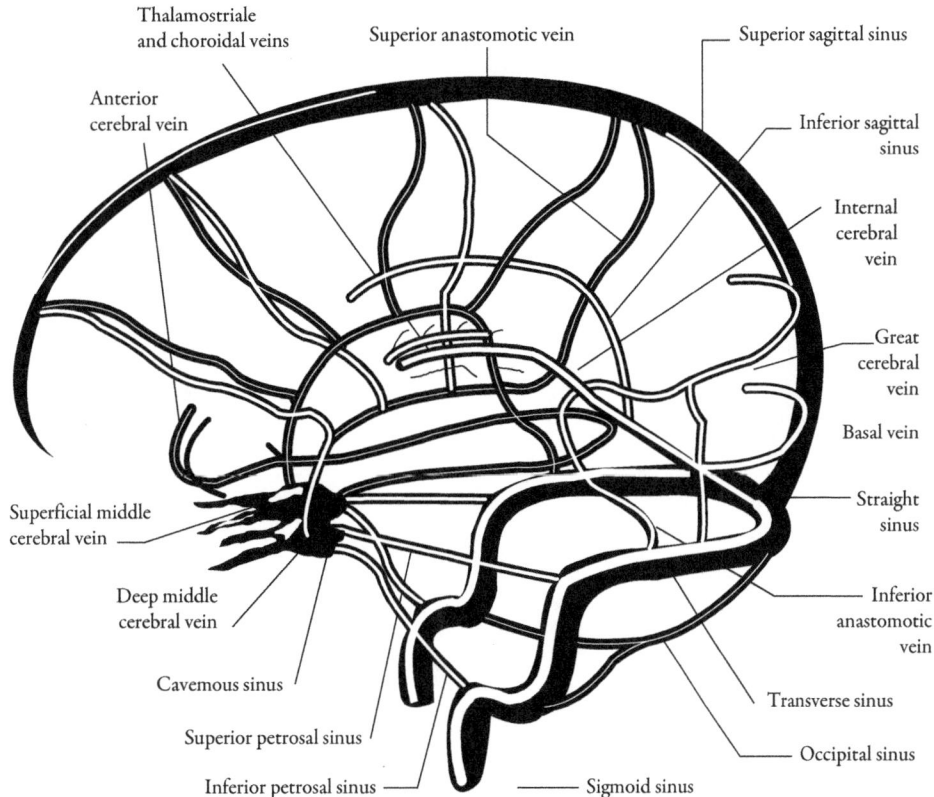

Thalamostriale and choroidal veins
Superior anastomotic vein
Superior sagittal sinus
Anterior cerebral vein
Inferior sagittal sinus
Internal cerebral vein
Great cerebral vein
Basal vein
Straight sinus
Superficial middle cerebral vein
Deep middle cerebral vein
Inferior anastomotic vein
Cavemous sinus
Superior petrosal sinus
Transverse sinus
Occipital sinus
Inferior petrosal sinus
Sigmoid sinus

**Figure 198.2.** Cerebral veins and venous sinuses.

during the parotidectomy surgery, which may stretch the ipsilateral internal carotid artery and kink the contralateral vertebral artery. In such case, the patient may be likely to have critically impaired cerebral circulation.[4] Intraoperative neuromonitoring techniques like transcranial doppler, intraoperative electroencephalogram (EEG), and near infrared cerebral spectroscopy (NIRS) can be used to assess for cerebral ischemia.[4] There are several arterial anastomoses on the surface of the brain, but these are rare within the brain parenchyma. Occlusion of rupture of an intraparenchymal artery will cause more damage than an incident on the surface of the brain.

## POSTOPERATIVE

Cerebral venous sinus thrombosis (CVST) is common after the surgeries. CVST is more common in the intracranial surgeries like brain tumor resection. Especially, the risk of CVST is very high when the surgery is to be performed in the close proximity of the venous sinuses. Certain tumors grow into the venous sinus, for example parasagittal meningioma, causing stenosis of sinus, and requires extra manipulation or repair of the sinuses. Sometimes, neurosurgeons ask anesthesiologists to limit the intravenous fluids to maintain a net-negative fluid balance. The net-negative balance is needed to reduce the cerebral edema. This leads to a hypovolemic state, which causes postoperative CVST.

## REFERENCES

1. Gould D, Fix J. *BRS Neuroanatomy.* 5th ed. Philadelphia, PA: Lippincott Williams & Wilkins; 2014:39–52.
2. Jacobson S, et al. *Neuroanatomy for the Neuroscientist.* 3rd ed. Springer; 2018:605–613.
3. Kim G, et al. The anatomy of the circle of Willis as a predictive factor for intra-operative cerebral ischemia (shunt need) during carotid endarterectomy. *Neurol Res.* 2002;24(3):237–240.
4. Bezzina M, Dent H. Anaesthetic management of a patient with compromised cerebral circulation. *Anaesth Cases.* 2017;5(1):49–52.
5. Benjamin C, et al. Postoperative cerebral venous sinus thrombosis in the setting of surgery adjacent to the major dural venous sinuses. *J Neurosurg.* 2019;131(4):1317–1323.

# Part XIV

# SPINAL CORD AND SPINE

# 199.

# VARIATIONS IN VERTEBRAL CONFIGURATION

*Douglas K. Rausch and Rany T. Abdallah*

## INTRODUCTION

The vertebral column functions to support the skull, protect the spinal cord, provide attachment points for the upper extremities, and transmit weight from the trunk to the lower extremities. It consists of 33 vertebrae (7 cervical, 12 thoracic, 5 lumbar, 5 sacral, and 4 coccygeal segments). This chapter will focus on key anatomical and functional differences between the cervical, thoracic, and lumbar vertebrae.

Vertebrae differ in shape and size at the various levels of the column. Typical vertebrae consist of a vertebral arch posteriorly, a vertebral body anteriorly, as well as 7 processes (4 articular, 2 transverse, 1 spinous). Two pedicles arise on the posterolateral aspects of each vertebra and fuse with the 2 laminae to encircle the vertebral foramen.[1] These structures form the vertebral canal, which contains the spinal cord, spinal nerves, and epidural space. The transverse processes arise from the laminae and project laterally, whereas the spinous process projects posteriorly from the midline union of the laminae.[2] A typical vertebra also contains 4 articular processes, 2 superior and 2 inferior, which contact the inferior and superior articular processes of adjacent vertebrae, respectively. The point at which superior and inferior processes meet is known as a facet, or zygapophyseal joint. These maintain vertebral alignment, control the range of motion, and are weight-bearing in certain positions.[3]

Refer to Figure 199.1 and Table 199.1 for a depiction and summary of the major characteristics of vertebrae.

## CERVICAL SPINE

The cervical vertebrae form a lordotic curve. Typical cervical vertebrae have unique features that distinguish them from typical thoracic or lumbar vertebrae. The most notable distinction is the presence of a foramen in each transverse process.[3] Vertebral arteries and veins travel through the foramina of C1–C6; however, C7's transverse foramina contain only accessory veins. An additional feature unique to cervical vertebrae is the bifid spinous process, which likely serves to increase surface area for various muscular attachments. Cervical vertebrae tend to have superior articular facets that face posteromedially. Lastly, cervical vertebrae are known to have the greatest intervertebral disc height, which increases the range of motion.

C1, C2, and C7 are considered atypical vertebrae due to their unique features. C1, also known as "atlas," is a ring-like bone that has no body or spinous process. It is formed by two lateral masses with facets that connect anteriorly to a short arch and posteriorly to a longer, curved arch. The superior articular facets of these masses contact the occipital condyles of the skull, and the inferior facets articulate with superior facets of C2. C2, also known as "axis," is distinct in that it contains bilateral masses to articulate with C1, a body, through which weight is transmitted through C3 and below, and an odontoid process, or "dens," on the superior aspect of the body. The dens articulates with the posterior surface of the anterior arch of C1.[3] C7, also known as "vertebra prominens," has a long, nonbifid spinous process that serves as a useful landmark for a variety of regional anesthesia procedures.[2]

## THORACIC SPINE

The thoracic vertebrae form a kyphotic curve. Typical thoracic vertebrae (T2–T10) have several features distinct from those typical of cervical or lumbar vertebrae and have the additional role of providing attachments for the ribs. The primary characteristic of the thoracic vertebrae is the presence of costal facets. There are 6 facets per thoracic vertebrae: 2 on the transverse processes and 4 demifacets. The facets of the transverse processes articulate with the tubercle of the associated rib. The demifacets are bilaterally paired and located on the superior and inferior posterolateral aspects of the vertebrae. They are positioned so that the superior demifacet of inferior vertebrae articulates with the head of the same rib that articulates with the inferior demifacet of a superior rib. Thoracic vertebrae have superior

## Cervical (3–6)

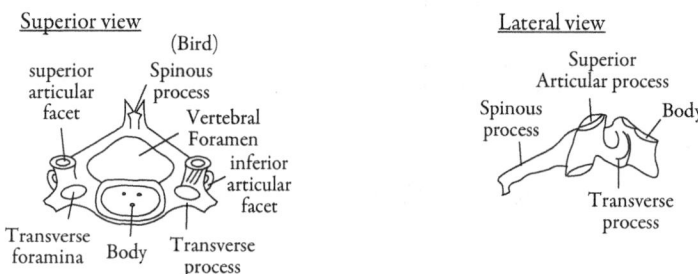

### Superior view
(Bird)

- superior articular facet
- Spinous process
- Vertebral Foramen
- inferior articular facet
- Transverse foramina
- Body
- Transverse process

### Lateral view

- Superior Articular process
- Spinous process
- Body
- Transverse process

## Thoracic (T5–T8)

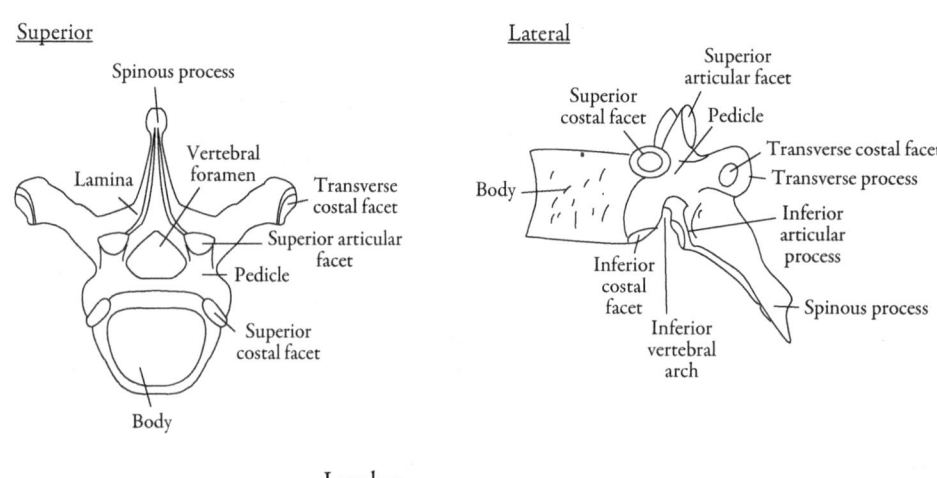

### Superior

- Spinous process
- Vertebral foramen
- Lamina
- Transverse costal facet
- Superior articular facet
- Pedicle
- Superior costal facet
- Body

### Lateral

- Superior costal facet
- Superior articular facet
- Pedicle
- Transverse costal facet
- Transverse process
- Body
- Inferior articular process
- Inferior costal facet
- Inferior vertebral arch
- Spinous process

## Lumbar

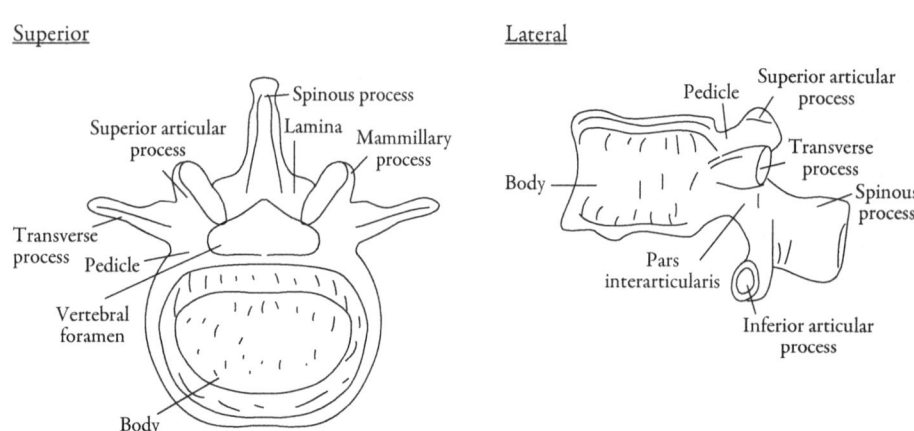

### Superior

- Spinous process
- Superior articular process
- Lamina
- Mammillary process
- Transverse process
- Pedicle
- Vertebral foramen
- Body

### Lateral

- Pedicle
- Superior articular process
- Transverse process
- Body
- Spinous process
- Pars interarticularis
- Inferior articular process

**Figure 199.1.** Depiction of cervical, thoracic, and lumbar vertebrae.

articular facets that face in a posterolateral direction. The spinous process is long and is directed posteroinferiorly. The main movement of the thoracic spine is rotation, and the intervertebral disc height is the shortest of the vertebral regions.[4]

There are three atypical vertebrae found in the thoracic region: T1, T11, and T12. The superior costal facets of T1 are "whole" costal facets. They alone articulate with the first rib; C7 has no costal facets. T11 and T12 are atypical in that they contain a single pair, a "whole" costal facet that articulates with the 11th and 12th ribs, respectively. They also lack facets on the transverse processes. Additionally, T12 is unique in that is represents a transition from thoracic to the lumbar vertebra.[4]

## LUMBAR SPINE

The lumbar vertebrae form a lordotic curve. Typical lumbar vertebrae have several features distinct from those typical of cervical or thoracic vertebrae. The most notable distinction is the presence of a large vertebral body. The spinous

| CHARACTERISTICS | CERVICAL | THORACIC | LUMBAR |
|---|---|---|---|
| Typical vertebrae | C3–C6 | T2–T10 | All |
| Body | Small; rectangular Uncinate processes | Larger than cervical; heart shaped; bears two costal facets | Large; kidney shaped |
| Pedicles | Small; superior and inferior vertebral notches | Large; no superior vertebral notch | Large; superior (small) and inferior vertebral notches |
| Spinous process | Short; bifid; projects directly posteriorly | Upper four: posteriorly directed Middle four: long and inferiorly directed Lower four: lumbar-like | Short; blunt; projects directly posteriorly |
| Vertebral foramen | Triangular; largest | Circular; smallest | Triangular; intermediate in size between cervical and thoracic |
| Transverse process | Contain foramina | Bears facets for ribs (except T11 and T12) | Thin and tapered |
| Superior and inferior articulating processes | Superior facets directed superoposteriorly Inferior facets directed inferoanteriorly | Superior facets directed posteriorly Inferior facets directed anteriorly | Superior facets directed posteromedially (or medially) Inferior facets directed anterolaterally (or laterally) |
| Movements allowed | Flexion and extension; lateral flexion; rotation; the spine region with the greatest range of motion | Rotation; lateral flexion possible but limited by ribs; flexion and extension prevented | Flexion and extension; some lateral flexion; rotation prevented |

process is short and thick, relative to the size of the vertebra, and projects perpendicularly from the body. The articular facets are markedly vertical, with the superior facets directed posteromedially and medially. The facets also have the unique feature of a curved articular surface. There is also the addition of the mammillary process on the posterior aspect of the superior articular process. The anterior aspect of the body of L5 has a greater height compared to the posterior. This creates the lumbosacral angle between the lumbar region of the vertebrae and the sacrum. The main movement of the lumbar spine is flexion and extension.[5]

## ANESTHESIA IMPLICATIONS

In the United States and most developed countries, there is an increase in the prevalence of spinal deformities such as spinal stenosis, scoliosis, hyperkyphosis, and hyperlordosis due to the increased aging population. Elderly patients present anesthetic challenges when neuraxial techniques are required. With advancing age, a diminishing thickness of intervertebral disks results in decreased height of the vertebral column. Thickened ligaments and osteophytes also contribute to difficulty in accessing both the subarachnoid and epidural spaces. The vertebral column serves as the landmark for a wide variety of regional anesthesia techniques. Therefore, it is important that an anesthesiologist can develop a three-dimensional mental image of the structures comprising the vertebral column.[2]

## REFERENCES

1. Standring S, ed. *Gray's Anatomy: The Anatomical Basis of Clinical Practice*. 40th ed. Edinburgh, New York: Churchill Livingston, Elsevier Health, 2008.
2. Orebaugh SL, Cruz Eng H. Neuraxial anatomy (anatomy relevant to neuraxial anesthesia). In: Hadzic A, ed. *Hadzic's Textbook of Regional Anesthesia and Acute Pain Management*, 2nd ed. McGraw-Hill. 318–327. https://accessanesthesiology.mhmedical.com/content.aspx?bookid=2070&sectionid=157600265. Accessed August 23, 2020.
3. Waxenbaum JA, et al. Anatomy, back, cervical vertebrae. [Updated July 27, 2020]. In: *StatPearls* [Internet]. Treasure Island. FL: StatPearls; 2020 Jan–. https://www.ncbi.nlm.nih.gov/books/NBK459200/.
4. Waxenbaum JA, et al. Anatomy, back, thoracic vertebrae. [Updated August 10, 2020]. In: *StatPearls* [Internet]. Treasure Island, FL: StatPearls; 2020 Jan–. https://www.ncbi.nlm.nih.gov/books/NBK459153/.
5. Waxenbaum JA, et al. Anatomy, back, lumbar vertebrae. [Updated August 10, 2020]. In: *StatPearls* [Internet]. Treasure Island, FL: StatPearls; 2020 Jan–. https://www.ncbi.nlm.nih.gov/books/NBK459278/

# 200.

# SPINAL NERVES

*Rany T. Abdallah and Jasmin Villatoro-Lopez*

## INTRODUCTION

The human body contains 12 cranial nerves and 31 pairs of spinal nerves that provide communication between the central nervous system (CNS) and the rest of the body. The spinal nerves carry motor, sensory, and autonomic signals between the spinal cord and the body. The spinal nerves correspond to a segment of the vertebral column: 8 cervical pairs (C1–C8), 12 thoracic pairs (T1–T12), 5 lumbar pairs (L1–L5), 5 sacral pairs (S1–S5), and 1 coccygeal pair.[1] Each nerve is composed from nerve fibers (fila radiculara) which extend from the posterior and anterior roots of the spinal cord. The roots then connect via interneurons. These root fibers join within the intervertebral foramina to form spinal nerves.[2]

The majority of the upper half of the cervical nerves construct the cervical plexus, specifically from the anterior rami of C1 to C5. The cervical plexus's sensory fibers provide cutaneous innervation to the scalp, neck, chest, and axilla. The motor branches assist in the movement of the neck and innervation of the diaphragm. They also provide motor innervation to the infrahyoid muscles and the sternocleidomastoid via the ansa cervicalis (C1 to C3).[2]

The ventral roots of C5–T1 form what is known as the brachial plexus, which is a highly complex network of nerves. These five nerve roots innervate about 50 muscles and skin in the upper extremities and pectoral region. The nerve fibers of the brachial plexus go along with autonomic fibers, mainly from T1, that regulate vasomotor control of the upper extremity and trunk, while a handful of other nerves in the plexus are solely muscular or cutaneous sensory nerves.[2]

The thoracic nerves are composed of 12 pairs of spinal nerves in the thoracic spine, each corresponding to a spinal segment. These nerves are responsible for cutaneous innervation of the skin, musculoskeletal system, and viscera. Most of the sympathetic trunk arises from the thoracic spine; therefore pre- and postganglionic sympathetic fibers will also be found within the thoracic spinal nerve network.[2]

The lumbosacral plexus is simply the lumbar and sacral plexi that share nerve root overlap. This plexus contains about 200,000 axons and provides all sensory and motor innervation to the lower extremity, with some innervation of the abdominal wall. Regardless of the connection via the lumbosacral trunk, the two plexi exist as a separate bundle anatomically. The lumbar plexus arises from primary branches of the anterior roots of the spinal nerves L1–L5, while the branches of the sacral plexus begin below the pelvic rim and are housed in the pelvic girdle.[2]

## CLINICAL FEATURES

Spinal nerve compression is a condition most commonly caused by gradual wear and tear on the bones of the spine, mostly known as osteoarthritis. Other causes may be sudden traumatic blows to the spine that fracture, dislocate, crush, or compress one or more of the vertebrae. Added damage usually occurs over days or weeks due to bleeding, swelling, inflammation, and fluid accumulation in and around the spinal cord.[5] One of the more severe spinal compressions is known as Cauda equina syndrome. It is a single- or double-level compression of the lumbosacral nerve roots that are located in the dural sac. The cauda equina nerve roots provide sensory and motor innervation of most of the lower extremities, the pelvic floor, and the sphincters.[2]

## DIAGNOSIS

Spinal cord compression can be diagnosed by through imaging, including X-rays, which may show bone growths called spurs that push against the spinal nerves. A computed tomography (CT) scan or magnetic resonance imaging (MRI) will give a more detailed look at the spinal cord and the structures that surround it. Imaging, such as these, is done if the patient presents with spinal cord compression symptoms, such as pain and stiffness in the neck, back, or lower back, burning pain that spreads to the extremities (sciatica), numbness, cramping, or weakness in the extremities, among other symptoms. Cauda equina may have many of the same symptoms; however, there are more severe symptoms that may indicate the presence of this syndrome. Those include sudden onset of bowel incontinence and bladder dysfunction, along with sensory abnormalities in the bladder or rectum.[2]

## TREATMENT

Spinal nerve compression can be treated with medications, physical therapy, injections, and in extreme cases, such as cauda equina syndrome, with surgical decompression.[3] Medications may include nonsteroidal anti-inflammatory drugs (NSAIDs) that will aid in relieving the pain and swelling. Steroid injections will also aid in reducing edema and inflammation. Physical therapy may include exercises to strengthen the back, abdominal, and leg muscles. Back braces may be provided to aid in supporting the back; a cervical collar may be of help as well.

## REFERENCES

1. American Society of Regional Anesthesia and Pain Medicine. The specialty of chronic pain management. American Society of Regional Anesthesia and Pain Medicine. https://www.asra.com/page/44/the-specialty-of-chronic-pain-management. Published August 13, 2020. Accessed August 25, 2020.
2. Kaiser JT. *Neuroanatomy, Spinal Nerves*. StatPearls. https://www.ncbi.nlm.nih.gov/books/NBK542218/. Published July 31, 2020. Accessed August 25, 2020.
3. AANS. *Cauda Equina Syndrome*. https://www.aans.org/en/Patients/Neurosurgical-Conditions-and-Treatments/Cauda-Equina-Syndrome. Published 2020. Accessed August 26, 2020.
4. Orendáčová J, et al. Cauda equina syndrome. *Progr Neurobiol*. https://www.sciencedirect.com/science/article/pii/S0301008200000654. Published April 10, 2001. Accessed August 26, 2020.
5. Mayo Clinic. *Spinal Cord Injury*. https://www.mayoclinic.org/diseases-conditions/spinal-cord-injury/symptoms-causes/syc-20377890. Published September 17, 2019. Accessed August 26, 2020.

# 201.

## BLOOD SUPPLY

*Rany T. Abdallah and Jasmin Villatoro-Lopez*

## INTRODUCTION

The spinal cord is located in the vertebral cavity and runs from the foramen magnum to the second lumbar vertebra (L2) where the conus medullaris ends.[1] The blood supply of the spinal cord derives from two sets of branches from the aorta:

- The first set is composed of the vertebral arteries that arise from the subclavian arteries. The vertebral arteries course cephalad bilaterally through the transverse processes of the upper six cervical vertebrae, entering the posterior fossa of the cranial cavity via the foramen magnum. The anterior spinal artery (ASA) is formed within the posterior fossa from a small ramus from each vertebral artery anastomosing in a Y-shaped configuration.[2]
- The second set comprises the branches of the segmental arteries. These arteries originate outside the vertebral column. They originate from branches of the vertebral arteries in the cervical region and from posterior intercostal arteries, lumbar arteries, and lateral sacral arteries in the rest of the cord.[2]

## ARTERIAL SUPPLY

The main blood supply of the spinal cord is via the single anterior spinal artery (ASA), which is formed by the vertebral arteries originating from the subclavian artery. The ASA provides blood to the anterior two-thirds of the spinal cord. Along with ASA, the two posterior spinal arteries (PSAs) provide blood to the posterior one-third of the spinal cord (Figure 201.1). The PSAs branch off from the posterior inferior cerebellar artery (PICA) or from the pre-atlantal vertebral arteries, which can also travel caudally down the spinal cord. Both the ASA and PSAs feed into additional arteries, called the segmental spinal arteries, throughout

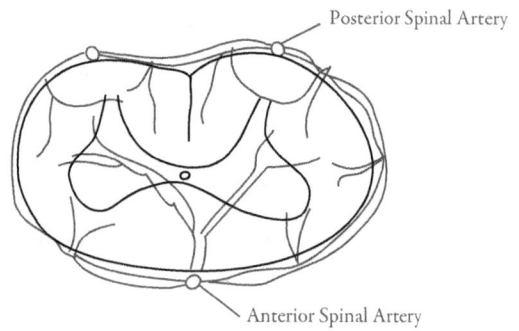

Posterior Spinal Artery

Anterior Spinal Artery

**Figure 201.1.** The spinal cord areas vascularized by the anterior spinal artery and by the posterior spinal arteries.

the spinal cord at each spinal level through the intervertebral foramen.[3]

The two ASA primarily supply the upper cervical spinal cord before anastomosing into a single ASA. The segmental medullary arteries coming from the vertebral artery are what supply blood to the mid-cervical spinal cord. The radiculomedullary arteries, arising from the cervicothoracic trunk C7 to T1, supply blood to the lower cervical through the upper thoracic spinal cord. The segmental spinal arteries supply the mid-thoracic area (T3–T9), while the Adamkiewicz artery (AKA), which branches off the left side of the descending aorta around T8–L2 and connects to the ventral side of the spinal cord so as to supply the anterior spinal artery, delivers to a large portion of the thoracolumbar region. Finally, branches of the internal iliac arteries supply the lumbosacral spinal cord.[3]

## VENOUS DRAINAGE

Briefly, the system in the vertebral canal comprises an epidural venous complex, and an irregular venous complex lying in the cord.[3] This complex has no valves and anastomoses freely. It consists of 6 veins: 3 anterior and 3 posterior veins.

## CLINICAL FEATURES

The Adamkiewicz artery is considered a watershed area, as it supplies blood to a large portion of the thoracolumbar region, as mentioned previously. This, however, may render this area to be prone to ischemia and infraction following severe hypotension, due to it being the last major artery feeding into the lumbar spinal cord. On account of the vascular anatomy, this may often lead to anterior spinal cord syndrome within the region of the lumbar spinal

cord, resulting in loss of motor and sensory function, along with pain.[3]

The diagnosis of anterior spinal cord syndrome may be determined via a spinal cord angiogram or magnetic resonance angiography of the spinal cord in patients who present with motor and sensory symptoms to evaluate for a true ischemic insult.[4]

The diagnosis for a vertebral artery dissection is determined through a catheter angiography. A "string sign," which is a long segment of narrowed lumen, is the most common findings in a catheter angiography. The artery may also show sudden tapering due to the occlusion of the lumen; in some cases, aneurysmal dilatations are also found.[5]

## TREATMENT

A successful long-term management of a spinal cord injury, such as anterior spinal cord syndrome, is very dependent on a comprehensive and effective rehabilitation. Patients may be required to undergo intensive physical therapy, occupational therapy, and psychological therapy. Along with this, management of spasticity, neuropathic pain, mobility impairment, and neurogenic skin, bowel, and bladder are recommended.[4]

So as to prevent thromboembolic (clotting) complications, it is recommended that patients have anticoagulation with intravenous heparin, followed with oral warfarin. This treatment may be completed regardless of the type of symptoms, lest there be contraindications, for instance, the presence of a large infarct with associated mass effect, hemorrhagic transformation of the infracted area, an intracranial aneurysm, or intracranial extension of the dissection.[4]

## REFERENCES

1. Colbert BJ, et al. *Anatomy and Physiology for Health Professions: An Interactive Journey.* 3rd ed. Boston: Pearson; 2015:179.
2. Purves D. The blood supply of the brain and spinal cord. In: *Neuroscience.* 2nd ed. https://www.ncbi.nlm.nih.gov/books/NBK11042/. Published January 1, 1970. Accessed August 19, 2020.
3. Gofur EM. Anatomy, back, vertebral canal blood supply. *StatPearls* [Internet]. https://www.ncbi.nlm.nih.gov/books/NBK541083/#:~:text=The main blood supply to part of the subclavian artery. Published July 27, 2020. Accessed August 19, 2020.
4. Klakeel M, et al. Anterior spinal cord syndrome of unknown etiology. *Proceedings (Baylor University Medical Center).* https://www.ncbi.nlm.nih.gov/pmc/articles/PMC4264724/. Published January 28, 2015. Accessed August 21, 2020.
5. Park K-W, et al. Vertebral artery dissection: Natural history, clinical features and therapeutic considerations. *J Korean Neurosurg Soc.* https://www.ncbi.nlm.nih.gov/pmc/articles/PMC2588305/. Published September 20, 2008. Accessed August 19, 2020.

# 202.

# SACRAL NERVES

*Jacob Topfer and Rany T. Abdallah*

## INTRODUCTION

The sacrum is a large bony structure that is made up by the fusion of 5 sacral vertebrae. It has articulation with the hip bones laterally at the sacroiliac junction. Specifically, the sacrum is divided by foramina on each side of the midline, while the median junction is traversed by a sacral canal.[1,2] Within the sacral canal lie adipose tissue, the cauda equina, including the filum terminale, epidural space, dura mater, arachnoid mater, and a thecal sac. Superiorly at the sacral base, the spinal nerves run through the sacral canal and pass inferiorly through the sacral hiatus.[3] This is where the terminal end of the filum terminale exists with S5 and the coccygeal nerve. In this chapter, we will focus on the 5 sacral nerves, namely the sacral elements of the lumbosacral plexus. The sacral nerves are importantly characterized by their triangular shape and their ability to provide sensory and motor innervation to portions of the lower extremity and perineum.

## SPINAL CORD ANATOMY

The spinal cord is proximally continuous with the medulla oblongata, and distally with the conus medullaris within the cauda equina, which makes the lumbar and sacral nerve roots.[2] In an adult lumbar spine, the cord typically will terminate at the level of the L1 vertebra, but can span as far as L3 in a child's spine. The cord traverses the spinal canal and is surrounded by three meningeal layers. The epidural space extends through the sacral canal to the sacral hiatus. This space contains fat, areolar tissue, lymphatics, blood vessels, and importantly, the nerve roots. Distally, the sacral canal contains the most caudal portion of the dural sac, typically terminating at S2 in adults. There are 31 pairs of spinal nerves (8 cervical, 12 thoracic, 5 lumbar, 5 sacral, and 1 coccygeal), and we will focus our attention here on the 5 sacral nerves.[2]

The cauda equina, which consists of the lumbar and sacral nerve roots, emerges from the spinal cord to give off two nerve roots at each spinal level. These roots will come out

of their respective dural sacs one level cephalad to the level at which they exit the spinal canal. The sacral nerve roots will exit through their respective intervertebral foramina within the sacrum.[3]

## SACRAL PLEXUS

The sacral plexus is typically discussed in conjunction with the lumbosacral plexus, due to the important overlay of function. This nerve plexus is formed by the union of the lumbosacral trunk (L4–L5) with the anterior rami of S1–S4 sacral nerves (Figure 202.1). It is characterized by its triangular-shaped nerves, with their proximal portions lying along the sacral foramina and distal vertex lying at the greater sciatic foramen.[1,4] The sacral nerves provide sensory and motor innervation to portions of the lower extremity, including but not limited to the hip, knee, and ankle joints. There are 12 peripheral nerves that are derived from the sacral plexus, including the pudendal nerve (S2–S4), the super and inferior gluteal nerves (L4–S1), the pelvic splanchnic nerves, the sciatic nerve (L4–S3), and the posterior femoral cutaneous nerves of the thigh (S1–S3)[1] (see Table 202.1).

The sciatic nerve is the largest and longest peripheral nerve in the body. Its nerve trunk is composed of the tibial nerve and the common peroneal nerve. They run together until the popliteal fossa, where they diverge from one another and become independent nerves. The common peroneal nerve innervates the dorsal surface of the foot and the dorsiflexors of the foot. The tibial portion of the sciatic nerve innervates the plantar flexors of the foot (gastrocnemius, soleus, popliteus, and plantaris). The posterior femoral cutaneous nerve is derived from the S1–S3 nerve root and provides the sensory innervation to the posterior thigh. Less discussed is the S5 nerve root, which typically runs along the coccygeal nerve. These nerves provide sensory and motor innervation to their dermatomes and partial innervation to certain pelvic organs.[1] Additionally, there is evidence of parasympathetic nervous system (PSNS) innervation leaving the central nervous system (CNS) from the S2–S4 nerves. The outflow of PSNS activity originates

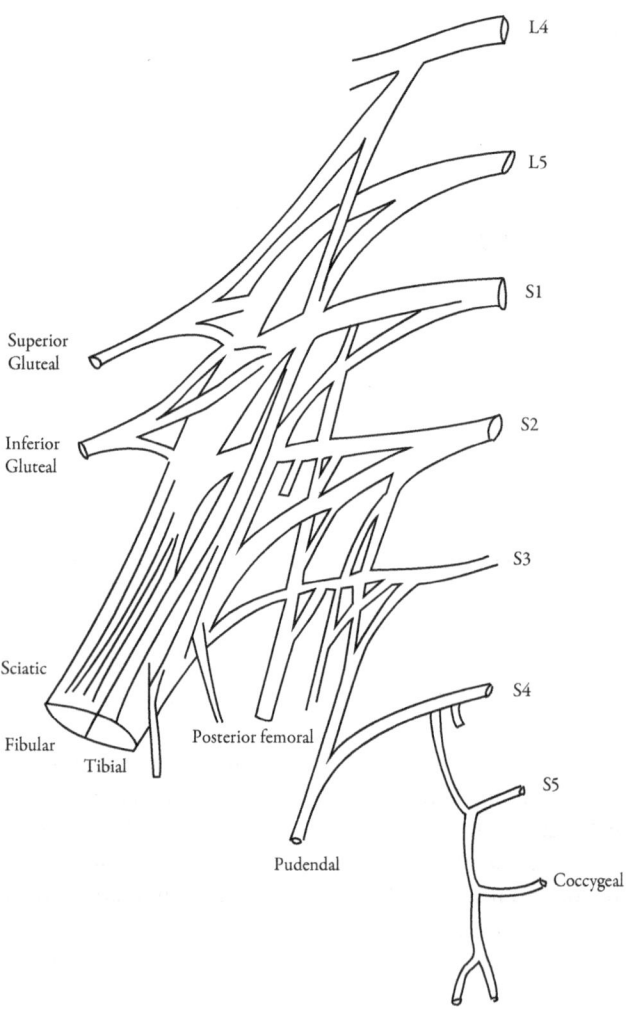

Figure 202.1. Lumbosacral plexus.

*Table 202.1* LUMBOSACRAL PLEXUS MAJOR NERVES

| SACRAL NERVE PLEXUS NERVES | SPINAL SEGMENTS | DISTRIBUTION |
|---|---|---|
| Superior inferior gluteal nerve | L4–S2 | Gluteus minimus, gluteus medius, tensor fasciae latae, gluteus maximus |
| Posterior femoral cutaneous nerve | S1–S3 | Skin of perineum; skin of the posterior thigh and leg |
| Sciatic nerve | L4–S3 | Semitendinosis, semimembranosus, biceps femoris, adductor magnus |
| Common peroneal nerve | | Biceps femoris short head, fibularis, tibialis anterior, toe extensor muscles, skin over the dorsal foot, lateral foot, and anterior surface of the leg |
| Tibial nerve | | Popliteus, gastrocnemius, soleus plantaris, tibialis posterior, long head of biceps femoris, toe flexor muscles, skin over the posterior surface of the leg |
| Pudendal nerve | S2–S4 | Urogenital diaphragm, external anal and urethral sphincter muscles, skin over the external genitalia and related muscles |

in the intermediolateral gray horns of these nerves and supplies the descending colon, rectum, uterus, and bladder.[4]

## CLINICAL CONSIDERATIONS

There are many pathologies of the sacral plexus that need to be considered when determining treatment modalities. These specific pathologic processes involve multiple, organ-specific medical specialties, such as neurology, urology, gynecology, gastroenterology, orthopedic surgery, and anesthesia, to name a few. A neurologic approach is required to combine diagnosis and management, and specifically, within anesthesia, the discipline of pain control.[5] Patients who present with sacral radiculopathies typically present with pain on the affected dermatome, allodynia, tingling, shock-like symptoms, numbness, and weakness, as well as urinary and bowel dysfunction.[5] More specific presenting symptoms of sacral nerve pathology include sciatica, gluteal pain with associated perineal, vaginal, or penile pain,

pudendal pain, vulvodynia, dysuria, painful ejaculation, refractory urinary and pelvic complaints.[5] Sole sacral nerve pathology without the inclusion of lumbar nerves is very rare due to its well-protected encapsulation by the pelvic wall. Etiologies of primarily sacral pathology include, but are not limited to, endometriosis, vascular entrapment, secondary to pelvic surgery, or pelvic tumors.[5]

## ANESTHESIA CONSIDERATIONS

Peripheral nerve blocks can be of great use for perioperative pain and chronic pain control. Lower extremity blocks and spinal cord stimulation are widely used modalities. In particular, sciatic nerve blocks and stimulation are used for pain relief in the lower extremity. It is appropriate for surgeries involving the posterior thigh, lower leg, foot and ankle, and is important for improvement of pain management perioperatively.[1] You can also perform a popliteal block of the sciatic nerve for foot and ankle surgery. Spinal cord stimulation may, however, be most effective for neuropathic pain. It is indicated for sympathetic-mediated pain, lesions, ischemic lower extremity pain due to PVD, and peripheral neuropathies.[1]

## REFERENCES

1. Vrooman BM, Rosenquist RW. Chronic pain management. In: Butterworth IV JF, et al., eds. *Morgan & Mikhail's Clinical Anesthesiology*, 6th ed. McGraw-Hill.
2. Manuel P, Miller RD. *Basics of Anesthesia*. 7th ed. Elsevier, 2018.
3. Tran DQ, et al. Lower extremity regional anesthesia: Essentials of our current understanding. *Reg Anesth Pain Med*. 2019;44:143–180.
4. Hwang G. Parasympathetic nervous system. In: Freeman BS, Berger JS, eds. *Anesthesiology Core Review: Part One Basic Exam*. McGraw-Hill.
5. Possover M, Farache C. Neuropelveological approach to pathologies of the sacral plexus. *J Clinical Neurol Neurosurg Spine*. 2018;1(1):115.

# 203.

# MENINGES

*Rany T. Abdallah and Jasmin Villatoro-Lopez*

## ANATOMY

The meninges are membranous layers surrounding the central nervous system (CNS). They are composed of three distinct layers: the outermost dura mater, the middle arachnoid mater, and the innermost pia mater. Cerebrospinal fluid (CSF) travels between these layers.1

The *dura mater* is a thick and dense collagenous membrane that is made of two layers. The first and outer layer (endosteal layer) serves as the periosteum of the internal surface of the skull. The second and inner layer (meningeal layer) is fused to the endosteal layer in most areas and is only separated at sites of dural venous sinuses in order to allow drainage of venous blood from the brain. The *arachnoid mater* is a thin, translucent membrane that contains a few layers of flattened cells. Beneath this membrane is the arachnoid trabeculae, a spongy connective tissue that is made of collagen fibers and fibroblasts. The *pia mater* has a fragile, single cell-layer membrane that closely adheres to the surface of the brain and spinal cord. The pia also contributes to the formation of the filum terminale internum, a whitish fibrous filament that extends from the conus medullaris to the tip of the dural sac. Additionally, blood vessels branch out from the subarachnoid space throughout the pia mater in the brain and are considered an extension of the pia mater.[1]

Both the dura and the arachnoid (jointly making the thecal sac) have typically been described as extending to the lower border of the S2 vertebra and beyond, well below the conus medullaris.

## CLINICAL CORRELATION

Developmental defects in the meninges are believed to cause two neurodevelopmental disorders in humans: Dandy-Walker malformation, and cobblestone lissencephaly. Both conditions can impair the function of the brain:[1]

- Dandy-Walker malformation (DWM) is caused by an enlargement of the posterior fossa, a cystic dilatation of the fourth ventricle and cerebellar hypoplasia. Some of the most frequent symptoms accompanied by DWM are signs of macrocrania, eye anomalies, spasticity, development delay, headaches, nausea, seizures, ataxia-walking difficulties, lethargy, and cranial nerve palsy.[2]
- Walker-Warburg syndrome affects the development of the muscles, brain (cobblestone lissencephaly), and eyes. In the most severe cases it may cause muscle weakness and atrophy beginning early in life.[3]

Tumors (e.g., meningiomas, neurofibromas) are frequently located in the intradural extramedullary compartment. Anomalous masses (tumors, infections, hematomas) may arise in any location in or around the spinal cord. Epidural masses, such as bone tumors or metastases, can move the dura locally and impinge on the spinal cord. Spinal cord compression may progress precipitously, possibly resulting in paraplegia or quadriplegia. Therefore, suspected spinal cord compression necessitates urgent workup as it can prevent catastrophic outcomes.[4]

## REFERENCES

1. Dasgupta K, Jeong J. Developmental biology of the meninges. In: *Genesis*. New York, NY: 2000. https://www.ncbi.nlm.nih.gov/pmc/articles/PMC6520190/.
2. Dandy-Walker malformation—Genetics Home Reference—NIH. U.S. National Library of Medicine. https://ghr.nlm.nih.gov/condition/dandy-walker-malformation. Published August 17, 2020.
3. Walker-Warburg syndrome—Genetics Home Reference—NIH. U.S. National Library of Medicine. https://ghr.nlm.nih.gov/condition/walker-warburg-syndrome#diagnosis. Published August 17, 2020.
4. Waxman SG. *Clinical Neuroanatomy*. 28th ed. McGraw-Hill Education.

# 204.

# CRANIAL NERVES

*Arun George and Shobana Rajan*

## INTRODUCTION

Cranial nerves (CN) I–IV arise from the midbrain or above, CN V–VIII arise from the pons, and CN IX–XII arise from the medulla (Figure 204.1).

## STRUCTURE AND FUNCTIONS

### OLFACTORY NERVE (CN I)

The afferent neurosensory cells of this nerve are in the roof of both nasal cavities. The efferent axons pass through the cribriform plate and synapse in the olfactory bulb at the base of the forebrain in the olfactory sulcus.

- Function: smell;
- Test: smell substances with eyes closed;
- Clinical finding with lesion: anosmia;
- COVID-19 has been associated with bilateral olfactory bulb edema and anosmia.

### OPTIC NERVE (CN II)

Rods and cones in the retina transmit signals from photoreceptors and transmit them to the retinal ganglion cells along the optic nerve which ascends through the optic canal. It synapses with fibers from the contralateral optic nerve at the optic chiasm. The temporal fibers decussate and join the fibers of the contralateral nasal field, which do not decussate. Optic radiations terminate in the visual cortex in the medial occipital lobe.

- Function: vision;
- Test: visual acuity and field;
- Clinical finding with lesion: amaurosis, homonymous hemianopsia.

### OCULOMOTOR NERVE (CN III)

The Edinger Westphal nucleus in the midbrain houses the neurons that control the pupillary muscles of the eye regulating constriction and dilation. All the extraocular muscles except the lateral rectus and superior oblique muscles are also innervated by this nerve.

- Function: eye movements, pupillary constriction, accommodation;
- Test: observation of tracking, doll's eye reflex;
- Clinical finding with lesion: diplopia, ptosis, mydriasis, loss of accommodation.

### TROCHLEAR NERVE (CN IV)

The nucleus of this nerve is located in the midbrain. This nerve exits the posterior portion of the brainstem and

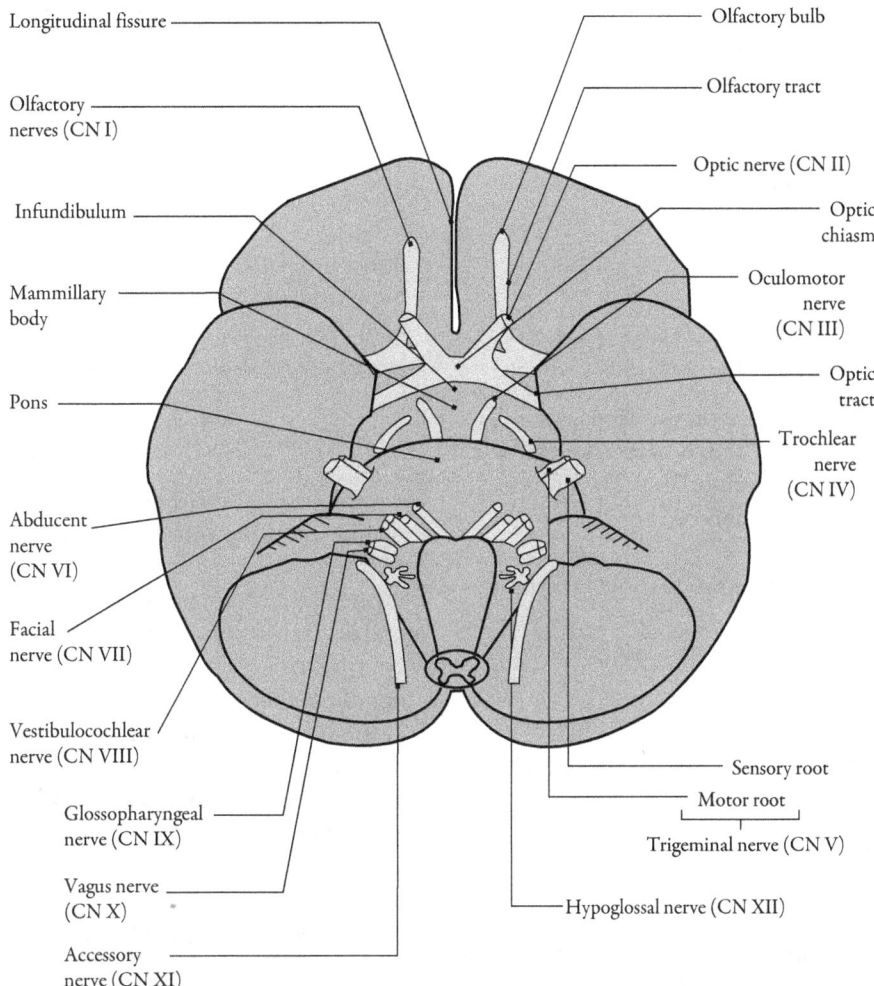

**Figure 204.1.** Superficial origin of the cranial nerves.
Reproduced with permission from Craven, J. Anatomy of the cranial nerves. *Anesth Intens Care Med.* 2010;11(12):529–534.

crosses to the contralateral side. CN IV is responsible for the movement of the superior oblique muscle.

- Function: eye movements;
- Test: observation of tracking, doll's eye reflex;
- Clinical finding with lesion: diplopia.

## TRIGEMINAL NERVE (CN V)

This is a mixed function nerve which supplies sensation to the face, nasal and buccal mucosa, and teeth. Its only motor function is the muscles of mastication. It is divided into the ophthalmic, maxillary, and mandibular divisions.

- Function: sensation of face, scalp, teeth, chewing movement;
- Test: facial sensation, corneal reflex, contract muscles of mastication;
- Clinical finding with lesion: numbness of face, weakness of jaw muscles.

## ABDUCENS NERVE (CN VI)

The nucleus of this nerve is in the middle of the pons adjacent to the floor of the fourth ventricle. After entering the cavernous sinus, it runs near the lateral aspect of the carotid artery. Hence, it may be impacted carotid artery disease.

- Function: eye movements; supplies the lateral rectus muscle;
- Test: observation of tracking, doll's eye reflex;
- Clinical finding with lesion: diplopia.

## FACIAL NERVE (CN VII)

This nerve has a larger motor component supplying the muscles of facial expression. A smaller sensory branch called the nervus intermedius carries special fibers for taste from the anterior tongue and palate and general sensory fibers from the external auditory meatus, soft palate, and the adjacent pharynx.

- Function: taste, sensation of palate, and external ear; lacrimal, submandibular, sublingual gland secretions, facial expression;
- Test: move eyebrows up and down, purse lips, show teeth;
- Clinical finding with lesion: loss of taste on anterior two-thirds of tongue, dry mouth, loss of lacrimation, paralysis of facial muscles.

## VESTIBULOCOCHLEAR (ACOUSTIC) NERVE (CN VIII)

The vestibulocochlear nerve is responsible for hearing, balance, and awareness of position. The cochlear and vestibular nuclei are located adjacent to each other in the brainstem, with the cochlear nucleus located more laterally.

- Function: hearing, equilibrium, spatial orientation;
- Test: test hearing;
- Clinical finding with lesion: deafness, tinnitus, vertigo, nystagmus.

## GLOSSOPHARYNGEAL NERVE (CN IX)

It supplies taste and general somatic sensation to the pharynx, posterior third of the tongue, part of the soft palate, and tympanic membrane. It also provides motor innervation to the stylopharyngeus muscle, which is responsible for swallowing and the gag reflex. Nerve fibers are derived from 3 brainstem nuclei: the nucleus ambiguus (motor function), inferior salivatory nucleus (salivation), nucleus tractus solitarius (taste).

- Function: taste, general sensation of the pharynx and ear, elevation of the palate, parotid gland secretion;
- Test: swallowing, gag reflex;
- Clinical finding with lesion: loss of taste on posterior one-third of the tongue, loss of sensation of pharynx, dry mouth.

## VAGUS NERVE (CN X)

It is a mixed nerve with motor, sensory, and parasympathetic functions that affect the cardiac, respiratory, and gastrointestinal systems. Vagus nerve efferent fibers carry parasympathetic innervation to the heart. The motor component innervates the laryngeal muscles and vocal cords.

- Function: sensation of pharynx, larynx and ear; swallowing; phonation; parasympathetic innervation impacts the cardiac, respiratory, and gastrointestinal systems;
- Test: swallowing, gag reflex;
- Clinical finding with lesion: tachycardia, dysphagia, hoarseness, palatal paralysis.

## SPINAL ACCESSORY NERVE (CN XI)

It has two components: a spinal part and a cranial part. The spinal component is a motor nerve that supplies the sternocleidomastoid and trapezius muscle. The cranial component of the accessory nerve provides motor control to the muscles of the soft palate, larynx and pharynx.

- Function: phonation; head, neck, shoulder movements;
- Test: head and shoulder movement.
- Clinical finding with lesion: hoarseness, weakness of head, neck, and shoulder muscles.

## HYPOGLOSSAL NERVE (CN XII)

The nerve arises from the hypoglossal nucleus in the medulla and innervates the intrinsic muscles of the tongue along with the genioglossus, styloglossus, and hyoglossus muscles. Damage to this nerve produces the well-known sign of ipsilateral deviation seen on protrusion of the tongue.

- Function: tongue movements;
- Test: tongue movement observation, tongue atrophy, fasciculations;
- Clinical finding with lesion: weakness, deviation, and wasting of tongue.[2]

## ANESTHETIC CONSIDERATIONS

### INTRAOPERATIVE CN MONITORING

Electromyography (EMG) recordings help assess the functional integrity of cranial nerves and detect changes related to intraoperative events.[3] Transcranial motor evoked potentials are used for monitoring motor nerve function. Spontaneous EMG is sensitive to irritation of the nerve root, such as retraction of spinal cord or nerve root, saline irrigation, and manipulation during surgery. The auditory brainstem response is the most resistant to anesthesia.[4]

### EYE BLOCKS

Retrobulbar blocks target the ciliary nerve, ciliary ganglion, and CN III, IV, and VI. Peribulbar blocks target the ciliary nerves, CN III and VI. The advantages of peribulbar block are as follows: there is less potential for intraocular or intradural injection; it is technically easier; and there is reduced risk of hemorrhage and injury to the optic nerve.

### AIRWAY

The larynx is innervated bilaterally by the superior laryngeal nerve and the recurrent laryngeal nerve, both branches of the vagus nerve. For awake fiberoptic intubations- superior laryngeal, transtracheal, and topicalization of the oropharynx.

## VAGAL STIMULATION

Stimulation of the CN X may produce cardiac effects, mainly bradycardia and even asystole with traction on the vagus nerve. Bezold-Jarisch reflex describes perioperative bradycardia with hypotension that results from activation of cardiac mechanoreceptors. The afferent limb of this reflex is the nonmyelinated, type C vagal fibers. Activation causes inhibition of sympathetic outflow, coupled with bradycardia, peripheral vasodilation, and hypotension.

## NAUSEA AND VOMITING

The reflex involved in nausea and vomiting is coordinated by the brainstem vomiting center, located in the lateral medullary reticular formation, and propagated chiefly via CN VIII and X.

## OCULOCARDIAC REFLEX

Decrease in heart rate is caused by pressure on the globe or traction of the ocular muscles. Afferent Limb- Trigeminal Nerve. Efferent Limb- Vagus Nerve. Immediately, notify the surgeon to stop orbital stimulation. Optimize oxygenation and ventilation, prevent light anesthesia. If arrythmia/bradycardia does not resolve, consider atropine 20 mcg/kg IV (or glycopyrrolate).

## PHARYNGEAL (GAG) REFLEX

Stimulus to posterior tongue, soft palate, or posterior pharyngeal wall causes bilateral pharyngeal muscle contraction. Afferent limb- CN IX, some contribution by CN X, via internal branch of superior laryngeal nerve. Efferent nerve X which can be blocked by topicalization.

## REFERENCES

1. Ng AL, et al. Cranial nerve nomenclature: Historical vignette. *World Neurosurg.* 2019 Aug 1;128:299–307.
2. Nadgir R, Yousem D. Cranial anatomy. In: Yousem D, Nadgir R, eds. *Neuroradiology: The Requisites.* 4th ed. Philadelphia, PA: Elseiver; 2017:1–39.
3. Roth M, Rakers L. Intraoperative neuromonitoring: Principles and considerations for perioperative nurses. *AORN J.* 2019 Jul;110(1): 11–26.
4. Ashram Y, Yingling C. Intraoperative monitoring of cranial nerves in neurontologic surgery. In: Flint P, Haughey B, eds. Cummings Otolaryngology: Head and Neck Surgery. 6th ed. Philadelphia, PA: Saunders; 2015:2778–2793.

# 205.

# CAROTID AND AORTIC BODIES AND CAROTID SINUS

*Kris Vasant and Muhammad Fayyaz Ahmed*

## INTRODUCTION

Chemoreceptors are necessary to maintain cardiopulmonary homeostasis by sensing variations in chemical concentrations. Peripheral chemoreceptors include the carotid and aortic bodies that lay within the arterial vasculature. The peripheral chemoreceptors work in concert with the central chemoreceptors that are located in the brainstem. The carotid bodies are located at the bifurcation of the internal and external carotid arteries bilaterally, while the aortic body chemoreceptors are located within the aortic arch. Peripheral chemoreceptors primarily sense the partial pressure of arterial oxygen ($PaO_2$) and are also involved in detecting alterations in the partial pressure of arterial carbon dioxide ($PCO_2$), pH, blood flow, and temperature.[1] The ventrolateral medulla and other brainstem locations house the central chemoreceptors that primarily sense alterations in hydrogen ion (H+) concentrations in the cerebrospinal fluid.[3]

## STRUCTURE AND FUNCTION

A closer look at the carotid bodies, which are the main peripheral chemoreceptors in the body, reveals that they have mostly ventilatory effects once stimulated, while aortic bodies mostly affect blood flow when stimulated.[1] At a microscopic level, the carotid body is made up of clusters of type I glomus cells, engulfed by type II cells composed of glial processes. The type I cells are responsible for transducing changes in arterial concentrations of oxygen, carbon dioxide, and acid/base disturbances, as well as temperature and flow.[2] Afferent signals from the carotid bodies are transmitted via cranial nerve IX (glossopharyngeal) to the brainstem, where central respiratory centers augment minute ventilation.[1] Afferent signals from the aortic bodies are transmitted via cranial nerve X (vagus) to the medullary centers and augment the parasympathetic nervous system, which can lead to bradycardia, increased bronchial tone, increased adrenal secretion, and increased blood pressure.[1]

## VENTILATORY EFFECTS

Both the carotid and aortic bodies have increase neural relay once $PaO_2$ levels begin to fall; specifically, when $PaO_2$ falls below 100 mmHg. However, it is not until $PaO_2$ levels decrease to 60–65 mmHg that a clinically significant alteration of minute ventilation occurs in healthy individuals, resulting in an increase in respiratory rate and/or tidal volume.[1] This is clinically relevant in patients with chronic obstructive pulmonary disease (COPD) who have chronically elevated $PCO_2$ levels and depend on hypoxic ventilatory drive for respiration—these individuals have $PaO_2$ levels in the 60s. Once their $PaO_2$ levels rise above the mid-60s, the ventilatory drive decreases until arterial $PaO_2$ levels fall and the ventilation threshold is stimulated.[1]

## CAROTID SINUS

The carotid sinus area is located cephalad to the bifurcation of the common carotid arteries bilaterally in the neck. The carotid sinus contains baroreceptors. Baroreceptors are stretch sensitive fibers, which play a role in the maintenance of blood pressure.

### STRUCTURE AND FUNCTION

Afferent signals from the carotid sinus are transmitted through cranial nerve IX (glossopharyngeal) to the medulla—specifically to the nucleus solitaries located in the cardiovascular center of the brainstem.[4] Once the stretch receptors are activated, typically with a systolic blood pressure greater than 170 mmHg, an afferent signal is transduced to the brainstem, which causes a decrease in sympathetic activity, leading to a decrease in inotropy, heart rate, and vasomotor tone, combining to decrease blood pressure.[4] The opposite effect occurs with a drop in blood pressure, in the aim to increase inotropy, heart rate, and vasomotor tone to increase blood pressure.

## ANESTHETIC CONSIDERATIONS

### PREOPERATIVE

Patients with a history of COPD should be restricted from getting benzodiazepines preoperatively if possible so as to avoid risk of hypoxia and apnea postoperatively.

### INTRAOPERATIVE

In response to a patient with a stable supraventricular tachycardia, the carotid sinus massage can be used as a first line to therapeutically induce the parasympathetic nervous system with an aim to terminate the arrhythmia. Occlusion of one carotid sinus can induce the baroreceptor firing as if responding to an acute response to hypertension, inducing a reflexive increased parasympathetic nervous system stimulation of the vagus nerve and resultant decrease in heart rate. If unsuccessful, the maneuver should be abandoned in favor of further advanced cardiovascular life support (ACLS) treatment per algorithm.

Patients with a history of orthotopic heart transplant lack response from carotid sinus activation due to loss of autonomic innervations to the heart. These patients have to be treated with direct-acting agents on the heart for bradycardia, such as isoproterenol, epinephrine, and norepinephrine.

Surgical stimulation of the carotid sinus during procedures on carotid can lead to atrioventricular block, bradycardia. or cardiac arrest. Prompt attention should be given to it by informing the surgeon to halt the stimulation and administering atropine if needed. The surgical area can also be infiltrated with local anesthetic to avoid further episodes.

### POSTOPERATIVE

In patients with COPD, volatile anesthetics, benzodiazepines, and opioids can depress the hypoxic ventilatory response by reducing the carotid body response to hypoxemia.[1] Since these patient have chronically increased $PaCO_2$, they are dependent on the hypoxic ventilatory drive for respiration. Residual anesthetic drugs after a general anesthetic can cause apnea, and these patients must be monitored closely in the post-anesthesia care unit. If possible, the use of opioids and benzodiazepines should be restricted.

Patients with bilateral carotid endarterectomy have denervation of their carotid bodies and do not have a functional ventilator response to hypoxia; hence they should be closely monitored after general anesthesia for apnea and hypoxia. In this case, the central chemoreceptors take over the function of maintaining ventilation. Unilateral carotid endarterectomy may lead to altered response to hypoxia.

## REFERENCES

1. Tamul OC, Ault ML. Respiratory function in anesthesia. In: Barash PG, Cullen BF, Stoelting RK, et al., eds. *Clinical Anesthesia*. 8th ed. Philadelphia, PA: Wolters Kluwer Health; 2017:361–383.
2. Toledo C, et al. Contribution of peripheral and central chemoreceptors to sympatho-excitation in heart failure. *J Physiol*. 2017;595(1):43–51.
3. Kavanagh BP, Hedenstierna D. Respiratory physiology and pathophysiology. In Miller RD, ed. *Miller's Anesthesia*. 8th ed. New York, NY: Elsevier/Churchill Livingstone; 2015:444-472.
4. Sun LS, et al. Cardiac physiology. In Miller RD, ed. *Miller's Anesthesia*. 8th ed. New York, NY: Elsevier/Churchill Livingstone; 2015:473-491.

# 206.

# GANGLIA, RAMI COMMUNICANTES AND SYMPATHETIC CHAIN

*Eric D. Friedman and Gunar G. Subieta-Benito*

## INTRODUCTION

The sympathetic nervous system is essential for life-sustaining functions and the preservation of well-being. Dysfunction of the system has repercussions varying from dysautonomia to pain. A thorough understanding of its anatomic relationships is paramount for the practitioner.

## PREGANGLIONIC PATHWAY

Within the seventh lamina of the thoracolumbar spinal cord gray matter at levels T1–L3 lies the origin of preganglionic sympathetic fibers. The cell bodies of these fibers form the intermediolateral column. These myelinated, type B, preganglionic fibers exit the spinal cord alongside motor fibers via the anterior spinal root, travel through the intervertebral foramina, and project onto the white rami communicans toward the paired paravertebral ganglia (or sympathetic chain), which extend from the cervical to the sacral spine. These presynaptic fibers travel a short distance from the central nervous system prior to synapse and thus are generally shorter than their postganglionic counterparts. Once the fibers reach a ganglion at the paravertebral chain, they may synapse with postganglionic cell bodies at the same spinal level, travel through the ganglion, extend superiorly or inferiorly, and synapse with a ganglion at a different spinal level, or they may travel to an unpaired prevertebral ganglion (anterior to the sympathetic chain) where they synapse and then innervate visceral organs. Preganglionic sympathetic fibers are cholinergic, produce acetylcholine (ACh), and act on ionotropic, ligand gated nicotinic receptors attached to postganglionic sympathetic cell bodies at the paravertebral ganglia and prevertebral ganglia. In the adrenal medulla, chromaffin cells, an embryologic derivative of neural crest cells, are analogous to postganglionic sympathetic cell bodies. Cholinergic transmission into the adrenal medulla activates a hormonal response by the chromaffin cells. They secrete norepinephrine (NE) and epinephrine (EPI) into the bloodstream, which compounds the sympathetic response. The multiple pathways undertaken by preganglionic sympathetic fibers, their interconnections with multiple ganglia, on top of the hormonal activation of NE and EPI by the adrenal gland, allow for synergism and amplification that

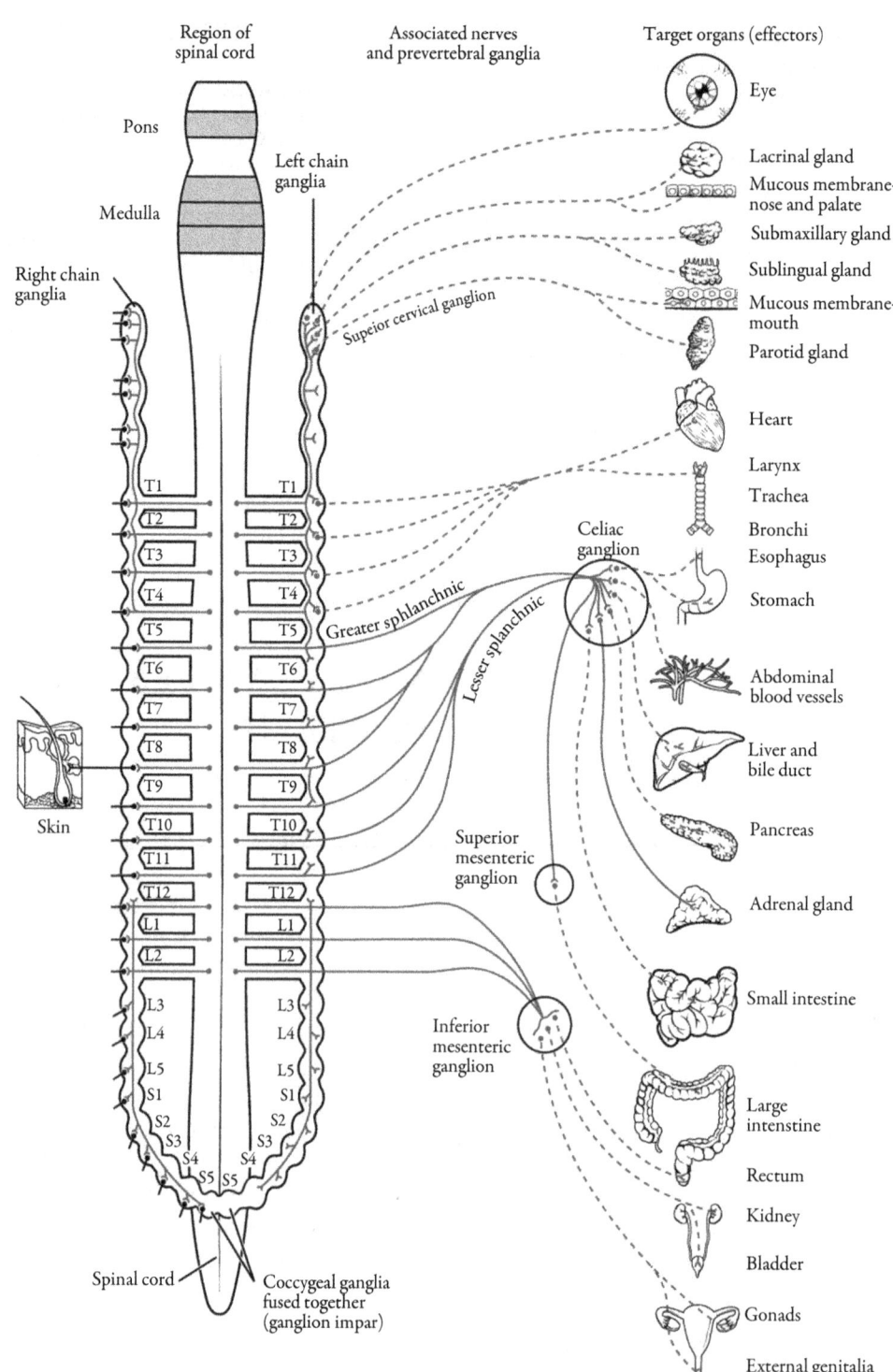

**Figure 206.1.** Schematic of the sympathetic nervous system. The network of axons course from the preganglionic cell bodies in the intermediolateral column of the thoracolumbar spinal cord to the paravertebral and prevertebral ganglia, where postganglionic cell bodies lie, to effector organs. Preganglionic fibers are the solid lines and postganglionic fibers are the dotted lines.

provide a graded sympathetic response to enviormental or intrinsic stressors.[1,2]

## POSTGANGLIONIC PATHWAY

Postganglionic sympathetic fibers emerge from the paravertebral ganglia, course through the gray rami communicans, and travel alongside spinal nerves to innervate downstream effector organs such as blood vessels in skeletal muscle, plus sweat glands and hair follicles in the skin. Postganglionic fibers emerging from the prevertebral ganglia directly innverate visceral effector organs. All postganglionic fibers act on G-protein coupled adrenergic receptors sensitive mostly to NE, except those that innervate sweat glands, which effect G-protein coupled muscarinic receptors sensitive to Ach. Transmission ceases once these neurotransmitters are metabolized in the synaptic cleft by either reuptake into the preganglionic or postganglionic nerve terminals, enzymatic breakdown of NE and EPI by monoamine oxidase (MAO) or catechol-O-methyltransferase (COMT), or in the case of Ach, hydrolysis by acetylcholinesterase or pseudocholinesterase in the synaptic junction.[3]

## GANGLIA

The paired paravertebral ganglia, fed by preganglionic fibers originating from the thoracolumbar spinal cord, extend superiorly and inferiorly from the cervical to the sacral spine. Both paravertebral ganglia converge at the coccyx as the ganglion impar.[4] Once preganglionic sympathetic fibers synapse with cell bodies in these ganglia, unmyelinated, type C, postganglionic fibers exit the paravertebral ganglia via the gray rami communicans and proceed to innervate effector organs. Blood vessel vasoconstriction is characteristic of the sympathetic response in the skin and gastrointestinal tract, whereas vasodilation is characteristic in skeletal muscle, and coronary and pulmonary circulation. The superior cervical ganglia and the stellate ganglia, composed of the inferior cervical ganglia and the first thoracic ganglia (C7, C8, T1), serve as the origin of postganglionic sympathietic fibers that innervate the head, neck and upper extremities. These fibers modulate pupillary response, lacrimation and salivation, as well as pilomotor, sudomotor and vasomotor functions of the skin, sweat glands and skeletal muscle in this region. Postganglionic cardioaccelerator, pulmonary bronchodilator, and esophageal smooth muscle inhibitory fibers originate in the proximal thoracic paravertebral ganglia (T1–T4), with contribution from the stellate ganglia observed in some cadaveric studies.[4]

The unpaired prevertebral ganglia, located in the prevertebral plexus adjacent to major branch points of the abdominal aorta, feed sympathetic innervation to abdominal and pelvic viscera. Presynaptic fibers that supply these ganglia are known as thoracic, lumbar, and sacral splanchnic nerves. These splanchnic nerves form the celiac, lumbar, and superior hypogastric plexus. Within the plexus network lies the celiac, superior mesenteric, aorticorenal, and inferior mesenteric ganglia. At these ganglia, presynaptic fibers synapse with cell bodies of postganglionic sympathetic fibers, which then travel to effector organs in the abdomen and pelvis. Sympathetic outflow to the celiac and superior mesenteric ganglia will inhibit gastrointestinal motility by relaxing intestinal smooth muscle, vasoconstricting splanchnic blood vessels and inhibiting pancreatic and biliary secretions (including insulin release). In the liver, sympathetic outflow enhances the conversion of glycogen into glucose. From the inferior mesenteric and aorticorenal ganglion, sympathetic outflow will constrict bladder and ureter smooth muscle, reduce renal blood flow resulting in renin secretion, contract uterine smooth muscle, contract smooth muscle in the vas deferens and prostate, and constrict vessels in the penile tissue (Figure 206.1).[2,3]

## ANESTHETIC CONSIDERATIONS

### NEURAXIAL ANESTHESIA

The application of local anesthetic (LA) to spinal nerve roots during epidural catheter placement or during intrathecal injection can inhibit preganglionic sympathetic fibers, leading to vasodilation in the periphery, which reduces systemic vascular resistance and manifests as hypotension. Cephalad migration of LA to the upper thoracic levels will cause inhibition of cardiac sympathetic outflow to the AV node and may result in bradycardia.

### INTRAOPERATIVE DRUG THERAPY

If an anticholinergic medication is given, parasympathetic tone can be decreased, resulting in sympathomimetic effects, since most organ systems in the body have dual autonomic innervation. For example, administration of the antimuscarinic drug glycopyrrolate for the purposes of reducing bronchial secretions will result in predominance of sympathetic tone in organs such as the heart (resulting in tachycardia) and the gastrointestinal tract (postoperative ileus).

### DISEASE STATES LEADING TO AUTONOMIC NEUROPATHY

Disease states such as diabetes can lead to autonomic neuropathy and can influence perioperative anesthetic management. The destruction of C fibers can result in loss of sympathetic tone, and manifests as orthostatic hypotension, loss of baroreceptor mediated reflex tachycardia, gastroparesis, and impotence.[3]

## SYMPATHETIC NERVE BLOCKS FOR CHRONIC OR ACUTE PAIN MANAGEMENT

Blockade of the sympathetic paravertebral and prevertebral ganglia with local anesthetic has been shown to be effective at addressing visceral or pelvic, ischemic, and neuropathic pain. Examples include a stellate ganglion block, celiac plexus block, lumbar sympathetic block, superior hypogastric plexus block, or ganglion impar block.[5]

## PERMISSION FOR GRAPHIC

The attached graphic is produced by OpenStax and is licensed under a Creative Commons Attribution License v4.0. Under the terms of this license, the graphic may be freely distributed in any format (including for commercial purposes) as long as the terms of the license are followed.

The terms of the license may be found here: https://creativecommons.org/licenses/by/4.0/

In summary, appropriate attribution and credit must be given, which is referenced under the caption.

## REFERENCES

1. Hwang G. Sympathetic nervous system. In: Freeman BS, Berger JS, eds. *Anesthesiology Core Review. Part One: BASIC Exam.* New York, NY: McGraw-Hill Education Medical; 2014:357–359.
2. Glick DB. The autonomic nervous system. In: Miller RD, et al., eds. *Miller's Anesthesia.* 7th ed. München: Elsevier Health Sciences; 2009:261–304.
3. Grecu L. Central and autonomic nervous systems. In: Barash PG, et al. *Clinical Anesthesia Fundamentals.* Philadelphia, PA: Wolters Kluwer; 2015:69–85.
4. Kommuru H, et al. Thoracic part of sympathetic chain and its branching pattern variations in South Indian cadavers. *J Clin Diagn Res.* 2014;8(12):AC09–AC12.
5. Vrooman BM, Rosenquist RW. Chronic pain management. In: Butterworth JF, et al., eds. *Morgan & Mikhail's Clinical Anesthesiology.* 6th ed. New York, NY: McGraw-Hill Education; 2018:1047–1110.

# 207.

# NOCICEPTION

*Richard Lennertz*

## INTRODUCTION

Pain is defined as "an unpleasant sensory and emotional experience associated with, or resembling that associated with, actual or potential tissue damage" according to the International Association for Pain. Though unpleasant, pain plays an important role in avoiding injury. Nociception is the process of perceiving pain. Nociceptors are specialized nerve fibers that convey painful stimuli to the spinal cord, where they are integrated and passed on to the brain. Injury changes nociception so that pain is exaggerated or perceived in the absence of potential tissue damage. These changes are adaptive while tissues heal and help to avoid further injury. However, changes in nociception become maladaptive and lead to chronic pain when they persist beyond the period of healing.

## MECHANISMS OF NOCICEPTION

Nociceptors are afferent nerve fibers that encode painful stimuli. Consistent with this purpose, nociceptors generate action potentials in response to intense, noxious stimuli. Nociceptors synapse onto second-order neurons in the dorsal horn. Spinal neurons integrate input from nociceptors with input from other sensory neurons and with descending input from the periaqueductal gray and rostral ventromedial medulla. Action potentials from spinal projection neurons propagate along spinal tracts to several regions of the brain. The somatosensory cortex generates the discriminatory component of pain including the location, modality, and intensity of the stimulus. Limbic regions such as the anterior cingulate cortex, insular cortex, and amygdala generate the affective

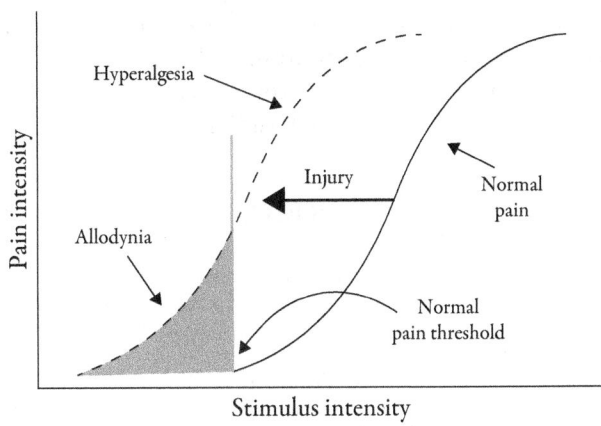

**Figure 207.1.** Hyperalgesia and allodynia compared to normal pain sensation. Injury increases the pain associated with noxious stimuli (hyperalgesia) and may decrease the pain threshold, so that normally innocuous stimuli become painful (allodynia).

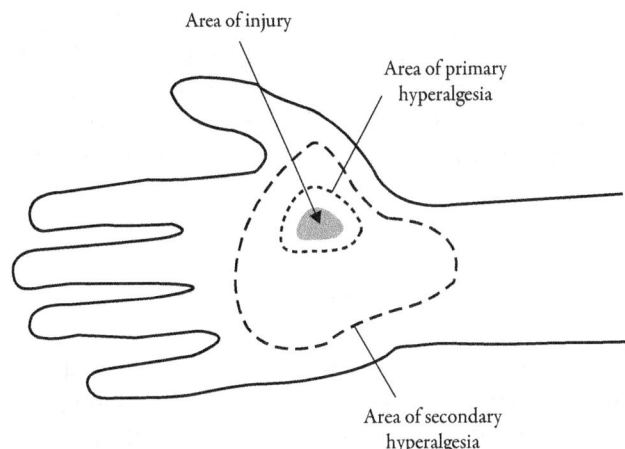

**Figure 207.2.** Primary and secondary hyperalgesia. Primary hyperalgesia occurs in the area of tissue injury and involves sensitization of nociceptors. Secondary hyperalgesia occurs in a larger area outside of the area of tissue injury and involves central sensitization.

component of pain. The affective component encompasses feelings of unpleasantness and the emotional response to pain.

Injury changes the perception of pain. Noxious stimuli become more painful (hyperalgesia) and innocuous stimuli may become painful (allodynia; Figure 207.1). Nociceptors become sensitized in response to injury due to the release of inflammatory mediators. This enhances their response to noxious stimuli or renders them responsive to innocuous stimuli. Sensitization also occurs within the central nervous system, and nerve fibers that normally convey the sensation of touch may convey the sensation of pain. Central sensitization is complex and plays an important role in the transition from acute to chronic pain.

## INFLAMMATORY PAIN

Tissue injury leads to inflammation and inflammatory pain. Inflammatory pain is characterized by two types of hyperalgesia. Primary hyperalgesia occurs within the area of tissue injury and primarily involves the sensitization of nociceptors (Figure 207.2). Nociceptors in injured tissue develop an augmented response to suprathreshold stimuli, become stimulated at a lower threshold, and may develop spontaneous activity. These changes occur in response to inflammatory mediators and correlate with subjective pain reports when microneurography is performed in humans. Secondary hyperalgesia occurs adjacent to the injured tissue and is mediated by central sensitization (Figure 207.2). In human studies, proximal nerve blocks prevent the development of secondary hyperalgesia if performed before an injury occurs. These studies support the rationale for using regional anesthesia for perioperative pain management.

Secondary hyperalgesia has been described according to "punctate hyperalgesia" to sharp stimuli and "stroking hyperalgesia" to gentle touch (allodynia). These appear to be mediated by different mechanisms. Punctate hyperalgesia typically manifests over a larger area and for a longer period than allodynia. Studies using selective nerve blocks suggest that nociceptors convey punctate hyperalgesia. However, low threshold nerve fibers that are not typically nociceptors mediate allodynia. In both situations, central sensitization strengthens input from peripheral nerve fibers onto secondary neurons in the spinal cord that convey pain to the brain.

## NEUROPATHIC PAIN

Injury to the nerve may lead to neuropathic pain. Patients often describe neuropathic pain as having a burning, lancing, or electric shock-like quality. Pain may coincide with diminished sensation, such as in anesthesia dolorosa or phantom limb pain. The mechanisms of neuropathic pain are less clearly understood than those of inflammatory pain and vary between types of nerve injury. Peripheral axons form a neuroma if disruption of the nerve sheath impairs regeneration. Nociceptors within neuromas are exquisitely sensitive and may develop spontaneous activity. Meanwhile, distal axon segments separated from the cell body undergo Wallerian degeneration. This active degradation process releases inflammatory mediators that sensitize surviving nociceptors. Low threshold nerve fibers may express neuropeptides similar to those expressed by nociceptors, a phenomenon referred to as "phenotype switching." Studies suggest that both nociceptor sensitization and central sensitization play a role in neuropathic pain following nerve injury. While acute deafferentation of the spinal cord or direct injury to the spinal cord can abolish pain sensation, pain may recur over time as plasticity occurs in the central nervous system.

## AUTONOMIC PAIN

The autonomic nervous system can influence nociception under certain conditions. Nociceptors are typically insensitive to norepinephrine released by the sympathetic nervous system, but may express α-adrenoreceptors in pathologic conditions such as complex regional pain syndrome (CRPS) type 1 and 2. In these syndromes, norepinephrine released by sympathetic nerves may directly activate nociceptors, a phenomenon described as sympathetic-sensory coupling. Abnormal sympathetic activity may indirectly influence nociceptors by causing local tissue hypoxia. The autonomic nervous system

also contributes to hyperalgesia during inflammation. Sympathectomy greatly diminishes hyperalgesia in response to inflammatory mediators such as bradykinin and nerve growth factor in animal studies.

## REFERENCES

1. Ringkamp M, et al. Peripheral mechanisms of cutaneous nociception. In: S McMahon, M Koltzenburg, I Tracey, D Turk, eds. *Wall & Melzack's Textbook of Pain*. 6th ed. Philadelphia, PA: Elsevier; 2013:1–30.
2. Bielefeldt K, Gebhart GF. Visceral pain: Basic echanisms. In: S McMahon, M Koltzenburg, I Tracey, D Turk, eds. *Wall & Melzack's Textbook of Pain*. 6th ed. Philadelphia, PA: Elsevier; 2013:703–717.
3. Devor M. Neuropathic pain: Pathophysiological response of nerves to injury. In: S McMahon, M Koltzenburg, I Tracey, D Turk, eds. *Wall & Melzack's Textbook of Pain*. 6th ed. Philadelphia, PA: Elsevier; 2013:861–888.
4. Gracely RH. Studies of pain in human subjects. In: S McMahon, M Koltzenburg, I Tracey, D Turk, eds. *Wall & Melzack's Textbook of Pain*. 6th ed. Philadelphia, PA: Elsevier; 2013:283–300.
5. Hurley RW, et al. Acute postoperative pain. In: M Gropper, L Eriksson, L Fleisher, J Wiener-Kronish, N Cohen, K Leslie, eds. *Miller's Anesthesia*. 9th ed. Philadelphia, PA: Elsevier; 2020:2614–2638.

# 208.

# PERIPHERAL NOCICEPTORS

*Richard Lennertz*

## INTRODUCTION

Nociceptors are afferent nerve fibers that encode painful stimuli. They generate action potentials in response to intense, noxious stimuli in a graded fashion. Action potential firing increases with the intensity of stimulation and correlates with the intensity of sensation in human studies. Nociceptors are pseudounipolar neurons. Their cell bodies reside in the dorsal root ganglia, sending one axon segment to the body and another to the dorsal horn of the spinal cord. While light-touch receptors may terminate in specialized

structures such as Pacinian corpuscles, nociceptors terminate as free nerve endings in the tissue. Some nociceptors respond to a wide range of touch, thermal, and chemical stimuli. Others respond to a single modality or may only respond to stimuli following tissue injury. These varied responses arise from a markedly heterogenous expression of ion channels and receptors. These ion channels produce "generator potentials" that depolarize the plasma membrane. Depolarizations that reach the "threshold potential" open voltage-gate sodium channels and initiate an action potential that travels along the axon to the spinal cord.

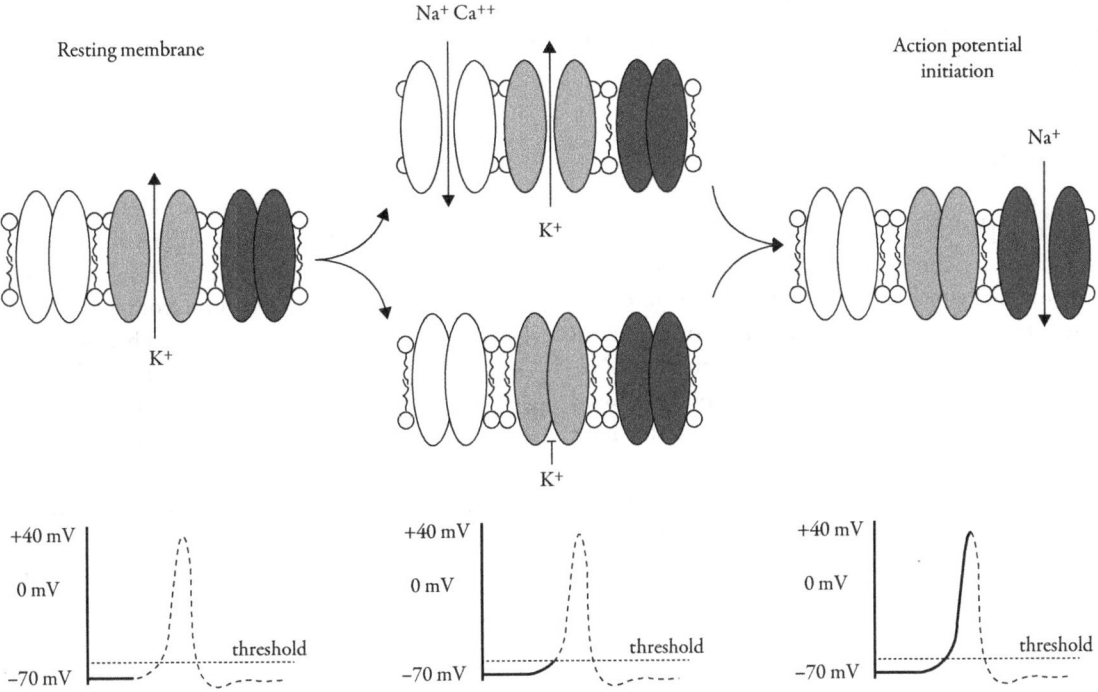

**Figure 208.1** Signal transduction leading to action potential generation. Potassium channel conductance maintains a hyperpolarized resting membrane potential (left). The opening of sodium and/or calcium channels (top arrow) or closing of potassium channels (bottom arrow) in response to a sensory stimulus depolarizes the plasma membrane (middle). If depolarization reaches a threshold potential, voltage-gated sodium channels open and initiate an action potential (right).

## CLASSIFICATION OF NOCICEPTORS

Nociceptors are classified according to their conduction velocity and response to physical stimuli. Unmyelinated nociceptors (C fibers) conduct action potentials more slowly than lightly myelinated nociceptors (A-delta fibers). Responses to mechanical, heat, and cold stimuli also differentiate nociceptors and provide insight into their function. Human studies correlate the activity of A-delta fibers with sharp pain. C fibers that are normally insensitive to mechanical stimuli become sensitive and contribute to the aching pain associated with tissue injury or sustained pressure. Although all C fibers were once considered to be nociceptors, primate and human studies have identified C fibers sensitive to light touch (but not heat) that do not appear to be nociceptors. Rather, these nerve fibers contribute to the sensation of pleasant touch and affiliative behavior.

Nociceptors can also be classified according to molecular markers. Peptidergic C fibers store and release neurohumoral peptides like substance P, calcitonin gene-related peptide (CGRP), and somatostatin. These peptides modulate the response to injury and inflammation. Both peptidergic and nonpeptidergic C fibers innervate the skin, but only peptidergic C fibers innervate muscle and viscera. These populations synapse onto separate layers of the spinal cord and signal to different regions of the brain. Many other molecular markers have been used to identify groups of nociceptors and assess their function.

## SIGNAL TRANSDUCTION

Action potential generation begins with the transduction of stimuli and depolarization of the plasma membrane. Research has identified ion channels that are sensitive to touch, thermal, and chemical stimuli. The transient receptor potential (TRP) family consists of nonspecific cation channels that respond to thermal and chemical stimuli. TRPV1 is activated by noxious heat, as well as the compound capsaicin found in spicy chili peppers. It is only expressed by nociceptors. Capsaicin creams reduce pain in some conditions by desensitizing nociceptors. The phosphorylation of TRPV1 by protein kinase C (PKC) may contribute to nociceptor sensitization during inflammation. The development of TRPV1 antagonists for analgesia has been hampered by side effects on thermoregulation. While TRPM8 responds to gentle cooling (and menthol), the mechanisms of noxious cold transduction remain elusive. The Piezo family consists of nonspecific cation channels that are sensitive to touch stimuli. The TRP and Piezo channels depolarize the plasma membrane by allowing the influx of sodium and calcium ions. However, the closure of potassium or chloride channels can also depolarize nociceptors (Figure 208.1).

## SIGNAL PROPAGATION

Depolarization of the plasma membrane must reach a certain threshold before the nerve fiber generates an action potential. Above the threshold potential, voltage-gated sodium channels ($Na_V$) open and generate an action potential that is propagated to the spinal cord. Some subtypes of $Na_V$ channels, such as $Na_V1.7$ and $Na_V1.8$, are highly expressed by nociceptors. $Na_V1.7$ gain-of-function mutations have been found in patients with erythromelalgia, and loss-of-function mutations have been found in some patients with congenital insensitivity to pain. $Na_V1.8$ channels are resistant to inactivation and allow nociceptors to convey pain signals at cold temperatures.

## SENSITIZATION

Many inflammatory mediators contribute to nociceptor sensitization. Hydrogen ions and ATP directly activate ligand-gated ion channels to depolarize the plasma membrane and increase intracellular calcium. Bradykinin, prostaglandins, and ATP activate G protein-coupled receptors (GPCRs). This leads to the production of second messenger molecules and the phosphorylation of ion channels (such as TRPV1) by protein kinases. Growth factors, cytokines, and chemokines also activate GPCRs on nociceptors or further stimulate the release of inflammatory mediators from immune cells. Nociceptor sensitization enhances their response to noxious stimuli, renders them responsive to less-intense stimuli, or leads to spontaneous activity.

## FATIGUE AND WIND-UP

Nociceptors themselves demonstrate fatigue, where prolonged stimuli elicit action potentials at a diminishing frequency. However, sustained input from nociceptors (0.5–5 Hz) elicits an increasing response from wide dynamic range neurons in the spinal cord. This phenomenon is called "wind-up" and results from the temporal summation of action potentials on the spinal neuron. As a result, sustained or repetitive stimuli may be perceived as increasingly painful. Wind-up typically occurs for the first seconds to minutes of a stimulus but contributes to long-term potentiation in spinal neurons and central sensitization. Of note, the perceptual correlate of wind-up is also referred to as "temporal summation."

## REFERENCES

1. Gold MS. Molecular biology of sensory transduction. In: S McMahon, M Koltzenburg, I Tracey, D Turk, eds. *Wall & Melzack's Textbook of Pain*. 6th ed. Philadelphia, PA: Elsevier; 2013:31–47.
2. Dawes JM et al. Inflammatory mediators and modulators of pain. In: S McMahon, M Koltzenburg, I Tracey, D Turk, eds. *Wall & Melzack's Textbook of Pain*. 6th ed. Philadelphia, PA: Elsevier; 2013:48–67.
3. Sandkühler J. Spinal cord plasticity and pain. In: S McMahon, M Koltzenburg, I Tracey, D Turk, eds. *Wall & Melzack's Textbook of Pain*. 6th ed. Philadelphia, PA: Elsevier; 2013:94–110.
4. Basbaum AI, et al. Cellular and molecular mechanisms of pain. *Cell*. 2009;139(2):267–284.

# 209.

# ASCENDING PATHWAYS AND DESCENDING INHIBITION

## *Richard Lennertz*

## INTRODUCTION

Multiple pathways carry pain signals from the body to the brain. Nociceptors convey pain signals to the dorsal horn of the spinal cord or sensory nuclei in the brainstem. Then, projection neurons carry pain (and temperature) information to the thalamus or brainstem nuclei. The thalamus largely receives discriminative information and communicates with the somatosensory cortex. The parabrachial nucleus (PB) receives affective information and communicates with limbic regions of the cortex. The rostral ventromedial medulla (RVM) and locus coeruleus (LC) also receive nociceptive input, and descending output from these areas strongly modulates nociceptive processing.

## SOMATIC AFFERENTS

Somatic pain from skin, muscle, and joints is well defined and localized. Unmyelinated nociceptors project to lamina I and II. Myelinated nociceptors project throughout lamina I–V (Figure 209.1, body). Somatic afferents innervate the spinal cord close to their spinal segment of entry. Somatotopy is maintained, as afferents from distal tissues project to the medial dorsal horn and proximal tissues project to the lateral dorsal horn. Trigeminal nociceptors have cell bodies that reside in the trigeminal ganglion and project to sensory nuclei in the medulla, particularly the trigeminal nucleus (Figure 209.1, head).

## VISCERAL AFFERENTS

Visceral pain is diffuse and strongly associated with the affective component of pain. Each organ receives innervation from two populations of nociceptors (Figure 209.1, viscera). Visceral afferents that follow the vagus nerve are sensitive to inflammatory mediators and noxious chemicals. The cell bodies of "vagal afferents" reside in the nodose and jugular ganglia. While most project to the solitary nucleus in the brainstem, a minority project to the upper cervical spinal cord and may contribute to somatic pain modulation. Visceral afferents that follow sympathetic nerves or parasympathetic nerves of the sacral plexus project to the spinal cord. These "spinal afferents" are sensitive to mechanical distention, ischemia, and inflammatory mediators. Their cell bodies reside in the dorsal root ganglia, and they project to lamina I, lamina II, lamina X, and the intermediolateral cell column in the dorsal horn. Visceral input spreads across multiple spinal levels and converges with somatic input onto second-order neurons in the dorsal horn. This physiology explains the diffuse nature of visceral pain and why visceral pain is often referred to other areas of the body.

## ASCENDING PATHWAYS

The spinothalamic tract (STT) is the dominant pathway for discriminatory pain, temperature, and itch sensation. Axons that form the STT cross midline within 1–2 spinal segments and ascend along the contralateral side of the spinal cord. Thus, lesions of the STT abolish pain and temperature sensation on the contralateral side of the body. Projection neurons from lamina I form the lateral portion of the STT, and projection neurons from lamina V and VII form the anterior portion (Figure 209.1, spinal cord). Caudal afferents within the lateral STT are organized lateral to rostral afferents. Projection neurons from sensory nuclei in the medulla form the trigeminothalamic tract. The trigeminothalamic tract crosses midline in the medulla and joins the anterior and lateral STT before synapsing in the thalamus. Ventral posterior nuclei of the thalamus relay signal to the primary and secondary somatosensory cortices (S1 and S2; Figure 209.1, cortex). These cortical areas interpret discriminatory components of pain such as location, modality, and intensity.

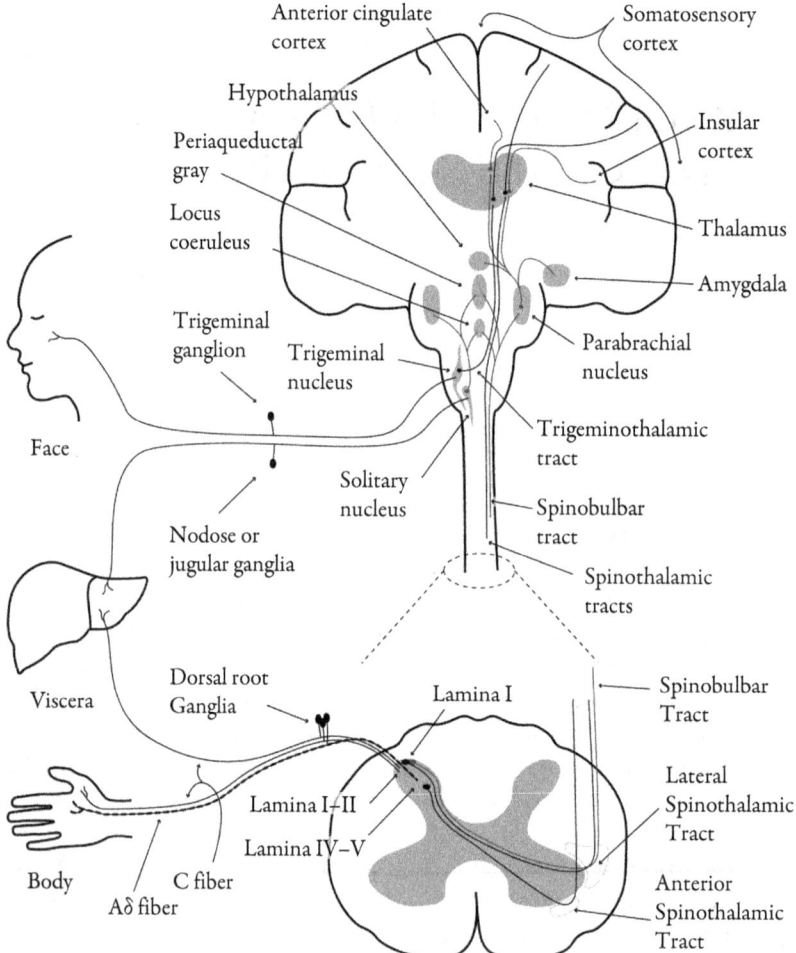

**Figure 209.1.** Ascending pain pathways. Nociceptors from the skin and some from the viscera project to the dorsal horn of the spinal cord. Nociceptors from the head project to the trigeminal nucleus. Some visceral nociceptors follow the vagus nerve and project to the solitary nucleus. Pain signals from the dorsal horn cross midline and form the contralateral spinothalamic and spinobulbar pathways. Pain signals from the trigeminal nucleus cross midline and form the contralateral trigeminothalamic tract. Pain signals from the solitary nucleus do not cross midline. The spinothalamic and trigeminothalamic pathways convey discriminatory pain signals to the somatosensory cortex. The spinobulbar pathway and solitary nucleus convey affective pain signals to multiple cortical regions. Spinal circuits, organization within cortical nuclei and cortical-cortical connections are generally not depicted.

The spinobulbar tract is the dominant pathway for affective pain and influences descending pain modulation. It ascends the spinal cord with the STT tract, but projects to separate regions: catecholamine cell groups in the ventrolateral medulla (including the locus coeruleus, LC), the parabrachial nucleus (PB), the periaqueductal gray (PAG), and the reticular formation. Input to the first three regions predominantly originates from projection neurons in lamina I. The PB nucleus projects to the hypothalamus, amygdala, and areas of the thalamus that relay to the insular, anterior cingulate, and prefrontal cortices (Figure 209.1, cortex). The catecholamine cell groups and PAG play important roles in descending pain modulation.

It is unclear whether a spinohypothalamic pathway exists in humans and contributes to affective pain.

## DESCENDING MODULATION

The PAG and the rostral ventromedial medulla (RVM) form a system that strongly modulates pain processing. The PAG projects to the RVM, particularly the nucleus raphe magnus, which projects to dorsal horn laminae that process nociceptive input (lamina I, II and V). Most projections from the RVM are gamma-aminobutyric acid (GABA)-ergic and some are serotonergic. Output from "ON-cells" in the RVM facilitates nociceptive signals, while output from "OFF-cells" inhibits them. An important mechanism of opioid analgesia is the inhibition of ON-cells and activation of OFF-cells. Serotonergic output from the RVM is not specifically associated with either ON- or OFF-cells and has mixed effects on pain processing in the dorsal horn. Both the PAG and RVM receive input from multiple areas of the cerebral cortex that are involved in emotional and autonomic regulation. Further, projections from the PAG to the thalamus and orbital frontal cortex may provide ascending modulation of pain signals.

The catecholamine cell groups (particularly the LC) also modulate pain processing. Noradrenergic output from the LC projects to the dorsal horn of the spinal cord. Noradrenergic input can either facilitate nociceptive signals via α-1 receptors or inhibit them via α-2 receptors. In the absence of injury, activation of the LC contributes to analgesia. Similarly, selective α-2 agonists produce analgesia via spinal α-2 receptors. Communication between the RVM and the LC appears to coordinate pain modulation.

## REFERENCES

1. Dostrovsky JO, Craig AD. Ascending projection systems. In: S McMahon, M Koltzenburg, I Tracey, D Turk, eds. *Wall & Melzack's Textbook of Pain*. 6th ed. Philadelphia, PA: Elsevier; 2013:182–197.
2. Apkarian AV, et al. Representation of pain in the brain. In: S McMahon, M Koltzenburg, I Tracey, D Turk, eds. *Wall & Melzack's Textbook of Pain*. 6th ed. Philadelphia, PA: Elsevier; 2013:111–128.
3. Heinricher MM, Fields HL. Central nervous system mechanisms of pain modulation. In: S McMahon, M Koltzenburg, I Tracey, D Turk, eds. *Wall & Melzack's Textbook of Pain*. 6th ed. Philadelphia, PA: Elsevier; 2013:129–142.
4. Villanueva L, Noseda R. Trigeminal mechanisms of nociception. In: S McMahon, M Koltzenburg, I Tracey, D Turk, eds. *Wall & Melzack's Textbook of Pain*. 6th ed. Philadelphia, PA: Elsevier; 2013:793–802.
5. Bielefeldt K, Gebhart GF. Visceral pain: Basic mechanisms. In: S McMahon, M Koltzenburg, I Tracey, D Turk, eds. *Wall & Melzack's Textbook of Pain*. 6th ed. Philadelphia, PA: Elsevier; 2013:703–717.

# Part XV

# RESPIRATORY SYSTEM PHYSIOLOGY

# 210.

# LUNG FUNCTIONS, CELLULAR PROCESSES, AND SURFACTANT

*Harsh Nathani and Antony Joseph*

## LUNG FUNCTIONS

The lungs are the foundational organs of the respiratory system—the primary function of which is to facilitate gas exchange from the environment into the bloodstream. The mechanics of the respiratory system allow for oxygen to be brought in through the upper airways, where it is humidified and warmed, through the bronchial tree into the alveoli. The alveoli are the primary site for gas exchange via diffusion where oxygen enters the bloodstream and carbon dioxide is eliminated.[1]

The lungs also have several nonrespiratory functions. The respiratory epithelium is lined with cilia which rhythmically carry mucus produced by goblet cells upward and expel bacterial and dust particles from within the airways. This mucociliary clearance is a significant barrier to airborne infections. Furthermore, the epithelial lining also contains immunoglobulin A, which also protects against respiratory pathogens. Within the lung there are also macrophages which engulf and destroy debris and pathogens via phagocytosis, and dendritic cells which help present antigens to the adaptive immune system cells.

The lung also has a role in maintaining homeostasis regulation of blood pressure as part of the renin-angiotensin system by catalyzing the conversion of angiotensin I to angiotensin II via ACE (angiotensin-converting enzyme), maintaining acid-base homeostasis by expelling carbon dioxide. They also play a role in the excretion of several endogenous and exogenous substances—prostaglandins, leukotrienes, serotonin, bradykinin, and drugs such as local anesthetics, propofol, opioids, and neuromuscular blocking agents. The lungs also are capable of filtering out particulate matter from the bloodstream, such as small clots and fibrin clumps, as they are a rich source of fibrinolysin activator and endogenous heparin and thromboplastin.[2]

## CELLULAR PROCESSES AND SURFACTANT

There are several cell lines present in the respiratory system. The lining of the respiratory tract from the trachea to the alveolar sacs consists of an epithelial lining made of primarily three cells: goblet cells, which secrete mucus; basal cells, which differentiate into other epithelial cells; and cilia cells, which are a significant component of the mucociliary escalator. The epithelium of the alveoli consists of the type 1 and type 2 pneumocytes. Type 1 pneumocytes make up much of the surface area of lungs and are the primary site of gas exchange. Type 2 pneumocytes secrete surfactant and play a role in acting as progenitor cells to replace damaged type 1 pneumocytes.[3]

## SURFACTANT

Surfactant is a complex mixture with unique phospholipid and protein composition that serves to reduce the surface tension of the alveoli, which reduces the propensity of the alveoli to collapse during expiration as per Laplace's law. Surfactant also increases pulmonary compliance and facilitates recruitment of collapsed airways. Surfactant is manufactured within the type 2 pneumocytes and is stored in lamellar bodies, which can first be appreciated at approximately 24 weeks gestational age of a fetus. Surfactant deficiency, whether through inadequate production or inactivation, has an important role in several respiratory diseases, especially in the neonatal population.[4]

Laplace law: $P \propto 2T/r$
P = alveolar membrane pressure
T = surface tension
R = alveolar radius

Suprfactant is also an opsonic agent that aids marchophages with the phagocytosis of *Staphylococcus aureus*.

## REFERENCES

1. Aung H, et al. An overview of the anatomy and physiology of the lung. In: *Nanotechnology-Based Targeted Drug Delivery Systems for Lung Cancer*. 2019:1–20.

2. Joseph D, et al. Non-respiratory functions of the lung. *Cont Educ Anaesth Crit Care Pain*. 2013;13(3):98–102.
3. Hogan B, Tata P. Cellular organization and biology of the respiratory system. *Nat Cell Biol*. 2019. doi:10.1038/s41556-019-0357-7
4. Chakraborty M, Kotecha S. Pulmonary surfactant in newborn infants and children. *Breathe*. 2013;9(6):476–488.

# 211.

# LUNG VOLUMES AND CAPACITY

*Muhammad Fayyaz Ahmed and Furqan Ahmed*

## INTRODUCTION

Lung volumes are vital parameters in clinical medicine since many physiological and pathological factors can change them. Lung capacities are a sum of two or more lung volumes. A spirometer is used to measure lung volumes by asking the person to breathe in and out, and measuring the displacement of the ball in the calibrated cylinder. Lung volumes are classified into static and dynamic lung volumes, depending on how the breaths are measured in a spirometer. Slow breaths measure static lung volumes, whereas fast breaths measure dynamic lung volumes.[1,2]

## STATIC LUNG VOLUMES

### TIDAL VOLUME (TV)

Tidal volume is the volume of air that moves into or out of the lungs with each resting inspiration or expiration, respectively. The average volume in a healthy adult is 500 ml.

### INSPIRATORY RESERVE VOLUME (IRV)

This is the volume of air that moves in the lungs when a person takes a maximal inspiration after a normal inspiration. The average volume in a healthy adult is 3000 mL.

## EXPIRATORY RESERVE VOLUME (ERV)

ERV is the volume of air that moves out of the lungs when a person takes a maximal expiration after a normal expiration. The average volume in a healthy adult is 1200 ml.

## RESIDUAL VOLUME (RV)

This is the volume of air remaining in the lungs after a maximal expiration. The average volume in a healthy adult is 1200 ml. Out of the four volumes, RV cannot be measured directly by spirometry since residual air does not move in or out of the spirometer. However, it can be measured indirectly by calculating the difference between functional residual capacity and expiratory reserve volume.

## INSPIRATORY CAPACITY (IC)

IC is the amount of air that moves in the lungs when a person takes a maximal inspiration after a normal expiration. It is the sum of TV (500 ml) and IRV (3500 ml). In a healthy adult, this is approximately 3500 ml.

## FUNCTIONAL RESIDUAL CAPACITY (FRC)

FRC is the amount of air remaining in the lungs after a normal expiration. It is the sum of ERV (1200 ml) and RV (1200 ml). Typically, it is around 2400 ml. FRC is the point at which the inward forces of the lung balance the outward forces of the chest wall without any involvement of respiratory muscles, and the respiratory system is in equilibrium. Since no respiratory muscle is involved, the intrinsic elastic properties of lung and chest wall determine the FRC. Many physiological and pathological factors can affect FRC. It increases with height, upright position, age, and obstructive lung disease. It decreases in obesity, female sex, pregnancy, supine position, restrictive lung disease, and diaphragmatic paralysis. As mentioned, RV cannot be measured directly with spirometry; thus FRC cannot be measured directly as well. Instead, methods such as body plethysmography, helium dilution, and nitrogen washout are used to measure FRC.[3]

## VITAL CAPACITY (VC)

VC is the amount of air that can be expired after a maximal inspiration. It is the sum of IC (3500 ml) and ERV (1200 ml). Typically, it is around 4700 ml.

## TOTAL LUNG CAPACITY (TLC)

Total amount of air in the lungs after a maximal inspiration. It is the sum of FRC (2400 ml) and IC (3500 ml). Typically, it is around 5900 ml.

## CLOSING CAPACITY (CC)

CC is the amount of air in the lungs at a point when the small airways start collapsing during expiration. It is the sum of residual volume and closing volume. In a healthy adult, the FRC is greater than CC; however, when the FRC decreases, the small airways close at the end of normal expiration, leading to atelectasis, hypoxemia, and V/Q mismatch.

## CLOSING VOLUME (CV)

This is the lung volume at which the small airways close. It is the difference between CC and RV. The lung volumes and capacities are summarized in Figure 211.1.

## DYNAMIC LUNG VOLUMES

### FORCED VITAL CAPACITY (FVC)

FVC is the amount of air that can be rapidly and forcibly expired after a maximal inspiration.

### FORCED EXPIRATORY VOLUME IN 1 SECOND (FEV1)

FEV1 is the volume of air that can be rapidly and forcibly exhaled in 1 second after a maximal inspiration.

Pathological conditions can affect the dynamic lung volumes, and changes can indicate lung disease. Specifically, the ratio of FEV1 to the FVC (FEV1/FVC) is an important indication of lung function. Normal ratio is 80% or greater. A ratio of <70% indicates an obstructive lesion such as asthma, chronic bronchitis, emphysema, and bronchiectasis.[2]

## ANESTHETIC CONSIDERATIONS

- The recommended TV intraoperatively in an average healthy adult is around 6–8 cc/kg of ideal body weight.
- Preoxygenating a patient before induction of general anesthesia is vital in every patient to gain safe apnea time for intubation. The idea is to denitrogenate the FRC and replace it with oxygen. In a healthy average adult, the

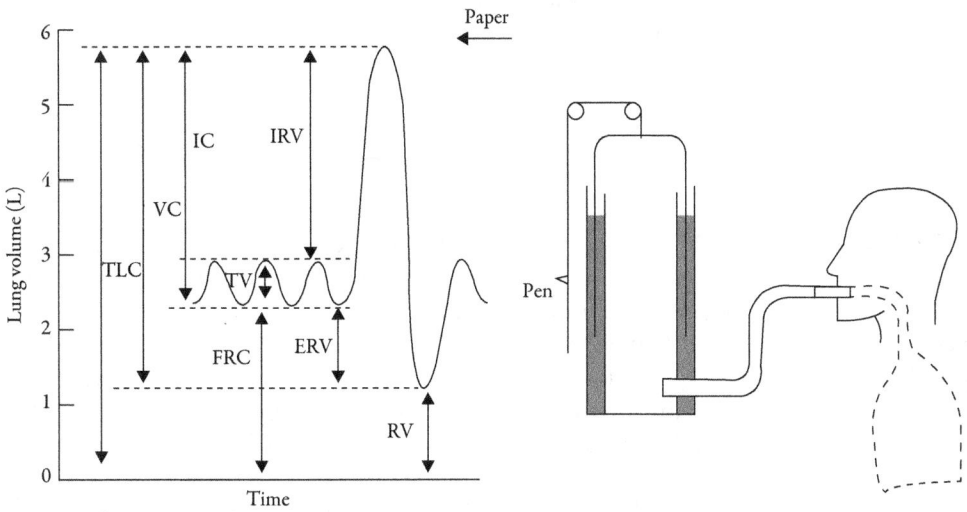

**Figure 211.1.** Lung volumes and capacities with spirometry.
Reproduced with permission from Feher J, *Quantitative Human Physiology*, Academic Press, 2017.

classic 3 minutes of preoxygenation are sufficient for an apnea time ($SpO_2$ >90%) of around 10 minutes.[5]
- In patients with lower lung volumes, positive end-expiratory pressure (PEEP) raises FRC above CC, decreasing intrapulmonary shunting and improving oxygenation.
- Obese patients present with restrictive pattern on spirometry, the FVC and FEV1 are decreased, but the FEV1/FVC ratio is preserved. The adipose tissue of the abdomen pushes the diaphragm cephalad, leading to a decrease in ERV more than RV and FRC. IRV increases in obesity. Therefore the TLC is either the same or mildly reduced. The fat content around the chest wall can cause significant reduction in chest wall compliance and can also cause mild reduction in lung compliance. During anesthesia of an obese patient, the FRC decreases significantly.
- In older patients, the elasticity of the lungs is lost, leading to increased lung compliance. On the contrary, the compliance of the chest wall decreases due to chest wall stiffness. Therefore, the net pulmonary compliance is unchanged. Geriatric patients also have increased alveolar and anatomic dead space, leading to increased

ventilation-perfusion mismatch. VC is decreased due to higher RV. IRV and ERV are decreased as well. CC is greater relative to the volume of lungs.
- In pregnancy, FRC decreases due to the gravid uterus displacing diaphragm cephalad. This also leads to decreased TLC and ERV. On the other hand, to fulfill the patient's and fetus's oxygen requirement, the TV and minute ventilation increase.

## REFERENCES

1. Kavanagh BP, Hedenstierna G. Respiratory physiology and pathophysiology. In Miller, RD, ed. *Miller's Anesthesia*. 8th ed. New York, NY: Elsevier/Churchill Livingstone; 2015:444–472.
2. Lutfi MF. The physiological basis and clinical significance of lung volume measurements. *Multidiscip Respir Med*. 2017;12(article number: 3).
3. Respiratory physiology and anesthesia. In: Butterworth IV JF, et al., eds. *Morgan & Mikhail's Clinical Anesthesiology*. 6th ed. New York, NY: McGraw-Hill; 2018:495–534.
4. Feher J. Lung volumes and airway resistance. In Feher J, *Quantitative Human Physiology*. 2nd ed. London: Academic Press, 2017:633–641.
5. Bouroche G, Bourgain JL. Preoxygenation and general anesthesia: A review. *Minerva Anestesiol*. 2015;81(8):910–920.

# 212.

# PULMONARY FUNCTION TESTS AND SPIROMETRY

*Vasu Sidagam*

## INTRODUCTION

The major types of pulmonary function tests (PFTs) are spirometry, spirometry before and after bronchodilators, lung volumes, and quantitation of diffusing capacity for carbon monoxide (DLCO). Measurement of maximal respiratory pressures and flow volume loops are useful in specific clinical conditions.

Spirometry measures the volume of air exhaled at specific time points during a forceful and complete exhalation after a maximal inhalation. The total exhaled volume, known as the

forced vital capacity (FVC), the volume exhaled in the first second, known as the forced expiratory volume in one second ($FEV_1$), and their ratio ($FEV_1$/FVC) are noted. "Predicted values" are determined by published studies of large numbers of healthy individuals. Lung volume measurements include vital capacity (VC), total lung capacity (TLC), functional residual capacity (FRC), and residual volume (RV).

In a patient with airway obstruction, an increase in the $FEV_1$ >12% and >200 ml is diagnostic of asthma. In chronic obstructive pulmonary disease (COPD), administration of bronchodilator sometimes leads to a significant change in

FEV₁, but reversal to normal spirometry rules out a diagnosis of COPD.[1] The peak expiratory flow (PEF, also known as a peak flow or peak flow rate) is the maximal rate that a person can exhale during a short maximal expiratory effort after a full inspiration. PEF is measured with a peak flow meter, although it can also be measured during spirometry. This measurement is useful in monitoring asthma symptoms. Normal values for PEF depend on sex, age, and height, similar to spirometric values. PEF is usually expressed as L/min.

For suspected respiratory muscle weakness, spirometry is obtained with the patient supine and sitting. Diaphragmatic weakness is suggested by a decrease in the supine VC >10%. Unilateral diaphragmatic paralysis may be associated with a decrease in VC of 15%–25%; bilateral diaphragmatic paralysis may be associated with a decrease in supine VC approaching 50%.

VC and TLC are the key lung volumes for determining restriction, defined as VC and TLC values <80% of those predicted; a reduced VC alone is not sufficient evidence of restriction because it can be caused by air trapping due to severe obstruction.[1] When flow rates during inspiration are added to these flow volume curves, "flow volumes loops" are obtained (Figures 212.1, 212.2, and 212.3).

In obstructive lung disease, the FEV₁/FVC ratio is <70%. If a patient has airway obstruction, FEV₁/FVC ratio is not useful for gauging the severity of disease, since the FVC also tends to decrease with increasing obstruction. The FEV₁, not the FEV₁/FVC ratio, should be used to monitor patients with asthma or COPD.

Air trapping is indicated when the FRC or RV is increased >120% of predicted; hyperinflation is indicated when the TLC is increased >120% of predicted. An elevation in TLC is suggestive of COPD. An improvement greater than 10% in FEV₁ after the use of bronchodilators indicates reversibility.

The effect of obesity on PFTs is reduction of FRC and expiratory reserve volume (ERV). FEV1 and FVC may be slightly reduced, but the ratio is usually preserved.

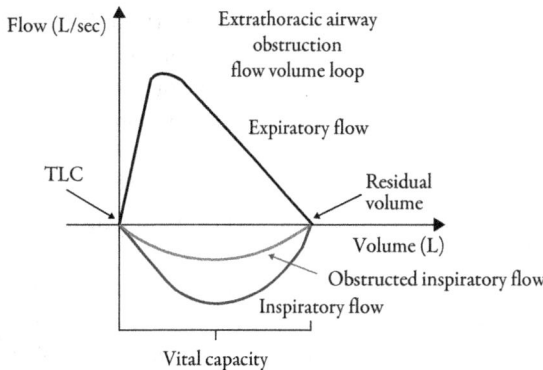

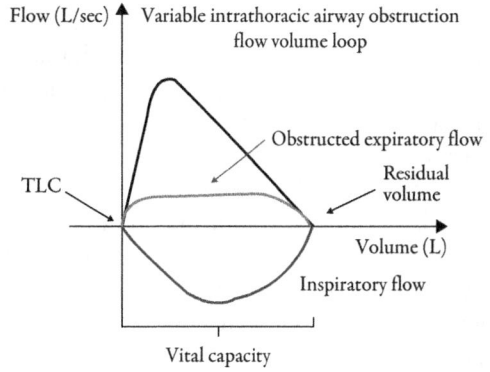

Figure 212.2. Flow volume loops in obstructive pathologies.

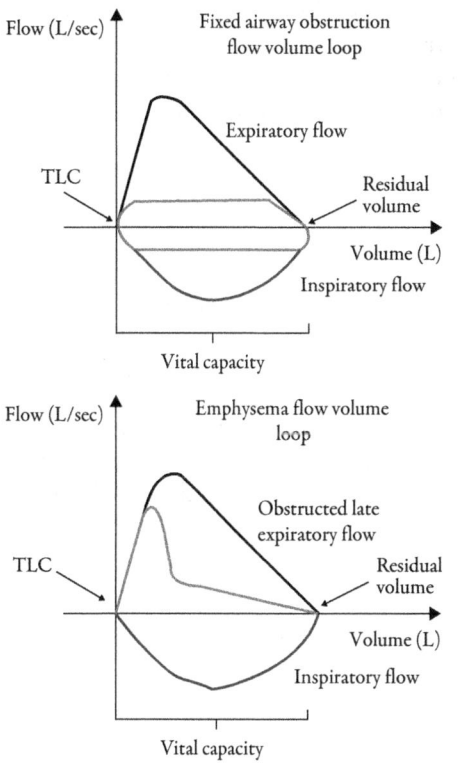

Figure 212.3. Flow volume loops in obstructive pathologies.

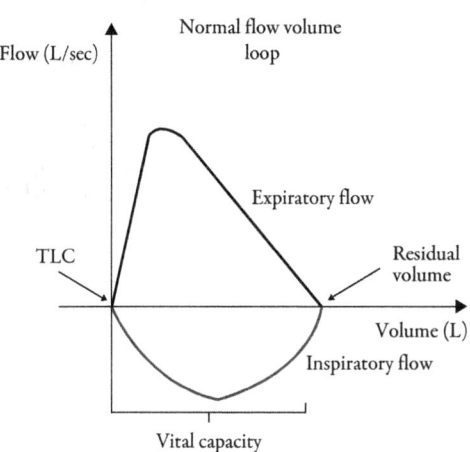

Figure 212.1. Normal flow volume loops.

Measurement of maximal inspiratory and expiratory pressures is indicated whenever respiratory muscle weakness is suspected clinically. Maximal expiratory pressure (MEP) is the maximal pressure measured during forced expiration after a full inhalation (TLC). Repeated measurements of maximal inspiratory pressure (MIP) and MEP are useful in following the course of patients with neuromuscular disorders.

Measurement of the single-breath diffusing capacity for carbon monoxide (DLCO, also known as transfer factor or TLCO) is used in the evaluation of restrictive and obstructive lung disease, as well as pulmonary vascular disease.

In restrictive disease, DLCO helps distinguish between intrinsic lung disease, in which DLCO is reduced, and other causes of restriction, like chest wall disease in which it is usually normal. Causes of high DLCO include supine position, exercise, fever, asthma, following bronchodilators, high altitude, polycythemia, alveolar hemorrhage, etc.[3] Causes of low DLCO include emphysema, anemia, post–lung resection, interstitial lung disease, sarcoidosis, pulmonary hypertension or acute PE, elevated carboxy hemoglobin.

The gold standard for measurement of TLC is body plethysmography.

Age-related changes include loss of elasticity, causing over-distension of alveoli. Closing capacity increases due to closure of small airways at normal tidal volumes. Dead space (both anatomical and physiological) is increased and chest wall rigidity also is increased. Those tests require the patient to perform at maximum effort. Forced expiratory flow from 75% to 25% of VC ($FEF_{25-75}$) is another spirography measurement that is less effort dependent.

In the maximum voluntary ventilation (MVV) test, the patient will breathe as quickly and deeply as possible through a pneumotachograph for 12 seconds. The exhaled volume is measured and multiplied by 5 to yield the maximal ventilation during 1 minute.

## ANESTHETIC CONSIDERATIONS

### PREOPERATIVE

In asthma, the risk of intraoperative bronchospasm is higher with upper abdominal surgery and proximity to recent asthma attack.[2] In COPD, PFTs do not reliably predict risk of postoperative pulmonary complications.[2] Patients with predicted postoperative (PPO) FEV1 and PPO DLCO >60% predicted do not need further testing and can undergo lobectomy or pneumonectomy without resulting in significant residual lung dysfunction.[3] In patients considered for lung resection surgery (PPO), FEV1 and PPO DLCO are the most important predictors of postoperative pulmonary complications.[3] In patients with anterior mediastinal masses, flow volume loops are helpful but unreliable.

### Diagnostic Modality of Choice Is CT Chest

Pregnancy, large intra-abdominal mass, and ascites impose a restrictive defect on PFTs. In morbid obesity the overall PFT pattern is of a restrictive nature.

### INTRAOPERATIVE

During spinal and epidural anesthesia, the relationship between closing capacity and FRC is unchanged.[2]

FRC of an obese patient under anesthesia decreases by 50% compared to 20% in a non-obese patient.[2]

In COPD patients with increased TLC, the goal of mechanical ventilation is to avoid dynamic hyperinflation and prevent development of auto-PEEP. This happens when positive pressure ventilation is applied and insufficient expiration time is allowed.[2]

Ketamine is the preferred induction drug in a hemodynamically unstable patient with asthma. Propofol is often used for hemodynamically stable patients.[2]

### POSTOPERATIVE

In COPD patients, lung regions with normal V/Q ratios can be replaced by atelectasis as a result of slow absorption of gas behind occluded airways, causing hypoxemia.[2]

## REFERENCES

1. Pellegrino R, et al. Interpretative strategies for lung function tests *Eur Respir J*. 2005;26(5):948.
2. Tao J, Kurup V. *Steolting's Anesthesia and Co-existing Disease*. 7th ed. 2018:15–32.
3. Brunelli A, Kim A. Diagnosis and Management of Lung Cancer, 3rd edition: ACCP guidelines. *Chest*. 2013;143(5)(Suppl):e166s–e190s.

# 213.

# STATIC, DYNAMIC COMPLIANCE AND AIRWAY RESISTANCE

*Ezra Shapiro and Ettore Crimi*

## INTRODUCTION

Physiologic work of breathing includes the inspiratory work to overcome both elastic and frictional forces. Elastic recoil is the natural tendency of the lungs to collapse and can be expressed in terms of elastance or its reciprocal, compliance. Frictional forces, also defined as non-elastic resistance, include the resistance to air flow of the conductive airways and the viscous tissue resistance of the lung and chest wall.[1,2]

## COMPLIANCE

*Compliance* is defined as the change in volume (V) per unit of pressure (P) change:

$$C = \Delta V/\Delta P$$

It is the inverse of *elastance*, defined as the ability of an elastic structure to return to its original form after being stretched by an external force. Compliance is a measure of lung distensibility. A stiff lung has low compliance and opposes to expansion with minimal volume changes despite a large change in pressure. The total compliance of the respiratory system is the sum of lung and chest wall compliance:

$$1/\text{Total Compliance} = 1/\text{Lung Compliance} + 1/\text{Chest Wall Compliance}$$

Lung compliance is calculated from changes in transpulmonary pressure (alveolar pressure − pleural pressure), primarily determined by the elastic recoil of the lung tissue. Chest wall compliance is calculated from changes in transpleural pressure (pleural pressure − atmospheric pressure), primarily determined by the elastic recoil of the chest wall. Normal total compliance is 100 ml/cmH$_2$O and decreases to 50–100 ml/cmH$_2$O in mechanically ventilated patients.[1]

Compliance can be static or dynamic. *Static compliance* is the compliance measured under static (zero flow) condition. Static compliance is a true measure of the distensibility of the respiratory system because at zero, flow changes in pressure are the result of changes in elastic recoil lung and chest wall without any influence of airway resistance. Static compliance can be calculated during mechanical ventilation at the end of inspiratory pause, assuming a full muscle relaxation, as:

$$\text{Cstat} = \text{Vt}/(\text{Pplateau} - \text{PEEP})$$

where Cstat is static compliance, Vt is tidal volume, Pplateau is plateau airway pressure, and PEEP is positive end-expiratory pressure[3] (Figure 213.1).

*Dynamic compliance* is the compliance measured during air flow and reflects the resistive and elastic properties of the respiratory system. While static compliance represents lung distensibility, dynamic compliance reflects both compliance and resistance. Dynamic compliance decreases when either lung stiffness or airway resistance increases. During mechanical ventilation, dynamic compliance is calculated as:

$$\text{Cdyn} = \text{Vt}/(\text{Ppeak} - \text{PEEP})$$

where Cdyn is dynamic compliance, Vt is tidal volume, Ppeak is plateau airway pressure, and PEEP is positive end-expiratory pressure[3] (Figure 213.1).

## CLINICAL IMPLICATIONS

Normal lung compliance is decreased in pulmonary edema, pneumothorax, atelectasis, fibrosis, pneumonectomy, and mainstem intubation. It is increased in emphysema. Chest wall compliance is decreased by abdominal distention, thoracic deformities, and by an increased muscle tone, as seen in patient-ventilator dyssynchrony.

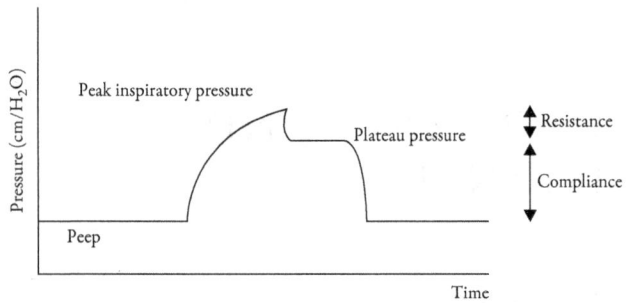

**Figure 213.1.** Airway pressure waveform analysis in mechanically ventilated patient can help in identifying changes in lung compliance and resistance.

Most pulmonary disorders reduce static compliance. In interstitial fibrosis, the excess of collagen deposition increases stiffness and decreases compliance. Pulmonary edema leads to a decreased lung compliance due to an alteration in surfactant properties. Furthermore, inappropriately high tidal volumes cause a decrease in static compliance secondary to overdistention.

A decrease of both static and dynamic compliance can be seen in pulmonary edema, consolidation, atelectasis, pleural effusion, and pneumothorax. An isolated decrease in the dynamic compliance with unchanged static compliance suggests an increase in airway resistance (e.g., bronchospasm, tube obstruction, mucous plug), when the gradient of the peak and plateau pressures is greater than 10.[4]

## RESISTANCE

Resistance is the pressure difference per unit rate of flow as per equation:

$$R = \Delta P / V$$

where R is resistance, ΔP is change in pressure, and V is the flow.

Resistance results from the friction of moving structures. Frictional forces, also called non-elastic resistance, are the second component of the total impedance to gas flow and include the resistance to air flow of the conductive airways, the viscous tissue resistance of the lung and chest wall, and the inertia of both gas and tissue. Resistance of the conductive airways is the most important factor.[2]

Gas flow in the respiratory tract is a function of pressure difference and resistance and can be laminar, turbulent, or mixed. Turbulent flow is related to gas density. Under ideal conditions, laminar flow in the airway is regulated by Hagen-Poiseuille's equation and is related to viscosity. From this equation, resistance can be expressed as:

$$R = 8 \times length \times viscosity / \pi \times (radius)^4$$

The radius is the most powerful determinant of airway resistance. If the radius is halved, the resistance increases 16-fold. Conductive airways greater than 2 mm in diameter are the major contributor of the resistance. Normal airway resistance is between 0.6 and 2.4 cmH$_2$O/L/sec. In intubated patient, airway resistance can increase up to 6 cmH$_2$O/L/sec depending on the endotracheal tube size: the smaller the internal diameter, the greater the resistance to flow.

In mechanically ventilated patients, airway resistance can be calculated from the airway pressure waveform using an end inspiratory airway occlusion (Figure 213.1), as per equation:[5]

$$Raw = Ppeak - Pplateau / V$$

## CLINICAL IMPLICATIONS

Any factor that decreases the radius of the airway increases airway resistance: bronchospasm, secretions, mucosal edema, foreign body in the respiratory tract, obstruction of the endotracheal tube. In patients with epiglottitis and airway obstruction, a combination of helium and oxygen can be used. This mixture of 80% helium and 20% oxygen is less viscous than air and decreases airway resistance.

## REFERENCES

1. Lumb AB, Thomas C. Elastic forces and lung volumes In: *Nunn's Applied Respiratory Physiology*. 9th ed. Editor: Elsevier; 2021:14–26.
2. Lumb AB, Thomas C. Respiratory system resistance. In: *Nunn's Applied Respiratory Physiology*. 9th ed. Editor: Elsevier 2021: 27–41.
3. Crimi E, et al. Bedside interpretation of ventilatory waveforms In: *Critical Care*. 5th ed. Editors: Wolters Kluver. Layon AJ. 2018: 1343–1356.
4. Bigatello L, Pesenti A. Respiratory physiology for the anesthesiologist. *Anesthesiology*. 2019;130:1064–1077.
5. Hess DR. Respiratory mechanics in mechanically ventilated patients. *Respir Care*. 2014;59:1773–1794.

# 214.

# PLEURAL PRESSURE GRADIENT, LAPLACE'S LAW, SURFACTANT, HYSTERESIS, AND FLOW-VOLUME LOOPS

*Ba Hoang Nguyen Pham and Jason Bang*

## PLEURAL PRESSURE GRADIENT

Inspiration and expiration are dependent on the pressure gradients exist between the atmosphere and the thoracic cavity. There are 4 basic thoracic pressures and 3 main pressure gradients that are involved in the breathing process. The thoracic pressures are:

- $P_m$ = mouth pressure or $P_{aw}$ = airway pressure
- $P_{alv}$ = alveolar pressure
- $P_{pl}$ = pleural pressure
- $P_{bs}$ = body surface pressure.

By convention, $P_m$ or $P_{aw}$ will be equal to the pressure of the outside atmosphere and is set at 0 (1 atmosphere) unless there is positive pressure applied. $P_{pl}$ is the negative pressure (relative to atmospheric pressure) that exists within the pleural cavity. It is generated by the opposing forces of the lungs and the chest wall. The value of $P_{pl}$ is usually around –5 cm $H_2O$ at functional residual capacity (FRC), although there are also variations between the lung zones, with highest or least negative in inferior parts and lowest or most negative in superior parts. $P_{alv}$ varies during the breathing cycle with the expansion and contraction of the thoracic cavity. $P_{bs}$ is generally at 0, equal to the atmospheric pressure.

The 3 main pressure gradients are:

- Transrespiratory pressure or transairway pressure
- Transpulmonary pressure
- Transthoracic pressure.

*Transrespiratory* or *transairway pressure gradient* are interchangeable terms and are the difference between $P_m$/$P_{aw}$ and $P_{alv}$.[1] It is the driving force for the movement of air during respiration. The transpulmonary pressure is obtained by subtracting $P_{alv}$ from $P_{pl}$. It is the gradient that keeps the lungs and alveoli opened. If transpulmonary pressure is negative (e.g., pneumothorax, $P_{pl}$ >0), there is a net force inward that makes the lung collapse. Transthoracic pressure is the gradient pressure between $P_{bs}$ and $P_{pl}$. It represents the pressure needed to expand or contract the lungs and the chest wall.

## LAPLACE'S LAW

Surface tension of the alveolus is the result of the attraction forces between the gas and the thin liquid layer lining the alveolus. It promotes the collapse of the alveolus. Laplace's law indicates that for an alveolus to remain open, there is certain pressure required which is directly proportional to the surface tension and inversely proportional to the radius of the alveolus. It is presented as:

$$P = 2T/r$$

where P is pressure, T is surface tension, and r is radius of the spherical alveolus.

According to Laplace's law, if the radius of an alveolus is small, the pressure within it will be higher than that of an alveolus with a larger radius. Therefore, when the two alveoli are connected, air from the smaller alveolus will move into the larger alveolus, further collapsing the smaller one.

## SURFACTANT

Surfactant is molecule synthesized by type II alveolar cells. It helps prevent the collapse of smaller alveolus into a larger one by disrupting the intermolecular forces between the liquid-gas interface, hence lowering the surface tension. In larger alveoli, the concentration of surfactant is diluted in comparison with the concentration in the smaller alveoli, which leads to the balancing of the surface tension forces. It is composed of approximately 80% phospholipids, 10% protein, and 10% neutral lipids.[2] The primary active component found in surfactant is the phospholipid, which mainly

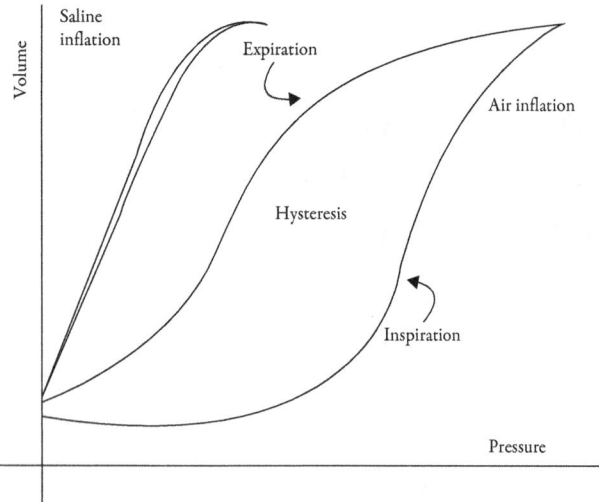

**Figure 214.1.** Static lung compliance volume-pressure graph.

consists of dipalmitoyl phosphatidylcholine (lecithin). In the fetus, surfactant can be synthesized as early as in week 24, and fully presents by week 34.[2] A lecithin:sphingomyelin ratio obtained from the amniotic fluid can be used to assess fetal lung function, with ratio greater than 2:1 indicating adequate lung maturity. The decrease in surfactant functioning level is associated with certain diseases like infant respiratory distress syndrome, adult respiratory distress syndrome, and chronic lung pathologies.

## HYSTERESIS

On a pressure-volume curve, there is a difference between inspiratory and expiratory compliance curve such that at any given pressure, lung volume during deflation will have a larger value than during inflation. This phenomenon is call hysteresis, where the energy invested during inspiration

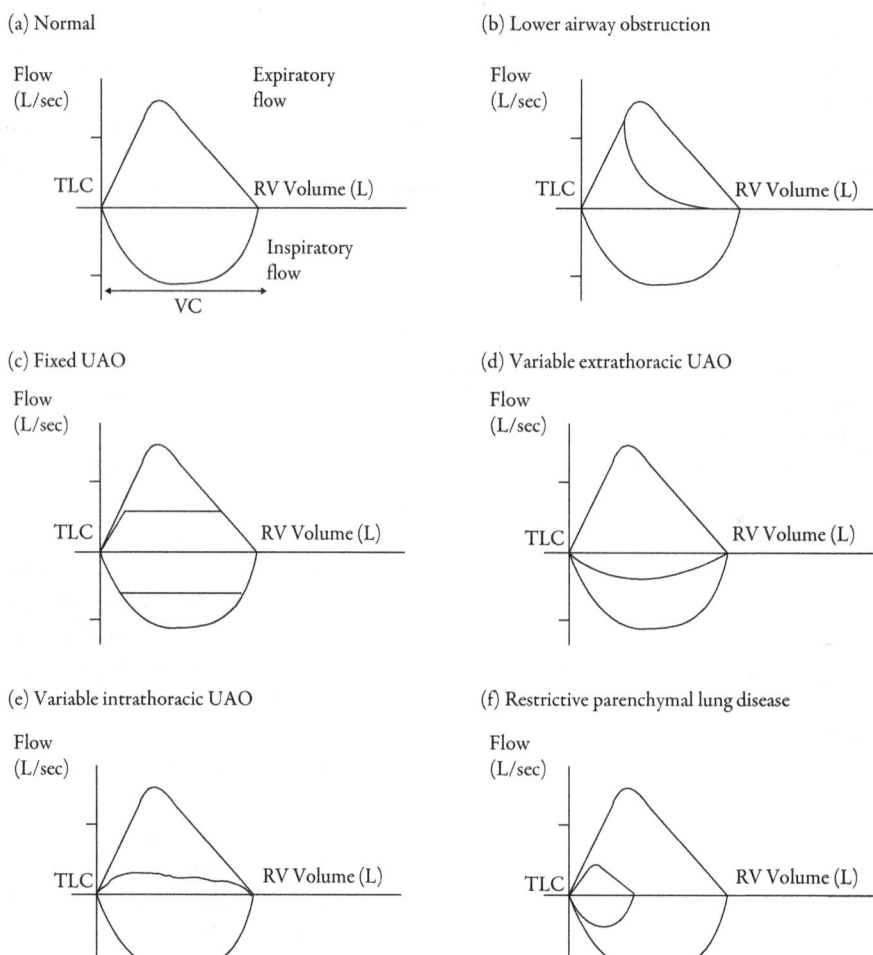

**Figure 214.2.** Flow-volume loops.

is not recovered in expiration.[3] Hysteresis presents in both static and dynamic compliance curves. In dynamic lung compliance curve, it is because airway resistance is proportional to flow rate. In static compliance curve, it is mainly due to the surface tension of the alveoli. This can be demonstrated through the saline-filled lungs and normal (air-filled) lungs experiment. On the pressure-volume graph, the saline-filled lungs will have almost identical inspiration and expiration curve due to no surface tension, while hysteresis is present in the compliance curve of the air-filled lungs (Figure 214.1).[4]

## FLOW-VOLUME LOOPS

The flow-volume loop is a plot recoded using a spirometer when the patient is asked to perform maximum force inhalation to total lung capacity, then forcibly and rapidly exhale to residual volume. The changes in the contour of the loop in comparison with the normal plot can help in the diagnosis of certain airway obstruction as well as lung-restrictive diseases (Figure 214.2). Although it is a valuable tool, the test is insensitive and heavily depends on the patient's effort.

- Lower airway obstruction (e.g., COPD, asthma): characterized by an effort-independent portion of the expiration curve that becomes concave;

- Variable intrathoracic obstruction (e.g., intrathoracic tracheomalacia, tumors): characterized by flattening of the expiratory curve;
- Variable extrathoracic obstruction (e.g., vocal fold paralysis, extrathoracic tracheomalacia, tumors): characterized by flattening of the inspiratory curve, the opposite to intrathoracic obstruction;
- Fixed upper airway obstruction (e.g., tracheal stenosis, goiter): characterized by peak limited and flattening of the inspiratory and expiratory flow rates;
- Restrictive lung disease (e.g., interstitial lung disease): characterized by a normal shape curve but diminished in size.

## REFERENCES

1. Wolfe D, Sorbello J. *Comparison of Published Pressure Gradient Symbols and Equations in Mechanics of Breathing*. [online] American Association for Respiratory Care. 2020. Available at: <http://rc.rcjournal.com/content/51/12/1450>.
2. Nkadi PO, et al. An overview of pulmonary surfactant in the neonate: Genetics, metabolism, and the role of surfactant in health and disease. *Mol Genet Metab*. 2009;97(2):95–101.
3. Escolar JD, Escolar A. Lung hysteresis: A morphological view. *Histol Histopathol*. 2004;19(1):159–166.
4. Harris RS. Pressure-volume curves of the respiratory system. *Respir Care*. 2005;50(1):78–99.

# 215.

# WORK OF BREATHING

*Ba Hoang Nguyen Pham and Jason Bang*

## INTRODUCTION

*Work of breathing* is defined as the energy spent to move air in and out of the lung during inspiration and expiration, respectively. During unassisted breathing, respiration has an active inspiratory and a passive expiratory phase. In the active phase, the inspiratory muscles (e.g., diaphragm and external intercostal muscles) work to overcome the elastic

forces of lung tissues that keep the lungs from expanding, and the frictional forces which hinder the movement of air into the tubular system of the lungs, whereas expiration is a passive process that utilizes the stored potential energy from the expanded lungs and the chest wall. During forced breathing, the accessory muscles of inspiration (e.g., scalene, sternocleidomastoid muscles) and the expiratory muscles (e.g., internal intercostal and abdominal muscles) are employed to help with the increased work of breathing.

The work of breathing is normally measured in Joules (J), while the power of breathing, which also takes into account the respiratory rate and flow rate, is expressed in Joules/min or Watts. At rest, work of breathing is around 0.35 J for a healthy person, and the power of breathing is about 2.4 J/min.[1] Even though during normal respiration, tidal breathing only uses less than 2% of the total basal metabolic oxygen consumption, it is not a very efficient process, as most of the energy spent is used generating heat. Certain conditions, such as obesity, congestive heart failure, or lung diseases, can significantly increase the work of breathing, and potentially lead to failure of extubation from excessive and nonsustainable work of breathing.[2] Ishaaya et al.[2] have demonstrated that work of breathing is higher immediately after extubation in comparison to breathing spontaneously through an endotracheal tube.

## DETERMINING THE WORK OF BREATHING

In the physics world, work is the product of force and displacement:

$$Work = force \times distance$$

where force = pressure × area; and distance = volume/area. Hence the work of breathing can be formulated as:

$$Work\ of\ breathing = pressure \times volume.$$

Campbell diagrams can be used to demonstrate the dynamic relationship between pleural pressure and lung volume during breathing.[3] The work of breathing is measured by finding the area on the pressure-volume curve:

Work of breathing can be broken down into elastic work (from lung and chest wall compliance) and resistive work (airway and tissue resistance). The elastic work done to inflate the lungs from functional residual capacity (FRC) with tidal volume is the area of the triangle shown in Figure 215.1. It is calculated by subtracting the area found under the lung compliance curve from the area under the chest wall compliance curve, as some of the work is done by the elastic recoil of the ribcage.

The inspiratory resistive work area in Figure 215.1 covers the work done to overcome both the airway and tissue resistance, as well as the resistance from external apparatus (e.g., ventilatory circuit, endotracheal tube). The expiratory resistive work is spent from the stored elastic potential energy during inspiration and embedded in the elastic inspiratory work of breathing area.

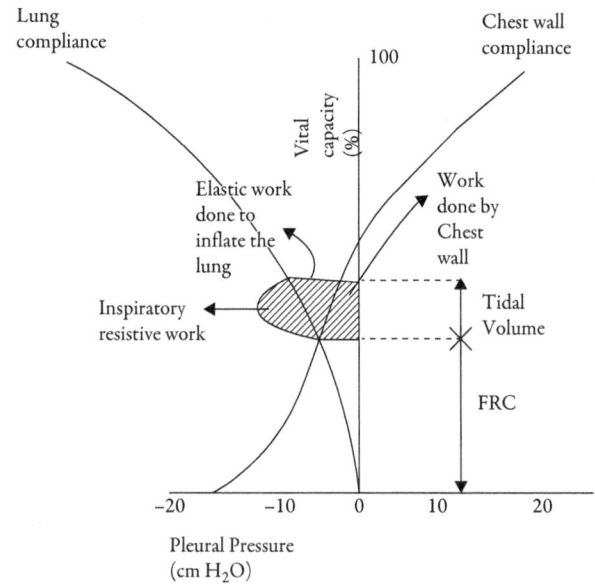

**Figure 215.1.** Pressure-volume graph.

In the clinical setting, to measure the work of breathing, esophageal pressure is measured and used as a substitution for the pleural pressure, and the slope of the chest wall compliance curve used is a theoretical value instead of a true measured value.[4]

## IMPROVING THE WORK OF BREATHING

In general, work of breathing is increased when there is an increase of resistive work, or a reduction of lung/thorax compliance. To minimize the resistive work, certain things can be done, such as:

- Decrease respiratory rate; as it is proportional to the flow rate, a decrease will in turn decrease the airway resistance.
- Increase laminar flow. This can be achieved by reducing the gas density, hence lowering the Reynolds number (an index to determine whether the flow is laminar or turbulent). Heliox, a mixture of helium and oxygen that is less dense than air, can be used with the goal of reducing airway resistance. It has been shown to help with decreasing the work of breathing in obstructive airway diseases like asthma or chronic obstructive pulmonary disease (COPD).[5]
- Increase airway radius with bronchodilators.

To help in reducing the elastic work:

- Increase positive end-expiratory pressure (PEEP) to maximize opened alveoli that can be ventilated.

• Optimize lung/tidal volume; when volume increases, elastic work also increases.

## REFERENCES

1. Mancebo J, et al. Comparative effects of pressure support ventilation and intermittent positive pressure breathing (IPPB) in nonintubated healthy subjects. *Eur Respir J.* 1995;8(11):1901–1909.
2. Ishaaya A, et al. Work of breathing after extubation. *Chest.* 1995;107(1):204–209.
3. Banner M, Jaeger M, Kirby R. Components of the work of breathing and implications for monitoring ventilator-dependent patients. *Crit Care Med.* 1994;22(3):515–523.
4. Cabello B, Mancebo J. Work of breathing. *Intens Care Med.* 2006;32(9):1311–1314.
5. Barnett T. 1967. Effects of helium and oxygen mixtures on pulmonary mechanics during airway constriction. *J Appl Physiol.* 1967;22(4):707–713.

# 216.

# REGULATION OF AIRWAY CALIBER

*Vadzim Lapkouski and Tatiana Jamroz*

## INTRODUCTION

In healthy humans, respiratory resistance is controlled by changing the airway caliber, mostly in small airways and bronchioles. This change is expected to alter only the airway component of respiratory resistance, but some studies show that contraction of bronchial smooth muscle also causes changes in tissue resistance. Interdependence exists between the airway diameter and lung tissue parenchyma in a way that airway constriction distorts the surrounding elastic tissue, altering its viscoelastic properties. Caliber of the airway may be reduced by either physical compression (leading to airway collapse) or by constriction of the bronchial muscle in the airway wall.[1]

## MUSCULAR CONTROL OF AIRWAY DIAMETER

Small airway dysfunction is one of the most important causes of obstruction in multiple pathological conditions.[1] The following 4 mechanisms are responsible for controlling muscle tone in small bronchi and bronchioles:

1. Neural pathway
2. Humoral (via blood) control
3. Direct physical and chemical effects
4. Local cellular mechanisms.

Even though they may be considered as discrete factors, there is considerable interaction between them, particularly in pathological states. Neural pathways are the most important ones in normal lung, with direct stimulation and humoral control being involved in some circumstances. Cellular mechanisms, particularly mast cells, are important in airway disease but have minimal influence under normal conditions.

## NEURAL PATHWAYS

Autonomic nerves mediate both contractions and relaxations of airway smooth muscle. Cholinergic-parasympathetic nerves mediate contractions, whereas adrenergic-sympathetic and/or noncholinergic parasympathetic nerves mediate relaxations. Sympathetic-adrenergic innervation of human airway smooth muscle is minimal or nonexistent, based on histological analyses, and plays little or no role in regulating airway caliber. It is interesting that in humans and in many other mammals, postganglionic noncholinergic parasympathetic nerves provide the only relaxant innervation of airway smooth muscle.[2]

## Parasympathetic System

This system is of major importance in the control of bronchomotor tone, and when activated can completely obliterate the lumen of small airways. Both afferent and efferent fibers travel in the vagus nerve, with efferent ganglia in the walls of small bronchi. Afferents start from receptors under the tight junctions of the bronchial epithelium and respond either to noxious stimuli acting directly on the receptors or from cytokines released by cellular mechanisms such as mast cell degranulation. Efferent nerves release acetylcholine, which acts at $M_3$ muscarinic receptors, causing contraction of bronchial smooth muscle, while also stimulating $M_2$ prejunctional receptors, leading to negative feedback on acetylcholine release. Bronchoconstriction is a result of stimulation of any part of the reflex arc. Resting tone is normally present to some extent and therefore may permit some degree of bronchodilation when vagal tone is reduced. With the reflex being not just a simple monosynaptic reflex, there is considerable central nervous system modulation of the response. Therefore, the brain itself plays a potentially significant role in controlling the degree of airway hyperresponsiveness in lung disease.

## Sympathetic System

In contrast to the parasympathetic system, the sympathetic system is poorly represented in the lung and has not yet proven to be of major importance in humans. Indeed, it is unlikely that there is any direct sympathetic innervation of the airway smooth muscle, although there may be a possible inhibitory effect on cholinergic neurotransmission.

## Noncholinergic Parasympathetic Nerves

The airways are provided with another autonomic control which is neither adrenergic nor cholinergic. This is the only potential bronchodilator nervous pathway in humans, although the exact role of these nerves is still unclear. The efferents supplied by the vagus nerve reach to the smooth muscle of the airway, where they cause slow (several minutes) and prolonged relaxation of bronchi. The neurotransmitter is vasoactive intestinal peptide (VIP), and it produces airway smooth muscle relaxation via enhancing production of nitric oxide (NO). Relaxation of the smooth muscle in the airway brought about by NO is not as well understood as its effect on vascular smooth muscle. It looks like NO has its effect even without crossing the cell membrane by some form of cell-surface interaction that activates guanylate cyclase to produce a second messenger (cyclic guanosine monophosphate) and following muscle relaxation. Interestingly, resting airway tone does involve bronchodilation by NO, but its mechanism is not clear.

## HUMORAL CONTROL

Even though sympathetic innervation is of a minimal significance on bronchial smooth muscle, there are a lot of β-2 adrenergic receptors responding to circulating

*Table 216.1* MEDIATORS INVOLVED IN ALTERATION OF BRONCHIAL SMOOTH MUSCLE TONE DURING AIRWAY INFLAMMATION

| SOURCE | BRONCHOCONSTRICTION | | BRONCHODILATATION | |
| | MEDIATOR | RECEPTOR | MEDIATOR | RECEPTOR |
| --- | --- | --- | --- | --- |
| Mast cells and other proinflammatory cells | Histamine | H1 | Prostaglandin E2 | EP |
| | Prostaglandin D2 | TP | Prostacyclin (PGI2) | EP |
| | Prostaglandin F2a | TP | | |
| | Leukotrienes C4 D4 E2 | CysLT1 | | |
| | PAF | PAF | | |
| C-fibers | Bradykinin | B2 | | |
| | Substance P | NK2 | | |
| | Neurokinin A | NK2 | | |
| | CGRP | CGRP | | |
| Endothelial and epithelial cells | Endothelin | ET b | | |

PAF: platelet-activating factor; CGRP: calcitonin gene-related peptide.

Reprinted with permission from Lumb AB, *Nunn's Applied Respiratory Physiology*. Elsevier; 2017:33–50.

adrenaline, and once again acting via complex second-messenger systems. It looks like basal levels of adrenaline do not contribute to bronchial muscle tone, but this mechanism plays an important role during exercise or sympathetic "stress response." Alpha-adrenergic receptors, which stimulation of may cause bronchoconstriction, are present in small amounts and are unlikely to be of clinical significance.

## PHYSICAL AND CHEMICAL EFFECTS

Direct stimulation of the airway's epithelium produces the parasympathetic reflex which causes bronchoconstriction. Physical factors involved in this response include mechanical stimulation of the upper airways during laryngoscopy and the presence of foreign bodies in the trachea or bronchi. Inhalation of particulate matter, an aerosol of water, or just cold air may also lead to bronchoconstriction, the latter being used as a simple provocation test. Many chemical substances may cause bronchospasm, including liquids with low pH such as gastric acid and gases such as ammonia, ozone, and nitrogen dioxide.

## LOCAL CELLULAR MECHANISMS

Lungs contain a variety of inflammatory cells, such as mast cells, macrophages, lymphocytes, eosinophils, and neutrophils, which play a crucial role in infection and inflammation. Different pathogens may stimulate these inflammatory cells, but some may also be activated by the previously mentioned direct physical factors. Having been activated, cytokine production causes amplification of the response, and it leads to a variety of mediators being released, resulting in bronchoconstriction (as shown in Table 216.1). Many of these substances are produced in healthy individuals, but patients with airway pathology are usually "hyper-responsive," putting them at increased risk for developing symptoms of bronchospasm.

## REFERENCES

1. Lumb AB. *Nunn's Applied Respiratory Physiology*. Edinburgh, New York: Elsevier; 2017:33–50.
2. Canning BJ. Reflex regulation of airway smooth muscle tone. *J Appl Physiol*. 2006;101:971–985.

# 217.

# VENTILATION/PERFUSION

*Andrea Farela and Tatiana Jamroz*

## INTRODUCTION

*Ventilation* can be defined as the exchange of gas between the atmosphere and the lungs through inspiration and expiration.

*Pulmonary perfusion* is the amount of blood that flows through the lung. The lung is unique in that it has a dual supply: pulmonary and bronchial circulation. The pulmonary circulation is responsible for delivering deoxygenated blood from the right ventricle to the gas-exchanging units within the lung, where oxygen crosses the alveolar and capillary endothelium into the red blood cells, and carbon

dioxide crosses from blood to the alveolus to return oxygenated blood into the left atrium for systemic distribution.[1,2]

Both of these—ventilation and pulmonary perfusion—are essential components of the normal function of the lung, but it is their ratio (V/Q) that determines adequate gas exchange[2] (Figure 217.1).

## CLINICAL SIGNIFICANCE

In a normal individual, the overall alveolar ventilation at rest is ~4L/min, and pulmonary blood flow is ~5L/min,

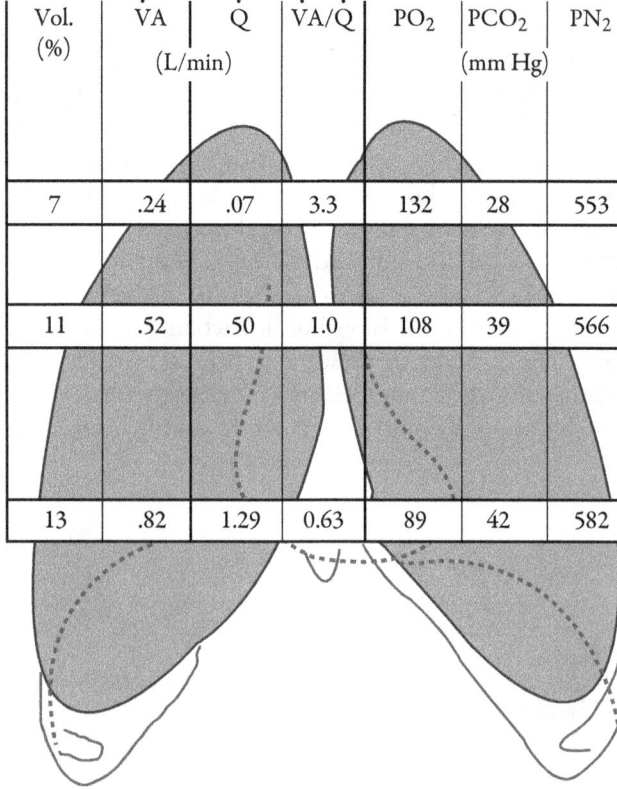

| Vol. (%) | V̇A (L/min) | Q̇ | V̇A/Q̇ | PO$_2$ | PCO$_2$ (mm Hg) | PN$_2$ |
|---|---|---|---|---|---|---|
| 7 | .24 | .07 | 3.3 | 132 | 28 | 553 |
| 11 | .52 | .50 | 1.0 | 108 | 39 | 566 |
| 13 | .82 | 1.29 | 0.63 | 89 | 42 | 582 |

**Figure 217.1.** Ventilation-perfusion ratio (V̇a /Q̇) and the regional composition of alveolar gas. Values for regional flow (Q̇), ventilation (V̇a), partial pressure of oxygen (P o $_2$), and partial pressure of carbon dioxide (P co $_2$) were derived from Fig. 217.2. Partial pressure of nitrogen (P n $_2$) represents what remains from total gas pressure (760 mm Hg including water vapor, which equals 47 mm Hg). The percentage volumes (Vol.) of the three lung slices are also shown. When compared with the top of the lung, the bottom of the lung has a low V̇a /Q̇ ratio and is relatively hypoxic and hypercapnic.

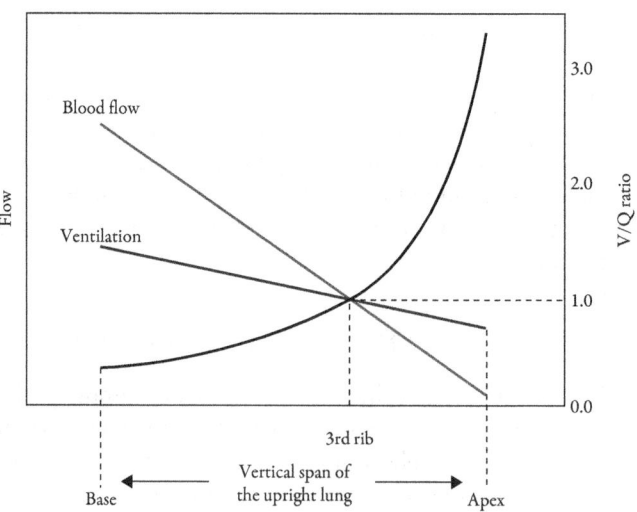

**Figure 217.2.** Distribution of ventilation and blood flow (left vertical axis) and the ventilation-perfusion ratio (V̇a /Q̇, right vertical axis) in normal upright lung. Both blood flow and ventilation are expressed in liters per minute per percentage of alveolar volume and have been drawn as smoothed-out linear functions of vertical height. The closed circles mark the V̇a /Q̇ ratios of horizontal lung slices (three of which are shown in Fig. 217.1). A cardiac output of 6 L/min and a total minute ventilation of 5.1 L/min were assumed.

Reprinted from Wilson WC, Benumof JL. Physiology of the Airway. In: Hagberg and Benumof's Airway Management, 5, 110–115. e4, (2018), with permission from Elsevier.

making the global ventilation/perfusion ratio ~0.8. This ratio is composed of a wide range of V/Q ratios across the lung that originate from the differences in ventilation and perfusion from the apex toward the base of the lung. The ideal V/Q ratio of 1 is believed to occur at the level of the third rib[1] (see Figure 217.2).[3]

Ventilation increase toward the base is slower compared to perfusion increase; therefore V/Q ratio at the apex of the lung will be higher than 1 (increased ventilation relative to blood flow), whereas at the base will be lower (increased blood flow relative to ventilation).

There are 4 main mechanisms for arterial hypoxemia, ventilation-perfusion mismatching being the most common in patients with respiratory system pathology.

Ventilation/perfusion mismatch occurs when compensatory mechanisms fail to be enough to maintain the balance of gas exchange during pathological states that cause increase of either dead space ventilation or shunt fraction.[1]

Such compensatory mechanisms are hypoxic pulmonary vasoconstriction and bronchiolar constriction. Hypoxic pulmonary vasoconstriction diverts blood flow from poorly ventilated to better ventilated areas of the lung, thereby decreasing the shunt fraction, whereas bronchiolar constriction decreases dead space ventilation.[1,4]

And thus, even though total alveolar ventilation might remain normal, it is unevenly distributed between the gas exchange units. The contribution of each of these units to the arterial blood is what will determine the actual PaO$_2$ and PaCO$_2$ values. An alveolar-arterial oxygen gradient will be observed secondary to the incomplete compensation between a relatively over-ventilated and an under-ventilated unit.

O$_2$ compensation is more difficult than CO$_2$ compensation, given the plateau on the upper portion of the oxyhemoglobin dissociation-curve. Hemoglobin is almost 100% saturated in over-ventilated areas; therefore the contribution of increased ventilation on oxygen content in blood will be minimal compared to changes in alveolar oxygen content.

On the other hand, CO$_2$ moves by diffusion, so as long as a gradient is maintained, this diffusion will continue to occur.[4]

Physiological dead space is constituted by anatomical and alveolar dead space.

Approximately 2 ml/kg Ideal body weight (IBW) is anatomic dead space ventilation, and it represents the ventilation of the airway portion that does not participate in gas change, this being from the oronaso-pharynx to the terminal and respiratory bronchioles. Anything that causes changes to the length of this area, such as endotracheal tubes, ventilator tubing between tracheal tube and Y-piece, or tracheostomy, causes alterations in anatomical dead space.[1]

Alveolar dead space occurs when there is ventilation of areas with poor or no perfusion.

During pathological states, the influence of disease over anatomic dead space is minimal; therefore alveolar dead space becomes the major determinant of overall physiologic dead space.[1,2]

This explains how a sudden drop in cardiac output is the primary cause of an acute increase of physiological dead space, since a drop in cardiac output will acutely decrease pulmonary blood flow, which means low perfusion in comparison to ventilation. Clinically, this can be observed during positive-pressure ventilation or positive airway therapy that diminishes venous return, which in turn causes a decrease in cardiac output and blood flow through the pulmonary vessels. Even though ventilation is improved with the positive pressure, there is a drop in perfusion, causing an increase in alveolar dead space. One way of avoiding or correcting this is by administration of intravenous fluid to maintain adequate venous return.

Physiological dead space remains usually a constant fraction of the tidal volume over a wide range of tidal volumes; therefore it is generally more useful to use the Dead space/Tidal volume $(V_D/V_T)$ ratio to describe it.

The Bohr equation is widely accepted as the definition of the physiological dead space:

$$V_D / V_T = (PaCO_2 - PACO_2 / PaCO_2)$$

or a modification of it where $PACO_2$ is substituted by $P\bar{E}CO_2$, which is the mixture of all expired gases measured over a period of time.

During spontaneous breathing $V_D/V_T$ IS 0.2–0.4, and 0.5 during positive pressure ventilation.

$V_D$ is increased with loss of perfusion to ventilated alveoli, increased airway pressure, extended neck, erect posture, rapid short inspirations, and increased age. $V_D$ is decreased with tracheostomy.

A typical example of pathology causing V/Q mismatch secondary to increased dead space is pulmonary embolism, regardless of etiology (thrombotic, fat, air, or amniotic). There are two important recognized mechanisms for the decrease in pulmonary blood flow in this state: (1) direct obstruction to blood flow, and (2) vasoconstriction induced by vasoactive substances like leukotrienes.

Acute lobar atelectasis, extensive acute lung injury, pulmonary edema and pneumonia are pathologic states that increase shunt fraction and therefore cause V/Q mismatch.[1]

Physiological shunt is caused by venous drainage of the myocardial (thebesian) and bronchial veins into the left side of the heart, and usually constitutes about 2%–3% of the cardiac output. In pathological states of complete cessation of ventilation in a region (due to atelectasis or consolidation, for example), shunt may range from 2% to 50% of the cardiac output. Low V/Q should not be confused with shunt. While shunt occurs when V/Q equals zero, there are 2 important differences between shunt and low V/Q:

1. Regions with low V/Q may present with narrowing airways and vasculature, which will reduce ventilation and blood flow in some regions and increase in others.
2. Increased $FiO_2$ will improve hypoxemia caused by low V/Q, but will have no effect on hypoxemia caused by shunt.[5]

## REFERENCES

1. Barash PG, et al. *Clinical Anesthesia.* 8th ed. Philadelphia, PA: Wolters Kluwer; 2017:15:372–376.
2. Cloutier MM. *Respiratory Physiology.* 2nd ed. Philadelphia, PA: Elsevier; 2019:7:90–98.
3. Hagberg CA. *Hagberg and Bernumof's Airway Management.* 4th ed. Philadelphia, PA: Elsevier; 2018:5:110–115.
4. Pardo M. *Basics of Anesthesia.* Philadelphia, PA: Elsevier; 2018:5:57–65.
5. Gropper, M. *Miller's Anesthesia.* 9th ed. Philadelphia, PA: Elsevier; 2020:13:354–383.

# 218.

# DISTRIBUTION OF VENTILATION

*Monnica Morales and Tatiana Jamroz*

## INTRODUCTION

To discuss how ventilation is distributed in the lung, we must first discuss compliance and pressure-volume relationships between the lung and chest wall.

At rest, lung and chest wall relationships are such that pressure in the pleural space (PPL) is negative because of the opposing forces of lung tissue favoring collapse and the chest wall trying to expand. This equilibrium state is *functional residual capacity* (FRC), the volume of air left in the lungs after normal expiration. Pressure inside the airways (PA) at this point equals atmospheric pressure at 0. The net pressure across the lungs (the airways and that of the pleural space) is termed *transpulmonary pressure* (PTP) (see Figure 218.1).

$$PTP = PA - PPL$$

As the diaphragm contracts during inspiration, pleural space pressures become more negative until the airway pressure becomes less than atmospheric pressure, favoring the passage of air into the lungs. When the alveoli fill sufficiently to where alveolar pressure equals atmospheric pressure (0), inspiration ends and no more movement of air occurs. It should be noted that when the alveoli are filled to their limit, they become less compliant and stiffer (it would require a greater change in pressure to achieve more volume). As the diaphragm relaxes, pleural pressures become less negative and alveolar pressures increase to greater than atmospheric pressure, favoring movement of air out of the lungs until equilibrium with atmospheric pressure occurs once again. This returns the lung to FRC and ends the respiratory cycle.[1] The change in volume over change in transpulmonary pressures that occurs is the lung's compliance. *Compliance* is defined as the amount of distension

(volume change) we can achieve for a given change in pressure.

Pleural pressure differences, termed *pleural pressure gradients*, exist in the lung due to a variety of reasons. These include gravity, density of the lung tissue (which can change in disease states, e.g., edema), compression from surrounding structures (the heart, abdominal organs causing cephalad displacement of the diaphragm in a supine patient), and the shape of the lung in the thorax favoring compression of tissues at the base; therefore, ventilation is also distributed differently.

## ANESTHETIC CONSIDERATIONS

In the upright position, gravity, lung tissue density, and shape favor expansion of the alveoli at the apex of the lung rather than the base. Pleural pressures are thus less negative at the base than at the apex. This makes alveoli at the base more compliant; they will see a greater change in volume for a change in pressure when the lungs fill with air. Both ventilation and perfusion are greater at gravity-dependent areas.[2] Therefore, distribution of ventilation will change with body position. During general anesthesia in a supine patient, the loss of muscle tone leads to loss of chest wall expansive forces and increase in airway pressures due to muscle relaxation. This ultimately leads to atelectasis, most pronounced in dependent areas, leading to the overall decrease in FRC and lung compliance known to occur in anesthetized patients. In the prone position, the shape of the lung in the thorax and decreased compression from surrounding structures (e.g., the heart) favors expansion of dorsal lung regions and more homogenous distribution of inspired gases than a patient would have in the supine position.[3]

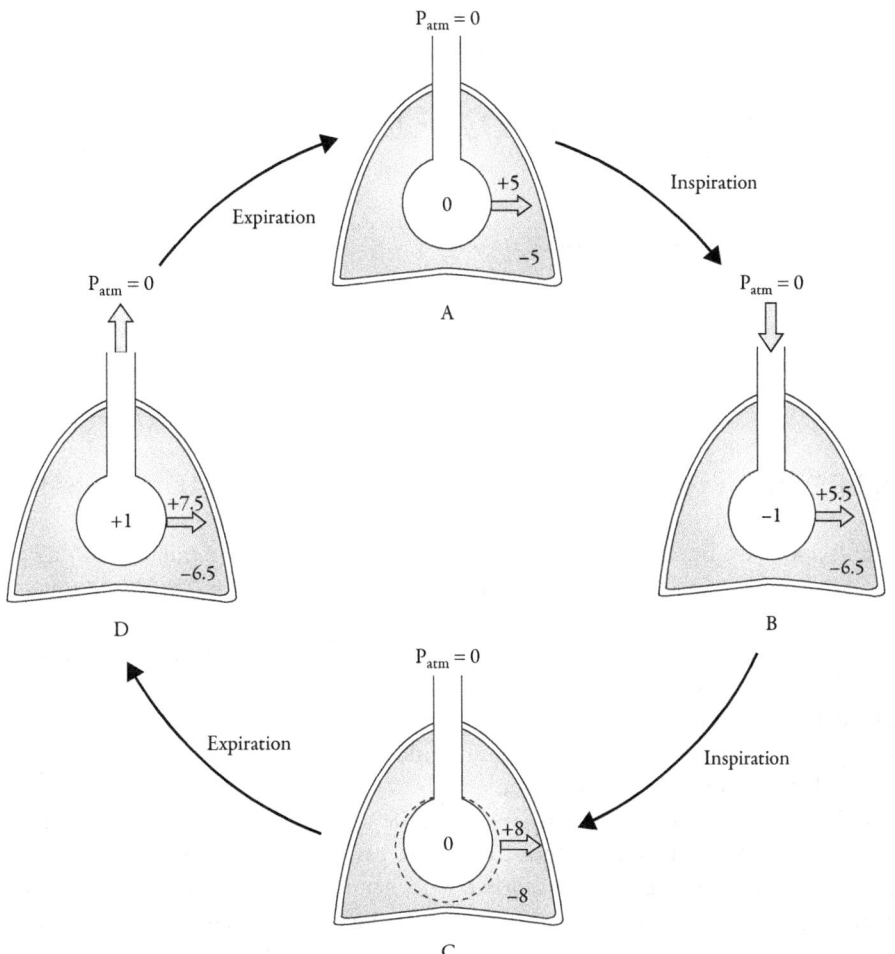

**Figure 218.1.** Pressures during normal breathing cycle. The numbers give pressures in cm $H_2O$ relative to atmospheric pressure ($P_{atm}$). The numbers over the *yellow arrows* give the magnitude of transmural pressures. The *wide blue arrows* show air flow into and out of the lungs. **A**, Rest; **B**, halfway through inspiration; **C**, end of inspiration; **D**, halfway through expiration.

# REFERENCES

1. Costanzo LS. Respiratory physiology. In: Linda S. Costanzo, ed. *Physiology*. 6th ed. Philadelphia, PA: Elsevier; 2018:189–243.
2. Barash PG. Ventilation and perfusion. In: Paul G. Barash, ed. *Clinical Anesthesia Fundamentals*. Philadelphia, PA: Wolters Kluwer Medical; 2015:27–31.
3. Gropper MA, et al. Respiratory physiology and pathophysiology. In: Michael A. Gropper, ed. *Miller's Anesthesia*. 9th ed. Philadelphia, PA: Elsevier; 2020:354–383.

# 219.

# DISTRIBUTION OF PERFUSION

*Gloria Rodriguez and Tatiana Jamroz*

## INTRODUCTION

The pulmonary circulation can be characterized as a low-pressure system when compared to the systemic circulation. This low vascular resistance results in a pulsatile flow through the capillaries. This lower vascular resistance also allows the existence of thinner capillaries and alveolar walls that facilitate the diffusion of gas exchange. Acute increases in pulmonary vascular pressures can lead to leaking of fluid into the alveoli, whereas slower increases stimulate vascular remodeling, which can lead to pulmonary hypertension.

The distribution of blood flow in the lungs is not uniform; for example, due to the effects of gravity and other factors, the bases of the lungs are better perfused as compared to the apices.

Based on the effects of gravity and alveolar expansion, the distribution of blood flow to the lungs can be divided into four different zones. These are so-called *West lung zones* (Figure 219.1). These zones are divided based on the principle that perfusion of the alveolus depends on the pressures in the pulmonary arteries ($P_{PA}$), pulmonary veins ($P_{PV}$) and alveolus ($P_{ALV}$).

- In zone I, $P_{ALV}>P_{PA}>P_{PV}$; this results in little to no perfusion, only ventilation, thus little gas exchange occurs. Zone I conditions are most likely to be seen during positive pressure ventilation or hemorrhagic shock.
- In zone II, $P_{PA}>P_{ALV}>P_{PV}$; perfusion occurs when $P_{PA}$ exceeds $P_{ALV}$ (i.e., intermittently during systole).
- In zone III, $P_{PA}>P_{PV}>P_{ALV}$; here pulmonary arterial pressure and pulmonary venous pressure always exceed alveolar pressure, thus there is perfusion throughout systole and diastole. Blood flow through this zone exceeds the blood flow at all other zones.
- Lastly, in zone IV, which is represented by the lowest portion at the bases of the lungs, $P_{PA}>P_{PV}>P_{ALV}$, but because of the effect of gravity and the increased interstitial pressure compressing the blood vessels, there is a significant increase in pulmonary vascular resistance and blood flow is reduced; here flow is governed by the gradient between alveolar and interstitial pressures.

## ANESTHETIC CONSIDERATIONS

Another important regulator of lung perfusion is the phenomenon known as *hypoxic pulmonary vasoconstriction* (HPV). This is a compensatory mechanism that diverts blood flow away from poorly ventilated, hypoxic regions toward better oxygenated regions and thus improving V/Q mismatch. Modern inhaled anesthetics, such as isoflurane and sevoflurane, have little effect on this phenomenon. Intravenous (IV) anesthetics do not inhibit HPV, but volatile anesthetics and potent vasodilators do. Inhaled nitric oxide (NO) is a specific pulmonary vasodilator that does not worsen HPV and often improves oxygenation by dilating blood vessels in areas of the lung that are already being ventilated.

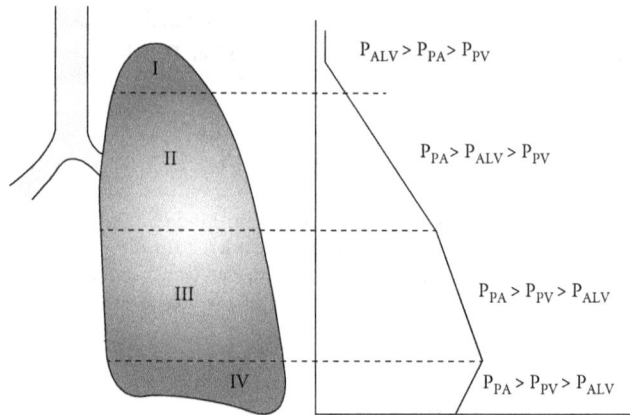

**Figure 219.1.** Vertical distribution of lung blood flow. The so-called zones I, II, III, and IV are indicated. In zone I there is no perfusion, only ventilation. In zone II, pulmonary artery pressure exceeds alveolar pressure which in turn exceeds venous pressure; the driving pressure is $P_{PA}-P_{ALV}$. In zone III, arterial and venous pressures both exceed alveolar pressure, and here the driving pressure is $P_{PA}-P_{PV}$. In the lung base, blood flow is decreased possibly because of increased interstitial pressure that compresses extra alveolar vessels. $P_{ALV}$, intraalveolar pressure; $P_{PV}$, pulmonary vein pressure; $P_{PA}$, pulmonary artery pressure.

Reprinted from from Kavanagh BP, Hedenstierna G. Respiratory Physiology and Pathophysiology in Miller's Anesthesia, 13, 354–383 (9th ed.). (2020) with permission from Elsevier.

**REFERENCES**

1. Miller RD. *Miller's Anesthesia*. Philadelphia, PA: Elsevier; 2020.
2. West's zones of the lungs. *Deranged Physiology*. November 2019. https://derangedphysiology.com/main/cicm-primary-exam/requi red-reading/respiratory-system/Chapter%20072/wests-zones-lung. Accessed on July 2020.
3. West JB, Dollery CT, Naimark A. Distribution of blood flow in isolated lung: Relation to vascular and alveolar pressures. *J Appl Physiol*. 1964;19(4):713–724.

# 220.

# ALVEOLAR GAS EQUATION

*Camila Teixeira and Tatiana Jamroz*

## INTRODUCTION

The alveolar gas equation (AGE) was created to estimate the partial pressure of oxygen inside the alveoli ($P_AO_2$). The $P_AO_2$ value needs to be estimated since it is not feasible to collect gases from the alveoli and have the sample analysis results, in the same way as arterial $PO_2$ results from blood gas analysis.

## ALVEOLAR GAS EQUATION

The alveolar gas equation may be expressed as:

$$P_AO_2 = (Patm - PH_2O)FiO_2 - \frac{P_ACO_2}{R}$$

where Patm is the atmospheric pressure (at sea level it is 760 mmHg), $PH_2O$ is partial pressure of water (around 47 mmHg), $FiO_2$ is the fraction of inspired oxygen, $P_ACO_2$ is the alveolar partial pressure of carbon dioxide (assumed to equal arterial $PCO_2$, normally in the range of 40–45 mmHg), and R is the respiratory quotient that correlates the amount of $CO_2$ produced to the amount of $O_2$ consumed. The R value usually ranges from 0.8 to 1.0 for a regular human diet, but can vary according to the type of diet and metabolic state.[1]

In a steady state, breathing 21% oxygen at sea level results in an alveolar $PO_2$ around 100 mmHg.

$$P_AO_2 = (760 - 47)0.21 - 40/0.8 = 99.7 \, mmHg$$

## CLINICAL RELEVANCE

The oxygen partial pressure in alveoli is closely linked upon each variable. The variation or manipulation of any variable quantity has a significant impact on $P_AO_2$ values, eliciting different clinical responses. Hyperoxygenation (when a patient is given 100% oxygen) preceding the intubation maneuver increases the $PO_2$ in the alveoli and plasma, and can be easily understood with the help of the AGE.

$$P_AO_2 = (760 - 47) \times 1 - (40/0.8) = 713 - 50 = 663 \, mmHg$$

In this case, under physiological conditions, the $P_AO_2$ rise could be clinically translated into more time to successfully intubate the patient before the $PO_2$ falls below 60 mmHg and the patient starts exhibiting signs of desaturation.

In addition, the alveolar gas equation is also helpful in estimating the alveolar and arterial $PO_2$ difference (A-a gradient). The alveolar $PO_2$ can be determined by the use of the AGE and the arterial $PO_2$ by the arterial blood gas analysis.

$$\text{A-a gradient} = P_A O_2 - PaO_2$$

Ideally, no A-a gradient would exist; however, the physiologic V/Q mismatch results in a physiologic difference between alveolar and arterial $PO_2$.[2] Physiologic A-a gradient values change with age and could be estimated using the following equation:

$$\text{A-a gradient} = (\text{Age} + 10) / 4$$

The A-a gradient has an important clinical application in regard of hypoxia etiology. The gradient calculation can help narrow the differential diagnosis in hypoxemic patients. Hypoxia is a result of inadequate oxygen delivery to the tissues. The oxygen delivery process can be interrupted at any of the following 3 points: airflow to the alveoli (ventilation); blood flow to the lung (perfusion); and gas exchange in the alveolar-capillary barrier (diffusion).[3]

The gradient can be classified as (1) normal or (2) elevated, and the result should be used as a complement to physical examination, guiding the physician whether to suspect a particular hypoxia leading dysfunction.

(1) Normal A-a gradient: present when both alveolar and arterial oxygen partial pressures are decreased. Hypoxia with normal A-a gradient can be corrected with supplemental oxygenation. Two etiologies are related: reduced oxygen tension (high altitudes) and hypoventilation. Hypoventilated patients exhibit hypoxia with low V/Q ratio and hypercapnia. Patients respond to supplemental oxygenation and diverse causes can be atributed, including:
  • Airway obstruction: asthma and COPD
  • Respiratory drive impairment: neurologic depression, sedation, coma
  • Restricted chest movements: obesity, massive ascites, chest wall fractures
  • Neuromuscular diseases: amyotrophic lateral sclerosis, muscular dystrophy
(2) Elevated A-a gradient: present when patients can ventilate (normal $P_A O_2$), but a pathology of the alveolar-capillary system affects the arterial oxygen level (low PaO2). This can be attributed to a diffusion defect (intersticial lung disease or pulmonary edema), a perfusion defect, or to a blood shunting (physiologic or anatomical). If a perfusion impairment is present, like in pulmonary embolism, the V/Q ratio is also increased. Physiologic shunt, like in atelectasis, occurs when blood reaches non-ventilated areas of the lung. Anatomical right to left shunt, as in ventricular septal defect, occurs when deoxygenated blood passes from the right to the left heart chamber. Usually, increasing FiO2 through supplemental oxygen therapy does not improve hypoxia in patients with right to left shunts.

## LIMITATIONS

The simplified alveolar gas equation is based on the assumption that the steady state condition is not violated. The elaborated version of the AGE has an extra term within brackets, which is given to compensate a larger $O_2$ uptake than $O_2$ elimination over the alveolar capillary membranes.[4]

$$P_A O_2 = PiO_2 - P_A CO_2 + \left[ P_A CO_2 \times FiO_2 \times \frac{1-R}{R} \right]$$

In cases of severe acidosis, carbon monoxide poisoning, or at low atmospheric pressure conditions, the equation could not reliably be applied. A low $PiO_2$ input in combination with $P_A CO_2$ and R fixed values could result in a negative $P_A O_2$ value. Therefore, AGE is not true for all conditions and could predict an absurdity.[5]

## REFERENCES

1. Sharma S, et al. Alveolar gas equation. In: *StatPearls* [Internet]. Treasure Island, FL: StatPearls; 2020 Jan.
2. Hantzidiamantis PJ, Amaro E. Physiology, alveolar to arterial oxygen gradient (Aa gradient). In: *StatPearls* [Internet]. Treasure Island, FL: StatPearls; 2020 Jan.
3. Bhutta BS, et al. Anoxia (hypoxic hypoxia). In: *StatPearls* [Internet]. Treasure Island, FL: StatPearls; 2020 May.
4. Miller RD. *Miller's Anesthesia*. 8th ed. Philadelphia, PA: Churchill Livingstone/Elsevier; 2015:446–448.
5. Cruickshank S, Hirschauer N. The alveolar gas equation. *Cont Ed Anaesth Crit Care Pain*. 2004;4:24–27.

# 221.

# DIFFUSION AND PULMONARY DIFFUSION CAPACITY

*Anna Moldysz and Archit Sharma*

## INTRODUCTION

Gas exchange in the lungs occurs in the distal airways and alveoli by passive diffusion. Oxygen is transported from the alveoli across the alveolar-capillary membrane into blood, where it binds to hemoglobin. Carbon dioxide diffuses from the plasma to the alveoli and is expired. The diffusion capacity, also called *transfer factor*, measures the capacity to transfer gas from alveolar spaces into the alveolar capillary blood. This occurs by passive diffusion and is a function of the pressure difference that drives gas, the surface area over which exchange takes place, and the resistance to gas movement through the membrane and into chemical combination with the blood.[1]

The diffusion capacity can be calculated according to the following equation:

$$\text{Diffusion capacity} = (SA \times \Delta P \times Sol)/(h \times \sqrt{MW})$$

SA = surface area of the membrane exposed to gas

$\Delta P$ = difference between partial pressure of gas in alveoli and partial pressure in blood

Sol = solubility of the gas in the membrane

h = membrane thickness

MW = molecular weight of the gas.

## DETERMINANTS OF DIFFUSION CAPACITY

*Surface area* is directly proportional to diffusing capacity and can be decreased by lung fibrosis, decreased lung volume such as post–lung resection, or lung tissue destruction as seen in emphysema.

The *pressure gradient* of the gas between the alveoli and blood is the driving pressure for passive diffusion. Therefore, a larger difference in partial pressure of gases will increase the diffusion rate. The pressure difference will vary along

the length of a capillary. In the setting of normal cardiac output, equilibrium is reached within 25%–30% of the capillary length. In the setting of stress or exercise, an increased cardiac output causes faster blood flow and the equilibrium is reached after a longer distance.

It is important to note that the plasma oxygen tension is determined only by dissolved oxygen. The majority of oxygen in blood is bound to hemoglobin, and therefore does not contribute to the partial pressure of oxygen. As a result, more oxygen can diffuse into the blood before equilibrium is reached. This also explains the susceptibility to hypoxemia in an anemic patient, as there is less oxygen bound.

An increased *solubility* of a gas in a membrane will increase the diffusion rate. This becomes relevant in the case of carbon dioxide, which is almost 30-fold more soluble than oxygen. Because of this, carbon dioxide diffusion is not significantly impaired in lung disease.

The *membrane thickness* is inversely proportional to diffusion capacity. In fibrotic membranes, this can prolong the equilibration process, and severely fibrotic membranes may prevent equilibrium from being reached, predisposing the patient to hypoxemia.

The *molecular weight* of the gas also affects diffusion capacity. The larger the molecule, the slower the rate of diffusion across the membrane.

## MEASUREMENT

Carbon monoxide is used for the clinical test of diffusing capacity because its extreme avidity for hemoglobin allows the back pressure to diffusion to be considered negligible.[2]

To perform this test, a patient maximally expires and then inhales 0.3% carbon monoxide to total lung capacity. This fills the lungs with dilute CO. This is fully exhaled after a 10-second breath hold, and the amount of exhaled CO is measured.[3] The difference between inhaled and exhaled CO is the CO taken up by blood or remaining the lung (in residual volume). The amount remaining in the lung can then be calculated if the CO is coadministered with an insoluble gas such as helium that remains in the lung and will not cross the alveolar-capillary membrane.

## IMPORTANCE OF DLCO

The pulmonary diffusion capacity can be thought of as a marker for pulmonary vascular health. It is a calculated, derived value that indirectly assesses the ability of the lungs to "transfer" oxygen to blood through the use of carbon monoxide. In general, a healthy individual has a value of between 75% and 125% of the average.[4] However, individuals vary according to age, sex, height, and a variety of other parameters.

A low DLCO could be due to impaired diffusion from cigarette smoking, emphysema, interstitial lung disease, decreased lung volumes, pulmonary edema, anemia, or pulmonary vascular disease such as pulmonary emboli or pulmonary hypertension.[5] Alternatively, DLCO can be increased by factors such as high altitude, lying supine, exercise, left to right cardiac shunt, polycythemia, pulmonary hemorrhage, asthma, or obesity.

## ANESTHETIC CONSIDERATIONS

### PREOPERATIVE

Measuring pulmonary diffusion capacity preoperatively can be useful in diagnosing preexisting pulmonary disease. A DLCO that is <45% predicted value is indicative of severe respiratory impairment. Notably, a patient's DLCO may be falsely decreased in the setting of severe restrictive or obstructive disease because of V/Q mismatching, increased distance from the terminal bronchioles to alveolar-capillary membranes, a decrease in alveolar surface area, or loss of capillary beds. In this case, it is important to adjust DLCO by alveolar volume, or DLCO/VA. A normal value would be >80% predicted.

### INTRAOPERATIVE

Patients who have decreased pulmonary diffusion capacity can quickly develop hypoxemia intraoperatively, and extra care should be taken to optimize other anesthetic conditions for prevention.

### POSTOPERATIVE

The predicted postoperative diffusing capacity for carbon monoxide is an important variable in lung resections, and a predicted diffusion capacity of less than 40% is considered high risk. These patients should be monitored very closely for signs of hypoxemia.

## REFERENCES

1. Morrell MJ. One hundred years of pulmonary function testing: A perspective on "The diffusion of gases through the lungs of man" by Marie Krogh. *J Physiol.* 2015;593(Pt 2):351.
2. Hughes JMB, Borland CD. The centenary (2015) of the transfer factor for carbon monoxide (TLCO): Marie Krogh's legacy. *Thorax.* 2015;70(4):391–394.
3. Ogilvie CM, et al. A standardized breath holding technique for the clinical measurement of the diffusing capacity of the lung for carbon monoxide. *J Clin Investig.* 1957;36(1):1–17.
4. ATS. Single breath carbon monoxide diffusing capacity (transfer factor): Recommendations for a standard technique. Statement of the American Thoracic Society. *Am Rev Respir Dis.* 1987;136:1299–1307.
5. Fernandez-Bonetti P, et al. Peripheral airways obstruction in idiopathic pulmonary artery hypertension (primary). *Chest.* 1983;83(5):732–738.

# 222.

# APNEIC OXYGENATION AND DIFFUSION HYPOXIA

*Ahmad Reza Parniani and Peggy White*

## INTRODUCTION

Apneic oxygenation is the process during which oxygen moves by mass flow from the upper airway into the alveoli when there is no respiratory effort. If oxygen is administered during apnea, there is an increase in the transfer of oxygen from the alveoli into the bloodstream, which results in a lower rate and extent of hypoxia.[1] In an apneic patient, the extraction of oxygen from the alveoli into the bloodstream results in subatmospheric alveolar pressure. This generates a pressure gradient that results in movement of the additional administered oxygen inside the alveolus. This is known as aventilatory mass flow, previously known as diffusion respiration or apneic diffusion of oxygenation. To facilitate apneic oxygenation, it is necessary to denitrogenate the lungs by breathing oxygen for a period of time before the onset of apnea. If no denitrogenation is done, the persistence of nitrogen in the lungs and rising levels of carbon dioxide diminish the pressure gradient available for transfer of oxygen into the alveolus, which results in a faster onset of hypoxia. Renitrogenation can be prevented by administering a fraction of inspired oxygen ($FiO_2$) of 1 for the duration of apnea.

## EFFICIENCY OF APNEIC OXYGENATION

In a recent meta-analysis and systematic review, apneic oxygenation was found to be associated with a higher peri-intubation oxygen saturation, higher first-pass intubation, and decreased occurrence of hypoxemia. The reduction of hypoxemia in patients who were urgently intubated might have resulted in more time for laryngoscopy, which would increase the first-pass success rate.[1]

## APNEIC OXYGENATION TECHNIQUES

Apneic oxygenation can be performed with any device that facilitates delivery of oxygen into the lungs. This includes a nasal cannula, facemask, nasopharyngeal catheter, endotracheal tube, supraglottic airway device, rigid bronchoscope, and front-of-neck catheter. Oxygen can also be administered through the side channels in direct laryngoscopes and videolaryngoscopes.

High-flow nasal oxygen (HFNO) is a fairly recent method for performing apneic oxygenation. It has advantages, including enhanced flushing of dead spaces and the ability to provide positive airway pressure, and it allows for heating and humidification of gases. HFNO also promotes washout of gases from anatomical dead space, as shown in previous studies. Positive airway pressure that is generated by HFNO results in an increase in end-expiratory lung impedance in patients breathing spontaneously. This is consistent with an increase in end-expiratory lung volume and functional residual capacity. For each 10-L increase in flow rate, there is an extra positive airway pressure of 0.5 to 1 $cmH_2O$. Furthermore, humidification and heating of the oxygen result in improved airway function by enhancing pulmonary compliance and gas flow. The humidification of oxygen also assists in the protection of ciliary function and prevention of bronchoconstriction from cold and dry gases.[2]

## BENEFITS AND APPLICATIONS OF APNEIC OXYGENATION

Apneic oxygenation can be used during airway management, urgent intubation, one-lung ventilation, and diagnosis of brain death.[2] Apneic oxygenation can also be used during airway management of obese patients. Obese patients often experience a faster onset of hypoxemia during apnea, which can be delayed by using apneic oxygenation. This is important because management of the airway in obese patients can be more challenging; having additional time before desaturation can provide an adequate opportunity to establish the airway.

## COMPLICATIONS OF APNEIC OXYGENATION

Carbon dioxide is not removed during apneic oxygenation, causing a decrease in pH that can result in cardiac dysrhythmias or arrest if continued. During the first minute of apnea, the rise in the partial pressure of carbon dioxide ($PaCO_2$) is approximately 6 mmHg. After the first minute of apnea, the average rate of increase in $PaCO_2$ is 3 mmHg/min.[3, 4] Based on a previous experiment, the potential limit of apneic oxygenation is estimated to be up to 15 minutes.[3] However, apnea should be kept to the minimum amount of time possible because of the risk of increasing respiratory acidosis and cardiac dysrhythmias.

## NITROUS OXIDE

Nitrous oxide ($N_2O$) is a sweet-smelling gas with a minimal alveolar concentration of 104%. It is mostly used as an anesthetic adjunct in combination with volatile anesthetics. It is stored in a cylinder that is condensed to 50 atmospheres, which equates to a pressure of 745 psi.

## DIFFUSION HYPOXIA

Patients can develop hypoxia during recovery from general anesthesia despite adequate ventilation. Hypoxia appears more frequently in patients who receive $N_2O$ as part of the anesthetic. The tissues and blood of a patient undergoing $N_2O$ anesthesia will absorb $N_2O$ from the lungs until the tension of the $N_2O$ throughout the body is at equilibrium.

Diffusion hypoxia is a consequence of rapid outgassing from the tissues of patients who receive $N_2O$. During the first 5 to 10 minutes after stopping $N_2O$ anesthesia, the flow of $N_2O$ into the alveoli from the blood can be several liters per minute. This flow can result in dilution of alveolar oxygen. Outgassing can also result in dilution of alveolar $PaCO_2$, which can result in hypoventilation. $N_2O$ has a higher solubility in blood than nitrogen; as a result, the excretion of $N_2O$ into the alveoli is faster than the uptake of nitrogen from alveoli into the blood.[5]

## REFERENCES

1. Oliveira JE, Silva L, et al. Effectiveness of apneic oxygenation during intubation: A systematic review and meta-analysis. *Ann Emerg Med.* 2017;70(4):483–494.e11.

2. Lyons C, Callagan M. Uses and mechanisms of apnoeic oxygenation: A narrative review. *Anaesthesia.* 2019;74(4):497–507.
3. Fraioli RL, et al. Pulmonary and cardiovascular effects of apneic oxygenation in man. *Anesthesiology.* 1973;39(6):588–596.
4. Eisenkraft JB, et al. Anesthesia for thoracic surgery. In: Barash PG, et al., eds. *Clinical Anesthesia.* 7th ed. Philadelphia, PA: Lippincott Williams & Wilkins; 2013:1057.
5. Forman SA, Ishizawa Y. Inhaled anesthetic pharmacokinetics: Uptake, distribution, metabolism, and toxicity. In: Miller RD, ed. *Miller's Anesthesia.* 8th ed. Philadelphia, PA: Saunders; 2015:656.

# 223.

# BLOOD GAS

## Nigel Knox and Michael Chang

## INTRODUCTION

Through compensatory mechanisms, the body is constantly striving to maintain a stable acid-base equilibrium. Information in regard to a patient's ventilation, oxygenation, and acid-base status may be interpreted from the information obtained with a blood gas, making this an integral part of the anesthesiologist's assessment. With review of the reported pH, partial pressure of oxygen ($PO_2$), partial pressure of carbon dioxide ($PCO_2$), bicarbonate ($HCO_{3-}$), base excess or deficit, and oxygen saturation, we are able to detect the presence and possible causes of acid-base and oxygenation disturbances. As an integral part of acute patient assessments, venous blood gas (VBG) interpretation has become more prominent. Given the recognized agreement between pH and $HCO_{3-}$ values derived from venous and arterial blood, integration of the clinical findings with VBG results is often sufficient to safely guide treatment decision-making.[1]

As an anesthesiologist, correct diagnosis of a metabolic or respiratory disorder will assist in providing the appropriate care or medication to a patient. Normal values and assessment of the variations can be seen in Table 223.1. With blood gas analysis, we have direct measurement of pH, $PO_2$, and $PCO_2$, which allows us to derive the oxygen saturation, $HCO_{3-}$ concentration, and base excess of the extracellular fluid. As normal values are directly measured, the $HCO_{3-}$ from a concurrent chemistry panel is often reviewed (correlation with time of sample collections should be performed). The reported values provide an insight into the patient's physiological response toward homeostasis at a point in time, yet a review and comparison with previous/repeat blood gas values are required to monitor and quantitate the response to changes in care.

## BLOOD GAS INTERPRETATION

Pulmonary gas exchange is a dynamic continuous process requiring maintenance of ventilation, diffusion, perfusion, and chemical reactions (oxygen ($O_2$) and hemoglobin, and carbon dioxide ($CO_2$) conversion to bicarbonate). Through blood gas interpretation we are able to ascertain the difference between inspired and mixed expired $O_2$ and $CO_2$ concentrations quantifying pulmonary function. Here we will address interpretation of blood gases in comparison to normal levels.[2]

### STEP 1. PH: ACID-BASE BALANCE

With the utilization of the Henderson-Hasselbalch equation we are able to calculate the patient's pH (pH = 6 . 1 +

**Table 223.1** BASELINE BLOOD GAS VALUES, AND VARIATION INTERPRETATION.
*ABG, ARTERIAL BLOOD GAS. VBG, VENOUS BLOOD GAS

| DIAGNOSTIC VALUE | ABG NORMAL RANGE | VBG NORMAL RANGE | VALUE ↓ | VALUE ↑ |
|---|---|---|---|---|
| pH | 7.35-7.45 | 7.30-7.40 | Acidosis | Alkalosis |
| $pCO_2$ | 35-45 mmHg | 44-48 mmHg | Alkalosis | Acidosis |
| $pO_2$ | 80-100 mmHg | 35-45 mmHg | Hypoxemia | Supplemental O2 |
| $HCO_3^-$ | 22-26 mEq/L | 24-30 mEq/L | Acidosis | Alkalosis |
| $SaO_2$ | > 95 % | 60-80 % | Hypoxemia | ▬▬▬▬▬ |

log $[HCO_3/(0.03 \times Paco)$. The identification of acidosis (pH <7.35), or alkalosis (pH >7.45) is then elaborated on to identify its etiology (▲$HCO_3$, metabolic or ▲$CO_2$, respiratory). With the variation in acid-base balance, the body compensates with increases in the opposing acid or base through ventilation ($CO_2$) or renal ($HCO_3$) effects. Despite these reactionary mechanisms, the primary buffer through H+ ion binding and release is hemoglobin.

## STEP 2. VENTILATION

Normal $PaCO_2$ ranges from 35 to 45 mmHg, with its primary controlling factor being ventilation. With hyperventilation we see a decrease in $CO_2$ levels, and subsequently create respiratory alkalosis. With hypoventilation, we see a decrease in $CO_2$ excretion and subsequent respiratory acidosis.

## STEP 3. OXYGENATION

With oxygenation we depend on a harmony of components that includes ventilation, perfusion, and pressure gradients. Through ventilation we identify the transport of a higher concentration of $O_2$ to pulmonary circulation to maintain a pressure gradient and allow diffusion based upon consistent perfusion. We must first identify the expected partial pressure of alveolar $O_2$ ($PAO_2$) to identify the efficacy of these processes in a patient. Through the alveolar gas equation we are able to estimate alveolar oxygen content. $PAO_2$ derived from the calculation can then be used to ascertain the degree of shunt present in a patient. With the $PAO_2$ calculated, we are able to determine the efficacy of pulmonary oxygenation by comparing it to the reported $PaO_2$, identifying the alveolar to arterial (A-a) gradient, as in the following equation:

Alveolar gas equation, $PAO_2$
$$= FiO_2 (Patm - pH_2O) - (paCO_2/RQ)$$

where $FiO_2$ is the fractional concentration of inspired oxygen; Patm is atmospheric pressure; pH20 is partial pressure of $H_2O$; and RQ is respiratory quotient, gas exchange ratio.

Given the normal physiologic V/Q mismatch in the lungs owing to apical and basilar perfusion and ventilation, there is a slight difference in oxygen tension between the alveoli and arterial blood.[3] This physiologic A-a gradient change is based on a patient's age, with the expected A-a gradient estimated with the following equation:

$$A-a \, gradient = (Age + 10)/4$$

The measured difference on the A-a gradient is used to diagnose the source of hypoxemia. In the setting of an increased A-a gradient and hypoxemia, the etiology is likely secondary to V/Q mismatch or diffusion compromise. However, with the identification of a normal A-a gradient and hypoxemia, etiology is subsequent to decreased inspired oxygen, or hypoventilation.

## REFERENCES

1. Kelly AM. Can VBG analysis replace ABG analysis in emergency care? *Emerg Med J.* 2016;33(2):152-154.
2. Wagner, P. The physiological basis of pulmonary gas exchange: Implications for clinical interpretation of arterial blood gases. *Eur Respir J.* 2015;45:227–243.
3. Hantzidiamantis PJ. Alveolar to arterial oxygen gradient (Aa Gradient). In: *StatPearls.* Treasure Island, FL: StatPearls; 2020 Jan. https://www.ncbi.nlm.nih.gov/books/NBK545153/.

# 224.

# OXYGEN TRANSPORT

*Michael Chang and Nigel Knox*

## INTRODUCTION

Oxygen is an essential component of life, contributing to aerobic respiration by acting as the terminal electron acceptor in the ATP-generating electron transport chain in the mitochondria at the cellular level. As such, it is easily overlooked as the most common drug administered during anesthesia and critical care medicine. At rest, the healthy adult consumes approximately 250 mL of oxygen per minute, and this may increase multiple-fold with exertion. In this chapter, we will discuss oxygen transport, the relationship between hemoglobin and oxygen binding, and anesthetic considerations relating to oxygen delivery.

## TYPES OF OXYGEN TRANSPORT

### DIFFUSIVE OXYGEN TRANSPORT

During inspiration, oxygen enters the alveolar sac and diffuses across the alveolar-capillary membrane, facilitated by the concentration gradient between the partial pressure of oxygen in the alveolar space and the deoxygenated pulmonary capillary blood. The oxygen carried in red blood cells then enters the systemic circulation to reach terminal capillaries. At this point, oxygen diffusion relies on the concentration gradient between the partial pressure of oxygen in the oxygenated capillary blood and the tissue bed.

### FICK'S LAWS OF DIFFUSION

Fick's First Law claims that particles move from an area of high concentration to an area of low concentration. The Second Law postulates how the concentration gradient changes with time. Altogether, these two laws can be combined into an equation that describes the rate of diffusion across a membrane barrier (Equation 1):

$$F = D * A(C1 - C2)/T$$

[Fick's Law F: rate of diffusion; D: diffusion constant permeability; A: surface area; C1-C2: concentration gradient/ difference in partial pressure; T: membrane thickness].

## CONVECTIVE OXYGEN TRANSPORT

This type of transport describes the energy-dependent movement of oxygen. In other words, this describes oxygen flowing through the tracheobronchial tree during inspiration or circulating through the vasculature. This is in contrast to the passive movement of oxygen during diffusion.

## OXYGEN TRANSPORT IN BLOOD

### DISSOLVED $O_2$ IN PLASMA

A minute amount of oxygen is dissolved in plasma and accounts for approximately 2% of the total $O_2$ content of blood. The concentration of the dissolved gas can be calculated by utilizing Henry's Law: the concentration of a dissolved gas is proportional to its partial pressure. Therefore, by applying the solubility of $O_2$ in blood, 0.003 mL $O_2$/100 mL blood/ mmHg, we can solve for the concentration of dissolved $O_2$ (Equation 2):

$$\text{Concentration of Dissolved } O_2 = 0.003 * PaO2$$

[$PaO_2$: arterial oxygen partial pressure].

### HEMOGLOBIN-BOUND $O_2$

Hemoglobin is a tetramer-molecule protein whose primary function is to carry oxygen molecules in red blood cells. It consists of four protein (globin) chains, each attached to an iron-porphyrin compound, which $O_2$ readily binds. The most common type of hemoglobin is HgbA, which consists of two alpha and two beta chains. Hgb A accounts for more than 95% of normal adult hemoglobin. Approximately 98% of the total $O_2$ content of blood is bound to hemoglobin.

There are other variants of the hemoglobin molecule, with different oxygen affinity profiles. These include methemoglobin, fetal hemoglobin, and hemoglobin S. Methemoglobinemia arises when the iron component of the hemoglobin is oxidized ($Fe^{2+} \rightarrow Fe^{3+}$), rendering it unable to bind oxygen. Fetal hemoglobin has a greater affinity for oxygen than adult hemoglobin, which facilitates $O_2$ movement from the mother to the fetus. Hemoglobin S is the abnormal hemoglobin variant that causes sickle cell disease.

## OXYGEN DISSOCIATION CURVE

The relationship between the oxygen content of blood and the saturation is linear. In contrast, there is a sigmoidal relationship between partial pressure and saturation. This is due to the increased affinity of the heme groups for oxygen with each successive $O_2$ molecule binding, which occurs at the steepest portion of the oxygen dissociation curve (ODC). The increased affinity is due to the alteration to the shape of the globin chain, causing an overall change in the quaternary structure of the hemoglobin.[1] Additional factors that affect the affinity for oxygen are shown in Table 224.1. Increased oxygen affinity can be demonstrated by a leftward shift of the ODC, whereas a rightward shift represents decreased oxygen affinity.

### 2,3-DIPHOSPHOGLYCERATE (2,3-DPG)

This is a byproduct of glycolysis in red blood cells, which is rapidly consumed under conditions of normal oxygen tension. However, during hypoxic conditions, the metabolism of 2,3-DPG is decreased, which results in accumulation within the cell. Furthermore, 2,3 DPG binds to the beta chains of deoxyhemoglobin and causes a reduction in $O_2$ affinity.[1] A clinical example of this phenomenon is living at high altitude under hypoxic conditions, leading

*Table 224.1* FACTORS AFFECTING OXYGEN DISSOCIATION CURVE

| LEFT SHIFT | RIGHT SHIFT |
| --- | --- |
| ↑ pH | ↓ pH |
| ↓ $PaCO_2$ | ↑ $PaCO_2$ |
| ↓ 2,3-DPG | ↑ 2,3-DPG |
| ↓ Temperature | ↑ Temperature |
| Met-Hgb | Hgb S |
| Fetal-Hgb | Sulf-Hgb |
| CO-Hgb | |

to accumulation of 2,3-DPG in the red blood cells. The ensuing decrease in $O_2$ affinity allows for efficient delivery of $O_2$ to the peripheral tissues.

### P50

This is the point on the ODC at which hemoglobin is 50% saturated. A change in this value can be used as a surrogate to identify changes in oxygen affinity. An increase in P50 reflects decreased affinity, and a decrease in P50 reflects increased affinity. The P50 of normal adult hemoglobin is 26.7 mmHg.

## OXYGEN CONTENT AND DELIVERY

Oxygen content or oxygen-carrying capacity is the amount of $O_2$ per volume of blood. Since the majority of $O_2$ transported in blood is bound to hemoglobin, the hemoglobin concentration is the main determinant of the oxygen content of blood. However, we must also account for the small amount of dissolved $O_2$ in the plasma (Equation 3):

$$CaO_2 = \underbrace{1.36 * Hgb * Percent\ Saturation}_{A} + \underbrace{0.003 * PaO_2}_{B}$$

[CaO2: arterial oxygen content; PaO2: arterial oxygen partial pressure; A: $O_2$ binding capacity (1g of hemoglobin can bind 1.36 mL O2); B: dissolved $O_2$ content].

Oxygen delivery is the amount of oxygen delivered to tissues each minute and is a product of cardiac ouput and oxygen-carrying capacity (Equation 4):

$$Oxygen\ Delivery = CO * CaO_2$$

[CO: cardiac output; CaO2: arterial oxygen content].

Of note, utilizing cardiac output as a surrogate for oxygenated blood flow to the tissues is a crude measurement of overall oxygen delivery. This equation does not reflect the regional differences of oxygen delivery to each tissue bed in the body, due to the variation in regional and local blood flow.

## ANESTHETIC CONSIDERATION

### PREOPERATIVE AND INTRAOPERATIVE

As illustrated by the oxygen content equation, the major determinant in affecting total oxygen delivery is the total hemoglobin concentration. Therefore, a higher transfusion threshold should be considered for patients with cardiac ischemic diseases.

Hypophosphatemia is overlooked compared to other electrolyte derangements. This is commonly seen in patients with sepsis. This can lead to a reduced concentration of 2,3-DPG in red blood cells, thereby decreasing the P50 of the ODC and facilitating tissue hypoxia. Additionally, older blood from a blood bank has reduced concentration of 2,3-DPG as compared to in vivo blood.[1]

## REFERENCES

1. Dunn J. Physiology of oxygen transport. *BJA Education*. 2016 Oct;16(10):341–348.
2. Costanzo L. *Respiratory Physiology*. 5th ed. Philadelphia, PA: Saunders Elsevier; 2014:214–217.

# 225.

# CARBON DIOXIDE TRANSPORT

## *Vasu Sidagam*

## INTRODUCTION

Carbon dioxide is the end product of cellular metabolism, and tissue carbon dioxide is the main source of plasma bicarbonate ($HCO_3$). This $HCO_3–H_2CO_3$ is one of the most important buffer systems that serves to maintain acid-base balance (pH) within normal ranges. Plasma $HCO_3$ level abnormalities provide important clues to acid-base disturbances and directly impact patient care decisions. Kidneys will attempt compensatory changes in acid-base disturbances either in primary metabolic or respiratory disorders by regulating the serum $HCO_3$ levels.

## TISSUE

This section explains the underlying pathways involved in the process.

About 200 ml of $CO_2$ is produced every minute and if not rapidly removed from the tissues, causes changes in local pH, thus impairing cellular functions.[1]

Blood carries the total $CO_2$ mainly in the form of plasma bicarbonate ($HCO_3$), which is about 90%. The remaining 10% of total $CO_2$ is made up of dissolved $CO_2$ (5%; in plasma and RBC) and carbamino compounds (5%; $CO_2$ binds to hemoglobin in RBC and proteins in plasma).

The carbonic acid and carbonate forms contribute negligibly and will not be discussed further.[2]

Under normal conditions, arterial blood $PCO_2$ is 40 mmHg. The total $CO_2$ content of the arterial blood is 48 ml/100 ml. As noted earlier, 43.2 ml of this is in the bicarbonate $HCO_3$ form (90%), 2.4 ml is in the form of dissolved $CO_2$ (5%), and 2.4 ml is in the form of carbamino compounds (5%).[2]

The partial pressure of $CO_2$ ($PCO_2$) at the tissues is about 46 mmHg, while the incoming arterial blood $PCO_2$ in the tissue capillaries is usually around 40 mmHg. Due to this pressure difference, $CO_2$ diffuses down the pressure gradient into the blood.[2]

As noted earlier, incoming arterial blood in the capillaries has a total $CO_2$ content of about 48 ml/100 ml. As the tissue is perfused, it picks up the diffused $CO_2$. Thus the mixed venous blood has a total $CO_2$ content of about 52 ml/100 ml, in effect picking up an incremental $CO_2$ of 4 ml/100 ml.[2]

Of this incremental $CO_2$ of 4 ml in the mixed venous blood, 70% travels as $HCO_3$, 20% travels as carbamino compounds (bound to hemoglobin), and 10% travels as dissolved $CO_2$ (in plasma and RBC).[2]

Thus it is clear that majority of total $CO_2$ transports as $HCO_3$ in arterial and venous blood, while carbamino compounds (hemoglobin bound) and dissolved $CO_2$ forms play a much bigger role in $CO_2$ transport in the venous blood in comparison to arterial blood.

## HOW IS THE TOTAL CO$_2$ CONVERTED TO HCO$_3$- AND OTHER FORMS OF CO$_2$?

Ninety percent of the total CO$_2$ which diffuses into the blood from the tissues enters into the RBC, and the remaining 10% stays in the plasma (Figure 225.1). Of the 90% of the total CO$_2$ which enters the RBC, the majority of it rapidly mixes with water (hydrolysis) to form H$_2$CO$_3$ which is then rapidly broken down to H+ and HCO$_3$-.The H+ is taken up by hemoglobin, thus buffering severe pH changes, and the HCO$_3$- diffuses out of the RB,C thus transporting in plasma as HCO$_3$. Chloride moves into the RBC in exchange for HCO$_3$ to maintain electrical neutrality. This is called chloride shift, or Hamburger effect.[3]

## WHY DOES SO MUCH MORE CO$_2$ CONVERT TO HCO$_3$- IN THE RBC COMPARED TO PLASMA?

This is because of the presence of enzyme carbonic anhydrase, which catalyzes the conversion almost 1000-fold. Please note that this enzyme is capable of converting CO + H$_2$O to HCO$_3$ and breaking down H$_2$CO$_3$ to HCO$_3$- + H+. Finally, it also can catalyze the reverse process of H$_2$CO$_3$ to CO$_2$ + H2O, which happens in the lung, thus allowing the release and exhalation of CO$_2$.

## NORMAL VALUES

The normal range of serum HCO$_3$ in arterial blood in adults at sea level extends from 21 to 27 meq/l, whereas corresponding range in peripheral venous blood is from 23 to 29 meq/l.[4] These ranges incorporate the fact that HCO$_3$ in women is about 1 meq/l lower than in men. The main reason that venous blood has a higher HCO$_3$ level is due to the fact that CO$_2$ transport from the tissues to lungs is mainly as HCO$_3$-.[4]

## MEASURED HCO$_3$- VS. CALCULATED HCO$_3$-

During blood gas analysis reporting, the HCO3 value provided is a calculated value based on pH and PCO$_2$ levels as applied in the Henderson Hasselbach equation.

In contrast to blood gas analyzer reports of calculated HCO$_3$, in the chemistry panel or metabolic panel obtained during routine daily patient care, the serum HCO$_3$ is a measured value. This measured serum bicarbonate value is in truth the total CO$_2$ (tCO$_2$), which includes dissolved form of CO$_2$ + HCO$_3$- form + carbamino form of CO$_2$.

Thus the chemistry panel–reported serum HCO$_3$ would be expected to be higher than calculated blood gas report value of HCO$_3$ by about 1–1.5 mg/l as it also measures the dissolved CO$_2$ form. The amount of dissolved CO$_2$ in serum can be estimated by multiplying PCO$_2$ by the solubility coefficient of CO$_2$ which is 0.0301 meq/mmHg at body temperature.[4]

Even though the dissolved CO$_2$ form is a minor component of the total CO$_2$, it is the only determinant of PCO$_2$ in the blood. The HCO$_3$ form and the carbamino form (hemoglobin-bound form) do not play any role in exerting partial pressure of CO$_2$ (i.e., PCO$_2$).

Please note that hemoglobin plays an important role in CO$_2$ transport by binding CO$_2$ to its free amino groups, though its role is not as critical as in O$_2$ transport.

## ANESTHETIC CONSIDERATIONS

### PREOPERATIVE

In patients presenting for surgery with serum HCO$_3$ levels <22 meq/l could mean severe illness and should be evaluated thoroughly for causes of metabolic acidosis like diabetic ketoacidosis, lactic acidosis, toxic alcohol ingestion, or severe gastrointestinal (GI) losses through diarrhea, advanced renal failure, etc.[5]

In patients presenting for surgery, high serum HCO$_3$ levels >26 meq/l could be seen in those with ongoing diuretic use or high gastric acid losses, either through severe vomiting or prolonged nasogastric drainage. In patients with primary hyperaldosteronism, low serum HCO$_3$- could be associated with hypertension.[5] Patients with chronic hypercapneic respiratory failure develop renal compensation by conserving HCO$_3$- and may have elevated serum HCO$_3$-.This could be a clue underlying pulmonary pathology.

Accurate measurement and accurate interpretation of serum HCO$_3$- is fundamental to assessing the patient's acid-base status, which is critical for normal body functions.

### INTRAOPERATIVE

A new development of low serum HCO$_3$- intraoperatively could mean developing metabolic acidosis from lactic acidosis. Causes could include inadequate resuscitation or low cardiac output. Excess saline administration causes a normal anion gap metabolic acidosis.

### POSTOPERATIVE

Low serum HCO$_3$ levels in patients recovering in the post-anesthesia care unit (PACU) will need evaluation for metabolic acidosis causes mentioned previously.

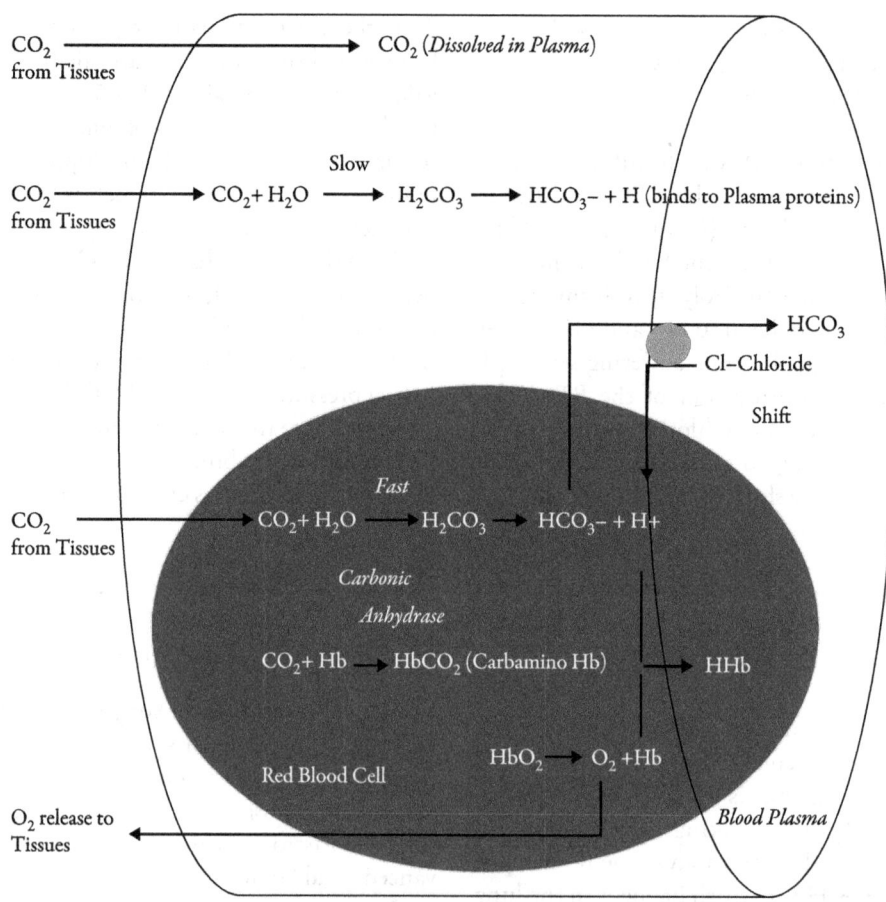

**Figure 225.1.** Carbon dioxide transport and role of RBC in $HCO_{3-}$ production.

## REFERENCES

1. GJ Arthurs, M Sudhakar. Carbon dioxide transport. *Cont Educ Anesth Crit Care Pain.* 2005;5(6):207–210.
2. Boron WF. Transport of oxygen and carbon dioxide in the blood. In: Boron WF, Boulpaep EL. *Medical Physiology: A Cellular and Molecular Approach.* 2nd ed. Pehiladelphia, PA: 672–684.
3. Hirsch CA. Gas exchange and transport. In: *Eagan's Fundamentals of Respiratory Care.* 10th ed. St. Louis, MO: 264–273.
4. Kraut JA, Madias NE. Re-evaluation of the normal range of serum total $CO_2$ concentration. *Clin J Am Soc Nephrol.* 2018 Feb 7;13(2):343–347.
5. Berend K, et al. Physiological approach to assessment of acid-base disturbances. 2014 Oct 9;371;(15):1434–1445.

# 226.

# SYSTEMIC EFFECTS OF HYPOCARBIA AND HYPERCARBIA

*Sarah C. Smith*

## INTRODUCTION

Carbon dioxide ($CO_2$) is produced by aerobic metabolism and is transported through the blood either in solution or bound to hemoglobin and other proteins. Carbonic acid ($H_2CO_3$) is formed intracellularly as $CO_2$ reacts with water, and is maintained in equilibrium with hydrogen ions ($H^+$) and bicarbonate ($HCO_3^-$) by carbonic anhydrase. Transport of $CO_2$ from the tissues to the alveoli is shown in Figure

226.1. To maintain $CO_2$ within the narrow range of 38–42 mmHg, chemoreceptors on central and peripheral neurons sensitive to both $CO_2$ and $H^+$ result in tight calibration of ventilation such that $CO_2$ is eliminated from the body at the same rate that it is produced. When ventilation is reduced, hypercarbia and respiratory acidosis result. More rarely, certain states, such as high fever, malignant hyperthermia, or thyrotoxicosis, may result in an increased production of $CO_2$, leading to hypercarbia. Conversely, increased

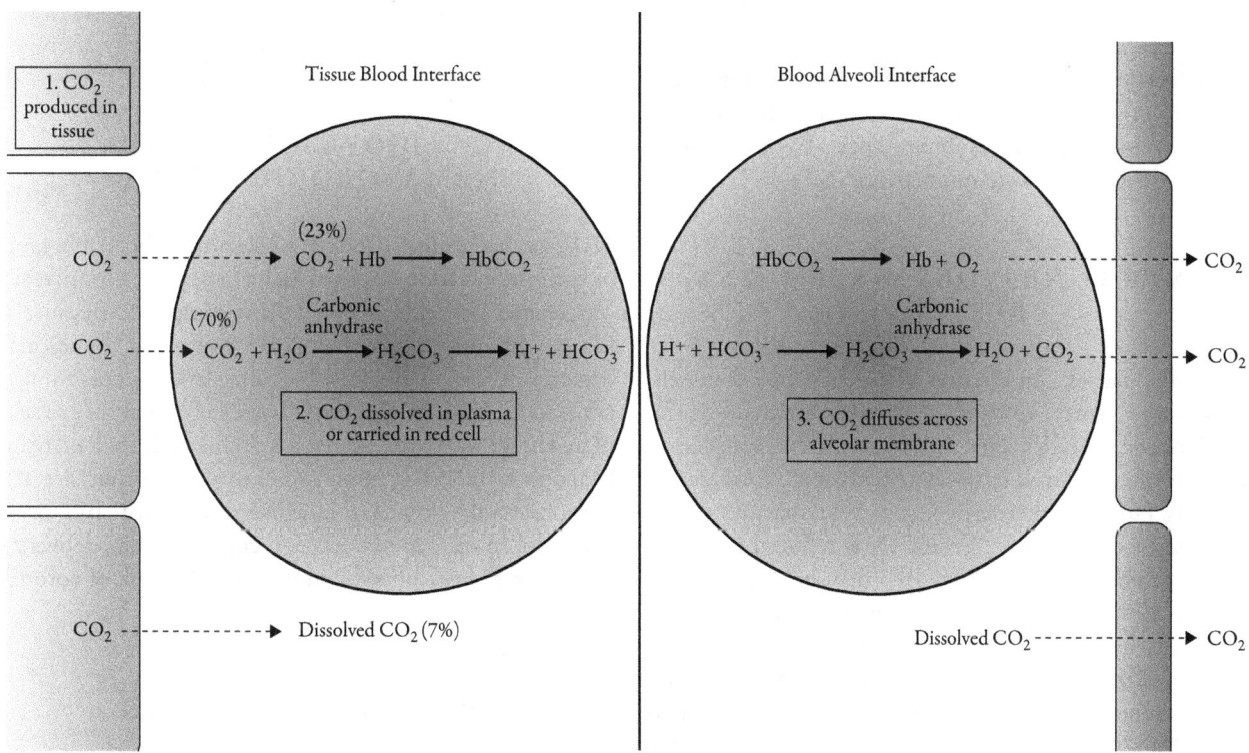

**Figure 226.1.** All tissues produce $CO_2$ through aerobic metabolism, which then diffuses across the cell membrane into the interstitial fluid and finally into the bloodstream across the capillary membrane. Approximately 7% of $CO_2$ remains dissolved in plasma, while the remainder diffuses into red cells. The majority of this (70%) is converted by carbonic anhydrase to $H_2CO_3$, which is maintained in equilibrium with H+ and $HCO_3^-$. Another 23% is bound to hemoglobin as carboxyhemoglobin. Once the blood arrives at the lung, $CO_2$ diffuses across the alveolar membrane to be exhaled and eliminated from the body.

*Table 226.1* EFFECTS OF HYPOCARBIA AND HYPERCARBIA

| | HYPOCARBIA | HYPERCARBIA |
|---|---|---|
| CNS | Neuronal excitability<br>Increased neuronal oxygen demand<br>Decreased CBF<br>Decreased ICP | Sympathetic stimulation<br>Increased cerebral blood flow<br>May protect against ischemia-reperfusion injury |
| Cardiovascular/<br>Hematologic | Vasoconstriction<br>Potential coronary vasospasm<br>Decreased perfusion of end organs and periphery<br>Leftward shift of hemoglobin/oxygen dissociation curve | Direct decrease of cardiac and vascular muscle, but offset by sympathetic activation<br>Increased heart rate, blood pressure, cardiac output, perfusion of end organs and periphery<br>Rightward shift of hemoglobin/oxygen dissociation curve |
| Pulmonary | Decreased pulmonary vascular tone<br>Decreased surfactant<br>Pulmonary edema<br>May exacerbate ischemia-reperfusion lung injury | Increased ventilation<br>Increased surfactant<br>Increased compliance<br>Augmented hypoxic vasoconstriction<br>Improved V/Q matching<br>Protective against ventilator-induced and neonatal lung injury<br>Increased pulmonary vascular tone |
| Other | Hypokalemia, hypocalcemia, hypophosphatemia<br>May be pro-inflammatory | Increased H+ excretion, Na+ absorption by kidney<br>Hyperkalemia<br>Anti-inflammatory |

ventilation, as occurs early in an asthma attack, at high altitudes, or in response to metabolic acidosis, will result in hypocarbia and a respiratory alkalosis. There are many systemic effects of hypo- and hypercarbia that are sometimes difficult to predict because they often occur within the context of coexisting acid-base abnormalities from metabolic processes.[1] These effects are summarized in Table 226.1.

## CENTRAL NERVOUS SYSTEM (CNS) EFFECTS

Hypocarbia causes constriction of cerebral blood vessels, leading to a decrease in cerebral blood volume and intracranial pressure (ICP). For this reason, hyperventilation therapy is often utilized in patients with acute intracranial pathology. However, there are negative effects of this strategy that must be considered.[2] If the $CO_2$ is reduced below 25 mmHg, cerebral blood flow (CBF) may be decreased as much as 50%, potentially impairing cerebral perfusion. Conversely, hypercarbia increases CBF by 1–2 mL/100g brain tissue/minute for every 1 mmHg increase in $CO_2$ above baseline. Additionally, hypocarbia leads to increased neuronal activity and oxygen consumption, leaving the brain vulnerable to ischemia. In animal models, hypocarbia has been shown to enlarge the area of injury in experimentally induced strokes and to worsen ischemia-reperfusion injury, while the opposite is observed with hypercarbia. It is also important to recognize that if deliberate hypocarbia is

sustained, CBF will approach normal within 4 hours as a result of compensatory mechanisms, such that rapid return of normocarbia can actually precipitate cerebral hyperemia.[1]

## CARDIOVASCULAR AND HEMATOLOGIC EFFECTS

Hypercarbia results in a rightward shift of the hemoglobin-oxygen dissociation curve, which corresponds to increased oxygenation of end organs and the periphery. Because acidosis generally worsens cellular functions, hypercarbia directly results in decreased cardiac and vascular muscle contractility, but this is generally offset by its ability to stimulate the sympathetic nervous system, such that increased heart rate, blood pressure, and cardiac output are usually observed.[3] Hypocarbia causes a leftward shift of the hemoglobin-oxygen dissociation curve, inhibits delivery of oxygen to the periphery, and increases the risk of coronary spasm and ischemia.[2]

## PULMONARY EFFECTS

Hypocarbia decreases pulmonary vascular resistance such that it can be a very effective strategy to mitigate acute pulmonary hypertension. However, hypocarbia decreases surfactant production and, if profound, can trigger bronchoconstriction.[2] Although hypercarbia increases pulmonary vascular tone, potentially exacerbating pulmonary hypertension, because it causes dilation of small airways, enhances hypoxic pulmonary vascular constriction, and increases surfactant production, it generally improves V/Q matching.[3] Hypercarbia has also been demonstrated as protective against ventilator-induced lung injury and neonatal lung injury, while hypocarbia can exacerbate ischemia-reperfusion-mediated lung injury.[1]

## METABOLIC, RENAL, AND INFLAMMATORY EFFECTS

Because hypo- and hypercarbia are generally associated with a respiratory alkalosis or acidosis, respectively, they trigger compensatory mechanisms in the kidney and cellular ion transporters, leading to alterations in electrolytes. Hypocarbia may result in hypokalemia, hypocalcemia, and hypophosphatemia, causing muscle cramps, tetany, and paresthesias.[2] Hypercarbia increases H+ secretion and Na+ absorption by the kidney and may be accompanied by hyperkalemia. There is substantial evidence from animal models and human clinical studies to suggest that hypercapnia suppresses inflammation, perhaps accounting for some of its protective effects in ischemia-reperfusions states and its ability to mitigate lung injury. However, there is some concern that this anti-inflammatory property could be potentially be deleterious in the presence of active infection. Because this has not been firmly established, the coexistence of an infection is not sufficient reason to discontinue lung-protective ventilation or permissive hypercapnia.[3]

## ANESTHETIC CONSIDERATIONS

### PREOPERATIVE

Recognizing the presence and etiology of hypo- or hypercapnia that may be present preoperatively is important so that systemic effects may be anticipated and managed as part of the anesthetic plan. Patients with obstructive sleep apnea or lung disease may have unrecognized chronic hypercarbia for which they have developed compensatory mechanisms. The perioperative goal for these patients should generally be to maintain their $CO_2$ at baseline rather than attempt for normocapnia.

### INTRAOPERATIVE

Hypo- or hypercarbia may develop intraoperatively either accidentally or deliberately to induce a desired systemic effect. For example, mild hypocarbia is often used to decrease intracranial pressure in neurosurgery; however, it is important not to do this to excess, in which case cerebral perfusion can be adversely compromised. In patients not being mechanically ventilated, hypercarbia may result due to the respiratory depressant effects of sedatives and opiates, or secondary to rebreathing of accumulated $CO_2$ under poorly positioned surgical drapes. Inattention to ventilation, exhaustion of $CO_2$ absorbent, or a faulty ventilator may cause hypercarbia even in patients with secured airways. Lung-protective ventilation will also result in hypercarbia, and the negative and positive systemic effects of this ventilatory strategy should be considered.[3] Another important cause of intraoperative hypercarbia is a result of deliberate insufflation of $CO_2$ to facilitate certain procedures, such as laparoscopic surgery or endoscopy.[4]

### POSTOPERATIVE

Extubated patients in the recovery area may experience hypercarbia due to the lingering respiratory depressant effects of anesthetics and analgesics. Alternatively, poorly controlled pain may cause hyperventilation and hypocarbia. Because monitoring of end-tidal $CO_2$ is not universal in anesthesia recovery areas, being aware of the patient's ventilatory status is important to avoid hypo- or hypercarbia and their accompanying systemic effects.[5]

## REFERENCES

1. Curley G, et al. Bench-to-bedside review: Carbon dioxide. *Crit Care*. 2010;14(2):220.
2. Godoy DA, et al. Hyperventilation therapy for control of posttraumatic intracranial hypertension. *Front Neurol*. 2017;8:250.
3. Kregenow DA, Swenson ER. The lung and carbon dioxide: Implications for permissive and therapeutic hypercapnia. *Eur Respir J*. 2002;20(1):6–11.
4. Murdock CM, et al. Risk factors for hypercarbia, subcutaneous emphysema, pneumothorax, and pneumomediastinum during laparoscopy. *Obstet Gynecol*. 2000;95(5):704 709.
5. Lam T, et al. Continuous pulse oximetry and capnography monitoring for postoperative respiratory depression and adverse events: A systematic review and meta-analysis. *Anesth Analg*. 2017;125(6): 2019–2029.

# 227.

# SYSTEMIC EFFECTS OF HYPEROXIA AND HYPOXEMIA

*Sarah C. Smith*

## INTRODUCTION

Oxygen homeostasis is maintained by chemoreceptors throughout the body that respond to increased or decreased oxygen tension by triggering physiologic adaptations that prevent end-organ ischemia. Some of these changes are immediate, while others, mediated by hypoxia inducible factors (HIFs), cause changes in gene transcription that take hours or days to manifest. Chemoreceptors responsible for the rapid adaptations are found in the carotid and neuroepithelial bodies of the arterial and pulmonary vasculature, respectively. When activated by hypoxia, these chemoreceptors inhibit potassium ($K^+$) channels, resulting in cell depolarization and the release of neurotransmitters, leading to downstream effects. While hypoxemia can result from low inspired oxygen tension, impaired gas exchange, or reduced oxygen-carrying capacity of the blood, hyperoxia is always iatrogenic, but nonetheless deleterious.[1] The systemic effects of hyperoxia and hypoxia are summarized in Table 227.1.

## SYSTEMIC EFFECTS OF HYPEROXIA

### CARDIOVASCULAR EFFECTS

A meta-analysis of 33 studies of hyperoxia in human subjects, including healthy volunteers as well as those with coronary artery disease (CAD), congestive heart failure (CHF), and sepsis, showed a variety of cardiopulmonary effects, with some variability between study populations. A decrease in heart rate (HR) and an increase in systemic vascular resistance (SVR) were observed in all groups except those with sepsis. This corresponded to a modest increase in blood pressure across groups, as well as a decrease in cardiac output (CO) among healthy volunteers and those with CAD and CHF.[2]

### PULMONARY EFFECTS

Hyperoxic acute lung injury (HALI) can develop after prolonged exposure to high concentrations of inspired oxygen due to formation of oxygen free radicals which exceed the

*Table 227.1* THE SYSTEMIC EFFECTS OF HYPEROXIA AND HYPOXIA

| | HYPEROXIA | HYPOXIA |
|---|---|---|
| Cardiovascular | ↓HR, ↑SVR, ↑BP (except in sepsis) <br> ↓CO | Acute: ↑ HR, ↑ BP, peripheral vasodilation, <br> ↓ CO/ stunned myocardium if severe or prolonged <br> Chronic: RV hypertrophy, pulmonary hypertension |
| Pulmonary | HALI <br> Neonates: ↓ surfactant production, <br> ↑ pulmonary edema and inflammation, <br> ↑ risk bronchopulmonary dysplasia | Acute: ↑ RR, pulmonary vasoconstriction, <br> pulmonary edema |
| CNS | Increased risk of poor neurologic outcome in critical illness/ post–cardiac arrest <br> May increase risk of cognitive deficits, periventricular leukomalacia, intraventricular hemorrhage in neonates | Acute: headaches, confusion, fatigue <br> Chronic: possible neurocognitive deficits, but generally subtle |
| Other | Hemolytic anemia (neonates) <br> ↑ risk of retinopathy of prematurity <br> Disruption of renal/vascular development (neonates) | Acute: rightward shift of oxygen hemoglobin desaturation curve, ↑ glycolysis <br> Chronic: ↑ basal metabolic rate, polycythemia, renal dysfunction |

body's normal antioxidant defense systems. In humans, risk of HALI is negligible below an $FiO_2$ of 60%, but increases as $FiO_2$ increases above 70%. The degree of injury is dependent on both $FiO_2$ and duration of exposure, but is generally only observed after days to weeks of oxygen therapy. Cellular damage from oxygen free radicals and inflammatory processes impacts the pulmonary vasculature as well as the alveolar endo- and epithelium. The presence of fever, exogenous catecholamines, and hypercarbia can exacerbate HALI, while hypothermia, sedatives, and antihistamines may be protective.[3]

## CNS EFFECTS

Hyperoxia in the critically ill and post–cardiac arrest has been associated with an increased risk of poor neurologic outcomes.[2]

## EFFECTS OF NEONATAL HYPEROXIA

Premature infants frequently require oxygen therapy after birth due to the immaturity of their lungs and insufficient surfactant production. However, there are a number of deleterious effects of hyperoxia in the newborn, including hemolytic anemia due to oxygen free radical damage of erythrocytes. In the lung, hyperoxia can impair surfactant production, increase pulmonary inflammation, and cause edema, eventually resulting in atelectasis, fibrosis, and an increased risk of bronchopulmonary dysplasia. Abnormal vascularization of the retina can result in retinopathy of prematurity and is exacerbated by hyperoxia. Animal studies have also suggested that hyperoxia in the neonatal period may disrupt glomerular and vascular development, increasing the risk of renal disease, hypertension, and other forms of cardiac dysfunction later in life. A potential negative influence on brain development is also a concern based on animal studies, which have shown an increased risk of intraventricular hemorrhage, periventricular leukomalacia, behavioral abnormalities, and memory deficits.[4]

# SYSTEMIC EFFECTS OF HYPOXIA

## CARDIOVASCULAR

Hypoxic activation of chemoreceptors results in stimulation of the sympathetic nervous system, causing an increase in heart rate and blood pressure. Cardiac output (CO) is generally maintained or increased unless severe hypoxia and cardiac ischemic impair contractile function. Some of this decrease in cardiac function is actually adaptive, as decreased myocardial contractility and oxygen consumption actually forestall cell death. The peripheral vasculature dilates as decreased intracellular ATP levels cause the opening of $K_{ATP}$ channels. This effect is most pronounced

in the heart and brain so that blood is preferentially delivered to these organs that are most intolerant of ischemia.[1]

## PULMONARY EFFECTS

Hypoxia results in an immediate increase in the respiratory rate due to activation of the sympathetic nervous system. Inhibition of $K^+$ channels in the smooth muscle of the pulmonary vasculature results in vasoconstriction and pulmonary hypertension, which, if sustained, results in right ventricular hypertrophy. Acute hypoxia may also cause pulmonary edema, as is typical in altitude sickness.[5]

## CNS EFFECTS

Acute hypoxia, as occurs when people rapidly ascend to a high altitude, has neuropsychological effects including difficulty concentrating, headaches, and drowsiness. It is unclear if those with chronic hypoxia have similar neuropsychological deficits.[5]

## METABOLIC, HEMATOLOGIC, AND RENAL EFFECTS

As less oxygen is available for metabolism, cells shift to using anaerobic processes for ATP production, primarily glycolysis.[1] Hypoxia results in an immediate rightward shift of the hemoglobin oxygen desaturation curve such that hemoglobin more readily releases oxygen to the tissues. Chronic hypoxia results in increased levels of erythropoietin produced by the kidney, increasing the hemoglobin concentration of the blood. Other effects on the kidney from chronic hypoxia include decreased renal perfusion, glomerular hypertrophy, proteinuria, and hyperuricemia. Subsequently, people living at high altitudes are more vulnerable to developing renal disease.[5]

# ANESTHETIC CONSIDERATIONS

## PREOPERATIVE

Patients with significant lung disease or right to left shunts may experience chronic hypoxia and can be anticipated to demonstrate a variety of subsequent systemic effects, including pulmonary hypertension, right ventricular (RV) failure, polycythemia, and renal dysfunction. Preoperative anesthesia assessment should focus on the degree and duration of the hypoxia, as well as systemic effects which may impact anesthetic management.

## INTRAOPERATIVE

Because monitoring of oxygen saturation is standard and ubiquitous, intraoperative hypoxia is usually recognized and addressed before systemic manifestations are apparent. Occasionally, periods of hypoxia during an invasive procedure must be tolerated, however, as during one-lung ventilation for thoracic surgery. During these episodes, the anesthesiologist must remain aware of the potential systemic effects, particularly pulmonary hypertension and potential RV dysfunction. As hyperoxia is also deleterious due to the effect of oxygen free radicals, unnecessarily high $FiO_2$ should also be avoided during general anesthesia, particularly in patients vulnerable to acute lung injury.

## POSTOPERATIVE

Patients requiring mechanical ventilation after general anesthesia should be maintained on an $FiO_2$ less than 70% whenever possible to avoid the deleterious effects of hyperoxia while also maintaining a satisfactory $PaO_2$. This is best accomplished with a lung protective ventilation strategy of low tidal volumes and titrated positive end-expiratory pressure (PEEP). Other methods to maximize oxygenation and minimize $FiO_2$ include aggressive pulmonary toilet, recruitment maneuvers, and keeping the head of the patient's bed elevated greater than 30°.

## REFERENCES

1. Michiels C. Physiological and pathological responses to hypoxia. *Am J Pathol.* 2004;164(6):1875–1882.
2. Smit B, et al. Hemodynamic effects of acute hyperoxia: systematic review and meta-analysis. *Crit Care.* 2018;22(1):45.
3. Kallet RH, Matthay MA. Hyperoxic acute lung injury. *Respir Care.* 2013;58(1):123–141.
4. Perrone S, et al. Oxygen use in neonatal care: A two-edged sword. *Front Pediatr.* 2016;4:143.
5. Hurtado A, et al. Cardiovascular and renal effects of chronic exposure to high altitude. *Nephrol Dial Transplant.* 2012;27 (Suppl 4):11–16.

# 228.

# BASIC INTERPRETATION OF ARTERIAL BLOOD GAS AND TEMPERATURE CORRECTION

*Erica Zanath and Mada Helou*

## INTRODUCTION

Biochemical reactions are sensitive to changes in hydrogen ion concentration, and therefore changes in pH can be dangerous.

## ACID-BASE DEFINITION

Multiple definitions are used to describe acids and bases.[1,2] According to the Bronsted-Lowry definition, an acid is molecule that can donate a proton (H+), and a base is a molecule that can accept a proton. The Arrhenius definition describes acids as molecules that react with water to form H+, and bases as molecules that react with water to form OH−.

Strong acids/bases almost irreversibly dissociate where as weak acid/bases reversibly dissociate to donate H+/accept H+.[1,2] A weak acid (HA) in solution behaves according to the following equation:

$$HA \leftrightarrow H+ + A-$$

Dissociation of this weak acid is described by:

$$K = [H+][A-]/[HA]$$

The Henderson-Hasselbalch equation[1,2] is then derived from the previous equation:

$$pH = pK + log([A-]/[HA])$$

When applied physiologically:

$$pH = pK' + ([HCO3-]/0.03\ PaCO2)$$

Therefore, the physiologic pH is directly proportional to changes in bicarbonate ion concentration and indirectly proportional to changes in the partial pressure of carbon dioxide.

Using the Henderson-Hasselbalch equation for acid-base analysis in biologic solutions is limited by their complexity. The strong ion difference (SID) can instead be used to account for variations in blood chemistry. SID is the difference between all strong cations and strong anions. A strong ion difference means unmeasured ions must be present.

## ACID-BASE DISTURBANCES

Disturbances in the normal acid-base balance can be defined as either acidosis or alkalosis.[1,2] Acidosis occurs when the primary disturbance decreases the pH, whereas alkalosis occurs when the primary disturbance increases the pH. A normal physiologic pH is 7.4. A blood pH <7.35 is acidemia, whereas a blood pH >7.45 is alkalemia.

An acid-base disturbance is further classified as respiratory or metabolic. A respiratory disturbance results from a change in the $PaCO_2$. A metabolic disturbance results from a change in the bicarbonate ion concentration. Mixed disorders occur when two disturbances exist simultaneously.

Therefore acid-based disorders are classified as: respiratory acidosis, respiratory alkalosis, metabolic acidosis, metabolic alkalosis, or mixed disorders.

Respiratory acidosis is defined as pH <7.35 resulting from an increase in $PaCO_2$ due to hypoventilation or increased $CO_2$ production. Respiratory alkalosis is defined as pH >7.45 resulting from a decreased in $PaCO_2$ due to hyperventilation from either central or peripheral stimuli. Metabolic acidosis is defined as pH <7.35 resulting from a decrease in $HCO_{3-}$. It is further separated into anion gap and non-anion gap pathologies. Anion gap measures the difference in major plasma cations and anions:[1,2]

$$Anion\ gap = [Na+] - ([Cl-] + [HCO3-])$$

A normal anion gap is 12 mEq/L. As the anion gap only accounts for measured ions, a change in the anion gap reflects a change in unmeasured ions. An elevated anion gap results from an increase in unmeasured anions or a decrease in

unmeasured cations. The causes of high anion gap metabolic acidosis are increased production or toxic ingestion.[1,2,3] The mnemonic "MUDPILES" is used to remember the typical causes: methanol, uremia, diabetic ketoacidosis, propylene glycol, isoniazid, lactic acidosis, ethylene glycol, and salicylates. Non-anion gap metabolic acidosis, a hyperchloremic acidosis, results from loss of bicarbonate from the gastrointestinal tract or kidneys.[1,2,4] The mnemonic "FUSED CAR" is used to remember typical causes: fistulas, ureteral diversion, saline infusion, exogenous acid, diarrhea, carbonic anhydrase inhibitors, adrenal insufficiency, and renal tubular acidosis. Metabolic alkalosis is defined as pH >7.45 resulting from an increase in $HCO_{3-}$ due to either decreased extracellular fluid or increased mineralocorticoid activity.

As normally physiologic function depends on a normal pH, the body has mechanisms to compensate for changes in acid-base status through buffers, respiratory compensation, and renal compensation.[1,2] Compensation via buffer systems occurs immediately. Physiology buffer systems include bicarbonate, hemoglobin, intracellular phosphates, and ammonia. Respiratory compensation starts within minutes and involves alteration in minute ventilation. Renal compensation starts within hours, with maximal compensation occurring within several days. It involves controlling bicarbonate reabsorption, bicarbonate formation, and elimination of hydrogen ions as phosphate and ammonia.

## BLOOD GAS ANALYSIS

Blood gas analysis should proceed in a stepwise approach.

1. Evaluate pH—acidemia vs. alkalemia.
2. Determine the primary disturbance—respiratory vs metabolic.
   a. Evaluate $PaCO_2$.
   b. Evaluate $HCO_{3-}$.
   c. If a primary metabolic acidosis exists, determine anion gap.
3. Determine if there is compensation. Determine if the compensation is appropriate.
4. Evaluate chronicity.

Table 228.1 summarizes the primary disturbance, compensation, and magnitude of compensation seen with each type of acid base disturbance.

### TEMPERATURE CORRECTION

Temperature has an important role in blood gas analysis. As temperature decreases, the solubility of gas molecules increases. This means that as temperature decreases, $O_2$ and $CO_2$ solubility increase and the partial pressures decrease.[2] However, bicarbonate ion concentration does not change

*Table 228.1* ACID-BASE DISTURBANCES AND ASSOCIATED COMPENSATIONS

| | PRIMARY DISTURBANCE | COMPENSATION | MAGNITUDE OF COMPENSATION |
|---|---|---|---|
| Acute respiratory acidosis | Increased $PaCO_2$ | Increased $HCO_{3-}$ | $HCO_{3-}$ increases 1 mEq/L per 10 mmHg $PaCO_2$ change |
| Chronic respiratory acidosis | Increased $PaCO_2$ | Increased $HCO_{3-}$ | $HCO_{3-}$ increases 4 mEq/L per 10 mmHg $PaCO_2$ change |
| Acute respiratory alkalosis | Decreased $PaCO_2$ | Decreased $HCO_{3-}$ | $HCO_{3-}$ decreases 2 mEq/L per 10 mmHg $PaCO_2$ change |
| Chronic respiratory alkalosis | Decreased $PaCO_2$ | Decreased $HCO_{3-}$ | $HCO_{3-}$ decreases 4 mEq/L per 10 mmHg $PaCO_2$ change |
| Metabolic acidosis | Decreased $HCO_{3-}$ | Decreased $PaCO_2$ | $PaCO_2$ decreases by 1.2 x $HCO_{3-}$ decrease |
| Metabolic alkalosis | Increased $HCO_{3-}$ | Increased $PaCO_2$ | $PaCO_2$ increases by 0.7 x $HCO_{3-}$ increase |

with temperature fluctuations; therefore pH consequently changes with temperature.

Blood gas analysis occurs at 37°C. If the patient is hypothermic with a temperature less than 37°C, heating the sample for analysis leads to an increase in reported $PaCO_2$ and a decrease in reported pH compared to the patient's actual $PaCO_2$ and pH—meaning the patient's $PaCO_2$ is lower and the patient's pH is higher.

There are two forms of blood gas analysis used: pH stat and alpha stat. pH stat is a temperature-corrected measurement that is often used during profound hypothermic states. The goal of this method is to maintain a constant pH by adding $CO_2$ to maintain $PaCO^2$ 40 mmHg. The advantage of pH stat is improved cerebral perfusion. The disadvantage of pH stat is an increased risk of microemboli related to increased amount of dissolved gas molecules in a hypothermic state, which then return to gaseous form with warming. Alpha stat is the method of blood gas analysis that uses the patient's uncorrected $PaCO_2$ and pH. Alpha stat management is based on the protonation state of histidine. As temperature changes, the protonation state of histidine remains constant. The goal of using alpha stat is to maintain electrochemical neutrality with a constant ratio of H+ to OH–.

## ANESTHETIC CONSIDERATIONS

Intraoperative ventilator management can affect acid-base balance as changes in minute ventilation alter the $PaCO_2$.[1,2] This may be useful in certain circumstances, for example in intracranial cases where hyperventilation can be utilized to decrease $PaCO_2$, which subsequently decreases cerebral blood flow.

Acid-base alterations can affect the expected physiologic function.[1,2] In conditions of acidosis, myocardial contraction is depressed. As acidosis progresses, response to catecholamines is diminished, further predisposing to cardiovascular decompensation.

## REFERENCES

1. Barash PG, et al. *Clinical Anesthesia*. 7th ed. Philadelphia, PA: Lippincott Williams & Wilkins; 2013.
2. Butterworth JF, et al. *Morgan and Mikhail's Clinical Anesthesiology*. 5th ed. McGraw-Hill; 2013.
3. Haber RJ. A practical approach to acid-base disorders. *The Western Journal of Medicine,* 1991;155(2).
4. Kraut JA, Madias NE. Differential diagnosis of nongap metabolic acidosis: Value of a systemic approach. *Clinical J Am Soc Nephrol.* 2012;7(4):671–679.

# 229.

# RESPIRATORY CENTERS

*Drew Cornwell and Lynn Kohan*

## INTRODUCTION

Control of ventilation occurs within an anatomical area referred to as the *respiratory center*. It is an anatomical collection of neurons within the medulla oblongata and the pons that work to maintain homeostatic balance of pH, $CO_2$, and oxygen throughout the varied metabolic demands encountered in normal and abnormal physiology. The medullary centers provide the most basic ventilatory control of inspiration and expiration. Additional influences of the respiratory pattern can be generated within the pons, cortical regions of the brain, and peripheral sites with significant cross-innervation (Figure 229.1). The sensitivity of respiratory centers can be augmented by physical conditioning, states of consciousness, comorbid respiratory disease, narcotics, and being under general anesthesia.

Peripheral chemoreceptors are present in the carotid bodies (cranial nerve IX) and aortic bodies (cranial nerve X); they stimulate the inspiratory center when $PaO_2$ decreases. The effect is greatest between 30 and 60 mmHg.

## MEDULLA

Two general areas, the dorsal respiratory (DRG) and ventral respiratory group (VRG), manage inspiration and expiration, respectively. Within the dorsum of the medulla, the DRG manages timing of the inspiratory rhythm as well as coordination of voluntary and involuntary respirations. Located near terminal afferent fibers of the glossopharyngeal (IX) and vagus (X) nerves, the signals generated from DRG neurons fire in a "ramping-up" pattern to increase efferent signaling over the course of 2–3 seconds until an abrupt termination of inspiration occurs.[1,2] The ventral respiratory group (VRG) within the ventral reticular formation of the medulla functions to coordinate expiration and prevent ataxic breathing by modulating the force generated by inspiratory muscles. The DRG and VRG balance and coordinate inspiration and expiration via negative feedback. As inspiratory effort generated by the DRG is slowed to eventual cessation by the VRG, which then prevents further activation of inspiratory musculature, provided by the primary mechanism of passive expiration. During times of increased demand, the VRG will stimulate muscles of expiration to shift from a passive to an active process. Conventional understanding termed the medulla as the "pacemaker" of the respiratory cycle, though it is now hypothesized that a group of neurons composes a central pattern generator responsible for the complex coordination. Overall, the medulla requires no afferent input to create the most primitive of ventilatory drive. When functioning in relative isolation the medulla would create "gasping" and ataxic breaths, as sometimes seen in patients

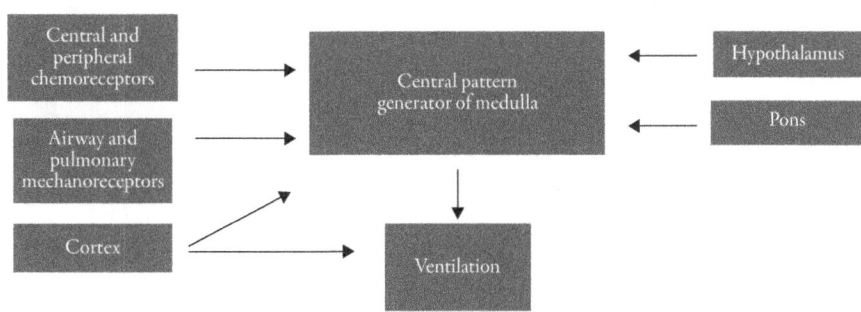

**Figure 229.1.** Select afferent and efferent pathways of the respiratory control center.

with traumatic or cardiovascular damage to surrounding neurological structures.

## PONS

Within the rostral pons, three groups of neurons, termed *inspiratory*, *expiratory*, and *phase-spanning* (previously referred to as the *pneumotaxic center*), fire in differing phases of ventilation to modulate the rate and pattern of breathing. Apneusis, the cessation of ventilatory effort when TLC is reached, is generated from these groups. As the understanding of the pontine role in the respiratory center evolves, it is no longer believed to be essential in the overall process.[1] Many afferent pathways from the cortex, hypothalamus, and nucleus tractus soltarius (NTS) converge on the pons, suggesting it primarily serves to coordinate and process the afferent signals prior to continuing to the medulla. In the lower pons, an apneustic center opposes actions of the pneumotaxic center, but plays no primary role under normal conditions.

## CORTICAL CONTROL

Cortical control of breathing is demonstrated by the conscious ability to hyper- and hypoventilate oneself. Neurons from cortical pathways bypass the respiratory center to permit coughing, talking, and singing. When partial pressure oxygen in artierial blood ($PaO_2$) or partial pressure carbon dioxide in arterial blood ($PaCO_2$) levels reach approximately 50 mmHg in an otherwise healthy individual, this conscious control is overwhelmed by the involuntary drive to generate a breath. This apneic threshold can be altered in clinical circumstances to raise or lower the point at which voluntary control is lost (see Chapter 231, "Carbon Dioxide Response Curves").

## NONCHEMICAL PERIPHERAL INFLUENCES

Mechanical forces play a notable role of afferent signaling to the respiratory center. Slow- and fast-adapting pulmonary stretch receptors from the lungs and airways produce afferent signal to the NTS. When anesthetized by neuraxial anesthesia, proprioceptive tendon spindles within the intercostal muscles can produce a sense of dyspnea, despite otherwise normal ventilation. Though incompletely demonstrated in humans, the Herring-Breuer reflex will trigger apnea in response to the overextension of lung parenchyma.[2] Pulmonary C-fibers lying in proximal capillaries influence the dyspneic breathing patterns that are seen with pulmonary edema and emboli, as well as the part of the ventilatory response to exercise.[1]

## ANESTHETIC CONSIDERATIONS

### PREOPERATIVE

Uncoordinated breathing patterns can be suggestive of brainstem pathology.

### INTRAOPERATIVE

Neuraxial anesthesia can invoke a sense of dyspnea in mothers, despite normal lung function, due to the blockage of intercostal proprioceptors.

## REFERENCES

1. Lumb A, Nunn J. *Nunn's Applied Respiratory Physiology.* 7th ed. Philadelphia, PA: Edinburgh: Churchill Livingstone/Elsevier; 2010:65–75.
2. West J, Luks A. *West's Respiratory Physiology.* 10th ed. Wolters Kluwer; 2015:278–290.
3. Barash P, et al. *Clinical Anesthesia.* 8th ed. Philadelphia, PA: Wolters Kluwer Health/Lippincott Williams & Wilkins; 2016:366–369.

# 230.

# CENTRAL AND PERIPHERAL CHEMORECEPTORS

*Drew Cornwell and Lynn Kohan*

## INTRODUCTION

Two sets of sensors function to provide input to the respiratory control center. Named based on relative location, the central and peripheral chemoreceptors function in different capacities to assist in maintenance of overall homeostasis. Chemoreceptors are specialized tissues that respond to changes in the chemical composition of blood and fluid.

## CENTRAL CHEMORECEPTOR

Embedded in the ventral medulla, central chemoreceptors sense minute-to-minute changes in extracellular fluid composition—specifically, pH changes within the cerebrospinal fluid (CSF). As the blood/gas-brain barrier prevents transmembrane movement of ionically charged bicarbonate and hydrogen ions, the system is dependent on the conversion to and transmembrane diffusion of carbon dioxide ($HCO_2$).

$$CO_2 + H_2O \leftrightarrow H_2CO_3 \leftrightarrow H^+ + HCO_{3-}$$

With a relatively acidotic pH of 7.32, the reduced buffering capacity of CSF makes it more sensitive to small changes in $CO_2$ concentration.[1] Elevations in $CO_2$ within the CSF lead to production of carbonic acid and an ultimate rise in [H]+, producing increased signaling to pacemaker neurons, which ultimately increases the rate of ventilation (Figure 230.1). This effect reaches peak levels within a matter of minutes and begins to wane after a number of hours after buffering of the CSF has occurred.[2]

Around 80% of the ventilatory response to changes in $CO_2$ levels occurs in receptors positioned near the glossopharyngeal (IX) and vagus (X) nerves (1).

Due to the acute rise of $CO_2$, respiratory acidosis has a more immediate impact on respiratory rate than that of metabolic acidosis. $PaO_2$ and pH are believed to have minimal impact upon central chemoreceptors

## PERIPHERAL CHEMORECEPTORS

Multiple peripheral receptors exist in locations such as the carotid and aortic bodies, as well as the lungs. Additional signaling is generated from the nose, joints, muscles, and in response to pain and temperature.

Located at the bifurcation of the common carotid artery with afferent signaling via the glossopharyngeal nerve (IV), the carotid bodies respond primarily to drops in arterial oxygen content. For their weight, the carotid bodies receive more blood flow per unit time than nearly any other organ in the body.[1] Carotid body function serves in situations of hypoxia to increase the respiratory rate (largest effect when $PaO_2$ between 30 and 60 mmHg). Minimal signaling occurs with $PaO_2$ >90 mmHg.[1-3]

Unlike the central receptors, the carotid bodies do respond directly to changes in arterial pH. As such, they play a greater role in the increased respiratory rate seen in the setting of metabolic acidosis. Response to changes in $PaCO_2$ does occur, but at 20% that of central receptors.

Aortic body receptors are positioned near the aortic arch with afferents via the vagus nerve (CN X). Receptors within the lungs respond to pulmonary stretch, triggering

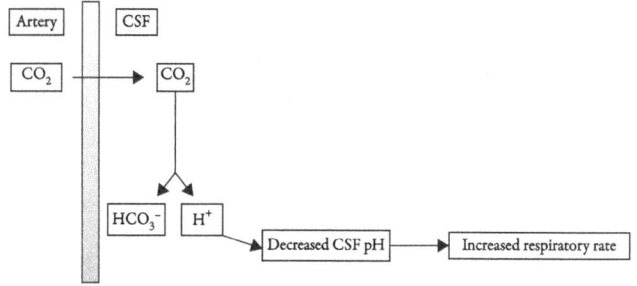

**Figure 230.1.** Effect of PaCO2 on rate of ventilation.

the Herring-Breur reflex. Rapidly acting receptors to irritants are implicated in bronchoconstriction as well as the asthmatic response to cold air. Juxtacapillary (J receptors) within alveolar walls respond to stimulation by producing dyspneic rapid-shallow breaths[3] and may play a role in patterns seen in conditions like pulmonary edema.

## ANESTHETIC CONSIDERATIONS

### PREOPERATIVE

Labs drawn on patients with preexisting pulmonary disease will often be noted to have elevated $CO_2$ levels on Basic metabolic panel, indicating a chronic compensation of respiratory acidosis.

### POSTOPERATIVE

Supplemental oxygen in patients with preexisting pulmonary disease can lead to bradypnea due to loss of "hypoxic-drive" of respiration.

## REFERENCES

1. West J. *Lectures in Respiratory Physiology.* [Online]. 2020. Available at: https://mhttps://meded.ucsd.edu/ifp/jwest/resp_phys/index.htmleded.ucsd.edu/ifp/jwest/resp_phys/index.html. Accessed April 16, 2020.
2. Barash P, et al. *Clinical Anesthesia.* 8th ed. Philadelphia, PA: Wolters Kluwer/Lippincott Williams and Wilkins; 2017:366–369.
3. Lumb, A. Non Respiratory Functions of the Lng. In Lumb A, ed. *Nunn's Applied Respiratory Physiology.* Elxeveier NY, NY; 2017:203–214.

# 231.

# CARBON DIOXIDE RESPONSE CURVES

*Drew Cornwell and Lynn Kohan*

## INTRODUCTION

The ventilatory response to changes in oxygen ($O_2$) and carbon dioxide ($CO_2$) tension sensed by the peripheral and central chemoreceptors can be illustrated through response curves. The $CO_2$ response curve is a graphical representation of the linear relationship between partial pressure of carbon dioxide ($PaCo_2$) and alveolar ventilation and its classical negative-feedback loop.[1] Physiologic and pharmacologic influences can alter this curve, though greater variations occur as influenced $CO_2$ than that of $O_2$ (Figure 231.1).[2]

## CARBON DIOXIDE RESPONSE CURVE

Ventilatory depression and its rise in $PaCO_2$ will demonstrate a linear increase in alveolar ventilation. Healthy

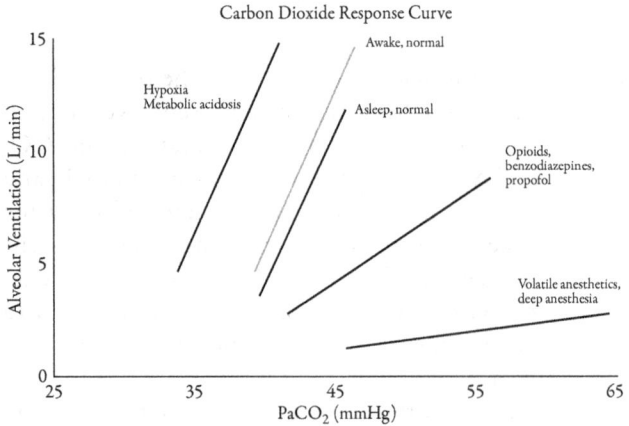

**Figure 231.1.** Carbon dioxide response curve and changes in response to physiological and pharmacological influences.

Reproduce with permission from Benner A and Sharma S. (2020), *Physiology, carbon dioxide response curve.* https://www.statpearls.com/.

and awake individuals who breathe $CO_2$ will show an increase in minute ventilation by an average of 3 L/min for every 1 mmHg increase of $PaCO_2$. Inhaled anesthetics of concentrations >1 MAC demonstrate a dose dependent rightward and downward shift in this response and with the near complete elimination of peripheral chemoreceptor response to $CO_2$.[3]

Clinically relevant changes in the $CO_2$ curve are seen with opioids and other CNS depressants (such as benzodiazepines and propofol) as a rightward shift and decrease in slope.

## OXYGEN INFLUENCE

Under normoxic conditions ($PaO_2$ 65–100 mmHg) there are minimal changes in the rate of ventilation by oxygen-sensing-chemoreceptors. At a constant partial pressure of oxygen ($PaO_2$), an upward and downward shift of hypoxic-drive curve can be seen in conditions of hypercapnia and hypocapnia, respectively.[4] This is primarily demonstrated in experimental models and is of minimal clinical significance.

Hypoxic conditions ($PaO_2$ <65 mmHg) do create a clinically significant leftward shift in the $CO_2$ response curve, similar to that seen during metabolic acidosis.[3]

The degree of hemoglobin oxygenation affects the position of the $CO_2$ dissociation curve. The lower the saturation of hemoglobin with $O_2$, the higher the $CO_2$ content for a given $PCO_2$. This is known as the Haldane effect.

## ANESTHETIC CONSIDERATIONS

### PREOPERATIVE

Administration of anxiolytic medications leading to apnea occurs because of the rightward shift in the $CO_2$ response curve.

### INTRAOPERATIVE

While nearing emergence at the end of a case, an anesthetic provider can utilize their knowledge of the $CO_2$ response curve to assist a patient to return to spontaneous ventilation. Apneic oxygenation with high fraction of inspired oxygen ($FiO_2$) can maintain a patient's $SpO_2$, though it may not provide sufficient ventilation to prevent hypercapnia.

## REFERENCES

1. West J. *Lectures In Respiratory Physiology*. [Online]. 2020. Available at: https://mhttps://meded.ucsd.edu/ifp/jwest/resp_phys/index.htmleded.ucsd.edu/ifp/jwest/resp_phys/index.html. Accessed April 16, 2020.
2. Benner A, Sharma S. Physiology, carbon dioxide response curve. Statpearls.com. https://www.statpearls.com/kb/viewarticle/18851. Published 2020. Accessed June 15, 2020.
3. Gropper M. *Miller's Anesthesia*. 8th ed. Philadelphia, PA: Elsevier 2020:540–571.
4. Duffin J. Measuring the ventilatory response to hypoxia. *J Physiol (Lond)*. 2007;584(1):285–293. doi:10.1113/jphysiol.2007.138883

# 232.

# NON-RESPIRATORY FUNCTION OF LUNGS

*Drew Cornwell and Lynn Kohan*

## INTRODUCTION

Beyond the role of ventilation and gas exchange, there are numerous non-respiratory functions of the lung that maintain normal physiology. These functions include defense against inhaled substances, filtration of endogenous and exogenous materials, drug extraction and metabolism, metabolism of hormones, and acting as a reservoir to the vascular system.

## DEFENSE

Physical barriers and immune function of the airways protect against inhaled physical and chemical materials.

A mucous covering of mucopolysaccharide gel that extends from the nose to the bronchioles is the first line of defense. Material trapped within this layer are removed and expectorated by the mucociliary elevator. Items in diameter of 2–5 micrometers make it to the smallest of airways.[1] Ciliary activity is parasympathetically controlled by the vagus nerve (CN X). Motility is slowed by smoking, dehydration, inspiration of dry gases, extreme temperature, and dysmotility conditions. Commonly administered anesthetics such as inhaled agents, local anesthetics, and atropine will slow activity. High-dose ketamine and fentanyl promote ciliary activity (2).

Immune activity is primarily mediated by pulmonary alveolar macrophages (PAM). Alveolar particles are engulfed by PAMs and deposited in either the mucociliary elevator or blood/lymphatic circulation for removal. When large quantities of noxious material are ingested by PAMs (such as from smoking), there is subsequent inflammation created by lysosomal products.[1] Long-term exposure leads to fibrosis and lung disease.

IgA immunoglobulin is found in high concentrations within bronchial secretions to fight respiratory infection.[1]

## FILTRATION

Endogenous materials (such as embolized blood, gas, and fat) as well as exogenous materials which have made it past primary defenses can be prevented from entering systemic circulation. Extensive pulmonary microcirculation maintains alveolar perfusion to a certain extent. Physically trapped blood clots are broken down by fibrinolysin, which is readily activated by pulmonary endothelium. A balance of coagulation is maintained by rich supplies of coagulation-inhibiting heparin and the coagulation-promoting activity of thromboplastin.[3]

## DRUG METABOLISM AND BINDING

A small and easily saturated cytochrome P450 system within the lungs serves as a site of extra-hepatic drug metabolism as well as the temporary extraction of drugs from circulation.[3] Intravenous (IV) anesthetic drugs such as propofol, fentanyl, diazepam, and local anesthetic amines are highly extracted by the lungs. While they are metabolized to a minimal extent, this extraction serves as a buffered

*Table 232.1* PULMONARY ENDOTHELIAL METABOLISM ON HORMONES WITHIN PULMONARY CIRCULATION

|  | UNCHANGED | ACTIVATED | REMOVED/ INACTIVATED |
|---|---|---|---|
| Peptide | Angiotensin II, vasopressin, oxytocin | Angiotensin I | Atrial natriuretic peptide |
| Arachidonic derived | Prostacyclin | Arachidonic acid | Leukotriene, $PGD_2$, $PGE_2$, $PGF_2$ |
| Purine derived | none | none | Adenosine, ATP/ ADP/AMP |
| Amine | Dopamine, epinephrine, histamine | none | Norepinephrine, serotonin |

Abbreviations: Prosstaglandin D (PGD); prostaglandin E (PGE); prostaglandin F (PGF); Anedosine triophosphate (ATP); adensoinde diphosphate (ADP); andosoine monophosphate (AMP).

release into systemic circulation after plasma concentration decreases.

Metabolic activity of the lungs is utilized for delivery of prodrugs which cannot be easily compounded for IV or PO administration.

## METABOLISM OF HORMONES

The pulmonary endothelium contains the most metabolically active cell types within the lungs. Hormones passing through pulmonary circulation can be either unchanged, activated, or entirely removed from circulation[4] (Table 232.1). This metabolic activity is responsible for the extremely short half-life seen in peripherally administered drugs like adenosine.

## VASCULAR RESERVOIR

Total pulmonary blood volume, as indexed to body surface area (BSA), is approximately 200–300 mL/m².[2] This means that about 10% of an adult's estimated blood volume is contained within pulmonary circulation at a given time, 25% percent of which is within the capillaries. This volume can be increased by as much as 50% when the highly compliant pulmonary beds are recruited during periods of increased demand. Valsalva maneuvers and changing from a supine to erect posture can increase and decrease pulmonary blood volume respectively.

## ANESTHETIC CONSIDERATIONS

### PREOPERATIVE

Ciliary function can be significantly compromised in smokers. Knowing when a patient last smoked can give insight on their ability to clear secretions.

### INTRAOPERATIVE

High-dose ketamine and fentanyl can promote ciliary function, producing a significant amount of secretions. Special attention should be paid to patients in the prone position, as this increased volume has the potential to impair the adhesive ability of tape securing endotracheal tubes.

## REFERENCES

1. Harada R, Repine J. Pulmonary host defense mechanisms. *Chest.* 1985;87(2):247–252.
2. Lumb AB. Chapter 12—Pregnancy, Neonates and Children. In: AB Lumb, ed. *Nunn's Applied Respiratory Physiology.* 8th ed. Elsevier; 2017:217–226.e1.
3. Joseph D, et al. Non-respiratory functions of the lung. *Cont Educ Anaesth Crit Care Pain.* 2013;13(3):98–102.
4. Chitkara R, Khan F. Endocrine functions of the lung. In: WB Essman, eds. *Hormonal Actions in Non-endocrine Systems.* Springer, Dordrecht; 1983:147–199.

# 233.

# PERIOPERATIVE SMOKING AND CAFFEINE USE

*David E. Swanson*

## INTRODUCTION

If the timing of the preanesthetic visit happens to allow, encouraging smoking cessation for 4 weeks prior to surgery can decrease the risk for the patient, and cessation for 8 weeks furthers this benefit. Wong's analysis countered prior teaching by showing that <4 weeks abstinence from smoking does not increase or reduce postoperative respiratory complications.[1] Attempts to quantitate effects of less than 4 weeks of cessation have not been as clear as Mills's demonstration of a relative risk reduction of 41% for prevention of postoperative complications and that each week of cessation increases the magnitude of effect by 19%.[2] Even if a patient stops smoking 48 hours prior to surgery, the carbon monoxide is eliminated from the body, making hypoxia theoretically less likely, but in as little as 8 hours after the last cigarette, the carbon monoxide level in the blood is halved. Carbon monoxide can increase carboxyhemoglobin.

Addiction is a disease that can be very challenging to manage. Nicotine is incredibly addictive, ranking right behind heroin and cocaine in some listings. It increases sympathetic tone. The addictive aspect of tobacco smoking is relevant to the perioperative period since it is a window of opportunity to encourage smoking cessation in this teachable moment. The discussion of smoking cessation during the preanesthetic evaluation can be a short, but very impactful use of time from a public health standpoint. Patients are often thinking about their health with an upcoming surgery more than at any other time in their lives. It can make a huge difference in the long-term health of a patient who quits because of your brief intervention.

Cessation interventions with more sessions, done face-to-face by nurses, as well as specific behavior-change techniques (discussing consequences, withdrawal symptoms, goals, regular monitoring by others, and later support) were associated with larger effects.[3] It is important to treat withdrawal in patients that will be admitted overnight. Older studies raised concern of increased cardiac mortality when nicotine replacement therapy (NRT) was used perioperatively. This has now been refuted in a large observational study showing that perioperative NRT is not associated with adverse outcomes after surgery. NRT is currently only prescribed to a small fraction of patients and should be prescribed routinely for smokers in the perioperative period.[4]

Not all aspects of perioperative smoking are bad. Smokers do have a decreased incidence of postoperative nausea and vomiting (PONV), preeclampsia, and death from cardiac events.

Caffeine has been touted as the most used psychoactive substance in the world, estimated as being used regularly by 80%–90% of adults around the world. Initially it increases blood pressure, plasma catecholamines, urine production, and gastric acid secretion. The problem of caffeine withdrawal on the day of surgery has lessened, as it has become common to allow clear liquids on the day of surgery. Withdrawal can cause headache, lack of energy, and fatigue. This should be high on the differential diagnosis of headache in the postoperative timeframe.

## CLINICAL FEATURES

Tobacco cigarette smoke is known to cause deleterious effects on the cardiovascular system, angiogenesis, and skin capillary perfusion by causing direct injury to blood vessel walls, increased platelet aggregation, microvascular thrombosis, and inflammation. Smoking decreases ciliary function in the bronchopulmonary tree and increases sputum production. While tobacco smoke has been extensively studied, with abundant knowledge of detrimental effects to humans, much less is known about the long-term effects of inhaling nicotine vapors. There is a growing body of literature that e-cigarettes present dangers in rodents, which implies similar long-term damage in humans. The inflammatory response to e-cigarette use increases neutrophil activation and mucus production, and decreased mucociliary clearance. It has been shown that the aerosolized nicotine-containing e-cigarette fluid increased airway hyperreactivity, distal airspace enlargement, mucin production, and cytokine and protease expression in mice, clearly indicating that e-cigarettes are just as toxic as tobacco cigarettes and that chronic exposure to nicotine vapor can cause significant lung damage.[5]

## DIAGNOSIS

A thorough history, including how many packs per day and for how many years, can guide postoperative planning, especially if a patient may be undiagnosed for chronic obstructive pulmonary disease (COPD).

## TREATMENT

Discussion of smoking cessation and management of bronchospasm and hypoxia are the keys to treatment.

## ANESTHETIC CONSIDERATIONS

### PREOPERATIVE

Have a heightened awareness for lung, coronary artery, and peripheral vascular diseases in smokers. After confirming current or recent cigarette smoking or vaping, offer cessation advice. If wheezes are detected on a pulmonary exam, preoperative bronchodilators with several puffs of albuterol or a nebulized treatment would be indicated. This is not just an issue for the smokers themselves. Children exposed to secondhand smoke have elevated respiratory perioperative adverse events and benefit from preoperative bronchodilator therapy.

### INTRAOPERATIVE

As the severity of the lung disease increases, the choice of anesthesia becomes increasingly important, with consideration for regional anesthesia (RA) as the sole anesthetic for lower extremity surgeries in the supine position. The special situation of patients with end-stage lung disease requiring shoulder surgery adds the extra risk of respiratory distress from phrenic nerve blockade, if interscalene block is used.

Coughing with induction and emergence is much more common in smokers. This can be minimized with induction by administering appropriate narcotics, assuring adequate depth of anesthesia prior to airway placement, and some claim benefit using atomized lidocaine of the trachea guided by direct laryngoscopy just prior to intubation. During general anesthetics, the end tidal carbon dioxide ($ETCO_2$) tracing can be useful in assessing the extent of diseased airways, acute bronchospasm, and response to bronchodilators. Volatile anesthetics are good bronchodilators. Keep in mind that desflurane is the least desirable in smokers. Nitrous oxide increases the chance of hypoxia, especially at emergence, due to diffusion hypoxia. This is readily detected by pulse oximetry, but smokers coughing with emergence may make it more difficult to correct quickly. Certain cases involving the head and neck in which coughing on emergence can lead to bleeding or increased intracranial or ocular pressures present an added challenge in smokers. Options to minimize this risk include intravenous lidocaine, proper intraoperative narcotic dosing, and deep extubation.

Many studies have been done looking at the hemostatic effects of caffeine. The role of energy drinks and coffee in the modulation of hemostasis is not completely understood, and may improve or worsen hemostasis likely depending on other bioactive compounds in the beverage.

## POSTOPERATIVE

Headache is a common problem postoperatively, and caffeine withdrawal is frequently the etiology. Caffeine has long been touted for mild post-dural puncture headaches (PDPH), but evidenced-based medicine offers little support of this practice. The risk of adverse events is low, but there are case reports of post-partum seizures related to caffeine for PDPH.

## REFERENCES

1. Wong J, et al. Short-term preoperative smoking cessation and postoperative complications: A systematic review and meta-analysis. *Can J Anesth.* 2012;59(3):268–279.
2. Mills E, et al. Smoking cessation reduces postoperative complications: A systematic review and meta-analysis. *Am J Med.* 2011;124(2):144–154.
3. Prestwich A, et al. How can smoking cessation be induced before surgery? A systematic review and meta-analysis of behavior change techniques and other intervention characteristics. *Front Psychol.* 2017;8:915.
4. Stefan MS, et al. The association of nicotine replacement therapy with outcomes among smokers hospitalized for a major surgical procedure. *Chest.* 2020;157(5):1354–1361.
5. Reinikovaite V, Rodriguez IE, Karoor V, et al. The effects of electronic cigarette vapour on the lung: direct comparison to tobacco smoke. *Eur Respir J.* 2018;51:1701661. https://doi.org/10.1183/13993003.01661-2017

# 234.

# SPECIAL CONSIDERATIONS IN PEDIATRIC OTOLARYNGOLOGY SURGERY

*Eric McDaniel and Ilana R. Fromer*

## INTRODUCTION

Pediatric Otolaryngology procedures are the most frequently performed surgeries in children. The majority of cases are booked as same-day elective procedures.

## TONSILLECTOMY AND ADENOIDECTOMY

### PREOPERATIVE CONSIDERATION

Adenotonsillectomy is the most commonly performed procedure in children. Indication for tonsillectomy and adenoidectomy (T&A) is either recurrent streptococcal pharyngitis or, most commonly, sleep disordered breathing (SDB), which occurs from tonsillar hypertrophy leading to partial or complete airway obstruction. Obstructive sleep apnea (OSA) affects up to 3% of children with peak age around 3–6 years.[1-3] Pediatric Sleep Questionnaire (PSQ) and STOP-BANG assessments are used to assess OSA in pediatric patients but fail to show the severity of OSA. Apnea Hypopnea Index (AHI) is also used to assess the severity of OSA in pediatric patients, but due to its high cost and poor access to polysomnography, most patients do not have sleep study results. Sequelae of OSA that may impact anesthesia include cardiac, respiratory, and pulmonary complications. Right ventricular dysfunction can lead to pulmonary hypertension or cor pulmonale, and left ventricular dysfunction can lead to systemic hypertension. It is important to note that cardiac changes can occur without significant OSA.[1]

## INTRAOPERATIVE CONSIDERATIONS

Inhalational induction is most commonly used, which causes a dose-related response to airway collapse. Very severe OSA or facial abnormalities will likely need peripheral intravenous access before induction. Obstructive sleep apnea occurs due to collapsible areas of the pediatric airway, which occurs at the tonsillar bed. Children are more resistant to collapse, requiring smaller airway pressures to maintain patency. Pediatric patients are susceptible to hypopnea and inspiratory flow problems, which causes them to spend larger amounts of time with low-flow inspiratory flows, causing partial airway collapse and snoring. This results in retained $CO_2$ compared to adults and an increased threshold for arousal. Adults need an AHI >40 for severe OSA classification, while in pediatrics it is only AHI of 10 due to the longer amount of time spent in partial airway obstruction.[3]

T&A is a painful procedure often requiring opioids; however, it is necessary to balance pain management with respiratory complications. These patients require half of the opiate dose for the same analgesic effect, which is thought to result from an increased arousal threshold, high retained $CO_2$, and increased arousal threshold from opiates themselves. Codeine should be avoided, as patient may be a hypermetabolizer and this may result in severe OSA while at home, leading to higher morbidity and mortality. Although there have been concerns that nonsteroidal anti-inflammatory drugs (NSAIDs) were associated with increased risk of bleeding, ibuprofen is effective and safe, with better pain scores than morphine. Use of adjuncts including ketamine, dexmedetomidine, dexamethasone, and local anesthetics to bathe the tonsillar bed are all useful in decreasing opioid requirements.[1,3] T&A is associated with an increased risk of postoperative nausea and vomiting (PONV), and it is recommended that all children undergoing this procedure be given dual antiemtic therapy with both ondansetron and dexamethasone.[3] Adequate and generous intravenous (IV) fluid administration is also recommended to help avoid PONV in the setting of dehydration.

## POSTOPERATIVE CONSIDERATIONS

Approximately 10% of children <4 years old have an unplanned admission following T&A, most commonly as a result of vomiting and dehydration rather than surgical complications.

Postoperative primary hemorrhage is usually within 6 hours post-surgery and, although infrequent, can be a serious complication.[1] Any child who has a respiratory complication in the immediate postoperative period is at greater risk of having a further event within the following 24-hour period and should be observed overnight. Inpatient versus outpatient observation also depends on the presence of craniofacial or neuromuscular disorder, upper respiratory infection (URI) in the last 2 weeks, history of

asthma, obesity, <3 years old, and severe OSA. If AHI is >30, they most likely need to go to the intensive care unit (ICU) for observation.[3] Guidelines for inpatient admission differ slightly by society, including AAP, AAOHNS, Nationwide, BSC. AAP recommends any child under 3 years old needs to be watched, and those with an AHI >24 are admitted overnight.

## COMMON EAR PROCEDURES

Middle ear procedures, including mastoidectomy, myringoplasty, and cochlear implantation, are some of the most common outpatient pediatric procedures. Length of surgery, access to the airway, coexisting syndromes, and facial monitoring are important preanesthetic considerations.[1] Many children with otitis media may have a coexisting or recent URI, so the decision to proceed must be based on the urgency of surgery. If the patient's temperature is normal, and behavior and diet are normal, with the absence of mucopurulent secretions or chest wheezing/rales, surgery should proceed as planned.

## INTRAOPERATIVE CONSIDERATIONS

Induction with inhalational sevoflurane or IV propofol are most common. Airway maintenance with either mask, LMA, or endotracheal tube will depend on length of surgery and access to airway during the procedure. Myringotomy tubes are often very quick procedures that do not necessitate intubation or PIV access. The airway is often maintained with a mask using sevoflurane and/or nitrous oxide. Longer middle ear surgeries are often performed with the head of the bed turned 180 degrees, and thus endotracheal intubation in order to safely secure the airway is preferred. Middle ear surgery is also associated with risk of PONV, necessitating dual antiemetic therapy with ondansetron and dexamethasone. If other risk factors are present, using total intravenous anesthesia (TIVA) and avoiding long-acting opioids should be considered to further reduce the risk of PONV.[1] If intraoperative facial nerve monitoring is required, care must be taken to avoid neuromuscular blocking agents.

## POSTOPERATIVE CONSIDERATIONS

Pain and PONV are the most common issues encountered in the post-anesthesia unit. Most commonly, acetaminophen and NSAIDs are used for pain management, and patients should resume PO fluids once awake in order to prevent dehydration and worsening of PONV. For myringotomy procedures performed without PIV access, pain medications are commonly given via the intramuscular or intranasal route.

# FLEXIBLE AND RIGID BRONCHOSCOPY

Both flexible and rigid bronchoscopies are used commonly in pediatric airway procedures, ranging from removal of aspirated foreign body to diagnosis and treatment of respiratory disease, including removal of secretions, treatment for atelectasis, and evaluation of airway for tracheomalacia, bronchomalacia, or airway compression from exterior structures. Occasionally bronchoscopic procedures in neonates and children may involve laser and jet ventilation techniques.

## FOREIGN BODY ASPIRATION

### PREOPERATIVE CONSIDERATIONS

Foreign body aspiration (FBA) is the leading cause of unintentional injury mortality in children; 80% of cases occur <3 years of age[4] and are removed by rigid bronchoscopy for control of airway as well as visualization and manipulation of the foreign body. Predisposing factors include improper dentition to chew food properly and immature swallowing coordination. Round foreign objects are more likely to cause airway obstruction, with nuts and seeds being common offenders. Diagnosis is made based on detailed history, clinical presentation, focused physical exam, and chest radiograph. Chest radiograph will show lung hyperinflation, atelectasis, and mediastinal shift away from affected lung; however, a normal chest radiograph does not rule out FBA.[1,4] Aspirated foreign bodies are an emergency, especially if the child is symptomatic. Although NPO (nothing by mouth) status is important, it can be unreasonable to wait if the child is deteriorating or showing signs of wheezing, stridor, decreased air entry, or desaturation. Food products expand with moisture and fragment into small pieces, oily substances can cause chemical pneumonitis, and sharp objects can cause trauma to the airway. Most foreign bodies are lodged in the right main stem bronchus.[4]

### INTRAOPERATIVE CONSIDERATIONS

The decision to keep the patients spontaneously breathing or not is a matter of debate, as there are pros and cons to both alternatives. Allowing the patient to breathe spontaneously decreases the risk for barotrauma and converting a proximal partial obstruction to a complete obstruction.[1,4]

However, if the procedure is expected to last long with deeper insertion of the bronchoscope, controlled ventilation may be preferred in order to blunt the reflexes of the patient and allow for better operating conditions, as well as preventing airway trauma that could result from coughing and resistance. If allowing the patient to breathe spontaneously, laryngeal tracheal anesthesia with lidocaine applied to the vocal cords and epiglottis can reduce hemodynamic and airway reactions and decrease the risk of laryngospasm.[4] Ventilation can be performed either through a port on the rigid bronchoscope, or using jet ventilation via a tracheal catheter.[1] Use of manual jet ventilation during rigid bronchoscopy in the nonobstructed lung can help minimize hypoxemia, especially in children prone to quick desaturation who are unable to maintain oxygen saturation while breathing spontaneously.[4]

## LASER SURGERY OF THE LARYNX

The use of lasers for procedures in the airway is also common in pediatric airway surgeries. It is most often used for laryngeal papilloma treatment, supraglottoplasty, or epiglottopexy for laryngomalacia and oral lesions. Laryngeal papillomas are the most common airway tumor in children, secondary to human papilloma virus (HPV), which can lead to serious airway obstruction and right-sided heart failure. Children present at age 2–4 years old, with a high rate of recurrence following surgical resection. Although endotracheal tubes (ETTs) specifically designed for use with lasers exist, they are often not available in smaller sizes and there is an increased risk of airway fire with standard tubes. Because of this, it is often preferred that either standard ETTs be intermittently inserted and removed during laser surgery or to keep the child un-intubated and spontaneously ventilating.[1] When lasers are used, it is important to cover the eyes of the patient and all personnel in the room. Airway fires are a real danger during the procedure, necessitating the use of fraction of inspired oxygen ($FiO_2$) <30% and avoiding nitrous oxide ($N_2O$), which potentiates combustion.

## PERITONSILLAR ABSCESS

Peritonsillar abscess is the most common cause of deep neck infections in children. Distorted anatomy, trismus causing limited mouth opening, and pharyngeal edema may make tracheal intubation difficult. Additionally, during intubation the abscess may be ruptured, releasing its purulence into the pharynx. It is essential to assess the airway preoperatively, watching closely for impending airway obstruction, and to verify the degree of mouth opening in order to prepare the most appropriate method of airway management. Postoperatively, inflammatory swelling can involve supraglottic structures and postextubation obstruction may occur. Dexamethasone should be considered intraoperatively and the patient should be observed closely in the postoperative period.

## REFERENCES

1. Harper P, et al. Update on ENT anaesthesia. *Anaesth Intens Care Med.* 2015;16(12):635–640.
2. Somerville N, Fenlon S. Anaesthesia for cleft lip and palate surgery. *Cont Educ Anaesth Crit Care Pain.* 2005;5(3):6–79.
3. Trucco F, et al. The McGill score in the diagnosis of Obstructive Sleep Apnoea in children with associated medical conditions. *Eur Respir J.* 2019 Sep;54(Suppl 63):PA4974. doi: 10.1183/13993003.congress-2019.PA4974
4. Kendigelen P. The anaesthetic consideration of tracheobronchial foreign body aspiration in children. *J Thorac Dis.* 2016;8(12):3803–3807.

# 235.

# RESPIRATORY AND CONGENITAL PEDIATRIC AIRWAY PROBLEMS

*Caroline Al-Haddadin and Alain Harb*

## HURLER

Hurler syndrome is a rare, genetically transmitted lysosomal storage disease, resulting in accumulation of acid mucopolysaccharides (MPS) in the nervous system. It is the prototype of MPS and its most severe form, with mortality around 20%. Incidence of difficult airway is high and increases with age. The main clinical features are an enlarged tongue, small mouth, thick profuse secretions, limited movement of the neck and perilaryngeal tissue. Treatment has increased life expectancy, but deposition of mucopolysaccharides continues as age advances. Most common associated conditions are sleep apnea, chest deformity, myocardial hypertrophy, pulmonary hypertension, nerve and tendon entrapment, and progressive mental retardation. Anesthetic management is challenging due to the deposition of mucopolysaccharides in the tongue, tonsils, adenoid, epiglottis, glottis, and trachea. Equipment related to managing difficult airways should include a flexible bronchoscope, and a video laryngoscope.[1] A pediatric anesthesiologist will ideally be managing the airway in a hospital equipped with an intensive care unit (ICU). Regional anesthesia is a safe alternative or adjuvant to children with MPS. Recovery after anesthesia is often slow and accompanied by periods of breath holding, apnea, bronchospasm, pulmonary hypertension, and negative pressure pulmonary edema. Early return of consciousness and airway reflexes is paramount.[2]

## PIERRE ROBIN

The clinical triad of micrognathia, glossoptosis, and airway obstruction defines the Pierre Robin sequence (PRS). Although clefting of the palate is common, it does not occur in all PRS. There is no clear genetic abnormality. It is an association with certain syndromes in two-thirds of cases, most commonly: Stickler, velocardiofacial, fetal alcohol syndrome, and Treacher-Collins syndrome. If these are suspected, a preoperative evaluation will include echocardiography. Patients may present with stridor, retractions, and cyanosis. Severe obstruction results in feeding difficulties, reflux, and failure to thrive. Airway obstruction treatment depends on the severity; it includes prone positioning, nasopharyngeal airways (NPA), tongue lip adhesion, mandibular distraction osteogenesis, and tracheostomy as part of a multidisciplinary approach. Prone positioning may relieve airway obstruction in as many as 70% of cases. Optimal surgical management remains controversial. Airway obstruction and OSA (obstructive sleep apnea) are predictors of intraoperative and postoperative complications. Patients who cannot tolerate supine positioning will be more difficult to mask ventilate and may require airway adjuncts such as oral pharyngeal airways, NPA, and laryngeal mask airways (LMAs). Several airway techniques can be used: LMA, fiberoptic scope, retrograde wire, or video laryngoscopes. In some patients an awake LMA insertion is a safe alternative.

General anesthesia may also be induced before securing the airway; however, maintaining spontaneous ventilation is essential and may be very difficult or impossible without airway adjuncts. If the airway remains obstructed, laryngoscopy should be performed for intubation. If intubation is not possible, follow the pediatric "cannot intubate, cannot ventilate" scenario. Using a paraglossal approach may be more effective than standard laryngoscopy. In addition to a volatile drug, anesthesia maintenance can be supplemented with an opioid and an α-2 agonist. PRS patients should be extubated awake, and an NPA can be placed to minimize airway obstruction.[3]

## TREACHER COLLINS

Treacher Collins syndrome (TCS), or mandibulofacial dysostosis, is a rare disorder of craniofacial development, due to mutations in the TCOF1 gene. It exhibits autosomal dominant inheritance with variable penetrance. It is a disorder of the first and second branchial arches, thus bilateral and symmetrical and restricted only to the head and neck. Direct laryngoscopy and intubation can be difficult because of maxillary, zygomatic, and mandibular hypoplasia combined with a small oral aperture, a high arched palate, and temporomandibular joint abnormalities. One should prepare for an anticipated difficult airway in all children with TCS, and it should be expected that direct laryngoscopy may become difficult with increasing age.[4]

## GOLDENHAR

Goldenhar syndrome, also known as oculo-auriculo-vertebral dysplasia, is characterized by a wide range of congenital anomalies, such as unilateral facial hypoplasia, micrognathia, oral cavity malformations, central nervous system malformations, cardiac malformations, and vertebral anomalies, and always causes difficult airway Male-to-female ratio is 3:2. Most cases are sporadic; familial cases are consistent with autosomal recessive, autosomal dominant, and multifactorial patterns of transmission. Gene location has not been identified. General anesthesia, with the use of an intubating LMA (I-gel™ supraglottic airway) for ventilation, then intubation with a cuffed tube by inserting a fiberoptic scope through the LMA, is the safest and most effective method. Other techniques might also be used, such as pediatric GlideScope, Airtraq, wire-guided intubation, and LMA; intubating LMA was also a good option. Surgical airway equipment and experts should be ready. Furthermore, intraspinal anesthesia may be difficult due to spine malformations. In addition, the presence of loose or protruding teeth, cystic hygroma or cysts in the mouth, mandibular size, and temporomandibular joint movement should be considered.

## CROUZON

Crouzon syndrome is a rare autosomal dominant disorder, caused by the mutation of the FGFR2 genes, also present in Apert syndrome, Pfeiffer syndrome, and Jackson-Weiss syndrome. Crouzon syndrome is characterized by craniofacial dysostosis, which includes a triad of skull deformities, facial anomalies, and exophthalmos. It is detected at birth or in infancy. These dysmorphic features either become more prominent or may show regression in deformity with advancing age. These include exophthalmos, hypertelorism, strabismus, hypoplastic maxilla, a beaked nose with a compressed nasal bridge, deformed lips, mandibular prognathism, optic atrophy, and visual disturbances. The worsening of these features can be a big sociocultural stigma; therefore, surgery to correct these craniofacial deformities is advised early on. Airway management can be safely performed by keeping the patient spontaneously breathing and intubating using a fiberoptic scope or video laryngoscope. Use of neuraxial anesthesia may circumvent the problems that Crouzon syndrome presents, but may be difficult to carry out, owing to vertebral fusion and the presence of scoliosis.

## CLEFT LIP AND PALATE

Cleft lip and palate (CLP) are one of the more common congenital malformations; more common in males and, strangely, cleft lips are usually left-sided. Patients may have middle ear infections, difficulty swallowing, and are at high risk of aspiration. Etiology is often unknown. CLP has a huge social impact on the patient and their family. Surgery, at 3 months of age for cleft lip repair and 6 months for cleft palate, aims to correct the anatomically obvious cleft lip, augment normal dento-alveolar development, and lead to effective palatal function. Associated anomalies are other defects of branchial arch development (e.g., ear or upper airway defects). They can also include heart, renal, or skeletal anomalies. CLP per se does not lead to upper airway obstruction; the most important group of CLP patients with airway problems are those with micrognathia, glossoptosis, and cleft palate, termed Pierre Robin sequence. A clear airway is obviously paramount and placing the infant prone suffice for milder forms. Next is to provide a nasopharyngeal airway. It is strongly recommended to maintain spontaneous ventilation during induction. The best practice is to induce anesthesia by inhalation. Intravenous (IV) lidocaine administration before intubation may decrease laryngospasm. Neuromuscular blocking agents are contraindicated if the ability to inflate the lungs is in doubt; spontaneous ventilation must be maintained. Difficult view at laryngoscopy is more common than difficult mask ventilation. Recovery is slow and associated with airway obstruction.

The child is extubated when fully awake. Laryngospasm, upper airway narrowing, blood clot, retained throat pack, tongue swelling from retraction, or inadequate mouth breathing are commonly seen. Careful insertion of a nasopharyngeal airway relieves upper airway obstruction and should not damage the palate repair. Mild laryngospasms can be treated with positive pressure ventilation, while severe laryngospasms can be treated with succinylcholine 0.3 mg/kg.

## REFERENCES

1. Patwari PP, Sharma GD. Common pediatric airway disorders. *Pediatr Ann.* 2019;48(4):e162–e168.
2. Gupta AK, et al. Hurler syndrome: Anaesthetic challenges and management. *Anestesia Pediatrica e Neonatale.* 2010;8(2).
3. Kumar A, et al. Pierre Robin sequence: A perioperative review. *Anesth Analg.* 2014 Aug;119(2):400–412.
4. Hosking J, et al. Anesthesia for Treacher Collins syndrome: A review of airway management in 240 pediatric cases. *Paediatr Anaesth.* 2012;22(8):752–758.

# Part XVI

# ANATOMY

# 236.

# NASAL ANATOMY AND PATHOLOGY

*Evan Falgoust and Alan D. Kaye*

## INTRODUCTION

The nose is a vital structure of the human body that plays an important role in everyday life ranging from respiration, olfaction, immune function, and anesthetic management. It is composed of an upper nasal bone with a lower cartilaginous portion. Openings in the nasal cartilage (connective tissue) on each side form the nostrils through which air moves through the nasal cavity. The nasal cavity is a compilation of structures that are bordered by a lateral wall on each side of the nasal septum. The cavity on each side of the septum contains three turbinates or conchae (inferior, middle, and superior), as well as a choana, which is an opening to the nasopharynx. This unique structure, known as the nose, provides vital functions to the human body, including adjusting the quality of external air that is inhaled, while also filtering the external particles and simultaneously receiving chemical stimuli via sensory free nerve endings.[1]

## ETIOLOGY AND DIAGNOSIS

The blood supply, cell type, and innervation are distinct components of the nose which aid the structure in performing its various function. The blood supply of nose receives branches from both the internal and external carotid arteries. Many of the branches form anastomoses near the anteroinferior nasal septum to create a structure known as Kiesselbach's plexus. This structure is composed of five terminal branches: the anterior ethmoidal artery, posterior ethmoidal artery, sphenopalatine artery, greater palantine artery, and superior labial artery.[2] This anastomotic arterial structure is the source of the majority of nosebleeds (epistaxis), and the mucosa overlying the structure is susceptible to changes in humidity and temperature, leading to greater susceptibility to nosebleeds. Epistaxis can be broken down into local and systemic etiologies that vary based on different factors. Common local causes of nosebleeds include factors such as trauma, structural deformities, infection, and lesions.

Rhinitis (coryza) is a disorder that can be characterized as irritation or inflammation of the nasal mucosa due to a variety of underlying causes, such as allergens, irritants, bacteria, or viral infection. The nasal mucosa consists of epithelium, basement membrane, and lamina propria. The epithelium is composed of several types of cells, including pseudostratified columnar, goblet, basal, and mucous cells.[3] When pathogens are able to effectively invade this mucosa, they are able to employ a variety of virulence factors in order to replicate and evade immune defense. While bacteria such as *Streptococcus pneumoniae*, *Staphylococcus aureus*, and anaerobic bacteria may be the cause of some of these "colds," the most common culprits of the common cold are human rhinoviruses (HRV). These viruses can contribute to airway inflammation and may lead to pulmonary exacerbations when in conjunction with cystic fibrosis, asthma, and chronic obstructive pulmonary disease (COPD).

Inflammation of the airway can also be problematic in the case of allergen-related sinusitis such that it can precipitate chronic rhinitis. The resulting inflammation is thought to potentially play a role in the formation of nasal polyps. Elevated levels of histamine and immunoglobin E (IgE) antibodies have been isolated around these nasal polyps with mast cells and eosinophilia found inside the polyps.[4] This suggestive evidence reveals a probable link between the chronic allergen-related inflammation and formation of nasal polyps. These smooth, round translucent masses are the cause of many patient complaints that encompass a variety of symptoms, such as congestion, hyposmia, rhinorrhea, epistaxis, and postnasal drip. Partial treatment and management for these lesions contains similar mechanisms to the etiologies mentioned previously.

## MANAGEMENT

The previously mentioned etiologies are commonly managed pharmacologically in the first step of treatment, but surgical treatment may be required in some persisting cases. In the case of epistaxis, it can typically be managed with the use of pressure for light nosebleeds, but management plans have been developed for severe cases where life-threatening bleeds may result in hematological instability. The aim of treatment for this etiology is to decrease blood pressure in order to cease further bleeding. This goal is often accomplished by pressure alone in the majority of treatments, but topical vasoconstrictors may be required in some cases. In life-threatening or recurrent cases, surgical treatment may be required to reduce the bleeding. This can typically be done by cauterization with silver nitrate or electrocoagulation.

The other nasal etiologies previously mentioned (rhinitis and polyps) have similar non-surgical management options. For rhinitis, the goal of treatment is to maximally reduce the inflammation with no adverse effects with the use of topical corticosteroids. This option is the conventional treatment if the rhinitis is not self-limited with short resolution, and the use of topical corticosteroids is common practice for nasal polyps as well, to reduce the size and increase the breathing airway. While many surgical treatments do exist for allergic rhinitis, individual options are directed toward the underlying nasal obstructive factor. While no single modality has become the standard of practice for every case involving allergic rhinitis, reduction of the inferior turbinate has become a commonly practiced intervention.[5] In the case of recurrent or large-sized polyps, the mainstay surgical treatment used is functional endoscopic sinus surgery (FESS) to perform polypectomy.

## REFERENCES

1. Freeman SC, et al. Physiology, nasal. In: *StatPearls* [Internet]. Treasure Island, FL: StatPearls; 2020 Jan.
2. Fatakia A, et al. Epistaxis: A common problem. *Ochsner J.* 2010;10(3):176–178.
3. Nasal vaccine delivery. In: Skwarczynski M, István T, eds. *Micro- and Nanotechnology in Vaccine Development.* William Andrew/ Elsevier; 2017:279–301.
4. Meymane Jahromi A, Shahabi Pour A. The epidemiological and clinical aspects of nasal polyps that require surgery. *Iranian J Otorhinolaryngol.* 2012;24(67):75–78.
5. Chhabra N, Houser SM. Surgical options for the allergic rhinitis patient. *Curr Opin Otolaryngol Head Neck Surg.* 2012;20(3):199–204.

# 237.

# PHARYNX

*Kayla Penny and Elyse M. Cornett*

## INTRODUCTION

The pharynx is a fibromuscular tube that is lined by mucous membrane that is posterior to the larynx and continuous with the esophagus. It extends from the base of the skull to the inferior border of the cricoid cartilage. The pharynx serves to conduct food to the esophagus and air to the larynx; thus, it consequently serves as a common channel for both swallowing and respiration. In anesthetized patients, air is most feasibly passed through the pharynx when the neck is extended.[1]

The external pharynx is bounded by musculature. The internal pharynx is commonly examined cross-sectionally and divided into three major subdivisions: the naso-pharynx, oropharynx, and laryngopharynx. The major anatomical landmarks of the external pharynx, as well as each internal subdivision, will be discussed in this chapter.

## EXTERNAL PHARYNX

### MUSCULATURE

The musculature apparatus of the pharynx comprises its exterior aspect and is divided into the circular and longitudinal muscles. The circular muscles are a group of three

*Table 237.1* CIRCULAR MUSCLES OF THE PHARYNX

| | ORIGIN | INSERTION | INNERVATION | BLOOD SUPPLY |
|---|---|---|---|---|
| Superior constrictor | Medial pterygoid plate, pterygomandibular raphe, lingula of the mandible | Median pharyngeal raphe, pharyngeal tubercle of the skull | CN X via the pharyngeal plexus | Ascending pharyngeal artery |
| Middle constrictor | Body and lesser horn of the hyoid bone | Median pharyngeal raphe | CN X via the pharyngeal plexus | Ascending pharyngeal artery |
| Inferior constrictor | Lateral surfaces of the thyroid and cricoid cartilages | Median pharyngeal raphe | CN X via the pharyngeal plexus, superior laryngeal nerve, recurrent laryngeal nerve | Ascending pharyngeal artery, superior thyroid artery, inferior thyroid artery |

overlapping muscles known as the pharyngeal constrictor muscles. Each constrictor muscle attaches posteriorly to the median pharyngeal raphe. Collectively, they serve as the posterior and lateral walls of the pharynx in which they function to narrow the pharynx when swallowing through a sequential top-to-bottom activation that propels food toward the esophagus.[2]

The longitudinal muscles of the pharynx are composed of three small accessory muscles. Each muscle has a separate origin, though they all insert onto the posterior pharynx on one of the circular muscles. When swallowing is initiated, the longitudinal muscles function to elevate the larynx and the pharynx. Details regarding the origin, insertion, innervation, and blood supply of the circular and longitudinal pharyngeal muscles are listed in further detail in Table 237.1 and Table 237.2, respectively.

## INTERNAL PHARYNX

### NASOPHARYNX

The nasopharynx is a region located above the soft palate and extends superiorly to the basal parts of sphenoid and occipital bones. It lies posterior to the nasal cavity. The anterior border of the nasopharynx communicates with the nasal cavity through the choanae. The lateral and posterior borders of the nasopharynx are defined by the superior pharyngeal constrictor muscles and the pharyngobasilar facia. The Eustachian tubes, specifically the cartilaginous portion known as the torus tubarius, open into the lateral walls of the nasopharynx at the pharyngeal ostium. This allows for communication between the pharynx and the middle ear. Located on the posterosuperior aspect of the nasopharynx are lymphoid aggregates known as the pharyngeal tonsils (adenoids).[3]

## OROPHARYNX

The oropharynx is bordered superiorly by the soft palate and inferiorly by the epiglottis. Its anterior aspect communicates with the oral cavity through the oropharyngeal isthmus, which is bound laterally by the palatoglossal arches. These muscular arches mark the boundary between the oral cavity and the oropharynx. Just posterior to the palatoglossal arches, the palatopharyngeal muscles form palatopharyngeal arches. Located in a space between the palatoglossal and palatopharyngeal arches is lymphoid tissue known as the palatine tonsils.[3]

## LARYNGOPHARYNX

The lowest section of the pharynx is the laryngopharynx. It extends from its superior border, the epiglottis, to its

*Table 237.2* LONGITUDINAL MUSCLES OF THE PHARYNX

| | ORIGIN | INSERTION | INNERVATION | BLOOD SUPPLY |
|---|---|---|---|---|
| Stylopharyngeus muscle | Styloid process of the temporal bone | Pharyngeal constrictors, thyroid cartilage | CN IX | Ascending pharyngeal artery |
| Palatopharyngeus muscle | Hard and soft palates | Pharyngeal constrictors, thyroid cartilage | CN X via pharyngeal plexus | Ascending pharyngeal artery |
| Salpingopharyngeus muscle | Eustachian tube cartilage | Pharyngeal constrictors | CN X via pharyngeal plexus | Ascending pharyngeal artery |

inferior border, composed of the posterior surface of the cricoid cartilage of the larynx. At the level of the cricoid cartilage, this segment of the pharynx joins with the esophagus. The anterior border of the laryngo pharynx is the posterior larynx, which protrudes into the oropharynx to form two lateral mucosal pouches known as the piriform sinuses. These sinuses rejoin at the level of the esophageal inlet.[4]

## VASCULAR SUPPLY

The blood supply of the pharynx comes mainly from various branches of the external carotid artery, with the inferior thyroid branch of the thyrocervical trunk contributing to a minor inferior portion. The ascending pharyngeal arises directly from the external carotid artery and contributes the vast majority of pharyngeal blood supply. The following external carotid arterial branches contribute pharyngeal branches to supply the remainder of the pharynx: maxillary, facial, lingual, and superior thyroid.

## INNERVATION

Sensory innervation of the pharynx varies depending on section. Sensation of the nasopharynx is received by cranial nerve (CN) $V_2$; CN IX provides sensation for the oropharynx; and CN X via the pharyngeal plexus for the laryngopharynx. CN X via the pharyngeal plexus also supplies motor innervation for all muscles of the pharynx, with the exception of the stylopharyngeus muscle, which is supplied by CN IX.[2]

## ANESTHETIC CONSIDERATIONS

In patients who are awake and not under anesthesia, the pharyngeal muscles contract in synchrony with the diaphragm, allowing the tongue to move forward with an open airway against the negative inspiratory pressure generated by the diaphragm.[5] Residual effects of both inhaled and neuromuscular blocking drugs can decrease pharyngeal tone and impair this pharyngeal function. When evaluating a patient for anesthesia, the anesthesiologist should consider the mouth opening, incisor distance, and pharyngeal anatomy (uvula, adenoids, etc.), as quantified in the Mallampati score (1–4), which helps determine whether the patient will be a difficult intubation. Postoperatively, support of the airway may be needed in patients who have a Mallampati score of 3 or 4. This can be accomplished through a continuous positive airway pressure (CPAP) face mask or a "jaw thrust maneuver" that opens the airway.[5]

## REFERENCES

1. O'Rahilly RF, et al. The pharynx and larynx. In: *Basic Huma Anatomy: A Regional Study of Human Structure*. 1st ed. Saunders; 1983.
2. Morton DA, Foreman BK, Albertine KH,]. Pharynx. In: Morton DA, et al., eds. *The Big Picture: Gross Anatomy*. 2nd ed. McGraw-Hill Education; 2019.
3. Arjun JS. Pharynx anatomy: Overview, gross anatomy, microscopic anatomy. Medscape. Gest, TR; November 18, 2013. Accessed August 24, 2021. https://emedicine.medscape.com/article/1949 347-overview.
4. Probst R, Grevers G, Iro H. Basic otorhinolaryngology. In: *Basic Otorhinolaryngology*. Georg Thieme Verlag; 2017.
5. The Mayo Foundation for Medical Education. *Faust's Anesthesiology Review*. 5th ed. Elsevier; 2020.

# 238.

# LARYNX

*Fatima Iqbal and Elyse M. Cornett*

## INTRODUCTION

The larynx is a 5-cm long structure at the C4 to C5 verte-brae level that bridges the oropharynx to the trachea. It is the area of the greatest resistance to the flow of air to the lungs and, as such, plays a crucial role in anesthetic airway management. Its three main functions include mainte-nance of a patent airway, prevention of aspiration of gastric or oral contents into the trachea, and vocalization.[1] The larynx's cartilaginous scaffold supports its intrinsic mus-cles and is interconnected by various joints, ligaments, and membranes (Figure 238.1).

## CARTILAGES

The larynx contains a total of 9 cartilages, with 3 of them unpaired and the remaining 6 occurring in pairs.[2]

### UNPAIRED CARTILAGES

The epiglottis is a leaf-shaped, elastic cartilage that covers the glottis during swallowing to prevent aspiration of

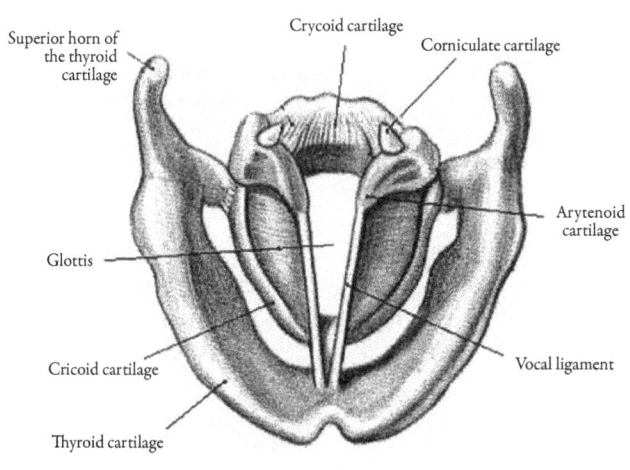

Superior horn of the thyroid cartilage
Crycoid cartilage
Corniculate cartilage
Arytenoid cartilage
Glottis
Cricoid cartilage
Vocal ligament
Thyroid cartilage

**Figure 238.1.** The larynx, viewed from above.

substances into the larynx. It is attached to the mid-line of the inner aspect of the thyroid cartilage via the thyroepiglottic ligament and to the body of the hyoid bone via the hyoepiglottic ligament. The mucous membrane cov-ering the upper anterior part of the epiglottis gives rise to the medial and lateral glossoepiglottic folds, while the aryepiglottic folds are mucosal folds on the posterior sur-face of the epiglottis.

The thyroid is a hyaline cartilage and the largest of all laryngeal cartilages, composed of two laminae that join an-teriorly to form the palpable laryngeal prominence, known as the Adam's apple. This is an important anatomical land-mark for percutaneous airway techniques and laryngeal nerve blocks.[3]

The cricoid forms a complete ring of hyaline cartilage around the airway at the C6 level and has a smaller diameter than the trachea. The broad portion posterior to the airway is the lamina, while the narrow anterior part is the arch. It connects to the first tracheal ring by the cricotracheal lig-ament, and to the thyroid cartilage via the cricothyroid ligament.

### PAIRED CARTILAGES

The arytenoid cartilages are pyramid-shaped, three-sided cartilages. Their bases articulate with the upper border of the cricoid lamina on both sides, while the apices articulate with the corniculate cartilages. The corniculate cartilages are small, cone-shaped cartilages that articulate with the apices of the arytenoid cartilage and are located in the pos-terior part of the aryepiglottic folds of the mucous mem-brane. The cuneiform cartilages are small, club-shaped cartilages in the aryepiglottic folds anterior to the cornicu-late cartilages and are not always present.

### LIGAMENTS AND MEMBRANES

The larynx contains both extrinsic and intrinsic ligaments. The extrinsic ligaments include the thyrohyoid mem-brane, hyoepiglottic ligament, and cricotracheal ligament.

The thyrohyoid membrane is a fibroblastic ligament that connects the hyoid bone and the superior border of the thyroid cartilage.[2]

The intrinsic ligaments include the conus elasticus and the quadrangular membrane. The conus elasticus is a submucosal membrane that extends from the anterior arch of the cricoid and attaches anteriorly to the thyroid cartilage and posteriorly to the vocal processes of the arytenoid cartilage. The thickened superior margin of the conus elasticus forms the vocal ligament. The quadrangular membrane is also a submucosal membrane whose thickened lower margin forms the vestibular ligaments (false vocal cords), which extend from the thyroid cartilage to the arytenoid cartilage above the vocal folds.[1,2]

## JOINTS

Joints of the larynx include the cricothyroid joint, the articulation of the inferior horns of the thyroid cartilage with articular facets on the outer posterolateral surface of the cricoid, and the cricoarytenoid joint, the articulation between the inferior surface of the arytenoid cartilage and the superior surface of the cricoid lamina.[1]

## INTERIOR OF THE LARYNX

### LARYNGEAL CAVITY

The laryngeal inlet marks the superior aspect of the laryngeal cavity and connects it to the pharynx. The cavity is tubular in shape, is lined with mucosa, and is made up of three portions: the vestibule, ventricle, and infraglottic cavity. The vestibule is the portion between the inlet and the vestibular folds. The ventricle is the space between the vestibular and vocal folds where the mucosa bulges laterally, while the infraglottic space is the area between the vocal folds and opening of the larynx into the trachea.[2]

## OTHER STRUCTURES

The rima vestibuli and rima glottidis are the openings between the vestibular folds and the vocal folds, respectively. Both openings are triangle-shaped, with the apex anterior and the base formed by the posterior wall of the laryngeal cavity. The piriform recesses are pockets present anterolaterally on both sides of the laryngopharynx, are bounded medially by the aryepiglottic folds, and laterally by the thyroid cartilage and thyrohyoid membrane, and are common sites for food to become stuck.[2]

## MUSCLES

Muscles of the larynx are divided into intrinsic and extrinsic muscles (Table 238.1).[2,4] The blood supply to the intrinsic muscles is from branches of the superior and inferior thyroid arteries, particularly the superior laryngeal artery from the superior thyroid artery and the inferior laryngeal artery and the cricothyroid artery from the inferior thyroid artery.

The extrinsic muscles are responsible for the elevation and depression of the larynx. They are grouped as suprahyoid and infrahyoid muscle, attaching either on the superior or inferior aspect of the hyoid bone, respectively. The infrahyoids (omohyoid, sternohyoid, and sternothyroid) are depressors, while the suprahyoids (stylohyoid, digastrics, mylohyoid, and geniohyoid), in addition to the stylopharyngeus, are elevators.[1]

*Table 238.1* INTRINSIC MUSCLES OF THE LARYNX

| | ORIGIN | INSERTION | ACTION | INNERVATION |
|---|---|---|---|---|
| Cricothyroid | Cricoid arch and the lower lamina of the thyroid | Lower lamina of the thyroid (superior belly) and inferior cornu (inferior belly) | Elongate vocal folds | External laryngeal nerve of superior laryngeal nerve |
| Posterior cricoarytenoid | Posterior cricoid cartilage | Muscular process of arytenoid cartilage | Abduct vocal folds | Recurrent laryngeal branch |
| Anterior cricoarytenoid | Lateral cricoid cartilage | Muscular process of arytenoid cartilage | Adduct vocal folds | Recurrent laryngeal branch |
| Thyroarytenoid | Interior surface of the thyroid cartilage | Anterolateral surface of the arytenoid cartilage | Relax and approximate vocal folds | Recurrent laryngeal branch |
| Aryepiglottic | Arytenoid cartilage | Epiglottis | Adduct aryepiglottic folds | Recurrent laryngeal branch |
| Arytenoid (transverse and oblique part) | Arytenoid cartilage | Opposite arytenoid cartilage | Adduct vocal folds | Recurrent laryngeal branch |

## INNERVATION

The vagus nerve (CN X) provides sensory and motor innervation to the larynx via its branches. The superior laryngeal nerve is a branch of the vagus nerve that further divides into two branches: the internal laryngeal nerve and external laryngeal nerve. The internal laryngeal nerve provides only sensory innervation to the area from the mucosa of the tongue and to the vocal cords, while the external laryngeal nerve provides motor innervation to the cricothyroid muscle and has no sensory component. The second branch of the vagus nerve is the recurrent laryngeal nerve, which enters the larynx in the groove between the esophagus and trachea. It provides motor innervation to all intrinsic muscles, other than the cricothyroid, and provides sensory innervation to the area between the vocal cords and the trachea.[2]

## VASCULAR SUPPLY

The superior and inferior laryngeal arteries are responsible for blood supply to the larynx. The superior laryngeal artery is a branch of the superior thyroid artery, which arises from the external carotid artery, while the inferior laryngeal artery is a branch of the inferior thyroid artery, which arises from the thyrocervical trunk, an offshoot of the subclavian artery. The superior laryngeal artery travels with the superior laryngeal nerve, entering the larynx through an aperture in the thyrohyoid membrane, while the inferior laryngeal artery accompanies the recurrent laryngeal nerve, entering the larynx in the groove between the esophagus and trachea.[2]

## ANESTHETIC CONSIDERATIONS

Cricothyrotomy is carried out by an incision in the cricothyroid membrane. However, a cricothyrotomy is contraindicated in cases of a disrupted laryngeal mucosa or skeletal fracture of the larynx, as it can exacerbate the injury.[1] It is also contraindicated in children younger than 6 years, as the cricoid cartilage is the narrowest part of the airway, and the isthmus of the thyroid gland reaches the cricothyroid membrane, placing it at risk for damage.[3]

The funnel-shaped pediatric larynx, with the cricoid its narrowest point, is also positioned higher and more anteriorly than the adult larynx. The infant epiglottis is narrow and retroflexed compared to the trachea, and so can pose a challenge for direct laryngoscopy.[5]

Damage to laryngeal nerves can occur as an iatrogenic consequence of procedures such as cricothyrotomy or thyroidectomy. Damage to the external laryngeal branch can result in hoarseness and loss of high-pitched sound production, while damage to the recurrent laryngeal nerve can result in vocal fold paralysis.[2,4] To avoid the possibility of recurrent laryngeal nerve injury, nerve function may be monitored during surgery using a unique endotracheal tube and recording electrodes, at the level of the larynx and vocal cords, respectively.[1]

## REFERENCES

1. Segura LG. Anatomy of the larynx. In: Trentman TL, et al., eds. *Faust's Anesthesiology Review*. 5th ed. Philadelphia, PA: Mayo Foundation for Medical Education and Research; 2020:113–114.
2. Vashishta R, et al. Larynx anatomy: Gross anatomy, functional anatomy of the larynx, laryngeal tissue [Internet]. *MedScape*. 2017. Available from: https://emedicine.medscape.com/article/1949369-overview#:~:text=The larynx is located within,and superior to the trachea.&text=Other functions of the larynx,acting as a sensory organ.
3. Bodenham AR, Mallick A. *Airway Management in the ICU*. 8th ed. Core Topics in Airway Management. Elsevier; 2011:262–273.
4. Suárez-Quintanilla J, et al. Anatomy, head and neck, larynx [Internet]. In: *StatPearls* [Internet]. 2020. Available from: https://www.ncbi.nlm.nih.gov/books/NBK538202/.
5. Harless J, et al. Pediatric airway management. *Int J Crit Illn Inj Sci*. 2014;4(1):65–70.

# 239.

# INNERVATION

*Sarah Lauve and Elyse M. Cornett*

## INTRODUCTION

The respiratory tract consists of the upper and the lower respiratory tract. The upper respiratory tract includes the nose, oral cavity, and pharynx. The lower respiratory tract consists of the tracheobronchial tree, which is the trachea, bronchi, and bronchioles. The larynx will be discussed separately because it is classified as part of both divisions. Understanding innervation of the respiratory tract is crucial because anesthetic agents affect ventilation and respiration.

## INNERVATION OF THE RESPIRATORY TRACT

### THE UPPER RESPIRATORY TRACT

The upper respiratory tract consists of the nose, the oral cavity, and the pharynx, the passage for air. The trigeminal nerve (V) provides sensory information to the nasal cavity via two branches: the ophthalmic nerve (V1) and the maxillary nerve (V2). The ophthalmic division of the trigeminal nerve branches into the anterior ethmoidal nerve, which innervates the anterior lateral wall of the nasal cavity. The posterior lateral wall is innervated by the posterior superior lateral nasal nerve, a branch of the maxillary nerve. The olfactory nerve innervates the olfactory epithelium, and the anterior ethmoidal, anterior superior alveolar, and nasopalatine nerves innervate the nasal septum.

The pharyngeal plexus is made up of branches of the vagus (X) nerve, glossopharyngeal (IX) nerve, and sympathetic nerve fibers from the superior cervical ganglion. The pharyngeal plexus is located posteriorly on the external layer of pharyngeal muscles and is responsible for all sensory and motor pharyngeal innervation.[1] All pharyngeal motor innervation is supplied by the cranial branch of the accessory nerve via the vagus nerve (X), except for the stylopharyngeus muscles, which receive motor input from the glossopharyngeal nerve (IX), and the tensor veli palatini, which receives motor input from the mandibular

division (V3) of the trigeminal nerve.[3] The external layer of pharyngeal muscles is innervated by laryngeal branches of the vagus nerve. The internal layer, excluding the stylopharyngeus, is innervated by pharyngeal branches of the vagus nerve. The glossopharyngeal nerve (IX), the maxillary division (V2) of the trigeminal nerve (V), and the vagus nerve (X) are responsible for supplying the pharynx with sensory information. The anterior and superior region of the nasopharynx receives sensory information from the maxillary division (V2) of the trigeminal nerve (V). The posterior region is innervated by the glossopharyngeal nerve (IX). All sensory information supplied to the oropharynx and laryngopharynx is from the glossopharyngeal nerve (IX).

### THE LARYNX

The vagus (X) nerve originates from the inferior vagal ganglion and innervates the larynx via two separate branches: the recurrent laryngeal nerve and the superior laryngeal nerve. The recurrent laryngeal nerve runs along the tracheoesophageal groove and innervates every intrinsic laryngeal muscle, except for the cricothyroid.[3] The recurrent laryngeal nerve supplies sensory information to all areas of the larynx located below the vocal cords. The superior laryngeal nerve divides into an external and internal branch. The external branch provides motor information to the cricothyroid muscle. The internal branch provides sensory information to all of the areas of the larynx located above the vocal cords.

### THE LOWER RESPIRATORY TRACT

The lower respiratory tract consists of the trachea, bronchi, and bronchioles (collectively referred to as the tracheobronchial tree), which is innervated by the autonomic nervous system through the vagus nerve (X). It sends autonomic afferent information and receives parasympathetic efferent and sympathetic efferent fibers through various pathways via the pulmonary plexus.[3] The pulmonary plexus innervates the lungs and lower respiratory tract and is located near the tracheal bifurcation and hila of each lung.[1] Cholinergic motor control of smooth muscles and glands in the tracheobronchial tree is conducted by efferent fiber pathways that are controlled by the vagus nerve (X). Adrenergic motor control of smooth muscle and glands in the tracheobronchial tree is conducted by efferent fiber pathways, which originate at levels T1/T2–T5/T6 of the spinal medulla and synapse in the cervical sympathetic ganglia and upper thoracic ganglia of the sympathetic trunk.[3]

## ANESTHETIC CONSIDERATIONS

### PREOPERATIVE

For regional anestheisa, a neurological exam is recommended as part of the preoperative assessment to document any neurological deficits prior to nerve block.[2] Autonomic neuropathies can affect the intraoperative course of anesthesia.[4] A patient with a known neurological disease should have strength and sensation evaluated, and should be asked about their history of stroke, nerve injury, medications, and mental status.[4] For a patient with a diagnosed seizure disorder, it is important to monitor hepatic and renal function, and to avoid any medications that induce seizures.[4]

### INTRAOPERATIVE

Intraoperative nerve blocks can reduce surgical stress response and thus lower the risk of stress-induced complications.[2] Neural blocks can be combined with regional anesthetics to generate good postoperative outcomes, but they must be implemented preoperatively and continued postoperatively. Common strategies include combining an epidural with local anesthetic and a low-dose opioid to improve postoperative analgesia, or using a local anesthetic in partnership with a continuous peripheral nerve block to reduce opioid side effects.[2]

### POSTOPERATIVE

Common postoperative neural complications include nerve injuries and hearing loss; however, other postoperative complications, such as hypoventilation and hypertension, can be neural in etiology.[4] Nerve injuries are a complication of regional and general anesthesia, caused by poor patient or limb positioning.[4] Peripheral nerve injuries are not dependent on positioning, yet may not be preventable. Risk factors for peripheral nerve injuries include hypotension, small body habitus, age, vascular disease, diabetes, and smoking.[1]

### REFERENCES

1. Moses KM, et al. *Atlas of Clinical Gross Anatomy*. 2nd ed. 2012.
2. Butterworth JF, Warnick DCM. *Morgan and Mikhail's Clinical Anesthesiology*. 2018.
3. Mills GH. Respiratory physiology and anaesthesia. *BJA CEPD Rev.* Published online 2001.
4. Bhatt H, et al. *First Aid for the Anesthesiology Boards*. McGraw-Hill Medical; 2010.
5. Netter FH, Rose D. Respiratory system (The Cibn Collection of Medical Illustrations, Vol. 7). *Anesthesiology*. Published online 1980.

# 240.

# VOCAL CORDS

*Warner Moore and Alan D. Kaye*

## INTRODUCTION

The vocal cords are composed of two sets of bilateral folds: true vocal cords and "false vocal folds." True vocal cords contain three types of tissue: stratified squamous epithelium, lamina propria, and the vocalis and thyroarytenoid muscles. The "false vocal folds" sit superiorly to the glottis and have been hypothesized to reduce translaryngeal flow, leading to an increase in sound intensity.[1] The vocal cords are attached anteriorly to the thyroid cartilage and posteriorly to the arytenoid cartilages. They vary in length and thickness depending on age and sex. At birth, vocal cords start off between 6 and 8 mm and lengthen upward to 16 mm as an adolescent. Males have thicker vocal cords, which can be contributed to testosterone produced by the testes during puberty. Through the release of testosterone, the vocal cords undergo changes to the musculature that produce a lower pitch. Another important element to note is the recurrent laryngeal nerve, a branch of the vagus nerve, which supplies innervation to the vocal cord muscles.

## DIAGNOSIS

The most common pathologic findings involving the vocal cords are laryngitis, polyps, and vocal cord paralysis. Acute laryngitis (inflammation of the vocal cords) can have numerous underlying causes from bacterial, viral, and fungal infections to gastrointestinal reflux, allergies, and smoking. Symptoms of acute laryngitis may include voice changes (hoarseness) and dry cough, which usually last no more than a week. If a patient presents with shortness of breath or stridor for over 3 weeks, the physician should consider a more serious disease process such as a malignancy. Some viral infections to keep in mind include rhinovirus, adenovirus, and the parainfluenza virus, especially in children as it is the leading cause of croup ("seal barking cough"). Bacteria affecting the vocal cords by superinfection are *Streptococcus pneumoniae* and *Haemophilus influenzae*, which presents with a diagnostic pearl "cherry" red epiglottis. Fungal infections, however, rarely cause acute laryngitis in immunocompetent patients and usually occur in the immunocompromised or individuals with inadequate inhaled steroid hygiene.

One prevalent virus that is known to cause laryngeal papillomatosis (vocal cord polyps) is human papilloma virus 6 and 11 due to its affinity for stratified squamous epithelium. The most common presenting symptom in both adults and children is hoarseness due to incongruent vocal cord vibrations. A serious complication to be aware of is an obstruction of the airway caused by rapidly growing polyps, especially in children with smaller tracheas. Laryngeal papillomas are often misdiagnosed as asthma or chronic bronchitis due to similarities in symptoms, so it is important to rule these polyps out via laryngoscopy. The two methods used are indirect laryngoscope using a fiberoptic telescope through the nose to view the vocal cords, or direct laryngoscope performed under general anesthesia to allow physicians to biopsy tissue samples if needed to view on a microscopic scale.

Another medical condition affecting the vocal cords is vocal cord paralysis, usually attributed to a defect in the recurrent laryngeal nerve (can be unilateral or bilateral). Leading causes are viruses, trauma to the neck, and numerous surgeries, including a thyroidectomy. Patients with this disorder present with breathy voice, reduced vocal range, vocal fatigue, aspiration, and shortness of breath. Videostroboscopy, a high-definition camera with a strobe light attached, allows for the visualization of vocal cord vibration in "slow motion" and vocal cord closure. There are cases where the vocal cords return to baseline within a year, and if not, surgical procedure may be explored. Some surgery options include bulk injections, thyroplasty (structural implant), or reinnervation of the damaged nerve. To assess how well a patient may recover, laryngeal electromyography (LEMG) can be performed to test the electrical currents passing through the vocal cord muscles. Significant neural degeneration on an LEMG predicts a poor prognosis associated with a worse functional outcome.[2]

## ANESTHETIC CONSIDERATIONS

### PREOPERATIVE

A baseline of vocal cord function should be established to compare postoperative as well as any potential airway complications. Prior radiation therapy, usually due to laryngeal cancer, is a risk factor physicians should be aware of due to difficult airway management. Complications include laryngeal edema due to previous radiation, causing an increased risk of hypotension during induction of anesthesia, and post-radiation tissue fibrosis that is unable to be relaxed by neuromuscular blocking agents.

### INTRAOPERATIVE

There are many anesthetic techniques used based on the vocal cord disorder present, including local anesthesia, intermittent apnea without endotracheal intubation, general anesthesia with a microdirect laryngoscopic tube, and jet ventilation. For minor procedures, local anesthetics are administered, and for light sedation, midazolam can be given. Dexmedetomidine, an alpha-2 adrenergic receptor agonist, is used perioperatively for its sedative sparing effects, reduced delirium, cardiovascular stabilizing effects, and lack of respiratory depression.[3] Propofol and etomidate are administered for general anesthesia, coupled with a muscle relaxant such as succinylcholine for intubation procedures.

### POSTOPERATIVE

Patients who were under general anesthesia should be monitored for stridor, laryngeal spasm, aspiration, and respiratory obstructions such as hematomas. Administration of dexamethasone may reduce edema, and 2–3 ml (1:1000) nebulized epinephrine can be administered to reduce the presence of stridor.[4] Continuous positive airway pressure support is also used to improve minor stridor until the anesthesia residues completely wear off. The use of heliox (21% oxygen in helium) is an option to reduce the work of breathing if minor airway obstruction develops for a short period of time. As always, equipment for emergent airway access should be available in the operating room until the patient is ready for discharge.

### REFERENCES

1. Zheng X, et al. A computational study of the effect of false vocal folds on glottal flow and vocal fold vibration during phonation. *Ann Biomed Eng*. 2009;37(3):625–642.
2. Guha K, et al. Role of laryngeal electromyography in predicting recovery after vocal fold paralysis. *Indian J Otolaryngol Head Neck Surg*. 2014;66(4):394–397.
3. Kaur M, Singh PM. Current role of dexmedetomidine in clinical anesthesia and intensive care. *Anesth Essays Res*. 2011;5(2):128–133.
4. English J, et al. Anaesthesia for airway surgery. *Cont Educ Anaesth Crit Care Pain*. 2006 Feb;6(1):28–31.

# 241.

# DIFFERENCES BETWEEN INFANT AND ADULT AIRWAY

*Susan Jeffers and Alan D. Kaye*

## ANATOMICAL DIFFERENCES

Neonate and infant airway anatomy and breathing patterns differ greatly from those of adults. Despite their small nasal passages, until about 5 months of age, neonates and infants are obligate nasal breathers.[1] Anatomically, important considerations include the proportionally larger head and tongue, and prominent occiput of neonates and infants.[2] These features can contribute to airway obstruction during mask ventilation. Children can also have prominent tonsils and adenoids, which can contribute to airway obstruction and make endotracheal tube placement more challenging.[1] The airway of infants and neonates is shorter than the airway of an adult. The larynx of adults is located at the C6 vertebral level, whereas in infants and neonates it can be found at the C4 vertebral level. In addition to being located more cephalad, the neonatal and infant larynx is located more anteriorly than the adult larynx.[2] The infant airway is shorter and narrower than the adult airway. The shape of the airway itself has also been noted to be different. The pediatric airway was often previously described as funnel shaped, while the adult airway is more cylindrical. Traditionally it has been taught that the narrowest portion of the airway also changes with age. It was previously accepted that the narrowest portion of the neonatal and infant airway is the cricoid cartilage, while the narrowest portion of the adult airway is the glottis.[3] Recent magnetic resonance imaging (MRI) studies and bronchoscopic evidence contradict this notion and indicate that pediatric airways are also cylindrical, with the narrowest portion being the laryngeal aperture at the vocal cords, as it is in adults.[2] Additionally, the vocal cords are not positioned perpendicular to the trachea, as they are in adults. The cords are situated in an anterior-inferior to posterior-superior fashion in infants.[1] This can make endotracheal tube insertion more challenging for the provider, as the angle can hinder passage of the endotracheal tube through the cords. The adult epiglottis is typically flatter than the epiglottis of a neonate or infant. The epiglottis in infants is larger and floppier than that of an adult and is more of an omega, U, or V shape.[2] The tissue structure of the neonatal and infant airway is much more compliant than the tissue comprising the adult airway.

## ANESTHETIC CONSIDERATIONS

The proportionately larger head of infants can easily contribute to airway obstruction. The large occiput can force the neck into a flexion position when supine, while the large tongue can readily fall back into the airway, both adding to possible airway obstruction. Positioning a pillow under the occiput, as one might do to achieve the sniffing position for an adult patient, can actually hinder laryngoscopy in a child.[2] No pillow or a small, properly positioned shoulder roll can help open the airway by positioning the neck into a more neutral position. The neck of neonates and infants is also much shorter than the neck of adults. This can make

laryngoscopy more challenging and is one of the reasons the use of a Miller blade is often favored.

The anatomically shorter airway of infants can predispose to endobronchial intubation if the provider is not careful in endotracheal tube placement. The tip of the endotracheal tube should only pass 1–2 cm past the glottis in infants in order to avoid accidental endobronchial intubation.[3] The formula used as a guideline to estimate endotracheal tube depth insertion is 12 + (age/2).[3] With initial placement and each positional change of the patient, the provider should inspect the tube for possible movement and listen to bilateral breath sounds.

Commonly used tube sizes are as follows:

- Premature (<2.5 kg): internal diameter (ID) 2.5
- Term neonate: ID 3
- 2–8 months: ID 3.5
- 8–12 months: ID 4
- 18–24 months: ID 4.5
- Older than 24 months: age (yrs)/4+4.

Endotracheal tube position follows the 1-2-3/7-8-9 rule (1 kg infant, 7 cm at lip). ID X3 gives the approximate position at the lip, add 2 to 3 cm for a nasotracheal tube.

The characteristically floppy and omega-shaped infant epiglottis makes using the Macintosh blade more challenging for laryngoscopy. The Macintosh blade requires the provider to insert the blade into the epiglottic vallecula and lift the epiglottis out of the way indirectly. This does not reliably yield a good view of the vocal cords in younger patients. Use of the Miller blade allows the provider to directly lift up the epiglottis in order to better visualize the cords.[1] The compliant structure of the neonatal and infant airway predisposes these patients to dynamic airway obstruction with the use of neuromuscular blocking agents and negative pressure ventilation.[1] Frequently, inhalational anesthetics are used for induction of neonates and infants and spontaneous ventilation is maintained.

## REFERENCES

1. Harless J, et al. Pediatric airway management. *Int J Crit Illn Inj Sci*. 2014;4(1):65–70.
2. Gottlieb EA, Andropoulos DB. Basics of anesthesia. *Pediatrics*. 2011;34:547–567
3. Chapter 42. Pediatric Anesthesia: 877–905. In: Butterworth JF, IV, Mackey DC, Wasnick JD, eds. *Morgan & Mikhail's Clinical Anesthesiology, 5e*. McGraw Hill; 2013.

# 242.

# STRUCTURES AND RELATIONSHIPS IN THE NECK AND CHEST

*E. Saunders Alpaugh and Alan D. Kaye*

## INTRODUCTION

The anatomic structures in the neck and the chest are complex and have a wide variety of pathology and anesthetic considerations. These structures consist of respiratory, cardiovascular, nervous, endocrine, and musculoskeletal systems. Compartmentalizing the neck and chest facilitates correct identification of important structures.

## NECK

The neck contains many critical structures (Figure 242.1). These structures play a major role with regard to cardiovascular, pulmonary, and nervous functions. The neck is divided into four compartments: vertebral, visceral, and two vascular compartments. The vertebral compartment contains the cervical vertebra and postural muscles. The visceral compartment contains the thyroid, parathyroid, and

thymus glands, and the larynx, pharynx, and trachea. The two vascular compartments contain the common carotid artery, internal jugular vein, and the vagus nerve, on each side of the neck.

## MEDIASTINUM

The mediastinum is divided into the superior, anterior, middle, and posterior compartments.

The superior mediastinum contains the following structures:

*Organs*: thymus, trachea, esophagus;

*Arteries*: aortic arch, brachiocephalic trunk, left common carotid artery, left subclavian artery;

*Veins and lymphatics*: superior vena cava, brachiocephalic veins, the arch of the azygos, thoracic duct;

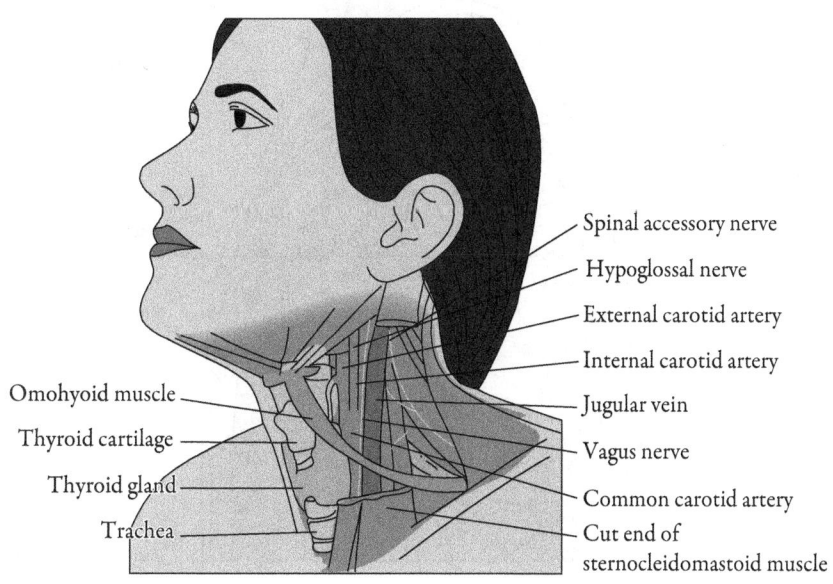

Figure 242.1. Major structures of the neck.

*Nerves*: left and right vagus, recurrent laryngeal, cardiac, left and right phrenic nerves.

The anterior mediastinum contains the following structures:

*Organs*: thymus;

*Arteries*: internal thoracic branches;

*Veins and lymphatics*: internal thoracic branches, parasternal lymph nodes;

*Nerves*: none.

The middle mediastinum contains the following structures:

*Organs*: the heart and its great vessel roots, trachea, and main bronchi;

*Arteries*: ascending aorta, pulmonary trunk, pericardiacophrenic arteries;

*Veins and lymphatics*: superior vena cava, pulmonary veins, pericardiacophrenic veins;

*Nerves*: phrenic, vagus, sympathetics.

The posterior mediastinum contains the following structures:

*Organs*: esophagus;

*Arteries*: descending thoracic aorta;

*Veins and lymphatics*: azygos hemiazygos veins, thoracic duct;

*Nerves*: vagus, splanchnic, sympathetic chain[1] (see Figures 242.2 and 242.3).

## RESPIRATORY SYSTEM

The respiratory structures in the neck and chest include the pharynx, larynx, trachea, and the bronchopulmonary segments. Within the neck, the airway contains the distal aspect of the distal pharynx, laryngopharynx, the larynx, and the proximal trachea. Along the airway are cartilaginous structures including the cricoid cartilage and the thyroid cartilage, which serve as anatomic landmarks to the anesthesiologist. The trachea is approximately 10 to 13 cm in length, originating at the inferior aspect of the larynx and terminating in the superior mediastinum at the carina. The bronchopulmonary tree begins at the carina and consists of 23 dichotomous branches. At the first division, the trachea will divide into the right and the left mainstem bronchi, before further dividing into secondary and tertiary bronchi. The tertiary bronchi will then form a bronchopulmonary segment supplying the different lobes of the lung. The right lung will contain the superior, middle, and inferior lobes, and the left lung will contain the superior and inferior lobes and the lingula.[2]

## CARDIOVASCULAR SYSTEM

The cardiovascular system has several major vessels originating in the thoracic cavity and extending into the neck.

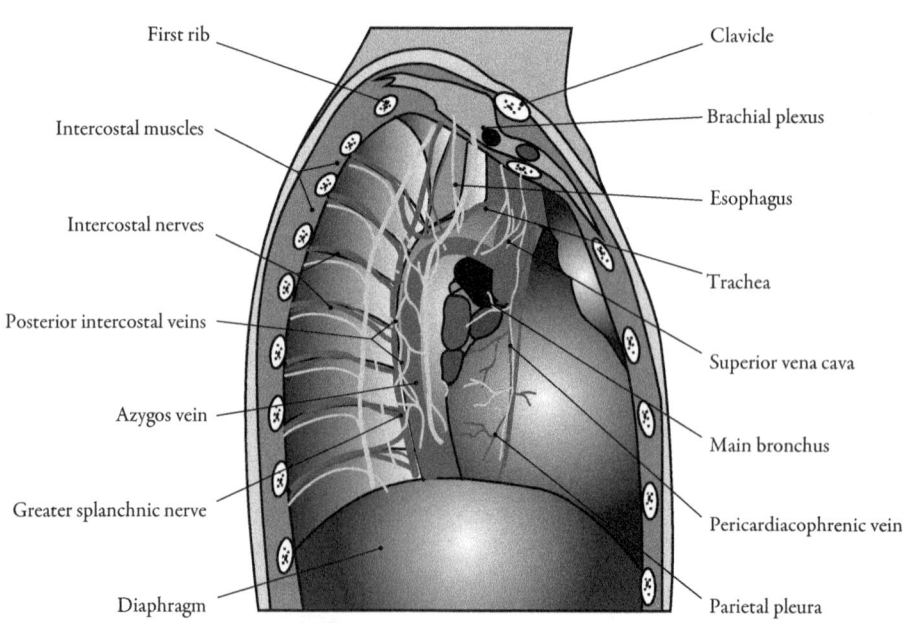

**Figure 242.2.** Major structures of the mediastinum.

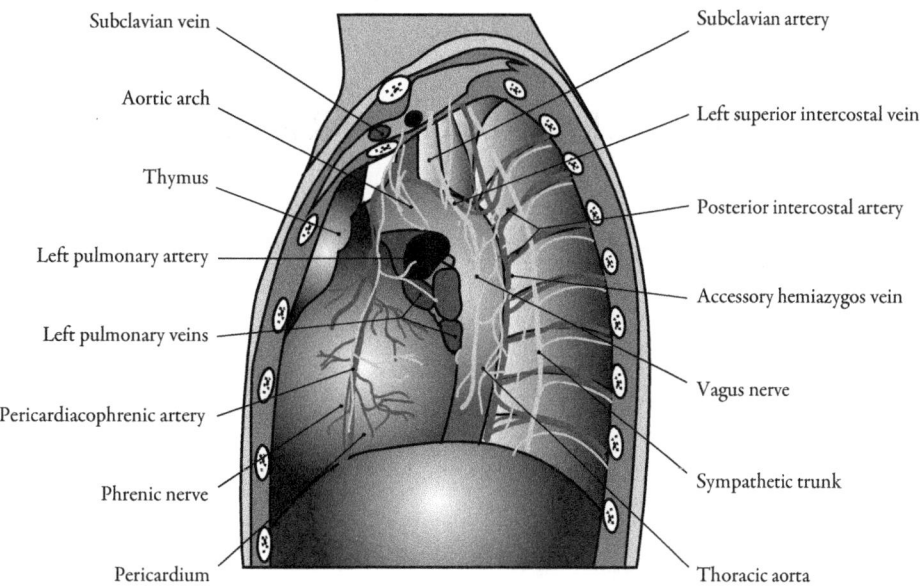

Subclavian vein
Aortic arch
Thymus
Left pulmonary artery
Left pulmonary veins
Pericardiacophrenic artery
Phrenic nerve
Pericardium

Subclavian artery
Left superior intercostal vein
Posterior intercostal artery
Accessory hemiazygos vein
Vagus nerve
Sympathetic trunk
Thoracic aorta

**Figure 242.3.** Additional major structures of the mediastinum.

Important arterial vessels in the mediastinum include the proximal aorta, the aortic arch, the primary vessels arising from the aortic arch, and the descending aorta. The heart will supply blood from the left ventricle through the aortic valve and into the proximal aorta. The aorta will turn at the aortic arch in the superior mediastinum and give off the three primary vessels. The vessels of the aortic arch include the innominate artery (IA), the left common carotid artery (LCCA), and the left subclavian artery (LSA). The descending aorta will redirect in the superior mediastinum and supply blood to major organs in the abdomen and lower extremities.[3]

## NERVOUS SYSTEM

The nervous structures within the neck and chest have a significant role for intrathoracic physiology. These nerves provide motor, sensory and autonomic function to a variety of organs. The autonomic fibers will induce sympathetic and parasympathetic physiologic changes on intrathoracic organs, including heart rate, blood pressure, bronchomotor tone, mucous production, vascular permeability, respiratory rate, and depth of breathing. The major nerves in the neck and chest include the vagus nerve, the phrenic nerve, the sympathetic trunk, and the nerves arising from the brachial plexus.[4]

## REFERENCES

1. Stoddard N, et al. Anatomy, thorax, mediastinum. In: *StatPearls* [Internet]. Treasure Island, FL: StatPearls; 2020 [cited October 2, 2020]. Available from: http://www.ncbi.nlm.nih.gov/books/NBK539819/.
2. Patwa HS, et al. Evidence-based guideline: Intravenous immunoglobulin in the treatment of neuromuscular disorders: Report of the Therapeutics and Technology Assessment Subcommittee of the American Academy of Neurology. *Neurology.* 2012 Mar;78(13): 1009–1015.
3. White HJ, et al. Anatomy, abdomen and pelvis, aorta—StatPearls—NCBI Bookshelf [Internet]. [cited October 2, 2020]. Available from: https://www.ncbi.nlm.nih.gov/books/NBK537319/
4. Bankenahally R, Krovvidi H. Autonomic nervous system: Anatomy, physiology, and relevance in anaesthesia and critical care medicine. *BJA Educ.* 2016 Nov 1;16(11).381–387.

# 243.

# MUSCLES OF RESPIRATION

*Lauren K. Eng and Alan D. Kaye*

The muscles utilized in respiration are classified as primary or accessory muscles. Specific muscles expand the thoracic cavity during inspiration and help compress the thoracic cavity during expiration.[1] The muscles of respiration are skeletal muscles, and they are both voluntary and involuntary.[1]

## PRIMARY MUSCLES

The primary muscles include primarily inspiratory muscles. The respiratory muscles that participate in inspiratory lung expansion include the diaphragm, external intercostal muscles, and parasternal internal intercostal muscles.[1] These muscles work in concert to expand the ribs and to increase negative pressure in the thoracic cavity.

The diaphragm is caudad to the lungs, and the center moves caudad while the lateral portion moves cephalad during inspiration. The relaxation of the diaphragm results in contraction of the thoracic cavity and exhalation. The diaphragm is responsible for 75% of volume expansion during quiet inspiration.[2] The intercostal muscles are located between the ribs as three layers of muscles; external intercostals, internal intercostals, and innermost intercostals.[2] The external intercostals contract during inhalation and relax during exhalation to expand and to contract the rib cage.[2] The parasternal intercostal muscles also participate in inhalation and expansion of the ribs.[2] During quiet or normal breathing, expiration occurs as a passive process related to elastic recoil of the lung and relaxation of primary muscles.

## ACCESSORY MUSCLES

The accessory muscles also include both inspiratory and expiratory muscles. Accessory muscles are employed when primary muscles do not adequately provide sufficient respiration.[2] These circumstances can arise through labored breathing from increased demand or pathological states.[2] During forced inspiration and expiration, the accessory muscles play a primary role.

The accessory muscles of inspiration include the scalenes, sternocleidomastoid, levator scapulae, trapezius, iliocostalis thoracis, subclavius, and omohyoid.[1] The accessory muscles of expiration include the interosseous intercostals, abdominal muscles, transversus thoracis, subcostalis, quadratus lumborum, iliocostalis lumborum, latissimus dorsi, and serratus posterior.[1]

## ANESTHETIC CONSIDERATIONS

### PREOPERATIVE

A physical exam should be performed to identify breathing mechanics that may unmask any potential pathology. Overutilization of accessory muscles may warrant further investigation.[3]

### INTRAOPERATIVE

Muscle relaxation is imperative during cases under general anesthesia to prevent contraction of respiratory muscles that may interfere with the operation.[4] Weak diaphragmatic contraction and accessory muscle activity during ventilator weaning is a sign the patient requires further mechanical ventilation.[4]

Additionally, it should be noted that regional nerve blocks can cause unintended anesthesia to primary or accessory muscles of respiration. This can have clinical implications when patients have limited reserve from chronic or acute disease states. Shortness of breath or inability to lie flat may limit the capacity of the patient to tolerate positioning required for surgery. For example, a supraclavicular or interscalene block may result in local anesthetic mediated cervical nerve root blockade and consequent anesthesia to the diaphragm. In high-risk patients with limited pulmonary reserve, this can easily be enough to compromise breathing and create additional anesthesia challenges.

## POSTOPERATIVE

Continue to monitor respiration, especially in patients who received regional nerve blocks that could impact/paralyze respiratory muscles and in patients who have respiratory conditions.

## REFERENCES

1. Roussos C, Macklem PT. The respiratory muscles. *N Engl J Med*. 1982. doi:10.1056/NEJM198209233071304
2. Derenne PJ, et al. The respiratory muscles: Mechanics, control, and pathophysiology—Part I. *Am Rev Respir Dis*. 1978. doi:10.1164/arrd.1978.118.1.119
3. Marsh MH, et al. Anesthesia, sedation, and the chest wall. *Int Anesthesiol Clin*. 1984. doi:10.1097/00004311-198402240-00003
4. Rehder K, Marsh HM. Respiratory mechanics during anesthesia and mechanical ventilation. In: *Comprehensive Physiology*. 2011. doi:10.1002/cphy.cp030343

# Part XVII

# PHARMACOLOGY

# 244.

# THE TRACHEOBRONCHIAL TREE

*E. Saunders Alpaugh and Alan D. Kaye*

## INTRODUCTION

The anesthesiologist must understand the anatomy and management of the tracheobronchial tree, which has significant importance for proper ventilation for a wide variety of procedural and surgical interventions. Establishing a patent airway and maintaining ventilation are critical roles for the anesthesiologist. The pathologies of the distal trachea and its surrounding structures are numerous and can alter the anesthetic approach to ventilation. Related to the advancement of thoracic interventions, anesthesiologists have developed more complex techniques for intraoperative management of the tracheobronchial tree.

## ANATOMY

The tracheobronchial tree originates at the distal edge of the larynx, below the cricoid cartilage, and is composed of the trachea, the bronchi, and the bronchioles. These structures allow for transport of inhaled and expired air from the surrounding environment to the lungs. The tracheobronchial tree consists of 23 generations of dichotomous divisions, beginning at the trachea and terminating at the alveoli. The trachea is a cartilaginous and membranous structure with a length of 10–13 cm. It originates at the level of the cricoid cartilage and travels through the superior mediastinum. At its distal portion it divides into the right and left mainstem bronchus at an anatomic structure called the carina. This occurs at the level of the fourth or fifth thoracic vertebrae or at the level of the sternal angle. The lumen of the trachea narrows as it heads toward the carina and has a diameter of 13–27 mm in men and 10–23 mm in women. The trachea is surrounded by 18–22 C-shaped cartilages, which do not completely encircle the trachea. These cartilaginous rings provide structural support to keep the trachea patent while allowing for some degree of flexibility during ventilation. Between each tracheal ring lies noncartilaginous tissue that has elastic properties to allow for expansion and contraction during inhalation and exhalation, respectively. The trachea is lined with psuedostratisfied ciliated columnar epithelium, which is seen throughout the majority of the respiratory tract. Along with these cells lie goblet cells that are responsible for mucus production. The cilia will then allow passage of mucus along with airway contaminants to move upward in the respiratory tract to facilitate excretion. Beneath the epithelial layer lie the submucosa, hyaline cartilage, and trachealis muscle, providing circulation and additional support.[1,2]

Once the trachea divides at the carina, the right main bronchus and left main bronchus form. The right main bronchus is larger in diameter, shorter in length, and takes a steeper angle than the left. Before separating into three lobar bronchi, the right main bronchus travels roughly 1.5–3 cm. The left main bronchus has a longer segment of approximately 4.5–5 cm before dividing into two lobar bronchi: the left lower lobe bronchus and the left upper lobe bronchus. Each bronchus will supply ventilation to a specific area called a bronchopulmonary segment. The lobar bronchi will separate into segmental bronchi, also called tertiary bronchi, before forming bronchioles and terminal alveoli.[2]

The blood supply to the trachea includes arterial branches from the inferior thyroid artery, subclavian artery, internal mammary artery, bronchial artery, and the innominate artery. The inferior thyroid artery will supply the proximal trachea, while the bronchial arteries supply the distal portion. The bronchial artery will also supply the carina, and right and left main bronchus. The tracheobronchial tree has venous drainage to the azygos and hemi azygos veins before returning to the superior vena cava and the right atrium.[3]

Innervation to the tracheobronchial tree includes nerve branches from the thoracic sympathetic chain and the inferior ganglion of the vagus nerve, which together form the pulmonary plexus. The presynaptic nervous fibers from the vagus nerve will provide parasympathetic nerves to the pulmonary plexus, while the postsynaptic nerves from the sympathetic chain will provide sympathetic nervous fibers. These nerves will have physiologic effects on the airway consisting of bronchomotor tone, mucus production, and vascular permeability.[5]

## ANESTHETIC MANAGEMENT

The anesthetic considerations of the tracheobronchial tree consist mainly of various ventilation techniques used during surgery. The anesthetic approach depends on the procedural and surgical interventions performed and their relations to the surrounding structures. While there are many airway devices used, endotracheal intubation is typically required for advanced surgical procedures. Endotracheal intubation utilizes an endotracheal tube (ETT) that is placed through the vocal cords and into the trachea proximal to the carina. Prior to intubation, preoperative airway assessment including mallampati classification, mouth opening, thyromental distance, dentition, as well as external features of the anatomy allows the anesthesiologist to choose optimal airway devices to facilatate placement of the ETT. Proper ETT placement can be confirmed with end tidal $CO_2$ capnography and auscultation of bilateral lung fields. It is important that breath sounds are heard equally on both sides to confirm that the ETT is not placed too distally and only ventilating through the right or left mainstem bronchus.[2]

For specific intrathoracic surgeries, the anesthesiologist can utilize single lung ventilation (SLV) to assist the surgeon's control and exposure to surrounding tissues. Separation of lung ventilation is commonly utilized with a double lumen tube placed directly to either the right or left mainstem bronchus and requires confirmation with the use of a small fiberoptic scope placed into the tube. The nonventilated lung will have a bronchial cusp inserted with an inflatable balloon to prevent any airflow to the lung. This allows the nonventilated lung to deflate, creating more intrathoracic space for the surgeon to obtain optimal exposure to the tissue of focus. Preoperatively, FEV1 and DLCO are commonly obtained to assess for postoperative complications and mortality, especially in elderly populations. Many patients undergoing surgery that requires SLV commonly have some degree of respiratory disease, and special precautions for these patients are required. Intraoperatively, physiologic shunting is present in the nonventilated lung, related to hypoxic vasoconstriction of the pulmonary capillaries. Normal shunt is 5%–8%. An easy formula to measure shunt is as follows:

$$Shunt = \frac{680 - PO2(on\ 1.0\,FiO2)}{20}$$

Postoperatively, extubation requires careful attention to respiratory depression, and in the case of continued ventilation requirements, the double lumen tube is switched out to a normal standard ETT.[1]

## REFERENCES

1. Bohringer C, et al. A synopsis of contemporary anesthesia airway management. *Transl Perioper Pain Med*. 2019;6(1):5–16.
2. Patwa A, Shah A. Anatomy and physiology of respiratory system relevant to anaesthesia. *Indian J Anaesth*. 2015 Sep; 59(9):533–541.
3. Drevet G, et al. Surgical anatomy of the tracheobronchial tree. *J Thorac Dis*; 2016 Mar;8(2):121–129.
4. Mehrotra M, Jain A. Single lung ventilation. [July 31, 2020]. In: *StatPearls* [Internet]. Treasure Island, FL: StatPearls; 2020 Jan–.
5. Amador C, et al. Anatomy, thorax, bronchial. [August 10, 2020]. In: *StatPearls* [Internet]. Treasure Island, FL: StatPearls; 2020 Jan–.

# 245.

# BETA (B) AGONISTS

*Sheridan Markatos and Larry Manders*

## INTRODUCTION

Adrenoceptors are part of the sympathetic nervous system and are stimulated by the catecholamines epinephrine and norepinephrine. $\beta_1$ receptors are located on the postsynaptic membrane of the heart, and agonism causes chronotropy, dromotropy, and ionotropy. $\beta_2$ receptors are located in smooth muscle, gland cells, and ventricular myocytes, and agonism causes smooth muscle relaxation. $\beta_3$ receptors are located in the gallbladder and brain adipose tissue, and agonism is believed to cause lipolysis, thermogenesis in brown fat, and bladder relaxation.[1] For the purposes of this review chapter, we will be focusing on $\beta_2$ receptors and agonists.

## MECHANISM OF BRONCHODILATION

Bronchodilation occurs when $\beta_2$ receptors are stimulated by epinephrine, and less so norepinephrine. Beta receptors are linked to $G_s$ proteins, consisting of an $\alpha$ subunit and a $\beta$ subunit. The $\alpha$ subunit dissociates from the $\beta$ subunit and is charged with GTP. This leads to the activation of adenylyl cyclase, resulting in an increase in the rate of synthesis of cAMP. The increase in cAMP then activates cAMP-dependent protein kinase A, leading to phosphorylation of Gq-coupled receptors and a cascade of intracellular signals.[2] Ultimately, there is a decrease in intracellular calcium that prevents contraction of the smooth muscles in the airway (see Figure 245.1).

## SHORT-ACTING B2 AGONISTS (SABAS)

SABAs are molecularly similar to epinephrine but have been modified to be selective $\beta_2$ agonists. Examples include albuterol, levalbuterol, metaproterenol, and pirbuterol. Albuterol is a 1:1 racemic mixture of R-albuterol and S-albuterol. The R-isomer is responsible for bronchodilation, and thus levalbuterol was developed as strictly an R-isomer. However, studies are inconclusive regarding levalbuterol's efficacy compared to albuterol.[3,4] They are the mainstay

of acute obstructive lung pathology including asthma and chronic obstructive pulmonary disease (COPD). Therefore, they are prescribed for use as needed, rather than scheduled. Albuterol is available as a metered-dose inhaler (MDI) or dry powdered inhaler (DPI) and is formulated as 90 mcg/attenuation. Dosing for acute asthma relief is 2 to 8 inhalations, depending on asthma severity, every 20 minutes for 3 doses. Dosing for COPD exacerbations is 1 to 2 inhalations every 1–4 hours as needed. Levalbuterol is also available as an MDI, and dosing for bronchospasm is 90 mcg every 4–6 hours as needed.

## LONG-ACTING B2 AGONISTS (LABAS)

Examples include formoterol, salmeterol, and vilanterol. The FDA warns against the use of LABAs as monotherapy, and thus they are used in combination with inhaled

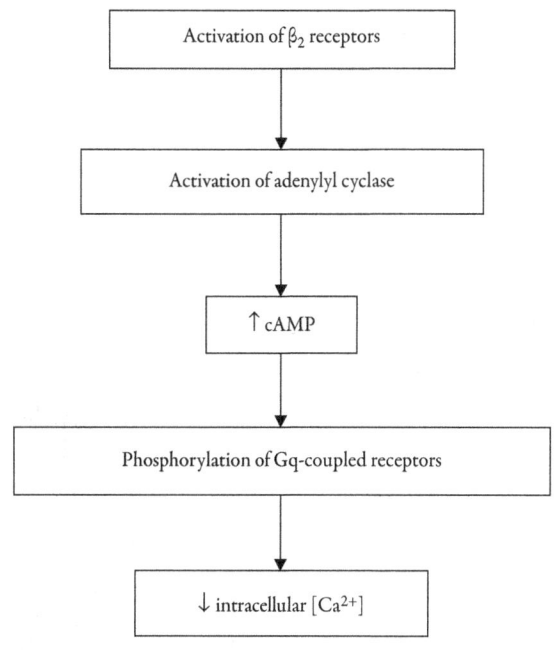

Figure 245.1. Mechanism of action

corticosteroids.[4,5] These are commonly utilized in long-term management of COPD in a scheduled fashion and not for acute perioperative therapy. An anesthesiologist should ensure that patients have continued and have not abruptly stopped LABAs perioperatively, as inappropriate discontinuance can increase risk of air constriction. Formoterol is no longer available in the United States. Salmeterol is available as a dry powder inhaler, and dosing for bronchospasm is 50 mcg every 12 hours. Vilanterol is only used in combination inhalers with anticholinergics or steroids.

## CLINICAL CONSIDERATIONS

Bronchospasm is an increase in bronchiolar smooth muscle tone, leading to increased airway resistance and wheezing. Intraoperatively this will also manifest as rapidly increasing peak inspiratory pressures, a slow increase in the height of the capnography wave form, and decreasing exhaled tidal volumes.[4] Bronchospasm occurs when vagal afferents in the bronchi are stimulated by histamine, cold air, inhaled irritants, and instrumentation such as laryngoscopy and endotracheal intubation.[1] The vagal activation leads to an increase in intracellular cyclic guanosine monophosphate (cGMP) and bronchoconstriction. When bronchospasm occurs intraoperatively, the first step is to increase the fraction of inspired oxygen ($FiO^2$) to 100% and deepen the level of anesthesia. Albuterol can be administered through the inspiratory limb of the circuit. It is important to consider that only 1%–3% of a dose of nebulized medication reaches the bronchi of a patient and therefore more metered doses of albuterol will need to be administered.[3,4]

## REFERENCES

1. Brunton L, et al., eds. *Goodman and Gilman's The Pharmacological Basis of Therapeutics.* 13th ed. New York, NY: McGraw-Hill Education; 2018.
2. Billington CK, et al. cAMP regulation of airway smooth muscle function. *Pulm Pharmacol Ther.* 2013;26(1):112–120.
3. Barisione G, et al. Beta-adrenergic agonists. *Pharmaceuticals.* 2010;3(4):1016–1044.
4. Hemmings HC, Egan TD, Emala CW. Pulmonary pharmacology. In: *Pharmacology and Physiology for Anesthesia.* 2nd ed. Philadelphia, PA: Elsevier, Inc; 2019.
5. Cazzola M, et al. β2-agonist therapy in lung disease. *Am J Respir Crit Care Med.* 2013;187:690.

# 246.

# ANTICHOLINERGICS

*Sheridan Markatos and Larry Manders*

## INTRODUCTION

Anticholinergics block the neurotransmitter acetylcholine in the brain and peripheral tissues. Inhaled anticholinergics, including ipratropium bromide and tiotropium bromide, are important medications in the management of chronic obstructive pulmonary disease (COPD) and severe asthma. They have slower onset of action than beta agonists and are therefore used for long-term management rather than acute exacerbations. Irritation of the upper airway with endotracheal tubes or suction catheters initiates an afferent irritant reflex arc. Vagal parasympathetic release of acetylcholine then binds to $M_3$-muscarinic receptors on smooth muscle in the small and medium airways, leading to bronchoconstriction.[1]

## MECHANISM OF ACTION

The M3-muscarinic receptor is bound to a Gq-coupled protein on the cell membrane of airway smooth muscles (Figure 246.1). When acetylcholine binds to the receptor,

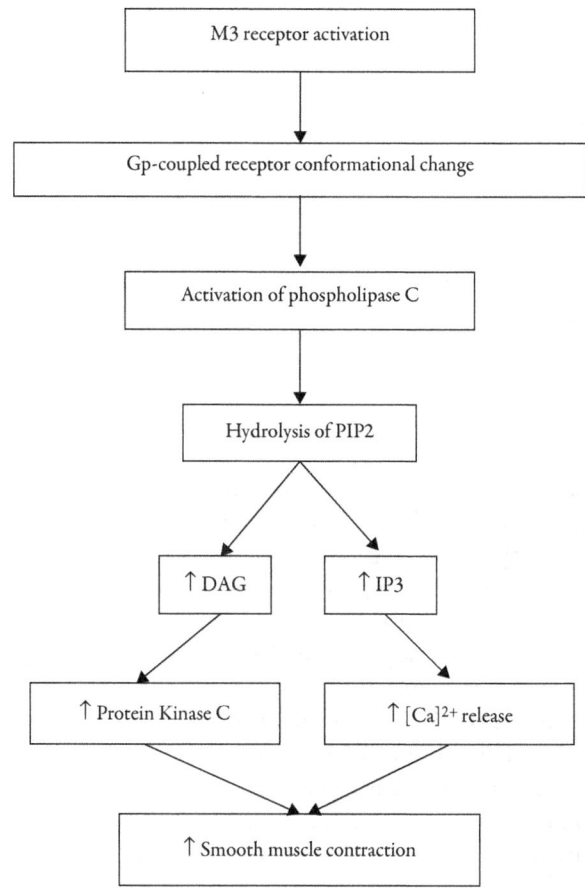

Figure 246.1. Activation of the muscarinic receptor.

the Gq-coupled protein receptor undergoes a conformational change that allows the alpha subunit to activate membrane-bound phospholipase C (PLC). PLC hydrolyzes phosphoinositol 4,5- bisphosphate ($PIP_2$) into 1,2-diacylglycerol (DAG) and inositol 1,4,5- trisphosphate ($IP_3$). Increased amounts of DAG lead to increased protein kinase C and cross-bridge cycling of smooth muscle. Increased

*Table 246.1* COMPARING BRONCHODILATION BY ANTICHOLINERGICS VS. BETA AGONISTS

| ANTICHOLINERGICS | BETA AGONISTS |
| --- | --- |
| Proximal large airways | Distal small airways |
| Reduces cholinergic tone, causing bronchodilation | Direct action on smooth muscle |
| Sustained activity | Rapid onset |

amounts of $IP_3$ triggers release of intracellular calcium from the sarcoplasmic reticulum.[2,3,4] Anticholinergics therefore block this signaling cascade to promote bronchodilation.

### IPRATROPIUM

Ipratropium, a derivative of atropine, is quick in onset with a shorter duration of action. It is available as a nebulizer or metered dose inhaler (MDI), which makes it more ideal in the perioperative setting compared to ipratropium.[5] The MDI dosing for acute asthma exacerbations is 140 mcg every 20 minutes for 3 hours. The MDI dosing for COPD is 2 inhalations 40 mcg 4 times daily.

### TIOTROPIUM

Tiotropium competitively binds to M1, M2, and M3 receptors; however, it rapidly dissociates from the M2 receptor. Compared to ipratropium, it is also longer acting.[3] Tiotropium is available as a dry powder inhaler or soft mist inhaler. The dosing of the soft mist inhaler for asthma and COPD is 2.5 mcg once daily and 5 mcg once daily, respectively. Dosing of the dry powder inhaler for COPD is 18 mcg once daily.

### SIDE EFFECTS

The most common side effect is dry mouth due to inhibition of mucosal secretions. Ipratropium does not cross the blood-brain barrier due to its quaternary structure and thus does not cause the central nervous system or ocular side effects seen in other anticholinergics (hyperthermia, mydriasis, facial flushing, delirium) (Figure 246.1).[2]

### REFERENCES

1. Hemmings H, Egan T. Pulmonary pharmacology. In: *Pharmacology and Physiology for Anesthesia*. 2nd ed. Philadelphia, PA: Elsevier; 2019.
2. Nishtala P, Mohammed S, Hilmer S. Anticholinergics: Theoretical and clinical overview. *Expert Opin Drug Safe*. 2016; ;753–768.
3. Goodman LS. *Goodman and Gilman's The Pharmacological Basis of Therapeutics*. New York, NY: McGraw-Hill; 1996.
4. Billington CK, Penn RB. M3 muscarinic acetylcholine receptor regulation in the airway. *Am J Respir Cell Mol* Biol. 2002;26(3): 269–272.
5. Yohannes AM, et al. Tiotropium for treatment of stable COPD: A meta-analysis of clinically relevant outcomes. *Respir Care*. 2011 Apr 1;56(4):477–487.

# 247.

# STEROIDS

*Neeraj Maheshwari and Larry Manders*

## INTRODUCTION

Steroids, in particularly glucocorticoids, are commonly utilized for the treatment of obstructive and reactive airway disease such as chronic obstructive pulmonary disease (COPD) and asthma. This chapter will discuss the mechanism of action, relative potencies of the common utilized steroids, and anesthetic considerations in the context of pulmonic conditions. A vast range of doses and treatment regiments have been described; this chapter will touch upon a few that are commonly utilized.

## MECHANISM OF ACTION

Inflammation is a normal physiologic response designed to protect injured tissue and promote their healing. Corticosteroids exert anti-inflammatory properties and serve to attenuate an exaggerated inflammatory response to an acute stressor. The anti-inflammatory effects of glucocorticoids are induced through the steroid-cell receptor complex that binds DNA and prevents the translocation of transcription factor NFκB, ultimately interfering with the genetic synthesis of pro-inflammatory mediators including prostaglandins, histamine, bradykinin, leukotrienes, and inflammatory cytokines.[2] Corticosteroids reduce the expression of phospholipase A2, decreasing the synthesis of arachidonic acid, prostaglandins, leukotrienes, and thromboxane A2. The anti-inflammatory effects of corticosteroids reduce smooth muscle hypertrophy, goblet cell hyperplasia, and thickening of the pulmonary basement membrane, all of which slow the progression of airway remodeling.[3] While the focus of the chapter revolves around glucocorticoids, also known as corticosteroids, Table 247.1 reviews the commonly utilized steroids, doses, and comparison of their glucocorticoid versus mineralocorticoid activity.

## ANESTHETIC CONSIDERATIONS

Corticosteroids may be indicated in specific pulmonary diseases that are characterized by chronic inflammation of any component of the airway, including bronchial asthma and COPD. Corticosteroids treat pulmonary disease by inhibiting bronchoconstriction, promoting bronchodilation, suppressing the immune response, and reducing airway and pulmonary inflammation.[4] The contraindications to corticosteroids include hypersensitivity, systemic fungal infection (or ophthalmic/skin infection if considering topical steroid use), idiopathic thrombocytopenic purpura, and intrathecal use.[2]) Acute side effects of corticosteroids include impaired wound healing, hyperglycemia, and increased risk of infection. Chronic side effects of these medications include downregulation of the hypothalamic-pituitary-adrenal (HPA) axis, loss of bone density, dermal atrophy, increased intraocular pressure (IOP), cataracts, redistribution of body fat, fluid retention, hypertension, acute psychosis, and a predisposition to diabetes and insulin resistance.[4]

## PREOPERATIVE

In patients with obstructive airway disease, the use of preoperative steroids (in addition to maintenance steroids the patient is already taking) is unlikely to provide any benefit unless started 2–3 days before surgery, with most treatment effects seen within 5 days. It has been shown that the use of albuterol vs. albuterol in addition to steroids decreases the incidence of wheezing in patients with reactive airway disease when initiated 5 days prior to intubation.[6] Different dosing regimens for uncontrolled COPD include 125 mg methylprednisolone, 100 mg hydrocortisone, or 30 mg prednisone daily.[3] Patients with a history of adrenal insufficiency or use of chronic steroid therapy should be questioned about current dose and duration of steroid therapy as well as previous adrenal crises, including triggering stressors and severity of episodes.[5]

## INTRAOPERATIVE

Complications of reactive airway disease, such as bronchospasm and mucus plugs, should be identified and

*Table 247.1* CORTICOSTEROID POTENCIES

| STEROID | GLUCOCORTICOID ACTIVITY | MINERALOCORTICOID ACTIVITY | EQUIVALENT DOSE (IV/PO) | HALF-LIFE (HRS) |
|---|---|---|---|---|
| Cortisol (hydrocortisone) | 1 | 1 | 20 | 8–12 |
| Cortisone | 0.8 | 0.8 | 25 | 8–12 |
| Prednisone | 4 | 0.8 | 5 | 18–36 |
| Prednisolone | 4 | 0.8 | 5 | 12–36 |
| Methylprednisolone | 5 | 0.5 | 4 | 18–36 |
| Dexamethasone | 30–40 | 0 | 0.5–0.75 | 36–54 |

treated quickly with appropriate acute interventions such as removing offending stimuli, deepening the anesthetic agent, administering an inhaled beta-2 agonist, or bronchoscopy. While a bolus of IV steroids, such as 125 mg IV methylprednisolone of 100 mg IV hydrocortisone, may be administered as an adjunct in the case of an asthma or COPD exacerbation before or during surgery, the steroids will take at least 4–6 hours to provide any effect.[4] Inhaled glucocorticoids can be considered in patients with asthma as well as other reactive airway states such as anaphylaxis.

## POSTOPERATIVE

The postoperative uses of steroids mirror the indications of the pre- and intraoperative settings. There utilization should be tailored to patient symptoms and should be used to decrease airway resistance resulting from their baseline disease and/or perioperative insult.

## REFERENCES

1. Holst JP. Steroid hormones: Relevance and measurement in the clinical laboratory. *Clin Lab* Med. 2004;24(1):105.
2. Marcela H, et al. Putting the brake on inflammatory responses: The role of glucocorticoids. *IUBMB Life* 2003;55(9):497–504.
3. James AL, Wenzel S. Clinical relevance of airway remodeling in airway diseases. *Eur Respir J.* 2007;30(1):134–155.
4. Ibrahim J, et al. Corticosteroids and Their Use in Respiratory Disorders. Al-kaf AG, ed. 2018: 47.
5. Woodcock T, et al. Guidelines for the management of glucocorticoids during the peri-operative period for patients with adrenal insufficiency: Guidelines from the Association of Anaesthetists, the Royal College of Physicians and the Society for Endocrinology UK. *Anaesthesia.* 2020;75(5):654–663.

# 248.

# LEUKOTRIENE MODIFIER DRUGS

*Adam Cruz and Larry Manders*

## INTRODUCTION

The leukotriene modifiers include montelukast, zafirlukast, and zileuton. These medications mitigate the effects and production of leukotrienes, proinflammatory mediators produced during inflammatory responses via arachidonic acid breakdown. As anti-inflammatory agents, the leukotriene modifiers are indicated for use in prophylaxis of asthma exacerbations and chronic asthma treatment.

## LEUKOTRIENE SYNTHESIS AND EFFECTS

Leukotrienes are synthesized in response to stimuli including complement, antigen, and cross-linked immunoglobin E (IgE).[1] This process begins with the breakdown of phospholipid from cell membranes into arachidonic acid, as outlined in Figure 248.1. End products include leukotriene B4 (LTB4) and the cysteinyl leukotrienes (CysLTs); the latter is known for having the most significant contribution to asthma pathogenesis. CysLTs include LTC4, LTD4, and LTE4.

The cysteinyl leukotrienes stimulate the G-protein coupled CysLT receptors, CysLT1 and CysLT2. In addition to pro-inflammatory signaling and chemotaxis, acute effects of CysLT1 include increased vascular permeability, bronchoconstriction, and airway mucus production.[1] Chronically, leukotrienes induce fibroblast proliferation, which may suggest that they contribute to airway remodeling in patients with chronic asthma.[2] CysLT2 has not been shown to contribute to bronchoconstriction, though its effects contribute to inflammatory responses and edema.

## MONTELUKAST AND ZAFIRLUKAST: LEUKOTRIENE RECEPTOR ANTAGONISTS, CYSLT1 ANTAGONISTS

The CysLT1 antagonists approved for use in the United States include montelukast and zafirlukast. CysLT1 antagonists are most commonly prescribed for prophylaxis and treatment of chronic asthma. These agents may also be prescribed for the treatment of allergic rhinitis. Montelukast dosing is 10 mg daily, while zafirlukast dosing is 20 mg 2 times daily.

## ZILEUTON: 5-LIPOXYGENASE INHIBITOR

Zileuton is a 5-lipoxygenase inhibitor that inhibits the conversion of arachidonic acid to leukotriene A4. By acting more "upstream" relative to the CysLT receptor antagonists, zileuton decreases the production of all leukotrienes. In a head-to-head comparison of montelukast versus zileuton, zileuton demonstrated slightly more improvement in peak expiratory flow rate 64.8 L/min vs. 40.6 L/min (P <0.001); adverse event rate was not significantly different between the groups.[3] Immediate release dosing for zafirlukast is 600 mg 4 times daily.

## ANESTHETIC CONSIDERATIONS

Typically indicated for the treatment of chronic asthma and persistent allergic rhinitis, the effects of leukotriene modifiers on alleviating symptoms and helping to lessen exacerbations in patients with asthma are overall favorable from an anesthetic standpoint. However, in patients with asthma who are

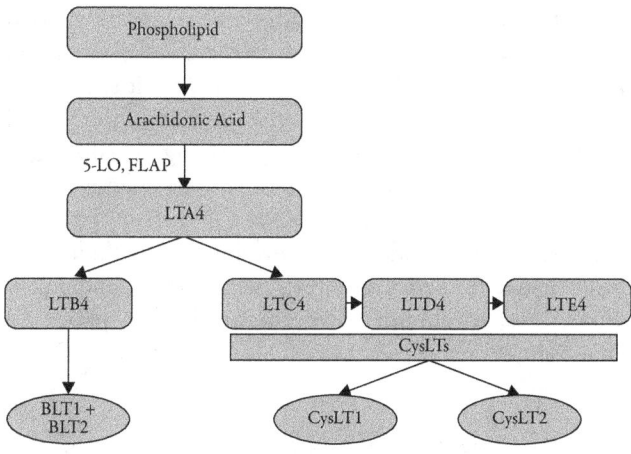

**Figure 248.1.** Synthesis of leukotrienes.
5-Lipoxygenase: 5-LO; 5-LO activating protein: FLAP; Cys-LT1 and Cys-LT-2: Cys-LT receptors.

not taking a leukotriene inhibitor, it is not recommended that an anesthesiologist begin treatment in the perioperative period. Montelukast now has a black box warning pertaining to the increased risk of neuropsychiatric side effects, a side effect that has long been studied.[4] Hypersensitivity to a leukotriene modifier is a contraindication to its use.

### PREOPERATIVE

There are no anesthetic contraindications to preoperative continuation of leukotriene modifiers. These medications should be continued in the perioperative period.

### INTRAOPERATIVE

There are no intraoperative considerations or adjustments necessary for patients taking leukotriene modifiers.

### POSTOPERATIVE

Postoperatively, known side effects of leukotriene modifiers may be considered. As noted previously, montelukast is known to demonstrate mood and behavior-related changes.[5] Both montelukast and zileuton carry headache and gastrointestinal upset as side effects.[3] Additionally, hepatotoxicity is a concern with zileuton. Transaminases should be monitored periodically in patients undergoing treatment with this medication.

### REFERENCES

1. Peters-Golden M, Henderson Jr WR. (2007). Leukotrienes. *N Engl J Med.* 2007;357(18):1841–1854.
2. Espinosa K, et al. CysLT1 receptor upregulation by TGF-β and IL-13 is associated with bronchial smooth muscle cell proliferation in response to LTD4. *J Allergy Clin Immunol.* 2003;111(5):1032–1040.
3. Kubavat AH, et al. A randomized, comparative, multicentric clinical trial to assess the efficacy and safety of zileuton extended-release tablets with montelukast sodium tablets in patients suffering from chronic persistent asthma. *Am J Ther.* 2013;20(2):154–162.
4. Haarman MG, et al. Adverse drug reactions of montelukast in children and adults. *Pharma Res Per.* 2017;5(5):e00341. https://doi.org/10.1002/prp2.341
5. Marschallinger J, et al. Structural and functional rejuvenation of the aged brain by an approved anti-asthmatic drug. *Nat Commun.* 2015;6(1):1–16.

# 249.

# MAST CELL STABILIZERS

## *Eric Reilly and Larry Manders*

### INTRODUCTION

There are two types of mast cells: connective tissue mast cells, which are found in the skin bowel submucosa and peritoneal cavity; and mucosal mast cells, which are found in mucosa such as in airways. Mast cells are key mediators in allergic diseases, and can be activated through both immunolglobin E (IgE) dependent and IgE independent mechanisms. For IgE dependent mechanisms, a mast cell is considered sensitized when IgE complexes are expressed on the surface of a mast cell. When an allergen comes into contact with the IgE complex on a sensitized mast cell, it starts a tyrosine kinase signaling cascade, which leads to a calcium influx and ultimately the release of chemical mediators such as histamine, prostaglandins, leukotrienes, cytokines, and chemokines. These mediators are responsible for the symptoms seen in primary, secondary, and idiopathic mast cell disorders—commonly grouped under the term *mast cell activation syndrome* (MCAS). Primary mast cell disorders refer to abnormal increases in tissue mast cells, such as in mastocytosis. Secondary disorders include normal mast cell activation in response to environmental triggers, such as asthma. Idiopathic disorders, such as anaphylaxis, do not specifically fit either primary or secondary definitions. Mast cell stabilizers, such as sodium cromoglycate, stabilize mast cells to inhibit the release of allergic mediators, thus providing symptomatic relief in primary, secondary, and idiopathic mast cell disorders.

## MECHANISM OF ACTION

There are many natural, semi-synthetic, and synthetic mast cell stabilizers which all have varying specific mechanisms of actions—many of them poorly understood. Some proposed mechanisms include blocking late phase chloride channels or blocking specific mediators in the tyrosine kinase pathway. Ultimately, the major mechanism is preventing mast cell degranulation in the presence of a trigger or allergen (see Figure 249.1).

### COMMON FORMULATIONS AND USES

Common mast cell stabilizers include sodium cromoglycate (cromolyn), ketotifen, pemirolast, and even some

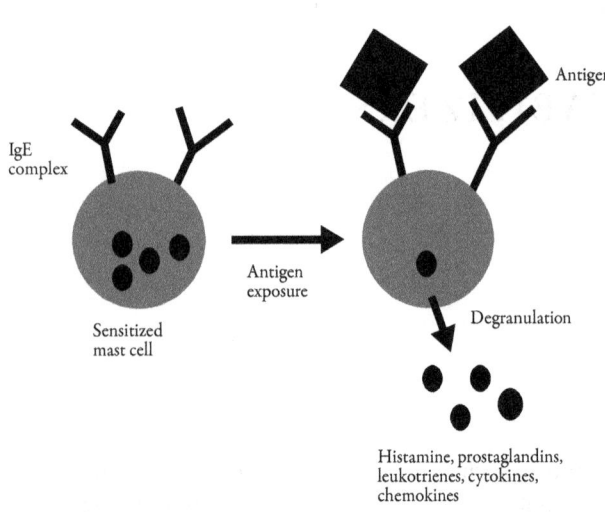

**Figure 249.1.** Mast cell sensitization and degranulation.

antihistamines such as olopatadine. They are often used in allergic reactions where mast cells are a key mediator, such as allergic rhinitis, allergic conjunctivitis, asthma, and mastocytosis. Cromolyn is the most commonly used formulation, with dosing usually starting at 200 mg 4 times daily and titrated down to the lowest effective dose. The only true contraindication is a hypersensitivity to cromolyn. Adverse effects are rare but can include diarrhea, headache, pruritus, myalgias, tinnitus, and many others. Dosages should be adjusted in both hepatic and renal failure.[1]

## ANESTHETIC CONSIDERATIONS

*Mast cell activation syndrome* (MCAS) is a generalized term to describe a wide array of mast cell disorders which can be primary (e.g., mastocystosis), secondary (e.g., asthma, rhinitis, physical urticaria), or idiopathic (e.g., angioedema, anaphylaxis) in nature. These conditions can cause symptoms in the perioperative setting such as flushing, pruritus, palpitations, dysrhythmia, hypotension, cough, seizures, psychosis, nausea, diarrhea, abdominal pain, and hypersensitivity reactions. Specific guidelines are poorly defined for the management of MCAS in the perioperative setting, but the avoidance of mast cell mediator release should be of greatest concern—especially in patients with a history of MCAS such as mastocytosis. The following perioperative recommendations should be taken into consideration when managing MCAS.

### PREOPERATIVE

Any scheduled outpatient medications to promote mast cell stability or prevent degranulation, such as mast cell stabilizers, should be continued until the day of surgery. Premedication with H1 and H2 receptor antagonists, and sometimes corticosteroids, is recommended prior to invasive procedures. Benzodiazepines can also help reduce potential mast cell activation triggers from anxiety.

### INTRAOPERATIVE

Operative time should be minimized. Drugs which can promote histamine release should be limited. These drugs include thiopental, morphine, meperidine, codeine, NSAIDs, atracurium, mivacurium, vancomycin, polymyxin B, adenosine, and protamine. In the event of an intraoperative reaction—such as anaphylactic or anaphylactoid, the suspected offending agent should be discontinued, followed by symptomatic and supportive treatments. These may include oxygen, H1 and H2 antagonists, mast cell stabilizers, corticosteroids, epinephrine, and airway protection.

If a patient is suspected of experiencing MCAS during surgery, a serum tryptase level or specific urinary markers (e.g., histamine metabolites, leukotriene E4) should be ordered. Additionally, the patient should undergo outpatient allergen skin tests to try to identify potential triggers. Supportive and symptomatic management should continue until the patient is stable.[2,3]

## REFERENCES

1. Finn DF, Walsh JJ. Twenty-first century mast cell stabilizers. *Br J Pharmacol.* 2005;170(1), 23–37.
2. Kumaraswami S, Farkas G. Management of a parturient with mast cell activation syndrome. *An Anesthesiologist's Experience: Case Reports in Anesthesiology.* 2018:1–5.
3. Dewachter P. Perioperative management of patients with mastocytosis. *Anesthesiology.* 2014;120(3):753–759.

# 250.

# IMMUNOGLOBULIN E (IGE) BLOCKERS (ANTI-IGE THERAPY)

*Eric Reilly and Larry Manders*

## MECHANISMS OF ACTION

Anti-IgE therapies can either limit immunoglobin E (IgE) production, neutralize free IgE in blood, or reduce the number of mediator-releasing effector cells. Novel drugs like quilizumab attempt to limit IgE production by suppressing IgE-producing B cells. Drugs like omalizumab bind and neutralize free IgE in the serum, thus preventing IgE binding to effector cells. Experimental fusion proteins, such as CTLA4Fcε, reduce the number of effector cells in an effort to limit IgE binding and subsequent preformed mediator release. Overall, by reducing mediator and cytokine release, anti-IgE therapies help reduce inflammation and additional sequelae, such bronchoconstriction in allergic asthmatics.[1]

## COMMON FORMULATIONS AND USES

Omalizumab is the anti-IgE agent which is most commonly used, FDA approved, and most supported by large clinical trials. Literature supporting omalizumab shows strong evidence for treating allergic asthma and chronic urticaria. The literature shows good evidence for omalizumab's effectiveness against allergic rhinitis and allergen immunotherapy; and fair evidence for its use in atopic dermatitis, food allergies, oral immunotherapy, and mast cell disorders. Omalizumab is approved by the FDA as an add-on for treating moderate-to-severe persistent allergic asthma refractory to inhaled corticosteroids and long-acting beta agonists in patients over 6 years old. Omalizumab is also approved by the FDA for treating chronic urticaria refractory to H1 antihistamines in patients over 12 years old. The drug is administered subcutaneously, with the dose varying widely based on body weight and pretreatment total IgE serum levels. The only true contraindication is a history of anaphylactic response to omalizumab. Adverse effects are rare but include hypersensitivity reactions and an increased risk of parasitic infections.[2]

## ANESTHETIC CONSIDERATIONS

Omalizumab is FDA approved for moderate-to-severe persistent allergic asthma and chronic urticaria. Given the drug's cost and relatively delayed onset of action, it is not an appropriate therapy for the acute asthma or allergic exacerbations which are commonly encountered in the perioperative setting. Thus, the main anesthetic considerations are for maintenance of outpatient therapies and preoperative optimization.

## PREOPERATIVE

Patients should be interrogated about their asthma history, including the details of their most recent exacerbations and how often they occur. If a smoker, the patient should be recommended to stop smoking at least 2 months in advance of the scheduled surgery. Patients should remain compliant with their outpatient asthma medications, including omalizumab, up until the day of surgery. Short courses of beta agonist inhalers or corticosteroids may also be appropriate on a case-by-case basis.[2]

## INTRAOPERATIVE

Anti-IgE therapy, such as omalizumab, does not currently have any literature support for intraoperative use. Scenarios where one may be tempted to use it, such as in acute bronchospasm, should be treated with appropriate rapid-acting medications such as beta agonists, corticosteroids, and epinephrine.[3]

## POSTOPERATIVE

Similar to intraoperative management, there is no recognized use for anti-IgE therapy in acute postoperative conditions. Patients should continue their home medication

*Table 250.1* PERIOPERATIVE STRATEGY FOR IGE ANTAGORIST THERAPY

| Setting | Role of Anti-IgE (Omalizumab) Therapy |
| --- | --- |
| Pre-operative | Continue current outpatient regimen up until the day of surgery, optimize conditions through smoking cessation, etc. |
| Intra-operative | No acute role |
| Post-operative | No acute role, scheduled outpatient medication should be resumed as soon as possible when clinically appropriate |

regimen, including anti-IgE therapy, as soon as clinically safe and possible in the postoperative period (Table 250.1).

## REFERENCES

1. Hu, J. et al. Anti-IgE therapy for IgE-mediated allergic diseases: From neutralizing IgE antibodies to eliminating IgE+ B cells. *Clin Transl Allergy.* 2018;8:27.
2. Stokes J. Anti-IgE treatment for disorders other than asthma. *Front Med.* 2017;4:152.
3. Woods BD, Sladen RN. Perioperative considerations for the patient with asthma and bronchospasm. *Br J Anaesth.* 2009 Dec;103:157–165.

# 251.

# PERIOPERATIVE USE OF ALCOHOL

*Lindsey Cieslinski*

## INTRODUCTION

During the initial evaluation of a patient, it is imperative to identify all risk factors, with the goal of mitigating potential negative outcomes prior to surgery. As an anesthesiologist, identifying substance use is a critical component of this risk reduction as part of the perioperative assessment and plan. When assessing a patient's alcohol consumption, is it important to understand the type and quantity of alcohol. Thus, a few definitions are pertinent for this discussion. A standard drink in the United states is defined as 14 grams of ethanol, which is equivalent to 12 ounces of beer, 5 ounces of wine, or 1.5 ounces of distilled spirits.[1,2] According to the National Institute on Alcohol Abuse and Alcoholism (NIAAA), *heavy alcohol use* is defined as more than 4 drinks on any day for men and more than 3 drinks for women. Binge drinking and heavy alcohol use are risk factors for alcohol use disorder.[2] Conversely, the NIAAA states that *low risk drinking* is defined as 3 or less drinks per sitting and no more than 14 drinks per week, for men. For women they recommend no more than 2 drinks per sitting, and no more than 7 drinks per week. *Alcohol abuse* is described as a distinct diagnosis with a pattern of repeated alcohol-related consequences involving health, relationships, and the legal system, without evidence of addiction. Conversely, *alcohol-dependent* individuals not only experience these same consequences, but also show signs of addiction: withdrawal symptoms, craving, and preoccupation with alcohol.[3]

Ethanol is metabolized by alcohol dehydrogenase to acetaldehyde, which is then metabolized by acetaldehyde dehydrogenase to $CO_2$ + $H_2O$ + acetate.

A recent epidemiologic study in the United States determined the prevalence of alcohol use disorders (AUDs), including alcohol abuse and dependence, to be 8.26%. Given these data, the likelihood for anesthesiologists to encounter AUD preoperatively is almost guaranteed.[3] Another study reveals increased morbidity among those with AUDs was observed after a diverse range of procedures, from

prostatectomy, ankle surgery, subdural hematomas, and abdominal surgery, to hysterectomy. Additional studies show the same increased morbidity in thoracic and vascular surgery patients, as well as a higher rate of readmission to the intensive care unit among those who abuse alcohol. Postoperative morbidity among these patients with AUDs most commonly includes infections. However, the need for ventilator support, bleeding disorders, and cognitive dysfunction can also occur.[3]

Infection and more seriously sepsis are, not surprisingly, a common complication because heavy alcohol use suppresses T-cell dependent activity, macrophage, neutrophil mobilization, and phagocytosis. Furthermore, delayed wound healing is seen due to alcohol's negative effects on the accumulation of collagen in the wound.[2] Alcohol increases bleeding risk by affecting the fibrinolytic and coagulation pathways, as well as causing quantitative and qualitative thrombocytopenia.

It is critical to evaluate chronic alcoholics for electrolytes abnormalities, particularly due to the potential for increased perioperative morbidity and mortality. Acid-base abnormalities commonly encountered include metabolic acidosis, often secondary to alcoholic ketoacidosis and respiratory alkalosis. One study found 40.5% of alcoholic patients had an acid-base disturbance, with 12.6% of those being a pure respiratory alkalosis and 25.3% with alcoholic ketoacidosis. The metabolic acidosis occurs due to metabolism of ethanol to lactic acid, resulting in a compensatory respiratory alkalosis. Additionally, alcohol withdrawal in chronic alcoholics causes central and sympathetic nervous system activation, leading to an increased respiratory drive resulting in a respiratory alkalosis. Classically, chronic alcoholism causes electrolyte disturbances including hypokalemia, hypomagnesemia, hyponatremia, and hyperuricemia. Common causes of these electrolyte disturbances can be from frequent vomiting, diarrhea, and malnutrition seen with chronic alcoholic abuse. Malnutrition alone causes hypokalemia, hypomagnesemia, and hyponatremia. The sequelae of alcoholism lead to gastrointestinal losses causing

**Table 251.1** COMORBIDITIES ASSOCIATED WITH CHRONIC ALCOHOLISM

| | |
|---|---|
| Neurologic | Dementia, polyneuropathies, Wernicke's encephalopathy, Korsakoff syndrome, withdrawal seizures |
| Respiratory | Aspiration pneumonia, COPD |
| Hematology | Coagulopathy, anemia, thrombocytopenia |
| Cardiovascular | Hypertension, cardiac arrythmias, congestive heart failure, cardiomyopathy |
| Gastroenterology | Esophageal varices, cirrhosis or hepatitis, pancreatitis, splenomegaly, ascites |
| Delirium tremens | Occur 48–72 hours after cessation of drinking. Manifest as hallucination, diaphoresis, hyperpyrexia, tachycardia, and hypertension. Lead to hypomagnesemia, hypokalemia, and respiratory alkalosis. Treated with benzodiazepines, thiamine, magnesium, and potassium. |

malabsorption. Renal shifts alter free water imbalance and decreased renal tubular electrolyte reabsorption, leading to dilutional hyponatremia. Hypomagnesemia occurs commonly with chronic diarrhea and increased renal magnesium excretion. Lastly, alcohol leads to hyperuricemia through several different uric acid metabolic pathways. Purines contained in beer are metabolized to uric acid, and ethanol metabolism increases lactate, which inhibits renal excretion of uric acid.[1] Ethanol also increases adenine degradation, producing xanthine and hypoxanthine, which are subsequently metabolized to uric acid.

It is important to combine the clinical picture with objective findings to aid in treatment and management of patients with AUD. Common diagnostic findings seen in alcoholism include macrocytic (megaloblastic) anemia, thrombocytopenia, transaminitis, elevated international normalized ratio (INR), and mild bilirubin. Electrocardiogram (ECG) findings can include premature ventricular contractions, heart block, QT prolongation, atrial fibrillation or flutter. An echocardiogram may show dilated cardiomyopathy, systolic or diastolic dysfunction, left ventricular hypertrophy, or valvular regurgitation. The decreased cardiac function seen in chronic abusers is thought to be secondary to alterations in cardiac conduction and myocyte contractility.[2]

Liver ultrasound will show evidence of cirrhosis and portal hypertension with heavy chronic alcohol use. When hepatic dysfunction progresses, a Child-Pugh score is used to assess the severity and prognosis. It can be combined with the Model for End-stage Liver Disease (MELD) score to determine priority for liver transplantation. Patients with cirrhosis are at a higher risk of the common postoperative complications seen with heavy alcohol use. The degree of risk depends on the type of surgery and also the severity of hepatic disease.[2] Table 251.1 lists potential findings that are not specific to chronic alcoholism but can be a consequence of the AUD.

## DISULFIRAM (ANTABUSE)

Disulfiram blocks the conversion of acetaldehyde by acetaldehyde dehydrogenase. Increase in levels of acetaldehyde causes nausea, vomiting, tearing, and potentially bronchoconstriction and cardiac arrhythmias. It has a half-life of 1–2 weeks. It can also block dopamine-beta- hydroxylase, which is essential for conversion of dopamine to norepinephrine, leading to perioperative hypotension.

## PERIOPERATIVE ANESTHETIC CONSIDERATIONS

An 8% prevalence of AUD makes encountering this preoperatively almost inevitable. Knowledge about AUD is advantageous for physicians to increase vigilance during the postoperative period and can potentially prevent complications.[3] For example, it is important to note that alcohol abuse may influence gastric emptying. Also, known or suspected heavy alcohol intake places a patient at higher risk for intraoperative awareness.[2] Acute alcohol ingestion decreases the MAC of anesthetic agents, while chronic alcoholism increases MAC.[1] Patients with alcohol dependence have an increased tolerance to many sedatives utilized as part of anesthetic management. These patients are at an increased risk of hepatic disease, which can impact the choice of anesthetics agents.[2]

## REFERENCES

1. Elisaf M, et al. Acid-base and electrolyte abnormalities in alcoholic patients. *Miner Electrolyte Metab.* 1994;20(5):274–28.1.
2. Boxhorn C. Substance use disorder and perioperative management. *Anesthesia Toolbox* [Online]. https://www.anesthesiatoolbox.com/. Published September 2, 2019.
3. Burnham EL. Identification of risky alcohol consumption in the preoperative assessment: opportunity to diagnose and intervene. *Anesthesiology.* 2008;109(2):169–170.

# 252.

# COCAINE PHARMACOLOGY

*Lindsey Cieslinski*

## INTRODUCTION

Cocaine is a powerful drug originating from the leaves of the *erthryoxylon coca* plant. It was first discovered by South American civilizations who utilized the coca leaves for religious, mystical, social, and medicinal purposes.[1] Known for its ability to increase stamina and to alleviate hunger and thirst, early on cocaine was described to have toxic effects with highly addictive capacity. Given cocaine's widespread use and abuse potential, the chemical and biological effects are important to understand for proper perioperative management.

Cocaine came into Western medicine as the first local anesthetic in 1884 and it remains unique due to its combined vasoconstrictive and local anesthetic properties. Today in modern medicine, cocaine can be used as a topical intranasal anesthetic agent for sinus surgery, or less commonly for awake intubation in a 4% solution.[2] The active coca alkaloids are hydrolyzed to obtain ecgonine, a tropane derivative, which is then benzoylated and methylated to the base-cocaine. More simply, cocaine is extracted from the coca leaf by mechanical degradation in the presence of a hydrocarbon solvent.[3] Peak plasma levels appear to be proportional to the dose regardless of the concentration; however, the time to peak concentration lengthened with increasing doses via potent vasoconstriction.[1] Cocaine's vasoconstrictive properties prolong the rate of absorption and delay its effect when absorbed through mucosal surfaces.[3] It is substantially absorbed from the upper respiratory tract, highest through tracheal and laryngeal mucosa.[1] In clinical studies, intranasal cocaine was rapidly absorbed with peak plasma concentration occurring within 30–60 minutes. Interestingly, higher peak plasma concentrations occurred in those patients with significant cardiac disease.[1]

Cocaine has 3 major metabolites: benzoylecgonine (BE), formed from spontaneous hydrolysis; ecgonine methyl ester (EME), formed from metabolism by plasma pseudocholinesterase; and norcocaine, formed from metabolism via N-demethylation by the p450 system.[3] Norcocaine is the only metabolite of cocaine with significant pharmacology activity.[1] A deficiency in pseudocholinesterase enzyme results in decreased metabolism and prolonged effects of this substance. Cocaine has a serum half-life of 0.5–1.5 hours.[3] EME and BE make up 80% of cocaine's metabolites and have a biological half-life of approximately 4 and 6 hours, respectively.[1] These metabolites are excreted in the urine and detected in the urine for 14–60 hours after administration.[1] Cocaine's volume of distribution is about 2.7 L/kg, and it is about 90% protein bound.[1]

Cocaine toxicity can manifest as overwhelming stimulation of the central nervous, respiratory, and cardiovascular systems, culminating in seizures, followed by profound depression and cardiorespiratory collapse.[1] Cocaine is an indirect sympathomimetic agent via presynaptic reuptake inhibition of neurotransmitters with binding sites in both the central and peripheral nervous system. It also increases the concentration of the excitatory amino acids' glutamate and aspartate in the brain.[2] It stimulates alpha-1, alpha-2, beta-1, and beta-2 adrenergic receptors through primarily increased levels of norepinephrine by inhibition of reuptake in the synaptic cleft.[3] Cocaine exhibits preferential alpha-receptor activity on the cardiac and peripheral vasculature.[3] The euphoric properties of cocaine derive from the inhibition of neural serotonin reuptake in the central nervous system (CNS). This pharmacologic effect of cocaine can precipitate serotonin syndrome.[2] Cocaine addiction has been linked to its effects on dopamine uptake. Shown in animal studies, effects on dopamine-containing neuronal systems traveling from the limbic region to the frontal cortex are strongly associated with cocaine addiction.[3] As a local anesthetic, cocaine blocks sodium channels, which can affect cardiac sodium channels. This can be seen clinical with prolongation of the QRS complex, along with negative inotropy.[3] At high concentration, cocaine's negative ionotropic effects may cause acute depression of left ventricular function and heart failure.[3]

Though cocaine has numerous physiologic effects, from an anesthetic perspective the more significant effects involve the CNS, peripheral nervous system, cardiovascular, and pulmonary system. Acute cocaine overdose can lead to various CNS symptoms, including tremors, restlessness, seizures, psychomotor agitation, headache, and more serious intracerebral hemorrhage.[3] The psychomotor agitation caused by cocaine intoxication can lead to hyperthermia where peripheral vasoconstriction prevents the body from dissipating the heat being generated from persistent agitation.[3] The degree of hyperthermia is directly related to the extent of the agitation and the ambient temperature. The mortality rate can be as high as 33%.[3] Generally speaking, respiratory drive is usually maintained. If rapid sequence induction is indicated for intubation, then the use of succinylcholine is relatively contraindicated, as cocaine is also metabolized by plasma psuedocholinesterases and when coadministrated can prolong the effects of cocaine and paralysis of succinylcholine.[2] Ketamine also markedly potentiates the cardiovascular toxicity of cocaine.[1]

Clinically important cardiovascular adverse effects include chest pain, hypertension, and tachycardia with the potential to cause arrhythmias, ventricular ectopy, and even cardiac arrest.[3] These cardiovascular effects are centrally mediated via direct action at myocardial receptors and sympathetic stimulation, causing arterial vasoconstriction, enhanced thrombus formation, increased myocardial oxygen demand, and increased vascular shearing forces.[3]

Chronic cocaine use can cause accelerated atherogenesis and left ventricular hypertrophy, which increases the risk of myocardial ischemia or infarction and can lead to dilated cardiomyopathy.[3] Intranasal and inhalational cocaine use is associated with pneumothorax, pneumomediastinum, and pneumopericardium resulting from valsalva. Cocaine is associated with exacerbation of reversible airway disease and bronchospasm.[3] Inhalational cocaine can injure the upper and lower airways, potentially complicating airway management.

## ANESTHETIC CONSIDERATIONS

Cocaine has numerous physiologic effects, with numerous potential drug interactions further challenging anesthetic management. It is important to be mindful that acute cocaine intoxication is a major risk factor for intraoperative awareness under general anesthesia and is associated with increased Minimum alveolar concentration requirements.[4] During general anesthesia, the fever and sympathomimetic effects of a cocaine overdose could mimic malignant hyperthermia.[1] Unpredictable but clinically significant interactions have been noted with virtually all classes of psychotropic drugs.[1] For cocaine-induced myocardial ischemia, it is not recommended to use beta blockers, based principally upon theoretical concerns of coronary artery vasoconstriction and severe systemic hypertension which can result from unopposed alpha-adrenergic stimulation.[5] It may potentiate the action of muscle relaxants. Use of pure beta blockers in patients intoxicated with cocaine can cause unopposed alpha stimulation and severe hypertension.

## REFERENCES

1. Fleming J, et al. Pharmacology and therapeutic applications of cocaine. *Anesthesiology*. 1990;73:518–531.
2. Sumner, C. Cocaine intoxication: Treatment. *OpenAnesthesia* [Online]. 2013. https://keywords.selfstudy.app/cocaine-intoxication-treatment/. Accessed August 12, 2020.
3. Nelson L, Odujebe O. Cocaine: Acute intoxication. *UpToDate* [Online]. https://www.uptodate.com/contents/search. Accessed June 20, 2020.
4. Inhaled anesthetics. In: Pardo MD, Miller RD, eds. *Basics of Anesthesia*. 6th ed. Philadelphia, PA: Elsevier; 2011:81–82.
5. Drug interactions. In: Barash PG, ed. *Clinical Anesthesia*. 7th ed. Philadelphia, PA: Wolters Kluwer; 2017:560.

# Part XVIII

# CARDIOVASCULAR SYSTEM PHYSIOLOGY

# 253.

# THE CARDIAC CYCLE

*Robert Pellicer and Alaa Abd-Elsayed*

## INTRODUCTION

The cardiac cycle is a series of physiological events in which blood moves through the chambers of the heart in alternating phases of systole and diastole. Blood is ejected from the heart during ventricular systole and is quantified as *stroke volume* (SV), the volume of blood pumped out of the left ventricle during a cardiac contraction. During ventricular diastole, the ventricles relax, allowing blood to enter from the atria. Movement of blood through the heart is dependent on pressure changes generated by the alternating contraction and relaxation of myocardium. These pressure changes create gradients between the chambers and the vasculature, allowing blood to flow through the heart and the body.

The cardiac cycle is generally described as having four phases: filling phase, isovolumetric contraction, ejection phase, and isovolumetric relaxation.

## FILLING PHASE

During the filling phase, blood enters the right and left ventricle from the atria. Atrial pressures increase as blood enters from the vena cava and pulmonary veins, eventually reaching the critical threshold of the atrioventricular (AV) valves, which causes them to open. Blood from the atria then enters the ventricles, initially falling down a pressure gradient that favors rapid ventricular filling; this rapid filling phase accounts for 75% of ventricular filling volume. The remaining 25% enters the ventricle during atrial systole, an active phase referred to as the "atrial kick."[1] The passive and active stages of the filling phase are associated with the "y" descent and the "a" wave on the central venous pressure (CVP) waveform, respectively (see Figure 253.1). The volume of blood in the ventricle at the end of the filling phase is the *end-diastolic volume.*

## ISOVOLUMETRIC CONTRACTION

At the beginning of systole, ventricular pressure rapidly increases, exceeding that of the atria. This causes the closure of the mitral and tricuspid valves. This closure corresponds to the first heart sound, S1. During isovolumetric contraction, the volume of blood in the ventricle remains unchanged as the force of myocardial contraction increases. The "c" wave of the CVP waveform is associated with the bulging of the tricuspid valve as right ventricular pressure increases during this phase.

## EJECTION PHASE

Ejection of blood from the ventricles occurs when ventricular pressures exceed aortic and pulmonary artery pressures, causing the aortic and pulmonic valves to open. The first part of the ejection phase is known as the *rapid ejection phase* as two-thirds of the end-diastolic volume is ejected from the ventricle during this time. The maximum ejection velocity of blood leaving the ventricles is reached early in the ejection phase, and as the pressure in the aorta reaches its maximum amplitude, the ejection velocity decreases.[2] This slowing of the ejection velocity corresponds to ventricular repolarization and the T wave of the ECG. The volume of blood that remains in the ventricle after the ejection phase is known as the *end-systolic volume.*

## ISOVOLUMETRIC RELAXATION

As ventricular pressures fall below aortic and pulmonary artery pressures, the semilunar valves close, which causes the second heart sound (S2). A physiologic splitting of the second heart sound may occur during inspiration due to increased filling of the RV secondary to decreased intrathoracic pressure and increased transit time across the

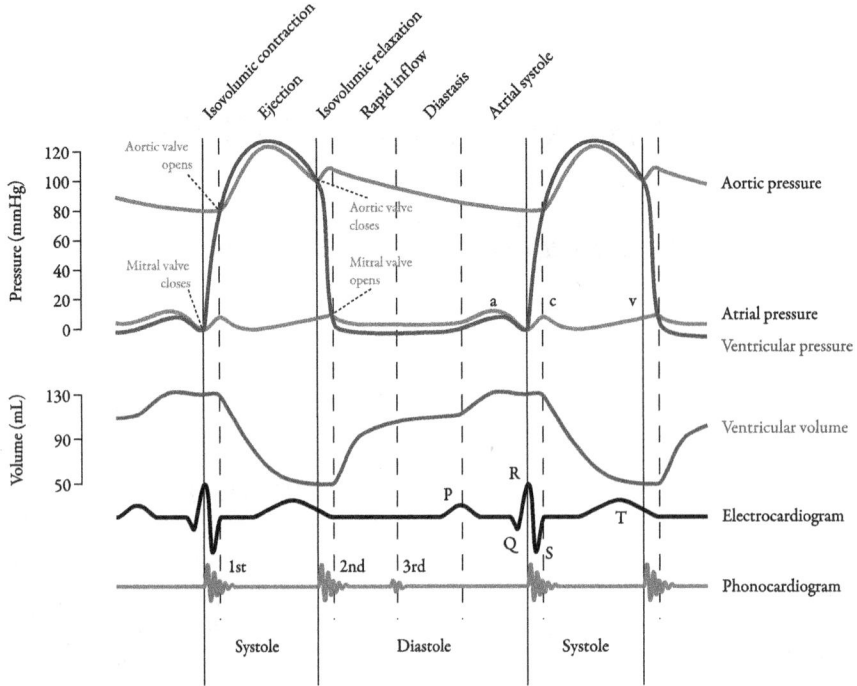

**Figure 253.1.** Wiggers diagram, showing the relationship between aortic, atrial, and left ventricular pressure and volume in relation to a standard ECG tracing.

adh30 revised work by Daniel Chang, MD, who revised original work of DestinyQx; Redrawn as SVG by xavax/CC BY-SA https://creative commons.org/licenses/by-sa/4.0)

pulmonic valve. As ventricular pressures decrease, ventricular volumes remain the same as all valves are closed. The rate of myocardial relaxation is termed *lusitropy*, and it is a function of the level of cytoplasmic calcium present in the cardiomyocytes. The volume of blood remaining in the ventricles at this time is the *end-systolic volume*. *Stroke volume* can be calculated from the *end-systolic volume* and *end-diastolic volume*:

$$SV = EDV - ESV$$

## THE CARDIAC CONDUCTION SYSTEM

The cardiac conduction system plays an integral role in maintaining appropriate intracardiac pressure gradients and ensuring synchronized contraction of the atria and ventricles.[3] The sinoatrial (SA) node, located in the right atrium, is the heart's pacemaker, spontaneously generating action potentials that lead to atrial contraction. Action potentials traveling away from the SA node eventually reach the atrioventricular (AV) node, where a brief delay in signal propagation prevents simultaneous contraction of the atria and ventricles. Leaving the AV node, action potentials travel along the His-Purkinje system (HPS), which contains the bundle branches and fascicles. The HPS ensures synchronized contraction of ventricular myocardium to ensure optimal cardiac output. Disruptions along the cardiac conduction system may significantly alter cardiac function by affecting heart rate, contractility, and cardiac output.

## REFERENCES

1. Larusso K, Elmoselhi A. The cardiac cycle. In: Elmoselhi A., eds. *Cardiology: An Integrated Approach.* McGraw-Hill. https://accessm edicine-mhmedical-com.ezproxy.library.wisc.edu/content.aspx?boo kid=2224&sectionid=171660329. Accessed April 25, 2020.
2. Mohrman D, Heller L. The heart pump. In: Mohrman DE, Heller L, eds. *Cardiovascular Physiology.* 9th ed. McGraw-Hill. https:// accessmedicine-mhmedical-com.ezproxy.library.wisc.edu/cont ent.aspx?bookid=2432&sectionid=190800576. Accessed April 3, 2020.
3. Glover B, Brugada P. *Clinical Handbook of Cardiac Electrophysiology.* 1st ed. Springer International; 2016:1–37.

# 254.

# CONTROL OF HEART RATE

*Emuejevoke Chuba and Muhammad Fayyaz Ahmed*

## INTRODUCTION

Heart rate (HR) is a key parameter of cardiovascular monitoring. The normal intrinsic HR for adults is 60–100 bpm. The normal HR is impacted by a number of factors such as age, exercise, stress, medication, and anxiety, among others. The HR for each age group can be calculated with the following formula:

$$Normal\ heart\ rate = 118\ beats/min - (0.57 \times Age)$$

HR is directly proportional to cardiac output when the stoke volume remains constant.

The HR is an intrinsic function of the sinoatrial (SA) node, which can be controlled by the autonomic system, reflex, and hormonal and local factors. [1]

## AUTONOMIC CONTROL

The HR is for the most part controlled by the autonomic nervous system (ANS). The ANS comprises parasympathetic and sympathetic nervous systems. The sympathetic nervous system consists of the $\alpha_1$, $\alpha_2$, $\beta_1$, and $\beta_2$ receptors. The parasympathetic nervous system consists of the muscarinic receptors with subtypes $M_1$–$M_5$. The parasympathetic nervous system predominates early in life, while the sympathetic nervous system is the most predominant in the adult. This disparity is the explanation for the bradycardia seen in children during laryngoscopy. Increased sympathetic activity leads to an increase in HR. The neurotransmitters epinephrine and norepinephrine, released from the sympathetic nerve endings in the SA, increase the HR through activation of the $\beta_1$ receptor. After cessation of sympathetic stimulation, the chronotropic response gradually returns to the control level. The parasympathetic activity is predominant during the resting phase of the heart. The neurotransmitter acetylcholine, released

at the vagal nerve endings, decreases the firing of the automatic cells of the SA node, which decreases the HR via activation of the $M_1$ receptor. [1,2,3]

## REFLEX CONTROL

### BARORECEPTOR REFLEX

The baroreceptors are located within the walls of the carotid sinus and the aortic arch. They are activated by changes in blood pressure. Increase in blood pressure increases the firing of the afferent nerves of the reflex, sending signals to the vasomotor centers in the brainstem via the glossopharyngeal and vagus nerves from the carotid sinus and aortic arch, respectively. In response, it increases parasympathetic activity, thus decreasing the HR and blood pressure.

### BAINBRIDGE REFLEX

Increase in venous return increases the right atrial pressure, which stretches and activates the atrial receptors. This sends signals to the medullary control centers to decrease the parasympathetic activity via the vagus nerve, leading to an increase in HR. [3]

## HORMONAL CONTROL

Common hormones controlling HR include thyroid hormones, growth hormone (GH), cortisol, and sex hormones. Hyperthyroidism increases the HR, resulting in tachycardia, while hypothyroidism decreases the HR, causing bradycardia. GH causes an increase in HR; hence acromegaly is associated with elevated HR, and GH deficiency causes decreased HR. Cortisol is a stress hormone, released during surgery, exercise, and other forms of stress. Cortisol increases the HR. Estradiol preferably induces the parasympathetic activity, while elevated testosterone levels increase HR. [1,3]

## LOCAL FACTORS

HR increases with inspiration and decreases with expiration. Thermoregulation affects HR variability. For every 1°C rise in temperature, the HR increases by 10 beats per minute. Cooling decreases the HR; hence it is used in most cardiac surgeries.[5]

## ANESTHETIC CONSIDERATIONS

- The HR can be estimated by palpation of the arterial pulse, most commonly the radial arterial pulsation; auscultation, usually at the apex of the heart; pulse oximeter; and the electrocardiogram (most commonly used in the operating room).

- Tachycardia >100 bpm in the operating room is common and can be associated with light anesthesia, pain, hypovolemia, inflammatory response, hypercarbia, hypoxia, and pulmonary embolus (Table 254.1). Rarely tachycardia can evolve into a severe rhythm in the absence of comorbidities. It should be managed with giving oxygen if hypoxic and performing continuous monitoring (electrocardiogram, blood pressure, oximeter, and capnography). Verify the presence of working intravenous access. If the patient has unstable signs, including altered mental status, hypotension, chest pain, or HR >150, perform synchronized cardioversion and consult cardiology if clinically indicated. If patient is stable, perform 12-lead electrocardiograph (EKG) and manage according to the morphology of the QRS complex (narrow vs. wide) and rhythm (regular vs. irregular).

- Bradycardia <60 bpm is also common under general anesthesia. Differential diagnosis includes bradycardia secondary to beta blocker taken before surgery. The stepwise approach to manage intraoperative bradycardia is as follows: Assess the surgical field for possible causes, such as occulocardiac reflex, stretching of carotid sinus, or traction on the omentum, and exclude physiological causes such as hypoxia and hypercarbia. Differential diagnosis for bradycardia is listed in Table 254.1. If the patient is unstable with severe hypotension or low ET $CO_2$, initiate CPR, deliver 100% fraction of inspired oxygen ($FiO_2$), secure airway and intubate if not intubated to assist with ventilation, administer fluid bolus, consider administering atropine and epinephrine bolus of 10–100 mcg if needed until trancutanous pacer is available. If the blood pressure is stable, and cardiac output is maintained with adequate perfusion, it is not indicated to treat bradycardia, and patient should be observed and cardiology consult may be considered.

- Esmolol is commonly used during emergence from anesthesia when patients have tachycardia and hypertension. Due to its short half-life of 9 minutes, it is ideal in the situation. An intravenous bolus can decrease HR, contractility, and occasionally blood pressure, improving the supply-to-demand ratio.

- Managing bradycardia in the heart transplant patient: The transplanted heart does not have baseline parasympathetic innervations, and hence the patients do not respond with increased contractility and tachycardia with hypovolemia and hypotension. It also does not respond to medication that works by blocking the parasympathetic system. Bradycardia is managed with drugs that act directly on the heart, such as isoproterenol, glucagon, epinephrine, and norepinephrine. Bradycardic reflex is also absent during carotid sinus massage, hypertension, and laryngoscopy.

*Table 254.1* DIFFERENTIAL DIAGNOSIS OF TACHYCARDIA AND BRADYCARDIA IN THE OPERATING ROOM

| HS | TS |
| --- | --- |
| - Hypoxia | - Tamponade |
| - Hypervagal | - Tension Pneumothorax |
| - Hypovolemia | - Trauma |
| - Hyperkalemia/Hypokalemia | - Thrombus—Pulmonary |
| - Hypothermia | - QT prolongation |
| - Hypoglycemia | - Toxins |
| - Malignant Hyperthermia | - Pulmonary HyperTension |

## REFERENCES

1. Cardiovascular physiology and anesthesia. In: Butterworth JF, et al., eds. *Morgan and Mikhail's Clinical Anesthesiology*. 6th ed. New York, NY: Lange Medical Books/McGraw Hill Medical; 2018:343–380.
2. Fatisson J, et al. Influence diagram of physiological and environmental factors affecting heart rate variability: An extended literature overview. *Heart Int*. 2016;11(1):e32–e40.
3. Sun LS, et al. Cardiac physiology. In: Miller RD, ed. *Miller's Anesthesia*. 8th ed. New York, NY: Elsevier/Churchill Livingstone; 2015:473–491.
4. Stauss HM. Heart rate variability. *Am J Physiol Regul Integr Comp Physiol*. 2003; 927–R931.
5. Levy MN, Martin PJ. Neural control of the heart. In: Sperelakis N, ed. *Physiology and Pathophysiology of the Heart: Developments in Cardiovascular Medicine*, vol 34. Boston, MA: Springer; 1984:337–354.

# 255.

# SYNCHRONICITY OF PRESSURE

*Muhammad Fayyaz Ahmed and Furqan Ahmed*

## INTRODUCTION

The cardiac physiology is largely dependent on the concept of pressure differences within the heart chamber and the major vessels. It consists of a sequential and synchronized series of electrical and mechanical events that takes place with every heartbeat. The events are characterized by phases of systole and diastole, which are further classified. Systole consists of isovolumetric contraction and ejection, whereas diastole consists of isovolumetric relaxation and ventricular filling. The contraction and relaxation cause a change in pressure in the chambers of heart which impacts valvular action. The trigger between these phases is a change in valvular action which is either valve opening or closing.[1,2]

## PRESSURE VOLUME LOOP

One way to represent pressure and volume relationship during a cardiac cycle is through the pressure volume loop.

The series of events are followed in a counterclockwise direction. Horizontal axis represents ventricular volume, whereas vertical axis represents left ventricular pressure. Depicted in Figure 255.1 are the events, which include valve action, volume, and pressure changes.

- Point A to B consists of the ventricular filling phase, which is the period between mitral valve opening and closing. During this phase the volume in the left ventricle increases, with minimal increase in the left ventricle pressure.
- Point B to C consists of the isovolumic contraction phase, which is the period between mitral valve closing and aortic valve opening. It consists of left ventricular contraction with no change in volume, thereby increasing pressure in the left ventricle until the opening of the aortic valve.
- Point C to D consists of the ejection phase, which is the period between aortic valve opening and closing. It consists of the ejection of a fraction of blood present in

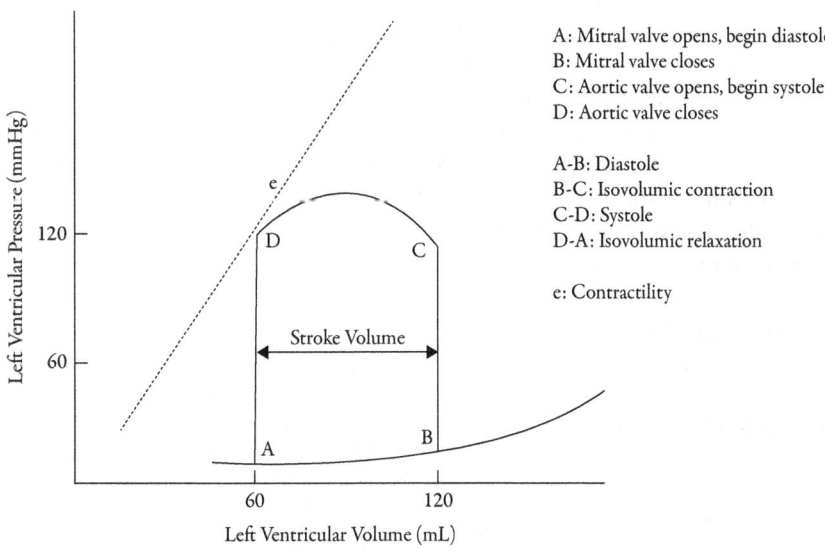

A: Mitral valve opens, begin diastole
B: Mitral valve closes
C: Aortic valve opens, begin systole
D: Aortic valve closes

A-B: Diastole
B-C: Isovolumic contraction
C-D: Systole
D-A: Isovolumic relaxation

e: Contractility

**Figure 255.1.** Pressure volume loop.
From: Loushin MK, et al. Mechanical aspects of cardiac performance. In: Iaizzo P, eds., *Handbook of Cardiac Anatomy, Physiology, and Devices.* Springer, Cham; 2015.

*Table 255.1* SUMMARY OF EVENTS DURING CARDIAC CYCLE

| | PHASE | SEMILUNAR VALVES | ATRIOVENTRICULAR VALVES | HEART SOUNDS | EKG* | RIGHT ATRIAL PRESSURE CURVE |
|---|---|---|---|---|---|---|
| 1 | Isovolumetric contraction | Closed | Closed | S1 | QRS | *c* |
| 2 | Ejection | Open | Closed | | | *x* |
| 3 | Isovolumetric relaxation | Closed | Closed | S2 | T | *v* |
| 4 | Ventricular filling | | | | | |
| 4a | Rapid filling | Closed | Open | S3** | | *y* |
| 4b | Reduced filling | Closed | Open | | | |
| 4c | Atrial systole | Closed | Open | S4** | P | *a* |

* = electrical events precede their respective phases
** = might be pathological.

the left ventricle, which is called the ejection fraction. The amount ejected is known as the stroke volume.
- Point D to A consists of the isovolumetric relaxation phase, which is the period between aortic valve closing and mitral valve opening. During this phase the volume does not change and the pressure in the left ventricle drops.[1,2]

## RIGHT ATRIAL PRESSURE CURVE

The right atrial pressure (RAP), or central venous pressure (CVP), can be measured using a catheter, and changes in it correspond to events in cardiac cycle. There are 3 peaks (*a*, *c*, *v*) and 2 descents (*x*, *y*). Peaks represent an increase in pressure, and descents represent a fall in pressure. The sequence of events is initiated with peak wave *a*, which represents atrial systole, followed by peak wave *c*, which occurs during isovolumetric contraction when a closed tricuspid valve bulges into the right atrium during. It is followed by descent *x*, which represents atrial relaxation during ejection phase. It moves to peak wave *v* by the filling of the right atrium against a closed tricuspid valve during the isovolumetric relaxation phase. It enters the last phase of descent *y*, which represents atrial evacuation into the ventricles during the ventricular filling phase.[1,2]

The described events are summarized in Table 255.1

## PRESSURES IN HEART CHAMBERS

Pressure differences between the chambers of the heart direct flow and valve action, and any changes can lead to

*Table 255.2* PRESSURE IN HEART CHAMBERS AND MAJOR VESSELS IN A HEALTHY INDIVIDUAL

| LOCATION | PRESSURE |
|---|---|
| Right atrium | <5 |
| Right ventricle | 25/5 |
| Pulmonary artery | 25/10 |
| PCWP | 4–12 |
| Left atrium | <12 |
| Left ventricle | 130/10 |
| Aorta | 130/90 |

PWCP = pulmonary capillary wedge pressure. Approximates left atrial pressure and can be measured directly using Swan-Ganz catheter.

Left ventricle: Coronary perfusion occurs only during diastole.

Right ventricle: Coronary perfusion occurs both during diastole and systole

pathologies. Table 255.2 depicts the pressures in the heart chambers in systole and diastole.[1,2]

## REFERENCES

1. Sun LS, et al. Cardiac physiology. In Miller RD, ed. *Miller's Anesthesia*. 8th ed. New York, NY: Elsevier/Churchill Livingstone; 2015: .
2. Cardiovascular physiology and anesthesia. In Butterworth IV JF, et al., eds. *Morgan & Mikhail's Clinical Anesthesiology*. 6th ed. McGraw-Hill; 2018:.
3. Loushin MK, et al. Mechanical aspects of cardiac performance. In: Iaizzo P, ed., *Handbook of Cardiac Anatomy, Physiology, and Devices*. Cham: Springer; 2015: .

# 256.

# IMPULSE PROPAGATION

*Nadeen Dakhlallah and Larry Manders*

## INTRODUCTION

The heart is a pump made up of muscle tissue. The heart's pumping capabilities are regulated by an electrical conduction system that coordinates contraction of the chambers of the heart. The main components of the heart's electrical conduction system are the sinoatrial (SA) node, atrioventricular (AV) node, bundle of His, bundle branches, and Purkinje fibers.

The SA node is considered the "anatomical pacemaker" of the heart, as it starts the sequence of impulses. It delivers an electrical gradient to the atria to facilitate contraction while subsequently sending a signal to the AV node, through the bundle of His, bundle branches, and Purkinje fibers.[1] An accumulation of these electrical impulses stimulates the ventricles to contract and push blood out to the rest of the body.

## ACTION POTENTIALS

Cardiac excitation involves a series of action potentials by individual cells and by communication of cells through intercellular gap junctions.[2] An action potential in non-pacemaker cardiac cells is characterized by an intracellular calcium gradient, followed by a fast inward flux of sodium ions, which depolarize the cellular membrane at a fast rate. When the sodium channels inactivate, the inward calcium current subsequently activates, which provides a depolarizing current. This depolarizing current supports the action potential plateau against the repolarizing action of the outward delayed potassium current.[3-4]

## SA NODE AND EXCITATION-CONTRACTION COUPLING

The SA node is a group of specialized pacemaker cells in the sulcus terminalis, located at the posterior junction of the right atrium and superior vena cava. The SA node generates action potentials that spread throughout the atria at a velocity of about 0.5 m/second.[3] The accumulation of action potentials throughout the cardiomyocytes depolarizes the atrial muscle, initiating contraction. This process is called excitation-contraction coupling.[3,5]

Excitation-contraction coupling is the process by which an action potential causes contraction and relaxation of a myocyte.[3] The steps of this process begin with an action potential traveling down the sarcolemma and into the transverse tubule system, depolarizing the cellular membrane. Voltage-sensitive dihydropyridine receptors open to allow calcium entry into the cell. This calcium influx triggers a release of calcium that is stored intracellularly. The calcium is stored in the sarcoplasmic reticulum and exits through ryanodine receptors. This free cytoplasmic calcium binds troponin, which induces a conformational change, exposing a site on the actin molecule that is able to bind to myosin ATPase.[3,5] This process supplies energy, allowing actin and myosin filaments to slide past one another, shortening sarcomere length. This process eventually slows and calcium is returned back into the sarcoplasmic reticulum by an ATP-dependent calcium pump, lowering calcium concentration in the cytoplasm and removing it from the troponin complex.[3,5] At the end of this cycle, a new ATP molecule binds the myosin head, and the length of the sarcomere is restored.

## STIMULATION FROM SA NODE THROUGH THE PURKINJE FIBERS

Once the SA node stimulates contraction of atrial muscle, the electrical signal reaches the AV node. The AV node is located in the posterior region of the interatrial septum. It consists of highly specialized cardiac tissue that slows the electrical propagation to about 0.05 m/sec. This slowing ensures that the heart has adequate time to complete atrial depolarization and contraction prior to stimulating the ventricles.[1]

The electrical impulses then travel through the bundle of His and through the left and right bundle branches along the interventricular septum. These specialized fibers conduct the electrical impulses at a fast rate of 2 m/sec. The bundle branches subsequently divide into an extensive system called the Purkinje fibers. The Purkinje fibers conduct impulses at a velocity of 4 m/sec throughout the ventricular tissue.[3] This system results in a rapid depolarization of ventricular myocytes throughout both ventricles.

## AUTONOMIC NERVOUS SYSTEM REGULATION

Impulse propagation in the heart is regulated by the autonomic nervous system. The influence of the autonomic nervous system is most evident at the AV node. Sympathetic stimulation increases conduction velocity at the AV node by increasing the rate of depolarization and action potentials propagation. Sympathetic stimulation also reduces the normal delay of action potential conduction through the AV node, reducing the time between atrial and ventricular contraction.[4] Sympathetic nerves release the neurotransmitter norepinephrine that binds to beta-receptors, leading to an increase in intracellular cAMP. Parasympathetic activation decreases the conduction velocity previously described. Acetylcholine binds to the muscarinic receptors in the heart, which decrease intracellular cAMP. This leads to slower depolarization of adjacent cells[1] (see Figure 256.1).

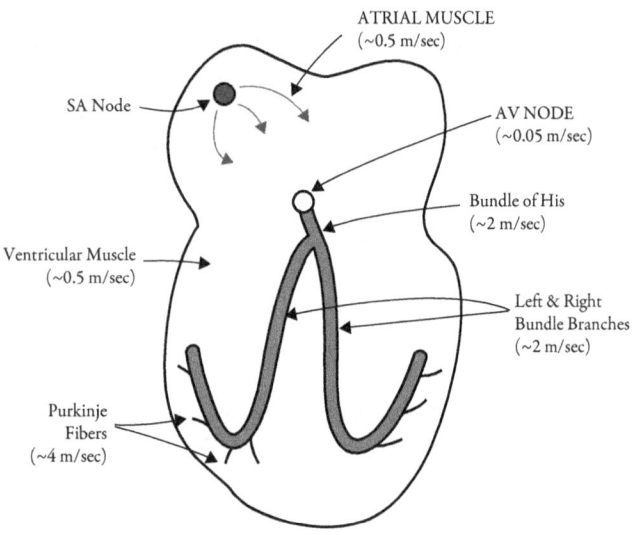

**Figure 256.1.** The cardiac conduction system for impulse propagation.

## ANESTHETIC CONSIDERATIONS

### PREOPERATIVE

Individuals with anatomical or functional disease of their SA or AV nodes may present with pacemakers in place. It is important to obtain a thorough history and physical and to understand why these devices are in place and what their underlying rhythm is. A chest X-ray can provide a great amount of insight, including whether the patient has a PPM or AICD in place and the position of the leads. It is important to have the device interrogated prior to the procedure to ensure it is functioning appropriately.

### INTRAOPERATIVE

Inhaled anesthetics are known for their cardio-depressant effects, most specifically their depression of SA node automaticity. Volatile agents have both antiarrhythmic and arrhythmogenic effects on the electrophysiological system. The antiarrhythmic effects may be secondary to depression of calcium influxes. The arrhythmogenic effects may be secondary to a potentiation of catecholamines with agents such as halothane. Opioids can decrease AV node conduction and subsequently slow impulse propagation down the Purkinje fibers. High blood concentrations of local anesthetics have been shown to depress electrical activity at the SA node and ventricular muscle.

### POSTOPERATIVE

Individuals with underlying electrophysiological disease require close monitoring of their rate and rhythm in the postoperative period. A postop electrocardiogram (EKG) may prove to be useful.

### REFERENCES

1. Podrid P. (2019). Enhanced cardiac automaticity. *UpToDate* [Online]. https://www.uptodate.com/contents/enhanced-cardiac-automaticity?search=purkinje%20fibers&usage_type=default&source=search_result&selectedTitle=1~36&display_rank=1#H123140. Accessed July 13, 2020.
2. Rice University. Cardiovascular system: Cardiac muscle and electrical activity. In *BC Open Textbook: Anatomy and Physiology*. 2013. Retrieved from https://opentextbc.ca/anatomyandphysiology/chapter/19-2-cardiac-muscle-and-electrical-activity/
3. Klabunde RE. Normal impulse conduction. 2008, December 13. Cvphysiology.com. https://www.cvphysiology.com/Cardiac%20Function/CF022. Accessed July 13, 2020.
4. Kléber AG, Rudy Y. Basic mechanisms of cardiac impulse propagation and associated arrhythmias. *Physiological Reviews*. 2004;84(2): 431–488.
5. Klabunde RE. Cardiac excitation-contraction coupling. 2008, December 13. Cvphysiology.com. https://www.cvphysiology.com/Cardiac%20Function/CF022. Accessed July 13, 2020.

# 257.

# NORMAL ECG AND ELECTROPHYSIOLOGY

*Nadeen Dakhlallah and Larry Manders*

## INTRODUCTION

The heart can be divided into a right and left pump, each consisting of an atrium and ventricle. The heart fills to eject blood to the rest of the body in a synchronized fashion. A series of electrical signals are generated that stimulate the muscle fibers of the heart to contract and relax, ensuring appropriate time for synchronous movement. An electrical potential (voltage) results in a directional flow (current) that can be quantified. This flow of current is large enough to be detected on the surface of the body as an electrocardiogram (ECG).

## NORMAL ECG

An ECG plots voltage on the vertical axis with time on the horizontal axis. Waves on an ECG graph are discussed in order of their occurrence (see Figure 257.1).

## P WAVE

This represents atrial depolarization. The right atrium depolarizes before the left atrium. The duration is normally less than 0.12 seconds, which can be quantified as 3 small boxes on ECG graph paper. The amplitude is less than 0.25 mv or 2.5 small boxes.[1]

## PR INTERVAL

This is measured from the beginning of the P wave to the first part of the QRS complex. It represents the time from atrial depolarization (P wave) to conduction through the AV node, bundle of His, and Purkinje fibers.[1-2] The duration is normally 0.12–0.20 seconds (3–5 small boxes), depending on sympathetic stimulation.[1] This interval can be decreased with high heart rates and increased with slow heart rates.

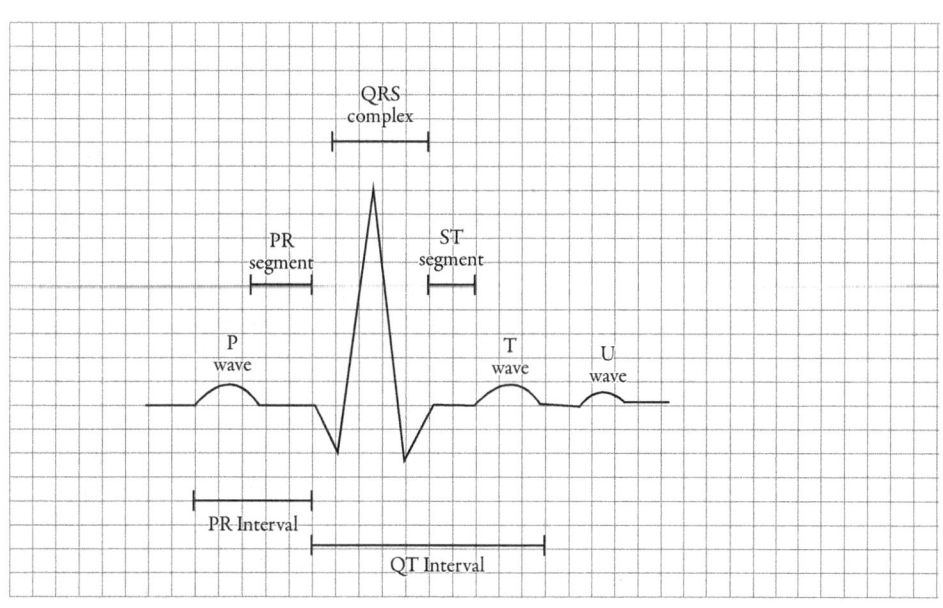

**Figure 257.1.** The normal electrocardiogram.

## QRS COMPLEX

This represents ventricular depolarization. The Q wave is a negative deflection on the ECG and is due to an initial septal depolarization. The next positive deflection is the R wave, which signifies depolarization of the left ventricle. Next, comes another negative deflection called the S wave.[1-2] This occurs secondary to terminal depolarization of the lateral wall. The duration of the QRS wave is 0.06 to 0.10 seconds (1.5 to 2.5 small boxes).[1] This complex is not influenced by heart rate.

## T WAVE

This represents ventricular repolarization. T waves have a slow, broad upstroke. This shape is because repolarization is slower than depolarization.[1]

## ECG AXIS

The normal ECG axis is between –30 and +90 degrees. Left axis deviation signifies QRS axis less than –30 degrees. Right axis deviation signifies QRS axis greater than +90 degrees.[1] Interpreting leads I, II, and aVF provides the easiest method of identifying ECG axis. A normal axis entails a QRS complex that is positive in leads I and II. A leftward axis entails a QRS complex that is positive in lead I but negative in lead II. A rightward axis entails a QRS complex that is negative in lead I but positive in aVF. Causes of a leftward axis include LVH, LBBB, and inferior wall myocardial infarction (MI). Causes of a rightward axis includes RVH, RBBB, left posterior fascicular block, and lateral wall MI.[1-2]

## ELECTROPHYSIOLOGY

All living cells have a resting membrane potential that is more negative intracellularly than extracellularly. The concentration of potassium inside the cell is higher than the concentration outside. On the contrary, the concentration of sodium, calcium, and chloride is higher outside the cell. This is made possible by a membrane bound $Na^+$-$K^+$ ATPase, which concentrates two K+ inside the cell, while pushing three $Na^+$ out.[2-3] When $K^+$ moves down its concentration gradient and out of the cell, a negative resting cell membrane potential is achieved. A normal ventricular cell has a resting membrane potential of –80 to –90 mV. In order to undergo depolarization, the cell membrane potential must become less negative and reach a threshold value of about +20 mV.[3]

## NON-PACEMAKER CARDIAC CELLS

An action potential in the non-pacemaker cardiac myocytes (atrial/ventricular cells, Purkinje conduction system) is

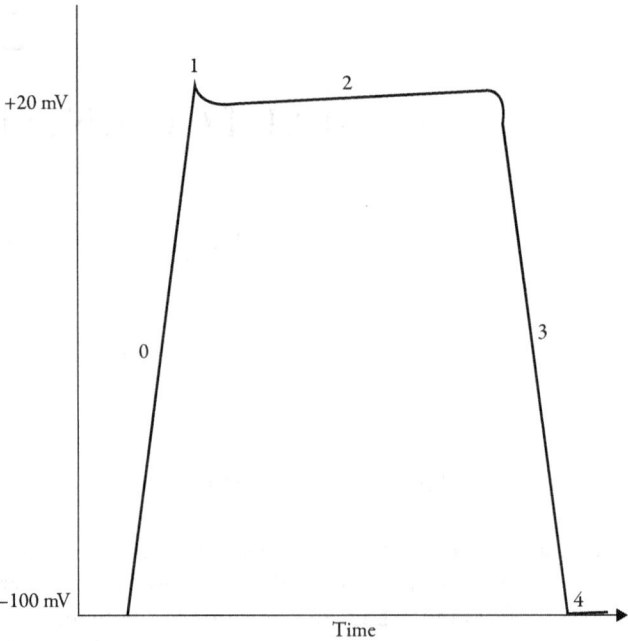

**Figure 257.2.** Non-pacemaker cardiac cell action potential.

achieved by the opening of voltage gated sodium channels, which allows $Na^+$ entry and decreased permeability to $K^+$ (phase 0, upstroke). The $Na^+$ channels are subsequently inactivated and followed by a transient increase in $K^+$ exiting the cell (phase 1, early rapid repolarization). Slow calcium channels are then activated which allow $Ca^{2+}$ entry (phase 2, plateau). Calcium channels are inactivated, and the cell develops increased permeability to $K^+$, allowing it to exit (phase 3, final repolarization).[3] The $Na^+$-$K^+$ ATPase pumps $K^+$ in and $Na^+$ out, restoring normal permeability and resting potential (phase 4, resting potential)[2] (see Figure 257.2).

## PACEMAKER CARDIAC CELLS

An action potential in the pacemaker cells of the heart (SA node, AV node) is different in the sense that they undergo spontaneous diastolic depolarization and have no true resting potential. Depolarization is initiated by voltage gated $Ca^{2+}$ channels rather than $Na^+$ channels (phase 0, upstroke). The slope of the upstroke is slower than in the non-pacemaker cells as there is a lack of $Na^+$ currents. Then, voltage gated $K^+$ channels open, increasing outward flow of $K^+$ (phase 3, repolarization).[3-5] Phase 4 is known as diastolic depolarization and accounts for the automaticity of the SA node to generate an action potential without neural input. Hyperpolarization-activated cyclic nucleotide gated channels are activated and allow intrinsic slow leakage of $Ca^{2+}$ into cells[3-4] (see Figure 257.3).

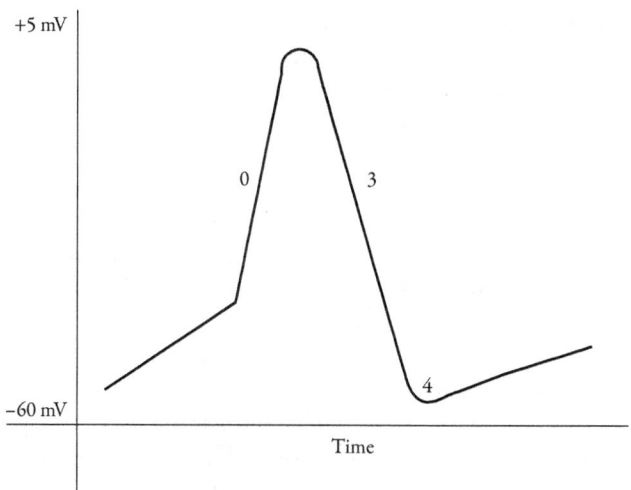
+5 mV

0     3

4

−60 mV

Time

**Figure 257.3.** Cardiac pacemaker cell action potential.

## ANESTHETIC CONSIDERATIONS

### PREOPERATIVE

The ACC/AHA guidelines recommend preoperative EKG in patients with at least one clinical risk factor undergoing vascular procedures. An EKG should also be obtained in individuals with coronary artery disease, peripheral artery disease, or other significant structural heart disease undergoing intermediate-risk procedures. A preop EKG has high utility when used for comparison postoperatively in a patient who has developed symptoms such as chest pain, palpitations, etc. The anesthesiologist should be skilled in interpreting an EKG, as abnormalities could warrant cancellation of an elective procedure or further work-up. Cancellation of an elective procedure is appropriate when an EKG demonstrates tall peaked T waves, acute ST segment elevation, new bundle branch block, or new acute axis deviation.

### INTRAOPERATIVE AND POSTOPERATIVE

An EKG is considered an ASA standard monitor. A peaked T wave is one of the first signs of ischemia. 75% of ischemic episodes can be detected by lead V5 alone, while lead V5 in addition to lead V4 will detect 90% of ischemic episodes. A combination of lead II, V4, and V5 increases the detection rate to 96%.

## REFERENCES

1. Prutkin J. ECG tutorial: Basic principles of ECG analysis. *UpToDate.* https://www.uptodate.com/contents/ecg-tutorial-basic-princip les-of-ecg-analysis?search=ekg&source=search_result&selectedTi tle=1~150&usage_type=default&display_rank=1. Published 2019. Accessed July 28, 2020.
2. Klabunde RE. Cardiac electrophysiology: Normal and ischemic ionic currents and the ECG. *Adv Physiol Educ.* 2017;41(1):29–37.
3. Jakoi E. Heart electrical activity. In: *Introductory Human Physiology.* www.lulu.com; 2015:1-5. https://web.duke.edu/histol ogy/MBS/Videos/Phys/Phys%204.1%20CV%20Heart%20Electri cal/Phys%204.1%20CV%20Heart%20Electrical%20NOTES.pdf
4. Klabunde R. Sinoatrial node action potentials. *CV Physiology.* https://www.cvphysiology.com/Arrhythmias/A004. Published 2008. Accessed July 13, 2020.
5. Feher J. Cardiac action potential. In: *Quantitative Human Physiology.* 2nd ed. Academic Press; 2017:528–536.

# 258.

# VENTRICULAR FUNCTION

*John Yousef and Larry Manders*

## INTRODUCTION

The heart consists of four chambers, two atria and two ventricles. The right side of the heart is a low-pressure system which, through the action of the right ventricle, pumps the blood incoming from the body and into the lungs. The left side of the heart is a high-pressure system that pumps oxygenated blood from the lungs and into the body. The average human has roughly 5 liters of intravascular blood volume which circulates through their body. Without the ventricles, especially the left, it would be impossible to transport oxygen and nutrients throughout the body.[1]

## STRUCTURE

Both the right and left ventricles consist of three layers—epicardium, myocardium, and endocardium, listed from outermost to innermost, respectively. The thickness of the ventricle, is primarily dependent on the myocardium. The left ventricular is thicker myocardium than the right, as it has to pump against a greater degree of afterload from the aorta and systemic vessels. Right ventricular pressures are approximately 75% lower due to the fact that the right ventricle only sees the afterload of the pulmonary system. Hypertrophy or increase muscle thickening beyond normal may occur in some disease states, just as systemic hypertension causes increase in muscle mass in the left ventricle and pulmonary hypertension on the right.[2-3]

On the inner portion of the ventricles, there are irregularities which are called trabeculae; they play a role in effective pumping via limiting the suction which is seen on flat surfaces, and also help prevent the inversion of the two atrial-ventricular valves (mitral and tricuspid valves). Another portion of the trabeculae, known as the moderator band, carries the right portion of the ventricular conduction system known as the bundle of His.[4]

Multiple valves exist within the heart to keep it functional and to prevent the mixing of oxygenated and deoxygenated blood. The valves are separated into three primary groups; atrioventricular valves, pulmonic valves, and aortic valves. Atrioventricular valves consist of the mitral and tricuspid valves, which are located between the left and right atria and ventricles, respectively. Pulmonic valves are located between the right ventricle and lungs, and aortic valves are located between the left ventricle and body. Over time, these valves may calcify, which can lead to stenosis or narrowing. If valves are damaged, symptoms such as difficulty breathing, chest pain, or edema in the lower extremities can arise due to inappropriate flow patterns.

## FUNCTION

As noted, the primary function of the ventricles is to receive blood via the atria and pump the received blood to either the lung or to the body. Pumping the blood is the phase of systole, and filling of the ventricles from the atria is in the phase of diastole. Each minute the human body has an average of 5 liters/minute pumping through the vessels, which is known as *cardiac output*. Cardiac output is dependent on stroke volume multiplied by heart rate. Stroke volume, the

amount of blood in one stroke, is roughly 70 milliliters in an average human, which can be calculated via an echocardiogram and by subtracting the blood at the end of each ventricular beat, known as the end-systolic volume.

Besides the cardiac output, stroke volume, and end-systolic volume, another important volume in cardiac function is the end-diastolic volume—the amount of blood left in the chamber at the end of filling, which is synonymous with preload. When there are higher end-diastolic volumes, there is a stroke amount of stroke volume due to increased sarcomere stretch in a mechanism known as the Frank-Starling mechanism.

The percent of blood which the left ventricle pumps is known as the ejection fraction (EF), and is commonly measured via echocardiography, magnetic resonance imaging (MRI), and cardiac catherization. Based on a 70-kg patient, the EF is formulated by dividing the stroke volume by the end-diastolic volume. The average EF is 55%–60%. Various pathologies can lead to elevated or decreased EFs. Elevated or even normal EFs are likely due to pathologies such as uncontrolled hypertension, leading to thickened left ventricular wall. Decreased EF is usually less than 50% and likely secondary to an ischemic event such as previous myocardial infarction. Patients with decreased EF can have a form of heart failure with reduced EF (HFrEF), in which a spectrum of symptoms can arise, with worsening symptoms as the EF reduces further. At an EF of 35%, there is worry that the patient's myocardium may become arrhythmogenic due to a lack of proper oxygen delivery, and it is recommended that the patient have placement of an implantable cardioverter-defibrillator (ICD), which provides electrical shock to change inappropriate rhythms such as ventricular tachycardia or fibrillation events.[2-4]

## ANESTHETIC CONSIDERATIONS

One of the primary considerations of ventricular function during anesthesia occurs during induction. A patient's heart rate and blood pressure may be extremely liable due to changes in intrathoracic pressure or decreased preloads with induction medications. Furthermore, should anatomic changes be present in the heart, such as ventricular hypertrophy or mitral stenosis, the ability to obtain and house appropriate preload may be reduced. These can cause catastrophic reduction in both systemic and myocardial prefusion and can be life-threatening.[3]

## REFERENCES

1. Stevenson WG, et al. Subcommittee on Electrocardiography and Arrhythmias of the American Heart Association Council on Clinical Cardiology. Heart Rhythm Society. Clinical assessment and management of patients with implanted

cardioverter-defibrillators presenting to nonelectrophysiologists. *Circulation*. 2004;110(25):3866–3869.

2. Van der Wall EE, Bax JJ. Different imaging approaches in the assessment of left ventricular dysfunction: All things equal? 2000; 1295–1297.

3. Olszowska M. Pathogenesis and pathophysiology of aortic valve stenosis in adults. *Polskie Archiwum Medycyny Wewnętrznej*. 2011;121(11).

4. Chapman BT. Left ventricular residual volume in the intact and denervated dog heart. *Circ Res*. 1965 Nov;17(5):379–385.

# 259.

# THE FRANK-STARLING LAW

*Youssef Daklallah and Larry Manders*

## INTRODUCTION

The Frank-Starling law is based on the relationship between the initial length of myocardial fibers and the force generated by myocardial contraction during systole. If myocardial fibers are first stretched and then stimulated to contract, the interaction between myosin and actin filaments is optimized. This stretching increases the number of cross bridges between the filaments, resulting in an increased force of contraction. Stretching also increases myocardial fibers' sensitivity to calcium, thus further increasing the force of contraction. Preload is the ventricular wall tension at the end of diastole and is approximated by end-diastolic volume or pressure. It is determined by blood volume, rhythm, and heart rate.[1-3] A patient's posture, pericardial pressure, intrathoracic pressure, and venous tone can affect the distribution of blood volume and therefore preload. The Frank-Starling law is the observation that increased preload increases cardiac output. Cardiac output is calculated as the product of heart rate and stroke volume. The three major factors that affect stroke volume are preload, afterload, and contractility.

The Frank-Starling curve (Figure 259.1) depicts the relationship between cardiac output and preload as long as afterload and contractility are held constant. In a normal heart (middle curve), a patient's cardiac output increases with increasing preload. Under states of increased contractility (top curve), like exercise or infusions of certain vasopressors, an increased cardiac output at any given preload can be seen when compared to normal circumstances. Conversely, in heart failure or cardiogenic shock, cardiac output will be

decreased at any given preload (bottom curve). In this setting, increasing preload can be detrimental and can result in significantly increased left ventricular end-diastolic pressure, leading to acute decompensation and pulmonary edema.[4] Notice the flatness of the heart failure curve depicting a decreased cardiac output response to increasing preload relative to a normal heart. The Frank-Starling curve has important clinical applications. For example, as seen in the figure, patients with the same left ventricular end-diastolic volume (points a, b, c) will have vastly different cardiac outputs depending on the level of cardiac contractility.[5]

## ANESTHETIC CONSIDERATIONS

According to the Frank-Starling law, reduced preload results in decreased contractility and lower cardiac output. This places patients at risk for hypotension. There are multiple causes of decreased preload in the preoperative, intraoperative and postoperative settings.

### PREOPERATIVE

In preoperative patients, reduced preload may be the result of absolute hypovolemia secondary to hemorrhage, diuresis, bowel prep, or long NPO (nil per os) times. In addition, a hemodynamically unstable patient may have relative hypovolemia secondary to abdominal compartment syndrome, pneumothorax, or cardiac tamponade. Finally, patients with congestive heart failure have a decreased response in cardiac output to preload changes, as depicted in Figure 259.1.[1-4]

When possible, identifying these factors and treating accordingly prior to entering the operating room can optimize patients for surgery. For example, administering a fluid bolus to a patient who has been NPO for 18 hours may improve preload, contractility, cardiac output, and decrease the severity of hypotension related to general anesthesia.

## INTRAOPERATIVE

In addition to unresolved preoperative causes of decreased preload, there are unique intraoperative events to consider. For example, abdominal insufflation of $CO_2$ in laparoscopic surgery can lead to compression of the inferior vena cava and decreased preload, thus resulting in decreased cardiac

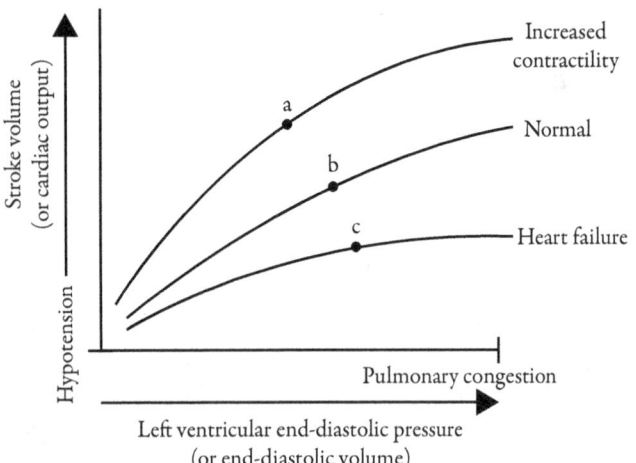

**Figure 259.1.** The Frank-Starling curve.

output and hypotension. Similarly, reverse Trendelenburg position, beach chair position, vasodilation secondary to general anesthesia, and sympathectomy due to neuraxial blockade may also reduce preload and contractility intraoperatively. Treating these events with fluid boluses, vasopressors, or changes in position may improve patients' position on the Frank-Starling curve.

## POSTOPERATIVE

In the postoperative setting, hypotension as a result of decreased preload may be due to numerous causes. These include but are not limited to occult bleeding, insufficient fluid management, or decreased venous tone. When managing a patient with postoperative hypotension, it is important to consider their position on the Frank-Starling curve (Figure 259.1) in order to help guide treatment options.

## REFERENCES

1. Butterworth JF, et al., eds. *Morgan & Mikhails Clinical Anesthesiology*. New York, NY: McGraw-Hill Education; 2018:353–355.
2. Delicce AV, Makaryus AN. Physiology, Frank Starling law. In: *StatPearls*. Treasure Island, FL: StatPearls; 2020.
3. Lilly LS. *Pathophysiology of Heart Disease: A Collaborative Project of Medical Students and Faculty*. 6th ed. Philadelphia, PA: Wolters Kluwer; 2016:222–224.
4. Sequeira V, van der Velden J. Historical perspective on heart function: The Frank-Starling law. *Biophys Rev*. 2015;7(4):421–447. doi:10.1007/s12551-015-0184-4
5. Sequeira V, van der Velden J. The Frank-Starling law: A jigsaw of titin proportions. *Biophys Rev*. 2017;9(3):259–267. doi:10.1007/s12551-017-0272-8

# 260.

# FORCE, VELOCITY, LENGTH, RATE OF SHORTENING

*Youssef Daklallah and Larry Manders*

## INTRODUCTION

Understanding cardiac performance is dependent on understanding myocardial contractility and inotropy. The

concept of inotropy is multifaceted. It is defined as the force of a cardiac muscle's contraction. Inotropy can be affected by multiple variables and disease processes that are relevant to any patient receiving an anesthetic. In this chapter we will define and discuss the relationships between the force of contraction, sarcomere length, velocity, and the rate of shortening.[1,2]

The development of myocardial contractile force is reliant on the calcium ion concentration in the myocyte cytoplasm, sarcomere length, velocity of sarcomere shortening, and the number of actin-myosin cross bridges. Multiple studies on cardiac muscle fibers have demonstrated links between length, force, and velocity. The Frank-Starling law observes changes in the force of myocardial contraction in response to changes in preload.[3] The force generated by myocardial contraction is dependent on the initial length of myocardial fibers. As stated in the previous chapter, the interaction between myosin and actin filaments is optimized by stretching. This increases the number of cross bridges between these filaments and therefore increases the force of contraction. The end result is that increased preload will increase the length of the sarcomeres and improve inotropy in the normal heart.

Myocardial fiber shortening velocity is defined as the speed of muscle contraction over time. The force of muscle contraction is inversely related to the shortening velocity. Intuitively this should make sense, as one can lift a feather at a much faster speed than a 50-pound object, which requires more force.[4] Otherwise stated, there is an inverse relationship between muscle tension and the rate of shortening of muscle fibers. This concept is known as the force-velocity relationship. Physiologically, as velocity of a muscle contraction decreases, more actin-myosin cross bridges have time to attach and generate an increased force. This is relevant to the anesthesia provider, as an increase in afterload will decrease the shortening velocity of myocardial fibers, which may decrease cardiac output.

## ANESTHETIC CONSIDERATIONS

A patient's cardiac output is dependent on the product of heart rate and stroke volume. Stroke volume depends on preload, afterload, and contractility. These factors are reliant on the physiologic function of sarcomeres. The relationship between the force of contraction, velocity, and length can be considered when administering any anesthetic.[5] As discussed earlier, any factor that changes a patient's preload or afterload will affect the relationship between force, velocity, and sarcomere length. Perioperatively, many pharmacologic, physiologic, and anatomic factors can play a role in this process. For example, a patient undergoing a liver transplant becomes hypotensive after suffering from massive blood loss. After transfusing 10 units of blood products, the patient is still hypotensive. Arterial blood gas results reveal that the patient is hypocalcemic, and after administering intravenous (IV) calcium the patient becomes normotensive. In this case, the patient initially suffered from decreased preload, causing a decreased length of sarcomeres and therefore a lower contractility. After transfusion of multiple blood products, calcium was chelated by citrate and inotropy was decreased. If hypocalcemia went unnoticed and the patient was given phenylephrine, afterload would be increased. In addition to the reflexive bradycardia seen with phenylephrine, this would decrease the rate of shortening (or velocity) of myocardial fibers and further decrease the patient's cardiac output.

## REFERENCES

1. de Tombe PP, ter Keurs HE. The velocity of cardiac sarcomere shortening: Mechanisms and implications. *J Muscle Res Cell Motil.* 2012;33(6):431–437. doi:10.1007/s10974-012-9310-0
2. Kobirumaki-Shimozawa F, et al. Cardiac thin filament regulation and the Frank-Starling mechanism. *J Physiol Sci.* 2014;64(4):221–232. doi:10.1007/s12576-014-0314-y
3. Muir WW, Hamlin RL. Myocardial contractility: Historical and contemporary considerations. *Front Physiol.* 2020;11:222. doi:10.3389/fphys.2020.00222
4. Sequeira V, van der Velden J. Historical perspective on heart function: The Frank-Starling law. *Biophys Rev.* 2015;7(4):421–447. doi:10.1007/s12551-015-0184-4
5. ter Keurs HE, de Tombe PP. Determinants of velocity of sarcomere shortening in mammalian myocardium. *Adv Exp Med Biol.* 1993;332:649–665. doi:10.1007/978-1-4615-2872-2_58

# 261.

# MYOCARDIAL CONTRACTILITY

*Daniel Tobes and Larry Manders*

## INTRODUCTION

Myocardial contractility represents the ventricles' ability to contract and eject blood. Although one technical definition is the "tension developed and velocity of shortening (i.e. the 'strength' of contraction) of myocardial fibers at a given preload and afterload," it is most easily thought of as the "squeeze" of the heart. It is one of the key contributors to EF (ejection fraction). There are two ways in which to modify contractility: in a length-dependent (increased preload) or length-independent fashion (inotropy).[1] This is in contrast to skeletal muscle, which can be altered by motor nerve activity. In short, contractility is dependent on the binding of myosin to actin, which is directly impacted by the myocardial intracellular $Ca^{2+}$ concentration.[1]

## STEPWISE APPROACH TO A MYOCARDIAL CONTRACTION

1. An action potential travels from the sinoatrial (SA) and atrioventricular (AV) nodes to the cardiomyocytes.[1]
2. This action potential activates $Ca^{2+}$ channels in the T-tubules, which leads to movement of $Ca^{2+}$ into the cell.
3. This $Ca^{2+}$ binds troponin-C on actin filaments, which reconfigures these filaments and exposes the myosin-binding site.
4. Myosin heads are now free to bind actin. This binding leads to adenosine triphosphate (ATP) hydrolysis, providing the energy for a conformational change (the "power stroke") in the myosin that acts to pull the actin filaments toward each other in the middle of the sarcomere. This is the muscle contraction.
5. After contraction, $Ca^{2+}$ exits the cell into the sarcoplasmic reticulum. This lower intracellular $Ca^{2+}$ concentration leads to unbinding of troponin-C, which then moves to cover the myosin-binding sites on actin, thereby ceasing contraction.

## INOTROPY

The concept of *inotropy* describes changes in cardiac contractility that occur in a length-independent manner. An increase in inotropy corresponds with an increased maximum velocity of fiber shortening, which leads to an increase in dP/dt during isovolumetric contraction.[2] Ultimately, the result of increased inotropy—with fixed preload and afterload—is a decrease in end-systolic volume and an increase in stroke volume.

## $CA^{2+}$ DEPENDENCE

Much of what impacts inotropy is the intracellular concentration of $Ca^{2+}$. After an action potential depolarizes the myocardial cell membrane, voltage-gated $Ca^{2+}$ channels (L-type) open to allow $Ca^{2+}$ into the cell. Myocardial cells utilize calcium-induced calcium release (CIRC) whereby this initial influx of $Ca^{2+}$ activates ryanodine receptors, leading to additional release of $Ca^{2+}$ from the sarcoplasmic

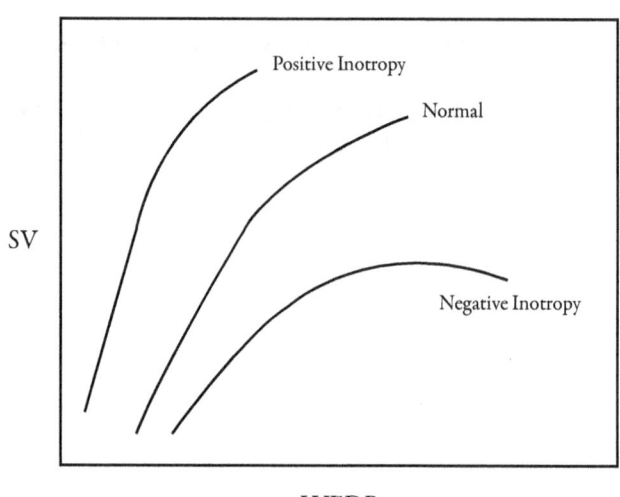

Figure 261.1. Relationship of inotropy on stroke volume and left ventricular end-diastolic volume.

reticulum (SR) into the cytoplasm. This massive increase in intracellular $Ca^{2+}$ is what allows activation of the actinomyosin complex.[2-4]

## GRAPHIC REPRESENTATIONS

Changes in inotropy shift the Frank-Starling curve. A decrease in inotropy shifts the Frank-Starling curve downward, corresponding to a decrease in stroke volume (SV) and an increase in left ventricular end-diastolic pressure (LVEDP) and volume (LVEDV).[2] An increase in entropy has equal, but opposite effects on SV and LVEDP (see Figure 261.1). Similarly, changes in inotropy lead to changes in ventricular pressure-volume loops. An increase in inotropy, leading to an increase in SV and a resultant decrease in LVEDP (and LVEDV), results in a left-shifted and widened loop. The dotted line at the end of systole represents the end-systolic pressure-volume relationship; this is utilized as a moniker for inotropy (see Figure 261.2).[2,4]

## ANESTHETIC CONSIDERATIONS

### BETA-1 RECEPTOR

Myocardium is flush with beta-1 adrenoceptors.[2] The activation of these receptors serves to increase contractility through multiple mechanisms. These receptors, which are coupled to Gs-proteins, activate adenylyl cyclase to make cAMP. This cAMP then serves to activate cAMP-dependent protein kinase A (PK-A), which activates the L-type $Ca^{2+}$, facilitating $Ca^{2+}$ influx into the cell. PK-A also serves to phosphorylate a protein on the SR, leading to increased $Ca^{2+}$ release from the SR through the ryanodine receipts. These increases in intracellular $Ca^{2+}$ cause an increase in inotropy.

### CARDIAC GLYCOSIDES

Digitalis inhibits $Na^+/K^+$-ATPase on the cardiac sarcolemma.[2] The resultant increase in intracellular $Na^+$ concentration leads to an increase in intracellular $Ca^{2+}$ by reducing the activity of the $Na^+/Ca^{2+}$ exchanger. This increase in intracellular $Ca^{2+}$ causes an increase in inotropy.

### PHOSPHODIESTERASE INHIBITORS (PDEI)

PDEi inhibit the breakdown of cAMP.[2] As described previously, an increase in cAMP concentration leads to an increase in $Ca^{2+}$ intracellularly. This increase in intracellular $Ca^{2+}$ causes an increase in inotropy.

### CALCIUM-SENSITIZING DRUGS

A newer class of drugs (e.g., Levosimendan) lead to an increase in troponin-C sensitivity to $Ca^{2+}$.[5] This causes more $Ca^{2+}$ to bind to troponin-C. This ultimately leads to increase inotropy.

## REFERENCES

1. Klabunde RE. *Myocardial Oxygen Demand.* Cardiovascular Physiology Concepts. https://cvphysiology.com/CAD/CAD003. Published April 2, 2007. Accessed July 12, 2020.
2. Kaplan JA, et al. Cardiac physiology. In: Pagel PS, Freed JK, eds. *Kaplan's Cardiac Anesthesia: For Cardiac and Noncardiac Surgery.* 7th ed. Philadelphia, PA: Elsevier; 2017:143–178.
3. Barash PG, et al. Cardiac anatomy and physiology. In: Pagel PS, Stowe DF, eds. *Clinical Anesthesia.* 8th ed. Philadelphia, PA: Lippincott Williams & Wilkins; 2017:277 300.
4. Muir WW, Hamlin RL. Myocardial contractility: Historical and contemporary considerations. *Front Physiol.* 2020;11: .
5. Nieminen MS, et al. Levosimendan: Current data, clinical use and future development. *Heart Lung Vessel.* 2013;5(4): 227–245.

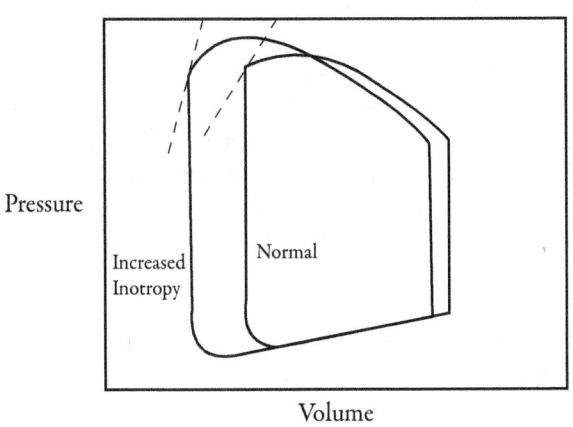

**Figure 261.2.** Intracardiac pressure volume loop.

# 262.

# MYOCARDIAL OXYGEN UTILIZATION/CONSUMPTION

*Daniel Tobes and Larry Manders*

## INTRODUCTION

Myocardial $O_2$ supply and demand exist at all times in a fragile balance. Situations where demand exceeds supply lead to myocardial ischemia. The heart has a relatively high $O_2$ consumption ($MVO_2$) compared with other organs due to its workload. $MVO_2$ can vary greatly based on the current workload of the heart; $MVO_2$ during heavy exercise exceeds that of any other organ in the body.

## $MVO_2$ IN RELATION TO BLOOD FLOW

The Fick principle (or equation) is able to relate $MVO_2$ to coronary blood flow (CBF) and the arterial blood oxygen content ($CaO_2$) and venous $O_2$ ($CvO_2$) content difference.[1,2]

$$CaO_2 = (Hb \times 1.39)(SaO_2) + (PaO_2)(0.003)$$

- Hb: hemoglobin
- $SaO_2$: oxygen saturation
- $PaO_2$: dissolved oxygen

$$CBF \propto (AoDBP - LVEDP)/R$$

- AoDBP: aortic diastolic blood pressure
- LVEDP: left ventricular end diastolic pressure
- R: total coronary resistance

$$MVO_2 = CBF \times (CaO_2 - CvO_2)$$

The equation can also be portrayed as

$$MVO_2 = (CBF \times CaO_2) - (CBF \times CvO_2)$$

to exhibit the difference between $O_2$ supply/delivery (CBF × $CaO_2$) and unused $O_2$ leaving the coronary vessels (CBF × $CvO_2$).[2] The Fick equation can accurately calculate a patient's $MVO_2$, but to obtain proper $CvO_2$ and CBF the patient must undergo a heart catheterization, which is not always practical. Parasympathetic stimulation causes direct coronary vasodilation, while sympathetically medicated coronary vasodilation results from increased myocardial oxygen consumption with production of local metabolites (that causes vasodilation).

## DETERMINANTS OF $MVO_2$

The overall main determinant of $MVO_2$ is myocyte activity. Therefore, to more thoroughly investigate we must decipher the determinants of myocyte activity: the tension they must overcome, the rate of development of said tension, and the rate at which this tension cycles. In short, these three factors are ventricular wall tension, inotropy, and heart rate.

## AFTERLOAD AND LAW OF LAPLACE (I.E., VENTRICULAR WALL TENSION)

Afterload, briefly defined as the "load the left ventricle (LV) must work against," is very difficult to properly imagine and measure in vivo. There are many complicated methods and formulas that are used to quantify or signify afterload, many of which are beyond the scope of this text. That being said, afterload is frequently thought of as the pressure in the proximal aorta and aortic root.[3] When discussing afterload for individual myocytes, the concept of wall tension ($\sigma$) must be addressed. The Law of Laplace relates wall tension or stress to ventricular pressure ($p$), ventricular radius ($r$), and ventricular wall thickness ($h$).

$$\sigma = pr / 2h$$

Increased wall tension leads to increased myocardial $O_2$ consumption.[3] Increased wall tension causes increased myocardial $O_2$ consumption because it increases the amount of work each myocyte has to perform. Increased chronic LV pressure (e.g., severe AS or chronic hypertension) leads to increased wall tension causing increased myocardial $O_2$ consumption. LV dilation, as seen in chronic AI or MR, leads to increased wall tension (and myocardial $O_2$ consumption) not only by an increase in LV radius, but also due to decreased wall thickness.

This concept also explains the development of hypertrophy. Concentric hypertrophy of the LV (increasing the ventricular wall thickness, $h$) is a vital compensatory mechanism to combat the increased LV wall tension from increased LV pressure. This increase in LV myocardial mass can predispose patients to ischemia due to increased $MVO_2$ because there are now more myocytes.

An increase in ventricular volume (as evidenced by an increase in SV or LVEDV) has a far lesser impact on wall tension than does an increase in radius. This has to do with the geometric relationship between volume and radius of spherical-like structures.

## INOTROPY

An increase in inotropy equates to an increase in the rate of development of the ventricular wall tension. This increased rate requires more adenosine triphosphate (ATP) hydrolysis and subsequently increased $O_2$ consumption by the myocytes. About 90% of myocardial $O_2$ consumption is for contractility, and the remaining 10% is used for maintaining cellular integrity and electrical activity.

## HEART RATE

Heart rate is directly proportional to $MVO_2$. A doubling of the heart will approximately double the $MVO_2$ because the myocytes will have to perform approximately double the amount of work in the same time they had previously.

## ANESTHETIC IMPLICATIONS

### CORONARY ARTERY DISEASE PATIENTS

One of the goals of care for patients with coronary artery disease (CAD) or having acute anginas symptoms is the reduction of $MVO_2$, as this will help to balance myocardial oxygen supply and demand/consumption, thereby decreasing existing ischemia or the risk of developing ischemia.[4,5] Effective methods of decreasing $MVO_2$ include a reduction in afterload, heart rate, or inotropy. Beta blockers accomplish all three of these goals, thus they are a mainstay of CAD treatment.

## REFERENCES

1. Klabunde RE. *Myocardial Oxygen Demand.* Cardiovascular Physiology Concepts. https://cvphysiology.com/CAD/CAD003. Published April 2, 2007.
2. Kaplan JA, et al. Cardiac physiology. In: Pagel PS, Freed JK, eds. *Kaplan's Cardiac Anesthesia: For Cardiac and Noncardiac Surgery.* 7th ed.). Philadelphia, PA: Elsevier; 2017:143–178.
3. Barash PG, et al. Cardiac anatomy and physiology. In: Pagel PS, Stowe DF, eds. *Clinical Anesthesia.* 8th ed. Philadelphia, PA: Lippincott Williams & Wilkins; 2017:277–300.
4. Rehman S, et al. Physiology, coronary circulation. *StatPearls* [Internet]. 2020. https://www.ncbi.nlm.nih.gov/books/NBK482413/.
5. Ramanathan T, Skinner H. Coronary blood flow. *Cont Educ Anaesth Crit Care Pain.* 2005;5(2):61–64.

# 263.

# SYSTOLIC AND DIASTOLIC FUNCTION

*Neal Al-Attar and Larry Manders*

## INTRODUCTION

In order to appropriately analyze systolic and diastolic function, it is important to understand the pressure-volume loop. End-diastole begins the cardiac cycle and is designated as point 1 on the graph. At this point, the mitral valve closes, and what follows is isovolumetric contraction. Once the left ventricle (LV) pressure is greater than the aortic pressure, the aortic valve opens at point 2, causing ejection of blood out of the LV and subsequent decreased volume.[1-3] When LV pressure is less than aortic pressure, the aortic valve closes (point 3). The mitral valve opens at a point during isovolumetric relaxation when LV pressure is less than left atrium (LA) pressure (point 4), allowing LV filling for the rest of diastole.[1]

Systolic function is determined by the amount of blood present prior to ventricular contraction (preload), the resistance of the downstream arterial tree that must be overcome by the LV ejection (afterload), and the force of contraction by the myocardial cells (contractility/inotropy).[1-3] These three variables determine how much blood volume is ejected from the LV in one cardiac cycle (stroke volume).

## PRELOAD

Preload is dependent on venous return, which is governed by venodilation or venoconstriction and fluid/blood loss. Although measuring the pre-contraction length of the myocyte sarcomere can most accurately determine LV preload, it is impractical to measure in vivo. Therefore, end-diastolic volume is most often used as a surrogate marker as it corresponds to pre-contraction lengthening of the sarcomeres.

## AFTERLOAD

Afterload is determined by size and compliance of arterial vessels, arteriolar tone, LV end-systolic wall stress, and the properties of blood as a hydraulic fluid. It is important to note that a major difference in measuring right ventricle (RV) versus LV afterload is the higher compliance of the RV compared to the LV, meaning that RV afterload is subject to greater variability compared to LV afterload. The most accurate way of calculating afterload is by measuring aortic input impedance, which is the continuous aortic pressure divided by the blood flow.[1] A higher impedance corresponds to a greater afterload. This method is not the most practical, however. Instead, the most clinically used estimate of LV afterload is calculating systemic vascular resistance (SVR), as defined in the following equation.[1]

$$SVR = \left[ \frac{(\text{Mean Arterial Pressure} - \text{Right Atrial Pressure})}{* \, 80 \, \text{dynes*sec*cm}^{-5} / \text{mmHg*min}^{-1} \text{*L}^1} \right]$$

## CARDIAC OUTPUT

Although terminal arteriolar resistance is a major factor of afterload, it does leave out the other three variables and therefore should not be used as a quantitative index, but more as an assessment of changes after vasoactive intervention.[1]

## CONTRACTILITY

The most commonly used estimation of LV contractility is by assessing LV ejection fraction (EF).[1-3] In the operating room, a quick method of EF assessment includes the fractional shortening and fractional area change (FAC). The examiner uses the midpapillary short axis to measure the diameter and area, respectively, at end-systole and end-diastole.[1]

## DIASTOLIC FUNCTION

Many of the anesthetics that we use today affect the LV's ability to relax and fill. Diastole is divided into four stages:

isovolumetric relaxation, early rapid filling, late slow filling, and atrial contraction.[4]

Isovolumetric relaxation is measured by the rate at which LV pressure declines over time.[1] Isovolumetric relaxation and early rapid filling are energy-dependent processes that involve the reuptake of cytosolic calcium back into the sarcoplasmic reticulum. This enables uncoupling of actin and myosin, resulting in a rapid decline in intracavity pressure and augments filling.[4] This early phase is often referred to as "LV suction."[4] This mechanism explains why patients with myocardial ischemia can be subject to increased LV filling pressures.[4,5]

Late slow filling is more a function of ventricular compliance.[4] It can be measured invasively or noninvasively by assessing changes in LV volume over time. Poorer ventricular filling due to decreased ventricular compliance will reflect as an increased end-diastolic pressure-volume relationship (EDPVR) slope on the pressure-volume loop. Stated simply, the slope of the EDPVR is the reciprocal of ventricular compliance. The duration between end-systole and mitral valve opening is called isometric volume relaxation time (IVRT). Using Doppler echocardiography, this variable is used in conjunction with the transmitral flow velocity pattern to assess LV relaxation.[1] The transmitral blood flow velocity has two peaks, an early "E" peak that represents LV filling, and a late "A" peak representing atrial contraction. Aging results in a less compliant heart, slowing of LV relaxation (E wave deceleration), and increasing A wave velocity, as this heart is more reliant on atrial contraction.[1,2]

## ANESTHETIC CONSIDERATIONS

### PREOPERATIVE

Patients with elevated LV afterload will compensate by increasing LV wall thickness, resulting in LV hypertrophy. However, this causes increased myocardial oxygen consumption, making patients more susceptible to myocardial ischemia. Therefore, afterload reduction in patients with heart failure is key to avoiding ischemic sequelae.[1]

### INTRAOPERATIVE

Special consideration should be taken when assessing EF via fractional shortening method in patients with mitral regurgitation, as measurement may reveal a falsely high EF because some of the blood flow is diverted upstream to the left atrium. LV relaxation is more dependent on afterload in the failing heart. Therefore, afterload reduction enhances LV relaxation time and improves ventricular filling.[1]

### POSTOPERATIVE

Evidence of ischemia should be assessed in these patients postoperatively. If there is any suspicion of ischemia (such as chest pain, arrhythmias, ST elevations/depressions, T wave inversions), a full cardiac workup should be completed. This includes ordering a 12-lead electrocardiogram (ECG) and serum troponins, in addition to routine labs.

## REFERENCES

1. Pagel P, Stowe D. Cardiac anatomy and physiology. In: Barash PG, ed. *Clinical Anesthesia*. Philadephia, PA: Wolters Kluwer; 2017:277–298.
2. Butterworth JF, et al. Cardiovascular physiology and anesthesia. In: *Morgan & Mikhail's Clinical Anesthesiology*. New York, NY: McGraw-Hill Education; 2018:343–379.
3. Feiner J. Clinical cardiac and pulmonary physiology. In Pardo MC, ed. *Basics of Anesthesia*. 7th ed. Philadelphia, PA: Elsevier; 2018:53–68.
4. Godfrey G, et al. Diastolic dysfunction in anaesthesia and critical care. *BJA Education*. 2016 Sep;16(9):287–291. https://doi.org/10.1093/bjaed/mkw007
5. Groban L, Kitzman D. Diastolic function: A barometer for cardiovascular risk? *Anesthesiology*. 2010;112(6):1303–1306.

# 264.

# CARDIAC OUTPUT

## FICK'S PRINCIPLE

*Jacqueline Sohn and Nicholas Pesa*

## INTRODUCTION

Cardiac output (CO) is defined as a volume of blood ejected by the heart per unit of time. It is calculated by multiplying stroke volume (SV) and heart rate (HR) (Equation 1). There are four factors that affect cardiac output: two intrinsic and two extrinsic factors to the heart. The intrinsic factors are heart rate and myocardial contractility, while the extrinsic factors are preload and afterload.[1] The heart rate is modulated by the autonomic nervous system through the spontaneous depolarization of the pacemaker cells in the sinoatrial (SA) node.[1,2]

$$CO = SV * HR$$

Eq. 1: CO: cardiac output (mL/min); SV: stroke volume (mL); HR: heart rate (beats/min).

The contractility (inotropism) refers to the myocardial cells' ability to shorten and generate force. It correlates with the changes in intracellular calcium concentration, and there are positive or negative inotropic agents that can either increase or decrease contractility.[1,2]

The preload is typically referred to as the left ventricular end-diastolic volume, which is the amount of blood in the left ventricle at the end of diastole before contraction.[1] This is dependent on the volume returned to the heart (venous return). Preload affects cardiac output, because the venous filling pressure affects stretching of the cardiac muscle fibers.[2] The Frank-Starling relationship describes the relationship between preload and contractility. It states that as the end-diastolic volume increases, the stroke volume ejected from the left ventricle also increases. This is a linear relationship until it reaches a critically high end-diastolic volume ($V_{max}$), where it does not increase anymore, because the myocardial muscle cells are stretched too far apart.

The afterload is typically thought of as aortic blood pressure, but it should actually be considered as the tension or stress on the ventricular wall during contraction. In other words, the afterload is the force that the left ventricle has to eject against.

## FICK'S PRINCIPLE

Cardiac output (CO) can be measured and calculated by using Fick's principle. Fick's principle is based on the idea of conservation of mass. In a steady state, the amount of oxygen returning back to the lungs through the pulmonary artery ($q_1$) and the rate of oxygen consumption ($q_2$) should be equal to the amount of oxygen leaving the lungs through the pulmonary vein ($q_3$) (Equation 2) (Figure 264.1).[1]

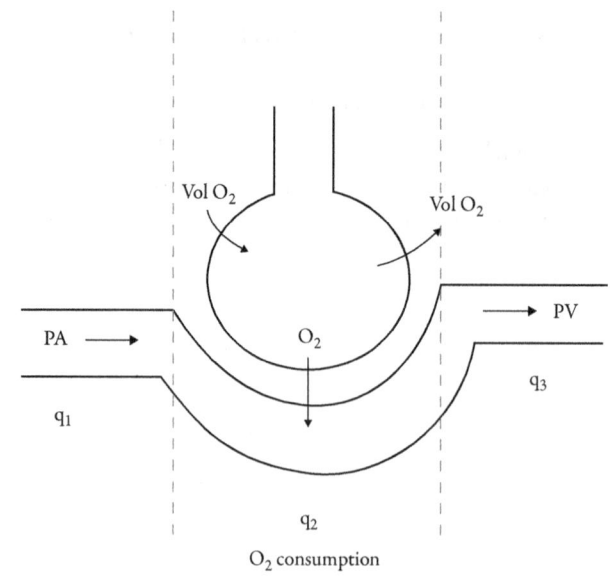

**Figure 264.1.** Fick's Principle is based on the conservation of the mass. In a steady state, the amount of oxygen through the pulmonary vein ($q_3$) should be equal to the sum of the amount of oxygen through the pulmonary artery ($q_1$) and the oxygen consumption ($q_2$). PA: pulmonary artery, PV: pulmonary vein.
Modified from Sun LS, Davis NA. Cardiac physiology. In: *Miller's Anesthesia*. 9th ed. Philadelphia, PA: Elsevier; 2020:384–404.

These variables depend on the blood flow (Q) to the area. Therefore, the amount of oxygen delivered to the pulmonary artery ($q_1$) is equal to the blood flow multiplied by the oxygen content in the pulmonary artery (Equation 3).[1] Likewise, the amount of oxygen leaving the pulmonary vein is equal to the blood flow multiplied by the oxygen content in the pulmonary vein (Equation 4).[1]

$$q_1 + q_2 = q_3$$

Eq. 2: $q_1$: the amount of oxygen returning back to the lungs through the pulmonary artery; $q_2$: the rate of oxygen consumption; $q_3$: the amount of oxygen leaving the lungs through the pulmonary vein.

$$q_1 = Q \times CaO_2$$

Eq. 3: $q_1$: the amount of oxygen returning back to the lungs through the pulmonary artery; Q: blood flow (cardiac output); $CaO_2$: oxygen content in the pulmonary artery.

$$q_3 = Q \times CvO_2$$

Eq. 4: $q_3$: the amount of oxygen leaving the lungs through the pulmonary vein; Q: blood flow (cardiac output); $CvO_2$: oxygen content in the pulmonary vein.

The oxygen consumption ($VO_2 = q_2$) can be thought of as the difference between the inspired and expired $O_2$ per unit time. This is accurately measured in a controlled setting using a water-sealed spirometer during exercise. However, in a clinical setting, it is typically assumed that the $O_2$ consumption at rest is 125 ml $O_2$/min per square meter of body surface area. This is an estimation, and it is important to note that there are variabilities depending on the person's age, gender, and physiological state. Thus, Equation 3 can be rearranged as follows: the rate of oxygen consumption ($VO_2$) is equal to the blood flow multiplied by the difference between the amount of oxygen leaving the lungs (pulmonary vein) and the amount of oxygen returning back to the lungs (pulmonary artery).[1,3]

$$VO_2 = Q \times (CaO_2 - CvO_2)$$

Eq. 5 (Fick's equation): $VO_2$: oxygen consumption (ml $O_2$/min); Q: blood flow, which is the cardiac output (L/min); $CaO_2$: oxygen content in pulmonary vein (oxygenated blood; ml $O_2$/100mL blood); $CvO_2$: oxygen content in pulmonary artery (deoxygenated blood; ml $O_2$/100mL blood).

The oxygen content of pulmonary artery, $CvO_2$, which represents deoxygenated blood, can be measured by obtaining a mixed venous blood sample from a pulmonary artery catheter. The oxygen content of arterial blood, $CaO_2$, can be calculated using the following equation (Eq. 6) and the values obtained from arterial blood gas measurement:

$$CaO_2 = (Hgb \times 1.34 \times SaO_2) + (0.0031 \times PaO_2)$$

Eq. 6 (oxygen content equation): Hgb: hemoglobin (g/dL); $SaO_2$: arterial oxygen saturation (%); $PaO_2$: arterial oxygen partial pressure (mmHg)

Thus, the cardiac output can be calculated by rearranging Fick's equation:

$$Q = \frac{VO_2}{CaO_2 - CvO_2}.$$

Fick's Principle can be further utilized to understand physiological conditions when there is a change in oxygen consumption or delivery and how that affects the mixed venous tension/saturation[4]. Mathematically, Equation 2 can be rearranged using the oxygen content equations for both arterial and venous. In these equations, the partial pressure of the dissolved oxygen in the arterial and venous system is negligible and can be removed to simplify the equation.

$$CaO_2 = (Hgb \times 1.34 \times SaO_2) + (0.0031 \times PaO_2)$$

$$CvO_2 = (Hgb \times 1.34 \times SvO_2) + (0.0031 \times PvO_2)$$

Therefore, by replacing those variables, Fick's equation can be rewritten as follows:

$$VO_2 = (Q \times 1.34 \times Hgb) \times (SaO_2 - SvO_2)$$

$$SvO_2 = SaO_2 - \frac{VO_2}{Q \times 1.34 \times Hgb}$$

Eq. 7: Rearranged Fick's equation that shows the relationship between variables and mixed venous saturation.

This equation shows that an increase in oxygen consumption ($VO_2$) will lead to decreased mixed venous saturation/tension. On the other hand, a decrease in cardiac output, hemoglobin, or arterial oxygen saturation will lead to a decreased mixed venous saturation/tension.

Fick's Principle can be used to calculate the cardiac output, and it can be further utilized to assess the relationship between mixed venous oxygen saturation/tension and other variables in the equation. A limitation of using Fick's equation is that it does not account for the oxygen consumption of the lungs and the $VO_2$ is an assumed value in a clinical setting.[3] Although the oxygen consumption of the lungs may be negligible in healthy patients, it can be significant in critically ill patients.[3]

## REFERENCES

1. Sun LS, Davis NA. Cardiac physiology. In: *Miller's Anesthesia.* 9th ed. Philadelphia, PA: Elsevier; 2020:384–404.
2. Costanzo LS. Cardiovascular physiology. In: *Physiology.* 6th ed. Philadelphia, PA: Elsevier; 2018:117–188.
3. Crystal GJ, et al. Cardiovascular physiology: Integrative function. In: *Pharmacology and Physiology for Anesthesia.* 2nd ed. Philadelphia, PA: Elsevier; 2019:473–519.
4. Shepherd SJ, Pearse RM. Role of central and mixed venous oxygen saturation measurement in perioperative care. *Anesthesiology.* 2009;111(3):649–656.

# 265.

# VENOUS RETURN

*Ryan Nowatzke and Larry Manders*

## INTRODUCTION

Veins (except for the pulmonary and umbilical vein, which carry oxygenated blood) return deoxygenated blood back to the heart. Veins have a thinner smooth muscle layer, one-way valves, higher capacitance for volume, and typically lower pressure systems compared to arteries. The venous system provides a huge reservoir for blood volume within the body, normally containing ~70% of total blood volume, and even more in pathological states, with ~25% of total blood volume within the splanchnic circulation.[1–4]

Blood coming out of the heart at any time must be met with blood returning to the heart; therefore cardiac output (CO) ≈ venous return (VR). If VR decreases, CO will quickly decrease as well, and vice versa.[3]

Using Ohm's law (Q = ΔP/R) (Q: flow; R: radius; ΔP: difference in pressure) we can apply this to hemodynamics using Q as CO, ΔP as the difference between mean arterial pressure (MAP) and central venous pressure (CVP), and R as the systemic vascular resistance (SVR). Therefore CO = (MAP – CVP)/SVR.[3]

Applying this concept to venous return, we can extrapolate that VR is determined by the driving pressure (difference between CVP and the pressure in the right atrium [RAP]), and the resistance of the vasculature. Therefore, if RAP/resistance to VR is increased (fluid overload, right-sided heart failure, or external compression/increased intrathoracic pressure), then the pressure gradient will be less, and VR will decrease. Likewise, factors increasing the resistance to return/tone in the venous systems (such as α-receptor agonists, compression in extremity skeletal muscles, etc.) will lead to increased CVP, which increases the pressure gradient, leading to increased blood return. Under normal physiologic circumstances, normal CVP is ~8–12 mmHg and RAP is ~<5 mmHg.[3]

As mentioned before, the venous system is a high capacitance system. It contains most of the body's blood volume. Because of its ability to "store" blood volume, when acute blood loss happens, it can compensate and mobilize this volume to maintain VR and CO. During the first stage of hypovolemic shock, there are no changes in vital signs, and one can lose up to ~15% of total blood volume (roughly 750 ml) = without any changes.[5] It is also worth noting that total blood volume per kilogram will differ based on age and gender, as seen in Table 265.1.

## Table 265.1 AVERAGE BLOOD VOLUMES BY AGE AND SEX

| AVERAGE BLOOD VOLUMES | ML/KG |
|---|---|
| Premature neonates | 95 |
| Full term neonates | 85 |
| Infants | 80 |
| Adult men | 75 |
| Adult women | 65 |

## MUSCLE ACTION, INTRATHORACIC PRESSURE, AND BODY POSITION

Changes in the venous pressure and pressure in the right atrium (RA)/pulmonary system will alter volume of blood return to the heart. If the resistance of the venous vasculature and/or external pressure on the veins increases, there will be a resulting decrease in the blood volume returned to the heart. Also, anything that changes the intrathoracic/intrapleural pressure (4 mmHg at rest) will result in changes on the external compression process on the vasculature.[4] It will also result in changes to RA/pulmonary pressure, leading to altered VR. Examples of some common factors that alter VR and their impact are listed in Table 265.2.

## ANESTHETIC CONSIDERATIONS

### PREOPERATIVE

- It is essential to understand each patient's total blood volume, starting volume status, and all underlying existing medical conditions that may alter venous and intracardiac pressures. This includes underlying heart failure, pulmonary hypertension, valvular disease, hepatic disease, and underlying pulmonary conditions.

### INTRAOPERATIVE

- It is important to understand changes in VR associated with spontaneous respirations versus positive pressure ventilation. During spontaneous respiration, VR will be augmented during inspiration secondary to negative intrathoracic pressure. During mechanical ventilation with positive pressure, inspiration will decrease VR secondary to compression of the vasculature. Increasing positive end-expiratory pressure will also result in decrease in VR.
- Alpha-1 agonists, as well as other venoconstrictors, will increase venous tone and improve VR, resulting

## Table 265.2 FACTORS AFFECTING VENOUS RETURN

| FACTOR | AFFECT |
|---|---|
| Skeletal muscle contraction (squatting, leg raise) | Extremity muscle contraction/exercise results in a compression of local veins of the extremities, increasing VR. |
| Inspiration cycle | During inhalation, transient pressure changes create a negative intrathoracic pressure from an expanding thoracic cavity (diaphragm contraction), increasing VR. |
| Expiratory cycle | During exhalation, the diaphragm relaxes, returning intrathoracic pressure gradient to baseline, resulting in decreased pressure gradient for VR. During forced exhalation, accessory respiratory muscles are also used, further decreasing VR and increasing thoracic cavity pressure. |
| Gravity/positioning | Gravity affects VR depending on the location of the RA in respect to most of the patients' blood volume (abdomen/pelvis/lower extremities). If the heart is below, such as in Trendelenburg position, driving pressure for VR is increased by the force of gravity. If the heart is above, such as in reverse Trendelenburg or standing position, gravity will promote pooling of blood in lower extremities and VR will decrease. |
| Sympathetic tone | Sympathetic activity (via $\alpha$-1 receptors) decreased venous compliance/results in contraction of venous system promoting VR. |
| Positive pressure ventilation | Leads to compression of veins, and increased RA pressure, causing a decrease in VR. |
| Valsalva maneuver | Forced expiration against a closed glottis in combinations of contracting accessory respiratory muscles leads to external compression on veins, as well as increased RA pressure from external compression, resulting in decreased VR. |

in increased cardiac output in patients with normal physiology.

### POSTOPERATIVE

- Patients with decreased VR will experience a decrease in cardiac output. Removal of the stress of surgery and/or adequately treating pain may result in decreased sympathetic stimulation, resulting in decreased venous tone.
- Patients attempting to ambulate after surgery must be watched carefully due to the decreased VR associated with moving from supine to standing position. This can create transient hypotension leading to syncope. This also may occur if patients perform a Valsalva

maneuver, usually while attempting to void or pass a bowel movement postoperatively. This is exaggerated in patients who are already hypovolemic.

## REFERENCES

1. Pang CC, Measurement of body venous tone. *J Pharmacol Toxicol Methods*. 2000;44(2):341–360.
2. Shen T, Baker K. Venous return and clinical hemodynamics: How the body works during acute hemorrhage. *Adv Physiol Educ*. 2015;39(4):267–271.
3. Young DB. Venous return. In: *Control of Cardiac Output*. U.S. National Library of Medicine. January 1, 1970. www.ncbi.nlm.nih.gov/books/NBK54476/.
4. Gelman S. Venous function and central venous pressure: A physiologic story. *Anesthesiology*. 2008;108(4):735–748.
5. Hooper N, Armstrong TJ. HemorrhagicaShock. In: *StatPearls*. Treasure Island, FL: StatPearls; 2019.

# 266.

# VESSEL FUNCTION

*John Yousef and Larry Manders*

## INTRODUCTION

Five types of vessels exist in the body to carry oxygenated blood to the tissues and take deoxygenated blood away from them. These are the arteries, arterioles, capillaries, venules, and veins. The exchange between cellular waste and nutrition takes place at the level of the capillaries. Substances such as water, oxygen, carbon dioxide, and glucose are supplied and removed.

## STRUCTURE

Larger vessels such as the arteries and veins consist of three layers, with the middle layer being the thickest layer. These three layers are the tunica intima, tunica media, and tunica adventitia. These three layers' presence and thickness vary throughout the vessels depending on the size. Tunica intima is the innermost layer and is made of a single layer of squamous cells and small layer of sub-endothelial tissue. Tunica media is the thickest layer and is primarily found in arteries and veins; it consists of elastic fibrous tissue, and some vessels have smooth muscle tissue which can control the diameter of the vessel.[1] Lastly, the tunica adventitia is the outer layer and thickest especially in the veins. It is primarily made of connective tissue and has capillaries which

supply the vessel with nutrition, especially the larger vessels. Arterioles will carry the blood flow from arteries and into capillaries. It is at the level of the arterioles where vascular resistance takes place due to their muscular walls. Capillaries are the smallest unit and consist of a single layer of endothelial cells; as mentioned earlier, this is where nutrients and waste are exchanged. Three forms of capillaries exist: continuous, fenestrated, and sinusoidal. Continuous capillaries allow only lipid-soluble material and small molecules to pass through and usually are found in the blood vessels.[1] Fenestrated and sinusoidal capillaries allow 60–80 nm and 30–40 micrometers to pass through, respectively. Fenestrated and sinusoidal capillaries are found in areas such as the renal glomerulus and spleen.

Beyond the capillaries is the venous system. The first step of returning the blood back to the heart is the venules, which have a diameter that ranges from 7 nanometers to 1 millimeter and contain about 25% of the total blood flow. Venules consist of an inner endothelium, middle muscular and elastic layer, and an outer fibrous layer.[2] Veins will take the blood from venules back to the heart. The larger veins in the body are the venae cava. Most veins have one-way valves which prevent reverse blood flow. These valves tend to fail with old age, leading to back-up of blood and causing varicose veins. Veins also consist of the three layers made of tunica intima, tunica media, and tunica externa. When compared to the tunica media of arteries, the veins' tunica media is much thinner.

## PHYSIOLOGY

Arteries can regulate their diameter via contraction known as vasoconstriction. Vasoconstriction is regulated via nerves, neurotransmitters, and hormones. Vasoconstriction will lead to clinical relevance in way of elevated blood pressure. Arterioles are the most influential determents of blood pressure, considering their innervation via the autonomic nervous system (ANS). The ANS consists of the sympathetic and the parasympathetic systems. Both the sympathetic nervous system causes vasoconstriction, primarily via working on alpha-1 receptors which use the neurotransmitter norepinephrine to active a G-coupled protein response, leading to an activation of phospholipase C, ultimately causing an increase in intracellular calcium release, resulting in constriction and an elevation in blood pressure (Figure 266.1).[3]

While most arterioles primarily have alpha-1 receptors, arterioles in the skeletal and pulmonary system have a high ratio of beta-2 receptors. When epinephrine activates these beta-2 receptors, it causes arteriole vasodilation for increased oxygenation of skeletal and pulmonary tissue in times of need.

Relaxation of arterioles will lead to a decrease in blood pressure. One of the primarily mechanisms of relaxation is via nitric oxide (NO), which is released from the endothelial cells. Production of NO is synthesized from L-arginine via the enzyme nitric oxide synthase. After NO is produced in the endothelial cells, it will diffuse to the smooth muscle with the arterioles to bind to the guanylate cyclase enzyme, which produces cyclic-GMP.[4] Cyclic-GMP causes a sequence of phosphorylation which leads to a decrease of intracellular calcium and thus muscle relaxation. Similar relaxation can also happen in the veins, and because the veins are much more compliant than the arteries and arterioles, this leads to pooling of blood volume within the veins and thus a decrease in blood pressure via decreasing volume back to the heart in the form of preload.

Besides NO and norepinephrine binding to receptors to lead to changes in blood pressure, other hormones and receptors may also lead to the same changes. Other hormones that may increase blood pressure include angiotensin II and endothelin, while hormones such as bradykinin, atrial natriuretic peptide, and prostacyclin may work via various mechanisms to decrease arterial constriction.

## ANESTHETIC CONSIDERATIONS

### PREOPERATIVE

In the preoperative setting, medications that work on vessels, such as hydralazine or angiotensin converting enzyme (ACE) inhibitors, should be stopped to prevent intraoperative hypotension, unless otherwise indicated.[3] If patients continue to take said medications, especially vasopressor agents such as phenylephrine, ephedrine, and vasopressin should be placed and ready to use prior to bringing the patient back to the operating room.[4,5] Preoperative blood pressure should also be taken and noted.

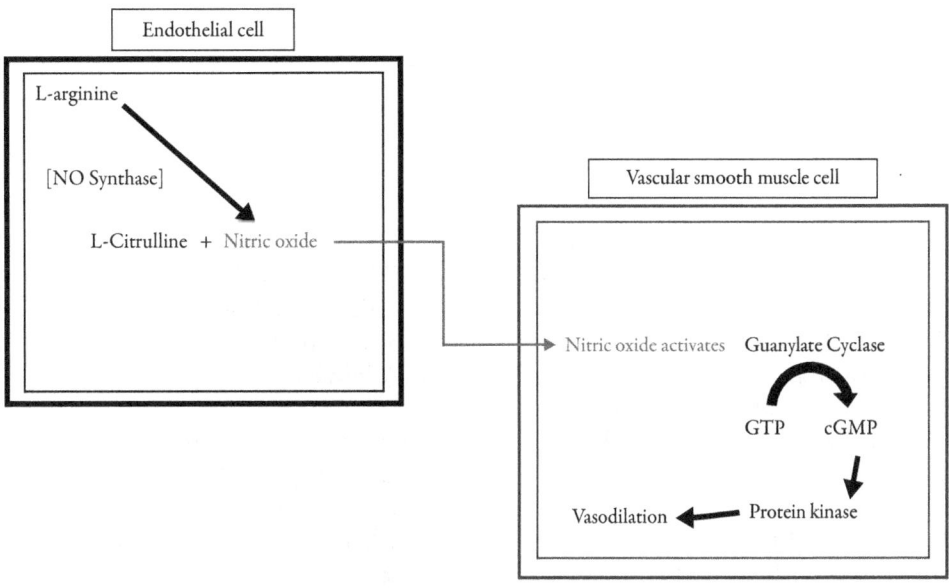

Figure 266.1. Intercellular regulatory pathway for vasodilation.

In the operating room, both intravenous (IV) and inhalation agents can result in profound hypotension, especially in patients who took ACE inhibitors or vasodilators (as mentioned previously). Also of note, local anesthetic delivered via neuraxial techniques can prevent sympathetic activity, thus decreasing alpha activation, leading to vasodilation. General anesthetics usually cause vasodilation via decrease in alpha activation as well as increase in beta activation within heart decrease cardiac output. Furthermore, venous pooling can contribute to decrease preload, which furthers the reduction in cardiac output.

## POSTOPERATIVE

Consequences of decreased vascular tone can clinically correlate to hypotension in the post-anesthesia care unit (PACU), increasing morbidity and mortality, particularly in patients with coronary artery disease or peripheral arterial disease.[5] Cardiac output in hypotensive patients is largely maintained by an increase in heart rate, which can be difficult for an older, sicker heart. Thorough physical assessment is important to rule out detrimental cardiovascular effects such as as myocardial infarction. Patients will usually respond to supportive treatment such as fluid boluses. If no response is achieved, it is likely that a stepwise fashion of alpha-1 vasoactive agents would need to be used to increase the patient's blood pressure, and admission to the hospital for close monitoring is needed.

## REFERENCES

1. Weiss L, ed., *Cell and Tissue Biology*. 6th ed. Baltimore, MD: Urban & Schwarzenberg; 1988:381.
2. Murad F. Cyclic guanosine monophosphate as a mediator of vasodilation. *J Clin Invest.* 1986;78(1):1–5.
3. Stoica EB, et al. Evaluation of molecularly imprinted thin films for ephedrine recognition. *Materiale Plastice.* 2019;56(4): 865–874.
4. Ahmad A, et al. Role of nitric oxide in the cardiovascular and renal systems. *Int J Mol Sci.* 2018;19(9):2605.
5. Calver A, et al. Nitric oxide and blood vessels: Physiological role and clinical implications. *Biochem Educ.* 1992;20(3):130–135.

# 267.

# BLOOD VOLUME AND DISTRIBUTION

*Neal Al-Attar and Larry Manders*

The average estimated blood volumes are shown in Table 267.1.

In general, patients who are otherwise healthy should be transfused only after blood loss is greater than 10%–20% of their blood volume. The transfusion point can be calculated by identifying the amount of blood loss necessary for the preoperative hematocrit to decrease to 30%. This can be calculated as follows:[1]

1. Estimate blood volume (EBV)
2. Estimate preoperative red blood cell volume: $(RBCV_{preop}) = EBV * Hemotocrit_{preop}$
3. Estimate red blood cell volume when the hematocrit (Hct) is 30%: $RBCV_{30\%} = EBV * 30\%$
4. Calculate red blood cell volume lost when Hct is 30%: $RBCV_{lost} = RBCV_{preop} - RBCV_{30\%}$
5. Allowable blood loss: $ABL = RBCV_{lost} * .3$

Blood flow and distribution are heavily dependent on cardiac output. The vessel-rich groups (brain, heart, liver, kidney, and endocrine organs) comprise 75% of the cardiac output. Muscle and skin account for ~20% of the cardiac output, and fat comprises ~5% of cardiac output. Bones, cartilage, hair, and teeth are termed the

**Table 267.1** ESTIMATED BLOOD VOLUMES BASED ON AGE AND SEX[1]

| AGE | ESTIMATED BLOOD VOLUME |
|---|---|
| Premature neonates | 95 cc/kg |
| Full-term neonates | 85 cc/kg |
| Infants | 80 cc/kg |
| Adult men | 75 cc/kg |
| Adult women | 65 cc/kg |

vessel-poor groups and account for <1% of the cardiac output.[1,2]

Distribution of blood volume in the systemic circulation is shown in Table 267.2.

The majority of blood volume is in the venous system. A sympathetic response to fluid or blood loss will cause an increase in venous tone, which will return more blood to the heart, increasing preload and augmenting cardiac output.1–3 The arterioles account for the biggest pressure drop of the vascular tree, about 50%. Although the pressure difference between mean arterial pressure and central venous pressure is calculated by systemic vascular resistance multiplied by cardiac output, as in the following equation, $MAP - CVP = SVR*CO$, it is important to remember that SVR is mostly determined by the tone of the arterioles and the CVP is negligible compared to MAP, so the CVP value is often dropped in this equation.[1]

Autoregulation is the process by which tissues beds regulate their own blood flow and is due to vascular smooth muscle stretch response and vasodilatory metabolites.[1,3] When tissue perfusion pressure is low, arterioles will dilate as a compensatory mechanism. If the perfusion pressure is too high, arterioles will constrict. Endothelium-derived factors can vasoconstrict (i.e., endothelins, thromboxane $A_2$) or vasodilate (i.e., nitric oxide, prostacyclins [$PGI_2$]), hence affecting the blood pressure and blood flow.

**Table 267.2** BLOOD VOLUME DISTRIBUTION IN THE SYSTEMIC CIRCULATION[1]

| | |
|---|---|
| Heart | ~5% |
| Lungs | ~10% |
| Arterial circulation | 15% |
| Capillaries | 5% |
| Venous circulation | 65% |

Additionally, systemic vasculature is subject to autonomic control. Alpha-1 adrenergic receptors cause vasoconstriction that is most active in the muscle, GI system, kidney, and skin. The alpha-1 receptors are least responsive in the brain and heart. Beta-2 adrenergic receptors are significant vasodilators and increase flow to skeletal muscle in response to exercise.[1] The aforementioned factors work to divert, alter, and regulate blood distribution, flow, and pressure to vital organs.

## ANESTHETIC CONSIDERATIONS

### PREOPERATIVE

Anticipation of intraoperative blood losses may necessitate a need for a preoperative hematocrit value in order to calculate the transfusion point by using the preceding formula.

### INTRAOPERATIVE

Induction of general anesthesia decreases venous tone, resulting in venodilation and subsequent hypotension.[1,3–5] A larger fluid infusion volume is required at this stage for maintenance of adequate tissue perfusion. Volatile agents used today all depress the *baroreceptor reflex*, the body's natural reflex to vasoconstrict or vasodilate in response to pressure changes sensed in the carotid arteries and aorta.[1] This often necessitates the need for external intervention by administering adrenergic agonists or antagonists intraoperatively.

### POSTOPERATIVE

A simple and noninvasive method for estimating the effectiveness of fluid resuscitation after surgery can be used in the postanesthesia care unit by observing the pulse oximeter variations during inspiration and expiration, or *pulse pressure variation*. During negative-pressure inspiration, venous return is increased due to negative intrathoracic pressure. Venous return is decreased during spontaneous expiration. The difference between the pulse pressure at maximum height and minimum height, divided by the mean pulse pressure, is the *pulse pressure variation*. A value >12% indicates a patient who may be dehydrated and therefore fluid responsive.[1]

## REFERENCES

1. Butterworth JF, et al. Cardiovascular physiology and anesthesia. In: *Morgan & Mikhail's Clinical Anesthesiology*. New York, NY: McGraw-Hill Education; 2018:343–379.

2. Barash PG. *Clinical Anesthesia*. Philadelphia, PA: Lippincott Williams & Wilkins; 2017.
3. Jacobsohn E, et al. The role of the vasculature in regulating venous return and cardiac output: historical and graphical approach. *Can J Anaesth*. 1997;44:849–867.
4. Kazama T, et al. Relation between initial blood distribution volume and propofol induction dose requirement. *Anesthesiology*. 2001;94(2):205–210.
5. Sano Y, et al. Anaesthesia and circulating blood volume. *Eur J Anaesthesiol*. 2005 Apr 1;22(4):258–262.

# 268.

# BLOOD PRESSURE

*Erica Zanath and Mada Helou*

## INTRODUCTION

Blood pressure monitoring is an essential component to every anesthetic; Standard II of the American Society of Anesthesiologts (ASA) requires that circulation be continually evaluated, with measurements at least every 5 minutes.[1] This is because blood pressure provides oxygen to vital organs, and alterations can lead to end organ damage. Normal blood pressure, outlined by the American College of Cardiology and the American Heart Association, is systolic blood pressure <120 mmHg and diastolic blood pressure <80 mmHg.[2]

## BLOOD PRESSURE MEASUREMENT

Blood pressure measurement is crucial during anesthesia delivery. Perioperatively, multiple factors can lead to significant hemodynamic changes; therefore careful monitoring and control of a patient's blood pressure can help to minimize fluctuations and subsequent adverse effects.

Blood pressure is the pressure generated in the arterial system as a result of cardiac contraction, and maintains perfusion to all vital organs.[3,4,5] Adequate perfusion is important for delivery of nutrients, including oxygen. Both hypotension and hypertension can be detrimental, causing end organ damage.

Blood pressure can be measured via both noninvasive and invasive methods. Commonly used noninvasive methods rely on a sphygmomanometer, an inflatable cuff with an attached pressure gauge. When using a cuff, it is important to choose an appropriate size; a cuff that is too small will produce a higher blood pressure, whereas a cuff that is too large will produce a lower blood pressure.[3,4,5] It is recommended that the length of the cuff is 80% of the patient's arm circumference and that the width of the cuff is 40% of the patient's arm circumference.[3,5]

The noninvasive methods of blood pressure measurement are palpation, Doppler, auscultation, oscillometry, and arterial tonometry.[3,4,5]

Palpation of a peripheral pulse during blood pressure cuff inflation and deflation allows for the determination of systolic blood pressure. To measure blood pressure in this manner: palpate the pulse, inflate the cuff until the pulse is no longer palpable, and deflate the cuff slowly until a pulse is once again palpated. The pressure at which the pulse can be palpated after cuff deflation is the systolic blood pressure. This method is not useful for determining diastolic blood pressure or mean arterial blood pressure (MAP).

Using the same technique described for palpation, a Doppler probe can be placed over the peripheral pulse to determine systolic blood pressure.

Blood pressure can be determined by auscultating Korotkoff sounds as a blood pressure cuff is deflated. Korotkoff sounds are those generated from the turbulent flow produced in the artery as blood flow returns. Typically,

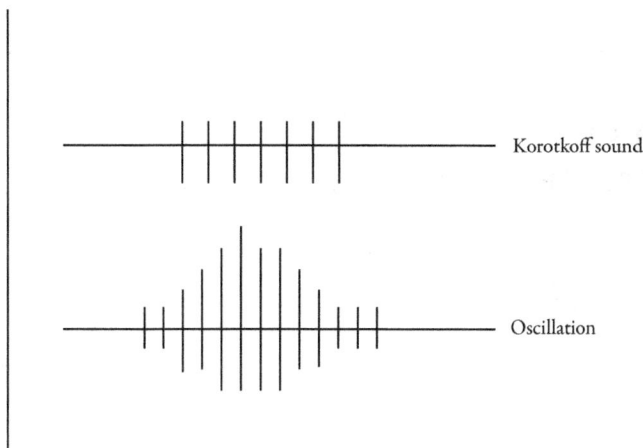

**Figure 268.1.** Comparison of Korotkoff sounds to oscillometry for determining blood pressure.

the blood pressure cuff is applied to the upper arm and inflated to a pressure at least 30 mmHg above the presumed systolic blood pressure. The cuff is slowly deflated (about 5 mmHg/second) while listening with a stethoscope over the brachial artery (distal to the cuff). The first Korotkoff sound heard is the systolic blood pressure.[3,4,5] As the cuff is further deflated, the sound produced will changed. The diastolic pressure is the pressure at which the Korotkoff sounds disappear, representing return to laminar flow.[3,4,5]

Oscillometry is a method of noninvasive blood pressure determination that uses an automated blood pressure cuff. In the same manner as described earlier, turbulent flow is produced in the artery as the cuff deflates. The cuff detects this turbulent flow as vibrations, or oscillations, which are then transduced to an electrical signal. The peak amplitude of oscillations corresponds to the mean arterial blood pressure.[3,4,5] Systolic and diastolic blood pressures are determined using a proprietary calculation. A visual depiction of Korotkoff sounds versus oscillometry for determining blood pressure is shown below in Figure 268.1.

Arterial tonometry is another noninvasive method that can be used for blood pressure determination.[4] This method uses a tonometer, a device with multiple pressures sensors, applied over a superficial artery. Blood pressure is continuously measured as the tonometer senses the pressure required to partially flatten the artery that it is placed over.

Invasive blood pressure monitoring is indicated in cases in which significant blood pressure alterations are expected, when there is a need for more frequent blood pressure monitoring than standard 3- to 5-minute noninvasive measurements, and when multiple arterial blood gases are needed.[3] Invasive blood pressure monitoring is the optimal method for monitoring.[4] This method relies on an arterial line connected to pressure tubing with a transducer. The pulsatile blood flow generated from cardiac contraction is transmitted via the pressuring tubing to the transducer, which converts the pressure to an electrical signal. Fourier analysis then produces an arterial waveform. The MAP is calculated by integrating the area under the curve.

Blood pressure measured via invasive arterial line requires that the transducer be placed at the level of the organ to be monitored.[3,4,5] This usually means placing the transducer at the level of the heart. The transducer can also be placed in line with the tragus to provide an estimate of the perfusion to the brain, the cerebral perfusion pressure.

In addition to the selection of the blood pressure monitoring method, the site of monitoring must be carefully selected.[3,4,5] Both patient and surgical factors should be considered. Patient factors include arm size, arm shape, history of mastectomy, and history of arterial-venous fistula or graft. Surgical factors include site of operation, surgical positioning, and expected length of the operation.

## ANESTHETIC CONSIDERATIONS

Preoperatively, it is important to measure a patient's blood pressure in order to determine the patient's baseline. Preoperative measurement allows the anesthesiologist to ensure that the patient's blood pressure is optimized for surgery. A blood pressure measurement >180 mmHg systolic and/or >120 mmHg diastolic is considered hypertensive urgency; when accompanied by symptoms of end organ damage, this constitutes hypertensive emergency.[2] Both hypertensive urgency and emergency should receive prompt attention.

Intraoperatively, blood pressure should be measured at least every 5 minutes. Many intraoperative factors can contribute to hypotension and hypertension, including medications administered, depth of anesthesia, and surgical stimuli.[3,4,5] Hypotension and hypertension can lead to end organ damage; therefore minimizing significant fluctuations is crucial to providing a safe anesthetic.

## REFERENCES

1. American Society for Anesthesiology. *Standards for Basic Anesthetic Monitoring.* 2015.
2. Whelton PK, et al. Guidelines for prevention, detection, evaluation, and management of high blood pressure in adults. *J Am Coll Cardiol.* 2017;71(19): .
3. Barash PG, et al. *Clinical Anesthesia.* 7th ed. Philadelphia, PA: Lippincott Williams & Wilkins; 2013.
4. Butterworth JF, et al. *Morgan and Mikhail's Clinical Anesthesiology.* 5th ed. McGraw-Hill; 2013.
5. Pardo MC, Miller RD. *Basics of Anesthesia.* 7th ed. Philadelphia, PA: Elsevier; 2018.

# 269.

# SYSTOLIC, DIASTOLIC, MEAN, AND PERFUSION PRESSURES

*Erica Zanath and Mada Helou*

## INTRODUCTION

Blood pressure measurements are reported as *systolic blood pressure, diastolic blood pressure,* and *mean arterial blood pressure.* Each of these terms represents a different force within the blood vessels during the cardiac cycle.

Blood pressure is generated by ejection of blood from the left ventricle into the arterial system, and is maintained by the tone in the blood vessels. Systolic blood pressure (SBP), or the blood pressure generated during systole, is the highest pressure within the arterial vasculature. As such, systolic blood pressure is related to the maximal force generated by cardiac contraction. Diastolic blood pressure (DBP) is the pressure in the arterial vasculature when the heart is relaxed, or in diastole.[1-3] Therefore, diastolic pressure is related to the resting tone in the blood vessels.

Mean arterial blood pressure (MAP) is the weighted average of the pressure in the blood vessels throughout the cardiac cycle. MAP is the blood pressure value that is measured during automated oscillometry; however, it is calculated during other forms of blood pressure determination (i.e., auscultation, invasive). To calculate MAP, one-third of the SBP is added to two-thirds of the DBP.[1,2,3]

$$MAP = (SBP + 2\,DBP)\,/\,3 = 1/3\,SBP + 2/3\,DBP$$

In the preceding equation, DBP is given more weight than SBP due to the relative time spent in diastole compared to systole during the cardiac cycle.

The location of blood pressure measurement affects the systolic and diastolic values obtained. Peripheral measurements (i.e., radial artery) will have exaggerated systolic and diastolic pressures (Figure 269.1) compared to those obtained in the aorta.[1] Additionally, the pulse pressure, the difference between SBP and DBP, becomes wider with peripheral measurements. The amplification of SBP at peripheral sites is attributed to pressure wave reflections, which are additive with respect to the initial blood pressure wave.

Perfusion pressure is a determinant of blood flow to the organ of interest.[1-3] To better understand perfusion pressure, it can be thought of in terms of pressure gradients. It is the pressure driving perfusion to an organ less the pressure resisting perfusion.

$$Perfusion\ pressure = MAP - Venous\ pressure$$

When considering the brain, the cerebral perfusion pressure is calculated as:

$$Cerebral\ PP = MAP - ICP\ \left(or\ CVP,\ whichever\ is\ greater\right)$$

$$ICP = Intracranial\ pressure$$

$$CVP = Central\ venous\ pressure$$

Similarly, the spinal cord perfusion pressure is calculated as:

$$Spinal\ Cord\ PP = MAP - CSFP$$

$$CSFP = Cerebral\ spinal\ fluid\ pressure$$

When considering the left ventricle, the coronary perfusion pressure is calculated as:

$$Coronary\ PP = DBP - LVEDP$$

$$LVEDP = Left\ ventricular\ end\ diastolic\ pressure$$

End organ perfusion pressures are important to understand when considering the management of patients with various pathologies.

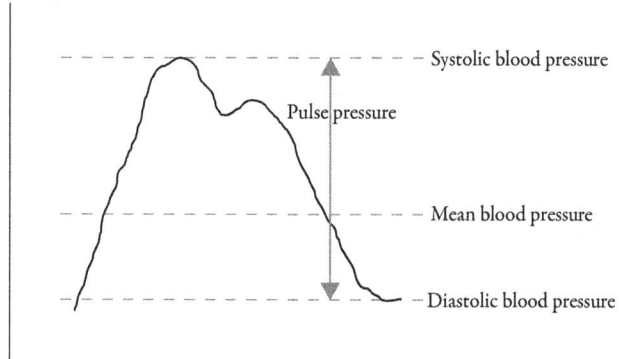

Figure 269.1. Systolic, diastolic, and mean blood pressures depicted on a standard arterial blood pressure waveform.

## ANESTHETIC CONSIDERATIONS

When managing an anesthetic, maintaining appropriate blood pressure levels is of prime importance. There are specific patient pathologies and specific operations that require consideration of the end organ perfusion pressures. For example, a patient with intracranial hypertension requires the clinician to strictly monitor and control blood pressure in order to preserve cerebral perfusion. Additionally, during the endovascular repair of a thoracic aortic aneurysm, spinal cord perfusion pressure is of critical importance, both intraoperatively and postoperatively, in order to prevent cord ischemia.[1] During an anesthetic this can be of increased importance given the reductions in blood pressure that often accompany general anesthesia.

## REFERENCES

1. Barash PG, et al. *Clinical Anesthesia*. 7th ed. Philadelphia, PA: Lippincott Williams & Wilkins; 2013.
2. Butterworth JF, et al. *Morgan and Mikhail's Clinical Anesthesiology*. 5th ed. McGraw-Hill; 2013.
3. Pardo MC, Miller RD. *Basics of Anesthesia*. 7th ed. Philadelphia, PA: Elsevier; 2018.

# 270.

# INTRACARDIAC, PULMONARY, AND VENOUS PRESSURES

*Adriana Martin and Surendrasingh Chhabada*

## INTRODUCTION

Each heart chamber has a normal range of pressure that will happen during the cardiac cycle. It is important to know the normal progression of pressures from central venous pressure (CVP) through the left ventricle end-diastolic pressure (LVEDP). *The gold standard to assess intracardiac pressures is invasive cardiac catheterization.*[1] Central venous pressure can provide right-sided values, and pulmonary artery catheter (PAC) can help estimate left-sided pressures. Table 270.1 presents the normal range pressure for each chamber and major vessels.

Knowing the normal values and normal waveform will help the anesthesiologist identify abnormalities and can aid in diagnosing pathologies, e.g., pulmonary hypertension, differential diagnosis in shock state, right and left heart failure, and compliance abnormalities (pressure-volume loop changes).

| CHAMBER | PRESSURE (MMHG) | CHAMBER | PRESSURE (MMHG) |
|---------|-----------------|---------|-----------------|
| CVP | 4–12 | Mean PA | 10–20 |
| RA | 1–8 | LA | 4–12 |
| RV | 15–25/1–8 | LV | 100–140/4–12 |
| PA | 15–30/8–15 | Aorta | 100–140/60–90 |

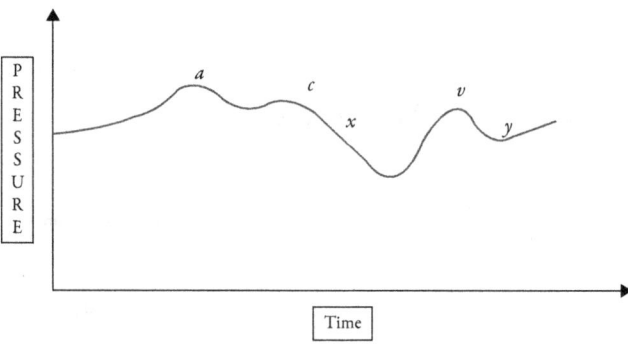

Figure 270.1. Normal central venous pressure waveform.

## CENTRAL VENOUS PRESSURE

### CVP MONITORING INDICATIONS AND USES

CVP provides estimation of right atrial pressure and is also a reflection of right ventricle (RV) preload in the presence of a normal tricuspid valve. CVP can help assess the volume status of the patient. The reliability of the CVP in assessing fluid responsiveness is a subject of debate, with a meta-analysis showing poor prediction value.[3] Besides hypervolemia, CVP can be elevated in a number of diseases involving the tricuspid valve, right ventricle (ischemia and cardiomyopathy), pulmonary valve, and pulmonary artery. High CVP can also evident in cardiac tamponade, congenital heart diseases with left to right shunt, and left-sided heart failure. Most anesthesiologists agree that the value of monitoring CVP will depend more on the trend than on the static number. It has also been demonstrated that right-sided pressures are poor indicators of left ventricular filling.

### CVP WAVEFORM COMPONENTS

The CVP waveform consists of three peaks (*a*, *c*, and *v* waves) and two descents (*x* and *y* descents) as shown in Figure 270.1. It is important to know what each of these peaks and descents represent and on what phase of the cardiac cycle they happen. Table 270.2 describes each one of these components.

### CVP WAVEFORM WITH DIFFERENT PATHOLOGIES

CVP will be affected by many factors, including heart rate, intrathoracic pressure changes, ventricular compliance changes, atrioventricular (AV) synchronicity, tricuspid valve pathologies, etc. *Atrial fibrillation will have absent "a" waves since atrial contraction will not happen in a synchronized way.* Table 270.3 lists multiple pathologies and their effects on the CVP waveform. *Advanced cardiac tamponade has a classic presentation of elevation and equalization of diastolic pressure in all heart chambers, including CVP and pulmonary capillary wedge pressure (PCWP).*[2] This occurs because rapid accumulation of fluid in the pericardium uniformly increases the pressure and transmits it to all chambers during the low-pressure phase (diastole) of the cardiac cycle.

Table 270.2 CVP WAVEFORM COMPONENTS: MECHANICAL EVENTS, CARDIAC CYCLE PHASES AND VALVE EVENTS

| WAVEFORM COMPONENT | MECHANICAL EVENT | PHASE OF CARDIAC CYCLE AND QRS | VALVE EVENT |
|--------------------|------------------|-------------------------------|-------------|
| a wave | Atrial systole/contraction | End of diastole—immediately after P wave | Mitral valve closes after the contraction |
| c wave | Bulging of the TV into the RA during RV contraction | Early systole—immediately after QRS | Aortic valve opens after isovolumetric contraction |
| x descend | Atrial diastole/relaxation | Mid-systole | |
| v wave | Atrial filling | Late systole—T wave | Aortic valve closes |
| y descend | Tricuspid valve opens—early ventricular filling | Early diastole | Mitral valve opens |

## Table 270.3 CVP WAVEFORM COMPONENT VARIATION WITH VARIOUS PATHOLOGIES

| PATHOLOGIES | CVP WAVEFORM CHARACTERISTICS |
|---|---|
| Atrial fibrillation | Loss of *a* wave<br>Prominent *c* wave |
| AV dissociation (3rd degree block) | Cannon *a* wave |
| Tricuspid stenosis | Tall *a* wave<br>Attenuation of *y* descent |
| Pulmonic stenosis and RV hypertrophy | Tall *a* wave |
| COPD with pulmonary hypertension | Tall *a* wave |
| Tricuspid regurgitation | Tall *v* wave<br>Junction of *c* and *v* wave<br>Loss of *x* descent |
| Right ventricular ischemia | Tall *a* and *v* waves<br>Steep *x* and *y* descent |
| Cardiac tamponade | Prominent *v* wave<br>Dominant *x* descent<br>Attenuated *y* descent |

## PULMONARY ARTERY CATHETERIZATION AND PRESSURE

Pulmonary artery catheters, also called Swan-Ganz catheters, are multi-lumen catheters available in different sizes that measure intracardiac filling pressures and can aid the diagnosis and management of numerous cardiovascular illnesses. The major hemodynamic indices measured are pulmonary artery and pulmonary artery occlusion pressure, right atrial and right ventricular pressure, cardiac output by thermodilution and Fick's principle and cardiac index, systemic and pulmonary vascular resistance, and mixed venous oxyhemoglobin saturation ($SvO_2$). CVP is measured from the proximal port. RV systolic and diastolic pressures are measured during catheter insertion using the distal tip of the catheter. It is important to note that the left-sided filling pressures are not directly measured; instead, they are indirectly estimated by the pulmonary artery occlusion pressure (PAOP).

### PAC INDICATIONS AND CONTRAINDICATIONS

The Swan-Ganz catheter can be used to measure important hemodynamic indices and aids in determining the hemodynamic status of critically ill patients. It is indicated for managing severely ill patients with pulmonary hypertension, cardiogenic shock, mixed shock states, and cardiac tamponade. Intraoperatively it has been used in cardiac surgery; liver, heart, and lung transplants; aortic surgery; and surgery in patients with severe cardiac pathologies. Although commonly used intraoperatively, there is no evidence of benefit or improved

outcomes of treatment guided by PAC when compared to standard of care.[4] Studies have not shown mortality benefits in patients receiving therapy guided by PAC. Contraindications can be related to the cannulation of a central vein or related to the advancement of the catheter into the pulmonary artery. *Right-sided endocarditis, presence of a right ventricular assist device, and right-sided mass are absolute contraindications.*[5] PAC is considered high risk in patients with severe pulmonary hypertension, Eisenmenger's physiology, left bundle branch block (LBBB), recently placed transvenous pacemaker leads, prosthetic or stenotic tricuspid or pulmonic valve, and persistent left superior vena cava (misplacement to the left atrium). Caution should be taken during placement due to the risk of arrhythmias. *When placing a PAC in a patient with a pre-existing LBBB there is a risk of causing complete heart block if damage to the conduction system in the right side of the heart.*

### INSERTION TECHNIQUE, WAVEFORMS, AND PAC WEDGING

To insert a PAC, first an introducer sheath is placed in a central vein. The PAC is then advanced inside the sheath until 20 centimeters. At that moment the balloon should be inflated and the catheter slowly advanced while observing the waveforms, as shown in Figure 270.2, and the electrocardiogram for any arrhythmias. Initially an RA pressure will be observed, with the components described in the CVP waveform section. Once in the RV, the systolic pressure will be higher with a low diastolic pressure. The systole will have a swift upstroke and downstroke, and the diastole will have a characteristic slow upstroke that represents ventricular filling and will finalize with an *a* wave that represents atrial contraction. Once the catheter has passed the pulmonic valve, a diastolic surge will be noticed (also called diastolic step-up), as well as a dicrotic notch representing pulmonary valve closure. Another difference is that diastole will be characterized by a downstroke instead of the upstroke present in the RV. Continue to advance the catheter to obtain a wedged pressure that will have a similar waveform to the RA. At the end of diastole there is cessation of forward blood flow and a static fluid column is presumed to exist from the LV to the tip of the catheter. *Once the wedge pressure is obtained, the balloon should be deflated and the catheter should be withdrawn a few centimeters. It is essential that the balloon is inflated whenever the catheter is being advanced and deflated whenever the catheter is being withdrawn.*

*The right internal jugular vein is the ideal site of placement because of the straight pathway to the heart.* The left subclavian vein is the second most ideal site. The right subclavian vein is the most difficult site to successfully insert a PAC.

### PULMONARY ARTERY PRESSURES

Waveform of the pulmonary artery is similar in morphology to that of the aorta, but the pressures are lower.

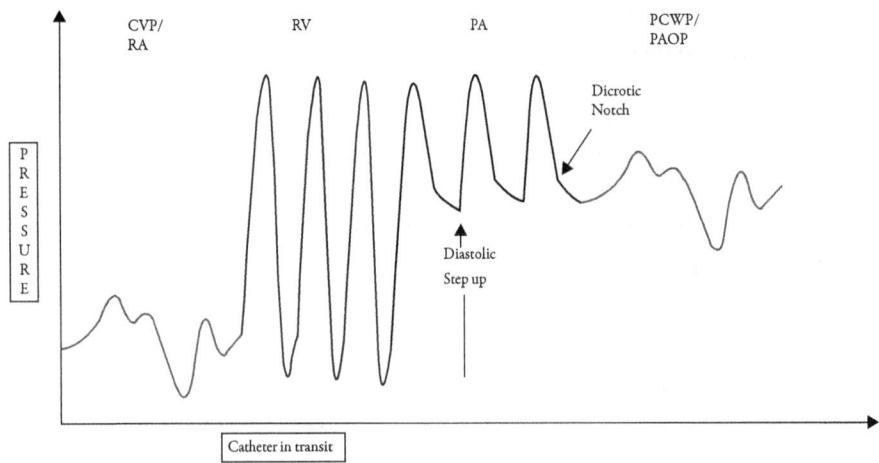

**Figure 270.2.** Normal pressure waveform during pulmonary artery catheter insertion from right atrium to wedge position.

The dicrotic notch represents closure of pulmonic valve. Normal pulmonary artery (PA) systolic pressures range from 15 to 30 mmHg, while PA diastolic pressures range from 8 to 15 mmHg. The mean PA pressure is typically 16 mmHg (10–22 mmHg). The mean PA pressure can be elevated by acute conditions (e.g., venous thromboembolism or hypoxemic-induced pulmonary vasoconstriction), or by chronic conditions (e.g., pulmonary hypertension [PH]). *Pulmonary hypertension is defined when mean pulmonary artery pressures are more than 25 mmHg.*

## PULMONARY CAPILLARY WEDGE PRESSURE

Pulmonary capillary wedge pressure (PCWP), also known as pulmonary artery occlusion pressure, is the pressure measured at the tip of the PAC when it is positioned in a peripheral branch of the PA, while the balloon is inflated. *For accurate reading, the catheter tip has to be placed in zone 3 of the lungs for measurement where there is a continuous column of blood between the catheter tip and the left atrium and the effect of alveolar pressure is minimal.* Normal values for PCWP range from 4 to 12 mmHg. PCWP is an estimation of left atrial pressure and, if no mitral pathology, it can be a reciprocal of left ventricle end-diastolic pressure (LVEDP). Wedge pressure can be a surrogate for LVEDP and LV preload (LVEDV) through the Frank-Starling mechanism. Multiple factors can underestimate or overestimate the PCWP, including mitral disease, aortic insufficiency (premature closure of mitral valve), lung pathologies like chronic obstructive pulmonary disease or respiratory failure (constriction of veins in hypoxic regions), positive pressure ventilation with high positive end-expiratory pressure, changes in ventricular compliance, atrial fibrillation, etc. The LVEDP is a function of chamber compliance and may be elevated when the left ventricle experiences excessive diastolic volume overload, as occurs, for example, with

mitral or aortic valvular regurgitation or high-volume shunting at or distal to the ventricular septum.

## PAC COMPLICATIONS

Complications can occur from establishing a central venous access or from the pulmonary catheterization itself. Complications of establishing central venous access include malpositioning, unintentional arterial puncture, neck hematoma, neuropathy, air embolism, and pneumothorax. Complications from the catheterization include dysrhythmias, increase in tricuspid regurgitation, right bundle-branch block and complete heart block, and PA rupture with life-threatening pulmonary hemorrhage. Serious complications specifically to PA catheterization (PA rupture, serious ventricular dysrhythmias, endocarditis) occur in 0.1%–0.5% of surgical patients. Complications of catheter residence include venous thrombosis, pulmonary embolism and infarction. There are also problems with the catheter itself, for example, balloon rupture and catheter knotting. Prolonged catheterization can also cause catheter-related sepsis and endocarditis.

## REFERENCES

1. Kubiak GM, et al. Right heart catheterization-background, physiological basics, and clinical implications. *J Clin Med.* 2019;8(9):1331.
2. Khandaker MH, et al. Pericardial disease: Diagnosis and management. *Mayo Clin Proc.* 2010;85(6):572–593.
3. Eskesen TG, et al. Systematic review including re-analyses of 1148 individual data sets of central venous pressure as a predictor of fluid responsiveness. *Intensive Care Med.* 2016;42(3):324–332.
4. Sandham JD, Hull RD, Brant RF, et al. A randomized, controlled trial of the use of pulmonary-artery catheters in high-risk surgical patients. *N Engl J Med.* 2003;348(1):5–14.
5. Kelly CR, Rabbani LE. Videos in clinical medicine: Pulmonary-artery catheterization. *N Engl J Med.* 2013;369(25):e35.

# 271.

# BARORECEPTOR FUNCTION

*Kris Vasant and Muhammad Fayyaz Ahmed*

## INTRODUCTION

Baroreceptors are stretch-sensitive fibers that function to maintain blood pressure within a normal range, specifically regulating the mean arterial pressure (MAP).[1] These peripheral stretch receptors are located in the aortic arch and in each carotid sinus.[2] The carotid sinuses are located bilaterally at the bifurcation of the common carotid arteries.[2] Complex autonomic nervous system neural loops that incorporate baroreceptors are responsible for the short-term regulation of MAP by altering heart rate, contractility, and systemic vasomotor tone.

## FUNCTION, LOCATION, AND EFFECTS

The integrated neural feedback loop is depicted as follows. Alterations in arterial blood pressure are sensed by peripheral baroreceptors located in the aortic arch and carotid sinus. The cardiovascular center in the medulla, known as the nucleus solitarius, receives afferent impulses via the glossopharyngeal and vagus nerves from the carotid sinus and aortic arch, respectively. The nucleus solitarius has two functionally separate areas that regulate blood pressure: lateral and rostral (increase blood pressure); central and caudal (lower blood pressure).[2] In general, the peripheral baroreceptors are activated when systemic blood pressure exceeds 170 mmHg; however, the reflex ceases to function when systemic blood pressure falls below 50 mgHg.[2] The efferent portion of the feedback loop from nucleus solitarius has projections that contain parasympathetic and sympathetic innervations to the heart, peripheral vasculature, and other organs that further modulate MAP, such as the kidneys and adrenals.[1] As an effect of this feedback loop, decreases in arterial blood pressure (less stretch of the baroreceptors) results in an increase in sympathetic tone (vasoconstriction), increased adrenal gland release of epinephrine (increased heart rate), and reduced vagal activity (increased cardiac contractility), which leads to a rise in arterial blood pressure.[3] Conversely, an increase in arterial blood pressure leads to increased baroreceptor stretch, causing inhibition of sympathetic tone (vasodilation), enhanced vagal activity (decreased cardiac contractility), leading to a fall in arterial blood pressure—an example of a negative feedback loop.

## VENOUS CONSIDERATIONS

In addition to arterial baroreceptors, venous baroreceptors also play an important role in the regulation of cardiac output. When baroreceptors in the venous circulation (right atrium and great veins) are stretched as a result of increased right atrial pressure, an increase in heart rate is seen; similarly decreased right atrial pressure decreases heart rate.[4] When venous baroreceptors are triggered, the effects on the heart rate are opposite to those seen when arterial baroreceptors fire. The four major determinants of cardiac output include heart rate, contractility, preload, and afterload. Venous baroreceptors monitor preload by sensing the right atrium stretch, and arterial baroreceptors monitor afterload by monitoring systemic arterial pressure, specifically MAP.[4] Just as preload and afterload have opposing effects on cardiac output, so do venous and arterial baroreceptors in response to stretch.

## ANESTHETIC CONSIDERATIONS

### CAROTID SINUS MASSAGE

In situations when a patient develops a stable supraventricular tachycardia (SVT), manual manipulation of carotid baroreceptors activates the reflex. This intervention can be used as a first-line treatment to terminate the arrhythmia. Manual pressure is applied at the level of the carotid sinus on one side of the neck only. This stimulates the carotid sinus baroreceptors to induce parasympathetic activity of the vagus nerve through the atrioventricular (AV) node— thus slowing the heart rate and possibly terminating the arrhythmia. If not successful in terminating the arrhythmia, advanced cardiac life support (ACLS) algorithm should be followed for further clinical care.

## BAINBRIDGE REFLEX

The Bainbridge reflex is seen with paradoxical slowing of the heart rate in response to a spinal anesthetic in an un-medicated patient. During a spinal anesthetic, blockage of the efferent cardiac accelerator fibers at the level of T1–T4 spinal nerves can occur, leading to unopposed vagal nerve activity. The resultant bradycardia, however, is more related to the development of arterial hypotension rather than a blockade of the cardiac accelerator fibers, often depicted as a high spinal.[4] Although arterial hypotension in teaching reflexively causes tachycardia, in an un-medicated patient, the venous baroreceptors are principal over arterial baroreceptors.[4] Hence, during a spinal anesthetic a reduction in venous pressure or preload results in a decrease in stretch of right atrial baroreceptors, leading to a decrease in heart rate. Important considerations to augment this potential response in patients include: adequate intravenous prehydration with fluids, use of drugs with inotropic activity such as ephedrine, anti-muscarinic agents including glycopyrolate, and even atropine with severe bradycardia.

## CAROTID ENDARTERECTOMY (CEA)

When open CEA is performed, many hemodynamic shifts must be anticipated. Surgical manipulation of the atheromatous plaque being removed and carotid sinus pressure by the surgeon can cause stimulation of baroreceptors, leading to a reflexive increase in vagal nerve stimulation, ultimately leading to hypotension and bradycardia requiring pharmacological intervention.[5] If discontinuation of manual manipulation or frequent disruption in the surgery occurs, infiltration of the carotid sinus with local anesthetic can be performed to relieve repetitive stimulation of the baroreceptor reflex.[5] Postoperative considerations that may be encountered include persistent hypertension due to denervation of carotid baroreceptors needed pharmacologic control.

## REFERENCES

1. Kougias P, et al. Arterial baroreceptors in the management of systemic hypertension. *Med Sci Monit.* 2010;16(1):RA1–8.
2. Sun LS, et al. Cardiac physiology. In Miller RD, ed. *Miller's Anesthesia.* 8th ed. New York, NY: Elsevier/Churchill Livingstone; 2015:473–491.
3. Cardiovascular physiology and anesthesia. In Butterworth JF, et al., eds. *Morgan and Mikhail's Clinical Anesthesiology.* 6th ed. New York NY: Lange Medical Books/McGraw Hill Medical; 2018:343–380.
4. Grecu, L. Autonomic nervous system anatomy and physiology. In Barash PG, et al. *Clinical Anesthesia.* 8th ed. Philadelphia, PA: Wolters Kluwer Health; 2017:333–360.
5. Bebawy JF, Pasternak, JJ. Anesthesia for neurosurgery. In Barash PG, et al. *Clinical Anesthesia.* 8th ed. Philadelphia, PA: Wolters Kluwer Health; 2017:1003–1028.

# 272.

# SYSTEMIC, PULMONARY VASCULAR RESISTANCE AND VISCOSITY

*Maria Huarte and Surendrasingh Chhabada*

## INTRODUCTION

Hemodynamics is the study of blood flow and the physics that determines flow through vessels. The human circulatory system consists of 2 circuits connected in series (systemic and pulmonary), each with its unique characteristics, and the heart that propels blood (the cardiac output) through them.

Flow (Q) through a blood vessel is determined by the pressure gradient between both extremes of the vessel ($\Delta$P) and the resistance of the vessel to the blood flow (R), such that:

$$Q = \Delta P / R$$

Hemodynamically, flow (L/min) is represented by the cardiac output (CO), ΔP is represented by the pressure difference between the arterial and venous sides (which will be different on the systemic vs. the pulmonary circuits) and R is represented by the vascular resistance.

Therefore: CO = (Mean arterial pressure – Mean venous pressure)/Vascular resistance

Also, Vascular resistance = (Mean arterial pressure – Mean venous pressure)/CO.

In normal physiologic conditions, in both the pulmonary and systemic circulation, arterial and venous pressures are maintained relatively constant; therefore flow is highly dependent on resistance.

Based on fluids dynamics, main factors that alter systemic vascular resistance (SVR) are represented by the Hagen-Poiseuille equation:

$$R = 8 \times l \times n / \pi \times r^4$$

(where: l = length of the vessel, n = viscosity of blood, $\pi$(pi) and r = radius of the vessel)

*Note that any change in radius has a magnified impact on resistance, and because of this, a large effect on flow.*

## SYSTEMIC VASCULAR RESISTANCE (SVR)

SVR refers to the resistance that the left ventricle (LV) must overcome to push blood through the systemic circulation to create flow. In other words, it is the amount of force exerted on the circulating blood by the vasculature of the body, and it is also referred to as *total peripheral resistance* (TPR). In the absence of aortic valve stenosis, it is the major contributor to the afterload of the LV. The systemic circulatory system includes all the vessels from the aorta to the right atrium, but it is at the level of the *arterioles* where most of the resistance is represented. Changes in radius at the arteriolar level allow for fine regulation of the resistance and therefore the flow.[1] Capillaries, despite being the smallest blood vessels, are not responsible for most of the SVR because there are so many in parallel. SVR is calculated by the following equation.

### CALCULATION

$$SVR = 80 \times (MAP - CVP)/CO$$

MAP: mean arterial pressure
CVP: Central venous pressure
CO: Cardiac output

And 80 is the factor that converts units into dyne/s/cm⁵ from pressure in millimeters of mercury (mm Hg) and CO given in liters per minute (L/min).

*Normal SVR values are 900–1500 dyne.s/cm.⁵*

### FACTORS THAT INFLUENCE SVR

- Length of the vessel (l): this is constant under normal conditions.
- Viscosity of blood (n): see later discussion.
- Vessel radius (r): *Changes in the diameter of a vessel are the most important quantitatively for regulating blood flow within an organ, as well as for regulating arterial blood pressure.* Constriction and dilation, particularly in small arteries and arterioles, enable organs to adjust their own blood flow to meet their metabolic requirements.
  Vessel radius can be altered in response to extrinsic (neural and hormonal) or intrinsic (myogenic) factors.[2]
  Neural extrinsic factors are represented by sympathetic vascular tone via adrenergic innervation; hormonal extrinsic factors can cause vasoconstriction (epinephrine, norepinephrine, dopamine, angiotensin II) or vasodilation (prostaglandins, NO, histamine, etc). *Neurohumoral influence is the primary regulator of the systemic vascular tone.*
  Intrinsic myogenic mechanism involved in local blood flow regulation causes vasodilation when blood flow decreases and vasoconstriction with increasing pressure.
- Other factors:
  Laminar vs turbulent flow: normal blood flow tends to be laminar (lower energy loss). When disrupted such as with stenotic valvular lesions, energy gets wasted as friction and *more energy is required for the same amount of flow*. In other words, turbulence increases resistance to flow.

### PULMONARY VASCULAR RESISTANCE (PVR)

Like SVR, PVR refers to the resistance that the right ventricle (RV) must overcome to push blood through the pulmonary circulation to create flow. This circuit is different from the systemic one in its regulation, normal pressures, and responses to drugs.

The pulmonary vascular bed is a low-pressure high-flow system, and the pulmonary (PA) pressure is normally around one-fifth of systemic pressure. The lung vasculature can accommodate and adapt to large volumes of blood keeping its low pressures. Consequently, the morphology of the RV reflects this difference. Resistance in the pulmonary circulation at rest is located one-third in the pulmonary arteries, one-third in the capillaries, and one-third in the pulmonary veins (*in contrast to the systemic circulation, in which 70% occurs at the arterioles*).[3]

## CALCULATION

$$PVR = 80 \times (MPAP - PCWP)/CO$$

MPAP: mean pulmonary arterial pressure
PCWP: Pulmonary capillary wedge pressure
CO: Cardiac output

*Normal PVR values are 50–150 dyne.s/cm$^5$*

## FACTORS THAT INFLUENCE PVR (AND PULMONARY BLOOD FLOW)

- Alveolar hypoxia/hyperoxia: hypoxic vasoconstriction of small pulmonary arterial vessels (HPV) is induced with low alveolar partial oxygen pressure (PAO$_2$). This local response allows the diversion of blood from poorly ventilated areas, enhancing V/Q matching. Global hypoxia (severe hypoventilation, high altitude) can cause significant HPV and life-threatening increase in PVR. Inversely, high inspired oxygen causes pulmonary vasodilation (reducing PVR), as seen during transition to extrauterine life. HPV can be impaired by potent inhaled anesthetic drugs and remains largely unaffected by commonly used intravenous drugs (propofol, opiates, and benzodiazepines).
- PCO$_2$: Hypercarbia increases PVR, while hypocarbia decreases it.
- Arterial pH: Alkalosis (metabolic and respiratory) reduces PVR.
- Lung volumes: compression of intra-alveolar vessels and dilation of extra-alveolar vessels at large lung volumes (with the opposite happening at low lung volumes) determine that very low or high lung volumes have higher PVR (*lowest PVR achieved at FRC*).[4]
- Sympathetic nervous system stimulation: increases both PVR and SVR. It is extremely important to *blunt sympathetic response in patients with pulmonary hypertension.*
- Hypothermia and polycythemia: increase PVR.
- Pulmonary intravascular pressure: PVR and pulmonary intravascular pressure are inversely related. *Recruitment* and *distension* of pulmonary capillaries are mainly responsible for the increase in pulmonary capillary volume maintaining a stable PVR during situations of increased CO such as exercise.[3,4]

Pathological enlargement of open capillaries is seen in left-sided heart failure with increased right atrial pressure and pulmonary veins, over time resulting in increased PVR (secondary to reactive smooth muscle hypertrophy and fibrosis of the pulmonary vasculature).[3]

## VISCOSITY

Viscosity is the intrinsic property of fluid related to the internal friction of adjacent fluid layers sliding past one another.[5] This corresponds to the informal concept of "thickness" if a fluid, and it is directly related to resistance (as per Hagen-Poiseuille equation) and inversely related to flow. Henceforth at any given driving pressure, *flow will be reduced with increased viscosity.*

Viscosity of plasma is 1.8 times that of water, and is increased to about 4 in whole blood by the addition of formed elements (red blood cells, platelets, and white blood cells). Red blood cells have the greatest effect on viscosity, making the *hematocrit* its main determinant. Patients with an abnormally elevated hematocrit (polycythemia), have as a consequence high blood viscosity and an increase in PVR with possible decreased organ perfusion.

Other factors influencing blood viscosity are *temperature* (viscosity increases 2% per degree Celsius of temperature decrease) and situations in which platelet aggregation or plasma protein interactions occur (clotting and low flow states), which increase viscosity.[5]

## REFERENCES

1. Cavagna G. Circulation of blood. In: Cavagna G. *Fundamentals of Human Physiology.* Cham, Switzerland: Springer; 2019:1–64. https://doi.org/10.1007/978-3-030-19404-8
2. Brown G, Desvarieux T. Blood pressures and resistances. In: Freeman BS, Berger JS, eds. *Anesthesiology Core Review, Part One: Basic Exam.* New York, NY: Mc Graw Hill; 2014:429–430.
3. Cloutier MM. The pulmonary circulation. In: Cloutier MM, *Respiratory Physiology.* 2nd. ed. Philadelphia, PA: Elsevier; 2019:74–89.
4. Widrich J, Shetty M. *Physiology, Pulmonary Vascular Resistance. StatPearls* [Internet]. https://www.ncbi.nlm.nih.gov/books/NBK554380/. Published January 2020.
5. Klabunde RE. Vascular function. In: Klabunde RE, *Cardiovascular Physiology Concepts.* 2nd ed. Baltimore, MD: Lippincott Williams & Wilkins; 2012:93–123.

# 273.

# CAPILLARY DIFFUSION, OSMOTIC PRESSURE, AND STARLING'S LAW

## *Andrew Hayden and Archit Sharma*

## INTRODUCTION

The administration of IV fluids is an integral component of anesthetic practice. To understand the physiologic effects of fluid administration, one must first understand the principles that govern fluid and electrolyte movement in the body.

*Diffusion* is a term that describes this motion and is defined as the process by which particles from a zone in which the gas exerts a high partial pressure move to a zone in which it exerts a lower partial pressure.

## DETERMINANTS OF DIFFUSION

**Fick's law** describes the factors that affect the diffusion rate of a gas through fluid.[1] The various factors are as follows:

- *Diffusion coefficient of the gas*, which is influenced by molecular size, temperature, fluid viscosity, and the density of the gas;
- *Partial pressure gradient* between the capillary and the alveolus, which is influenced by alveolar gas mixture and solubility of the gas;
- *Blood-gas barrier thickness*, which is influenced by age and disease (e.g., pulmonary fibrosis);
- *Surface area of the pulmonary gas exchange surface*, which is influenced by age and disease (e.g., emphysema), pulmonary blood flow and blood volume, and V/Q matching;
- *Protein-gas binding*, which determines the affinity of hemoglobin and oxygen.

**Henry's law** states that the amount of dissolved gas in a liquid is proportional to its partial pressure above the liquid. Hence it is the inherent differences between different gases that determine their solubility. Carbon dioxide is inherently more soluble than oxygen, and thus diffuses much faster than oxygen into liquid.[2] The *more* *soluble* a gas is, the *faster* it will diffuse through a liquid medium, for example across the alveolar membrane and into capillary blood.

## OSMOTIC PRESSURE

*Osmosis* is the net diffusion of water across a membrane from areas of high to low *water* concentration (in other words, from areas of low to high *solute* concentration). Whenever there is a higher concentration of solutes on one side of a cell membrane, water will diffuse across that membrane until the water (and thus solute) concentration on both sides are equal.

*Osmotic pressure* is the osmotic force within the intravascular compartment exerted by proteins such as albumin and other macromolecules, which counteract capillary hydrostatic forces in determining net fluid flux across the endothelium.[3] Patients with hypoalbuminemia are therefore at risk for edema formation and relative hypovolemia, both of which lead to *hypoperfusion*.

The term *osmolality* is defined as the number of osmoles present in one kilogram of solvent and may be used to describe solutions containing many different particles. In the body, serum osmolality is estimated by the following equation:

$$\text{Serum osmolality} = (2 \times \text{Na}) + (\text{glucose}/18) + (\text{urea}/2.8)$$

*normal body osmolality ~ 280 mOsm per kilogram*

To determine the physiologic effect of administration of a particular fluid, one must understand the fluid's *tonicity*, as described in Figure 273.1. The ability of an extracellular solution to make water move into or out of a cell by osmosis is known as its *tonicity*.[4] A solution's tonicity is related to its *osmolarity*, which is the total concentration of all solutes in the solution.

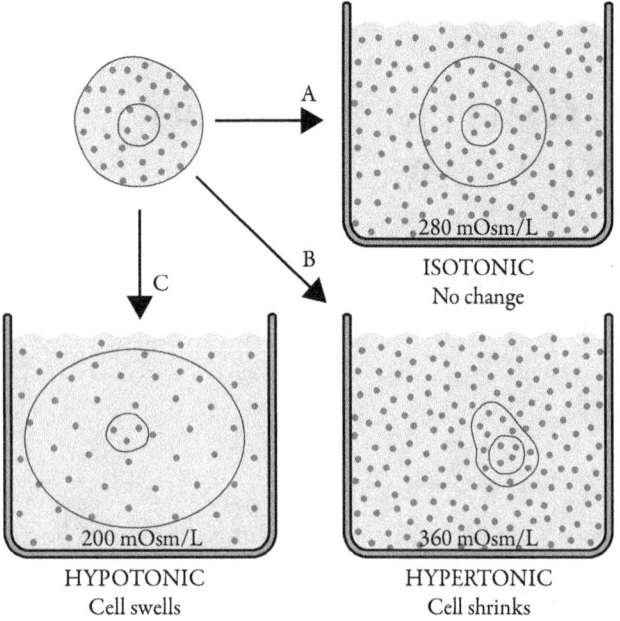

Figure 273.1. Various types of tonicity, producing different actions on cell size.

*Table 273.1* OSMOLALITY OF COMMONLY USED INTRAVENOUS FLUIDS

| FLUID | OSMOLALITY |
| --- | --- |
| Normal saline (0.9% NaCl) | 308 |
| ½ Normal saline (0.45% NaCl) | 154 |
| Hypertonic saline (1.8% NaCl) | 616 |
| Lactated ringer | 273 |
| Plasmalyte | 294 |

If a cell is placed into a solution with an osmolality of 280 mOsm/kg (the same as the body's normal osmolality), the cell with neither shrink nor swell, as the intracellular and extracellular water concentrations are equal; thus, the solution is said to be *isotonic*. If a cell is placed in a *hypotonic* solution, water will diffuse into the cell, causing cellular swelling. Conversely, a *hypertonic* solution would cause water to diffuse out of the cell, causing cellular shrinkage. Physiologic tonicity is normally maintained by hypothalamic osmoreceptors. However, there is a variety of clinical scenarios that warrant the manipulation of this tonicity via the administration of specific intravenous fluids. The osmolality of various intravenous fluids has been provided in Table 273.1.

## STARLING'S LAW

Broadly, there are two primary forces (termed *Starling forces*) that govern net fluid movement across capillary membranes: hydrostatic pressure and oncotic pressure.[5] Hydrostatic pressure is the pressure exerted by a fluid at equilibrium. Oncotic pressure (or colloid osmotic pressure) is the pressure exerted by plasma proteins that serves to prevent significant loss of fluid from the intravascular compartment. Figure 273.2 shows these forces in action. **Starling's Law** states that the fluid movement due to filtration across the wall of a capillary is dependent on the balance between the hydrostatic pressure gradient and the osmotic pressure gradient across the capillary. The balance of these forces allows calculation of the net driving pressure for filtration.

Hence, fluid moves into the extravascular space at the arteriolar end of the capillary secondary to the higher hydrostatic pressure and is subsequently reabsorbed at the venous end of the capillary due to an increased oncotic pressure. The sum of these forces (or net filtration) is summarized by the Starling equation:

$$J = K_f([P_c - P_{if}] - [\pi_p - \pi_{if}])$$

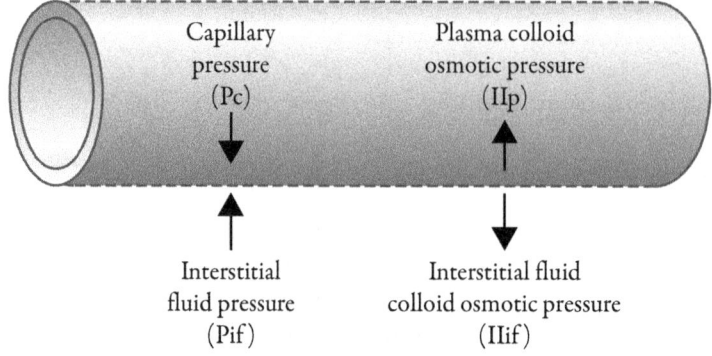

Figure 273.2. Starling forces in action: sum total of capillary hydrostatic pressure and osmotic pressure.

J is the transcapillary flow, $K_f$ is the filtration coefficient, $P_c$ is the capillary hydrostatic pressure, $P_{if}$ is the interstitial hydrostatic pressure, $\pi_p$ is the capillary oncotic pressure, and $\pi_{if}$ is the interstitial oncotic pressure.

## ANESTHETIC CONSIDERATIONS

### PREOPERATIVE

Diffusion of oxygen, which is relatively insoluble, depends on a gradient for oxygen between the alveolus and the capillary and on the time of contact of blood and alveolar air, hence the rationale for preoxygenation with 100% oxygen before induction. Carbon dioxide diffuses readily because of its high solubility.

### INTRAOPERATIVE

Isotonic solutions are used intraoperatively to increase the extracellular fluid volume due to *blood loss, surgery, dehydration,* and *fluid loss.*

### POSTOPERATIVE

Gases like nitrous oxide, nitrogen, and inert gases diffuse and equilibrate rapidly, and if adequate amount of oxygen is not provided at the end of an inhalational anesthetic, can dilute alveolar oxygen, producing "diffusion hypoxia."

### REFERENCES

1. Jaynes DB, Rogowski AS. Applicability of Fick's law to gas diffusion. *Soil Sci Soc Am J.* 1983;47(3):425–430.
2. Goldstick TK, et al. Diffusion of oxygen in plasma and blood. In: *Oxygen Transport to Tissue—II.* Boston, MA: Springer; 1976:183–190.
3. Krogh A, et al. The movement of fluid through the human capillary wall in relation to venous pressure and to the colloid osmotic pressure of the blood. *J Clin Invest.* 1932;11(1):63–95.
4. Shackford SR, et al. (1992). Intravenous fluid tonicity: Effect on intracranial pressure, cerebral blood flow, and cerebral oxygen delivery in focal brain injury. *J Neurosurg.* 1992;76(1):91–98.
5. Taylor AE. Capillary fluid filtration: Starling forces and lymph flow. *Circ Res.* 1981;49(3):557–575.

# 274.

# PRE- AND POST-CAPILLARY SPHINCTER CONTROL IN SHOCK

*Rollin Cook and Archit Sharma*

## INTRODUCTION

With each heart contraction, blood is ejected in the aorta. From the aorta, blood flows into the arteries and arterioles and, ultimately, to the capillary beds. As it reaches the capillary beds, the rate of flow is dramatically slower than the rate of flow in the aorta. This slow rate of travel through the capillary beds assists with gas (especially oxygen and carbon dioxide) and nutrient exchange. This blood is then carried by the venules that form the veins, back to the heart, and constitutes the normal circulatory system in the body.

## ANATOMY OF THE MICROCIRCULATION

<Heart→Aorta→Arteries→Arterioles→Metarterioles→ **Pre-capillary sphincter**→Capillaries→**Post-capillary sphincter**→Venules→Veins- Vena Cava→Heart>

The microcirculation refers to the smallest blood vessels in the body: the smallest arterioles, the metarterioles, the pre-capillary sphincters, the capillaries, and the small venules. Capillaries tend to arise abruptly from much larger vessels, the metarterioles. The arterioles contain vascular smooth muscle and are the major site of systemic vascular resistance.

The blood entering some capillary beds is controlled by small muscles called *pre-capillary sphincters*. A sphincter is a ringlike band of muscle that surrounds a bodily opening, constricting and relaxing as required for normal physiological functioning. If the pre-capillary sphincters are open, the blood will flow into the associated branches of the capillary bed. If all of the sphincters are closed, then the blood will flow directly from the arteriole to the venule through the thoroughfare channel, and this is known as a *shunt*. After the blood has passed through the capillary beds, it enters the venules through *the post-capillary sphincter*, then travels to the veins, and finally the two main venae cavae (singular, vena cava) that take blood back to the heart.

## ARTERIAL INFLOW

In skeletal muscle and other tissues, a large number of capillaries remain closed for long periods due to contraction of the *pre-capillary sphincter*. These capillaries provide a reserve flow capacity and can open quickly in response to local conditions such as a fall in partial pressure of oxygen ($pO_2$) when additional flow is required.[1] If the pre-capillary sphincters dilate, blood flows in the true capillaries and contributes to the exchange with the tissue cells. If the pre-capillary sphincter contracts, blood flows into the metarteriole and the thoroughfare channel, bypassing the true capillaries and the cells.

## VENOUS OUTFLOW

Venules are the smallest veins and receive blood from capillaries. They also play a role in the exchange of oxygen and nutrients for water products. There are *post-capillary sphincters* located between the capillaries and venules. The venule is very thin-walled and easily prone to rupture with excessive volume.

The smooth muscle of the metarterioles and the pre-capillary sphincters contracts and relaxes regularly, causing intermittent flow in the capillaries: this is known as *vasomotion*. A local drop in $pO_2$ is the most important factor causing relaxation of the pre-capillary sphincters.

## FUNCTION OF MICROCIRCULATION

The principal function of the microcirculation is to permit the transfer of substances between the tissues and the circulation. Substances involved include water, electrolytes, gases ($O_2$, $CO_2$), nitrogenous wastes, glucose, lipids, and drugs. Without the regulation, the cardiac output required to provide indiscriminate continuous perfusion would be too great to be sustainable.

## REGULATION OF MICROCIRCULATION

There are two primary mechanistic theories regarding the function of pre- and post-capillary sphincters in normal physiologic conditions.[2] These mechanisms are thought to vary by tissue type.[3] Both of the prevailing theories hinge on the observation that pre-capillary sphincters are either fully open or closed, and the number of open sphincters and duration of which the sphincter is open is proportional to the metabolic requirement of the tissue. The term for cyclical opening and closing of the sphincter is *vasomotion*.

1. *Vasodilator theory* is the idea that a greater rate of metabolism of nutrients and/or oxygen in tissue results in formation of vasodilatory substances within the tissue cells. The substances would then diffuse through the tissue to their site of action (i.e., pre-capillary sphincters). Possible vasodilatory agents include ions like K+, H+, adenosine, adenosine phosphate compounds, $CO_2$, and histamine. After causing vasodilation, the increased blood flow to the tissue would decrease the concentration of the vasodilatory substance, hence acting as a feedback loop, restoring function back to normal.

2. *Oxygen/nutrient demand theory* is the idea that smooth muscle surrounding vessels and in the pre-capillary sphincters requires oxygen for contraction. In the absence of oxygen, the sphincter or smooth muscle is no longer able to contract, and as a result, relaxes and dilates, increasing flow to the capillaries. The number of pre-capillary sphincters that would open up is directly proportional to the degree of requirement of nutrition by that particular tissue. One can assume that once the nutrients are adequately replaced, the pre-capillary sphincters would contract again. If there was a positive oxygen balance, then the pre-capillary sphincters would stay in a contracted state, until the oxygen and nutrients were used up.

The truth is that most likely a combination of both these mechanisms exists, which lends control to microvascular function, transport of oxygen, and nutrients to different organs of the body.[4]

## SHOCK AND THE MICROCIRCULATORY DYSFUNCTION

*Shock* is defined as a state of cellular and tissue hypoxia due to either reduced oxygen delivery, increased oxygen consumption, inadequate oxygen utilization, or a combination of these processes. The various etiologies of shock have a complex impact on the function of the microcirculation and pre- and post-capillary sphincters. This is an ongoing area of research, as the function of microvasculature has been linked to patient outcomes in critically ill patients, and practical methods of monitoring microcirculation are evolving. Typical symptoms of shock include elevated but weak heart rate, low blood pressure, and poor organ function, typically observed as low urine output, confusion, or loss of consciousness. There are four subtypes of shock with differing underlying causes and symptoms: hypovolemic, cardiogenic, obstructive, and distributive, and all shock states lead to inadequate substrates for aerobic cellular respiration. In the early stages, this is generally caused by an inadequate tissue level of oxygen. The typical signs of shock are low blood pressure, a rapid heartbeat, and signs of poor end-organ perfusion or decompensation (such as low urine output, confusion, or loss of consciousness).

The *initial* stage of shock is characterized by hypoxia and anaerobic cell respiration, leading to lactic acidosis. At this initial state, since there is inadequate circulating volume and hence inadequate perfusion, both the pre-capillary sphincters and the post-capillary sphincters relax, to flood the capillary bed with blood and nutrients.[5] Should the cause of the crisis not be successfully treated, the shock will proceed to the progressive stage, in which the compensatory mechanisms begin to fail.

In this *second* stage, the pre-capillary sphincters are relaxed, but the post-capillary sphincters resist relaxation and are closed, leading to pooling of blood in the capillary bed. As anaerobic metabolism continues, increasing the body's metabolic acidosis, the arteriolar smooth muscle and pre-capillary sphincters relax. Blood remains in the capillaries, leading to leakage of fluid and protein into the surrounding tissues. As fluid is lost, blood concentration and viscosity increase, causing blockage of the microcirculation.

Microcirculatory damage can be caused by ischemia, reperfusion, inflammation, and hypoxia, resulting in endothelial and glycocalyx and red blood cell (RBC) damage. Activation of leukocytes induces rolling, adhesion, and ultimately extravasation to the tissue, which further accelerates the inflammation. Decreased vascular permeability causes vascular leakage and edema formation. The prolonged vasoconstriction will also cause the vital organs to be compromised due to reduced perfusion. If the bowel becomes sufficiently ischemic, bacteria may enter the bloodstream, resulting in the additional complication of endotoxic shock.

## CONCLUSION

Pre- and post-capillary sphincters, along with the microcirculation, are important considerations as critical care medicine continues to advance. They play a vital role in regulating the flow of blood through the microcirculation. Restoring the hemodynamic balance in a physiologic form is the way to resolve the shock state; this is fluid administration in the case of hypovolemic and septic shock, increasing cardiac output with inotropes or mechanical assist devices (ECMO) in cardiogenic shock, and treating infections in septic shock.

## REFERENCES

1. Mellander S, Lewis DH. Effect of hemorrhagic shock on the reactivity of resistance and capacitance vessels and on capillary filtration transfer in cat skeletal muscle. *Circ Res*. 1963:13(2);105–118.
2. Bateman RM, et al. Bench-to-bedside review: Microvascular dysfunction in sepsis—hemodynamics, oxygen transport, and nitric oxide. *Crit Care*. 2003 Oct;7(5):359–373.
3. Sakai T, Hosoyamada Y. Are the precapillary sphincters and metarterioles universal components of the microcirculation? An historical review. *J Physiol Sci*. 2013;63(5):319–331. doi:10.1007/s12576-013-0274-7
4. Altura BM. Chemical and humoral regulation of blood flow through the precapillary sphincter. *Microvasc Res*. 1971;3(4):361–384.
5. Chambers R. Blood capillary circulation under normal conditions and in traumatic shock. *Nature*. 1948:162(4126):835–837.

# 275.

# VISCOSITY AND RHEOLOGY

## *David Padilla and Archit Sharma*

## INTRODUCTION

*Viscosity* is an intrinsic property of fluid related to the internal friction of adjacent fluid layers sliding past one another, which contributes to the resistance by Poiseuille's equation. It states that the flow (Q) of fluid is related to a number of factors: the viscosity (n) of the fluid, the pressure gradient across the tubing (P), and the length (L) and diameter(r) of the tubing.

$$Q = \pi \, p \, r^4 / 8\eta \, l$$

Therefore, a vessel having twice the length of another vessel will have twice the resistance to flow. Similarly, if the viscosity of the blood increases 2-fold, the resistance to flow will double. In contrast, a 2-fold increase in radius decreases resistance by 16-fold.

*Rheology* is the study of the flow of matter, primarily in a liquid or gas state, but also as "soft solids" or solids under conditions in which they respond with plastic flow rather than deforming elastically in response to an applied force. It primarily deals with flow of non-Newtonian fluids and viscoelastic substance. A Newtonian fluid (like water) is one where viscosity is not dependent on shear stress.

A non-Newtonian fluid (like paint or blood) is one where the viscosity does change with shear stress. At very low velocity gradients, there is intense aggregation and rouleaux formation between red blood cells, resulting in a higher viscosity. However, as the velocity gradient or intensity of shearing action is increased, these aggregates are more vigorously broken up and the blood becomes "thinner."

The viscosity of blood is dependent on hematocrit at every level of shear rate, with a higher hematocrit making it harder to move blood. Anemia reduces the total peripheral resistance by making the blood thinner and hence less viscous. The acute physiologic response to this is an increase in cardiac output, such that the arterial pressure remains reasonably constant. To some extent, this increase in blood flow offsets the decrease in the oxygen-carrying ability of the blood consequent to the lowered hematocrit. $O_2$ delivery is maximal in the hematocrit range from 35% to 45%.[1]

The science of rheology and the characterization of viscoelastic properties in the production and use of polymeric materials has been critical for pharmacists working in the manufacture of several dosage forms, such as simple liquids, ointments, creams, pastes, etc.

## FLUID VISCOSITY

Flow is inversely proportional to the viscosity of the fluid. Increasing viscosity decreases flow through a catheter. Viscosity of commonly infused intravenous solutions range from 1.0 centiPoise(cP) to 40.0 cP (reference: viscosity of water is 1.002 cP).

Viscosity of common infusions:

- Lactated ringers: 1.0 cP
- Hetastarch: 4.0 cP
- 5% albumin: 40.0 cP.

It is notable that the viscosity of blood increases with increasing hematocrit and decreasing temperature, hence one of the rationales for fluid warmers: warming and diluting blood prior to administration increases flow rates. Although plasma is mostly water, it also contains other proteins like albumin and fibrinogen and hence at 37°C, it is about 1.8 times more viscous than water at the same temperature; therefore, the relative viscosity ($\eta_r$) of plasma compared to water is about 1.8.[2]

Increasing red cell hematocrit increases relative viscosity in a nonlinear manner. Patients with an abnormal elevation in red cell hematocrit (polycythemia) have much higher blood viscosities. In fact, increasing the hematocrit from 40% to 60% (a 50% increase) increases the relative viscosity from 4 to 8 (a 100% increase). Increased viscosity increases the resistance to blood flow and thereby increases the work of the heart and impairs organ perfusion.

Another important factor that influences blood viscosity is temperature. When blood gets cold, it becomes "thicker" and flows more slowly. Viscosity increases about 2% for each degree Centigrade decrease in temperature. For example, if a person's hand is exposed to a cold environment and the fingers become cold, the blood temperature in the fingers falls and viscosity increases, which together with sympathetic-mediated vasoconstriction decreases blood flow in the cooled region. If clotting mechanisms are stimulated in the blood, platelet aggregation and interactions with plasma proteins occur. This leads to entrapment of red cells and clot formation, which dramatically increases blood viscosity.

The factors that determine when turbulent flow commences can be combined to form an equation which calculates the Reynolds number.

$$\text{Reynolds number} = v * \rho * d / \eta$$

where $v$ = velocity; $\rho$ = density; $d$ = diameter; $\eta$ = viscosity.

When the Reynolds number is less than 2000, there is laminar flow; when the Reynolds number is greater than 4000, flow will be turbulent. Hence, within the body, whenever a tube divides (e.g., bronchi, blood vessels) or narrows, velocity of the fluid increases, making turbulent flow likely to occur.

## ANESTHETIC CONSIDERATIONS

### PREOPERATIVE

Carotid plaque leads to increased velocity and hence turbulent flow as the Reynolds number exceeds 4000, and that is why a carotid bruit can be auscultated due to this turbulent flow.

### INTRAOPERATIVE

Intraoperatively, when blood velocity is lowered, viscosity is the highest, and this produces a higher risk of developing a deep vein thrombus (DVT).[3] During cardiopulmonary bypass in cardiac surgery, when the patient is cooled to decrease myocardial oxygen demand, blood viscosity increases, and the patient has to be hemodiluted down to a lower hematocrit to maintain the same flow.[4]

### POSTOPERATIVE

In infants that have polycythemia and respiratory distress syndrome, the increased viscosity is thought to lead to increased blood sludging and impaired circulation, and these infants have improved circulation and perfusion after phlebotomy and exchange transfusion where the hematocrit is decreased.[5]

## REFERENCES

1. Crowell JW, Smith EE. Determinant of the optimal hematocrit. *J Appl Physiol.* 1967;22(3):501–504.
2. Gordon RJ, et al. Potential significance of plasma viscosity and hematocrit variations in myocardial ischemia. *Am Heart J.* 1974;87(2):175–182.
3. Hume M, et al. *Venous Thrombosis and Pulmonary Embolism*, Vol. 15. Cambridge, MA: Harvard University Press; 1970.
4. Gordon RJ, et al. Changes in arterial pressure, viscosity, and resistance during cardiopulmonary bypass. *J Thorac Cardiovasc Surg.* 1975;69(4):552–561.
5. Kontras SB. Polycythemia and hyperviscosity syndromes in infants and children. *Pediatr Clin North Am.* 1972;19:919–933

# 276.

# REGIONAL BLOOD FLOW AND ITS REGULATION

*Anureet Walia and Archit Sharma*

## INTRODUCTION

The heart and major vessels are responsible for generating flow (cardiac output) and pressure (arterial blood pressure) adequate for the needs of the body. However, different organs and regions within organs need differing blood flow dependent upon current, past, and future metabolic needs.

Blood is a fluid and is therefore governed by the laws of fluid mechanics. Therefore, flow is governed by the Hagene-Pouiseille equation, provided flow is laminar.

$$Q = P\pi R^4 / 8\eta L$$

where Q is flow (vol/time), P is the pressure gradient across the cylinder (vessel), R is the radius of the cylinder, L is the length of the cylinder, and $\eta$ is the viscosity.

In other words, the resistance to flow in a vessel is directly proportional to its length and inversely proportional to the fourth power of the radius. Hence, a change in the radius is a key mechanism to control flow.

## REGULATION MECHANISMS

The function of blood flow is to transport materials to and from tissues. In many regions of the body, the main transport function is to meet the local metabolic demands. In several other regions, however, the primary purpose of the circulation is to provide a large flow rate for the processing of the physicochemical constituents of the blood, and the blood flow is in excess of that needed to meet the local metabolic demands.[1] The kidneys regulate the balance of water and solutes, the lungs regulate the blood gases, and the skin regulates heat balance. In these specific areas, the ratio of blood flow to oxygen consumption ($V_B/O_2$) is in excess of the amount needed to maintain just the metabolic needs of an organ. The blood flow and oxygen consumption in a given region determine the difference in $O_2$ content between the arterial and venous blood ($\Delta A - \dot{V}O_2$).

Therefore, the A-VO$_2$ difference is inversely related to the ($V_B/O_2$) ratio.

*Intrinsic* mechanisms of local blood flow regulation contribute to the precise matching of a tissue's metabolic needs to the quantity of blood flow delivered by the microcirculation. These mechanisms (vasodilatory mechanism, oxygen deficiency mechanism, and myogenic mechanism) are dependent on the specific organ system. Local blood flow can also be regulated by factors *extrinsic* to the local tissues, which include neural mechanisms or hormones which affect the contraction of arterioles and pre-capillary sphincters through the autonomic nervous system.

Broadly, there are two major means of local regulation of blood flow, which are described in the following:

1. *Metabolic control*, which consists of metabolites and chemical agents released from surrounding tissue that act on the blood vessels. For example, as tissue metabolism increases, oxygen is used up and the amount of available oxygen decreases, driving down the pH and triggering a release in adenosine, which triggers the blood vessel to vasodilate.
2. *Myogenic control*, which originates from the wall of the blood vessel itself and consists of both muscle reflexes and products released from endothelial cells that line the vessel. These endothelial products include nitric oxide (NO) and endothelin-1 that are released in response to either chemical stimuli, like histamine, or increased shear stress on the blood vessel. While NO causes vasodilation, endothelin-1 causes vasoconstriction.

The following are examples of different types of local blood flow regulation, by specific organ systems (Table 276.1). In each case, there is a specific type of intrinsic regulation occurring in order to maintain or alter blood flow to that given organ alone, instead of creating a systemic change that would affect the entire body.

*Table 276.1* REGIONAL DISTRIBUTION OF THE TOTAL CARDIAC OUTPUT

| ORGAN SYSTEM | PERCENTAGE OF BLOOD FLOW |
|---|---|
| 1. Coronary | 5 |
| 2. Cerebral | 15 |
| 3. Splanchnic | 25 |
| 4. Renal | 22 |
| 5. Cutaneous | 8 |
| 6. Muscular | 17 |
| 7. Other regions | 8 |
| Total Systemic Circ. | 100 |

- *Cerebral* circulation is highly sensitive to changes in partial pressure of carbon dioxide ($pCO_2$), as well as the hydrogen ion concentration. Both of these factors affect pH and, in turn, the balance between vasodilation versus vasoconstriction in the brain.[2] So, the blood vessels found specifically in the brain respond to changes in dissolved $CO_2$ levels. Low $pCO_2$ levels, or hypocapnia, can cause cerebral vasoconstriction and vice versa.
- *Coronary* circulation is controlled at the local level primarily by metabolic control mechanism. More specifically, it is regulated by adenosine, a local vasodilator produced by neighboring cells.[3] Therefore the heart is influenced by a form of metabolic control through the effects of paracrine signaling.
- *Renal* circulation is primarily controlled by tubule-glomerular feedback, which is a system of organ-specific autoregulation that directly affects renal blood flow.[4]
- *Pulmonary* circulation undergoes hypoxic vasoconstriction, which is a unique mechanism of local regulation in that the blood vessels in this organ react to hypoxemia, or low levels of dissolved oxygen in the blood, in the opposite way as the rest of the body.[5] The blood vessels in the lungs vasoconstrict to decrease blood flow in response to low oxygen.
- *Splanchnic* circulation, which supplies blood to several gastrointestinal organs, is influenced by gastrointestinal hormones and metabolites, such as vasodilatory kinins, released from the cells lining the intestines, bile acids from the gallbladder, and byproducts of digestion.
- *Skeletal* muscle is influenced by multiple factors. First, metabolites that are produced by active muscle use can alter skeletal muscle tone. Second, skeletal muscle can undergo hyperemia, which is a mechanism of local blood flow, leading to an increase in blood flow to the affected skeletal muscle.
  - *Active hyperemia* is one subtype, which occurs in response to increased metabolic demand, meaning high oxygen requirements within the tissue. It follows the principle of metabolic control, with the release of vasodilatory substances in response to increased oxygen demand.
  - *Reactive hyperemia* is the second subtype, which occurs after a short interruption, or arrest, in blood flow. In response to the blood flow interruption, a temporary compensatory vasodilation occurs as soon as blood flow has resumed, due to release of vasodilatory substances like adenosine, which are released in response to the blood flow interruption.

## REFERENCES

1. Coleman TG, et al. Control of cardiac output by regional blood flow distribution. *Ann Biomed Eng.* 1974;2(2):149–163.
2. Sato A, Sato Y. Regulation of regional cerebral blood flow by cholinergic fibers originating in the basal forebrain. *Neurosci Res.* 1992;14(4):242–274.
3. Tune JD, et al. Matching coronary blood flow to myocardial oxygen consumption. *J Applied Physiol.* 2004;97(1):404–415.
4. Gurbanov KO, et al. Differential regulation of renal regional blood flow by endothelin-1. *Am J Physiol Renal Physiol.* 1996 Dec 1;271(6):F1166–1172.
5. Bergofsky EH. Mechanisms underlying vasomotor regulation of regional pulmonary blood flow in normal and disease states. *Am J Med.* 1974;57(3):378–394.

# 277.

# REGULATION OF CIRCULATION AND BLOOD VOLUME

*Kirk Dressen and Archit Sharma*

## INTRODUCTION

The distribution of blood flow in any particular organ or tissue of the body is primarily controlled by local tissue mechanisms in proportion to metabolic needs. Three mechanisms ensure adequate blood flow, blood pressure, and perfusion: *neural, endocrine,* and *autoregulatory* mechanisms.[1]

## NEURAL CONTROL

Neural regulation of blood pressure and flow depends on the cardiovascular centers located in the medulla oblongata, which respond to changes in blood pressure (BP) and concentration of oxygen and carbon dioxide.

### AUTONOMIC NERVOUS SYSTEM

Flow between different areas of the body is largely regulated by the autonomic nervous system via control of systemic arterial pressure and heart function. Both sympathetic and parasympathetic impulses originate from an area in the brain called the *vasomotor center* occupying the medulla and lower third of the pons. Separate vasoconstrictor (that excite sympathetic preganglionic vasoconstrictor neurons), vasodilator (that inhibit vasoconstrictor activity), and sensory areas (that provide reflex control of circulation via vagus and glossopharyngeal nerves) in this center have been identified. Additionally, the hypothalamus, amygdala, hippocampus, and many parts of the cerebral cortex have been shown to excite or inhibit this vasomotor center.[2] The *cardioaccelerator* centers stimulate cardiac function by regulating heart rate and stroke volume via sympathetic stimulation from the cardiac accelerator nerve. The *cardioinhibitor* centers slow cardiac function by decreasing heart rate and stroke volume via parasympathetic stimulation from the vagus nerve. The *vasomotor* centers control vessel tone or contraction of the smooth muscle in the tunica media, changing systemic vascular resistance and cardiac output.

*Baroreceptors* are stretch receptors located within thin areas of blood vessels and heart that respond to the degree of stretch caused by the presence of blood. The *aortic sinuses* are found in the walls of the ascending aorta just superior to the aortic valve, whereas the *carotid sinuses* are in the base of the internal carotid arteries. When blood pressure rises too high, the baroreceptors fire at a higher rate and trigger parasympathetic stimulation of the heart. When blood pressure drops too low, the rate of baroreceptor firing decreases, hence increasing cardiac output.[3]

*Chemoreceptors* also monitor levels of oxygen, carbon dioxide, and hydrogen ions (pH), and thereby contribute to vascular homeostasis. For example, an increase in carbon dioxide and hydrogen ion levels (falling pH) causes the chemoreceptors to respond by stimulating the cardioaccelerator and vasomotor centers, increasing cardiac output and constricting peripheral vessels.

## ENDOCRINE CONTROL

Endocrine control over homeostatic mechanisms involves the secretion of epinephrine and norepinephrine, as well as several hormones that interact with the kidneys in the regulation of blood volume.

### CATECHOLAMINES

Epinephrine and norepinephrine are released by the adrenal medulla and enhance and extend the body's sympathetic or "fight-or-flight" response. They increase heart rate and force of contraction, while temporarily constricting blood vessels to organs not essential for fight-or-flight responses and redirecting blood flow to the liver, muscles, and heart.[4]

### ANTIDIURETIC HORMONE (ADH)

Another hormone important in regulating extracellular fluid volume is ADH or vasopressin, which is secreted by the cells in the hypothalamus and stored in the posterior pituitary, where it is stored until released upon nervous stimulation. It increases water permeability of the distal tubule, collecting tubule, and collecting duct epithelia, leading to increased water reabsorption. Several different natriuretic hormones also help regulate blood volume.

## ATRIAL NATRIURETIC PEPTIDE (ANP)

Specific cardiac atrial cells secrete a peptide called ANP, in response to atrial stretch during conditions of fluid overload and elevated atrial blood pressure. ANP inhibits both renin secretion and the resorption of sodium and water, primarily in the renal collecting duct, causing a decrease in blood volume and blood pressure.

## RENIN-ANGIOTENSIN-ALDOSTERONE SYSTEM (RAAS)

In conjunction with pressure natriuresis and diuresis, both nervous and hormonal mechanisms regulate renal excretion to exert control on body fluid. Increases in reflex sympathetic activity from conditions such as hemorrhage produces several effects: constriction of renal arterioles to reduce glomerular filtration rate, an increase in salt and water reabsorption through activation of alpha-adrenergic receptors on the renal tubular epithelial cells, and stimulation of the RAAS. Decrease in renal blood flow leads to secretion of renin from juxtaglomerular cells of the kidney. This further leads to conversion of angiotensin I to angiotensin II and formation of aldosterone. Angiotensin II is a powerful hormone that imparts three effects: stimulates aldosterone secretion from the zona glomerulosa cells of the adrenal cortex; constricts efferent renal arterioles to increase filtration fraction and net tubular resorption; and directly stimulates sodium resorption at the proximal tubule, thick ascending loop of Henle, and collecting tubule. Aldosterone acts in the cortical collecting tubule to increase sodium reabsorption and potassium excretion. Conversely, when sodium intake is higher than normal, downregulation of the renin-angiotensin-aldosterone system works to reduce the increase in extracellular fluid and arterial pressure.[5]

## AUTOREGULATORY CONTROL

Autoregulation requires neither specialized nervous stimulation nor endocrine control. These are the self-regulatory mechanisms that allow each region of tissue to adjust its blood flow and perfusion via chemical control of sphincters and myogenic responses. Precapillary sphincters are opened in response to decreased oxygen concentrations; increased

$CO_2$ concentrations; increasing levels of lactic acid, potassium ions, or hydrogen ions (falling pH); further leading to nitric oxide (NO) production and vasodilation.

When blood flow is low, the vessel's smooth muscle is only minimally stretched. In response, it relaxes, allowing the vessel to dilate and thereby increase the movement of blood into the tissue. Conversely, when the flow is high, the smooth muscle will contract in response to the increased stretch, prompting vasoconstriction that reduces blood flow.

## ANESTHETIC CONSIDERATIONS

### PREOPERATIVE

In congestive heart failure, stimulation of the sympathetic nervous system and the renin-angiotensin-aldosterone system can increase blood volume by 15%–20%, while extracellular fluid can increase by as much as 200%.

### INTRAOPERATIVE

In patients presenting with hypovolemic shock, such as massive hemorrhage, homeostatic mechanisms try to increase perfusion by increasing heart rate and vascular resistance, due to low intravascular volume. However, restoration of intravascular volume to normal is the treatment strategy in shock.

### POSTOPERATIVE

Neurogenic shock is a form of vascular shock that occurs with cranial or spinal injuries that damage the cardiovascular centers in the medulla oblongata, leading to hypotension, usually after an intracranial hemorrhage or brainstem stroke.

### REFERENCES

1. Harrison TR, et al. The regulation of circulation: VIII. The relative importance of nervous, endocrine and vascular regulation in the response of the cardiac output to anoxemia. *Am J Physiol-Legacy.* 1927;83(1):284–301.
2. Guyenet PG. The sympathetic control of blood pressure. *Nature Rev Neurosci.* 2006;7(5):335–346.
3. Guazzi M, Zanchetti A. Carotid sinus and aortic reflexes in the regulation of circulation during sleep. *Science.* 1965;148(3668):397–399.
4. Lohmeier TE. The sympathetic nervous system and long-term blood pressure regulation. *Am J Hypertens.* 2001;14(S3):147S–154S.
5. Hall JE, Hall ME. *Guyton and Hall Textbook of Medical Physiology.* Elsevier Health Sciences; 2020.

# 278.

# BASICS OF CARDIOPULMONARY RESUSCITATION

## Donnie Laborde

## BASIC LIFE SUPPORT

The term *basic life support* (BLS) refers to airway maintenance and support of breathing and circulation. Early intervention or activating emergency medical services (EMS) and initiating cardiopulmonary resuscitation can greatly improve a patient's outcome. The sooner BLS can be initiated, the better the outcome. When initial assessment, airway maintenance, ventilation, and chest compressions are combined, the term *cardiopulmonary resuscitation* (CPR) is used.[1,2]

## INITIAL ASSESSMENT

Initial assessment is the first step in BLS. Check for responsiveness by conducting a tap and shout method and asking, "Are you ok?" If the individual is unresponsive, activate EMS and get an automatic external defibrillator (AED), if available. Simultaneously, within 5–10 seconds, check for pulse and abnormal breathing (e.g., lack of breathing or gasping). If there is a pulse, rescue breathing at the rate of 1 breath every 5–6 seconds with a pulse check every 2 minutes is necessary. If there is no pulse, begin chest compressions at the ratio of 30 compressions to 2 breaths.

## CHEST COMPRESSIONS

In adults, the required compression rate is 100–120 per minute with a depth of 2 inches, or 5 cm. Allow complete chest recoil after each compression. High-quality chest compressions are vital. The circulation of blood is a result of increasing the intrathoracic pressure, not just direct pressure on the heart. This pressure takes several compressions to build up a "prime" and to maintain circulation. This is one reason why manual CPR will give you only 25%–35% of normal cardiac output and coronary effusion. If a provider gets tired and compressions become weak or slow, you will lose this prime; therefore, it is recommended that every 2 minutes providers should rotate to ensure adequate chest compressions. The target compression fraction must be at least 60%, with a goal of 80%. Interruption of chest compressions must be limited to less than 10 seconds to maximize coronary perfusion and blood flow.

## AUTOMATED EXTERNAL DEFIBRILLATOR (AED)

The AED should be utilized as soon as it is available. If an AED is utilized within 2 minutes of cardiac arrest, survival rate improves by approximately 50%. When possible, continue chest compressions and breaths while another provider is powering on the AED and attaching pads. No person should be touching the patient when the AED indicates it is analyzing a heart rhythm. If a shock is advised, verbally announce to "stand clear" and then deliver a shock. Continue CPR compressions and ventilation at a 30:2 ratio, immediately following the shock. Every 2 minutes the AED will begin to analyze the heart rhythm again. If there is a nonshockable rhythm, resume CPR immediately for 2 minutes, until prompted by AED to allow a rhythm check.

## CARDIAC ARREST

Essentially, in cardiac arrest, there is no circulation of blood providing oxygen to the cells of the body. If any cell is without oxygen for up to 6 minutes, the cells begin to necrose. CPR is an attempt to get necessary air into the lungs and is accompanied by chest compressions to circulate the blood and carry it to the cells of the body. This is why, for every minute we fail to respond to cardiac arrest, there is a 10% less chance of survival due to cellular death. Get the oxygen in and circulated! The central nervous system (CNS) does not contain myoglobin and cannot store any extra oxygen. Any decreased cerebral circulation for more than 10 minutes may cause permanent neural damage. This is why chest compressions are the most important tool we have in BLS and should not be interrupted for more than 10 seconds.

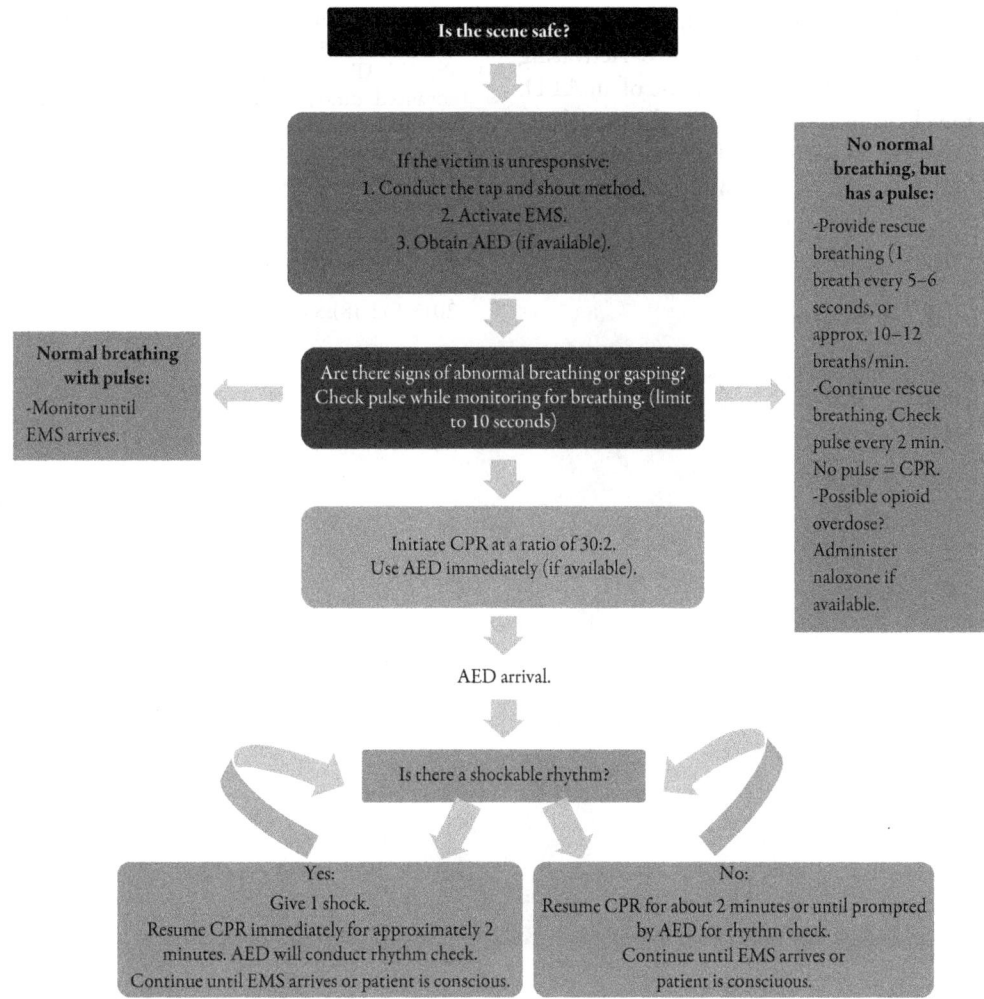

**Figure 278.1.** The BLS adult cardiac arrest algorithm.

From: Kleinman ME et al. Part 5: Adult basic life support and cardiopulmonary resuscitation quality: 2015 American Heart Association guidelines update for cardiopulmonary resuscitation and emergency cardiovascular care. *Circulation.* 2015;132(18):S414–435.

If a patient is unconscious with abnormal or absent breaths, it is reasonable to assume cardiac arrest. The American Heart Association (AHA) recommends for a layperson, untrained in CPR, to provide chest-compression-only CPR.[3] If there is a suspected spinal injury, one hand should be placed on either side of the patient's head for stabilization purposes. The use of immobilization devices by lay rescuers may be harmful. The airway of an unconscious person who is breathing normally is at risk of both tongue obstruction and aspiration of mucus or vomit. Placing the victim on their side will prevent these issues and allow for these fluids to drain from the mouth. This position is known as the recovery position and has been used by providers for years.[3]

## COMMON ERRORS

There are common errors that providers encounter when administering BLS. One of the most common errors is inadequate compression. One way to check your rate of compressions is to notice if you have completed 5 cycles of 30 compressions with 2 breaths within the 2-minute necessary time frame. Additionally, the depth should be at least 2 inches, or 5 cm. Another common error is hyperventilation. If hyperventilation occurs, the blood $PCO_2$ (partial pressure of carbon dioxide) levels may decrease to the levels where the central chemoreceptors are not stimulated. $PO_2$ (partial pressure of oxygen) levels to the brain are already decreased due to the fact that even high-quality chest compressions are only about 25%–35% of the normal oxygen delivery to the body and brain. In the CNS, the levels of blood $PCO_2$ are the primary stimulus for effective breathing rate and depth.

## BLS SKILL REVIEW

The techniques involved in BLS need to be taught, learned, and remembered by the providers.[1,2] Annual or bi-annual BLS skill reviews will likely be mandated by the providers' employer. This is essential in maintaining skills in the event of an emergency. At present, survival rate improvement rests in the hands of increased education in CPR. Activating EMS, alongside initiation of BLS with the use of an AED, is imperative in the chain of survival. While the guidelines for BLS are intended for adults, these skills can be used to increase survival rates in infants and children, as well (see Figure 278.1 for the BLS algorithm).

# REFERENCES

1. Handley AJ. Basic life support. *Br J Anaesth*. 1997;348:g1730. doi:10.1136/bmj.g1730.

2. Nolan JP. Basic life support. *Curr Opin Anaesthesiol*. 2008;21(2):194–199. doi:10.1097/ACO.0b013e3282f49cb4.

3. Panchal AR et al. American Heart Association focused update on advanced cardiovascular life support: Use of advanced airways, vasopressors, and extracorporeal cardiopulmonary resuscitation during cardiac arrest: An update to the American Heart Association Guidelines. *Circulation*. 2019;140:e881–e894.

4. Kleinman ME, et al. Part 5: Adult basic life support and cardiopulmonary resuscitation quality: 2015 American Heart Association guidelines update for cardiopulmonary resuscitation and emergency cardiovascular care. *Circulation*. 2015;132(18):S414–435.

# Part XIX

# ANATOMY

# 279.

# CORONARY CIRCULATION

*Keith A. Andrews and Mada Helou*

## INTRODUCTION

Coronary arterial and venous anatomy is a complex system of vessels that carry blood to and from the myocardium, since the blood contained in the heart chambers does not perfuse the myocardium itself. The left and right main coronary arteries arise from the aorta via ostia (small openings) behind the right and left aortic valve cusps. Hence, the third aortic cusp is named the non-coronary cusp. The left main artery divides into anterior descending and circumflex branches. The right coronary artery also travels in the atrioventricular groove on the right side of the heart, terminating in the posterior descending artery (PDA) in the majority of the population. *Coronary dominance is dictated by which coronary artery, right or left, gives rise to the PDA.* Following myocardial perfusion, deoxygenated blood returns to the right atrium via the coronary sinus and the anterior cardiac veins, with a small amount of blood returned directly into the heart chambers, including the left ventricle, by way of the thebesian veins.[1-3] Italicized elements of this chapter represent high-yield information for the Anesthesia Basic exam (see Figure 279.1).

## ARTERIAL SUPPLY

The left main coronary artery courses anterior and caudad over the cardiac surface, primarily as the left anterior descending (LAD) and circumflex arteries. The LAD is notable for perfusion of the following regions: most of the ventricular septum, anterior left ventricle, most of the right and left bundle branches, and partial supply to the left ventricular anterolateral papillary muscle.[1] This vessel terminates at the inferior aspect of the cardiac apex.[2] Along its course, it has several perfusing branches, most typically the first diagonal, first septal perforator with three to five additional septal perforators, some right ventricular branches, and frequently two to six additional diagonal branches. At its termination, the LAD provides collateral circulation to additional areas of the right ventricle via the

circle of Vieussens and even to the posterior descending artery from the right-sided circulation.[1,2]

*Critically, the regions supplied almost exclusively by the LAD are represented by leads V3–V5 on standard ECG; therefore aberrancy in these leads suggests pathology in the LAD.*

The left circumflex artery (LCX) courses posteriorly around the heart in the left atrioventricular (AV) sulcus, terminating near the obtuse margin of the left ventricle. In a minority of the population (10%–15% of individuals) it continues around the crux of the heart as the posterior descending artery, making that portion of the population "left-heart dominant."[1,3] The LCX is notable for perfusing the left atrium, posterolateral left ventricle, anterolateral papillary muscles of the left ventricle, and the sinoatrial (SA) node. Along its course, it typically has the following perfusing branches: SA nodal branch in 40%–50% of the population, left atrial circumflex branch, anterolateral marginal branch, and posterolateral marginal branches. It terminates in either the distal circumflex artery or as the posterior descending in left-dominant individuals, as described previously.[1]

*Of vital clinical importance is the representation of the LCX perfused regions via leads I and aVL on standard ECG.*

The right coronary artery (RCA) emerges between the pulmonary trunk and the right atrium before coursing over the coronary surface in the right AV sulcus. Along its course it typically has many perfusing branches, including the conus artery, SA nodal artery (50%–60% of individuals), anterior right ventricular branches, right atrial branches, acute marginal branch, AV nodal and proximal bundle branches.[1,3]

Of particular relevance, the posterior descending artery (PDA) comes from the RCA in 85%–90% of the population, providing blood supply to the AV node and making right-sided coronary dominance the most common configuration. The PDA then travels past the cardiac apex in the posterior AV sulcus, terminating as either the left ventricular branch or to anastomose with the LCX.[1]

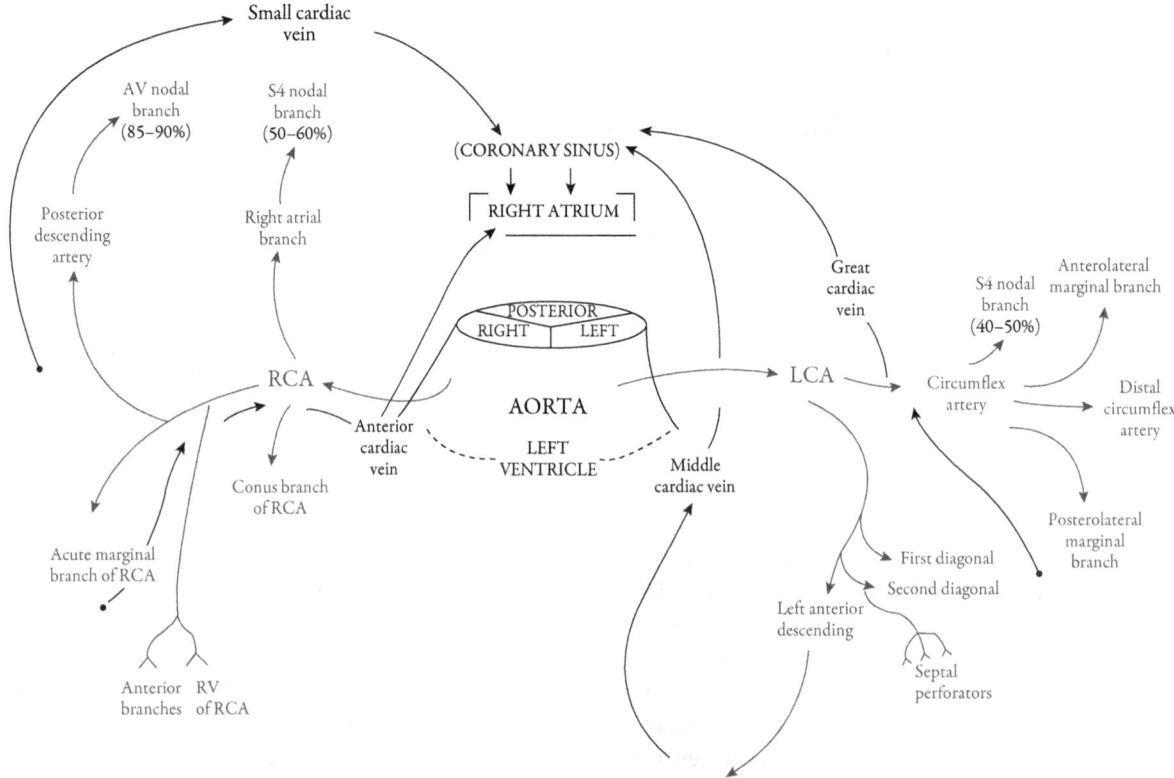

**Figure 279.1.** Simplified drawing of coronary arteries and veins.

*Lastly, the RCA is represented by leads II, III, and aVF on standard ECG.*

## VENOUS RETURN

There are three primary systems for draining freshly perfused myocardium and returning deoxygenated blood to circulation. The largest is the coronary sinus, which is located in the posterior AV groove. The coronary sinus effectively drains the left ventricle and left atrium via the great, middle, and small cardiac veins, posterior veins of the left ventricle, and left oblique atrial vein. The coronary sinus empties into the right atrium.[1]

The anterior cardiac vein travels along with the RCA to drain the right ventricular wall, entering directly into the right atrium. Lastly, the thebesian veins, accounting for only approximately 15% of coronary venous drainage, drain into both the right atrium and left ventricle. Consequently, a small portion of deoxygenated blood is sent to the systemic circulation from the left heart, bypassing the pulmonary circuit.[1]

## REFERENCES

1. Ramakrishna H. *Faust's Anesthesiology Review.* 4th ed. Philadelphia, PA: Elsevier Saunders; 2015:119–122.
2. Winchester DE, Pepine CJ. Nonobstructive atherosclerotic and nonatherosclerotic coronary heart disease. In: Fuster V, et al., eds. *Hurst's The Heart.* 14th ed. McGraw-Hill; 2017. https://accessmedicine.mhmedical.com/content.aspx?bookid=2046&sectionid=176555511. Accessed May 10, 2020.
3. Cardiovascular physiology and anesthesia. In: Butterworth IV JF, et al., eds. *Morgan & Mikhail's Clinical Anesthesiology.* 6th ed. McGraw-Hill; 2018. https://accessmedicine.mhmedical.com/content.aspx?bookid=2444&sectionid=193559221. Accessed September 10, 2020.

# 280.

# DIGOXIN

*Carlos M. Perez-Ruiz and Ali Abdullah*

## INTRODUCTION

Digoxin is one of the oldest cardiovascular medications used today. Digoxin is classified as a cardiac glycoside and was initially approved by the Food Drug Administration (FDA) in 1954.[1] The glycosides are composed of two portions: a sugar and a cardenolide (hence the name "glycosides").[2] Digoxin causes increased availability of intracellular calcium by inhibiting the sodium-potassium ATPase on the cell membrane of cardiac myocytes.[3] This leads to an increase in cytosolic $Na^+$, thereby decreasing the activity of $Na^+$–$Ca2^+$ exchange and indirectly resulting in an increase in intracellular $Ca2^+$ available to interact with actin and myosin (Figure 280.1).[3]

## INDICATIONS AND THERAPEUTIC USES

In clinical practice, the indications for digoxin include anti-arrhythmic and heart failure support (Table 280.2).

*Table 280.1* CARDIAC GLYCOSIDES

| CARDIAC GLYCOSIDES | |
| --- | --- |
| Digitalis | • Derived from purple foxglove flower (*Digitalis purpurea*).<br>• Prescribed for heart failure |
| Digoxin | • Derived from (*Digitalis lanatus*), more reliable pharmacokinetic and remains major form of cardiac glycosides used today.<br>• Mainly eliminated by the kidneys |
| Digitoxin | • Is a secondary glycoside extracted from *Digitalis purpurea*.<br>• It has a longer half-life than digoxin<br>• Toxic effects, which are similar to those of digoxin, are longer lasting<br>• More highly protein bound than digoxin<br>• Mainly eliminated via hepatic metabolism |

*Table 280.2* THERAPEUTIC USES OF DIGOXIN AND INDICATIONS

| INDICATIONS | THERAPEUTIC USES OF DIGOXIN |
| --- | --- |
| Arrhythmias | Decreased AV nodal conduction<br>Decreased ventricular rate in atrial flutter and fibrillation |
| Heart failure | Increased inotropy<br>Increased ejection fraction<br>Decreased preload<br>Decreased pulmonary congestion/edema |

*Table 280.3* PHARMACOKINETICS OF DIGOXIN

| | PHARMACOKINETICS EFFECTS |
| --- | --- |
| Absorption | Oral bioavailability 60%–80% |
| Distribution | After drug administration, a 6–8-hour tissue distribution phase seen<br>*Volume of Distribution*: Large (~ 640 L/70 kg): binds to skeletal muscle<br>Digoxin crosses both the blood-brain barrier and the placenta. |
| Metabolism | Only a small percentage (13%) of a dose of metabolized. Metabolism via hydrolysis, oxidation, and conjugation. Does not induce or inhibit the cytochrome P-450 system. |
| Elimination | First-order kinetics elimination<br>90% renal excretion<br>Normal renal function: half life 36–48 hours |

*Table 280.4* PHARMACODYNAMIC EFFECTS OF DIGOXIN

| PHARMACODYNAMIC EFFECTS |
| --- |
| *Onset of Action (Intravenous)*: ~30 minutes<br>*Time to Peak Effect (Intravenous)*: 1–5 hours<br>*Onset of Action (Oral)*: ~30 min to 2 hours<br>*Time to Peak Effect (Oral)*: 2–6 hours<br><br>*Hemodynamic Effects (Short- and Long-term)*:<br>1) Increases: Cardiac output, left ventricular ejection fraction<br>2) Lowers: Pulmonary artery pressure, pulmonary capillary wedge pressure and systemic vascular resistance |

## PHARMACOKINETICS AND PHARMACODYNAMICS

### MECHANISM OF ACTION

Digoxin is a potent inhibitor of cellular Na+/K+–ATPase. Inhibiting the Na$^+$/K$^+$–ATPase causes an increase in intracellular sodium concentration, leading to an accumulation of intracellular calcium via the Na$^+$-Ca$^{++}$ exchange system. In the heart, increased intracellular calcium causes more calcium to be released by the sarcoplasmic reticulum (SR), thereby more calcium available to bind to troponin-C (TnC), which increases contractility (inotropy) (Figure 280.2).

### TOXICITY

Therapeutic levels of digoxin are *0.8–2.0 ng/mL*. The toxic level is *>2.4 ng/mL*.

Digoxin has a *narrow therapeutic window*, and prevention of toxicity depends on understanding the pharmacokinetics and the risk factors for toxicity.

### ECG CHANGES

Digoxin can cause a multitude of dysrhythmias due to (Figure 280.1):

1. Increased automaticity (increased intracellular calcium): manifests with premature atrial beats or premature ventricular beats, which are considered an early sign of overdosing. At higher levels, atrial and ventricular tachyarrhythmias may occur.
2. Diminished impulse contraction (increased vagal effects at AV node): lengthening PR interval which may progress to atrioventricular block.
- Younger patients more likely to develop bradycardia
- Elderly patients and patients with severe myocardial dysfunction are more prone to developing ventricular dysrhythmias and atrial ectopy.
- The degree of blockade is potentiated by concomitant use of beta blockers and calcium channel blocking agents.

### SIGNS AND SYMPTOMS OF DIGOXIN TOXICITY

- Confusion
- Irregular pulse
- Loss of appetite
- Nausea, vomiting, diarrhea
- Vision changes (unusual), including blind spots, blurred vision, changes in how colors look, or seeing spots.

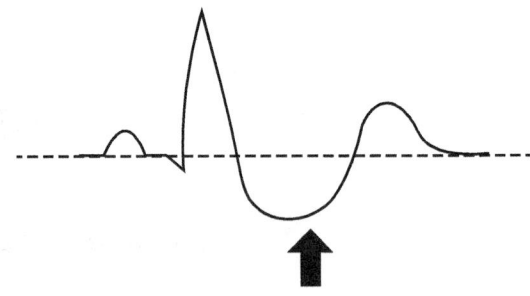

**Figure 280.1.** EKG changes

### ECG FEATURES OF DIGOXIN TOXICITY

- Frequent PVCs (most common abnormality), including ventricular bigeminy and trigeminy
- Sinus bradycardia
- Slow atrial fibrillation
- Any type of AV block (1st degree, 2nd degree, and 3rd degree)
- Ventricular tachycardia, including polymorphic and bidirectional VT.

### RISK FACTORS FOR DIGOXIN TOXICITY

The risk factors for digoxin toxicity include: advanced patient age, renal failure (including chronic kidney disease), electrolyte disturbances (hypokalemia), metabolic disorders, and drug interactions.

### MANAGEMENT

Treatment of digoxin toxicity relies on normalizing plasma potassium levels and minimizing arrhythmias by avoiding potential risk factors. Life-threatening digoxin toxicity can be treated with *anti-digoxin antibodies*.[3] These polyclonal antibodies form 1:1 complexes with digoxin that are rapidly cleared from the body.[3] Fab fragments of these antibodies (i.e., the portion of the antibody that interacts with antigen) have been shown to be less immunogenic than anti-digoxin immunoglobin G (IgG) and have a larger volume of distribution, more rapid onset of action, and increased clearance compared to the intact IgG.[3]

Supportive care of digoxin toxicity includes the following:

- Hydration with IV fluids
- Oxygenation and support of ventilatory function
- Discontinuation of the drug and correction of any electrolyte imbalances (correct hypokalemia; concomitant hypomagnesemia may result in refractory hypokalemia)

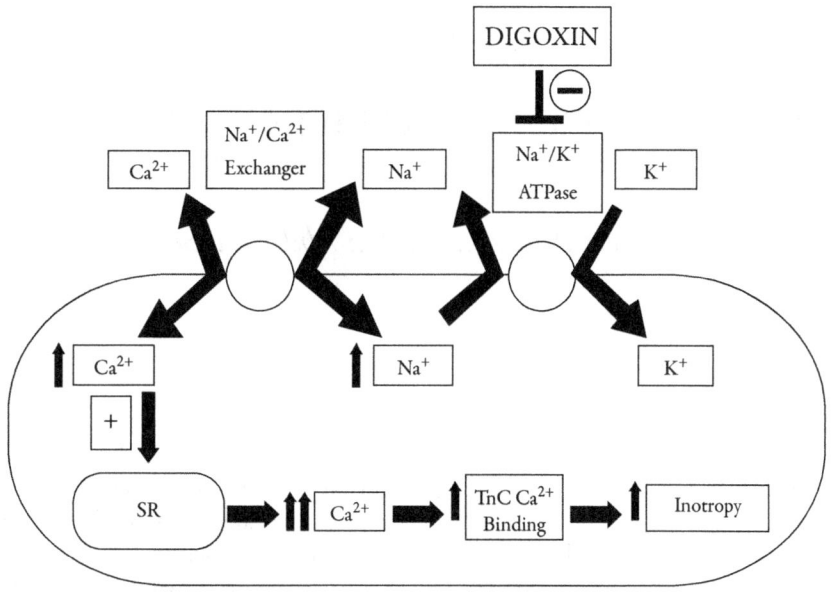

**Figure 280.2.** Mechanism of action of Digoxin

- Treatment with digoxin Fab fragments is indicated for a K+ level greater than 5 mEq/L
- Hemodialysis may be necessary for uncontrolled hyperkalemia.

### DIGOXIN IMMUNE FAB

Digoxin immune Fab is considered the first-line treatment for significant dysrhythmias from digitalis toxicity.[4] Other indications for its use include the following:

- Ingestion of massive quantities of digoxin (in children, 4 mg or 0.1 mg/kg; in adults, 10 mg)
- Serum digoxin level greater than 10 ng/mL in adults at steady state (i.e., 6–8 hours after acute ingestion or at baseline in chronic toxicity)
- Hyperkalemia (serum potassium level greater than 5 mEq/L)
- Altered mental status attributed to digoxin toxicity
- Rapidly progressive signs and symptoms of toxicity.

### ANESTHETIC CONSIDERATIONS

Patients should take their prescribed digoxin dose on the day of surgery. A preoperative digoxin level in patients who are compliant and asymptomatic is not indicated.

1. Monitoring serum digoxin level is particularly important in patients with chronic renal dysfunction or rapidly changing renal function, patients with electrolyte disturbances (e.g., hypokalemia and hypomagnesemia), and in noncompliant patients.
2. During surgery, electrolyte disturbances need to be evaluated and corrected.
3. Use caution with diuretics, which may predispose to electrolyte disturbances and arrhythmias.
4. New cardiac arrhythmias intraoperatively may require ruling out digoxin toxicity.

### REFERENCES

1. Giardina, EG. Treatment with digoxin: Initial dosing, monitoring, and dose modification. In: Post T, ed. *UpToDate*. Waltham, MA: UpToDate; 2020. https://www.uptodate.com/contents/treatment-with-digoxin-initial-dosing-monitoring-and-dose-modification.
2. FDA. Approved drug products: Lanoxin (digoxin) prescribing information. https://www.accessdata.fda.gov/drugsatfda_docs/label/2019/020405s015lbl.pdf. Published August 2009.
3. Amstrong EJ, Rocco TP. Pharmacology of cardiac contractility. In: Golan DE, et al., eds. *Principles of Pharmacology*. 2nd ed. Baltimore, MD: Lippincott Williams & Wilkins; 2008:335–338.
4. Patel V, et al. Digitalis toxicity. *Medscape*. https://emedicine.medscape.com/article/154336-overview. Published January 4, 2017.
5. Whayne TF Jr. Clinical use of digitalis: A state of the art review. *Am J Cardiovasc Drugs*. 2018 Dec;18(6):427–440.

# 281.

# HEART CONDUCTION SYSTEM

*Robert Pellicer and Alaa Abd-Elsayed*

## INTRODUCTION

The cardiac conduction system is a specialized collection of cells that generate and propagate action potentials throughout the heart in order to facilitate the synchronized contraction of myocardium. The system consists of the sinoatrial (SA) node, the atrioventricular (AV) node and the His-Purkinje system. Impulses initiated in the SA node contribute to synchronized atrial contraction and propagation of action potentials toward the AV node. The P wave of the electrocardiogram (ECG) corresponds to depolarization of the atria. When the action potential reaches the AV node, there is a brief delay prior to further propagation of the impulse. This delay corresponds to the PR interval of the ECG and is important in preventing simultaneous contraction of the atria and ventricles. After the AV node, the signal propagates down the bundle of His, which branches into the right and left bundle branches, toward the Purkinje fibers (Figure 281.1). The Purkinje fibers are specialized conduction cells that rapidly carry the cardiac impulse from the bundle branches to the ventricular myocardium to trigger ventricular contraction. Depolarization of the ventricles is rapid, lasting 0.06–0.10 seconds, and corresponds to the QRS complex of the ECG. The cardiac conduction system is regulated by the autonomic nervous system, which allows modulation of the speed of electrical conduction in order to meet the demands of varying metabolic states. Sympathetic nerves are distributed to all parts of the heart, especially the ventricular muscle. Parasympathetic nerves are distributed via the vagus nerve mainly to the SA and AV nodes and to a lesser extent to the atria.

## SINOATRIAL NODE

The sinoatrial node is a specialized collection of pacemaker cells located in the right atrium. The main function of the SA node is to initiate a cardiac action potential that will propagate along the length of the cardiac conduction system to initiate myocardial contraction. The rhythmogenicity of the SA node can be attributed to the pacemaker current (also referred to as the "funny current"), a spontaneously generated current mediated by specialized hyperpolarization-activated cyclic nucleotide-gated (HCN) channels.[1] These channels primarily dictate potassium permeability across the membrane and are regulated by cyclic nucleotides cCMP and cAMP. The inward sodium-potassium current is activated by hyperpolarization of cardiac myocytes in the diastolic voltage range and may be modulated by beta adrenergic and M2 muscarinic receptor stimulation. While other regions of the conduction system also have pacemaker potential (AV node, Purkinje fibers), the higher inherent rate of the SA node inhibits these regions from acting as pacemakers.

## ATRIOVENTRICULAR NODE

The AV node is located in the interatrial septum near the coronary sinus and regulates electrical conduction propagated toward the ventricles from the SA node. One of the primary functions of the AV node is to delay signal propagation long enough to allow the atria to empty prior to ventricular contraction. This delay is represented by the PR interval of the ECG and is 120–200 ms in length. The intrinsic pacemaker rate of the AV node is 40–60 bpm, which is generally slower than the SA node. If electrical conduction from the SA node is disrupted, the AV node will take over as pacemaker, setting a slower ventricular rate. Recent studies suggest that certain cardiac disease processes may contribute to AV node remodeling that may increase the risk of arrhythmias, including complete heart block. These data suggest a new mechanism of cardiac remodeling that involves altered expression of cardiac ion channels, rather than fibrosis and sclerosis.[2]

## HIS-PURKINJE SYSTEM

After leaving the AV node, signal propagation proceeds to the bundle of His, where it is transmitted to the right and left bundle branches along the interventricular septum.

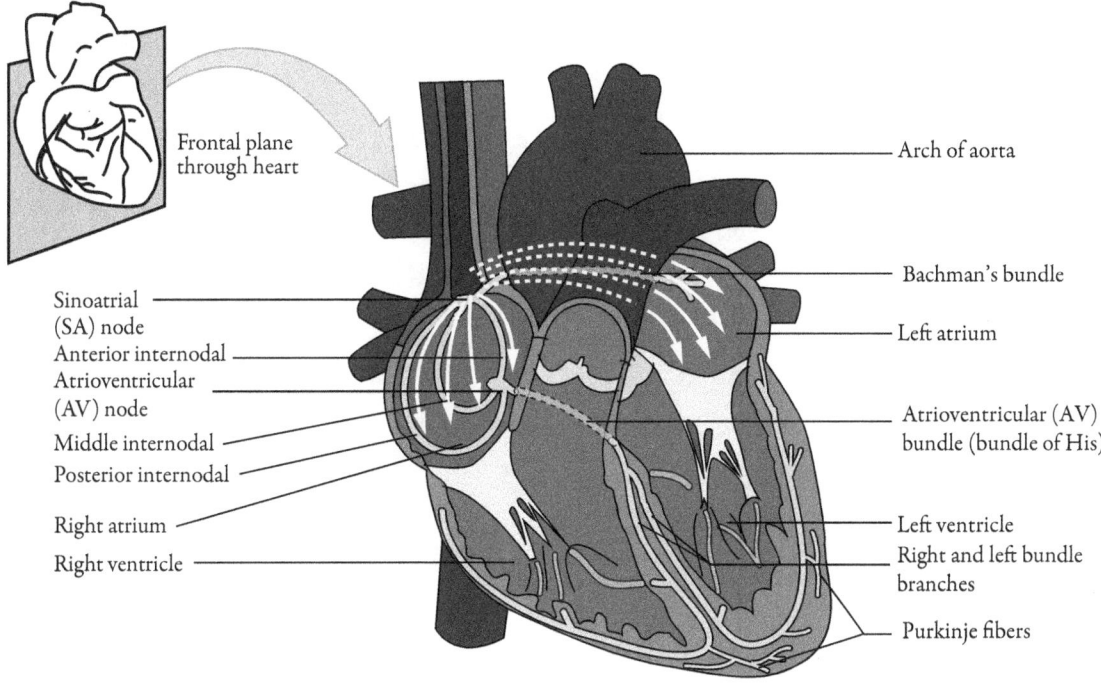

**Figure 281.1.** Diagram of heart with elements of cardiac conduction system.
OpenStax College/CC BY (https://creativecommons.org/licenses/by/3.0).

The bundle branches contain fascicles that allow action potentials to propagate more effectively to distal areas of the myocardium. The fascicles and bundle branches terminate into Purkinje fibers, which carry the action potential to the ventricular myocardium. Synchronized ventricular contraction is dependent on effective signal propagation along the fascicles and bundle branches. If these electrical connections are disrupted, ventricular depolarization may be prolonged and ventricular contraction may be impaired. Bundle branch blocks and fascicular blocks are characterized by altered electrical conduction from the bundle of His to the Purkinje fibers. Characteristic ECG findings include a prolonged QRS and altered QRS morphology.

## CONDUCTION REGULATION

Autonomic regulation of the heart is mediated by preganglionic sympathetic fibers arising from T1–T4 and parasympathetic innervation via the vagus nerve. The adult resting heart rate is around 65–75 beats/minute and reflects predominant parasympathetic tone at the SA node. Different physiologic states may alter the balance of autonomic input, causing signal propagation to increase or decrease throughout the cardiac conduction system.

Beta-1 adrenergic receptors are present in the SA node, AV node, and on atrial and ventricular cardiac myocytes.

Beta-1 stimulation increases heart rate by modulating sodium, potassium, and calcium permeabilities in the SA node. During periods of exercise or stress, increased sympathetic neural activity increases cAMP levels in the SA node, which leads to increased opening of the HCN channels, leading to increased chronotropy.

Muscarinic receptors in the SA and AV nodes mediate parasympathetic activity and, when stimulated, become hyperpolarized due to increased potassium conductance. This slows action potential generation at the SA node and decreases signal conduction through the AV node. Cardiac muscarinic receptors are primarily located in the SA node, AV node, and atria. While parasympathetic activity may alter atrial contractility, it does little to modulate ventricular contractility. Therefore, any decrease in cardiac output that may occur with increased parasympathetic activity is the result of decreased atrial contractility.[3]

## REFERENCES

1. DiFrancesco D. The role of the funny current in pacemaker activity. *Circ Res.* 2010;106(3):434–446.
2. Temple IP, et al. Atrioventricular node dysfunction and ion channel transcriptome in pulmonary hypertension. *Circ Arrhythm Electrophysiol.* 2016;9(12).
3. Gordan R, et al. Autonomic and endocrine control of cardiovascular function. *WJC.* 2015;7(4):204.

# Part XX

# PHARMACOLOGY OF
# PHOSPODIESERASE III INHIBITORS

# 282.

# PHOSPHODIESTERASE III INHIBITORS (INOTROPIC DILATORS)

*Muin Haswah and Igor Kolesnikov*

## INTRODUCTION

Phosphodiesterases (PDEs) are a class of enzymes that hydrolyze and terminate the intracellular actions of cyclic monophosphate secondary messengers, including cyclic adenosine monophosphate (c-AMP) in a variety of tissues. Of relevance to this review, the human myocaridum contains PDE III isoenzyme that is bound to the sarcoplasmic reticulum (SR) and is responsible for cleaving active c-AMP to its inactive metabolite adenosine monophosphate. Therefore, inhibition of the PDE III isoenzyme leads to an increase of intracellular c-AMP (Figure 282.1). Increased cAMP level mediates the phosphorylation of protein kinases, which in turn activates intracellular cardiac calcium. This calcium influx from the SR during phase 2 (the plateau phase) of the cardiac action potential leads to a positive inotropic effect of PDE3 inhibitors, as they will increase the force of cardiac contraction (increased inotropy).[2] Increased diastolic calcium storage will also lead to its systolic release during contraction. As such, an increased reflux of calcium into the SR following the plateau phase is responsible for the observed positive lusitropic effect, demonstrating that PDE III inhibiting agents increase myocardial relaxation speed.

PDE III inhibitors possess several other mechanisms of actions and have a variety of outcomes. They can act as vasodilators through mediation of cyclic guanosine monophosphate (c-GMP) in vascular smooth muscle. Mean arterial, venous, and coronary pressures may be modestly reduced or augmented during infusions of this drug, unless preload is supplemented with another agent. These actions are anti-ischemic in patients with coronary disease undergoing heart surgeries. Additionally, improved mixed venous admixture may be observed through its reduction in myocardial oxygen consumption.

An increased lusitropy is depicted on the myocardial pressure-volume loop as a rightward shift of the diastolic filling phase and a reduction in the slope, following Frank-Starling laws. Positive lusitropy will deliver a reduced left ventricular end-diastolic pressure with increased volumes during this phase. This effect will also increase coronary perfusion pressure.[3] Isovolumetric contraction will therefore occur resulting in greater inotropy, at a point where there is greater left ventricular end-diastolic volume, and subsequently giving greater stroke volumes with improved myocardial relaxation.

Milrinone is the most commonly used PDE III inhibitor for our review. Milrinone is a bypyridine derivative, an isoenzyme PDE III inhibitor. This inhibition decreases the hydrolysis of c-AMP, leading to increased intracellular concentration of c-AMP in the myocardium and vascular smooth muscle. Increased intracellular concentration of c-AMP (and to a lesser effect on c-GMP) results in stimulation of protein kinases

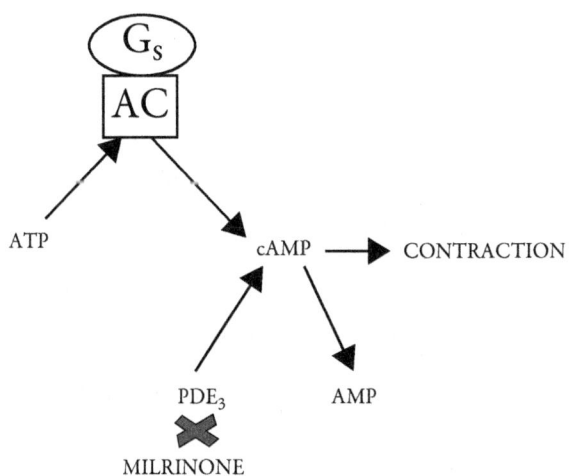

**Figure 282.1.** Cardiac muscle.
Abbreviations: G$_s$: G$_s$ protein; AC: adynyl cyclase; PDE$_3$: phosophodiesterase III; cAMP: cyclic adenosine monophosphate.

that phosphorylate substances responsible for the up-take, storage, and release of calcium from the SR during excitation-contraction coupling. Milrinone enhances the effects of catecholamines, which also increase c-AMP concentrations through beta-adrenergic stimulation. Milrinone is a derivative of amrinone (also known as imamrinone).[2] It has 20–75 times the inotropic potency of the parent compound amrinone. It is available in an IV and PO formularions.

## ANESTHETIC CONSIDERATIONS

Milrinone increases cardiac index, while decreasing systemic vascular resistance and cardiac filling pressures. Heart rate is generally unchanged. In patients with CHF, milrinone does not significantly increase myocardial oxygen consumption. There is a balanced arterial and venous dilation with a corresponding fall in systemic and pulmonary vascular resistances, and analogous left and right heart-filling pressures. Cardiac output increases due to the stimulation of myocardial contractility and the decrease in left ventricular afterload.[1]

- Adult intravenous (IV) dosing: 50 mcg/kg IV over 10 min, followed by 0.375–0.75 mcg/kg/min infusion. This is not to exceed 1.13 mg/kg/day.
- Onset time: 5–15 min
- Elimination half-time: 2.7 hours (up to 20 hours on Continuous Veno-Venous Hemofiltration (CVVH) renal replacement therapy)
- Metabolism/Excretion: greater than 70% will be protein bound. Excretion is hepatic (<15%) and renal (80% excreted unchanged, as majority is not metabolized).

## CLINICAL CONSIDERATIONS

In setting of severe renal dysfunction (GFR <50 ml/min), careful attention should be given to reduce the dose or avoid it entirely.[3,5]

## SIDE EFFECTS

Side effects include arrhythmia, tachycardia, hypotension, thrombocytopenia by inhibiting platelet aggregation (most commonly with amrinone), hypokalemia, tachyphylaxis, elevated transaminase levels, and increased arterial hypoxemia through an intrapulmonary shunt.[3,5]

## CONTRAINDICATIONS

Contraindications include obstructive cardiomyopathy, hypovolemia, tachycardia, ventricular aneurysm, and usage while breastfeeding.[2]

## COMMON PDE III INHIBITING MEDICATIONS

These include the following:

- *Heart failure*: milrinone, amrinone, inamrinone, enoximone;
- *Peripheral arterial disease (PAD)*: ciloztazol, dipyridamole.
- *Non-specific PDE inhibition used in PAD and obstructive lung disease*: theophylline, aminophylline.[2,4]

## CARDIOVASCULAR EFFECTS

Cardiovasuclar effects include positive inotropy, chronotropy, inodilation, increased lusitropy, increased ejection fraction, increased stroke volume, increased contractility, increased cardiac index and output, decreased afterload, pulmonary vasodilation and systemic vasodilation through reducing systemic and pulmonary vascular resistance, decreased preload, improved diastolic relaxation, and synergistic effect with adrenergic agents.[1,4]

## CLINICAL USE

PDE III inhibiting medications are used in combination with adrenergic agonists to wean patients following cardiac bypass surgeries. Commonly used for patients with comorbid pulmonary hypertension undergoing cardiac surgery to improve vasodilation or those with peripheral arterial disease.[2,4]

## REFERENCES

1. Kikura M, et al. The effect of milrinone on hemodynamics and left ventricular function after emergence from cardiopulmonary bypass. Anesth Analg. 1997 Jul;85(1):16–22.
2. Flood P, et al. *Stoelting's Pharmacology & Physiology in Anesthetic Practice*, 5th ed. Wolters Kluwer; 2014.
3. Barash P, et al. *Clinical Anesthesia*, 7th ed. Wolters Kluwer; 2015:243–244.
4. Levy JH, et al. Intravenous milrinone in cardiac surgery. Ann Thorac Surg. 2002 Jan;73(1):325–330.
5. Miller R, et al. *Miller's Anesthesia*, 8th ed. Churchill Livignstone; 2015:870, 1705.

# 283.

# ANTIARRHYTHMICS

*Greta Nemergut*

## INTRODUCTION

The Vaughan-Williams classification of antiarrhythmics is based on where the drug has its primary effect on the phases of the action potential (AP) of a myocardial cell.[1,2] There are four classes of antiarrhythmic drugs based on this model. Modifications and updates have been added to the model that further explain the mechanisms of the drugs as they relate to actions on ion channels and receptors and consider potential new drug pipelines.[2] A new class, class 0, has been proposed that includes a new drug and new mechanisms of action. This chapter will review how antiarrhythmics exert their primary action and which drugs fall in each class of antiarrhythmics.

## ACTION POTENTIAL

Action potential of the cardiac cell starts and finishes at phase 4, resting potential. Class II antiarrhythmics work at this phase. Phase 0 is depolarization and results from an influx of sodium ions. Class I antiarrhythmics exert their action at this phase. Depolarization is followed by repolarization, in Phases 1, 2 and 3, when other ion shifts occur (potassium and calcium) making the membrane more negative. Class III agents work on phase 1 and 3, while Class IV agents work on phase 2[1,2] (Figure 283.1).

## ANTIARRHYTHMIC CLASSES

There are four primary classes of antiarrhythmic drugs. However, a new class, class 0, has been added, the introduces a new mechanism of action and drug product. The classes of antiarrythmics, their mechanisms of action, and included drug products are described below. Table 283.1 provides a summary of the classes and each drug that included in the class.

## CLASS 0

This newer class includes the pacemaker channel HCN4 modulators that affect the pacemaker current $I_f$. Heart rate is reduced due to prolongation of diastolic repolarization and slowing the firing of the sinoatrial (SA) node.[1,2] The sole drug in this class is ivabradine.

## CLASS I: SODIUM-CHANNEL BLOCKERS

These drugs are divided into three subgroups based on their kinetics. The primary action is blocking sodium channels and inhibiting Phase 0, depolarization.[1,2]

Class Ia drugs (quinidine, procainamide, disopyramide) block sodium channels as well as potassium channels, to a lesser degree. They have anticholinergic effects that reduce contractility.[1,2] These drugs have not shown mortality benefits and are not widely used in current practice.[1]

Class Ib (lidocaine, mexiletine) work on inactivated sodium channels in the depolarized tissues. They work best on tachyarrhythmias.[1,2]

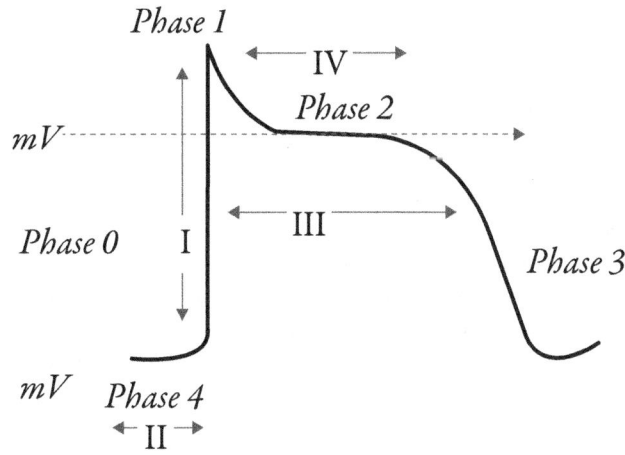

**Figure 283.1.** Phases of action potential of the cardiac cell.

**Table 283.1** ANTIARRHYTHMIC CLASSES

| CLASS | DRUGS |
|---|---|
| Class 0: HCN channel blockers | Ivadrabine |
| Class I: Sodium channel blockers | Ia: quinidine, disopyramide, procainamide<br>Ib: lidocaine, mexiletine<br>Ic: propafenone, flecainide |
| Class II: Beta blockers | Nonselective: carvedilol, propranolol, nadolol<br>Selective: atenolol, bisoprolol, betaxolol, esmolol, metoprolol |
| Class III: Potassium channel blockers | Amiodarone, dronedarone, dofetilide, ibutilide, sotalol |
| Class IV: Calcium channel blockers | Verapamil, diltiazem |

**Table 283.2** ROUTES OF ADMINISTRATION

| INTRAVENOUS FOR ACUTE USE | ORAL FOR CHRONIC USE |
|---|---|
| Beta blockers (esmolol, atenolol, metoprolol) | Beta blockers (carvedilol, propranolol, nadolol, atenolol, bisoprolol, betaxolol, metoprolol) |
| Calcium channel blockers (verapamil, diltiazem) | Calcium channel blockers (verapamil, diltiazem) |
| Sodium channel blockers<br>Ia (procainamide)<br>Ib (lidocaine) | Sodium channel blockers<br>Ia (quinidine, disopyramide)<br>Ib (mexiletine)<br>Ic (flecainide, propafenone) |
| Potassium channel blockers (ibutilide, amiodarone) | Potassium channel blockers (sotalol, dofetilide, amiodarone, dronaderone) |

Class Ic drugs (flecainide, propafenone) block open sodium channels, slowing conduction. They remain on the sodium channels for some time and have use-dependent kinetics, resulting in increased activity at a faster heart rate. This characteristic contributes to their antiarrhythmic effects, but can also be a reason for their proarrhtymic effects in some patients with structural heart disease. They also block potassium channels, and propafenone has beta-blocker activity.[1,2]

## CLASS II: BETA BLOCKERS

This class of antiarrhythmics work primarily via beta blockade inhibiting sympathetic activity and controlling heart rate. Beta blockers can be non-selective, binding to both beta-1 (myocardial) and beta-2 (pulmonary) receptors, and selective, where they bind primarily to beta-1 receptors. They also increase adenylyl kinase activity and cyclic adenosine monophosphate (cAMP), reducing the SA node pacemaker rate.[1,2]

## CLASS III: POTASSIUM CHANNEL BLOCKERS

This class works on potassium channels and lengthens the AP duration. The drugs included are: amiodarone, dronedarone, ibutilide, dofetilide, sotalol. The drugs have other antiarrhythmic effects as well. Sotalol also exerts beta blockade, and at doses of less than 160 mg it does not show any class III effects; amiodarone and dronedarone block

sodium channels (similar to a Class Ib agent), calcium channels, potassium channels, and adrenergic receptors. Ibutilide enhances the slow delayed inward sodium current and blocks potassium channels.[1,2]

## CLASS IV: CALCIUM CHANNEL BLOCKERS

This class includes the nondihydropyridines, verapamil, and diltiazem. These drugs work by increasing the refractory period of the atrioventricular (AV) node and control sinus rate. They are also used to prevent or stop SVTs that are dependent on the AV node.[1,2] Other calcium channel blockers, the dihydropyridines (e.g., amlodipine) do not have antiarrhythmic activity.

## ROUTE OF ADMINISTRATION

Antiarrhythmics are available in intravenous (IV) and oral forms, to allow for acute and chronic use. The drugs classes and available forms are listed in Table 283.2.

## REFERENCES

1. Mankad P, Kalahasty G. Antiarrhythmic drugs: Risks and benefits. *Med Clin N Am* 2019;103:821–834.
2. Makielski JC, Eckhardt LLL. Cardiac excitability, mechanisms of arrhythmia, and action of antiarrhythmic drugs. In: Levy S. ed. *UpToDate.* Waltham, MA: UpToDate. https://www.uptodate.com August 2020.

# 284.

# VASOPRESSORS AND INOTROPES

*Jacqueline Sohn and Nicholas Pesa*

## INTRODUCTION

Activation of α-, β-, or dopamine-adrenergic receptors lead to various cardiovascular effects. $\beta_1$-adrenergic receptor activation in particular can lead to various effects in the heart, including positive chronotropy (increase in heart rate), positive dromotropy (increase in conduction velocity), positive inotropy (increase in contractility), and positive lusitropy (better ability of the myocardium to relax).[1] *Inotropes* refer to pharmacological agents that produce increased contractility of the heart. *Vasopressors* are agents that increase vascular tone by causing vasoconstriction. Although different, it is important to note that some of the adrenergic agonists have both vasopressor and inotropic effects. These adrenergic agents can be categorized by either their structures or their function. Structurally, there are natural catecholamines, which are derived from β-phenylethylamine and normally made in the body, synthetic catecholamines, and synthetic non-catecholamines.[1] For non-catecholamines, they can be divided into groups depending on their function: sympathomimetics, phosphodiesterase (PDE) inhibitors, and others (e.g., digoxin).

## PHYSIOLOGY

The common mechanism of action for positive inotropic drugs is to increase intracellular calcium in myocardium and the effectiveness of calcium interaction with troponin C, and faster removal of calcium after contractions.[1] Catecholamines mediate their effects through $\alpha_1$-, $\beta_1$-, $\beta_2$-adrenergic receptors, and dopaminergic receptors.[2] These adrenergic receptors are G-protein coupled receptors. Stimulation of $\beta_1$- and $\beta_2$-adrenergic receptors lead to activation of $G_s$-GTP unit, resulting in increased cyclic adenosine monophosphate (cAMP) and increased cytosolic calcium (Figure 284.1). This increase in intracellular calcium results in positive inotropy and positive chronotropy of the heart.[1,2] Stimulation of $\beta_2$-adrenergic receptors also cause smooth muscle relaxation such as bronchodilation. Activation of $\alpha_1$-adrenergic receptors leads to activation of $G_q$-GTP

unit. This leads to hydrolysis of phosphatidylinositol 4,5-bisphosphate ($PIP_2$) by phospholipase C (PLC) into diacylglycerol (DAG) and inositol triphosphate ($IP_3$). $IP_3$ increases cytosolic calcium by releasing intracellular storage, and DAG activates protein kinase C.[1,2] These effects lead to smooth muscle contraction and vasoconstriction.

## SPECIFIC AGENTS

### ENDOGENOUS CATECHOLAMINES

#### Epinephrine

Epinephrine is a naturally occurring catecholamine that is synthesized, stored, and released in adrenal medulla. It works non-selectively on adrenergic receptors α, $\beta_1$, and $\beta_2$. However, at lower doses (0.01–0.05 μg/kg/min), its effects are more β-receptor dominant, whereas at higher doses, its effects are more α-receptor dominant.[1,3] Its clinical use includes treatment of anaphylaxis, severe asthma

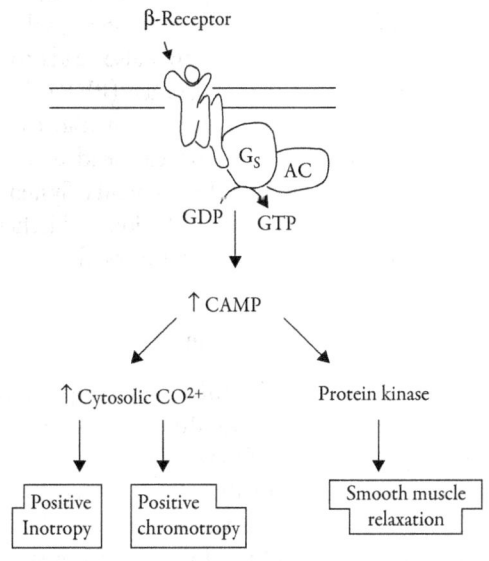

**Figure 284.1.** β-adrenergic receptor pathway.
AC: adenylyl cylase. $\beta_2$-adrenergic receptors also have $G_i$-GTP action, which is not depicted here.

or bronchospasm, cardiac arrest, and cardiogenic shock. In anaphylaxis, epinephrine is used for its $\alpha$ and $\beta$-adrenergic effects. Through $\alpha$-adrenergic receptors, mean arterial pressure (MAP) is increased by vasoconstriction of small arterioles and precapillary sphincters.[3] Activation of $\beta$-adrenergic receptors cause bronchodilation and stabilization of mast cells, which decreases the release of inflammatory mediators such as histamine and tryptase.[1] For cardiac arrest, high-dose epinephrine is used for its $\alpha$-adrenergic effects to increase MAP and increase cerebral perfusion pressure.[1] For cardiogenic shock or low cardiac output state, epinephrine can be useful for its $\beta_1$-adrenergic receptor activation leading to increased inotropy. Epinephrine cannot cross the blood-brain barrier and lacks action on the central nervous system. Other effects include increased liver glycogenesis and adipose lipolysis ($\beta_1$), inhibition of insulin secretion ($\alpha_1$), mydriasis, hepatosplanchnic vasoconstriction, and hypercoagulability.[1,3]

## Norepinephrine

Norepinephrine, like epinephrine, is also a naturally occurring sympathetic neurotransmitter. It has both $\alpha_1$ and $\beta_1$ effects, but greater $\alpha_1$ than $\beta_1$-adrenergic effects; it has almost no $\beta_2$-adrenergic effects. Therefore, it is considered to be a predominantly vasoconstrictive agent. However, it is commonly included in the discussion of inotropes, because of its $\beta_1$-adrenergic effects. Norepinephrine is the first-line drug for sepsis, because of its potent vasoconstrictor effects to increase MAP and total peripheral vascular resistance.[1,3] Its effect is minimal on cardiac output due to increase in resistance against ventricular ejection.[1] Heart rate remains unchanged or decreased due to almost no $\beta_2$-adrenergic effects and also due to reflex-bradycardia, which is a baroreceptor-mediated vagal activity.[1,2,3] Due to vasoconstriction mediated by the $\alpha_1$-adrenergic receptor activation, there is decreased blood flow to the kidney, mesenteric, splanchnic, and hepatic vessels. Furthermore, this also leads to an increase in pulmonary vascular resistance (PVR). Excessive vasoconstriction from norepinephrine can lead to various adverse effects. Severe hypertension can lead to increased cardiac demand, causing myocardial ischemia. Systemic vasoconstriction can also cause hypoperfusion and ischemia in renal, mesenteric, splanchnic, peripheral vessels.[1,3]

## Dopamine

Dopamine is another naturally occurring catecholamine that activates $\beta_1$- and $\alpha_1$-adrenergic receptors, and $D_1$-dopaminergic receptors. Dopamine is used to increase cardiac output mostly via its direct $\beta_1$-adrenergic receptor activity. Dopamine has high variability, even in healthy patients, in its net effect. At high doses, it directly stimulates $\beta_1$-adrenergic receptors and also increases norepinephrine release from the sympathetic nerve terminals. At even higher doses, $\alpha_1$-adrenergic receptor activity predominates, resulting in generalized peripheral vasoconstriction. At low dose, dopamine can increase renal blood flow and induce natriuresis and diuresis. However, this "renal dose dopamine" is not recommended because it did not show any efficacy in preventing acute renal failure.[1,2,3] Dopamine is associated with sinus tachycardia and dose-related ventricular arrhythmias more than dobutamine or epinephrine. It can also lead to myocardial ischemia due to tachycardia, increased contractility, increased afterload, and possible coronary artery vasospasm. Furthermore, at high doses, it can lead to decreased splanchnic perfusion and gut ischemia, and reduced ventilatory response to hypoxemia. Dopamine infusion can decrease pituitary hormone functions and immune functions, because dopamine is an endogenous neurotransmitter in hormonal regulation and in the immune system.

## SYNTHETIC CATECHOLAMINE

### Dobutamine

Dobutamine is a synthetic catecholamine that directly acts on $\beta$-receptors. Its activity on $\beta_1$-adrenergic receptors is much more potent than on $\beta_2$-receptors. Dobutamine is often used for diagnostic perfusion imaging (dobutamine-induced stress echocardiography) to noninvasively assessed reversible myocardial ischemia.[1,3] It can also be used in patients with decreased cardiac output, such as in congestive heart failure or while weaning from cardiopulmonary bypass.[2] Similar to epinephrine, dobutamine also has a potential to cause tachycardia and arrhythmias leading to myocardial ischemia in susceptible patients.

### Isoproterenol

Isoproterenol is a synthetic catecholamine derived from dopamine. It acts on $\beta$-adrenoreceptor non-selectively. It has very low affinity for $\alpha$-adrenergic receptor and has almost no $\alpha$-adrenergic effects. It increases chronotropy and inotropy through $\beta_1$-adrenergic receptor activation. Its effect on $\beta_2$-adrenergic receptor causes arterial vasodilation, leading to decreased systemic vascular resistance (SVR). This can further lead to decrease in left ventricular (LV) preload, reduced coronary perfusion pressure, and decreased diastolic filling time.[1] It fell out of favor for use due to its potential to cause tachyarrhythmias and acute myocardial ischemia or subendocardial necrosis.

## SYMPATHOMIMETICS

### Ephedrine

Ephedrine is a synthetic sympathomimetic agent that has both indirect and direct actions. Its indirect activity stimulates release of endogenous norepinephrine, resulting in both α- and β-adrenergic effects, which are further magnified by its direct activity on α- and β-adrenergic receptors. It leads to increase in MAP, myocardial contractility, heart rate, and cardiac output.[1,3] Tachyphylaxis, or ceiling effect, occurs with repeated doses, most likely due to depletion of endogenous norepinephrine storage. Ephedrine can cross the blood-brain barrier, which can lead to agitation and insomnia. It can also cause urinary retention in patients with prostatic hypertrophy and precipitate a hypertensive crisis in patients who are taking monoamine oxidase inhibitors (MAOIs).[1]

## Phenylephrine

Phenylephrine is a direct selective $\alpha_1$-adrenergic receptor agonist.[1,4] Although very similar to epinephrine structure, it has a missing hydroxyl group on the phenyl ring, which makes it very selective on the $\alpha_1$-adrenergic receptor.[1] Activation of $\alpha_1$-adrenergic receptor leads to increased venous and arterial vasoconstriction, leading to increase in both LV preload and afterload. Therefore, baroreceptor-mediated reflex bradycardia occurs very commonly. It also increases pulmonary artery pressures through pulmonary arterial constriction.[1] These effects can potentially lead to decreased cardiac output in a heart that has impaired LV function or is dependent on afterload, but in a normal heart cardiac output is unchanged.[1] Phenylephrine is frequently used in hypotension with normal or elevated heart rate and in obstetric anesthesia.

## VASOPRESSORS USED IN OBSTETRICS ANESTHESIA

### Methoxamine

Methoxamine is a similar drug to phenylephrine. It is a pure $\alpha_1$-adrenergic receptor agonist that causes an intense vasoconstriction leading to reflex bradycardia. Similar to phenylephrine it has no β-adrenergic receptor activity. It was used for hypotension after spinal anesthesia, but it is no longer used. It has concerns for causing decreased uterine blood flow, and some animal studies show negative effects on fetal acid-base status.[4]

### Mephentermine

Mephentermine is a similar drug to ephedrine. It has agonist action on both α- and β-adrenergic receptors both directly and indirectly. It is widely used in developing countries for hypotension after spinal anesthesia, because of its ease of use and economical advantage. It has been shown that mephentermine is as effective as phenylephrine in hypotension after spinal anesthesia, but tachyphylaxis develops rapidly with its use.[4]

## Metaraminol

Metaraminol is also another agent that is similar to ephedrine and mephentermine. Like the other drugs, it has agonist action on both α- and β-adrenergic receptors, both directly and indirectly. It has much more significant direct effect on vascular α-adrenergic receptors.[4] Furthermore, as expected, tachyphylaxis develops due to its indirect effect through the release of norepinephrine.

## OTHERS

### Aminophylline

Aminophylline is a combination of theophylline and ethylenediamine that is commonly used for severe acute bronchial asthma, chronic bronchitis, and emphysema.[5] Aminophylline releases theophylline once in the body, and although not completely understood, there are three ways that theophylline works to achieve its effects: inhibition of phosphodiesterase, antagonist action on adenosine receptor, and activation of histone deacetylase.[5] Its mild inotropic effect most likely results from the inhibition of phosphodiesterase (type III and IV), but aminophylline is rarely used for its inotropic effects. Its mild adverse effects are similar to the effects of caffeine, but severe adverse effects can lead to cardiac arrhythmias and seizures.[5]

### Glucagon

The receptor that glucagon binds to is a G protein-coupled receptor that is also present in the heart.[6] It can activate $G_s$-protein receptor cascade, which will increase cAMP and intracellular calcium. Therefore, there are reports of a high level of exogenous glucagon being associated with positive cardiac inotropy and chronotropy.[6] There also reports of high-dose glucagon leading to increased catecholamine levels and its subsequent effects, and there are animal studies that show possible PDE-inhibitor effects of glucagon leading to positive inotropy.[6] However, these are all limited data, and further investigations are needed that include dosage, long-term effects of increased glucagon levels, and other systemic adverse effects caused by glucagon.[6]

### Digoxin

Digoxin is known as cardiac glycosides. It selectively binds to the $Na^-K^+$ ATPase on sarcolemma of cardiac cells and reversibly inhibits the enzyme.[3] This indirectly increases calcium availability leading to increased inotropy.[1] Increases in parasympathetic activity, in addition to its effect on the $Na^-K^+$ ATPase, can lead to alterations in electrophysiology, including delayed conduction through the atrioventricular

(AV) node and bradycardia.[1,3] It has a narrow therapeutic range which can worsen in the setting of hypokalemia.[3] Digoxin toxicity can be treated with correction of the electrolytes, administration of drugs to treat dysrhythmias, or insertion of temporary pacemaker. In a life-threatening toxicity, digoxin antibodies can be used to decrease the digoxin concentration.[3]

## Levosimendan

Levosimendan is the only drug in its class, which is a myofilament calcium sensitizer. It causes positive inotropy and vasodilating effects by increasing the calcium sensitivity of the actin-myosin apparatus.[1] There are three mechanisms. First, levosimendan binds to troponin C (TnC), which prolongs the interaction between actin and myosin filaments, leading to increased myocardial contractility.[1] Second, it also acts as a potent PDE III inhibitor, which leads to positive inotropic and lusitropic effects.[1] Lastly, it

also opens ATP-dependent potassium channels, leading to the vasodilatory effects.[1] Levosimendan has a prolonged effect, because its metabolite (OR-1896) also has activities similar to levosimendan.[1]

## REFERENCES

1. Pagel PS, Grecu L. Cardiovascular pharmacology. In *Clinical Anesthesia.* 8th ed. Phildelphia, PA: Wolters Kluwer; 2017:301–332.
2. Glick D. Autonomic nervous system. In *Basics of Anesthesia.* 6th ed. Philadelphia, PA: Elsevier; 2011:66–77.
3. Stoelting RK, et al. Sympathomimetic drugs. In *Stoelting's Handbook of Pharmacology and Physiology in Anesthetic Practice.* 3rd ed. Philadelphia, PA: Wolter Kluwer Health; 2015:352–375.
4. Nag DS, et al. Vasopressors in obstetric anesthesia: A current perspective. *World J Clin Cases.* 2015;3(1):58–64.
5. Zafar Gondal A, Zulfiqar H. Aminophylline. In: *StatPearls* [Internet]. Treasure Island, FL: StatPearls; 2020 Feb 21. Available from: https://www.ncbi.nlm.nih.gov/books/NBK545175/
6. Petersen KM, et al. Hemodynamic effects of glucagon: A literature review. *J Clin Endocrinol Metab.* 2018 May; 103(5):1804–1812.

# 285.

# ANTIANGINAL DRUGS

*Vasu Sidagam*

## INTRODUCTION

Angina occurs due to imbalance between myocardial blood supply and demand (Figure 285.1). In this chapter, 3 commonly used classes of medications for therapy in acute and chronic stable angina—nitrates, beta adrenergic blockers (BBs), and calcium channel blockers (CCBs)—are discussed. In addition, new antianginal agents like ranolazine and ivabradine are mentioned. Certain newer antianginal drugs like nicorandil and trimetazidine are used in Europe and elsewhere as second-line antianginal drugs but are not available in the United States, and they will not be discussed further.

## NITRATES

Nitroglycerin (GTN), isosorbide dinitrate (ISDN), and isosobide mononitrate (ISMN) are commonly used medications.

The GTN tablet is administered sublingually. Onset of action is within 1–3 min and is faster if given by sublingual spray. Its prime use is in acute angina (see Figure 285.1 for mechanism of antianginal effect). It can also be used in cocaine-induced ischemic chest pain, but be aware, as it can worsen preexisting tachycardia. It has extensive first-pass metabolism in the liver, so it is not suitable for oral therapy or chronic stable angina. Isosorbide dinitrate

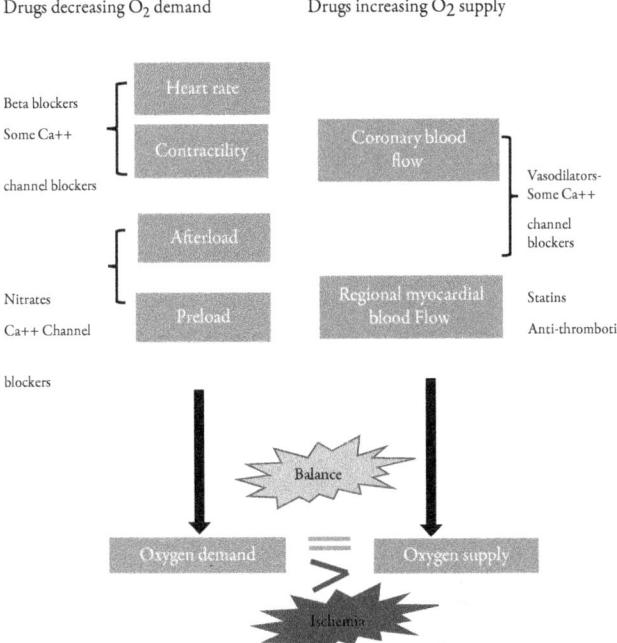

Drugs decreasing O₂ demand

Drugs increasing O₂ supply

Beta blockers
Some Ca++

channel blockers

Heart rate

Contractility

Coronary blood flow

Vasodilators-
Some Ca++

channel
blockers

Afterload

Nitrates

Ca++ Channel

Preload

Regional myocardial
blood Flow

Statins

Anti-thrombotics

blockers

Balance

Oxygen demand

=
>

Oxygen supply

Ischemia

**Figure 285.1.** Drug modification of myocardial oxygen balance.

and its metabolites isosorbide 2 mononitrate and ISMN have a half-life of 4–6 hours and can thus be used for both stand-by and sustained therapy. Unlike the previous two nitrates, ISMN cannot be used for acute angina relief, as its onset of action is too slow.[1]

Nitrates preferentially dilate large venous and arterial vessels more than small resistance vessels. Thus they do not cause coronary steal phenomenon. Nitrates are first choice in vasospastic angina or prinzmetal angina, along with CCBs, and second choice in the prevention of exertional angina.[1]

Nitrates work normally in cardiac transplant patients; however, compensatory tachycardia will not be present in the early post-transplant period. Tachyphylaxis or tolerance is a function of dosage and frequency of use. Nitrate-free interval of more than 8 hours allows a return of efficacy.[1]

Contraindications for nitrate therapy include severe aortic stenosis, hypertrophic obstructive cardiomyopathy (even if there is no gradient), acute right ventricular infarction, hypotension, and use of phosphodiesterase (PDE) inhibitors within the prior 24 hours (Figure 285.2). Use with caution in patients with neuraxial anesthesia.2

## BETA ADRENERGIC BLOCKERS (BBS)

Beta blockers (BBs) are the drugs of choice for chronic angina, as they reduce anginal episodes and improve exercise tolerance. Common BBs used are atenolol, propranolol,

metoprolol, esmolol, labetalol, etc. They reduce myocardial work and oxygen demand by decreasing heart rate, blood pressure, and myocardial contractility. BB-mediated decrease in heart rate also increases myocardial blood flow.

Increased collateral blood flow and redistribution of blood flow to ischemic areas may occur with beta blockade. At the microcirculatory level, O₂ delivery improves and O₂ dissociates easily from hemoglobin after beta blockade.[3]

BBs are the only antianginal drugs proven to prevent reinfarction and to improve survival in patients who had a myocardial infarction.[4] BBs should not be used in vasospastic or prinzmetal angina. They are ineffective and induce coronary vasospasm due to unopposed alpha receptor activity. Abrupt discontinuation of BBs can cause exacerbation of angina and increase risk of sudden death.[1]

## CALCIUM CHANNEL BLOCKERS

They include the dihydropyridine group (amlodipine and nifedipine) and non-dihydropyridine group (diltiazem and verapamil).

They are coronary vasodilators which produce dose-dependent reduction in myocardial O₂ demand, contractility, and blood pressure.[3] The dihydropyridine group does not have any negative ionotropic and chronotropic effects, and they are not effective as antiarrhythmic drugs.[3]

Diltiazem and verapamil have negative ionotropic effects and are contraindicated in patients with systolic dysfunction. Verapamil should not be combined with BBs due to adverse effect on heart rate and contractility.[3]

Diltiazem can be combined with a BB in patients with normal ventricular function and no conduction abnormalities. Amlodipine and BBs have complimentary actions of reducing coronary blood flow and myocardial oxygen demand; whereas the former decreases blood pressure and dilates coronary arteries, the latter slows heart rate and decreases contractility.[3] Peripheral edema and constipation are known side effects of CCBs.

## NEW ANTIANGINAL AGENTS

Ranolazine is used as antianginal drug in chronic stable angina when BBs are inadequate or not tolerated.

It can be combined with a BB for symptoms relief if initial BB monotherapy is unsuccessful.

The mechanism of action is prevention of both intramyocardial cell calcium overload and the subsequent increase in diastolic tension due to inhibition of late inward sodium channel. Thus its antianginal effect occurs independently of reductions in heart rate or blood pressure or coronary blood flow.

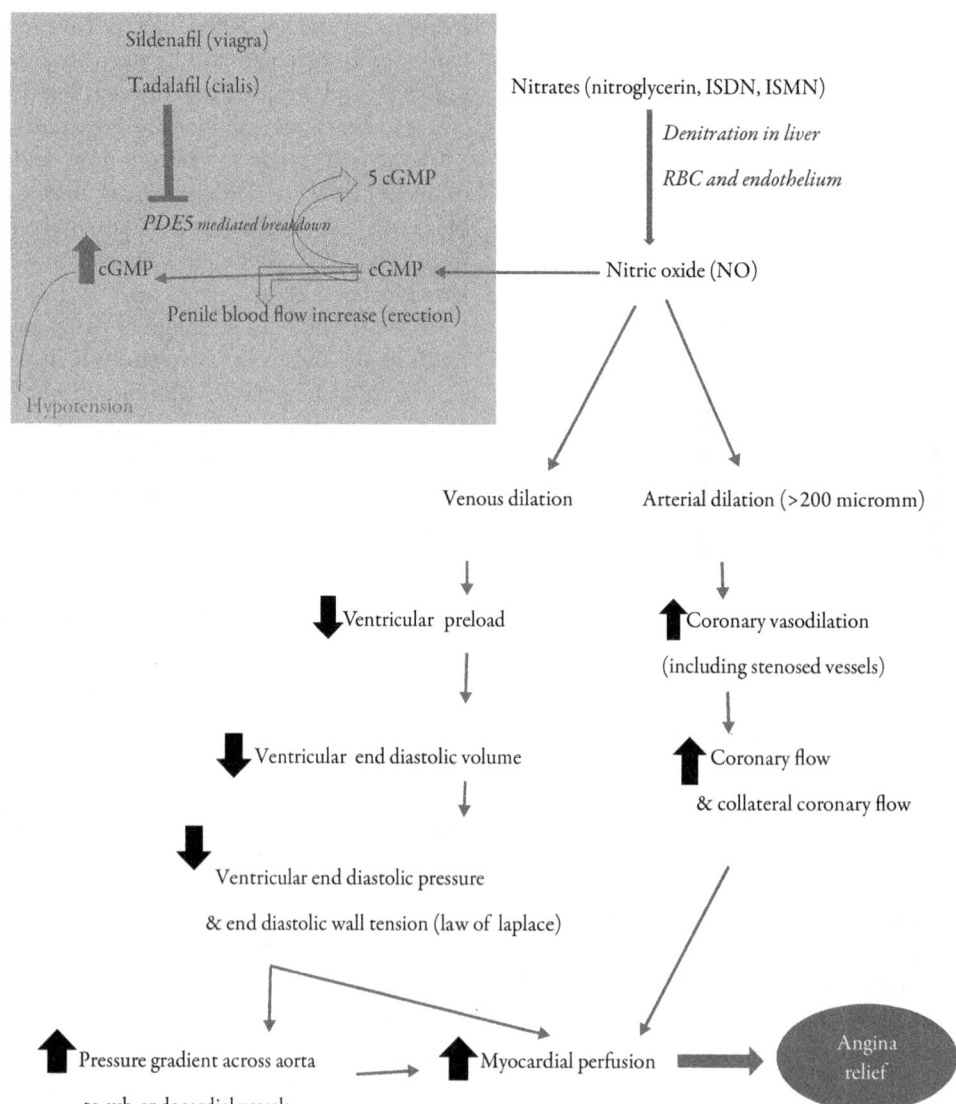

**Figure 285.2.** Mechanism of anti-anginal effects of nitrates and interaction with PDE5 inhibitors causing hypotension.

QT prolongation can occur. It is contraindicated in liver cirrhosis and preexisting QT prolongation.[1]

## IVABRADINE

This is a new antianginal drug which is a specific sinus nodal pacemaker current inhibitor, thus lowering heart rate. It increases exercise capacity and reduces anginal frequency and severity.[4] It is currently only recommended for use in patients with angina and clinical heart failure. Its antianginal effect in solely due to decreased heart rate.[1]

## REFERENCES

1. Eschenhagen T. Treatment of ischemic heart disease. In: *Goodman & Gilman's The Pharmacological Basis of Therapeutics.* 13th ed. 489–506.
2. Shear T, Katz J. Coronary artery disease. In *Kaplan's Essentials of Cardiac Anesthesia for Noncardiac Surgery.* 16–32.
3. Antman EM, Loscalzo J. Ischemic heart disease. In *Harrison's Principles of Internal Medicine.* 20th ed. Vol. 2. 1850–1872 .
4. Teo KK, et al. Effects of prophylactic antiarrhythmic drug therapy in acute myocardial infarction: An overview of results from randomized controlled trials. *JAMA.* 1993;*270*(13): 1589.285.285.

# 286.

# ANGIOTENSIN-CONVERTING ENZYME INHIBITORS AND ANGIOTENSIN RECEPTOR BLOCKERS

*Laurence Ohia and Jacob Guzman*

## INTRODUCTION

Angiotensin-converting enzyme inhibitors (ACEIs), along with angiotensin receptor blockers (ARBs) and direct renin inhibitors, antagonize the renin-angiotensin-aldosterone-system (RAAS) and, as such, are effective in treating hypertension, and prolonging survival in heart failure, acute myocardial infarction, and coronary artery disease; as well as slowing down progression of chronic kidney disease secondary to diabetic nephropathy. ACEIs inhibit the angiotensin-converting enzyme (ACE), also known as kininase II and peptidyl

dipeptidase, which is involved in the conversion of angiotensin I to angiotensin II in the RAAS, and in bradykinin degradation.

ACEIs lowers the level of circulating angiotensin II, aldosterone, and increases the level of bradykinin, a direct vasodilator involved in the formation of prostaglandins (Figure 286.1). ARBs inhibit the action of angiotensin II on AT1 receptors, bringing about vasodilation and inhibiting secretion of aldosterone. ARBs are as cardioprotective and renal protective as ACEIs, as well as having similar adverse effects. ARBs are commonly prescribed for patients with adverse reactions to ACEIs.

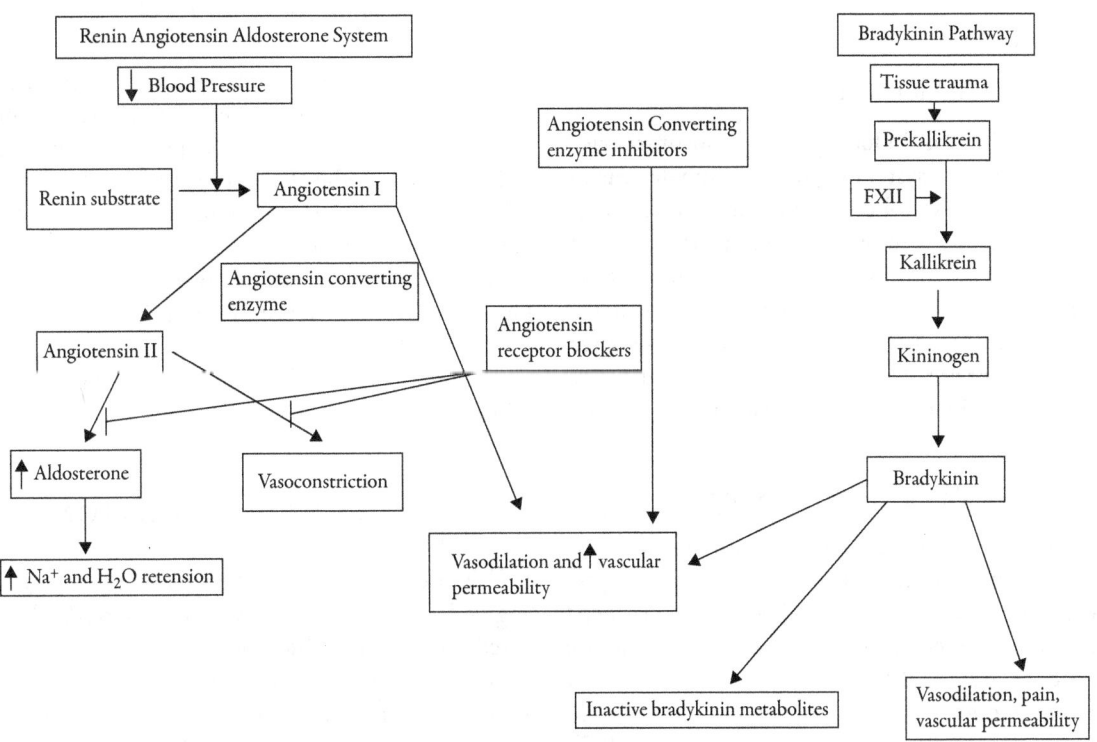

**Figure 286.1.** Sites of action of ACEIs and ARBs on the RAAS and bradykinin system.

## PHARMACOKINETICS

ACEIs are classified into 3 groups based on chemical structure: sulfhydryl-containing ACE inhibitors, such as captopril; dicarboxylic-containing ACEIs related to enalapril, such as benazepril, moexipril, quinapril, lisinopril, ramipril, trandolapril, and perindopril; and phosphorus-containing ACEIs like fosinopril.

ACEIs are metabolized in the liver via ester hydrolysis to the active diacid form and are usually excreted in urine. Reduced plasma clearance of ACEIs is seen in patients with impaired renal function and, as such, drug dosages are reduced in these patients. Benazepril and fosinopril are excreted in the biliary system.

## CLINICAL INDICATIONS

### HYPERTENSION

ACEIs lower the systemic vascular resistance by causing systemic arteriolar dilation and increased compliance of large arteries without any compromise in stroke volume and cardiovascular reflexes in response to posture and exercise. Systolic and diastolic blood pressures are in turn lowered in many hypertensive states, except for hypertension due to primary hyperaldosteronism/Conn syndrome. The renal vessels are particularly sensitive to angiotensin II, so reduced levels increase renal perfusion via dilation of the afferent and efferent arterioles. Glomerular filtration rate (GFR) remains unchanged, but the filtration fraction is reduced.

### HEART FAILURE

Angiotensin II effects in inducing acute venoconstriction via sympathetic nervous system stimulation and decreasing arterial compliance in systolic dysfunction are reversed by ACE inhibition, resulting in reduction in cardiac afterload, ventricular wall stress, pulmonary artery pressure, pulmonary capillary wedge pressure, left atrial and ventricular filling volume and pressure, and renovascular resistance. Natriuresis is promoted, causing a contraction in excess body fluid, and exercise tolerance is increased.

### ISCHEMIC HEART DISEASE

ACEIs are among therapy used in patients for post-MI (myocardial infarction) management, but they may also be preventive against new MI, as noted in studies[1,2] where reduced incidence of MI was reported in patients with heart failure who received ACEIs. ACEIs given before surgery confer myocardial protection by reducing troponin release in patients undergoing coronary artery bypass graft (CABG), as seen in a study reported by Benedetto et al.[3]

## KIDNEY DISEASES

ACEIs exert their renal protective effects through various mechanisms. ACEIs prevent glomerular injury by decreasing glomerular capillary pressure via dilating the renal efferent arterioles and lowering systemic blood pressure. Mesangial cell proliferation and matrix formation are stimulated by exposure to significant amounts of filtered plasma proteins, as seen in proteinuria; and by angiotensin II, which is a growth factor for mesangial cell proliferation. ACEIs block expansion of the mesangium by enhancing the selective permeability of the filtering membrane to proteins and reducing circulating levels of angiotensin II, which in turn delay progression of chronic kidney disease.[4]

## ADVERSE EFFECTS

Dry cough, bronchospasm, angioedema, and other symptoms like skin rashes are due to inhibition of bradykinin metabolism by ACEIs. ARB use does not result in as much incidence of dry cough compared to ACEIs. Angioedema, although rare, is the most significant adverse effect and can affect many parts of the body, including the intestine, but of most concern is when it affects the airway (e.g., the larynx, tongue, and glottis), with securing of the airway being the priority.

ACEIs can cause hyperkalaemia and hyponatremia due to decreased aldosterone secretion. At-risk groups include history of chronic kidney disease, use of potassium-sparing diuretics, potassium supplements, beta blockers, nonsteroidal anti-inflammatory drug (NSAID) use, and in heart failure.

Acute renal failure can be induced by ACEIs, especially in conditions like bilateral renal artery stenosis due to vasodilation which reduces renal perfusion pressure. Heart failure patients who depend on the RAAS could also develop changes in renal function, with elevation of creatinine and urea in the blood.

Neutropenia, thrombocytopenia, anemia, and agranulocytosis have been reported with ACEI use, especially in patients with collagen vascular diseases like systemic lupus erythematosis and scleroderma, renal failure, and heart failure.

## CONTRAINDICATIONS

ACEIs are contraindicated in patients with a history of angioedema or hypersensitivity related to ACEIs treatment, hereditary or idiopathic angioedema.

ACEIs and ARBs are category D drugs and as such are contraindicated in pregnancy, especially in the second and third trimesters. ACEIs reduce utero-placental blood flow, and induce fetal hypotension by inhibiting fetal

RAAS, resulting in impaired fetal renal function and oligohydramnios. Exposure of the fetus to ACEIs during the second and third trimester is associated with intrauterine growth retardation, premature labor, pulmonary hypoplasia, limb contractures, respiratory distress syndrome, skeletal deformations, renal failure, skull hypoplasia, and death.

## ACEIS/ARBS ANESTHESIA CONSIDERATIONS

Blood pressure is typically sustained by the sympathetic nervous system (SNS), the RAAS, and vasopressin, which all act by increasing intracellular calcium concentration in vascular smooth muscles. Anesthesia induction reduces the SNS influence on the cardiovascular system, leaving the RAAS via angiotensin II and vasopressin to counterbalance this offset. ACEIs and ARBs block the effects of RAS, leaving only vasopressin which is less effective on the systemic vascular capacitance to maintain blood pressure. This leads to severe episodes of hypotension during anesthesia, which can be corrected by fluid resuscitation and administering vasopressors like ephedrine and phenylephrine. The incidence of hypotension during anesthesia in patients whose ACEIs have been maintained until the day of surgery is above 75%. Many studies recommend holding ACEIs and ARBs 24 hours before surgery due to the risk of hypotension requiring aggressive fluid resuscitation and vasopressors after anesthesia induction.[5]

## REFERENCES

1. Pfeffer M, et al. Effect of captopril on mortality and morbidity in patients with left ventricular dysfunction after myocardial infarction. *N Engl J Med*. 1992;327(10):669–677.
2. Jong P, et al. Effect of enalapril on 12-year survival and life expectancy in patients with left ventricular systolic dysfunction: A follow-up study. *Lancet*. 2003;361(9372):1843–1848.
3. Benedetto U, et al. Preoperative angiotensin-converting enzyme inhibitors protect myocardium from ischemia during coronary artery bypass graft surgery. *J Cardiovasc Med (Hagerstown)*. 2008;9:1098–1103.
4. Lozano-Maneiro L, Puente-García A. renin-angiotensin-aldosterone system blockade in diabetic nephropathy: Present evidences. *J Clin Med*. 2015;4(11):1908–1937.
5. Nabbi R, et al. Case report: Refractory hypotension during general anesthesia despite preoperative discontinuation of an angiotensin receptor blocker. F1000Research. 2013;2:12.

# 287.

# VASODILATORS

*Stefan Besada and Christina T. Nguyen*

## INTRODUCTION

Use of vasodilators in anesthetic practice may be useful for patients with acute or chronic hypertension. Altered physiology under anesthesia, poorly compliant vascular anatomy characteristic of elderly patients, diastolic dysfunction, non-adherence to preoperative antihypertensive therapy, and various other factors may complicate intraoperative blood pressure management. In this chapter, we will discuss the selection of the appropriate intraoperative antihypertensive therapy.

## NITROVASODILATORS

Nitrovasodilators work similarly to endogenous nitric oxide (NO) that is produced by vascular endothelium: by stimulation of guanylate cyclase in vascular smooth muscle cells, which converts guanosine triphosphate to cyclic GMP, resulting in phosphorylation of proteins involved in the regulation of free intracellular calcium and smooth muscle cell contraction and relaxation.[1-5]

## NITROPRUSSIDE

Nitroprusside works by relaxing arteriolar and venous smooth muscle, causing a reduction in preload and afterload. It is very potent, and thanks to its favorable pharmacokinetics, easily titratable. It has a rapid onset (1–2 minutes) and a short duration of action (2 minutes). It is administered as a bolus at 1–2 mcg/kg, and as a continuous infusion at 0.5–10 mcg/kg/min. Of note, its molecular structure's $Fe^{2+}$ ion reacts with sulfhydryl (–SH) groups in red blood cells, releasing cyanide.[4] High nitroprusside doses can result in cyanide toxicity, which may manifest as arrhythmias, tachyphylaxis, metabolic acidosis, and increased mixed venous partial pressure of oxygen ($PaO_2$) Treatments and supportive measures are 100% fraction of inspired oxygen ($FiO_2$) inhaled amyl nitrite, intravenous sodium nitrite, sodium thiosulfate, and hydroxocobalamin.[1,2,5]

## NITROGLYCERIN

Nitroglycerin is a venodilator (works at venule level), that effects smooth muscle relaxation through the same nitric oxide mediated mechanism described previously.[3-5] Its pharmacokinetics are similar to that of nitroprusside—onset within 2 minutes, and recession within 5 minutes.[1] Its primary use is treatment of myocardial ischemia,[4] which is accomplished by reduction of preload, resulting in decreased myocardial oxygen demand.[2] It is also used to combat acute hypertension and cardiogenic pulmonary edema. It is rapidly metabolized by the liver into nitrite, which can convert hemoglobin to methemoglobin. Although rarely encountered in practice, said methemoglobinemia is treated with methylene blue.[5] Unlike with nitroprusside, there is no concern for cyanide toxicity; thus it is preferred over the former in obstetric patients.[1]

## HYDRALAZINE

Hydralazine is a direct vasodilator that relaxes vascular smooth muscle at the arteriolar level by a poorly understood mechanism. Its onset is comparatively slow at circa 15 minutes at doses of 5–20 mg, and its duration of action of 2–4 hours[1] makes it unfavorable in the operating room. Hydralazine's afterload reduction results in a baroreceptor-mediated reflexive tachycardia that can be harmful to patients with coronary artery disease.[2] The tachycardia can be overcome by concomitant administration of β-1 adrenergic antagonists, but caution should be exercised, as these can lead to excessive hypotension.

## ADRENERGIC ANTAGONISTS

Alpha- (α-) and β-adrenergic antagonists bind to adrenoreceptors, preventing their activity; α- blockers (oral phenoxybenzamine and IV phentolamine) have limited intraoperative use. They are almost exclusively used in the management of pheochromocytoma.[1] Phentolamine is also used to prevent tissue necrosis in the case of extravasation of α agonist.[3] Mixed antagonists (labetalol) and β-adrenergic antagonists (esmolol) have greater utility in the operating room.

## ESMOLOL

Esmolol is a selective β-1 blocker that owes its ultrashort duration of action (onset at 1 minute, half-life of 9 minutes) to its hydrolysis by red blood cell esterases. It is commonly bolused at a dose of 0.5 mg/kg to attenuate the sympathetic surge resulting from laryngoscopy, intubation, or surgical stimulation.[3] Given its short half-life, it is easily titratable, making it a suitable infusion (dosed at 50–300 mcg/kg/min following a 0.5 mg/kg loading dose),[1] commonly used for blood pressure control in thyroid storm[5] and heart rate control in atrial fibrillation.

## LABETALOL

Labetalol is a mixed antagonist with anti-α and anti-β receptor activity with a ratio of α:β blockade of circa 1:7. This allows it to reduce peripheral vascular resistance without a concomitant reflexive tachycardia, making it a suitable agent for patients with coronary artery disease who depend on an optimized myocardial oxygen supply-to-demand ratio. Dosed at 2.5–20 mg, its onset is rapid (within 5 minutes), but with a terminal half-life of 5.5 hours[1] it is not very practical in the operating room, perhaps with the exception of hypertensive emergencies or type A aortic dissection[2] in addition to its utility in treating *postoperative* hypertension.

## DOPAMINE AGONISTS

Of the dopamine agonists in use, the one used in hypotensive therapy is fenoldopam. Unlike dopamine, it does not exhibit any α or β receptor activity, and is thus not a pressor, but rather a natriuretic and a diuretic.

## FENOLDOPAM

Fenoldopam relaxes arteries by D1 dopamine receptor agonism, as well as moderate α-2 adrenoreceptor agonism.[3] Its short half-life of 5 minutes makes it a good choice for use in the operating room. As opposed to nitroprusside, it preserves, indeed increases, renal blood flow. Given this, it would seem that it offers a true renal protective effect, but studies regarding said effect are mixed.[1-5] It is worth remembering that its use can result in increased intracranial and intraocular pressures; thus caution is advised in patients with cerebral masses/edema, or glaucoma, respectively.[3]

## CALCIUM CHANNEL BLOCKERS

Dihydropyridine calcium channel blockers inhibit, as their name implies, influx of calcium through voltage-sensitive L-type calcium channels found in vascular smooth muscle, thereby causing vasodilation.[1,4] They act primarily on arteries and have little effect on veins due to the relative preponderance of L-type receptors in arteries compared to veins.[3]

### NICARDIPINE

Nicardipine is an almost pure arteriolar dilator, with no significant effect on cardiac conduction or myocardial contractility, whereas other calcium channel blockers have negative chronotropic, dromotropic, and inotropic effects.[1,2] It has a fast onset (<10 minutes), and a terminal half-life of 2–4 hours,[5] making it less useful for acute bouts of hypertension and instead more suitable for sustained perioperative hypertension. It is also a coronary vasodilator, making it useful to dilate arterial grafts during coronary artery bypass grafting.[2] Unlike nitroprusside, labetalol, or hydralazine, a reflex tachycardia is *not* generally observed.

### CLEVIDIPINE

Clevidipine is a relatively novel agent that works by the same mechanism as nicardipine, but owing to its short duration of action and a corresponding half-life of only 2 minutes,[5] it is easily titratable. The pharmacokinetics are analogous to that of esmolol, in that it is hydrolyzed into inactive metabolites by serum esterases.[1] Unlike some of the other agents described previously (e.g., nitroprusside), clevidipine is *not* known to exhibit tachyphylaxis or rebound hypertension.[2] Its high cost is one of the main reasons preventing widespread use.

## REFERENCES

1. Barash PG, et al. *Clinical Anesthesia.* 7th ed. Philadelphia, PA: Wolters Kluwer Health; 2013.
2. Barash PG, et al. *Clinical Anesthesia Fundamentals.* Philadelphia, PA: Wolters Kluwer Health Adis (ESP); 2015.
3. Butterworth JF, et al. *Morgan & Mikhail's Clinical Anesthesiology.* New York, NY: McGraw-Hill; 2013.
4. Faust RJ, et al. *Anesthesiology Review.* 4th ed. Philadelphia, PA: Elsevier; 2015.
5. Shafer SL, et al. *Stoelting's Pharmacology and Physiology in Anesthetic Practice.* Philadelphia, PA: Wolters Kluwer Health; 2015.

# 288.

# ELECTROLYTES

*Lindsey Cieslinski*

## INTRODUCTION

Electrolyte homeostasis is essential to cellular and organ function. Cellular fluid shifts associated with the physiological response to surgical stress have significant implications on fluid management.[1] Fluid compartments are divided into intracellular fluid volume (ICF) and extracellular (ECF). The ECF consists of 80% interstitial fluid and 20% plasma.[3] Sodium is the major cation in the ECF, while $K^+$ is the main contributor to the ICF.[3] Chloride is the main anion in the ECF. Sodium levels are mediated by antidiuretic hormone (ADH), aldosterone, and corticosteroids. Potassium is regulated by aldosterone and steroids. While $Ca^{2+}$ and $Mg^{2+}$ are important for vascular tone, $Ca^{2+}$ is needed for ionotropy and peripheral vasoconstriction. $Mg^{2+}$ antagonizes the effect of $Ca^{2+}$ on the vasculature, plays a vital role in ATP production, and is a cofactor for DNA.[3] This chapter will discuss the essential electrolytes $Na^+$, $K^+$, $Ca^{2+}$, $Cl^-$, and $Mg^{2+}$ while focusing on combining basic science content with clinical application.

Sodium is a major determinant of extracellular osmotic pressure and volume.[3] ECF volume and total body water regulate sodium balance; thus correction of sodium irregularities is important. The urine and plasma osmolarity help distinguish the diagnoses for electrolyte disturbances.[1]

Hypernatremia is defined as sodium >145 mmol/L. It has a wide variety of causes, but clinical symptoms are identical, including mental status changes, hyperreflexia, and seizures. Hypovolemic hypernatremia is commonly caused by loss of bodily fluids.[4] Normovolemic hypernatremia is usually due to diabetes insipidus (DI) with high urine output. If caused by reduced ADH secretion, it is central DI. If there is abnormal renal response to ADH, it is nephrogenic DI.[3] Urine osmolality can differentiate the diagnosis: urine <200 mOsm/L with central DI, and 200–500 mOsm/L in nephrogenic DI.[4]

Hyponatremia, defined as $Na^+$ <135, may present with mental status changes, lethargy, cramps, decreased deep tendon reflexes, and seizures.[3] Na+ <120 is potentially life-threatening, with 50% mortality rate.[2] Volume status and urine sodium can help distinguish the origin of hypotonic hyponatremia. When due to renal losses, $Na^+$ urine >20 mEq/L causes include diuresis, cerebral salt wasting, and adrenal insufficiency. If $Na^+$ urine <10 mEq/L, it is likely extrarenal.[4] Euvolemic hyponatremia is due to adrenal or thyroid insufficiency, postoperative stress, mediations, and syndrome of inappropriate antidiuretic hormone (SIADH). Urine sodium and osmolality for SIADH reveal a urine $Na^+$ >

Extracellular potassium is primarily maintained by oral intake and renal elimination Extracellular potassium is tightly controlled, accounting for only 2% of total body potassium.[4] Potassium is dependent on acid-base balance, insulin sensitivity, $Na^+/K^+$ adenosine triphosphate-dependent exchange channels, and catecholamine levels.[2]

Significant clinical effect of hyperkalemia involves the cardiac conduction system at 6.0–6.5 mEq/L with electrocardiogram (ECG) changes of prolonged PR interval, QRS widening, ST segment elevation, and peaked T waves.[2] Initial treatment includes stabilization of the myocardium with calcium gluconate, then a decrease in serum $K^+$ via intracellular sequestration with insulin and glucose, and lastly, total body $K^+$ reduction. Removal in renal failure is most effective via hemodialysis.

Hypokalemia is usually asymptomatic until 2.5 mEq/L, at which point anorexia, nausea, muscle weakness, paralytic ileus, and conduction abnormalities may be apparent.[1]

Associated ECG changes include prolonged QRS interval, T wave flattening, and development of prominent U waves. Hypokalemia can be via transcellular shifts or total body depletion, commonly divided into extrarenal losses or renal losses. To help differentiate the cause, analyze the urine chloride.[4]

Maintain of calcium concentration involves parathyroid hormone and calcitonin, which regulates calcium and phosphorus by the kidneys, bones, and intestines through negative feedback.[5] Symptomatic hypocalcemia is a medical emergency. Major clinical effects of hypocalcemia are neuromuscular excitability and cardiovascular depression. Severe hypocalcemia is associated with a prolonged QT, bradycardia, peripheral vasodilation, decreased cardiac contractility, hypotension,[2] and, less commonly, Chvostek's and Trousseau's sign. Causes of hypocalcemia include hypoparathyroidism, $Ca^{2+}$ chelation via blood transfusion, renal insufficiency, and respiratory alkalosis.

Hypercalcemia is rare but usually due to malignancy, hyperparathyroidism, or medication.[3] Signs include lethargy, vomiting, abdominal pain, urinary stones, shortened QT interval, nephrocalcinosis, polyuria, and confusion.[3] It produces hypercalciuria, which causes osmotic diuresis. Patients require treatment if symptomatic.

Chloride is important in maintaining acid-base balance, renal tubular function, and gastric acid formation.[1] Regulation of chloride is passively related to sodium and inversely related to bicarbonate.[1] In the proximal tubules, chloride is excreted with ammonium ions to eliminate hydrogen ions in exchange for sodium.[1] Electrochemical neutrality is maintained when bicarbonate diffuses into the plasma and chloride shifts into the cell.[1] Clinically it is important to recognize that excessive normal saline resuscitation can result in hyperchloremic metabolic acidosis. This is due to a decrease in strong ion difference where renal excretion of $Na^+$ occurs in preference to $Cl^-$ and $H^+$.[1]

Magnesium is primarily an intracellular ion. Depletion is multifactorial, including decreased intake, impaired absorption, increased gastrointestinal and renal losses.[5] Magnesium indirectly affects vascular contractility via inhibition of catecholamine release from the adrenal medulla and peripheral adrenergic terminals, resulting in decreased vasoconstriction.[4] Hypomagnesemia may cause neuromuscular excitability, mental status changes, and seizures. ECG changes include a prolonged QT interval and ectopy.[5] Magnesium is a treatment for *torsades de pointes* and digoxin toxicity. Magnesium is an antiarrhythmic due to L-type calcium channel antagonism.[4] Hypermagnesemia commonly develops in the setting of renal failure or excessive magnesium intake, as in pre-eclampsia.[2] Neurologic and cardiac manifestations begin to occur when serum level exceeds 5mg/dL; commonly, hyporeflexia, sedation, and weakness.

EGC changes seen include prolonged PR interval and widened QRS complex.

## ANESTHETIC CONSIDERATIONS

Importantly, electrolyte disturbances can alter MAC requirements. Hypernatremia increases MAC requirements, while hyponatremia decreases MAC requirements.[5] Hypokalemia, hypocalcemia, and hypermagnesemia electrolyte disturbances potentiate neuromuscular blockade.[3] Massive transfusion can be a source of hypocalcemia and hyperkalemia. There are many drugs that can be a source of electrolyte disturbances.

## REFERENCES

1. Rassam SS, Counsell DJ. Perioperative electrolyte and fluid balance. *Cont Educ Anaesth Crit Care Pain.* 2005 Oct;5(5):157–160.
2. Trentman TL, et al. *Faust's Anesthesiology Review*, 5th ed. Amsterdam: Elsevier; 2020:105–107.
3. Patel AM, et al. *BASIC Essentials: A Comprehensive Review for the Anesthesiology BASIC Exam.* Cambridge: Cambridge University Press; 2019:175–183.
4. Fluids and electrolytes, magnesium, inhaled anesthetics keywords. *OpenAnesthesia*, www.openanesthesia.org/. In: Miller R, Pardo M. *Basics of Anesthesia.* 7th ed. Philadelphia, PA: W. B. Saunders; 2018.
5. Gragossian A, et al. Hypomagnesemia. [Updated September 6, 2020]. In: *StatPearls* [Internet]. Treasure Island, FL: StatPearls; 2020 Jan–.https://www.ncbi.nlm.nih.gov/books/NBK500003/.

# 289.

# NON-ADRENERGIC VASOCONSTRICTORS

*Albert Lee and Nathan Schulman*

## INTRODUCTION

Anesthesiologists must possess an intimate knowledge of the vasoactive agents that are ubiquitous in the operating room and intensive care unit. Though many common vasopressors and inotropes modulate adrenergic pathways, this chapter will discuss the physiologic mechanisms and dosing of non-adrenergic vasopressors in addition to their associated complications. Lastly, it will briefly discuss available literature specifically regarding angiotensin II and vasopressin in instances of refractory shock.

## VASOPRESSIN

Vasopressin produces intense peripheral vasoconstriction through its action on smooth-muscle V1 receptors. There is no action on β-adrenergic receptors. Activation produces vasoconstriction in the skin, muscle, intestine, and fat tissue to a higher degree compared to coronary and renal vessels, and in contrast produces cerebrovascular dilation.

Advantages include its potency and its ability to remain effective in severe acidosis.

Vasopressin is used for different forms of vasodilatory shock, such as sepsis, vasoplegia after cardiopulmonary bypass, and for patients taking angiotensin-converting enzyme inhibitors or angiotensin receptor blockers who develop refractory hypotension under general anesthesia.[1] Adult dose range for vasopressin is 1–6 units/hr.

## METHYLENE BLUE

A multitude of vasoactive agents target various processes in the nitric oxide (NO)-cyclic guanosine monophosphate (cGMP) pathway, an endogenous nitrovasodilator system. The pathway involves formation of endogenous NO by nitric oxide synthase (NOS). NO, by interacting with the enzyme guanylate cyclase (sGC), increases cGMP production, leading to smooth muscle relaxation and vasodilation. States such as sepsis and cardiopulmonary bypass lead to increased NO production due to increased NOS.

Methylene blue interacts with this pathway at two points: (a) direct inhibition of nitric oxide synthase, and (b) inhibition of sGC. Both result in a decrease in cellular cGMP, resulting in improved vascular tone.

To the anesthesiologist, methylene blue will most likely be used in one of three scenarios: (a) a dye during surgeries, (b) methemoglobinemia, or (c) vasoplegia. Vasoplegia most commonly treated with methylene blue are those associated with cardiac surgery and cardiopulmonary bypass, liver transplant surgeries, and sepsis. It is important to note that although studies involving methylene blue have demonstrated increased blood pressures, they have yet to demonstrate improved oxygen delivery or a mortality benefit. For vasoplegia, the typical dose of methylene blue is 1.5–2 mg/kg.[2]

The anesthesiologist should be aware that methylene blue can temporarily interfere with the measurement of oxygen saturation. The FDA warns against using methylene blue in patients taking serotonin reuptake inhibitors, serotonin-norepinephrine reuptake inhibitors, or certain tricyclic antidepressants given the concern for serotonin syndrome. It should be avoided in patients with glucose-6-phosphate dehydrogenase deficiency, as it can precipitate hemolytic anemia.

## ANGIOTENSIN II

The renin-aldosterone-angiotensin system is critical for the regulation of volume and systemic vascular resistance. Hypovolemia and hypotension lead to renin release by the juxtaglomerular apparatus. This results in a cascade of reactions that lead to the production of angiotensin II (Ang II), which exerts its physiologic function on angiotensin-receptor type 1 (AT-R1) and type 2 (AT-R2). AT-R1 activation leads to a multitude of downstream hemodynamic effects, including vasoconstriction, aldosterone secretion by the adrenal zona glomerulosa, vasopressin release, and cardiac remodeling. Other less desirable effects, such as increased vascular permeability and increased production of pro-inflammatory mediators, have also been implicated with AT-R1 activation. AT-R2 activation is less understood, though experimental data suggest its downstream effects counteract and regulate those of AT-R1 receptor activation through vasodilation and decreases in systemic vascular resistance.

Synthetic Ang II has largely been studied in the setting of refractory distributive shock (discussed in the following). Doses in this setting ranged from approximately 5 *nanograms*/kg/min to 40 ng/kg/min.[3]

## COMPLICATIONS OF VASOPRESSOR USE

Non-adrenergic vasopressors carry significantly less risk of dysrhythmia, myocardial ischemia, and hyperglycemia compared to their adrenergic counterparts given the lack of β agonism. However, complications still exist largely in the form of hypoperfusion due to excessive vasoconstriction (SVR >1300 dynes x sec/cm^5) paired with inadequate perfusion, usually in the setting of inadequate volume resuscitation or cardiac output. Extreme peripheral vasoconstriction may manifest as dusky fingers and toes, progressing to necrosis and auto-amputation if unaddressed. Individuals with baseline peripheral vascular disease are at risk of developing acute limb ischemia. Compromising renal and splanchnic perfusion increases the risk of renal insufficiency, gastritis, shock liver, and gut ischemia with subsequent bacterial translocation, resulting in bacteremia. Nonetheless, the clinical scenario may require prioritizing the maintenance of a global mean arterial pressure to save the patient's life, despite evidence of local tissue hypoperfusion.

## VASOPRESSIN AND SEPSIS

Numerous studies have sought the ideal vasopressor hierarchy in sepsis. The Surviving Sepsis campaign currently recommends norepinephrine as the first-line vasopressor in septic shock, based on numerous trials mostly comparing norepinephrine to dopamine. However, due to the relative vasopressin deficiency present in septic patients, vasopressin has emerged as another vasopressor of interest. The VASST trial was an RCT that compared norepinephrine alone to norepinephrine plus vasopressin in patients with septic shock, but failed to demonstrate a mortality benefit in an intention-to-treat analysis. The VANISH trial compared norepinephrine and vasopressin both with and without hydrocortisone, primarily measuring kidney failure-free days. Though the vasopressin group demonstrated fewer days utilizing renal replacement therapy, overall primary outcomes did not reach statistical significance. In the absence of additional large, robust studies comparing vasopressin to other agents, the Surviving Sepsis campaign currently recommends vasopressin as a supplementing vasopressor in addition to norepinephrine to achieve target MAP (mean arterial pressure) goals.[4]

## ANGIOTENSIN II: A NOVEL AGENT

The ATHOS-3 (2017) RCT investigated the ability of angiotensin II versus placebo to increase MAP on patients with refractory septic/vasodilatory shock, defined as receiving more than 0.2 mcg/kg/min of norepinephrine or equivalent vasopressor. The study demonstrated that angiotensin II significantly increased MAP, defined as an increase of 10 mmHg or an increase to at least 75 mmHg. Despite significant improvement in Sequential Organ Failure Assessment (SOFA) scores in the angiotensin II cohort, 28-day mortality did not differ between angiotensin II and placebo groups.[5] Angiotensin II is currently FDA approved for use in refractory vasodilatory shock, though further comparative studies against other vasopressors are lacking before recommendation as a second- or third-line agent.

## REFERENCES

1. Butterworth J IV. Cardiovascular drugs. In: Hensley F, ed. *A Practical Approach to Cardiac Anesthesia.* 5th ed. Philadelphia, PA: Lippincott Williams & Williams; 2013:23–88.
2. Hosseinian L, et al. Methylene blue: Magic bullet for vasoplegia? *Anesth Analg.* 2016;122(1):194–201.
3. Antonucci E, et al. Angiotensin II in refractory septic shock. *Shock.* 2017;47(5):560–566.
4. Rhodes A, et al. Surviving sepsis campaign: International guidelines for management of sepsis and septic shock. *Crit Care Med.* 2017;45(3):486–552.
5. Khanna A, et al. Angiotensin II for the treatment of vasodilatory shock. *N Engl J Med.* 2017;377(5):419–430.

# Part XXI

# GASTROINTESTINAL AND HEPATIC SYSTEMS

# 290.

# HEPATIC FUNCTION AND METABOLISM

*Faraz Mahmood and Florian Hackl*

## INTRODUCTION

The liver serves various metabolic functions, most notably the metabolism of carbohydrates, fats, and proteins.[1] Additionally, the liver has an essential role in the synthesis of proteins, including albumin and most coagulation factors. Hepatocytes also form bile acids, facilitating lipid absorption.[2] Liver functions extend to drug transport and metabolism.[3] Clinicians must be able to understand these various functions and how to monitor varying degrees of hepatocellular injury, dysfunction, as well as the resultant altered drug metabolism.

## SYNTHETIC FUNCTION

### ALBUMIN

Albumin, a serum protein formed by the liver, is critically important in maintaining plasma oncotic pressure, as well as serving as a carrier for steroids, fatty acids, and thyroid hormones. The average adult liver synthesizes about 15 g of albumin per day to maintaining a plasma albumin concentration of 3.5–5.5 g/dL.[3] Albumin exerts its osmotic effect from its large molecular weight and negative charge that attracts positively charged molecules and thus water into the intravascular space. Hypoalbuminemia can occur with liver disease, resulting in fewer drug-binding sites, subsequently increasing drug plasma concentration (*free*) and drug sensitivity. Drugs that are transported by albumin include: methadone, alfentanil, thiopental, warfarin, and furosemide, among others.[4] Acute hepatic failure is unlikely to significantly alter albumin concentrations, as the plasma half-life of albumin is ~21 days.[3]

### COAGULATION FACTORS

The liver is responsible for the production of most coagulation factors (except factors II, IV, and VIII), as well as anticoagulant proteins C and S and antithrombin III.[3] Vitamin K, absorbed by bile secretion into the gastrointestinal tract, plays an important role in the production of factors II, VII, IX, and X. It facilitates post-translational modification to allow participation in the clotting cascade (vitamin K dependent gamma-carboxylation of glutamic acid residues).[1] With hepatocellular dysfunction and decreased bile acid formation, the intestinal absorption of lipid soluble vitamins (A, D, E, and K) is impaired, resulting in vitamin K deficiency and coagulopathy.[2]

## HEPATIC METABOLISM

### PROTEIN METABOLISM

Hepatic protein metabolism includes processes such as deamination and transamination. The non-nitrogenous parts of protein are converted into glucose or lipids for energy. The enzymes used for these pathways include aspartate- and alanine-aminotransferase (AST and ALT) and are commonly assayed for assessment of liver function and damage.[1] The end products of amino acid degradation, such as ammonia and other nitrogenous waste products, are converted to the less toxic urea, which is readily excreted by the kidney. Accumulation of ammonia in the serum results in central nervous system dysfunction known as hepatic encephalopathy.[2]

### DRUG METABOLISM

Hepatic microsomal enzymes are essential to the metabolism of most drugs. Enzymatic alteration may inactivate the drug compounds, while others that are administered as prodrugs may require this transformation to be activated. The goal of metabolism is to convert these lipid-soluble compounds into water-soluble metabolites and facilitate excretion, which is divided in 3 phases of reactions. Phase I reactions introduce polar groups onto the substrates via oxidation, hydrolysis, or reduction. Cytochrome P450 enzymes (CYP), among others, are responsible for phase I reactions. The CYP3A4 subfamily metabolizes more than half of all anesthetic drugs, such as opioids (alfentanil, sufentanil, fentanyl), benzodiazepines, and local anesthetics (lidocaine, ropivacaine). Phase II reactions conjugate metabolites with charged molecules, preventing the diffusion across membranes and facilitating transport. Phase III reactions are involved in excretion of metabolites. [4]

Hepatic clearance of drugs depends on the metabolizing capacity of the liver, which can be altered by liver disease or induction of enzymes. Induction of these hepatic enzymes increases metabolism of most anesthetic drugs and subsequently results in lower plasma levels.[3] The induction of CYP isoenzymes can occur in response to chronic treatment with phenytoin, rifampin, isoniazid and with chronic alcohol abuse. Cirrhosis of the liver is associated with a prolonged elimination half-life of certain drugs (i.e., morphine, alfentanil, diazepam, lidocaine, pancuronium, and vecuronium).[1]

## HEME METABOLISM

Fetal erythrocyte production occurs exclusively in the liver. In adults, the liver is responsible for 20% of heme synthesis. Heme is synthesized from glycine and succinyl-CoA catalyzed by ALA-synthase, which is the rate-limiting step in this pathway, regulated by feedback inhibition by its own end product, heme.[3] Bilirubin is the end product of heme degradation, mainly by the reticuloendothelial system. Bound to plasma albumin, bilirubin is transported to the liver, where it is extracted and conjugated for secretion in the bile.[4]

## CLINICAL CONSIDERATIONS

### EVALUATION OF SYNTHETIC HEPATIC FUNCTION

Serum albumin levels are used to assess the liver's biosynthetic capacity. Prothrombin time (PT) is a test used to evaluate the extrinsic coagulation cascade, which is affected by reductions of factors VII, X, V, and prothrombin. It can be used to measure the consequences of decreased hepatic synthetic activity and is considered the primary qualitative measure of synthetic function of the liver. Factor VII has the shortest half-life of all coagulation factors with 3–6 hours. However, PT does not become abnormal until more than 80% of liver synthetic capacity is lost.[3]

## EFFECTS OF LIVER DISEASE ON ANESTHETIC DRUG ADMINISTRATION

Liver disease can affect the pharmacokinetics of anesthetic drugs by changing drug metabolism, protein binding, and volume of distribution. For instance, many hydrophilic medications have a larger volume of distribution requiring larger loading doses to obtain a desired effect.[2] Inversely, these drugs require lower maintenance doses as a result of decreased hepatic clearance. In particular, benzodiazepines are highly protein bound and have a low hepatic extraction, resulting in increased potency and a prolonged duration of action. Hepatic clearance of induction doses of propofol, etomidate, and ketamine are similar in patients with liver disease and healthy patients.[3] Succinylcholine metabolism can be prolonged by a decrease in pseudocholinesterase; however, this is often clinically insignificant.[1] Advanced liver disease has been shown to result in prolonging the duration of action of amino-steroid nondepolarizing neuromuscular blockers (i.e., rocuronium) of biliary excretion.[4] As a result, the initial dose required to achieve an effect is increased, while the maintenance doses are decreased. Exceptions are atracurium and cis-atracurium that are metabolized by Hoffmann degradation, which is not altered by liver disease.[3]

## REFERENCES

1. Ramsay MA. Morgan and Mikhail's Clinical Anesthesiology. Hepatic Physiology and Anesthesia. In: Butterworth JF, et al., eds. *Morgan and Mikhail's Clinical Anesthesiology*. 5th ed. New York, NY: McGraw-Hill; 2013:691–706.
2. Malhotra V, Pamnani A. Basics of Anesthesia. Renal, Liver, and Biliary Tract Disease. In: Miller RD, Pardo MC, eds. *Basics of Anesthesia*. 6th ed. Philadelphia, PA: Elsevier; 2011:448–462.
3. Murray MJ. Stoelting's Pharmacology and Physiology in Anesthetic Practice. Gastrointestinal Physiology. In: Flood P, et al., eds. *Stoelting's Pharmacology and Physiology in Anesthetic Practice*. 5th ed. Philadelphia, PA: Lippincott Williams & Wilkins; 2014:669–681.
4. Steadman RH, Braunfeld MY. Clinical Anesthesia. The Liver: Surgery and Anesthesia. In: Barash PG, et al., eds. *Clinical Anesthesia*. 8th ed. Philadelphia, PA: Lippincott Williams & Wilkins; 2017:1298–1326.

# 291.

# ENHANCED RECOVERY AFTER COLORECTAL SURGERY

*Patrick Torres and Hussam Ghabra*

## INTRODUCTION

Enhanced Recovery after Surgery (ERAS) refers to a set of multimodal and multidisciplinary protocols that aim to improve outcomes, decrease hospital length of stay, and reduce perioperative complications.[1,2] A wide range of providers is required to participate in order to successfully implement such protocols, including surgeons, anesthesiologists, nursing staff, physical and occupational therapists, and social workers, in addition to the patient, who is an active participant.

There is a multitude of literature describing ERAS protocols, especially in colorectal and gynecologic surgery. The protocols span the length of the preoperative, intraoperative, and postoperative periods. They usually consist of 15–20 elements, with each individual component contributing to the overall improved experience surrounding the procedure.[3] Research is ongoing to try to identify the specific contribution of various elements to a successful ERAS. Overall, strong evidence indicates that high compliance with ERAS protocols results in decreased hospital length of stay, reduced complications, and reduced (or no difference in) readmission rates.[1]

## ANESTHETIC CONSIDERATIONS

### PREOPERATIVE

1. Medical optimization: includes evaluation of patient's coexisting comorbidities and interventions directed toward optimizing the patient for surgery (e.g., cardiovascular, pulmonary, renal, etc.).[2,4]
2. Patient education: surgical and anesthetic management of their upcoming surgery to minimize anxiety and set expectations aiming at early recovery and discharge.
3. Fasting guidelines: allowing clear liquids up to 3 hours prior to surgery to minimize dehydration and hypoglycemia. Some protocols encourage carbohydrate-rich drinks the night before and on the morning of surgery up to 3 hours prior to surgery to ensure that the patient is in an anabolic state perioperatively, in addition to decreasing postoperative insulin resistance. However, data about carbohydrate-rich drinks are limited.
4. Preemptive analgesia: using preoperative acetaminophen and nonsteroidal anti-inflammatory drugs (NSAIDs) or COX-2 inhibitors (e.g., celecoxib).
5. Bowel preparation: which includes mechanical preparation and oral antibiotics.
6. Ileus prevention: by reducing opioids and the use of alvimopan (should be started preoperatively to be effective).

### INTRAOPERATIVE

1. Premedication: the routine use of benzodiazepines should be avoided to minimize postoperative adverse reactions (e.g., drowsiness, cognitive dysfunction, and delayed recovery).[2,4]
2. Anesthetic agents: short-acting anesthetic agents are recommended, such as sevoflurane and desflurane. Total intravenous anesthesia (TIVA) is another alternative. Intermediate-acting neuromuscular blocking agents (NMBAs) such as rocuronium are preferred, with the use of a peripheral nerve stimulator to reduce the incidence of residual muscle weakness postoperatively. Analgesia is best achieved with opioid-sparing techniques, including the use of regional anesthesia, which includes epidural analgesia for open cases and interfascial blocks such as transversus abdominis plane (TAP) or erector spinae plane (ESP) blocks for laparoscopic cases. Another alternative described in the literature is the use of ketamine (whether as a bolus on induction or as an infusion).
3. Mechanical ventilation: the recommended tidal volumes are 6–8 mL/kg of ideal body weight (IBW) with a peak end-expiratory pressure (PEEP) of 5 cm $H_2O$. Fraction of inspired oxygen ($FiO_2$) of 0.4–0.5

and plateau pressure of ≤16 mmHg is desired, to the extent possible.

4. Fluid management: several ERAS protocols recommend a restrictive fluid strategy aiming for zero-balance by replacing only fluids lost in surgery. If maintenance fluids are used, they should be limited to 2 mL/kg/hr for laparoscopic surgery and 3 mL/kg/hr for open surgery. Some protocols advocate for goal-directed fluid therapy (GDFT) with small boluses of 250 mL (of either crystalloids of colloids) to treat hypotension.

5- Temperature monitoring and regulation: with the goal of maintaining normothermia (≥35.5°C) to mitigate coagulopathy, adverse cardiac events, and surgical site infection.

6- Postoperative nausea and vomiting (PONV) prophylaxis: the routine use of ondansetron and dexamethasone is recommended. If the patient has a history of PONV, a transdermal scopolamine patch or intravenous haloperidol can be added. For high-risk patients, total intravenous anesthesia (TIVA) can be considered.

## POSTOPERATIVE

1. Pain control: this can be achieved with regional anesthesia (epidural analgesia or interfascial blocks) and scheduled multimodal analgesic medications (oral acetaminophen and NSAIDs/COX-2 inhibitors). Intravenous opioids can be used at small doses in the post-anesthesia care unit (PACU). Oral opioids can be available for breakthrough pain on an "as needed" basis. Patient-controlled analgesia (PCA) with opioids should be avoided as much as possible.[2,4]

2. Fluid management: crystalloids can be continued postoperatively at a rate of 1 mL/kg/hr, but

with the plan to discontinue them after 6 hours postoperatively or after 300 mL of oral intake, whichever occurs first. If the patient is hypotensive and it is deemed that the cause is hypovolemia, it can be treated with small boluses of 250 mL at a time.

3. Nutrition: diet should be resumed within a few hours postoperatively, starting with clear fluids without the need to wait for traditional markers of presence of bowel sounds, flatus, or bowel movement. If the patient is tolerating clear liquids by postoperative day 1, the diet should be advanced as tolerated.

4. Nasogastric tube should be avoided in elective colorectal surgery.

5. Peritoneal drains should also be avoided in elective colorectal surgery as their use has demonstrated no morbidity or mortality benefit.

6. Urinary catheters must be removed as soon as possible (as soon as in the operating room) to allow for early ambulation.

7. Early discharge: the criteria for discharge in many protocols consists of 2 elements: if the patient is able to tolerate oral diet meeting their nutritional needs and if their pain is well controlled.

## REFERENCES

1. Berian J, Ko C, Ban K. Does implementation of Enhanced Recovery after Surgery (ERAS) protocols in colorectal surgery improve patient outcomes? *Clin Colon Rectal Surg*. 2019;32(02):109–113.
2. Bordeianou L, Cavallaro P. Implementation of an ERAS pathway in colorectal surgery. *Clin Colon Rectal Surg*. 2019;32(02):102–108.
3. Ricciardi R, et al. Enhanced recovery after colorectal surgery. In: Post TW, ed., *UpToDate*. Waltham, MA: UpToDate; 2020.
4. Joshi GP. Anesthetic management for enhanced recovery after major surgery (ERAS) in adults. In: Post TW, ed., *UpToDate*. Waltham, MA: UpToDate; 2020.

# 292.

# ANATOMY OF THE GASTROINTESTINAL AND HEPATIC SYSTEMS

*Timothy F. Flanagan and Florian Hackl*

## GI SYSTEM ANATOMY AND HISTOLOGY

The gastrointestinal (GI) system consists of the esophagus, stomach, and small and large intestine. Contraction of smooth muscle sphincters and 3–12 peristaltic movements per minute facilitate mixing and passage of the GI content. Mechanical activity of the GI tract is stimulated by stretch and parasympathetic nervous system activation, whereas a sympathetic nervous system stimulation decreases activity.

## ESOPHAGUS

The esophagus extends from the cricopharyngeal sphincter ($C_6$ level) to the gastroesophageal junction. An inner circular muscle layer is surrounded by an outer longitudinal layer. The upper one-third of the inner circular muscle is striated, while the lower two-thirds are smooth.[1] The upper esophageal sphincter (UES) prevents air from entering the esophagus. Most anesthetics, except ketamine, will reduce UES tone. The lower esophageal sphincter (LES) has a resting tone of 10–15 cmH$_2$O and is the major barrier to reflux, which occurs when LES pressure is less than intragastric pressure. Vagal denervation does not significantly affect LES tone; however, reduced tone is seen with obesity and hiatal hernia.[1] Decreased LES tone in pregnancy is mainly progesterone-mediated.[2]

## STOMACH

The stomach is divided into cardia, fundus, body, and pylorus. The cardia is the entrance into the stomach, followed by the superior gastric portion, referred to as the fundus. The body of the stomach is followed by the pylorus, separating it from the duodenum. About 2 liters of gastric secretions, with a pH 1.0–3.5, are produced daily.[1]

Gastric body parietal cells are stimulated by histamine and acetylcholine to secrete hydrochloric acid and intrinsic factor, essential for absorption of vitamin B$_{12}$ in the ileum. Pepsinogen, secreted by Chief cells in the gastric body, is essential for protein digestion.[3] Gastrin is secreted by G cells in the antrum.

## THE INTESTINES

The small intestine consists of duodenum, jejunum, and ileum and is the main site of fluid and nutrient absorption. Mucosal folds and microvilli create an absorptive area of approximately 250m². Mucus-secreting Brunner glands, within the duodenum, protect the intestinal wall from damage by acidic gastric fluid. Sympathetic stimulation inhibits secretion, contributing to peptic ulcer formation in the duodenum. Epithelial cells in the small intestine contain digestive enzymes such as peptidases, disaccharidases, and lipases. Bile and pancreatic enzymes enter the duodenum via the ampulla of Vater. Flow is facilitated by the hormone-regulated sphincter of Oddi. Cholecystokinin, glucagon, and secretin decrease, whereas somatostatin and opioids increase sphincter tone. Biliary spasms are treated with glucagon or naloxone.

Absorption of water and electrolytes is the predominant function of the colon. Irritation of its mucosa, as seen with bacterial infections, causes increased secretion of water, mucus, and electrolytes, resulting in diarrhea. The vagus nerve supplies the colon up to the splenic flexure, causing segmental contraction of the proximal part of the colon. Sympathetic supply is provided by $T_{6-10}$, decreasing colonic motility with stimulation. Neostigmine increases colonic activity, while narcotics decrease both activity and tone.[1] Blood supply of the colon up to the splenic flexure is provided by ileocolic artery, whereas descending and sigmoid colon are supplied by the inferior mesenteric artery, making the splenic flexure an area of limited blood supply, susceptible to ischemia.

## ANESTHETIC CONSIDERATION

### Drugs Affecting LES Tone

The LES controls the passage of food between the esophagus and the stomach. Gastric barrier pressure, calculated as LES pressure minus intragastric pressure, is the main factor in preventing reflux. A number of drugs (Table 292.1) used in anesthetic practice can alter the LES tone.

## HEPATIC ANATOMY AND HISTOLOGY

The liver is divided topographically into 4 lobes (left, right, caudate, and quadrate) and functionally into 8 segments with independent biliary drainage, portal venous, and hepatic arterial supply. The falciform ligament separates the left from the right lobe. The coronary-, triangular-, and falciform ligaments attach the liver to the anterior abdominal wall and diaphragm.[1] The portal vein provides 75% of the hepatic blood flow, with the remaining 25% contributed by the hepatic artery.[2] $O_2$ delivered to the liver is equally divided between portal vein and hepatic artery.[4]

Blood flows past hepatocytes via sinusoids from branches of the portal vein and hepatic artery to the central veins, which join to form hepatic veins, ultimately draining into the inferior vena cava (IVC).[3] The endothelial cells lining the hepatic lobule are fenestrated to facilitate diffusion. Hepatocytes are located close to bile canaliculi, merging to form the common hepatic duct. The cystic duct from the gallbladder joins the common hepatic duct, together forming the common bile duct, which is joined by the main pancreatic duct, prior to entering the duodenum at the papilla of Vater.[3]

On a cellular level, hepatocytes are responsible for most metabolic and synthetic functions and represent 60%–80% of the liver parenchyma.[5] Non-parenchymal liver cells

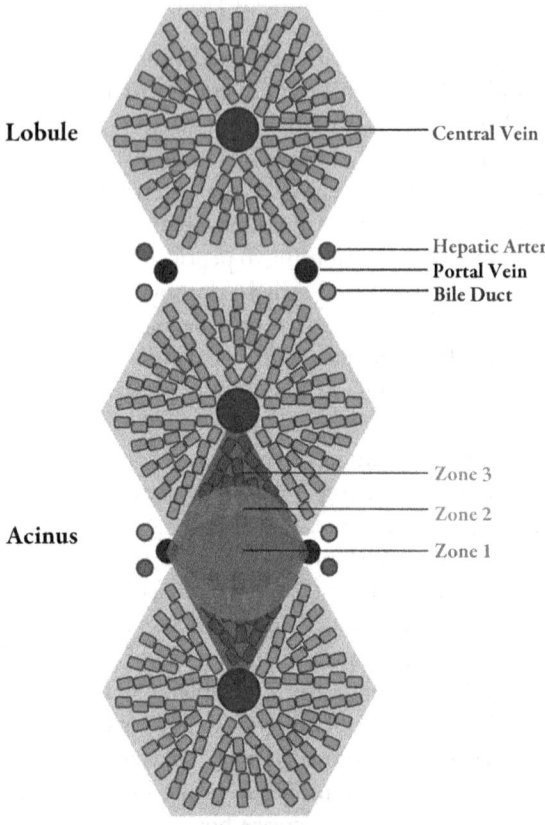

**Figure 292.1.** Histological units of the liver can be classified by the anatomic, hexagon-shaped hepatic lobule with hepatocytes radiating outward from a central vein and the portal triad (hepatic artery, portal vein, and bile duct) in the periphery, or the functional liver acinus with 3 different zones of varying metabolic activity according to the proximity of the arterial blood supply.

*Table 292.1* DRUGS AFFECTING THE LES TONE

| | |
|---|---|
| **Increase LES Tone** | |
| | Metoclopramide |
| | Domperidone |
| | Prochlorperazine |
| | Cyclizine |
| | Edrophonium |
| | Neostigmine |
| | Succinylcholine |
| | Pancuronium |
| | Metoprolol |
| | Alpha-adrenergic stimulants |
| | Antacids |
| Histamine | |
| **Decrease LES Tone** | |
| | Atropine |
| | Glycopyrrolate |
| | Dopamine |
| | Sodium nitroprusside |
| | Nitroglycerins |
| | Tricyclic antidepressants |
| Benzodiazepines (diazepam, oxazepam, triazolam) | |
| | Beta-adrenergic stimulants |
| | Opioids |
| | Thiopental |
| Meperidine | |
| | Verapamil |
| | Inhalational agents (dose dependent) |

include stellate cells, sinusoidal endothelial cells, Kupffer cells (macrophages), dendritic cells, and lymphocytes.[3]

Histologically, the anatomic lobule is differentiated from the functional acinus (Figure 292.1). At the center of the lobule lies the central hepatic vein, with branches of the portal vein, hepatic artery, and bile ducts in the periphery. In contrast, the hepatic acinus is formed by 3 different metabolic zones (Figure 292.1). Zone 1 (periportal) is an area of high metabolic activity with low susceptibility to ischemia, in close proximity to the hepatic artery. The $PaO_2$ and nutritional content of the blood decreases from zone 1 to zone 3. Zone 2 serves as an intermediate zone. Zone 3 (pericentral) is the primary site for glycolysis, lipogenesis, and detoxification of drugs and toxins. Necrosis of zone 3 is the hallmark seen in acetaminophen toxicity.[1]

## ANESTHETIC CONSIDERATIONS

### Portal Hypertension

A portal venous pressure 5 mmHg greater than IVC pressure is defined as portal hypertension, most commonly due to intrahepatic causes such as alcoholic or viral cirrhosis and non-alcoholic fatty liver disease.[4] Pre-hepatic causes include thrombus, portal vein narrowing, or splenomegaly. Post-hepatic causes are right-sided heart failure, restrictive pericarditis, and hepatic vein outflow obstruction.[3] Portal hypertension results in varices, connecting the portal vein with the systemic circulation.[2] Clinically significant varices, located in esophagus, stomach, duodenum, and rectum, can lead to massive bleeding within the GI tract.[4]

## REFERENCES

1. Steadman RH, Braunfeld MY. Clinical Anesthesia. In: Barash PG, et al., eds. *Clinical Anesthesia*. 8th ed. Philadelphia, PA: Lippincott Williams & Wilkins; 2017:1298–1326.
2. Malhotra V, Pamnani A. Basics of Anesthesia. In: Miller RD, Pardo MC, eds. *Basics of Anesthesia*. 6th ed. Philadelphia, PA: Elsevier; 2011:448–462.
3. Murray MJ. Stoelting's Pharmacology and Physiology in Anesthetic Practice. In: Flood P, et al., eds. *Stoelting's Pharmacology and Physiology in Anesthetic Practice*. 5th ed. Philadelphia, PA: Lippincott Williams & Wilkins; 2014:669–681.
4. Hevesi ZG, Hannaman M. Stoelting's Anesthesia and Co-Existing Disease. In: Hines RL, Marschall KE, eds. *Stoelting's Anesthesia and Co-Existing Disease*. 6th ed. Philadelphia, PA: Elsevier; 2012:274–286.
5. Theise ND. Robbins and Cotran Pathologic Basis of Disease. In: Kumar V, et al., eds. *Robbins and Cotran Pathologic Basis of Disease*. 9th ed. Philadelphia, PA: Elsevier; 2015:821–882.

# Part XXII

# RENAL SYSTEM

# 293.

# RENAL AND URINARY SYSTEMS/ELECTROLYTE BALANCE

*Lindsey Cieslinski*

## INTRODUCTION

The kidney is made up of approximately 1 million nephrons, each composed of 10 parts which are organized and compartmentalized to optimize the flow within the nephron. The organization is as follows: afferent arterioles → glomerulus → bowman's capsule → efferent arterioles → proximal convoluted tubules → descending limb of loop of Henle → ascending limb of loop of Henle → distal convoluted tubule → collecting duct. Each segment of the nephron has a specific purpose and fundamental role to fulfill. These parts will be discussed, along with their most significant contribution to the nephron unit, from a basic sciences perspective.

The glomerulus is responsible for filtration; the amount of filtered fluid will depend on the counterbalancing forces of hydrostatic and oncotic pressure.[2] Glomerular filtration rate (GFR) is the single best indicator of renal functioning renal mass.[1] It can be estimated by inulin due to the fact that it is freely filtered without being secreted or reabsorbed. Once the fluid filtered from the glomerulus exits the bowman's capsule, it enters the proximal tubule (PT). The PT is the major site of reabsorption. The PT reabsorbs a large proportion of water, $Na^+$, amino acids, phosphate, and glucose via gluconeogenesis. Importantly, the PT regulates acid-base balance by synthesizing buffers ($NH_3/NH_4^+$). The fluid then moves into the loop of Henle which works to concentrate the urine. This is accomplished via a countercurrent mechanism dependent upon solute transport processes and specific anatomical arrangement of the loops of Henle and vasa recta, where fluid flow occurs in opposite directions.[2] The thin descending limbs are close to the ascending limbs in what is described as a hairpin loop configuration to facilitate multiplication. The descending limb is permeable to water, while the ascending limb of the loops are impermeable to water in order to maintain a hypertonic medullary interstitium. Next, the distal convoluted tubule (DCT) secretes $K^+$ while chloride, calcium, and magnesium are reabsorbed. The DCT also is the site of action for the thiazide class of diuretics and amiloride.[3] Finally, we reach the collecting duct where salt

and water are transported via aldosterone and antidiuretic hormones (ADH) receptors. Within this segment, exertion of $NH3/NH_4^+$ and reabsorption of bicarbonate take place to aid acid-base balance. The kidneys work to compensate for an acid-base disturbance by either increasing the reabsorption of bicarbonate, in the case of metabolic acidosis; or, for metabolic alkalosis, the opposite, where bicarbonate secretion is increased to balance the alkalosis.

Twenty percent of the total cardiac output flows through the kidneys, and of this, 80% goes to the cortex, while 20% to the medulla.[3] Renal blood flow (RBF) is maintained by autoregulation to keep a glomerular capillary pressure of approximately 60–70 mmHg, for a constant filtration rate and thus a proportionate salt loss. Regulation of RBF occurs via intrinsic and extrinsic mechanisms. Intrinsic autoregulation occurs via myogenic mechanism and tubuloglomerular feedback mechanism. The tubuloglomerular feedback works by the tubular fluid composition in the distal tubule (macula densa cells) affecting the afferent arterioles (juxtaglomerular apparatus). Myogenic receptors regulate afferent arteriolar tone by vasoconstriction to protect the glomerulus from too high blood pressure, and by vasodilation to allow greater blood flow to the glomerulus in times of hypotension. Both mechanisms are impaired when mean arterial pressure (MAP) drops to less than 70 mmHg, potentially resulting in hypoperfusion of the cortex and oliguria.[1] The segment of the nephron most susceptible to ischemia is the thick ascending loop of Henle. The renin-angiotensin system (RAS) has both intrinsic and extrinsic regulatory properties. Extrinsic RBF is by renal nerves and circulating vasoactive hormones.[4]

Numerous hormones function within the nephron. Adenosine inhibits renin release and works as a vasodilation on efferent arterioles and vasoconstriction on afferent arterioles[2] to decrease GFR. Aldosterone and arginine vasopressin/ADH work within the nephron via different mechanisms, but with a shared goal to reabsorb NaCl and increase extracellular fluid volume.[5] ADH is released in response to increasing plasma osmolality, and by binding to

V2 receptors in the collecting duct it allows increased water permeability and reabsorption. Renin and angiotensin II respond to volume depletion to maintain blood pressure and intravascular volume.[2] As an opposing hormonal release to angiotensin II, atrial natriuretic peptide releases in response to atrial stretch to decrease volume by inhibition reabsorption of $Na^+$.[3] The kidneys also play a major role of calcium homeostasis; in fact, 99% of filtered $Ca^{+2}$ is reabsorbed, mostly by the PT. The kidneys are the site for the final hydroxylation reaction required to produce active vitamin D. Parathyroid hormone release in response to decreased plasma concentration of ionized calcium works to promote the formation of calcitriol in the kidney while decreasing reabsorption of phosphate. Erythropoietin stimulates erythropoiesis in response to decreased tissue oxygen tension.[4]

## ANESTHETIC CONSIDERATIONS

Renal failure can lead to electrolyte abnormalities such as hyponatremia, hyperkalemia, hyperphosphatemia, hypermagnesemia, and hypocalcemia.[2] Uremic patients should be considered as full stomach and therefore at risk of aspiration.[1] Furthermore, it is important to be cautious in patients with renal dysfunction as they will have impaired clearance of drugs; examples include morphine and nondepolarizing muscle relaxants. Certain drugs are particularly harmful to the kidneys, including but not limited to: aminoglycosides, amphotericin B, and radioactive contrast.

There are some drugs that impair renal autoregulation: angiotensin-converting enzyme inhibitors, angiotensin receptor blockers, and nonsteroidal anti-inflammatory drugs (NSAIDs). For example, ketorolac impairs prostaglandin activity, which can result in a decreased GFR, decreased RBF, and increased renal vascular resistance.[4] Increased intra-abdominal pressure during laparoscopy can mimic an abdominal compartment syndrome, compressing the kidneys and resulting in oliguria. Aortic cross clamping is dangerous, regardless of where the clamp is located.[1] Cardiopulmonary bypass is associated with acute renal failure, with incidences generally ranging from 2% to 7%.[1] Transurethral (TURP) syndrome results from excessive absorption of irrigation solution, which typically consists of a slightly hypotonic, non-electrolyte solution. This can result in severe hyponatremia, presenting as altered mental status.

## REFERENCES

1. Marieb, EN. The urinary system. *Essentials of Human Anatomy and Physiology*. 8th ed. San Francisco, CA: Pearson/Benjamin Cummings; 2006:502–520.
2. Farag EE, et al. *Basic Sciences of Anesthesia*. 1st ed. Cham, Switzerland: Springer; 2018:379–401.
3. Trentman TL, et al. *Faust's Anesthesiology Review*. Amsterdam: Elsevier; 2020:95–107.
4. Stoelting RK, Miller RD, editors. *Basics of Anesthesia*. 5th ed. Philadelphia: Churchill Livingstone; 2007.
5. Modak RK. *Anesthesiology Keywords Review*. Philadelphia, PA: Wolters Kluwer Health/Lippincott Williams & Wilkins; 2013:297.

# 294.

# RENIN-ANGIOTENSIN-ALDOSTERONE SYSTEM

*Marwa El-Sabbahy and Karim Fikry*

## INTRODUCTION

As noted in the Chapter 295 on kidney anatomy, the renin enzyme is secreted by the juxtaglomerular cells (JGC), which lie adjacent to the afferent arteriole. This occurs in response to a decrease in sodium chloride (NaCl) levels at

the macula densa in the setting of hypoperfusion of the kidneys. Renin causes angiotensinogen to be cleaved into angiotensin I, which is then converted to angiotensin II via the angiotensin converting enzyme (ACE). Angiotensin II will then initiate a number of events, including arteriolar vasoconstriction, as well as release of aldosterone, to counteract the hypoperfusion. Angiotensin also plays a direct role in increasing Na and water reabsorption via a direct effect on the proximal tubule.

Renin-angiotensin systems exist in various tissues throughout the body, including the kidneys, adrenal gland, cardiovascular system, and nervous system, where it may be involved in local regulation of vascular tone (Figure 294.1).

## RENIN

When a decrease in renal blood flow occurs with a decrease in the effective circulating volume (ECV), the JGCs convert prorenin into renin, which is then released into the circulation. Renin acts on angiotensinogen released from the liver, cleaving this into angiotensin I, and the latter is then converted to angiotensin II via ACE, which is located in the lung tissue, as well as the kidneys.[1] As noted in the Introduction to this chapter, the main stimulus for renin release is that of a low NaCl level sensed at the macula densa, which indicates a low extracellular fluid volume and the need to expand this volume with retention of Na and water. An Na-K-2Cl cotransporter in the cells of the macula densa is regulated by the delivery of NaCl. With an increase in extracellular fluid volume due to the effects of renin, there is more avid reabsorption of Na via this cotransporter, with subsequent negative feedback on renin release.

*Clinical pearl*: Hypertension may be treated using direct renin inhibitors, an example of which is aliskiren.[2] This is not a commonly used agent, however, and is not considered to be a first-line anti-hypertensive.

## ANGIOTENSIN II

This is a potent vasoconstrictor, which at the level of the kidneys primarily exerts its effect on the efferent arteriole of the kidney, although it does cause vasoconstriction of the afferent arteriole as well. Increasing resistance in the efferent arteriole will lead to an increase in the intraglomerular pressure, thereby increasing the glomerular filtration rate (GFR) of the kidney. At the same time as the GFR increases, the flow of plasma reaching the peritubular capillaries is reduced, leading to a reduction in the hydrostatic pressure in this capillary bed, with a subsequent increase in the oncotic pressure. This encourages reabsorption of tubular fluid. As you may imagine, this is imperative in the setting of decreased renal blood flow due to hypovolemia/hypotension (such as occurs in blood loss or shock). In addition, angiotensin II reduces the medullary blood flow in the vasa recta, which leads to elevated urea and NaCl in the medulla and also increases tubular fluid reabsorption.

Furthermore, angiotensin II leads to a direct increase in Na reabsorption via the proximal tubules, as well as the release of aldosterone from the zona glomerulosa of the adrenal cortex. The latter causes an increase in Na reabsorption via the distal convoluted tubules and the cortical collecting tubules. Both of these mechanisms lead to an increase in extracellular volume, thereby enhancing renal blood flow. As noted in Chapter 295 on kidney anatomy, there exist principal cells in the collecting ducts. These cells are acted upon by aldosterone, which stimulates the reabsorption of Na and the subsequent secretion of potassium (K). Aldosterone binds to mineralocorticoid receptors in the kidney tubules, which leads to the formation of an Na/K ATPase and an Na channel (ENaC) to facilitate the preceding electrolyte handling.

*Clinical pearl*: In hypertensive patients, aldosterone antagonists, such as spironolactone, may be utilized. This class of diuretic medication antagonizes the action of aldosterone at the mineralocorticoid receptors. In the kidneys, which is their main site of action, this causes an

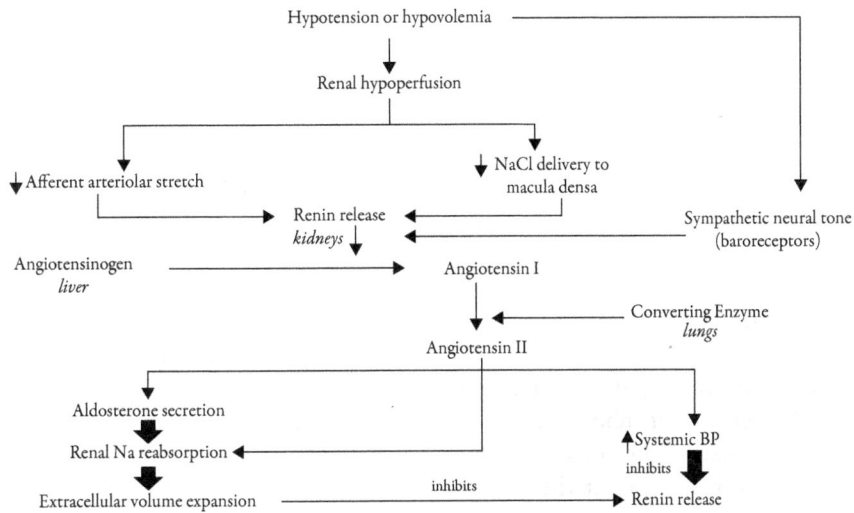

Figure 294.1. Renin-Angiotensin System.

increase in both Na excretion as well as K reabsorption. A common side effect is that of hyperkalemia. Hyperkalemia may cause cardiac arrhythmia due to decrease in conduction velocity in the myocardial tissues, and requires close monitoring.

The release of antidiuretic hormone (ADH) from the posterior pituitary gland is also directly influenced by angiotensin II. ADH stimulates the reabsorption of water via the kidneys.

It is important to note that angiotensin II is the major bioactive product of the renin-angiotensin axis, and is capable of inducing vasoconstriction in all of the body's arteriolar beds.

*Clinical pearl*: In the setting of hypertension, one of the most commonly used classes of antihypertensives is the ACE inhibitors (ACEi).[3] An example is the commonly used drug lisinopril. These reduce formation of the highly potent angiotensin II. Alternatively, the angiotensin II receptor antagonists (ARB) may be used to inhibit binding of angiotensin II to its receptor sites. An example of a commonly used ARB is losartan. It is important to note that one of the most common side effects of both the ACEi and ARB is hyperkalemia. The ACEi and ARB should not be used in combination therapy due to the potential for cumulative side effects. Furthermore, ACE is responsible for the hydrolysis of bradykinin. Therefore, ACEi will increase the levels of bradykinin, which is a vasodilator. A dry cough is thought to be due to the elevated bradykinin.

## ANESTHETIC CONSIDERATION

Continued use of ACEi and ARB through the perioperative period can lead to prolonged hypotension if the patients undergo general anesthesia, especially with large blood or fluid shifts. Withholding these anti-hypertensives 24 hours before surgery should be considered whenever possible for elective procedures.[4]

## REFERENCES

1. Patel S, et al. Renin-angiotensin-aldosterone (RAAS): The ubiquitous system for homeostasis and pathologies. *Biomed Pharmacother*. 2017;94:317–325
2. Békássy ZD, et al. Aliskiren inhibits renin-mediated complement activation. *Kidney Int*. 2018;94(4):689–700.
3. Heran BS, et al. Blood pressure lowering efficacy of angiotensin converting enzyme (ACE) inhibitors for primary hypertension. *Cochrane Database Syst Rev*. 2008;2008(4):CD003823.
4. Hollmann C, et al. A systematic review of outcomes associated with withholding or continuing angiotensin-converting enzyme inhibitors and angiotensin receptor blockers before noncardiac surgery. *Anesth Analg*. 2018;127(3):678–687.

# 295.

# ANATOMY OF THE KIDNEY

*Marwa El-Sabbahy and Karim Fikry*

## INTRODUCTION

The kidney is a complex and fascinating organ composed of glomeruli or filters, and a network of tubules. These are encompassed in the larger context of the cortex or outer "shell" and the medulla. The filtrate forms at the glomerulus and flows into the proximal tubule through the thin descending loop of Henle (inside the medulla) and back into the cortex via the thick ascending limb. From here, the loop of Henle connects to the distal convoluted tubule, and then the cortical collecting tubule, which spans both the cortex and medulla. The final destination of flow in the medulla is the papilla. Each distinctly named anatomical part of the tubular system lends itself to particular functions. The end result is the maintenance of a concentrated urine and homeostasis of the extracellular environment. The renin-angiotensin system is also regulated by the kidney, and this will be discussed in Chapter 294.

## GLOMERULUS

The glomerulus is formed of a network of capillaries branching from the afferent arteriole. They are located in Bowman's capsule and are supported structurally by the mesangium, which is composed of mesangial cells. Blood flow is directed from the afferent arteriole, through the capillary tuft, and then out of the glomerulus via the efferent arteriole. The juxtaglomerular apparatus is next to the glomerulus, and consists of the macula densa, granular or juxtaglomerular cells (JG), and the mesangium.[1] The macula densa lies in the wall of the distal convoluted tubule (DCT), at the point where this wall contacts the arteriolar bed of the glomerulus. This allows for regulation of the afferent arteriole based on changes in the sodium chloride (NaCl) levels in the DCT. The JG cells produce renin in response to the NaCl levels at the macula densa.

## TUBULES

The proximal tubule is located in the cortex and reabsorbs ~50% of the filtered sodium and water, as well as most of the filtered glucose, phosphate, and amino acids. These organic solutes are transported in coordination with the primary transport of sodium, and this process is aptly named *secondary active transport*. The proximal tubule is also responsible for ~90% of the reabsorption of bicarbonate via the sodium-hydrogen exchange mechanism. Both the apical and basolateral membranes of the tubule have water transmembrane channels or aquaporins, which render them highly permeable to water.

*Clinical pearl*: Inhibition of the carbonic anhydrase enzyme located in the proximal tubule allows for excretion of bicarbonate and excess water.

The thin descending and ascending limbs of the loop of Henle are located in the medulla, and the thick ascending limb is located in the cortex. A significant percentage of NaCl is also reabsorbed in the ascending limb of the loop of Henle; however, this limb is impermeable to water due to absence of the previously mentioned aquaporins. There is an Na-K-2Cl cotransporter in the apical membrane which allows this reabsorption of Na and Cl to occur.

*Clinical pearl*: When a loop diuretic is administered, it will act at the level of the thick ascending limb of the loop of Henle to impede Na and Cl reabsorption.[2]

The distal tubule is anatomically the closest in proximity to the glomerulus, and lies next to the macula densa of the juxtaglomerular apparatus in the cortex of the kidney. The presence of a Na-Cl cotransporter allows for <10% of total NaCl reabsorption. It is important to note that the distal tubule is also the site of calcium (Ca) reabsorption via apical vitamin D dependent channels, as well as Ca excretion via a basolateral Na-Ca exchange channel.

The connecting tubules lie adjacent to the distal convoluted tubules, and merge to form the collecting tubules, which then flow into the outer and inner medullary tubules, reaching deeper into the medulla of the kidney. The cortical collecting ducts contain principal cells and type A and B intercalated cells. The principal cells and the cells of the inner medullary collecting tubule are the sites of Na reabsorption. The intercalated cells and cells of the outer medullary collecting tubules regulate acid-base balance. Na channels in the apical membrane are regulated by hormones, including the atrial natriuretic peptide and aldosterone, which in turn influence the handling of K via an Na-K ATPase in the basolateral membrane. This regulation is discussed in Chapter 294. The collecting tubules are generally impermeable to water, unless an increase in antidiuretic hormone release causes the activation of vasopressin 2 receptors in the apical membrane of the collecting duct, leading to insertion of aquaporins.[3]

The papillary ducts are the most distal portion of the medullary collecting ducts, and converge at the apex of the renal pyramid. The papillary ducts then exit the pyramids at the renal papillae, where the filtrate empties into a minor calyx as urine.

*Clinical pearl*: Osmolarity is highest at the apex of the renal pyramid at 1200 mOsm, which leads to significant water reabsorption at this anatomical point.

## VASCULATURE

The kidney has a very rich blood supply branching from the efferent arterioles of the juxtamedullary nephrons, which are close in proximity to the medulla. These branches consist of the vasa recta and the peritubular capillaries. The vasa recta are a series of blood vessels which enter the medulla as the straight arterioles and ascend to the cortex as the straight venules, and lie parallel to the loop of Henle. The straight venules also join the interlobular veins to form venous arcades, which run along the sides of the renal pyramids. The peritubular capillaries, on the other hand, surround the tubules in the cortex of the kidney.

## REFERENCES

1. Perlewitz A, et al. The juxtaglomerular apparatus. *Acta Physiol (Oxf)*. 2012;205(1):6–8
2. Brater DC. Pharmacology of diuretics. *Am J Med Sci*. 2000;319(1):38–50
3. Schrier RW. Aquaporin-related disorders of water homeostasis. *Drug News Perspect*. 2007; 20(7):447–453

# 296.

# DIURETICS

*J. Brown and Maria F. Ramirez*

## INTRODUCTION

Diuretics are a class of medications that increase urinary output by reducing sodium chloride reabsorption at different sites along the renal nephron. Common indications include hypertension, congestive heart failure, cerebral edema, pulmonary edema, and the management of electrolytes disorders. Diuretics are categorized by either their mechanism of action or by their primary site of action in the nephron. Preoperatively all diuretics should be held on the morning of surgery in order to avoid dehydration while NPO (*nil per os*). Electrolyte imbalances associated with prolonged diuretic use require careful attention, as the anesthesia management could potentially be complicated by ventricular arrhythmias secondary to hypokalemia and hypomagnesemia for example.

## PROXIMAL TUBULE DIURETICS

Acetazolimide inhibits the activity of carbonic anhydrase (enzyme that converts $CO_2$ + $H_2O$ $HCO_3$ + $H^+$), which decreases the rate of hydrogen ($H^+$) formation and increases the excretion of sodium ($Na^+$), potassium ($K^+$), bicarbonate ($HCO_3$), and water ($H_2O$). In the eye, acetazolamide decreases aqueous humor formation and thus lowers the intraocular pressure in patients with glaucoma. Other indications include acute mountain sickness prophylaxis and anticonvulsant therapy for patients with refractory seizures. Acetazolimide may cause hypokalemia, hyponatremia, and hyperchloremic metabolic acidosis. Acetazolimide is also a sulfonamide and can lead to allergic reactions.[1]

## OSMOTIC DIURETICS

Mannitol produces diuresis because it is filtered by the glomeruli and is poorly reabsorbed by the nephron. This leads to increased tubular osmolality and associated excretion of water. Mannitol also causes the release of renal prostaglandins, promotes renal vasodilatation, and increases tubular urine flow. Mannitol is widely used for the management of elevated intracranial pressure and cerebral edema. It is also used in neurosurgery to optimize visualization during intracranial procedures. There is little evidence to support the use of mannitol for other indications such as renal protection in renal and cardiac surgery or renal transplantation where adequate hydration has shown to be effective. Side effects include risk of heart failure and pulmonary edema in patients with poor cardiac function secondary to the initial intravascular expansion (Table 296.1). Other side effects include hypotension, metabolic acidosis, hypernatremia, hypokalemia, high serum osmolality with neurologic complications, and renal failure (renal vasoconstriction plus intravascular depletion).[2]

## LOOP DIURETICS

Loop diuretics include furosemide, bumetanide, torsea-mide, and etacrynic acid. They reversibly inhibit the $Na^+$-$K^+$-$2CL^-$ symporter, located at the thick ascending loop of Henle, and inhibit sodium, chloride, and potassium reabsorption. Loop diuretics also increase the excretion of calcium and magnesium. Indications include cerebral edema, hypertension, edema associated with congestive heart failure, cirrhosis, and nephrotic syndrome. Side effects include hypovolemia, hypokalemia, hypomagnesemia, metabolic acidosis, hypercalcemia, hyperuricemia, ototoxicity, and acute renal failure. Among the different classes of diuretics, pre- and intraoperative use of loop diuretics has been associated with postoperative acute kidney injury. This effect could be secondary to greater intravascular depletion with loop diuretics than with other agents.[3]

## DISTAL CONVOLUTED TUBULE DIURETICS

Hydrochlorothiazide is the most common thiazide in clinical use. Other thiazides include metolazone, clorothiazide, and indapamide. Thiazides inhibit $Na^+$ $Cl^-$ cotransport in

*Table 296.1* DIURETICS: MECHANISM OF ACTION AND SIDE EFFECTS

| CLASS | NAME | MECHANISM OF ACTION | SIDE EFFECTS |
|---|---|---|---|
| Proximal Tubule Diuretics | Acetazolamide | - Inhibits activity of carbonic anhydrase<br>- Decreases rate of H+ formation<br>- Increases excretion Na+, K+, HCO3 and H20 | - Hypokalemia<br>- Hyponatremia<br>- Hyperchloremic metabolic acidosis<br>- Allergic reactions from sulfa component |
| Osmotic Diuretics | Mannitol | - Filtered by glomeruli, poorly absorbed<br>- Increased tubular osmolality<br>- Release of renal prostaglandins | - Renal vasodilation<br>- Increased tubular urine flow<br>- Initial intravascular expansion may cause CHF or pulmonary edema<br>- Hypotension<br>- Metabolic acidosis<br>- Hypernatremia<br>- Hypokalemia<br>- ↑ serum osmolality |
| Loop Diuretics | Furosemide, Bumetanide, Torseamide, Etacrynic acid | - Reversibly inhibits Na+-K+-2CL- symporter at thick ascending loop of Henle<br>- Inhibits Na+, K+, 2CL- reabsorption<br>- Increase excretion of Ca, and Mg | - Hypovolemia<br>- Hypokalemia<br>- Hypomagnesemia<br>- Metabolic acidosis<br>- Hypercalcemia<br>- Hyperuricemia<br>- Ototoxicity<br>- Acute Renal Failure |
| Distal Convoluted Tubule Diuretics | Hydrochlorothiazide Metolazone Clorothiazide Indapamide | - Inhibits Na+Cl- cotransport in renal convoluted tubule<br>- Increased Na+ and Cl- delivery to distal nephron | - Hypochloremic metabolic alkalosis<br>- Hyponatremia<br>- Hyperuricemia<br>- Hyperglycemia<br>- Hypokalemia |
| Distal Collecting Duct Diuretics | Spironolactone Amiloride Triamterene | - Competitive inhibitor of the aldosterone receptor<br>- Decreased Na+ and water reabsorption<br>- Decreased K+ excretion<br>- Inhibit luminal Na+ reabsorption and K+ and H+ secretion | - Hyperkalemia<br>- Hyperchloremic metabolic acidosis |
| Dopaminergic Agonist | Fenoldopam | - Selective DA1 agonist<br>- Decrease systemic vascular resistance<br>- Increase renal blood flow, diuresis, natriuresis | - Severe hypotension<br>- Tachycardia<br>- Headache<br>- Nausea |

the renal distal convoluted tubule, which leads to a greater $Na^+$ and Cl- delivery to a more distal portion of the nephron. Thiazides are commonly used for the treatment of hypertension, diabetes insipidus, and edema associated with heart failure, cirrhosis, and renal failure. Thiazides are commonly withheld before surgery due to concerns with intraoperative hypotension. Side effects are hypochloremic metabolic alkalosis, hyponatremia, hyperuricemia, hyperglycemia, and hypokalemia. Hypokalemia could possibly prolong the action of nondepolarizing neuromuscular blockade.

## DISTAL COLLETING DUCT DIURETICS

Spirolactone, amiloride, and triamterene are potassium-sparing diuretics that work in the cortical collecting tube.

Spirolactone is a competitive inhibitor of the aldosterone receptor, which leads to decreased $Na^+$ and water reabsorption and decreased $K^+$ excretion. Spirolactone is used for treating primary hyperaldosteronism, essential hypertension, congestive heart failure, and edema. Amiloride and triamterene inhibit luminal $Na^+$ reabsorption as well as potassium and hydrogen secretion. Potassium-sparing medications have minimal diuresis and hypertensive properties and are mainly used to conserve potassium in patients who are using thiazide or loop diuretics. Side effects include hyperkalemia and hyperchloremic metabolic acidosis.[4]

## DOPAMINERGIC AGONIST

Fenoldopam is a selective dopamine receptor type 1 $(DA_1)$ agonist that causes a decrease in systemic vascular resistance while simultaneously increasing renal blood flow, diuresis, and natriuresis. Fenoldopam has no effect on $DA_2$, α or β adrenoreceptors and it is currently used for the treatment of severe hypertension. Several meta-analyses have suggested a nephroprotective effect in critically ill patients with or at risk of acute kidney injury (AKI); however, recent randomized controlled trials found that fenoldopam does not prevent deterioration of renal function in patients with early AKI after cardiac surgery and has no impact on renal replacement therapy or mortality. Side effects include severe hypotension, tachycardia, headaches, and nausea.[5]

## REFERENCES

1. Kassamali R, Sica DA. Acetazolamide: A forgotten diuretic agent. *Cardiol Rev.* 2011;19(6):276–278.
2. Zhang W, et al. Mannitol in critical care and surgery over 50+ years: A systematic review of randomized controlled trials and complications with meta-analysis. *J Neurosurg Anesthesiol.* 2019;31(3):273–284.
3. Oh SW, Han SY. Loop diuretics in clinical practice. *Electrolyte Blood Press.* 2015;13(1):17–21.
4. Funder JW. Spironolactone in cardiovascular disease: An expanding universe? *F1000Res.* 2017;6:1738.
5. Sun H, et al. Does fenoldopam protect kidney in cardiac surgery? A systemic review and meta-analysis with trial sequential analysis. *Shock.* 2019;52(3):326–333.

# 297.

# DOPAMINERGIC DRUGS

## Vasu Sidagam

## INTRODUCTION

This chapter discusses commonly used dopaminergic drugs. It describes dopamine metabolism, enzymes involved in the process, and the basic pharmacology of the drugs used to influence the dopaminergic system for therapy.

These can be generally categorized as the following classes:

1. *Dopamine*: used as carbidopa/levodopa, extended-release preparations of the same combination called Rytary and an intestinal gel form called Duopa.
2. *Catechol-o-methyl transferase (COMT)/Monoamine oxidase-B (MAO-B) inhibitors*: includes entocapone and tolcapone: COMT inhibitors; selegiline and rasagiline: MAO-B inhibitors.
3. *Non-ergot dopamine agonists*: ropinirole, pramipexole, rotigotine, and apomorphine
4. *Ergotamine-derived dopamine agonists*: bromocriptine, cabergoline.

The first 3 classes of drugs are used to treat Parkinson's disease. Ropinirole in addition is used in the treatment of restless leg syndrome. Drugs in the fourth class are considered the drugs of choice for medical therapy for hyperprolactinemia of any cause, including prolactinomas.

## DOPAMINE

It is a catecholamine synthesized in dopaminergic neurons from tyrosine and stored, released, and metabolized by enzymes called catechol-o-methyl transferase (COMT) and monoamine oxidase-B (MAO-B). These neurons are in the substantia nigra of the midbrain and provide innervation to the striatum (caudate and putamen). Actions of dopamine are mediated by dopamine receptors of which D1 and D2.[1]

It is formulated as levodopa (l-DOPA); combined with carbidopa it is called levodopa/carbidopa. Levodopa if administered alone is rapidly decarboxylated by aromatic amine decarboxylase (AADC) enzyme in the intestinal mucosa to dopamine and less than 1% of the dopamine reaches the central nervous system (CNS) as it cannot cross the blood-brain barrier (BBB) (Figure 297.1). Carbidopa inhibits the AADC in the peripheral tissues, and when

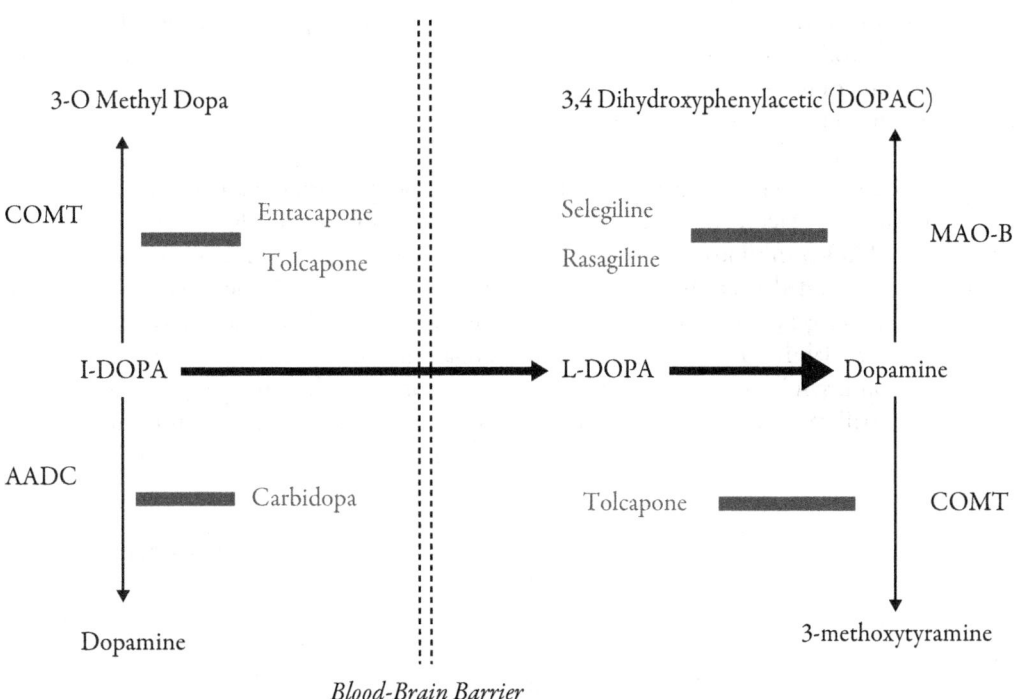

**Peripheral tissues**                    **Central Nervous System**

3-O Methyl Dopa                    3,4 Dihydroxyphenylacetic (DOPAC)

COMT          Entacapone        Selegiline                    MAO-B
              Tolcapone          Rasagiline

I-DOPA ──────────────→ L-DOPA ──────→ Dopamine

AADC          Carbidopa        Tolcapone                    COMT

Dopamine                    3-methoxytyramine

*Blood-Brain Barrier*

**Figure 297.1.** Metabolism of levodopa and sites of enzyme inhibition. Red lines indicate corresponding enzyme inhibition.

the drug reaches CNS it is converted to dopamine with higher availability for clinical effect. Patients may have bradykinesia and stiffness as the dose wears out ("off" period). Increasing the dose and frequency will help, but this can result in dyskinetic movements ("on" period). Some patients may fluctuate between being "off" and having no beneficial drug effect and being "on" but with dyskinetic movements. Some patients with Parkinson's disease compulsively take increasing doses of dopaminergic drugs despite worsening severe drug-related dyskinetic movements. This is called *dopamine dysregulation syndrome*. It could be associated with impulse control disorders like pathologic gambling.

Two new formulations of levodopa intended to address the "off" phenomenon have been approved: Rytary carbidopa/levodopa extended-release capsules, and Duopa as an intestinal gel administered through a gastrostomy a pump which reduces "off" time.

## COMT/MAO-B INHIBITOR DRUGS

These drugs which inhibit COMT not only increase the T1/2 of levodopa, but also increase the fraction of levodopa available for CNS entry. Tolcapone is longer acting and inhibits both the peripheral tissue COMT and CNS system COMT.

## NON-ERGOT DOPAMINE RECEPTOR AGONISTS

These are direct dopamine receptor agonists and are used along with carbidopa/levodopa for Parkinson's disease. Apomorphine is used as on-demand rescue medication for "off" period or as a bridge to wearing-off effect between scheduled levodopa doses; it is administered subcutaneously by injection pen.

## ERGOTAMINE-DERIVED DOPAMINE AGONISTS

Bromocriptine interacts with dopamine D2 receptors to inhibit prolactin. It decreases tumor size in more than 50% of prolactinomas. Cabergoline has a higher selective D2 receptor than bromocriptine and also has a longer half-life of 65 hours. It is the drug of choice for prolactinomas. Cabergoline has been linked to valvular heart disease.

## ANESTHETIC CONSIDERATIONS

### PREOPERATIVE

Dopaminergic medications for Parkinson's disease should be continued on day of surgery to reduce the risk of drooling or aspiration or chest wall rigidity leading to ventilation impairment. Duopa is administered through a feeding tube if the patient is kept nil per oral (NPO).

Abrupt withdrawal of levodopa may worsen Parkinson's disease symptoms and can cause an acute severe illness with tachycardia, hypertension, hyperthermia, and mental status changes. This syndrome has sometimes been called Parkinsonism hyperpyrexia syndrome. Surgery and infection are also known precipitating factors for this syndrome.

For patients taking MAO-B inhibitors like selegiline and rasagiline, it is recommended that they be stopped at least 1–2 weeks before surgery. These drugs interact with opioids, contribute to labile blood pressures, and can increase risk of serotonin syndrome. Even if surgery is emergent or urgent, it is still recommended to stop these medications.[4]

activity should be avoided in those patients taking MAO-B inhibitors like selegiline or rasagiline. Meperidine, in particular, is contraindicated although tramadol, methadone. This particular interaction can cause agitation. Rigidity, diaphoresis hyperpyrexia, and even serotonin syndrome. Morphine, codeine, oxycodone, and buprenorphine do not have serotonin reuptake inhibitor activity.[4]

Levodopa/carbidopa is known to cause hallucinations and confusion, especially in the elderly and those with cognitive impairment.[2] Treatment of postoperative delirium with some antipsychotics like haloperidol or olanzapine may worsen rigidity and tremors, as these drugs are anti-dopaminergic.[4] For treatment of postoperative nausea and vomiting, drugs like metoclopramide and promethazine are avoided because of the dopamine antagonistic actions and associated extra-pyramidal actions.

## INTRAOPERATIVE

Ketamine should be used cautiously due to potential interactions between levodopa and its sympathomimetic activities. Fentanyl and alfentanil are known to inhibit dopamine release and may worsen muscular rigidity.[5] Propofol produces dyskinesias and ablation of resting tremors at the same time.

## POSTOPERATIVE

When treating postoperative pain, opioids should be minimized. Opioids with serotonin reuptake inhibitory

## REFERENCES

1. Roberson ED. Treatment of central nervous system degenerative disorders. In: *Goodman & Gilman's Pharmacological Basis of Therapeutics.* 13th ed. New York, NY: McGraw Hill Medical; 2018:328–333.
2. Olanow CW. Parkinson's disease. In: *Harrisons' Principles of Internal Medicine.* 20th ed. New York, NY: McGraw Hill Medical; 2018:3120–3122.
3. Aminoff MJ. Nervous system disorders. In: Papadakis M, ed. *Current Medical Diagnosis and Treatment.* 54th ed. New York, NY: McGraw Hill Medical; 2015:988–991.
4. Katus L, Shtilbans A. Perioperative management of patients with Parkinson's disease. *Am J Med.* 2014;127(4):275–280.
5. Friese MB, et al. Neurologic disease and anesthesia. In: *Cotrell and Patel's Neuroanesthesia.* 6th ed. Elsevier; 2017:400–402.

# Part XXIII

# HEMATOLOGIC SYSTEM

# 298.

# ALTERNATIVES TO BLOOD TRANSFUSION

*Stacey Watt and Jennifer Lamb*

## INTRODUCTION

Patients undergoing both elective and emergent surgical procedures often experience some amount of blood loss while in the operating room. In healthy patients undergoing minor procedures, small amounts of blood loss are typically well tolerated and do not require replacement with blood transfusions. However, with significant or ongoing surgical blood loss, maintaining hemodynamic stability can become a serious intraoperative issue, particularly in patients with multiple complex comorbidities.

Although allogeneic blood transfusion is a commonly used treatment strategy for intraoperative blood loss, current practice supports minimizing blood transfusions to the degree of anemia that an individual patient can tolerate.[1,2] This individualized, multimodal approach to transfusion has evolved from knowledge that receiving a blood transfusion is not without risk, despite significant improvements in donor blood screening and pre-transfusion testing. Known complications from blood transfusions include transmission of infection, allergic and immune transfusion reactions, volume overload, and electrolyte imbalances. Thus, it is the responsibility of the anesthesiologist to have a thorough understanding of existing alternatives to blood transfusion in order to adhere to the relatively restrictive transfusion practice endorsed by most clinical guidelines.[3]

The anesthesiologist must additionally be prepared to encounter patients who decline blood transfusion in all situations, even if life-threatening. This is most commonly encountered in patients who are members of the Jehovah's Witnesses, a religious group that refuses blood transfusion based on the group's interpretation of Christian scripture. Other patients may refuse blood transfusion due to personal or cultural beliefs regarding the practice. It is important for the anesthesiologist to be equipped for these situations, particularly when preparing for surgical procedures in which substantial blood loss is likely.

## PREOPERATIVE PATIENT OPTIMIZATION TO REDUCE LIKELIHOOD OF BLOOD TRANSFUSION

### PREOPERATIVE LABORATORY EVALUATION

- Complete blood count (CBC) or baseline hemoglobin measurement
- Blood type and screen
- Coagulation testing.

### CORRECTION OF PREOPERATIVE ANEMIA

- Numerous studies have identified a correlation between preoperative anemia and increased postoperative morbidity and mortality.
  - This effect is especially pronounced when hemoglobin levels drop below 7–8 g/dL.[4]
- Three potential mechanisms are responsible for anemia:
  1. Decreased red blood cell (RBC) production
     - Examples: iron deficiency (most common cause of anemia), $B_{12}$/folate deficiency, anemia of chronic disease
  2. Increased RBC destruction
     - Examples: hemolytic anemia, intravascular hemolysis
  3. Blood loss
     - Occult malignancy
     - Surgical/trauma-related losses
- Treatment of preoperative anemia
  - Iron replacement for iron-deficiency anemia
  - $B_{12}$/folate supplementation
  - Administration of erythropoietin (EPO)
    - Full response may take up to 2 weeks.
    - Indications: renal deficiency, chronic disease, anemic patients who cannot receive blood transfusions.

## PREOPERATIVE AUTOLOGOUS BLOOD DONATION

- Preoperative autologous blood donation allows patients to donate units of their own blood for later use during an elective surgery.
- Remains uncommon secondary to hospital logistical issues/increased costs
- Indicated for patients who cannot receive allogenic transfusions (rare RBC antibodies, Jehovah's Witnesses).

## DISCONTINUATION OF ANTICOAGULANTS AND ANTIPLATELET AGENTS

- Drugs that increase the likelihood for significant intraoperative blood loss should be discontinued prior to surgery when possible.
    - Includes anticoagulants (i.e., warfarin, anti-Xa agents) and antiplatelet drugs (i.e., aspirin, clopidogrel)
- Decision and timing of discontinuation should be determined after consultation with surgeon and indicated specialists.

## INTRAOPERATIVE STRATEGIES TO REDUCE LIKELIHOOD OF BLOOD TRANSFUSION

### METHODS OF SURGICAL HEMOSTASIS

- Utilization of electrosurgical devices
- Use of topical hemostatic agents

- Note: biologically active agents (thrombin/fibrin sealants) may be sourced from human tissue, thus are potentially inappropriate for patients who decline blood transfusion.

## ACUTE NORMOVOLEMIC HEMODILUTION (ANH)

- Practice of withdrawing a predetermined amount of patient's own blood immediately prior to surgery and replacing with volume equivalent of crystalloid
    - Dilution of circulating blood volume decreases net amount of RBCs lost during surgical procedure.
    - Collected blood is returned to patient intraoperatively as required, obviating the need for allogenic transfusion
    - ANH requires careful patient selection and is generally avoided in patients with preexisting anemia or certain comorbidities.
    - Jehovah's Witnesses will typically accept ANH, as long as the autologous blood transfusion is maintained in a continuous circuit.

## INTRAOPERATIVE BLOOD SALVAGE

- Technique to recover lost surgical blood for reinfusion back into the patient
    - Blood suctioned from surgical field undergoes centrifugation and filtration prior to being returned to the patient (Figure 298.1).
    - Generally accepted by Jehovah's Witnesses provided that blood is maintained in continuous circuit.

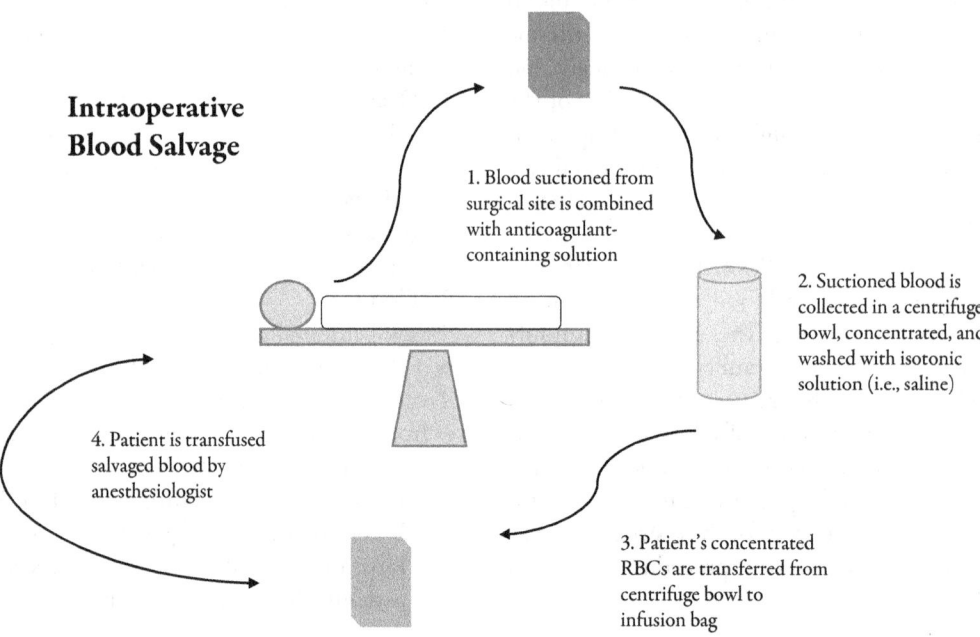

**Intraoperative Blood Salvage**

1. Blood suctioned from surgical site is combined with anticoagulant-containing solution

2. Suctioned blood is collected in a centrifuge bowl, concentrated, and washed with isotonic solution (i.e., saline)

3. Patient's concentrated RBCs are transferred from centrifuge bowl to infusion bag

4. Patient is transfused salvaged blood by anesthesiologist

**Figure 298.1.** Intraoperative blood salvage as a strategy to minimize need for allogeneic blood transfusions.

## INTRAOPERATIVE BLOOD PRESSURE MANAGEMENT

- High blood pressures can result in increased blood loss from the surgical field.
- Normotension can be maintained with a variety of antihypertensive and/or anesthetic drugs.

## AVOIDANCE OF INTRAOPERATIVE HYPOTHERMIA

- Lower body temperature causes impaired platelet aggregation and clot formation.
- Strategies to maintain intraoperative normothermia include:
  - Forced-air warming devices (i.e., Bair Hugger™)
  - Warming of intravenous fluids.

## AUGMENTATION OF SYSTEMIC HEMOSTASIS

- Antifibrinolytic agents: may be used prophylactically to reduce the risk of surgical bleeding as well as treatment for the actively bleeding patient
  - Examples: tranexamic acid (TXA) and epsilon-aminocaproic acid (EACA).

## MANAGEMENT OF COAGULOPATHY

- Emergency reversal of anticoagulation agents
  - May be required for non-elective procedures with significant life-threatening bleeding
- Intraoperative replacement of deficient coagulation factors
  - Deficiencies can occur secondary to significant blood loss or consumptive coagulopathy.
  - Intraoperative coagulation assessment: fibrinogen testing, thromboelastography (TEG).

## MANAGEMENT OF INTRAVASCULAR VOLUME DERANGEMENT

- Crystalloid: given as replacement in a 1.5:1 ratio
- Colloid: (i.e., albumin) usually administered in a 1:1 ratio

- Hydroxyethyl starch solutions (HES) are typically avoided in the bleeding patient due to concerns regarding impairment of hemostasis.
- Albumin is accepted by some Jehovah's Witnesses; specific patient wishes should be clarified prior to surgery.

## CONSIDERATIONS FOR THE ANESTHESIOLOGIST

- Identification and treatment of preoperative anemia is an important strategy for avoiding blood transfusion during elective surgery.
- Throughout the surgery, focus should shift toward minimizing surgical blood loss, as well as reclaiming a maximum percentage of what is lost by necessity.
- Strategies for minimizing surgical blood loss include acute normovolemic hemodilution (only suitable for patients without preexisting anemia), topical and systemic hemostatic agents, and maintenance of intraoperative normotension and normothermia.
- Intraoperative blood salvage allows the anesthesiologist to recover blood lost from the surgical site for autologous reinfusion into the patient.
- Specific patient wishes regarding blood products should be clarified prior to departure for the operating room, as they often differ between individuals of a particular culture or religion.

## REFERENCES

1. Practice guidelines for perioperative blood management: An updated report by the American Society of Anesthesiologists Task Force on Perioperative Blood Management. *Anesthesiology*. 2015;122(2):241–275.
2. Franchini M, et al. Patient blood management: A revolutionary approach to transfusion medicine. *Blood Transfus*. 2019;17(3): 191–195.
3. Shander A, Goodnough LT. From tolerating anemia to treating anemia. *Ann Intern Med*. 2019;170:125–126. doi: https://doi.org/10.7326/M18-3145
4. Desai N, et al. Perioperative patient blood management to improve outcomes. *Anesth Analg*. 2018;127(5):1211.

# 299.

# BLOOD TRANSFUSIONS

*Elaine A. Boydston*

## INTRODUCTION

Blood products available for transfusion include whole blood and fractionated blood components including packed red blood cells (PRBCs), platelets, fresh frozen plasma (FFP), and cryoprecipitate. The various components available are summarized in Table 299.1. This chapter will give an overview of the indications and benefits of blood transfusion as well as discuss the risks, complications, and alternatives.

## PACKED RED BLOOD CELLS

Packed red blood cells (PRBCs) are stored units of concentrated erythrocytes prepared by centrifuging whole blood and removing the plasma. One unit is 250–300 mL in volume and has a hematocrit of 55%–60%. Each unit will raise the hematocrit by 3% (or hemoglobin by 1 g/dL). PRBCs can be stored refrigerated for up to 42 days when mixed with preservatives, including an anticoagulant (citrate), dextrose (for energy), adenine (ATP-precursor), and a pH-buffer (usually phosphate). PRBCs are indicated to increase the oxygen-carrying capacity of blood, increase oxygen delivery to organs, and promote cardiac output until bleeding can be controlled.[1] PRBCs must be given according to ABO-compatibility to avoid a hemolytic transfusion reaction. If the recipient has antibodies against other RBC antigens (detected via the "screen" portion of the "type and screen"), the donor unit must be compatible with these antibodies as well.

*Table 299.1* SUMMARY OF AVAILABLE BLOOD PRODUCTS

| COMPONENT | VOLUME | EFFECT | STORAGE/USE | COMMENTS |
|---|---|---|---|---|
| PRBCs | 250–300 mL | Increase hemoglobin by 1 g/dL or hematocrit by 3% per unit | Stored at 1–6 °C for up to 42 days with citrate, phosphate, dextrose, adenine (CPDA) preservative | • ABO/Rh specific<br>• May have significant minor RBC antigens<br>• "Storage lesion" impacts efficacy and life span |
| FFP | 150–250 mL | Increase coagulation factors by 2–3% per unit | Stored at <–20°C for up to 1 year<br>Must be used within 5 days once thawed if stored at 4°C | • ABO group specific<br>• Takes 30 minutes to thaw<br>• Greatest risk of TRALI, citrate toxicity |
| Platelets, whole blood derived | 200–300 mL *(50 mL per unit pooled to form one "dose" of 4–6 units)* | Increase platelets by 5–10K per unit (or ~50K per "dose") | Stored at 24°C (room temp) for up to 5 days<br>Transfused slowly at room temperature (not through fluid warmer) | • No need for ABO compatibility<br>• Do give as Rh matched to women<br>• Recipient anti- HLA antibodies may impact life span<br>• Greatest risk of bacterial contamination |
| Platelets, apheresis | 200–400 mL | Increase platelets by 50K per unit | | |
| Cryoprecipitate | 60–90 mL *(~10 mL per unit of FFP pooled from 10 units to form one dose)* | Increase fibrinogen by 50–100 mg/dL | Stored at <–20°C for up to 1 year<br>Once thawed, must be used within 4–6 hours | • No need for ABO or Rh compatibility due to small amount of plasma transfused |

## PLATELETS

Platelets can be derived from donor whole blood (1 "dose" of platelets consists of 4–6 "units" pooled from individual donors) or from a single donor via apheresis. One "dose" of platelets has a volume of 200–400 mL and will increase the platelet count by 50 000. Platelets are indicated for microvascular bleeding due to thrombocytopenia, to "reverse" anti-platelet medications, and bleeding with evidence of platelet dysfunction (abnormal viscoelastic tests or platelet function assay). Platelets do not have to be ABO-compatible; however, women should receive Rh-matched platelets to avoid Rh-immunization.

## FRESH FROZEN PLASMA

Plasma is the fluid portion of whole blood. It contains all the coagulation factors (pro-thrombotic and anti-thrombotic) needed to create a clot. One unit of fresh frozen plasma (FFP) has a volume of 150–250 mL. The recommended dose to correct coagulopathy or reverse warfarin is 15–30 mL/kg (average of 4 units for adults). FFP is indicated for microvascular bleeding in the setting of an elevated INR (≥2), urgent warfarin reversal, coagulation factor deficiencies when specific concentrates are not available, and heparin resistance (e.g., anti-thrombin-III deficiency) in patients requiring heparinization.[2] FFP must be transfused in an ABO-compatible fashion since plasma may contain preformed antibodies against A and B antigens; however, it does not need to be Rh-compatible or cross-matched.

## CRYOPRECIPITATE

Cryoprecipitate is the fraction of plasma that precipitates when FFP is thawed and centrifuged, and contains factors VIII, XIII, I (fibrinogen), and Von Willebrand factor.[3] It can be stored for up to a year frozen; however, once thawed, it must be given within 4–6 hours. Cryoprecipitate contains 5 times more fibrinogen than FFP and is the agent of choice if fibrinogen <100 mg/dL. Other indications include as part of a massive transfusion protocol or bleeding in patients with hemophilia A or Von Willebrand disease when specific concentrates are not available.[3] If viscoelastic testing indicates normal fibrinogen activity with fibrinolysis, anti-fibrinolytic therapies may be indicated.

## TRANSFUSION RISKS AND COMPLICATIONS

Blood transfusion comes with serious risks; thus it is important to have strict indications for transfusions. The top 4 fatal complications of transfusions include transmission of blood-borne pathogens, hemolytic transfusion reactions, transfusion-related acute lung injury (TRALI), and transfusion-associated circulatory overload (TACO). Other complications include febrile nonhemolytic transfusion reactions, alloimmunization to minor blood-cell antigens, immunosuppression due to transfusion-related immunomodulation (TRIM), and metabolic and physiologic effects from blood preservation and storage.[4] These complications are discussed in detail in other chapters.

## RBC STORAGE LESION

As PRBCs are stored, glucose is broken down to lactate and hydrogen ions accumulate, lowering the pH. Stimulation of the sodium-potassium exchanger causes extracellular accumulation of potassium.[4] Levels of 2,3-DPG decrease, causing a "left shift" of the oxy-hemoglobin dissociation curve (donor RBCs may be less efficient at offloading oxygen), and the membrane becomes more fragile, causing RBC hemolysis and release of free hemoglobin.[4] The life span of transfused RBCs is reduced, averaging 35–42 days (normal is 100–120 days). Together, these changes may cause metabolic and physiologic derangements, particularly in patients receiving multiple units or older blood, including hyperkalemia, acidemia, pulmonary vasoconstriction, toxicity from free hemoglobin including kidney damage and oxidative stress, and hypocalcemia from chelation of calcium by citrate.[4]

## MASSIVE TRANSFUSION

Massive transfusion (MT) implies transfusion of greater than 1 blood volume (10 units) in 24 hours, or more than 4 units in one hour.[5] MT is most common in trauma, but also may be needed in management of ruptured aortic aneurysms, liver transplantation, and obstetric hemorrhage. Institutions usually have their own massive transfusion protocol (MTP) whereby packages of blood products are dispensed in a predetermined sequence until lab tests can guide further component therapy. Typically, type-O RBCs and type-AB plasma are given ("universal donor"), and the ratio of products is generally 1:1:1 or 2:1:1 PRBC to FFP to platelets.[5]

## TRANSFUSION ALTERNATIVES

At times, blood transfusion may be indicated but unavailable (due to patient refusal or inability to source compatible blood due to antibodies); thus alternatives may be needed. Autologous cell salvage (cell saver) is a process whereby blood is collected from the operative field, mixed with anticoagulant, concentrated, then washed or filtered and returned to the patient. In pre-deposit autologous blood donation (PABD), patients donate 2–3 units in the 6 weeks prior to surgery; then the patient's own blood is given back to them during or after surgery. Acute normovolemic hemodilution (ANH) is similar to PABD; however, the patient's own whole blood is removed on the same day as surgery, generally after induction of anesthesia but prior to anticipated blood loss. ANH reduces the total number of RBCs and coagulation factors lost during bleeding; then the blood is given back to the patient. The specific benefits, indications, and contraindications of these methods are beyond the scope of this chapter.

## REFERENCES

1. Rossaint R, et al. The European guideline on management of major bleeding and coagulopathy following trauma: Fourth edition. *Crit Care.* 2016;20:100.
2. Murad MH, et al. The effect of plasma transfusion on morbidity and mortality: A systematic review and meta-analysis. *Transfusion.* 2010;50(6):1370–1383.
3. Nascimento B, Goodnough LT, Levy JH. Cryoprecipitate therapy. *Br J Anaesth.* 2014;113(6):922–934.
4. Yoshida T, Prudent M, D'alessandro A. Red blood cell storage lesion: Causes and potential clinical consequences. *Blood Transfus.* 2019;17(1):27–52.
5. Holcomb JB, et al. The Prospective, Observational, Multicenter, Major Trauma Transfusion (PROMMTT) Study: Comparative effectiveness of a time-varying treatment with competing risks. *JAMA Surg.* 2013;148(2):127–136.

# 300.

# IMMUNOSUPPRESSIVE AND ANTI-REJECTION DRUGS

*Madiha Syed and Nicole Palm*

## INTRODUCTION

Each organ transplanted carries a unique immunogenic risk and may present challenges in preventing rejection. Many immunosuppressive therapies are utilized, which carry their own risks relevant to perioperative medicine.

## PHASES OF ORGAN REJECTION

- *Hyperacute*: within 24 hours of transplantation
- *Acute*: within the first postoperative weeks
- *Chronic*: months to years after transplantation.

## TYPES OF IMMUNOSUPPRESSION

- *Induction*: highly immunosuppressive, administered to reduce circulating T-cells; commonly high-dose glucocorticoids with polyclonal antibodies or IL2 inhibitors;
- *Maintenance*: intended to prevent acute and chronic rejection while balancing infection risk;
- *Antirejection*: treatment of rejection with aggressive immune-suppressing therapies to prolong graft survival.

## INDUCTION AGENTS

Induction agents are given perioperatively prior to transplantation. Lymphocyte-depleting regimens are used in higher immunologic risk cases or when delays in maintenance immunosuppression initiation are desired; IL2-antagonists are used in lower-risk cases.[1]

### DEPLETING REGIMENS

Polyclonal antibodies (thymoglobulin and ATGAM) are active against more than 50 cell-surface receptors on various cell types, and use induces rapid depletion of T-lymphocytes, B-cell, and NK cells. This broad spectrum of binding leads to direct cell death. While ATGAM has similar activity to thymoglobulin, it has demonstrated reduced efficacy and increased adverse effects comparatively.

## NON-DEPLETING REGIMENS

The most common monoclonal antibody target is interleukin-2. By binding IL2 and inhibiting activated T cells, basiliximab and dacilizumab inhibit activity without depletion of cell lines.

# MAINTENANCE IMMUNOSUPPRESSION

The most common maintenance regimen is a calcineurin inhibitor (CNI) and an antimetabolite with or without glucocorticoids. Some patients may be adjusted to an mTOR inhibitor or belatacept from a CNI long term, based on side effects and characteristics unique to the transplanted organ.[2]

## CALCINEURIN INHIBITORS

CNIs are the backbone of immunosuppression and are administered lifelong in most patients. They require monitoring with serum trough levels.

## GLUCOCORTICOIDS

Glucocorticoids at high doses bind DNA target transcription factors, including activator protein 1 and NF-κB. In general, an intraoperative high dose is given and quickly tapered in the postoperative period. For patients in whom glucocorticoids remain part of the maintenance regimen, consider perioperative stress dosing due to chronic adrenal insufficiency.

## ANTI-METABOLITES

Mycophenolic acid and azathioprine interfere with DNA synthesis and block T and B cell proliferation.

## MOTOR INHIBITORS

Sirolimus and everolimus inhibit target of rapamycin and IL2-driven T-cell proliferation. They delay wound healing and graft function and therefore are not added to an immunosuppressive regimen until months after the index transplantation. Therapeutic level monitoring is indicated.

## BELTACEPT

This is a selective co-stimulation blocker on T cells that can be used in place of a CNI in kidney transplantation.

*Table 300.1* ORGAN-SPECIFIC CONSIDERATIONS

| | |
|---|---|
| Heart | Minimize steroids with non-rejection graft dysfunction |
| Lung | High infection and rejection risk, err to immunosuppression |
| Liver | Minimally immunogenic, can often reduce maintenance regimen |
| Intestine | Limited enteral absorption of agents |
| Kidney/pancreas | Judicious use of nephrotoxic therapies, minimize CNI and glucocorticoid maintenance. |

## ACUTE REJECTION

Therapies directed at acute rejection require knowledge of the pathophysiology of rejection: cellular (T-cell) versus antibody-mediated (B-cell). Depleting agents can be used to treat cellular rejection. For antibody-mediated rejection, rituximab, a monoclonal antibody against CD20 on B cells can be used, Plasmapheresis, can be a valuable treatment strategy for the removal of circulating antibodies (Table 300.1).

## ADVERSE EFFECTS

Patients receiving immunosuppressive agents are at increased risk of acquiring infections or reactivation of viral infections. Table 300.2 shows the adverse effects of commonly used agents.

*Table 300.2* ADVERSE EFFECTS OF IMMUNOSUPPRESSANT AGENTS

| MEDICATION | SIDE EFFECTS |
|---|---|
| Cyclosporine | Hypertension, hyperlipidemia, nephrotoxicity, neurotoxicity |
| Tacrolimus | Nephrotoxicity, neurotoxicity, hyperglycemia/ post-transplant diabetes mellitus |
| Sirolimus | Cytopenia, hyperlipidemia |
| Azathioprine | Pancreatitis, lymphoma |
| Steroids | Hyperglycemia, hyponatremia, osteoporosis, hypertension |
| Mycophenolate mofetil | GI toxicity, anemia, neutropenia |
| Polyclonal antibodies | Leukopenia, thrombocytopenia, fever/ chills from cytokine release, opportunistic infections |
| Monoclonal antibodies | Allergic reactions, fever, rashes, diarrhea |

## DRUG INTERACTIONS WITH PERIOPERATIVE MEDICATIONS

Immunosuppressive agents can have interactions with medications and anesthetic agents. Cyclosporine can prolong the effect of muscle relaxants; studies show that the effects of vecuronium and pancuronium were prolonged in patients receiving cyclosporine. It can also increase the analgesic effects of fentanyl.[3]

Tacrolimus and cyclosporine are processed by the cytochrome P-450 system, and metabolism can be impacted by drugs that affect the P-450 system. Cyclosporine and tacrolimus can increase blood levels of benzodiazepines. Patients receiving tacrolimus or cyclosporine <4 hours prior to surgery may have subtherapeutic levels due to decreased absorption and reduction in gastric emptying that can occur with inhalational anesthetics.

Neostigmine can cause bradycardia and cardiac arrest in cardiac transplant recipients despite concomitant antimuscarinic agent administration.

No adverse effects with local anesthetics (bupivacaine or ropivacaine) have been reported in transplant recipients.

## PERIOPERATIVE MANAGEMENT

### PREOPERATIVE EVALUATION

Evaluation should focus on:

1. Graft function;
2. Presence of rejection;
3. Presence of infection;
4. Evaluation of other organ systems that might be impacted by immunosuppression or dysfunction of the transplanted organ.

Transplant recipients have a higher risk of atherosclerotic heart disease; changes in functional capacity or heart failure should prompt an evaluation of left ventricular (LV) function. Standard premedication can be used similar to nontransplant patients.

### INTRAOPERATIVE MANAGEMENT

- Regional and general anesthesia have been successfully utilized in transplant recipients. If a regional anesthetic is planned, clotting and platelet count should be assessed. Anti-thymocyte globulin and azathioprine can cause thrombocytopenia.
- Orotracheal intubation is preferred over nasal to prevent translocation of bacteria from the nasal passages to the lower respiratory tract.
- Invasive monitors should be placed only if clinically indicated and with strict sterile precautions.
- If renal and hepatic function is normal, there is no contraindication to any anesthetic.
- Transplant patients may undergo multiple surgeries and can develop tolerance to opioids; patients may need higher doses of opioids.
- NSAIDs are avoided in this population due to risk of gastrointestinal (GI) bleed, and renal and hepatic dysfunction.

### POSTOPERATIVE MANAGEMENT

- Immunosuppression regimen should be reinstated in the postoperative period.
- Close monitoring of graft function, drug levels, and renal and hepatic function should be continued, and medications modified if there is renal or hepatic insufficiency.
- Significant reduction of tacrolimus and cyclosporine can occur with dilution from large-volume infusions or cardiopulmonary bypass. Frequent monitoring of drug levels and redosing may be required.[4]

### REFERENCES

1. Mahmud N, et al. Antibody immunosuppressive therapy in solid-organ transplant: Part I. *MAbs*. 2010;2(2):148–156. doi:10.4161/mabs.2.2.11159
2. Halloran PF. Immunosuppressive drugs for kidney transplantation [published correction appears in *N Engl J Med*. 2005 Mar 10;352(10):1056]. *N Engl J Med*. 2004;351(26):2715–2729. doi:10.1056/NEJMra033540.
3. Kostopanagiotou G, et al. Anesthetic and perioperative management of adult transplant recipients in nontransplant surgery. *Anesth Analg*. 1999;89(3):613–622.
4. Brusich KT, Acan I. Anesthetic considerations in transplant recipients for nontransplant surgery, organ donation and transplantation: Current status and future challenges. In: Tsoulfas G, ed., *IntechOpen*. July 25, 2018. doi: 10.5772/intechopen.74329. Available from: https://www.intechopen.com/books/organ-donation-and-transplantation-current-status-and-future-challenges/anesthetic-considerations-in-transplant-recipients-for-nontransplant-surgery.

# 301.

# TRANSFUSION INDICATIONS

*Courtney L. Scott and Elaine A. Boydston*

## INTRODUCTION

Anesthesiologists are major users of blood products, and therefore blood transfusion is an important topic in anesthesia. Recommendations to guide transfusion practice exist from several anesthesia and critical care societies. The decision to transfuse should be goal-directed and based on objective criteria depending on the individual clinical scenario. Here we will discuss general transfusion principles and details about each blood component.

## RED BLOOD CELLS

Indications for transfusion of packed red blood cells (pRBCs) include the treatment of symptomatic anemia in order to increase oxygen-carrying capacity of the blood and to increase oxygen delivery to vital organs.[1] Remember that arterial oxygen content $(CaO_2)$ and therefore oxygen delivery to tissues $(DO_2)$ is primarily determined by the hemoglobin level and the oxygen saturation (as per the following equation).[1]

$$Ca_{O2} = (1.39 \times Hgb \times Sa_{O2}) + (Pa_{O2} \times 0.03)$$
$$D_{O2} = CO \times Ca_{O2}$$

($Ca_{O2}$ : Oxygen carrying capacity; Hgb : Hemoglobin; $Sa_{O2}$ : Oxygen saturation; $Pa_{O2}$ : Arterial oxygen concentration; $D_{O2}$ : Oxygen delivery; CO : Cardiac output)

A single unit of pRBCs has a volume of approximately 250–300 mL and a hemoglobin concentration of about 20 gm/dL. One unit is expected to increase an average adult's hemoglobin by about 1 gm/dL. The decision to transfuse should be based on signs and symptoms of organ ischemia, the existence of or potential for ongoing blood loss, the

volume status of the patient, and patient-specific risk factors for complications due to inadequate tissue oxygenation such as coronary artery disease or cerebrovascular disease.[1]

Historically, a hemoglobin level of 10 g/dL was considered the "lowest acceptable level"; however, a growing recognition of transfusion-related complications has led to the re-evaluation of transfusion practices. Transfusion is reasonable in most perioperative patients with a hemoglobin less than 7gm/dL, but it is widely accepted that increasing the hemoglobin level above 10 g/dL will not substantially increase oxygen delivery or improve tissue oxygenation further.[1] The Society of Thoracic Surgeons and Society of Cardiovascular Anesthesiologists recommend transfusions in patients with a hemoglobin between 7 and 10 g/dL with "critical noncardiac end-organ ischemia," active blood loss, or clinical indication of tissue hypoxia. Signs of tissue hypoxia include unstable vital signs, $SVO_2$ <50%, lactic acid >2 mmol/L, and signs of end-organ dysfunction.[1]

Often, acute blood loss will not be immediately reflected in the hemoglobin measurement because the dilutional effect from compensatory mechanisms, including resuscitation with crystalloid, is not apparent for several hours.[2] Thus, in the perioperative setting, the decision to transfuse red blood cells should be based on the individual patient's intravascular volume status, evidence of shock, duration and extent of the anemia, cardiopulmonary parameters, and the risk of ongoing hemorrhage, and the clinician must rely on hemodynamics and clinical situation while also anticipating potential blood loss intraoperatively.[2]

## FRESH FROZEN PLASMA

Fresh frozen plasma (FFP) is the fluid portion from whole blood, and contains all the coagulation factors for hemostasis. FFP is given to correct coagulopathy due to inherited or acquired factor deficits. Approximately 15cc/kg of FFP will raise factor activity levels by 10%–20% (Table 301.1).[3]

## Table 301.1 INDICATIONS FOR TRANSFUSION OF FRESH FROZEN PLASMA (FFP)[3]

| CLINICAL SETTING | INDICATIONS |
|---|---|
| Massive transfusion | Correct dilutional coagulopathy |
| | Signs of microvascular bleeding |
| Correction of congenital or acquired deficiencies of clotting factors | When specific factor concentrates are unavailable |
| Liver disease resulting in elevated INR | If active bleeding |
| | In preparation of surgery or invasive procedures |
| Reversal of anticoagulant therapy | In the presence of major bleeding/intracranial hemorrhage |
| | In preparation of surgery that cannot be delayed |
| Active bleeding in DIC | Correct consumptive coagulopathy |
| Reconstitution of whole blood for exchange transfusions | |
| Replacement fluid for apheresis in thrombotic microangiopathies | Thrombotic thrombocytopenic purpura |
| | Hemolytic uremic syndrome |

## Table 301.2 INDICATIONS FOR TRANSFUSION OF PLATELETS[4]

| INDICATION | CRITERIA |
|---|---|
| Thrombocytopenia | If no signs of bleeding, if platelets <10 000 |
| | If elevated risk of bleeding, if platelets <20 000 |
| | Prior to surgery if platelets <50 000 |
| Platelet dysfunction with bleeding | Reversal for antiplatelet medications |
| | After cardiopulmonary bypass |
| | Trauma |
| Massive transfusion | One unit of platelets for every 2–5 units of pRBCs |

The longer whole blood is stored (refrigerated), the more dysfunctional the clotting factors and platelets become.[2] When whole blood is not available in the setting of trauma or need for massive transfusion, the recommended ratio of blood products to avoid coagulopathy is generally 1:1:1 or 2:1:1 pRBC:FFP:platelets. These ratios have been shown to decrease mortality and increase hemostasis in these patient populations.[2]

## PLATELETS

Thrombocytopenia can present as acute or chronic and in the setting of acquired or congenital disease states. Platelets can be transfused as a pooled concentrate from 4–6 donor units or an apheresis unit from a single donor.[4] There are many recommendations for general guidance of management for thrombocytopenia depending on the clinical scenario (Table 301.2).

## CRYOPRECIPITATE

Cryoprecipitate is the fraction of plasma that precipitates when FFP is thawed. It contains fibrinogen, fibronectin, von Willebrand Factor, factor VIII, and factor XIII.[2] Each unit will increase fibrinogen by approximately 50 mg/dL.[2] Transfusion is indicated to treat microvascular bleeding when fibrinogen is less than 150gm/dL, and for bleeding prophylaxis for patients with hemophilia A, Von Willebrand's disease, or congenital dysfibrinogenemias when specific factor concentrates are not available.[2]

## WHOLE BLOOD AND RATIOS OF PRODUCTS IN MASSIVE TRANSFUSION

Whole blood has all the components of blood present in vivo and is not fractionated into individual blood components.[1]

## ANESTHETIC CONSIDERATIONS

### PREOPERATIVE

Part of the preoperative evaluation should include assessing patients for the presence of or risk factors for anemia, thrombocytopenia, or coagulation abnormalities. If the procedure is elective, this may warrant deferring the surgery until the patient can be better optimized hematologically. If the surgery is urgent or emergent, planning for the necessary blood products to be available can occur.

### INTRAOPERATIVE

Intraoperative management of bleeding and anemia is often variable and will depend on the clinical situation. In the setting of acute blood loss, laboratory values may not immediately reflect the degree of anemia or coagulopathy; therefore, hemodynamic instability and signs of end organ ischemia may be indications for transfusion. Otherwise, laboratory values, point of care viscoelastic tests, and arterial blood gas analyses can direct transfusion goals.

### POSTOPERATIVE

Bleeding may continue into the intensive care unit or other postoperative phase; therefore, ensuring the patient is adequately resuscitated for hemostasis and hemodynamic stability while avoiding over-transfusion is important to allow a safe transition of care.

## REFERENCES

1. Barash PG. *Clinical Anesthesia*. Philadelphia, PA: Wolters Kluwer; 2017.
2. Gropper MA, Miller RD. *Miller's Anesthesia*. Philadelphia, PA: Elsevier; 2020.
3. Liumbruno G, et al.; Italian Society of Transfusion Medicine and Immunohaematology (SIMTI) Work Group. Recommendations for the transfusion of plasma and platelets. *Blood transfusion = Trasfusione del sangue*. 2009;7(2):132–150.
4. Squires JE. (2015). Indications for platelet transfusion in patients with thrombocytopenia. *Blood transfusion = Trasfusione del sangue*. 2015;13(2):221–226.

# 302.

# COMPLICATIONS OF TRANSFUSIONS

*Courtney L. Scott and Elaine A. Boydston*

## INTRODUCTION

Anesthesiologists are one of the largest users of blood products; thus, it is important to be well versed in the risks and benefits of transfusion. In this chapter, we will discuss transfusion reactions and infectious risks associated with blood products.

## NON-HEMOLYTIC TRANSFUSION REACTIONS

A. *Febrile non-hemolytic transfusion reactions* (FNHTR) are among the most common transfusion reactions.[1,2] FNHTRs usually presents within 4 hours of transfusion with an increase in temperature of 1°–2°C, chills, myalgias, rigors, and headache.[2] Recipient antibodies (due to a previous transfusion or pregnancy) react with white blood cells present in the donor blood product and induce release of pyogenic cytokines. Leukocyte reduction processes can mitigate this reaction by reducing the number of leukocytes present in the donor blood.[1]

B. *Mild allergic reactions* causing urticaria and hives (but not fever) also may occur due to recipient mast cell and basophil degranulation (releasing histamine) in response to contact with foreign proteins present in the donor blood.[2]

C. *Anaphylaxis* can occur (as common as 1:20,000 transfusions) and is one of the most lethal types of non-hemolytic transfusion reactions.[2] Typically, anaphylaxis occurs in a patient with immunoglobin A (IgA) deficiency (with IgE antibodies against IgA) who receives a transfusion containing IgA proteins.[3] The signs/symptoms and treatment are the same as other types of anaphylaxis. One must stop the transfusion immediately and give supportive care with steroids, antihistamines, epinephrine, and advanced cardiac life support. Patients with IgA deficiency should only receive blood from IgA-deficient donors or blood that has been washed to remove plasma proteins.[1]

## HEMOLYTIC TRANSFUSION REACTIONS (HTR)

HTRs are life-threatening reactions due to donor blood incompatibility, leading to hemolysis and destruction of red blood cells.[2]

A. *Acute hemolytic transfusion reactions* are immediate and are due to ABO-incompatibility or to complement-fixing alloantibodies resulting in intravascular hemolysis.[1] The cause is almost always wrong blood product administration due to laboratory or human error. Symptoms include fever, chills, hypotension, tachycardia, bronchospasm, nausea, shortness of breath, flank pain, and red/brown-colored urine and bleeding due to disseminated intravascular coagulation (DIC).[3] Signs and symptoms may be nonspecific and can easily be missed under general anesthesia. Treatment includes stopping the transfusion, supportive care to maintain blood pressure and watch for development of DIC, and treatment to maintain urine output and prevent kidney damage from free hemoglobin (such as bicarbonate to alkalinize the urine).[3]

B. *Delayed hemolytic transfusion reactions* occur due to extravascular hemolysis via the reticuloendothelial system that occurs after a lag time of usually 2–21 days due to an anamnestic response in the recipient after being re-exposed to a minor red blood cell antigen.[2]

## INFECTIOUS TRANSFUSION COMPLICATIONS

Donor blood is screened for all major blood-transmittable viral illnesses, making their transmission via blood transfusion extremely rare today.[1] Apart from extremely common viruses such as CMV and EBV (which pose a risk typically only for immunocompromised individuals), bacterial contamination remains the infectious greatest risk associated with blood transfusion. The incidence of positive bacterial culture is as high as one in 3000; however, the risk of death due to sepsis is much lower (one in 200 000–500 000) due to the low bacterial load. Platelets are most commonly implicated due to their storage at room temperature (Yersinia is the most common bacterial pathogen).[1] Table 302.1 shows the relative risks of infectious pathogens associated with blood transfusion.

*Table 302.1* RELATIVE RISK OF TRANSMISSION OF VARIOUS TRANSFUSION-RELATED INFECTIOUS PATHOGENS

| PATHOGEN | RISK |
| --- | --- |
| HIV | 1:18 million to 1:2.3 million |
| Hepatitis A | 1:1 million |
| Hepatitis B | 1:280 000 to 1:350 000 |
| Hepatitis C | 1:1.8 million |
| Cytomegalovirus | 1:10 to 1:30 |
| Bacterial contamination | 1/3000 |

## TRANSFUSION-RELATED ACUTE LUNG INJURY (TRALI)

TRALI is a transfusion reaction that occurs within the first 6 hours following transfusion and results in non-cardiogenic pulmonary edema.[2] The symptoms resemble acute respiratory distress syndrome (ARDS), and diagnosis requires excluding other causes of pulmonary edema. The pathogenesis is thought to be secondary to leukocytes in the recipient's pulmonary vasculature that react to leukocyte antibodies present in the blood product and damage the pulmonary capillary endothelium.[3] The risk of TRALI increases with blood products from multiparous females, with increasing transfusions, and plasma-containing blood products including whole blood. TRALI remains the leading cause of transfusion-related mortality and the treatment is supportive.[1]

## TRANSFUSION-ASSOCIATED CIRCULATORY OVERLOAD (TACO)

In contrast to TRALI, pulmonary edema in TACO is due to circulatory overload from over-transfusion or transfusion of individuals who are sensitive to intravascular volume (such as heart failure with a reduced ejection fraction).[1] Other findings include evidence of left-sided heart failure, elevated brain natriuretic peptide (BNP), a positive fluid balance, and elevated central venous pressure.[3]

## TRANSFUSION-RELATED IMMUNOMODULATION (TRIM)

Blood transfusions can result in immunosuppression to be due to the large number of foreign antigens with differing implications for various patient populations.[2] In oncological patients, TRIM can increase the risk of cancer recurrence or distant metastasis following surgical resection. In contrast, for patients receiving solid organ transplants, TRIM may improve allograft survival due to decreased cellular-mediated rejection; however, this benefit does not outweigh the risks of transfusion and thus the decision to transfuse blood should not be based on this possible effect alone.[2]

## MASSIVE TRANSFUSION

Some transfusion risks and complications are related to the overall number of total blood products given.

### CITRATE TOXICITY

When blood products are stored, several preservatives are added to increase the shelf life. Citrate is an anticoagulant-preservative that binds calcium. With large numbers of transfusions, citrate toxicity may result, leading to profound hypocalcemia and hypotension from decreased systemic vascular resistance and decreased cardiac contractility.[1] These effects may be magnified in highly susceptible patient populations such patients with liver cirrhosis, those receiving liver transplantation, and pediatric patients.[3]

## METABOLIC DERANGEMENTS (RBC STORAGE LESION)

The longer packed red blood cells (pRBCs) are stored, the more anaerobic metabolism occurs, leading to increased lactate and free hydrogen molecules, lowering the pH.[1] Potassium also leaks out of the RBCs. Hyperkalemia and acidosis may result from massive transfusion, especially in patients who are less able to compensate for these effects, such as patients with impaired renal function.[3]

## HYPOTHERMIA

When a large number of cold (4°C) blood products are administered rapidly, hypothermia may result, further worsening tissue hypoxia and coagulopathy.[1]

## REFERENCES

1. Barash PG. *Clinical Anesthesia*. Philadelphia, PA: Wolters Kluwer; 2017.
2. Faust RJ, Cucchiara RF. *Anesthesiology Review*. New York, NY: Churchill Livingstone; 2002.
3. Gropper MA, Miller RD. *Miller's Anesthesia*. Philadelphia, PA: Elsevier; 2020.

# 303.

# BLOOD PRESERVATION AND STORAGE

*Stacey Watt and Prince Bonsu*

## INTRODUCTION

Since the formation of the first Institute of Blood Transfusion in 1926 in Moscow by Professor A. Bogdanov, there have been many techniques developed to efficiently expedite the processing and storing of blood products for future use. The objective of this chapter is to address the different components for blood preservation and storage.

The collection of blood from donors undergoes a rigorous screening process prior to storage. Blood is most often stored as a liquid at about 4°C, but can also be frozen for prolonged storage.[1] Prior to storage, anticoagulants and preservatives are used in order to provide nutrients, prevent clotting, and help maintain the overall viability of the red blood cell (RBC) during storage. Acid citrate dextrose (ACD) is one of the earliest anticoagulants used in blood storage, but citrate phosphate dextrose (CPD), along with the additive adenine (CPDA-1), is in use now.

## PRESERVATION SOLUTIONS

The most common preservation solution components used today include sodium citrate, citric acid, dextrose, double dextrose, sodium phosphate, and adenine. Each of these components plays a critical role within the solution. Sodium citrate is a calcium-chelating (binding) agent that interferes with the calcium-dependent steps in the clotting cascade and prevents coagulation.[2] Rapid transfusion of stored blood causes citrate to bind to calcium, leading to a transient decrease in ionized calcium in the patient. Transient decreases in ionized calcium can then lead to prolonged QT intervals and cause an increase in left ventricular end-diastolic pressure, as well as arterial hypotension. However, ionized calcium levels return to normal within 5 minutes of cessation of transfusion. Citrate can also cause a metabolic alkalosis following a large-volume transfusion once it is metabolized by the liver to bicarbonate.

## 2,3-DPG

Dextrose provides energy in the form of ATP for the RBCs. Both phosphate and citric acid act as a buffer. When used as a preservative solution, the acidic pH of ACD is incapable of maintaining levels of 2,3-DPG in stored blood. ACD allows blood to have a shelf life of 21 days. Other preservative solutions, such as CPD and citrate phosphate double dextrose (CP2D), also allow blood to have a shelf life of 21 days. However, the alkaline pH of CPD helps maintain the levels of 2,3-DPG in stored blood and as such is more commonly used than ACD solutions. The level of 2,3-DPG in stored blood determines the ease with which oxygen is unloaded from RBCs to tissues. An increase in 2,3-DPG shifts the oxygen dissociation curve to the right and facilitates easy unloading of oxygen to tissues (decreased affinity for hemoglobin), while a decrease in 2,3-DPG levels means the opposite (leftward shift in the oxygen dissociation curve with a P50 value less than 26) (Figure 303.1).

The addition of the additive adenine to CPD (CPDA-1) helps provide ATP needed by the stored blood. In addition, CPDA-1 prolongs the shelf life of blood by 2 weeks; 35 days in total. After the removal of plasma from stored blood, its shelf life can further be prolonged to 42 days by combining any of the preservative solutions with a mixture of adenine, glucose, and saline. The three different additive solutions currently used in the United States are Adsol (AS-1), Nutricel (AS-3), and Optisol (AS-5)1.

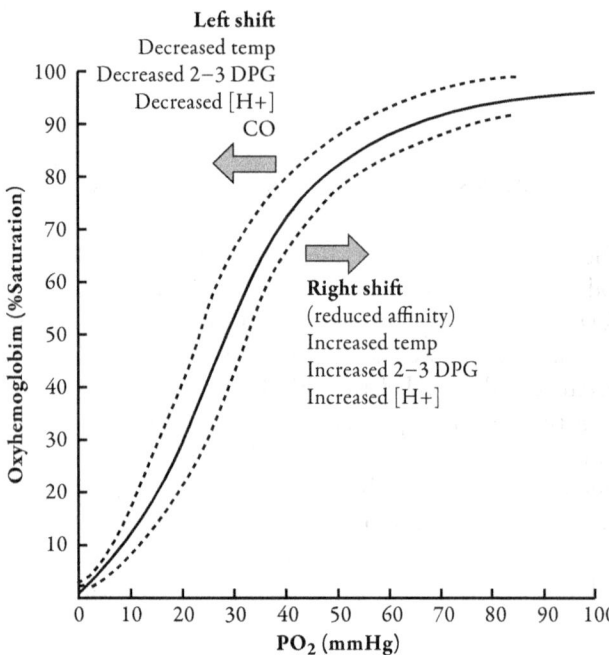

**Figure 303.1.** Oxyhemoglobin dissociation curve.

## STORAGE TIME

Storage time is defined as 70% viability of transfused erythrocytes 24 hours after transfusion, and this connotates a successful transfusion. Erythrocytes that survive longer than 24 hours after transfusion appear to have a normal life span.[1] Storage time can be increased by adding a cryoprotective agent such as glycerol to blood that has been collected and frozen at −65°C or at −120°C. When 40% glycerol is used, collected blood can be frozen at −65°C vs. −120°C when 20% glycerol is used. Regardless of what percentage of glycerol used, frozen blood can be stored for up to 10 years from the time of collection.

Blood is regularly stored at 4°C. At this temperature, platelets undergo irreversible shape changes and lose functionality and viability. The optimal temperature for platelet storage is 22°C ± 2°C, or room temperature.[1] However, since platelets need to be stored at room temperature in order to maintain functionality, they are prone to bacterial growth which could potentially lead to sepsis and death if transfused. This limits their storage time to 5 days at 22°C. The limited storage time also ensures that the platelets are not overly acidotic because pH continues to decrease secondary to platelet metabolism.

## ANESTHETIC CONSIDERATIONS

### PREOPERATIVE

If blood transfusion is anticipated, have units available and stored on site at a temperature of 4°C.

*Table 303.1* PROPERTIES OF WHOLE BLOOD AND PACKED RED CELL CONCENTRATES STORED IN CPDA-1

| PARAMETER | 0 | DAYS OF STORAGE 35 (WHOLE BLOOD) | 35 (PACKED CELLS) |
|---|---|---|---|
| pH | 7.55 | 6.73 | 6.71 |
| Plasma hemoglobin (mg/dL) | 0.5 | 46 | 246.0 |
| Plasma potassium (mEq/L) | 4.2 | 17.2 | 76.0 |
| Plasma sodium (mEq/L) | 168 | 153 | 122 |
| Blood dextrose (mg/dL) | 440 | 282 | 84 |
| 2,3-Diphosphoglycerate (μM/mL) | 13.2 | 1 | 1 |
| Percent survival* | — | 79 | 71 |

*Non-hemolyzed cells.

## INTRAOPERATIVE

All blood products except platelets should be kept cold prior to usage. Platelets can be kept at room temperature.

## POSTOPERATIVE

All unused blood products should be returned to the blood bank.

## REFERENCES

1. Miller RD. *Miller's Anesthesia*. New York, NY: Elsevier/Churchill Livingstone; 2014.
2. Barash PG, Cullen BF, and Stoelting RK. *Clinical Anesthesia*. Philadelphia, PA: Lippincott; 1989.
3. Hardwick J. Blood storage and transportation. *ISBT Science Series*. 2008;3:177–196. https://doi.org/10.1111/j.1751-2824.2008.00196.x

# 304.

# BLOOD FILTERS AND PUMPS

*Anand Prem and Suwarna Anand*

## INTRODUCTION

Blood product administration during intraoperative care of the surgical patient is an essential component of anesthetic management, particularly in the setting of trauma and acute blood loss. As the overall infectious risk of blood transfusion has reduced with more effective donor screening through nucleic acid testing, the noninfectious risks of transfusion have gained attention as risk factors for both morbidity and mortality. These include immune mediated reactions such as febrile nonhemolytic transfusion reactions, transfusion-related immunomodulation, alloimmunization and refractoriness to platelet transfusion, transfusion-related acute lung injury (TRALI), graft versus host disease (GVHD), transfusion-associated cardiac overload (TACO), and metabolic derangements such as hyperkalemia, citrate toxicity, hypothermia, and infusion of *microaggregates*.[1-4] Leukoreduction of blood products using filters or irradiation to remove white blood cells (WBCs) from red blood cells (RBCs) and platelets has reduced the risk of most of the immune-mediated reactions. Whenever blood products are stored, *microaggregates* of cellular debris, fibrin, platelets, as well as RBCs and WBCs, form. These *microaggregates* were thought to play a role in the development of acute respiratory distress syndrome (ARDS), though a direct causal link has not been established. The routine use of blood filters in blood administration sets has reduced the risk of these *microaggregate* infusions.

## BLOOD ADMINISTRATION SETS AND FILTERS

Blood products are typically transfused within 4 hours after release from the blood bank to minimize the risk of bacterial overgrowth. Standardized blood product infusion sets are required for infusion of all blood products, except hematopoietic precursor cells. While the external design varies between manufactures, they all share three main components: *inline filters*, *drip chambers*, and *tubing* that connects to an existing intravenous (IV) line.[1]

The *inline filters* of all blood product infusion sets have pore sizes between 170 and 260 microns to remove *microaggregates* before transfusion. Smaller aggregates of cellular debris and fibrin strands found in autologous blood salvaged from cardiac surgery procedures require filters of 20–40 microns.

The *drip chamber* allows control of the infusion rate and avoids infusion of air.

Prior to starting the transfusion, the *infusion set* and *tubing* are primed with either normal saline or the blood component being transfused.

Cell-saver or RBC salvage devices are used in surgeries where large-volume blood loss is expected. The salvaged blood is combined with an anticoagulant, centrifuged in a storage chamber, washed, and passed through a *microfilter* before transfusion back to the patient. Studies show that this practice reduces the need for allogenic packed red blood cell (PRBC) transfusion in adults and children during cardiac surgery and major trauma.[1,2]

Filters for leukoreduction are rarely used, with the trend toward universal pre-storage leukoreduction of blood products. Leukocyte removal filters use a different technology than red cell and platelet filters and are therefore not interchangeable. As these filters are specifically designed for gravity drip use, it is important to follow the manufacturer's special priming directions.

Specialized platelet administration sets contain the same integral mesh filter (170–200 microns) with a smaller lumen and smaller priming volume, but platelets can be given through a standard blood administration set.

Pediatric blood sets similarly contain an integrated 170–200 micron filter but are designed for small-volume transfusions with a smaller prime volume.

Fresh frozen plasma (FFP) requires a 170—200 microns filter.[1,3]

## CHANGING THE ADMINISTRATION SET

After completing a transfusion, flushing the line with saline is not recommended, as it may flush microaggregates through the filter into the patient. To prevent bacterial growth, after multiple units are transfused, the administration set should be changed every 12 hours. This also reduces the risk of incompatible fluids or medications causing hemolysis of residual blood cells.

## COADMINISTRATION OF FLUIDS AND BLOOD COMPONENTS

Traditionally, the only compatible fluid to prime the tubing and dilute blood products was 0.9% normal saline, besides compatible plasma and 5% albumin. Calcium-containing fluids like lactated ringer's solution were considered incompatible due to the theoretical concern that the high calcium concentration could chelate and overwhelm the ability of the citrate anticoagulant in the blood component, leading to clot formation. Studies have since refuted this concept, citing lack of clinical or experimental evidence of clot formation as long as a 2:1 ratio of PRBC to lactated ringer's dilution is maintained and the transfusion is not administered over a prolonged period.[2]

Hypotonic or hypertonic solutions should be avoided because of the risk of osmotic hemolysis.

## INFUSION PUMPS

Blood infusion pumps specifically approved for this purpose are certified to not cause shear stress–induced hemolysis.[1] These are either gravity driven or electronic infusion devices programmed to deliver a precise infusion rate, of particular importance in neonates where volumes transfused need to be precisely monitored. Some can be used with standard infusion sets, while others require special software. Infusion pumps should be regularly maintained in accordance with manufacturer's guidelines to ensure optimal function. Any pump malfunction must be reported to the manufacturer to allow hardware or software updates to prevent recurrence.

## INFUSION RATES

Optimal infusion rates differ with each blood component and depend on urgency of the transfusion and the patient's ability to tolerate the increase in intravascular volume. Patients with poor cardiac and renal status, prone to fluid overload, require close monitoring with lower infusion rates.

PRBCs, platelets, and plasma units are infused over 1–2 hours. Cryoprecipitate can be given after thawing, as rapidly as tolerated.

In *neonates and children*, the theoretical concern that increased flow rates cause intraventricular hemorrhage and electrolyte imbalances has little supporting evidence.[2] Transfusions are usually administered over 2–4 hours with infusion rates ranging from 5 ml/kg/h for PRBCs to 10–20 ml/kg/h for platelets and 15 ml/kg/h for FFP. If component transfusion is likely to last longer than 4 hours, "split half units" can be obtained from the blood bank to maintain component viability.

## BLOOD WARMERS

During massive blood transfusion protocols or when patients have cold agglutinins in their blood, warmers are used to warm the blood prior to transfusion, as pRBCs are typically stored at 4°C. Warming is not required for platelets which are stored at 22°C, while FFP and cryoprecipitate are thawed to 37°C prior to release from the blood bank. There is no evidence to suggest that infusion of platelets or FFP through a blood warmer is harmful. Rapid administration of cold blood products can lead to significant core hypothermia, precipitating arrhythmias, cardiac arrest, coagulopathy, and reduced red cell oxygen delivery to the tissues.[1,2,5] To avoid this, validated and approved blood warmers with temperature control and inline monitors should be used. Blood products are never to be warmed in a microwave or by immersion under hot water, as this can precipitate hemolysis or bacterial contamination. Rapid infusion devices have the ability to both warm blood and infuse it at very high rates of up to 500 ml per minute. Earlier versions were associated with a risk of air emboli, but recent enhanced safety features prevent this.

## REFERENCES

1. McClelland DBL, ed. *Handbook of Transfusion Medicine.* 4th ed. London, England: The Stationery Office; 2007.
2. Barash PG, et al. *Clinical Anesthesia,* 7th ed. Philadelphia, PA: Wolters Kluwer Health; 2013:408–444.
3. De Biasio L, Rymer T. Clinical guide to transfusion. *Blood Administration.* 2017;9:1–9.
4. Bianchi M, et al. Leukoreduction of blood components: An effective way to increase blood safety? *Blood Transfus.* 2016;14(2):214–227.
5. Rennie I, et al. Best practice in the use of blood warmers. *Nurse 2 Nurse.* 2002;2:11.

# 305.

# EFFECTS OF COOLING AND HEATING

*Madiha Syed and Pinxia Chen*

## INTRODUCTION

Temperature is frequently monitored under anesthesia in an attempt to maintain core temperatures within normal range. The human body maintains an average core temperature of 36.5–37.5°C via signals to the hypothalamus. However, the thresholds for vasoconstriction and shivering are significantly reduced under anesthesia, which can lead to hypothermia. Although sweating is the best maintained thermoregulatory mechanism during anesthesia, hyperthermia can also develop.[1]

## EFFECTS OF COOLING

Hypothermia, defined as core body temperature <36°C, can occur under general, neuraxial, and monitored anesthesia care. Heat loss can occur via radiation, convection, conduction, and evaporation (Table 305.1).[1,2] As body temperature decreases below 36°C, there is an increased incidence of deleterious effects on the body, such as decreased minimum alveolar concentration, decreased drug metabolism, decreased oxygen delivery to tissues, and increased time to emergence. Cold-mediated impairment of immune function and decreased oxygen delivery from vasoconstriction increase risk of wound infections and hinder wound healing. Coagulopathy can arise initially from alterations in platelet morphology, function, and aggregation; as temperatures drop below 33°C,

effects on coagulation enzyme activity can occur.[1] Effects on the cardiovascular system range from bradycardia and decreased cardiac output to tachyarrhythmias such as atrial fibrillation, ventricular fibrillation, and ventricular tachycardia. Intraoperative hypothermia is also associated with higher risk of postoperative cardiac events.[2,3]

Although physiological effects of hypothermia generally are considered harmful, they can also be beneficial. There is an 8% reduction in metabolic rate with each °C decrease in temperature.[1] Reductions in the cerebral metabolic rate and the release of neurotransmitters and pro-inflammatory cytokines can be protective against cerebral ischemia and hypoxia. Therapeutic hypothermia, or targeted temperature management, can improve outcomes after cardiac arrest. Hypothermia can also decrease

*Table 305.1* METHODS OF HEAT LOSS[1,2]

| | DEFINITION | % TOTAL HEAT LOSS |
|---|---|---|
| Radiation | Transfer of heat by infrared rays | ~60% |
| Convection | Transfer of heat by passing air currents | ~15% |
| Conduction | Transfer of heat from direct contact between surfaces | |
| Evaporation | Transfer of heat during water vaporization | ~22% |

cerebral blood flow which, if severe enough, can result in neurologic deficits.[1,2]

## ANESTHETIC CONSIDERATIONS

Intraoperative hypothermia can occur due to impaired thermoregulatory mechanisms under anesthesia. The major mechanism of hypothermia in both general and neuraxial anesthesia is the redistribution of body heat from the core to the periphery, which occurs in the first 30–60 minutes of anesthesia induction.[2,3] Further causes of heat loss are detailed in Box 305.1.

### PERIOPERATIVE PREVENTION AND MANAGEMENT

1. Assess patients for risk of perioperative hypothermia.
2. Intraoperative temperature monitoring for general anesthesia >30 minutes duration, deep sedation, and neuraxial anesthesia in patients felt to be at risk for hypothermia.[4]
3. Temperature monitoring at core sites (nasopharynx, distal esophagus, tympanic membrane, bladder, rectum, and pulmonary artery).[1]

---

**Box 305.1** CAUSES OF INTRAOPERATIVE HEAT LOSS[1-4]

Environmental
- Low ambient temperature
- Cold surgical cleansing solution
- Exposure during patient positioning

Anesthetic drugs
- Vasodilation: volatile anesthetics, propofol, morphine, meperidine
- Impaired thermoregulation: fentanyl and its derivatives, neuromuscular blocking agents
- General anesthesia induced reduction of metabolic rate
- Neuraxial anesthesia (vasodilation and impaired shivering)

Patient factors
- Elderly patients (decreased effective vasoconstriction and basal metabolism)
- Young children (increased body surface area to body mass ratio)
- Trauma and burn patients
- Presence of shock
- Preoperative hypothermia

Cold intravenous fluids and blood
Ventilation with dry gases

Surgical factors
- Prolonged duration of procedure
- Body cavity exposure
- Large surgical wound area

---

4. Heating and humidification of airway gases
5. Utilizing low flow rates
6. Passive and Active Warming
   6.1. Passive Warming[2-4]
        6.1.1. Raising ambient temperature
        6.1.2. Utilizing closed or semi-closed anesthesia systems
        6.1.3. Passive insulation (covering patients with blankets, surgical drapes, reflective coverings)
   6.2. Active Warming[2-4]
        6.2.1. Warming intravenous fluids and blood
        6.2.2. Cutaneous warming (forced air warming, circulating water mattresses, heat lamps).

### EFFECTS OF HEATING

Intraoperative hyperthermia is less common than hypothermia; however, it can have more deleterious effects compared to a similar degree of hypothermia. Hyperthermia is defined as a body temperature >38.5°C (101.3°F). Severe hyperthermia is any body temperature >40°C (104°F).

Fever is a specific type of hyperthermia caused by a change in the internal thermostat set point. It occurs due to the action of circulating interleukins and cytokines on the vagus nerve, which leads to a release of prostaglandin E2 in the hypothalamus. This increases the set point.[4]

Animal studies in mammals show that temperatures above 41°–42°C produce disruption of protein and RNA synthesis, disruption of the phospholipid bilayer, and inhibition of enzymatic activities, resulting in substantial cellular damage and possibly cellular death. It can increase metabolic demand and cardiovascular stress, which may be poorly tolerated in patients with limited reserves. Heat stress, however, can also lead to induction of heat shock proteins that may have a protective response. This can be seen in infections where fever and inflammation are an integral part of the immune response.[5]

Common causes of hyperthermia are detailed in Box 305.2. Passive heating occurs more frequently in infants and children due to an immature sweating response.

### PERIOPERATIVE CONSIDERATIONS

1. Evaluation of vital signs, review of history and physical exam prior to operating room (OR).
2. Use of appropriate temperature monitors: core vs. near-core sites.
3. Management: stop active warming devices and fluid warmers. Lower ambient temperature. Targeted therapy for the cause of hyperthermia, i.e., dantrolene for malignant hyperthermia.

4. Cooling (Noninvasive vs. Invasive)
    4.1. Noninvasive
        4.1.1. Evaporative cooling: decreasing ambient temperature, misting with water and blowing ambient room air with fans
        4.1.2. Immersive ice bath
        4.1.3. Ice packs (whole body vs. strategic [axilla and groin])
    4.2. Invasive
        4.2.1. Gastric lavage
        4.2.2. Peritoneal lavage
        4.2.3. Iced water rectal lavage.

### Refractory Hyperthermia

Most cases of severe hyperthermia are controlled with immersive cooling. For refractory cases options include:

    a. Cardiopulmonary bypass
    b. Intermittent hemodialysis
    c. Intravascular cooling catheters.

### REFERENCES

1. Barash PG. *Clinical Anesthesia.* 6th ed. Philadelphia, PA: Wolters Kluwer/Lippincott Williams & Wilkins; 2009.
2. Diaz M, Becker DE. Thermoregulation: Physiological and clinical considerations during sedation and general anesthesia. *Anesth Prog.* 2010 Spring;57(1):25–32.
3. McSwain JR, et al. Perioperative hypothermia: Causes, consequences and treatment. *World J Anesthesiol.* 2015 Nov 27;4(3):58–65.
4. Bindu B, et al. Temperature management under general anesthesia: Compulsion or option. *J Anaesthesiol Clin Pharmacol.* 2017 Jul–Sep;33(3):306–316.
5. Repasky E, Issels R. Physiological consequences of hyperthermia: Heat, heat shock proteins and the immune response. *Int J Hyperth.* 2002 Nov–Dec;18(6):486–489.

# 306.

# PREPARATION FOR TRANSFUSION

*Paul K. Cheng and Tariq M. Malik*

### INTRODUCTION

This chapter discusses issues related to blood product preparation before transfusion, including use of uncrossmatched blood, autologous blood, and designated donor blood products. Anesthetic considerations for transfusion in the perioperative period are also reviewed.

### TYPE AND SCREEN VS. TYPE AND CROSS

The goal of both type and screen and type and cross prior to blood transfusion is to find compatible blood for transfusion and avoid complications (detailed elsewhere in this book).

**Table 306.1** BLOOD TYPES AND COMPATIBLE ALLOGENEIC BLOOD PRODUCTS

| BLOOD GROUP | ANTIGEN ON ERYTHROCYTE | RHESUS (RH) FACTOR ON ERYTHROCYTE | PLASMA ANTIBODIES | COMPATIBLE RED BLOOD CELLS | COMPATIBLE PLASMA (FFP) |
|---|---|---|---|---|---|
| A+ | A | Present | Anti-B | A+, A–, O+, O– | A+, AB+ |
| A– | A | Absent | Anti-B, anti-Rh | A–, O– | A+, A–, AB+, AB– |
| B+ | B | Present | Anti-A | B+, B–, O+, O– | B+, AB+ |
| B– | B | Absent | Anti-A, anti-Rh | B–, O– | B+, B–, AB+, AB– |
| AB+ | AB | Present | None | All types | AB+ |
| AB– | AB | Absent | Anti-Rh | AB–, A–, B–, O– | AB+, AB– |
| O+ | None | Present | Anti-A, anti-B | O+, O– | O+, A+, B+, AB+ |
| O– | None | Absent | Anti-A, anti-B, anti-Rh | O– | Everyone |

## TYPE AND SCREEN

*Blood typing* identifies the antigens located on the membrane of erythrocytes (A, B, and Rh) and the antibodies which naturally form in situ against whichever antigens are not present on the erythrocyte. Antibodies to D, C, E, c, e, M, N, S, s, Pi, Le, K, Fy, and Jk are among those regarded as clinically significant. Rh-negative patients do not naturally have Rh antibodies but can develop these antibodies upon exposure to Rh-positive blood (through pregnancy or transfusion). There are about 45 Rh antigens in this system, but Rh-D is the most immunogenic and clinically significant, and this is the only one routinely tested.[1,2] A summary of ABO typing and the compatible allogeneic red blood cells (RBCs) and plasma are presented in Table 306.1. Of note, platelets express ABO antigens on their surface, but matching is not required as very little plasma is transfused (60 ml) with a standard platelet pack. Incompatibility, however, will decrease the effectiveness of transfused platelets. For cryoprecipitate, ABO matching is not required (only 15 ml plasma per unit).

Process:

1. Duration: 45 minutes
2. Three-step process:
   a. Cell-typing: to detect RBC surface antigens, recipient RBCs are mixed with commercially available known antibodies.
   b. Serum-typing: recipient serum is mixed with RBCs with known ABO antigens.
      Steps (a) and (b) identify the ABO-Rh type of the recipient.
   c. Screening: Recipient serum is mixed with commercially available O RBCs with uncommon antigens to help identify non-ABO system antibodies which may be present due to transfusion history. If positive, it will delay finding compatible blood.[1,2]

## TYPE AND CROSS

The donor RBCs are mixed with recipient plasma to ensure compatibility. A comparison of type and screen versus type and cross-match is presented in Table 306.2.

### UNCROSS-MATCHED BLOOD

a. In emergencies, give uncross-matched blood, ABO type-specific RBC if known; otherwise give O-negative RBC.[3]

## AUTOLOGOUS BLOOD

a. Blood collected from the patient (there are 3 variations, described in the following)

**Table 306.2** TYPE AND SCREEN VS. TYPE AND CROSS-MATCH

| | TYPE AND SCREEN | TYPE AND CROSS-MATCH |
|---|---|---|
| What is it? | • ABO typing<br>• Screen common antibodies | • ABO typing<br>• Mix donor and patient blood samples; check compatibility |
| Things to consider | • Initial transfusion test<br>• Screens for common, not rare, antibodies in recipient serum | • Usually after type and screen<br>• More time-consuming<br>• Check both common and rare antibodies |
| When to order? | • Unlikely to need transfusion but blood products should be available for backup | • Likely to need transfusion intraoperatively<br>• Should be done before all transfusions except in emergencies |

b. Avoids issues in giving allogeneic blood
c. Needs planning and good health; more expensive.

## PREOPERATIVE AUTOLOGOUS DONATION (PAD)

The simplest form and requires the least equipment. Patients donate RBCs in advance to be stored and used for their own surgery. Patients usually need hemoglobin of 11 g/dL to be eligible for PAD and can donate 6–10.5 ml/kg blood every 5–7 days, with the last unit collected 72 hours before surgery.[1] It reduces the number of patients requiring allogeneic blood transfusions and reduces the volume of allogeneic blood transfused per patient.[2,4] Recombinant human erythropoietin (rHuEPO) can be an effective means for increasing the amount of blood that can be collected from the patient before surgery. Risks include clerical error, cardiovascular overload, bacterial infection, and transfusion-related immunomodulation.[2]

## INTRAOPERATIVE AND POSTOPERATIVE BLOOD SALVAGE

This is the most expensive type of autotransfusion. Blood recovered intra- or postoperatively can be processed and transfused back. It is contraindicated when there is infection/pus, spilled bowel contents, foreign substance in the wound (as antibiotic irrigation, microfibrillar collagen hemostat), or malignancy. Cell-washing devices remove platelets and coagulation factors from salvaged blood; this represents a problem only when at least one blood volume has been retransfused. Risks include dilutional coagulopathy, reinfusion of excessive anticoagulant such as heparin, hemolysis, air embolism, and disseminated intravascular coagulation.[1,2,4]

## ACUTE NORMOVOLEMIC HEMODILUTION (ANH)

During ANH, 1–2 units of blood are extracted from the patient via venipuncture immediately before surgical incision and are stored for transfusion back to the patient at the end of surgery. Blood is replaced by crystalloid (3:1 ratio) or colloid (1:1 ratio). This is helpful when the recipient has multiple antibodies.[2]

## DESIGNATED/DIRECTED DONORS

Designated/directed donors are relatives or friends of patients who donate blood products specifically to that patient prior to surgery.[2] It is helpful when patients have rare blood types or need an uncommon phenotype of blood product.[5] There is a higher risk of graft versus host disease with directed donations coming specifically from blood relatives given their similar HLA haplotype. These units must be irradiated before transfusion to minimize the risk of GVHD.[2,5]

## ANESTHETIC CONSIDERATIONS

### PREOPERATIVE

- Identify risk factors for needing blood product transfusion.
- Discuss risks and benefits of transfusion.
- Order type and screen versus type and cross.
- If autologous blood or directed donation requested, make arrangements.

### INTRAOPERATIVE

- Confirm ABO blood type, screen, and cross-match prior to transfusion unless emergency situation, where you can use uncross-matched blood.
- If relevant, use autologous blood and designated donor blood products prior to allogenic.

### Special Considerations for PRBC Transfusion

- Irradiated blood used in
  - Malignancies, immunosuppressed, BMT
  - Directed donation from relative
  - Neonates/premature babies.
- CMV negative blood indicated in
  - Immunosuppressed
  - Antepartum transfusion/pregnant patient
  - Neonates.
- Washed RBC, volume-reduced platelets
  - If recipient is IgA deficient (to lower or remove IgA dose by removing donor plasma).
- Fresh RBC in hyperkalemic population if
  - Patient is neonate
  - On extracorporal membrane oxygenation (ECMO)
  - End-stage renal disease (ESRD).

### POSTOPERATIVE

- Monitor for bleeding and any signs of transfusion reaction.
- Consider postoperative recovery of autologous blood.

## REFERENCES

1. Miller RD. Blood Therapy. In: Miller RD, et al., eds. *Basics of Anesthesia*. 6th ed. Philadelphia, PA: Elsevier/Saunders; 2011.
2. Carabini LM, Ramsey G. Hemostasis and transfusion medicine. In: Barash PG, et al., eds. *Clinical Anesthesia*. Philadelphia, PA: Lippincott; 2013.

3. Yazer MH, et al.; Trauma, Hemostasis, Oxygenation Resuscitation Network (THOR) Working Party. Use of uncrossmatched erythrocytes in emergency bleeding situations. *Anesthesiology.* 2018;128(3): 650–656.
4. Management ASoATFoPB. Practice guidelines for perioperative blood management: an updated report by the American Society of Anesthesiologists Task Force on Perioperative Blood Management. *Anesthesiology.* 2015;122(2):241–275.
5. Dorsey KA, et al. A comparison of human immunodeficiency virus, hepatitis C virus, hepatitis B virus, and human T-lymphotropic virus marker rates for directed versus volunteer blood donations to the American Red Cross during 2005 to 2010. *Transfusion.* 2013;53(6):1250–1256.

# 307.

# ANESTHETIC CONSIDERATIONS FOR REACTIONS TO TRANSFUSIONS

*John Rose*

## INTRODUCTION

Transfusion-related reactions occur in approximately 1% of all blood product administrations, and can range from mild fevers to disseminated intravascular coagulopathy (DIC) and death.[1] They can be immune related, including nonhemolytic reactions (febrile reactions, allergic reactions, anaphylactic reactions, transfusion-related acute lung injury, immunomodulation) and hemolytic reactions (acute hemolytic reactions, and delayed hemolytic reactions), or nonimmune related caused by infections, hypervolemia, coagulopathy, hypothermia, and citrate toxicity. In this chapter, the pathophysiology, clinical presentation, and anesthetic considerations for these reactions are thoroughly examined.

## ANESTHETIC CONSIDERATIONS

### PREOPERATIVE

Obtaining a type and screen or cross-match is vital. Blood typing is carried out by mixing the patient's red blood cells (RBCs) with known antisera and by mixing patient serum with RBCs of known antigen type.[2] This redundant check ensures that the patient's blood type is correctly identified, and reduces the likelihood that a transfusion reaction will occur.

In an antibody screen, patient serum is combined with a panel of known reagents composed of various RBC antigens. If the antibody screen is positive, any blood product given to the patient should be screened beforehand to prevent the transfusion of that specific antigen. In a cross-match, the patient's serum is mixed with RBCs of a donor unit to test for agglutination.[5] If the cross-match between donor RBC and patient serum is negative, it is a positive indicator that those blood products can be safely transfused.

### INTRAOPERATIVE

Intraoperatively, transfusion reactions can present in several different ways. A summary of the pathological processes, presentations, and treatments for each of these reactions can be seen in Table 307.1.

### Febrile Transfusion Reactions

Being acutely febrile can signify many different pathological processes, and infection and hemolysis must be considered. If temperature should rise more than 2°C, the unit should be cultured and blood cultures should be taken from the patient.[1] If all other potential causes of fever have been excluded, antipyretics should be administered and the patient should be closely monitored.

**Table 307.1** A SUMMARY OF THE PATHOLOGICAL PROCESSES, PRESENTATIONS, TREATMENTS, AND POSTOPERATIVE CONSIDERATIONS FOR FEBRILE, ALLERGIC, ACUTE HEMOLYTIC, AND DELAYED HEMOLYTIC TRANSFUSION REACTIONS

| TYPE OF REACTION | MECHANISM OF ACTION | SYMPTOMS | TREATMENT | POSTOPERATIVE CONSIDERATIONS |
|---|---|---|---|---|
| Febrile transfusion reaction | Recipient antibody reaction to donor granulocytes and platelets. | Increase in temperature of 1°C within the first four hours of transfusion. | Administered antipyretics, rule out more serious causes of fever | Consider administering leukoreduced blood products in future transfusions. |
| Allergic transfusion reaction | Immune resposne to nonspecific donor proteins can lead to mild reactions. Anti-IgA antibodies in IgA-deficient patients can lead to anaphylactic reactions. | Mild reactions include urticaria, pruritis, edema. Severe reactions can result in frank anaphylaxis. | Mild reactions can be managed with antihistamines. Anaphylaxis should be treated promptly with epinephrine, antihistamines, steroids, and bronchodilators. | Consider administering washed blood products in future transfusions. |
| Acute hemolytic transfusion reaction | Recipient antibody production to ABO incompatible blood products | Fever, tachycardia, hypotension, shock, hemoglobinemia, and DIC | Immediately stop transfusion, report the event to the blood bank, administer fluid resuscitation, vasopressor support, and replace platlets and coagulation factors as necessary. | A thorough assessment of institutional transfusion practices should take place to correct the error leading to the acute hemolytic reaction. |
| Delayed hemolytic transfusion reaction | Recipient antibody production to minor antigens in donor blood (not ABO) | Jaundice, weakness, and fever | Typically no treatment is required. | Trend serial hematocrits to ensure that significant hemolysis does not occur. |

## Allergic Transfusion Reactions

Mild allergic responses include erythema, urticaria, and itching, and can be well managed with antihistamines. Anaphylactic responses are rare, and typically present with acute respiratory distress and severe hypotension. These reactions should be promptly treated by halting further blood product administration and giving epinephrine, antihistamines, bronchodilators, and intravenous steroids.

## Acute Hemolytic Transfusion Reactions

Acute hemolytic transfusion reactions will often present quickly after transfusing an ABO-incompatible blood product. The patient can develop fever, hypotension, hemoglobinuria, increased bleeding, DIC, or cardiovascular shock. If this occurs, the transfusion must be stopped immediately and the blood bank should be notified. Treatment includes fluid resuscitation and vasopressor administration. Fresh frozen plasma and platelets may be required if there is concern for DIC.

## Delayed Hemolytic Transfusion Reactions

Although delayed hemolytic transfusion reactions typically present weeks after transfusion, an amnestic response to a previously encountered blood antigen can sometimes appear within hours.[3] Patients typically present with fever, mild jaundice, and transient hemoglobinuria. Treatment typically is not required, and postoperative monitoring with serial hematocrits is all that is necessary. However, if severe hemolysis occurs, treatment is similar to that of an acute hemolytic reaction.

## POSTOPERATIVE

In patients with allergic transfusion reactions, washed blood products can be administered in future transfusions to minimize symptoms. In patients with a history of febrile transfusion reactions, giving leukoreduced blood products can significantly reduce this type of reaction from occuring.[1] In delayed hemolytic transfusion reactions, following serial hematocrits can ensure that the patient does not become severely anemic.

For patients with acute hemolytic transfusion reactions, supportive care in an intensive care unit (ICU) setting is often warranted. A thorough self-assessment within the institution concerning how the event occurred is necessary to ensure that the clerical or procedural error does not happen in the future. Acute hemolytic events are typically caused by clerical errors, such as misidentifying blood products.[3]

## REFERENCES

1. Castillo B, et al. *Transfusion Medicine for Pathologists: A Comprehensive Review for Board Preparation, Certification, and Clinical Practice.* Amsterdam, Netherlands: Elsevier; 2018.

2. Barry CL. Immunohematology and transfusion medicine. *Lab Med.* 2019;4(3):591–607.
3. Sesok-Pizzini DA. Chapter 28: Acute and delayed hemolytic transfusion reactions. In: Academic Press; 2001:247–252.

# 308.

# SYNTHETIC AND RECOMBINANT HEMOGLOBINS

*Samuel Tillmans and Stacey Watt*

## INTRODUCTION

Synthetic and recombinant hemoglobin may well play a vital role in the future of anesthesiology and beyond. Hemoglobin is the main component of red blood cells (RBCs), normally making up 34% of the cell content. The development of these synthetic and recombinant hemoglobins has led to a class of artificial blood called hemoglobin-based oxygen carriers. With blood bank shortages, the possibility of contamination of donor blood, cross-match issues, donor blood storage problems, shelf-life limitations, and ethical concerns regarding transfusion to certain patients, these new synthetic and recombinant hemoglobins have the potential to drastically alter the landscape of blood transfusion medicine in anesthesiology and elsewhere. Beyond the possibility of just solving our current blood donor/transfusion issues, we may actually develop a blood product that could be superior to human donor blood in certain aspects.

## ISSUES WITH HUMAN DONOR RED BLOOD CELLS

- Short shelf life of human donated blood
  - Current solutions of donated packed red blood cells (pRBCs) have a shelf life of around 42 days and must be refrigerated.
- Contaminants exist in the human blood bank.
  - Viral infections (COVID, hepatitis, HIV, ebola), bacterial infections (*Staphylococcus epidermidis* and *Bacillus cereus*), and protein infections (Creitzfieldt-Jakob disease)
- Incompatibility of donor and patient blood types limits the use of human red blood cell transfusion.
- Limitations of donors due to religious beliefs (e.g., Jehovah's Witnesses)
- Insufficient blood supply and shortages. Currently, there is no blood substitute available in the United States.

Recombinant hemoglobin
- Although there is no current blood substitute, one promising product is recombinant hemoglobin.
- These are typically a hemoglobin molecule that is produced via transgenic *Escherichia coli*, then further developed physiologically via protein engineering through site-specific mutagenesis.[1]
- There are other models of producing recombinant hemoglobin aside from *E. coli*.
- Possibly limitless production supply.
- Barriers to production
  - Extremely low yield of functional recombinant hemoglobin when produced
  - Generally, 7% of the total cell protein content has functional hemoglobin, and this is under ideal conditions in a very controlled experiment.[3]
  - Very expensive process, as the total cost of synthetic and recombinant hemoglobin is >$200/g when factoring in all costs, compared to around $2/g for human hemoglobin.[2]

Conjugated and polymerized hemoglobin
- Outside of recombinant hemoglobin, *conjugated hemoglobins* and *polymerized hemoglobin* are the other two most likely acellular hemoglobin sources of artificial blood.
- Conjugated hemoglobins are produced through the use inert polymers such as polyethylene glycol to attach to the surface of hemoglobin molecules.
- Conjugated hemoglobins have shown to have longer circulatory times.[5]
- Chemical modification goal is to stabilize hemoglobin in a tetrameric form to keep it intravascular and prevent renal accumulation.
- Hemoglobin in this process is derived from human or bovine RBCs.
- Issues remain with hemoglobin staying in tetrameric state long term.
- Polymerized hemoglobin is produced through a process of using extract hemoglobin from RBCs, and then mixing into an electrolyte solution. The polymerized hemoglobin is then protected against breakdown. This theoretically should result in less nephrotoxicity and liver toxicity.
  - Process to produce polymerized hemoglobin essentially intermoleculary cross-links hemoglobin molecules to increase the overall molecular size.
  - Like conjugated hemoglobin, the hemoglobin used is also derived from bovine or human RBCs.
- One of the main drawbacks in these two types of hemoglobin-based oxygen carriers (HBOCs) is the inability to convert $Fe(3+)$ to $Fe(2+)$.

Cellular HBOCs
- Cellular HBOC blood substitutes are derived by different materials used to encapsulate hemoglobin:
  - Nanoparticles
  - Liposome layers.
- Advantages
  - Less nitrous oxide scavenging
  - Prolong half-life
  - Smaller size than RBC allows bypass of blockages, and allows reductase to also be encapsulated preventing accumulation of methemoglobin.
  - The encapsulation also increases circulatory time.
- Disadvantages of HBOCs
  - Immunogenicity from cellular/liposomal structure
  - Expensive to produce
  - Hard to produce
  - Oxidative damage
  - Side reactions.

Advantages and Disadvantages to synthetic and recombinant hemoglobins
- The main advantages of these synthetic and recombinant hemoglobin/Hbs are lack of infectious agents/pathogens, longer shelf life, universally compatible, and adjustable supply.
- Generalized problems of synthetic and recombinant hemoglobin-based oxygen carriers:
  - Nitric oxide scavenging
    - Hemoglobin normally binds nitrous oxide; however, hemoglobin free in plasma can cross the endothelium and more easily bind nitrous oxide.
    - This leads to vasoconstriction via interrupting the nitric oxide vasoregulation.
    - Causes hypertension and pulmonary hypertension.
  - Lower P50
    - Free hemoglobin binds tighter to oxygen
    - Essentially a left shift in the $O_2$-Hb dissociation curve
  - HBOCs have a P50 of 10–16 vs. 26–28 in RBCs.
    - Separation of hemoglobin from 2,3-DPG
    - Hemoglobin dimers, due to hemoglobin tetramer degradation, bind much more tightly to oxygen.
  - Rapidly excreted renally
    - Free hemoglobin is degraded into smaller molecule, allowing rapid renal excretion.
  - Degradation from tetramer into dimer into monomer hemoglobin species
    - Shorter half-life
    - Possible kidney damage and renal failure through obstructing the renal tubules due to the smaller size after degradation.
- Side effects in clinical trials
  - Hypertension, gastrointestinal side effects (abdominal pain, esophageal spasm, diarrhea), kidney damage, pancreatic and liver enzyme elevation, hemostasis, hemoglobinuria, and stroke.[4]
- Current status of HBOCs
  - Because of these side effects and safety concerns regarding hemoglobin crossing the blood vessel wall, nitric oxide scavenging, and oxidative reactions,[4] these substitutes are not yet approved for use in the United States or the European Union.

## REFERENCES

1. Moradi S, Jahanian-Najafabadi A, Roudkenar MH. Artificial blood substitutes: First steps on the long route to clinical utility. *Clin Med Insights Blood Disord*. 2016;9:33–41. Published 2016 Oct 27. doi:10.4137/CMBD.S38461. https://www.ncbi.nlm.nih.gov/pmc/articles/PMC5084831/
2. Frost AT, Jacobsen IH, Worberg A, Martínez JL. How synthetic biology and metabolic engineering can boost the generation of artificial blood using microbial production hosts. *Front Bioeng Biotechnol*. 2018;6:186. Published 2018 Nov 30. doi:10.338d9/fbioe.2018.00186
3. Mozafari M, et al. Artificial blood—a game changer for future medicine: Where are we today? *J Blood Disord Transfus*. 2015;6:8–10.
4. Alayash AI. Blood substitutes: Why haven't we been more successful? *Trends Biotechnol*. 2014;32:177–185.

# 309.

# MASSIVE TRANSFUSION PROTOCOL

*Alina Genis*

## INTRODUCTION

Massive transfusion is the replacement of a large blood volume in a short period of time in responsive to uncontrolled hemorrhage, historically in the setting of trauma. Trauma patients typically experience a complex multisystem trauma-induced coagulopathy that is initiated prior to reaching the hospital. In adults, massive transfusion is defined as the transfusion of greater than 10 packed red blood cell (pRBC) units within 24 hours, transfusion of more than 4 RBC units in 1 hour with anticipated need for further blood product transfusion, or the replacement of >50% of total blood volume (TBV) by blood products within 3 hours. In the pediatric population, massive transfusion is defined as transfusion of 100% of TBV within 24 hours, transfusion support to replace ongoing hemorrhage of greater than 10% TBV per minute, or replacement of more than 50% TBV by blood products within 3 hours.

## INDICATIONS

Besides significant trauma leading to acute blood loss, massive transfusion is indicated in non-trauma patients with significant hemorrhage or lack of hemostasis, including those with gastrointestinal bleeding, ruptured abdominal aortic aneurysm, bleeding during surgery, cardiac surgery, liver transplantation, and obstetric hemorrhage. The purpose of the massive transfusion is to maintain cardiac output, oxygen carrying capacity, and hemostatic potential. The development and maintenance of a massive transfusion protocol (MTP) requires multidisciplinary input from various departments, including blood bank, transfusion medicine, emergency medicine, trauma and surgery, intensive care unit (ICU), and anesthesiology.

## PATHOPHYSIOLOGY

Traumatic injury and massive acute blood loss are often associated with trauma-induced coagulopathy which can result in challenges with obtaining hemostasis. The severity of trauma-induced coagulopathy is directly related to the severity of the injury.[1] Typically, injured endothelial initiates the process of hemostasis through the exposure of various subendothelial components. Primary hemostasis involves the formation of a platelet plug and vasoconstriction. This is followed by secondary hemostasis through the activation of coagulation factors to generate fibrin clot. Fibrinolysis also plays a significant role in hemostasis.

Various physiologic changes in trauma patients interfere with the normal functioning of the coagulation system. Uncontrolled hemorrhage is associated with excessive consumption of coagulation factors and platelets, as well as dilutional coagulopathy due to administration of large volumes of fluid. In addition, hemodynamic instability in these patients can result in acidosis, which attenuates thrombin generation and platelet function. Often, trauma patients are hypothermic, partially due to the administration of large volume resuscitation without adequate prewarming. Hypothermia is detrimental in this setting; it further reduces the enzymatic activity of coagulation proteins and decreases platelet function. Hyperfibrinolysis can often contribute to trauma-induced coagulopathy by accelerated degradation of fibrin. Hypoperfusion from hemorrhagic shock has been shown to activate protein C, which limits coagulation by inactivating factors V and VIII and enhancing fibrinolysis within 30 minutes of injury prior to the administration of any blood products.[2] In the setting of trauma, coagulopathy has been shown to be an independent predictor of early mortality.[1] Trauma-induced coagulopathy can be attenuated by the avoidance of hypothermia, acidosis, and dilution.

## PROTOCOLS

Massive transfusion protocols are institution dependent, but many involve predetermined ratio-driven guidelines. The earliest studies that evaluated the transfusion of pRBCs, fresh frozen plasma (FFP), and platelets in equal ratios came from the military setting. The goal was to mimic the transfusion of whole blood and limit the dilutional effects of transfusing higher ratios of pRBCs compared to FFP and platelets. Military studies demonstrated the mortality and survival benefits of transfusing blood products in more equivalent ratios. These were followed by superior prospective civilian studies that supported the survival benefits. The majority of level one trauma centers in the United States utilize protocols which target transfusing blood products in a 1:1:1 ratio. The aim is to switch to goal-directed strategy as laboratory information becomes available. Viscoelastical hemostatic assays such as thromboelastography (TEG) or rotational thromboelastometry (ROTEM) can be utilized to help guide transfusion.

## ADJUNCT THERAPIES

Components besides pRBCs, FFP, and platelets have been studied and incorporated into massive transfusion protocols at various institutions. Factor concentrates do not require cross-matching but can increase the risk of thromboembolic events. The CRASH-2 (Clinical Randomization of an Antifibrinolytic in Significant Hemorrhage 2) study demonstrated the benefits of administering transexamic acid (TXA) as a part of MTP. Early treatment (<3 hours from injury) significantly reduced the risk of death due to any cause by 10%, and reduced risk of death due to bleeding by 15%. There were no adverse events, particularly thromboembolic events, associated with administration of TXA. Anti-fibrinolytics have also been studied in the settings of postpartum hemorrhage and cardiothoracic surgery, which have demonstrated similar benefits.

Cryoprecipitate is a pooled human blood product that contains fibrinogen, factor VIII, factor XIII, vWF, and fibronectin. Although fibrinogen is a critical component for clot formation and sufficient clot strength, cryoprecipitate has not been shown to decrease in-hospital mortality in trauma patients. Recombinant FVIIa was not shown to reduce mortality in patients with refractory traumatic hemorrhage, but may reduce need for massive transfusion in patients with penetrating trauma. Unfortunately, multiple studies have demonstrated an increased incidence of thromboembolic events associated with recombinant FVIIa.

Prothrombin complex concentrates (PCC) are purified coagulation factors that include factors II, VII, IX, and X. PCC is commonly utilized for emergent warfarin reversal, as it contains all 4 vitamin K–dependent coagulation factors as well as proteins C and S. PCC is recommended for acute warfarin reversal over FFP due to the ease of storage, small infusion volume, and viral inactivation. Novel direct oral anticoagulants (NOACs) are increasing being utilized as anticoagulation agents for a variety of indications. NOACs introduce a new challenge for reversal in the setting of emergent hemostasis. These agent-specific reversal agents are expensive and can be short-acting. Idarucizumab, a monoclonal Fab fragment that specifically binds to dabigatran, is approved for emergent reversal. Andexanet reverses rivaroxaban or apixaban for approximately 3 hours. PCC has been used off-label for management of life-threatening bleeding in patients taking NOACs.

## COMPLICATIONS

The incorporation of an MTP introduces benefits such as a decrease in the amount of each blood component transfused, shorter turnaround times, and lower hospital expenses. However, MTPs have not been shown to have a significant effect on mortality. Although transfusing large amounts of blood products to an exsanguinating patient can be life-saving, it comes with its own risks that should be anticipated. Hypocalcaemia can result from large amounts of citrate inadvertently given in massive transfusions. Citrate is converted to bicarbonate, leading to metabolic alkalosis if renal function is impaired. Citrate accumulation in the setting of hepatic failure can lead to citrate toxicity and hypotension. Other electrolyte imbalances include hyperkalemia secondary to cell lysis or leakage during cell storage. Massive transfusion can also result in hypothermia, and blood warmers should be utilized to avoid hypothermia, which can lead to further coagulopathy, arrhythmias, and increased rates of surgical site infections. Transfusion-associated circulatory overload (TACO), particularity in those with preexisting cardiac disease, and transfusion-related acute lung injury (TRALI) are also potential risks of massive transfusion.

## REFERENCES

1. Misgav M, Martinowitz U. Trauma-induced coagulopathy: Mechanisms and state of the art treatment. *Harefuah*. 2011;150(2): 99–207.
2. Brohi K, et al. Acute traumatic coagulopathy. *J Trauma*. 2003;54: 1127–1130.
3. Muirhead B, Weiss ADH. Massive hemorrhage and transfusion in the operating room. *Can J Anaesth*. 2017;64(9):962–978.
4. Davenport RA, Brohi K. Cause of trauma-induced coagulopathy. *Curr Opin Anesthesiol*. 2016 Apr;29(2):212–219.
5. Holcomb JB, et al; PROPPR Study Group. Transfusion of plasma, platelets, and red blood cells in a 1:1:1 vs a 1:1:2 ratio and mortality in patients with severe trauma: the PROPPR randomized clinical trial. *JAMA*. 2015 Feb 3;313(5):471–482.

# 310.

# ANTICOAGULANTS, ANTITHROMBOTICS, AND ANTIPLATELET DRUGS

*Patrick Torres and Hussam Ghabra*

## INTRODUCTION

Hemostasis is conventionally divided into primary hemostasis and secondary hemostasis. Primary hemostasis is achieved when platelets adhere to the site of endothelial injury to form a "plug." Von Willebrand factor (vWF) promotes platelet adhesion and aggregation through glycoprotein (GP) receptors. Serotonin, thromboxane $A_2$ ($TxA_2$), and adenosine diphosphate (ADP) further enhance vasoconstriction (serotonin and $TxA_2$) and platelet aggregation ($TxA_2$ and ADP). Secondary hemostasis is achieved when the "platelet plug" results in activation of intrinsic, extrinsic, and common coagulation pathways (Figure 310.1), with the end goal of thrombin

converting fibrinogen to fibrin (to form a clot), which further activates factor XIII to cross-link fibrin monomers.[1]

Different medications are available for clinical use and they interfere with either primary or secondary hemostasis.

## ANTIPLATELETS 5

### CYCLOOXYGENASE (COX) INHIBITORS

*Drugs included:* aspirin, nonsteroidal anti-inflammatory drugs (NSAIDs), celecoxib.

*Mechanism of action:* small doses of aspirin irreversibly inhibit COX-1 (responsible for maintenance of gastric lining,

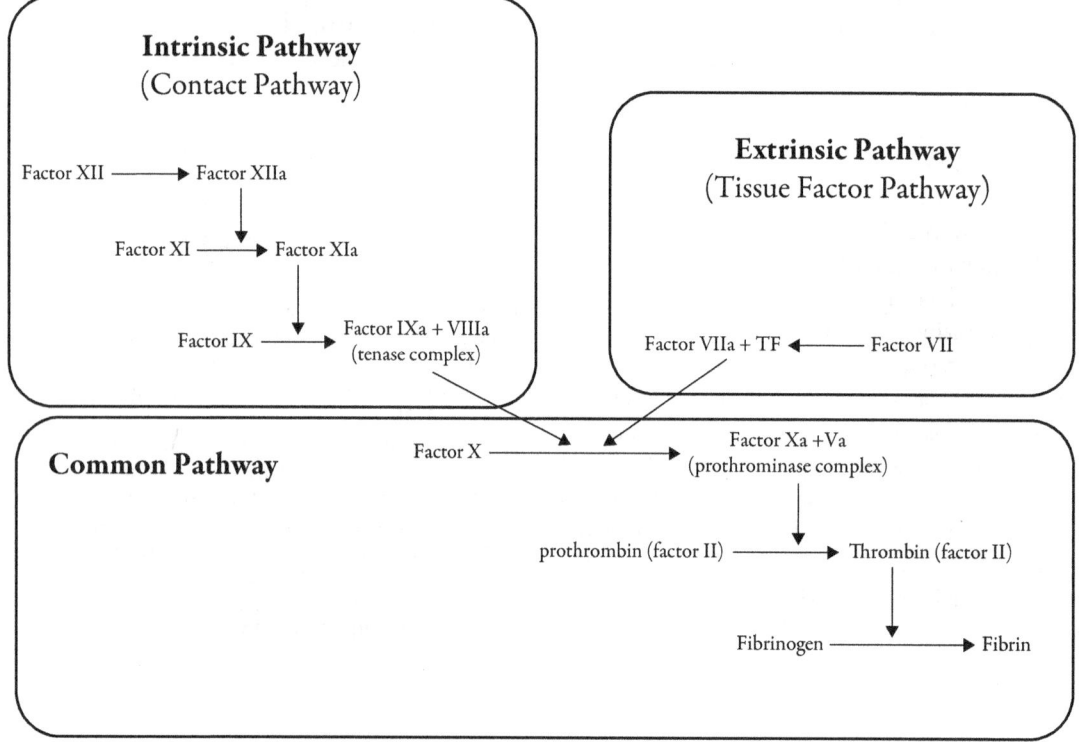

**Figure 310.1.** Coagulation cascade.

renal blood flow, and the formation of thromboxane $A_2$). Large doses of aspirin inhibit both COX-1 and COX-2 (responsible for synthesis of prostaglandins mediating inflammation and pain).

*Platelet function:* normalizes 7–10 days after discontinuation of aspirin.

## P2Y12 RECEPTOR ANTAGONISTS

*Drugs included:* clopidogrel, prasugrel, ticagrelor, and ticlodipine.

*Mechanism of action:* These drugs inhibit the P2Y12 receptor which further limits the expression of GPIIb/IIIa, resulting in inhibition of platelet adhesion and aggregation. It is important to mention that clopidogrel has a wide interindividual variability, resulting in treatment failure in patients who are CYP2C19-poor metabolizers.

*Platelet function:* normalizes 7 days after discontinuation of clopidogrel and 14–21 days after discontinuation of ticlodipine.

## GPIIB/IIIA ANTAGONISTS

*Drugs included:* abciximab, eptifibatide, tirofiban

*Mechanism of action:* These drugs irreversibly bind the GIIb/IIIa receptors, thereby inhibiting binding by fibrinogen or vWF. This leads to interference of platelet cross-linking and platelet-derived thrombus formation.

*Platelet function:* normalizes 24–48 hours after discontinuation of abciximab (irreversible antagonism) and 8 hours after discontinuation of eptifibatide and tirofiban (competitive, reversible antagonism) (Table 310.1).

*Table 310.1* ANTIPLATELETS

| ASRA RECOMMENDATIONS FOR HOLDING PRIOR TO NEURAXIAL[3] | |
|---|---|
| **COX Inhibitors** | |
| *Aspirin* | None |
| *NSAIDs* | |
| *Celecoxib* | |
| **P2Y12 Receptor Antagonists** | |
| *Clopidogrel* | 5–7 days |
| *Prasugrel* | 7–10 days |
| *Ticagrelor* | 5–7 days |
| *Ticlopidine* | 10 days |
| **GPIIb/IIIa Antagonists** | |
| *Abciximab* | 24–48 hours |
| *Eptifibatide* | 4–8 hours |
| *Tirofiban* | 4–8 hours |

# ANTICOAGULANTS

## UNFRACTIONED HEPARIN (UFH)

UFH binds antithrombin (AT) and indirectly inhibits factor Xa and factor IIa (thrombin). It is monitored using activated partial thromboplastin time (aPTT) or activated clotting time (ACT). UFH can be administered intravenously or subcutaneously. The advantages of using heparin are short half-time and the ability to fully reverse the drug with protamine. The major disadvantage, in addition to bleeding and osteoporosis, is heparin-induced thrombocytopenia (HIT). HIT is a life-threatening complication with a mortality rate ranging 20%–30%. Antibodies are triggered by the complex formed by heparin and platelet factor 4 (PF4), resulting in thromboembolic events and potential death. A decrease in platelet count by more than 50% or a platelet count less than 100 000 cells/μL should prompt HIT testing.[1]

## LOW MOLECULAR WEIGHT HEPARIN (LMWH)

LMWH inactivates factor Xa and partially inactivates thrombin.[1] It has excellent subcutaneous bioavailability with no monitoring needed; however, factor Xa levels can be obtained if necessary. It has less incidence of HIT and osteoporosis compared to UFH. Protamine is partially effective in reversing LMWH.[1]

## ULTRA-LOW MOLECULAR WEIGHT HEPARIN (FONDAPARINUX)

Fondaparinux is a pure factor Xa inhibitor. Its use is discouraged in patients with renal failure.[1]

## WARFARIN (COUMADIN)

A vitamin K antagonist, warfarin inhibits the synthesis of vitamin K dependent coagulation factors (thrombin, factor VII, factor IX, and factor X, in addition to protein C and S). Disadvantages of warfarin include the need for close INR monitoring, drug-food interactions, and drug-drug interactions (e.g., cytochrome P450 inducers and inhibitors).[1] Warfarin half-time is 40 hours and its anticoagulant effect takes 48–72 hours, so bridging with other agents is needed in patients with high-risk of thrombosis. Warfarin is contraindicated in pregnancy due to fetal teratogenicity.

## DIRECT THROMBIN INHIBITORS

This class includes *bivalirudin, argatroban, desrudin* (all in IV forms), and *dabigatran* (oral form).[2] They can be monitored using either aPTT or ACT. There is no antidote for direct thrombin inhibitors except dabigatran (idarucizumab, which can be used in cases of emergency). Bivalirudin is metabolized by plasma proteases and renally excreted. It is the drug of choice in both renal and hepatic dysfunction.

## DIRECT FACTOR XA INHIBITORS

Rivaroxaban, apixaban, edoxaban, and betrixaban directly inhibit factor Xa.[2] They all come in oral forms with no available parenteral factor Xa inhibitor. They are administered at fixed doses with no monitoring required. They are metabolized in the liver and are excreted renally. Direct factor Xa inhibitors can be reversed using andexanet alfa, which was approved by the FDA in 2018 (Table 310.2).

## ANESTHETIC CONSIDERATIONS

### PERIOPERATIVE MANAGEMENT OF ANTICOAGULATION

Perioperative discontinuation of anticoagulation increases the risk of thrombosis, while continuation increases the risk of bleeding with surgery and invasive procedures. The decision should be individualized for each patient, and clinical judgement should be based on careful weighing of risks and benefits.

### PREOPERATIVE

The patient should consult with primary care physician, surgeon, and expert consultants (hematologist, cardiologist, etc.), in addition to the perioperative anesthesiologist, to estimate their thromboembolic risk versus bleeding risk, to determine timing for discontinuation of anticoagulation, and to decide if bridging is needed (for very high-risk patients, e.g., mechanical heart valves). An inferior vena cava filter may be considered in select patients.[4] Delaying the surgery should be considered if feasible.

### INTRAOPERATIVE

The anesthesiologist should be aware of the patient's anticoagulation status and its implications on different anesthetic techniques, including neuraxial and regional anesthesia. The American Society of Regional Anesthesia and Pain Medicine (ASRA) has a detailed evidence-based guideline regarding all available anticoagulants.[3]

### POSTOPERATIVE

Anticoagulation should be restarted as soon as possible when it is believed that hemostasis has been achieved (usually ~2–3 days postoperatively, maybe sooner for very high-risk patients).[4]

*Table 310.2* ANTICOAGULANTS

| MEDICATION | COAGULATION FACTOR INHIBITED | MONITORING | REVERSAL | ASRA RECOMMENDATIONS PRIOR TO NEURAXIAL[3] |
|---|---|---|---|---|
| UFH | Xa and thrombin (indirect, through antithrombin) | aPTT | Protamine | Prophylactic: 4–6 hours (low dose), 12 hours (high dose) Therapeutic: 24 hours |
| LMWH | Xa and thrombin (partially and indirectly, through antithrombin) | None required (but can monitor anti-Xa levels) | Protamine (partially) | Prophylactic: 12 hours Therapeutic: 24 hours |
| Fondaparinux | Xa (indirectly, though antithrombin) | None required (but can monitor anti-Xa levels) | None | No recommendation |
| Warfarin | II, VII, IX, and X | PT, INR | FFP, vitamin K, prothrombin complex concentrate (PCCs) | 5 days and a normalized INR |
| Bivalirudin, argatroban, desrudin, dabigatran | Thrombin (direct) | aPTT, activated clotting time (ACT) | Idarucizumab (for dabigatran only) | Avoid neuraxial for most (hold up to 5 days for dabigatran) |
| Rivaroxaban, apixaban, edoxaban, betrixaban | Xa (directly) | None required | Andexanet alfa | 72 hours |

# REFERENCES

1. Onishi A, et al. *Front Biosci (Landmark Ed)*. 2016 Jun; 1372–1392.
2. Leung LLK. Direct oral anticoagulants (DOACs) and parenteral directacting anticoagulants: Dosing and adverse effects. In: Post TW, ed., *UpToDate*. Waltham, MA: UpToDate; 2020.
3. Horlocker TT, et al. Regional anesthesia in the patient receiving antithrombotic or thrombolytic therapy. *Reg Anesth Pain Med*. 2018;43(3):263–309.
4. Douketis JD, Lip GYH. Perioperative management of patients receiving anticoagulants. In: Post TW, ed., *UpToDate*. Waltham, MA: UpToDate; 2020.
5. Muluk V, et al. Perioperative medications management. In: Post TW, ed., *UpToDate*. Waltham, MA: UpToDate; 2020.

# Part XXIV

# ENDOCRINE AND METABOLIC SYSTEMS

# 311.

# HYPOTHALAMUS

## Zack Powers and Chris Giordano

### NORMAL PHYSIOLOGY

The hypothalamus is a funnel for communication within the hypothalamic-pituitary axis, recapitulating signals from higher brain inputs, the autonomic system, and endocrine feedback loops that can direct specific hormone release from the pituitary gland. Endocrine glands influenced by the hypothalamus include the thyroid, adrenal, and gonads. The hypothalamus also regulates the exocrine mammary gland in addition to influencing growth and free water retention. Non-endocrine function of this gland also involves thermoregulation, hunger/satiety, and effects on the autonomic system.[1]

The hypothalamus ("below the thalamus") is supratentorial and below the third ventricle, which is part of the diencephalon that also contains the pituitary. The optic chiasm is just below the hypothalamus but above the pituitary gland. Blood supply is robust, coming from branches of the anterior cerebral, anterior communicating, posterior communicating, posterior cerebral, and basilar arteries supplying the hypothalamic-hypophyseal portal venous system. The venous system is further broken down into the primary and secondary plexus. Arterial supply from the superior hypophyseal artery supplies the primary plexus in the hypothalamus, which traverses the pituitary stalk to the secondary plexus in the anterior pituitary. This portal construct is crucial, allowing hypothalamic hormones to reach the anterior pituitary in high concentrations required for effective communication.[4]

The hypothalamus receives and consolidates input from higher cortical function and also releases hormones to the anterior and posterior pituitary. The hypothalamic-hypophyseal portal venous system transports hormones released directly from neurons into the bloodstream to the anterior pituitary, including thyrotropin-releasing hormone (TRH), growth hormone-releasing hormone (GHRH), corticotrophin-releasing hormone (CRH), prolactin-releasing hormone (PRH), and gonadotropin-releasing hormone (GnRH). The posterior pituitary receives oxytocin and vasopressin from the hypothalamus via axons. The supraoptic nuclei and paraventricular nuclei of the hypothalamus are responsible for the release of these hormones directly into nerve terminals in the posterior pituitary. Other efferent pathways from the hypothalamus include connections to the reticular center via the dorsal longitudinal fasciculus affecting circadian rhythm (Figure 311.1).[4]

### ANESTHETIC CONSIDERATIONS

The hypothalamus can be directly impacted by intracranial procedures, most commonly from tumor resections. Benign tumors, such as craniopharyngiomas, can develop directly in the hypothalamus, or metastatic pathology from lung or breast carcinomas may be involved.[3]

Damage to the hypothalamus, specifically in the supraoptic or paraventricular nuclei or supraopticohypophyseal tract, can lead to reduction of vasopressin, causing central diabetes insipidus (CDI). Transsphenoidal surgery is the most common approach that results in CDI, and the most commonly associated tumor is craniopharyngioma. Intraoperatively, this can manifest as polyuria and hyponatremia, although most cases of polyuria in this setting are not due to CDI but a medication-induced osmotic diuresis.[3]

Surgical manipulation of the hypothalamus can also result in hyperthermia. Intraoperative hyperthermia as a result of physical manipulation is a diagnosis of exclusion. Communication with the surgery team is appropriate if this becomes a concern, but other diagnoses should be considered as well (Table 311.1).[2]

Pathology of the hypothalamic-pituitary axis may affect safe anesthetic delivery depending on the extent of damage to the hypothalamus. If hypothalamic-releasing hormones are jeopardized, the clinical outcome will affect the anterior pituitary and downstream regulation. A disruption in CRH will lead to adrenal insufficiency and potential hemodynamic instability or adrenal crisis. Loss of TRH can result in myxedema coma. Alteration of the posterior hypothalamus could result in CDI. Pathologic effects on other afferent and efferent pathways of the hypothalamus can damage communication with the reticular system, potentially altering circadian rhythm or causing extreme sleepiness. Other outcomes could be hyperthermia or autonomic fluctuations.[3]

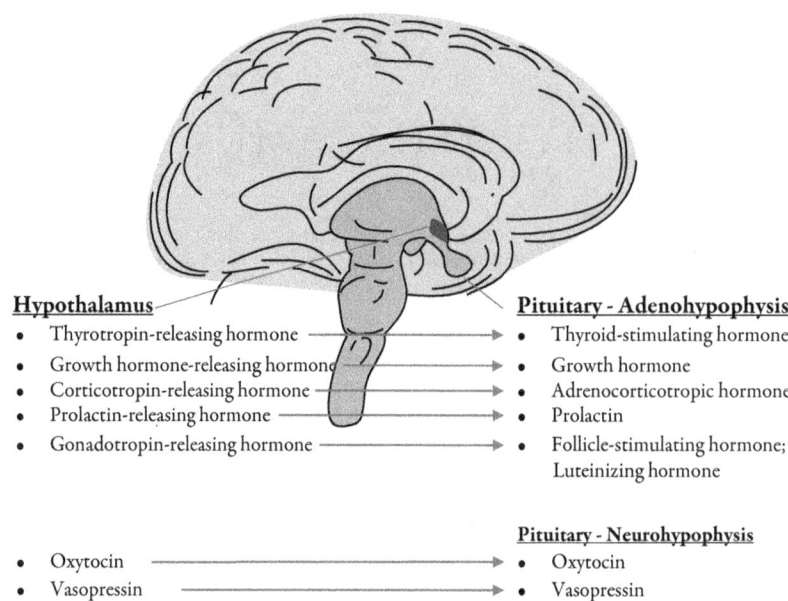

**Hypothalamus**
- Thyrotropin-releasing hormone
- Growth hormone-releasing hormone
- Corticotropin-releasing hormone
- Prolactin-releasing hormone
- Gonadotropin-releasing hormone

**Pituitary - Adenohypophysis**
- Thyroid-stimulating hormone
- Growth hormone
- Adrenocorticotropic hormone
- Prolactin
- Follicle-stimulating hormone; Luteinizing hormone

**Pituitary - Neurohypophysis**
- Oxytocin
- Vasopressin

- Oxytocin
- Vasopressin

**Figure 311.1.** The hypothalamus is attached to the pituitary via the pituitary stalk. Most communication between the hypothalamus and the pituitary is via hormones traveling in relatively high concentration in the pituitary portal blood system to the anterior pituitary (adenohypophysis). These hormones include thyrotropin-releasing hormone (TRH), which activates thyroid-stimulating hormone (TSH), growth hormone-releasing hormone (GHRH) activating growth hormone (GH), corticotropin-releasing hormone (CRH) activating adrenocorticotropic hormone (ACTH), prolactin-releasing hormone (PRH) activating prolactin, and gonadotropin-releasing hormone (GnRH) activating follicle-stimulating hormone and luteinizing hormone. The posterior pituitary receives oxytocin and vasopressin (antidiuretic hormone or ADH) directly from the nerve axons from the hypothalamus via the supraopticohypophyseal tract.

Reproduced with permission from Welt C. Hypothalamic-pituitary axis. In: *UpToDate*. Waltham, MA: UpToDate. https://www.uptodate.com/contents/hypothalamic-pituitary-axis.

*Table 311.1* DIFFERENTIAL DIAGNOSIS OF INTRAOPERATIVE HYPERTHERMIA

| HYPERTHERMIA: DIFFERENTIAL DIAGNOSIS | PRESENTATION/EVALUATION | INTERVENTION |
|---|---|---|
| Fever/sepsis | History or concern for infection | Antipyretic, antibiotics as appropriate |
| Decreased heat dissipation | Excessive active warming or drapes | Heat reduction or active cooling |
| Dehydration | Poor volume intake, tachycardia, hypotension, elevated PPV | Volume resuscitation |
| Febrile non-hemolytic reaction | Recent blood transfusion | Antipyretic |
| Direct manipulation of hypothalamus | Surgical intervention hypothalamus | Active cooling, communicate with surgery team |
| Thyroid storm | Tachycardia, hypotension, arrhythmia, altered mentation. Evaluate thyroid hormone levels | Beta Blocker, thionamide, iodine/radiocontrast, glucocorticoids |
| Neuroleptic malignant syndrome | Antipsychotic history, altered mentation, rigidity, dysautonomia | Stop offending agent, supportive care |
| Anticholinergic medications | History of administration causing dysregulation of the hypothalamus | Active cooling, antipyretic, hemodynamic support |
| Malignant hyperthermia | Increased end title carbon dioxide, tachycardia, acidosis, muscle rigidity, myoglobinuria | Stop volatile anesthetics, actively cool, administer dantrolene |

Mechanisms of insult include acute injuries such as traumatic brain injury, tumor resection, or a cerebral vascular accident. Conversely, mechanisms may be gradual, such as targeted radiation therapy, infiltrative lesions, or subtle infections. Radiation-induced deficiencies tend to be dose dependent. In children, 18 Gy of radiation to the hypothalamic-pituitary axis can increase the risk of growth-hormone deficiency, and doses of 30–40 Gy threaten production of luteinizing hormone, follicle-stimulating hormone, thyroid-stimulating hormone, and adrenocorticotropic hormone. Furthermore, effects of radiation may be dormant for several years.[3]

## REFERENCES

1. Grecu L. Autonomic nervous system anatomy and physiology. In: Barash PG, et al., eds. *Clinical Anesthesia*. 8th ed. Philadelphia, PA: Wolters Kluwer; 2017:334–335.
2. Luthra A, et al. Intraoperative hyperthermia: Can surgery itself be a cause? *Indian J Anaesth*. 2016;60:515–517.
3. Snyder, P. Causes of hypopituitarism. In: *UpToDate*. Waltham, MA: UpToDate. https://www.uptodate.com/contents/causes-of-hypopituitarism. Updated September 24, 2019.
4. Welt C. Hypothalamic-pituitary axis. In: *UpToDate*. Waltham, MA: UpToDate. https://www.uptodate.com/contents/hypothalamic-pituitary-axis?. Updated April 30, 2019.

# 312.

# PITUITARY GLAND

*Thomas Keith Jenkins and Chris Giordano*

## PREOPERATIVE

### PITUITARY HORMONES

The pituitary gland is an endocrine gland in the base of the brain. The pituitary is about the size of a pea and is located in the sella turcica of the ethmoid bone and attached anteriorly to the hypothalamus. The hypothalamic-pituitary axis influences most other endocrine systems and the gland produces multiple hormones (Table 312.1).

### PITUITARY ADENOMAS

Pituitary tumors are found in 0.1% to 0.2% of adults and have a variety of presentations. Microadenomas normally have substantially more hormone production and thus present with syndromes consistent with the hypersecreting hormone. Macroadenomas, on the contrary, often have minimal hormone production and present with mass effects such as headaches, vomiting, and changes in vision.

Prolactinoma is the most common pituitary adenoma (32% to 66%), and these tumors characteristically present with galactorrhea. Prolactinomas are routinely treated with dopamine agonists to block production and do not always require surgical resection. Acromegaly is seen in growth hormone-secreting tumors, which constitute 8% to 16% of pituitary adenomas. Acromegaly leads to anatomical changes, including macroglossia and swelling of pharyngeal structures that can lead to difficult airways. These patients often develop obstructive sleep apnea and diabetes, and they are at increased risk for developing cardiac diseases (e.g., coronary artery disease, cardiomyopathies, and valvulopathies). Cushing disease results from adrenocorticotropic hormone (ACTH)-producing tumors, which account for 2% to 6% of pituitary adenomas. The hypercortisolism leads to central obesity along with classical moon face with buffalo hump, obstructive sleep apnea (with possible myopathy of airway muscles), cardiac disease, diabetes, and hyperlipidemia. Patients with these symptoms may require petrosal sinus sampling to distinguish pituitary versus ectopic adenoma. The syndrome of inappropriate antidiuretic hormone secretion (SIADH) is rarely seen as a result of hypersecreting pituitary tumors. Rather, it is more commonly seen as an effect of medications and ectopic tumors producing antidiuretic hormone (ADH), typically small cell carcinoma of the lung. The primary symptoms of SIADH are decreased urine output and altered

*Table 312.1* OVERVIEW OF HORMONES PRODUCED BY THE PITUITARY GLAND

| ANTERIOR PITUITARY | FUNCTION | DYSFUNCTION |
| --- | --- | --- |
| Adrenocorticotropic hormone | - Stimulates release of cortisol by adrenal glands | - Elevation causes Cushing syndrome<br>- Deficiency causes secondary adrenal insufficiency |
| Growth hormone | - Stimulates cell growth and reproduction<br>- Increases IGF-1 and blood glucose | - Elevation causes acromegaly<br>- Deficiency causes stunted growth and osteoporosis |
| Luteinizing hormone | - Stimulates ovulation in females and testosterone production in males | - Elevation is often a sign of infertility |
| Follicle-stimulating hormone | - Stimulates maturation of germ cells | - Elevated in females undergoing menopause |
| Thyroid-stimulating hormone | - Stimulates thyroid to produce T3 and T4 | - Deficiency causes central hypothyroidism<br>- Most other thyroid problems arise in the thyroid gland |
| Prolactin | - Stimulates lactation | - Elevated levels cause lactation and loss of libido |
| **Posterior pituitary** | | |
| Vasopressin (antidiuretic hormone) | - Constricts arterioles (V1 receptor)<br>- Increases free water absorption in kidneys (V2 receptor) | - Elevation causes syndrome of inappropriate antidiuretic hormone secretion (SIADH)<br>- Deficiency causes diabetes insipidus |
| Oxytocin | - Stimulates uterine contraction<br>- Promotes social bonding | - Elevated level used to induce labor |

mental status, with laboratory findings of hypo-osmolality. Treatments include fluid restriction (approximately 800 mL/day), demeclocycline, or conivaptan (vasopressin 2 antagonist). Elevated levels of ADH are also seen in nephrogenic diabetes insipidus as the body attempts to compensate for the insensitivity of kidneys to ADH.

Clinically nonfunctioning tumors account for the remaining adenomas and can present with signs of mass effects or hypopituitarism. Compression of the optic chiasm (cephalad to the sella turcica) classically leads to bitemporal hemianopsia, which is the loss of peripheral vision bilaterally. As an adenoma grows and compresses the surrounding tissue, it impairs hormone release, leading to hypopituitarism.

## INTRAOPERATIVE

### HYPOPHYSECTOMY AND PANHYPOPITUITARISM

Hypophysectomy refers to the surgical removal of the pituitary gland and is the definitive treatment for symptomatic adenoma. A transsphenoidal resection is performed endoscopically through the nose and sphenoid sinus/air cells and has improved recovery time compared to open resections. Anesthesia for hypophysectomy requires consideration of tumor symptoms (as discussed earlier) and the endotracheal tube with smooth, rapid emergence to allow for neurological testing. Complete removal of the pituitary gland will lead to panhypopituitarism postoperatively, and patients will require lifelong hormone replacement. Other causes of panhypopituitarism include traumatic brain injury, radiation, and stroke.

Symptoms of panhypopituitarism can be understood based on the missing hormones. Hypothyroid symptoms such as fatigue, weight gain, and cold insensitivity can be seen with low thyroid-stimulating hormone. Sexual dysfunction, amenorrhea, or erectile dysfunction are consequences of low luteinizing hormone/follicle-stimulating hormone. Patients with diabetes insipidus because of low ADH present with polyuria, polydipsia, and hypernatremia. This is treated primarily with free access to water and possible ADH replacement. Secondary adrenal failure from low ACTH is one cause of adrenal crisis, which is characterized by low blood pressure, hypoglycemia, hyponatremia, hyperkalemia, nausea, and altered mental status. The details of hormone replacement therapy are beyond the scope of this chapter, but patients with an impaired hypothalamic-pituitary-adrenal axis will likely require stress-dose steroids.

## REFERENCES

1. Barish PG et al. *Clinical Anesthesia*. 8th ed. Philadelphia, PA: Wolters Kluwer; 2017.
2. Butterworth JF, et al. *Morgan and Mikhail's Clinical Anesthesiology*. 5th ed. New York, NY: McGraw-Hill; 2013.
3. Elsayed SA, et al. Physiology, pituitary gland. In: *StatPearls* [Internet]. 2020 Jan–.https://www.ncbi.nlm.nih.gov/books/NBK459247/.
4. Peterfreund RA, Hyder O. Anesthesia for trassphenoidal pituitary surgery. In: *UpToDate* [Internet]. December 18, 2018. https://www.uptodate.com/contents/anesthesia-for-transsphenoidal-pituitary-surgery
5. Molitch ME. Diagnosis and treatment of pituitary adenomas: A review. *JAMA*. 2017;317(5):516–524.

# 313.

# THYROID GLAND

*Jauhleene Chamu and Angela Johnson*

## PHYSIOLOGY

The thyroid gland produces the hormones T3, T4, and calcitonin, responsible for neurologic and somatic development in infants and metabolic activity in adults. T3 and T4 influence metabolic rate by binding mitochondrial receptors to increase nutrient breakdown and production of ATP. They also affect fertility, increase susceptibility to catecholamines, and regulate heat production. Thyrotropin-releasing hormone (TRH) from the hypothalamus stimulates the anterior pituitary to produce thyroid-stimulating hormone (TSH). TSH stimulates the thyroid gland to produce more T3 and T4. TRH, TSH, T3, and T4 comprise a negative feedback system so elevated levels inhibit further release of TSH.[5] Free T3 and T4 diffuse across lipid bilayers of cells; however, most is protein bound. When free levels are low, bound T3 and T4 are released to diffuse into their target cells. T3 is more active than T4, so those cells often convert T4 to T3 peripherally.[5]

The thyroid is responsible for production of calcitonin from parafollicular or C cells interspersed between follicles. Calcitonin decreases blood calcium concentrations by inhibiting osteoclasts, stimulating osteoblasts, decreasing intestinal absorption of calcium and increasing excretion of calcium in urine.[4]

## HYPERTHYROIDISM

### ETIOLOGY

Hyperthyroidism is the production of excess thyroid hormones. Intrinsic thyroid disease accounts for most cases (Table 313.1). Diagnosis is by low TSH and high-normal levels of T3 and/or T4. The hypermetabolic state resulting from tissue exposure to excess thyroid hormone is thyrotoxicosis.[3]

### SYMPTOMS

Thyrotoxicosis has physiologic repercussions on multiple organ systems (Table 313.1). The "apathetic" seen in the elderly presents mainly with cardiac manifestations as atrial fibrillation, and while the catecholamine levels are normal, the receptors are upregulated.

## TREATMENT

In thyrotoxicosis, catecholamine receptors are upregulated. Beta-adrenergic blockers (e.g., propranolol and nadolol) antagonize this response. They, along with glucocorticoids, inhibit conversion of T4 to T3. Propylthiouracil and methimazole inhibit thyroid hormone synthesis and peripheral conversion of T4 to T3. Iodine or iodinated contrast solutions inhibit synthesis and secretion of thyroid

*Table 313.1* HYPERTHYROIDISM ETIOLOGY AND PHYSIOLOGIC EFFECTS

| | |
|---|---|
| Primary Causes | Low TSH, elevated free T3 and T4 |
| | Grave's disease, multinodular toxic goiter, autonomous toxic adenoma |
| Secondary Causes | Elevated TSH, free T3 and T4 |
| | TSH producing pituitary adenoma, thyroid hormone resistance, gestational thyrotoxicosis |
| Organ Systems | Physiologic Effects |
| Cardiovascular/ Hematologic | Tachycardia, a-fib, heart block,↑ contractility, ↑ stroke volume and cardiac output, high output CHF, Anemia, neutropenia, thrombocytopenia |
| Pulmonary | Tachypnea, hypercarbia, ↑ oxygen consumption, ↓ vital capacity and compliance, pulmonary edema |
| Neurologic | Anxiety, tremors, diaphoresis, insomnia, muscle weakness, confusion, delirium, seizure, coma |
| Gastrointestinal | Diarrhea, cachexia |

Reproduced with permission from Ferri FF. Hyperthyroidism. In: *Ferri's Clinical Advisor.* 2020;742–743.e2.

hormone (Wolff-Chaikoff effect). These treatments are temporary, and permanent treatments of radioactive iodine and surgical resection are often recommended.[2] Lithium can be used in patients with iodine allergy.

## THYROID STORM

Decompensated severe thyrotoxicosis can result in thyroid storm. It is precipitated by infection, trauma, surgery, rapid withdrawal of iodine therapy, and antithyroid medications. It presents with tachycardia, hyperpyrexia, diarrhea, vomiting, irritability, congestive heart failure, shock, delirium, and coma. It should be differentiated from malignant hyperthermia, sepsis, neuroleptic malignant syndrome, pheochromocytoma, drug reaction, or light anesthesia. Treatment includes oxygenation, hydration, cooling, beta-blockade, anti-thyroid medications, decreasing active thyroid hormone, and supportive measures.[2] Aspirin should be avoided as an antipyretic because it displaces bound thyroid hormone, increasing free thyroid hormone levels.[4]

## SPECIAL CONSIDERATIONS IN PREGNANCY

Chronic use of iodine in pregnancy is contraindicated as it can case fetal goiter and hypothyroidism. Antithyroid medications cross the placenta but can be used in small doses. Use of propranolol is controversial due to the risk of fetal complications. Thyrotoxicosis of pregnancy usually improves in the second and third trimesters. Surgery after the first trimester can be an alternative option to medications.

## HYPOTHYROIDISM

### ETIOLOGY

Hypothyroidism results from inadequate production of thyroid hormone from the thyroid gland (primary) or TRH from the hypothalamus (secondary). Causes include autoimmune disease, thyroidectomy, radioactive iodine, antithyroid medications, iodine deficiency, or hypothalamic-pituitary axis failure. It is diagnosed by elevation of TSH (in primary hypothyroidism) or reduced total T3 (Table 313.2).[2]

### SYMPTOMS

Neonatal hypothyroidism can result in cretinism. Symptoms are multisystemic, with gradual onset unless associated with radioiodine or thyroid surgery (Table 313.2).[4]

### TREATMENT

Hypothyroidism is treated with synthetic, long-acting T4, levothyroxine. Treatment may take weeks to demonstrate a physiologic response.

*Table 313.2* HYPOTHYROIDISM ETIOLOGY AND PHYSIOLOGIC EFFECTS

| | |
|---|---|
| Primary | ↑ TRH & TSH, ↓ T4 |
| | Iodine ↓, Hashimoto's and subacute thyroiditis, surgery, genetic, drugs (lithium, amiodarone, anti-thyroid) |
| Secondary (hypopituitarism) | ↓TRH, low/low normal TSH, ↓T4 |
| | Adenoma, ablative therapy, pituitary destruction |
| Tertiary | Delayed TRH, ↓/↑ TSH, ↓ T4 |
| | Hypothalamic dysfunction |
| Organ System | Physiologic response, increased sensitivity to depressant drugs, slow metabolism |
| Cardiovascular/ Hematologic | Bradycardia, ↑QT interval, ↑SVR, ↓ cardiac contractility/ output, CHF, baroreceptor defect, higher warfarin dosing ↑factors II, VII, X; ↓factor VIII |
| Pulmonary | ↓ Respiratory drive, ↓ muscle strength, OSA, atelectasis, ↓ lung volumes, impaired ventilatory response to hypoxemia and hypercarbia. |
| Neurologic | Lethargy, muscle weakness, poor concentration |
| Gastrointestinal | Constipation, weight gain |
| Renal | ↓Renal perfusion and drug clearance, ↓sodium and creatinine clearance, ↑ADH, ↓ANF |

Reproduced with permission from Smith RP. Hypothyroidism. In: *Netter's Obstetrics and Gynecology.* 2018;47:99–101.

## MYXEDEMA COMA

Severe hypothyroidism, marked by impaired mentation, hypoventilation, hypothermia, hyponatremia, and congestive heart failure, is called *myxedema coma*. It is life-threatening and patients should be admitted to an intensive care unit for monitoring, resuscitation, and administration of intravascular thyroid hormone. Caution should be taken with administration, as rapid replacement can result in myocardial ischemia and arrhythmia. Hydrocortisone is often concomitantly given to rule out adrenal insufficiency.[3]

## ANESTHETIC CONSIDERATIONS

### PREOPERATIVE

Patients with thyroid disease should be euthyroid prior to elective surgery. If thyroid disease is suspected, thyroid function tests should be obtained. Patients deemed euthyroid within the last 6 months do not need additional testing.

If surgery is urgent, patients should receive medical therapy to correct their thyroid disorder as time permits.[4] When emergency surgery is required in those with moderate to severe hypothyroidism, invasive monitoring and intensive care unit (ICU) should be considered. The hyperdynamic state of hyperthyroidism may be controlled with an esmolol infusion in emergency settings. Thyroid replacement and antithyroid medications should be continued the day of surgery.[2]

Airway examination is paramount. Cancerous, obstructive, or substernal goiters should be investigated with advanced imaging, particularly when respiratory symptoms are present to evaluate location, size, extent of tracheal or vascular compression, and tissue infiltration.[4]

## INTRAOPERATIVE

Patients with thyroid disease may be hypovolemic and predisposed to hypotension on induction. Hypothyroid patients often have blunted baroreceptor reflexes. In hyperthyroid patients, avoid a sympathetic response to laryngoscopy and surgical stimulation, monitor temperature and cardiovascular function, and provide eye protection. Thyrotoxicosis is associated with an increased incidence of myopathies and myasthenia gravis, so neuromuscular blockers should be administered with caution.[2] Thyroid disease does not affect MAC; however, volatiles may cause hypoventilation in hypothyroid patients, so a secure airway is recommended.

With hyperthyroidism, avoid the use of anticholinergics as they interfere with sweating and can potentially increase heart rate. Thiopental has been proposed to be the induction agent of choice due to its antithyroid activity. Succinylcholine or nondepolarizing relaxants produce less cardiac effects and can be used for intubation.

Standard monitors are adequate for thyroid surgery. Recurrent laryngeal nerve monitoring may be requested, requiring avoidance of neuromuscular blockade.[2] Consider awake fiberoptic intubation for symptomatic, invasive, or substernal goiters. Remifentanil infusion, lidocaine, and dexmedetomidine can prevent hypertension or cough during emergence, preventing hematoma formation.[4]

## POSTOPERATIVE

Surgery can trigger thyroid storm. Hypothyroid patients may experience delayed emergence, requiring prolonged mechanical ventilation. Opioids should be used sparingly in this population.[1]

Thyroid surgery poses risk for postoperative airway complications. The recurrent laryngeal nerves (RLN) provide sensory function to the subglottic region and motor function to all muscles of the larynx except the cricothyroid muscle, allowing for vocal cord abduction and adduction.[5] The RLN transverses the tubercle of Zuckerkandl, posterior to each thyroid lobe, and can be damaged during surgical dissection, resulting in uni- or bilateral vocal cord paralysis. Laryngeal/vocal cord edema and tracheomalacia can also cause stridor and respiratory distress.[5] Steroids, racemic epinephrine, reintubation, or emergency tracheostomy may be necessary. Respiratory distress accompanied by neck swelling suggests hematoma and emergent surgical evacuation should be considered. Hypocalcemia results from removal of parathyroid glands. Symptoms range from parasthesias to respiratory distress, so calcium should be repleted.

## REFERENCES

1. Stathatos N, Wartofsky L. Perioperative management of patients with hypothyroidism. *Endocrinol Metab Clin N Am.* 2003; 32:503–518.
2. Butterworth, J. et al. Anesthesia for patients with endocrine disease. In: *Morgan & Mikhail's Clinical Anesthesiology.* McGraw-Hill Education. 2018; 5:733–736.
3. Chiaghana C, Awoniyi C. Hypothyroidism, hyperthyroidism, complications of thyroid surgery. In: *Anesthesiology Core Review.* McGraw-Hill Education. 2016; 393–399.
4. Furman W, Robertson A. Anesthesia for patients with thyroid disease and for patients who undergo thyroid or parathyroid surgery. In: Cowley M, ed. In: *UpToDate.* Retrieved March 15, 2020.
5. Salvatore B, et al. Thyroid gland. *Anat Physiol.* 2018; 10.1016/B978-0-12-801238-3.96022-7.

# 314.

# PARATHYROID ANATOMY AND PHYSIOLOGY

*Rosemary Prejean and Alan D. Kaye*

## INTRODUCTION

The parathyroid glands are responsible for secreting parathyroid hormone (PTH), which has a vital role in regulation of calcium levels in the blood, both directly and indirectly, via production of vitamin D (calcitriol). PTH carries out three separate actions in order to increase serum calcium: increased release from bone, increased reabsorption from the kidney, and activation of 1α-hydroxylase in the kidney, producing metabolically active 1,25(OH)2D from the inactive 25(OH)D form to increase calcium absorption in the gut. Calcitonin produced by the thyroid gland opposes the effects of PTH by inhibition of bone resorption and increased excretion of calcium by the kidneys.[1] Thus, calcium homeostasis is maintained by the interaction of PTH, vitamin D, and calcitonin.

## ANATOMY

The parathyroid glands are four small, ovoid-shaped glands, weighing an average of 35–40 milligrams (see Figure 314.1).[2] There are typically two superior parathyroid glands found 1 cm above the intersection of the recurrent laryngeal nerve with the inferior thyroid artery at the posterior aspect of the thyroid lobe.[2] The two inferior parathyroid glands can be commonly found anterior to the recurrent laryngeal nerve within 1 cm inferior, lateral, or posterior to the inferior pole of the thyroid.[2] The parenchyma consists of two types of cells: chief cells and oxyphil cells. The chief cells are responsible for synthesizing and secreting PTH, while the oxyphils cells carry an unknown function.[3]

## PTH RELEASE

PTH release is controlled by the plasma calcium concentration: any decrease in blood calcium will lead to an increased PTH secretion, and any increase in blood calcium will inhibit PTH release. The inverse relationship of PTH and calcium is expressed in a sigmoidal curve, whereas any small variation of serum ionized calcium produces a large variation in serum PTH concentration within minutes.[4,5] Short-term mediation of calcium control is enforced by this direct, rapid manipulation of PTH, while long-term maintenance of calcium balance is carried out indirectly by 1,25(OH)2D-mediated intestinal calcium absorption.[1]

## CALCIUM EFFECT ON PTH RELEASE

The chief cells of the parathyroid glands are where PTH is continuously synthesized as a prepropeptide in the endoplasmic reticulum before being converted to pro-PTH in the

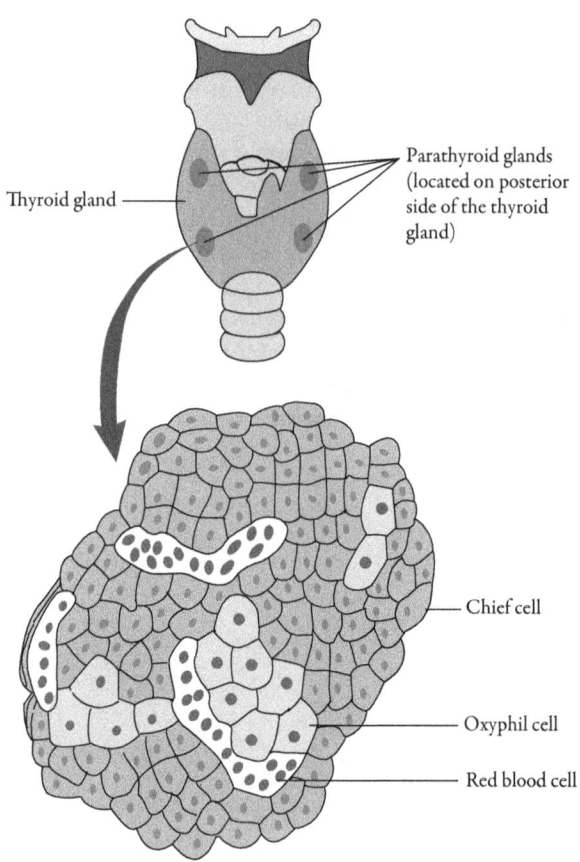

Figure 314.1. Anatomical location and parenchyma of parathyroid glands.

Golgi apparatus; pro-PTH is then changed to the mature form of PTH that is packaged into secretory vesicles.[1,5] The chief cells possess a transmembrane calcium sensing receptor (CaSR) coupled to guanine nucleotide-binding proteins ($G_{q/11}$, $G_i$, $G_{12/13}$). With increased levels of calcium in the body, these G-coupled proteins incite inhibitory intracellular cascades leading to decreased PTH release and increased PTH degradation.[5] With acutely decreased levels of calcium, the inactive CaSR is not stimulated to begin this second messenger system for PTH degradation, and there is a biphasic wave of PTH release. With longer exposure to hypocalcemia, there is also an increase in new hormone synthesis from stabilization of PTH mRNA for gene expression.[1]

## PHOSPHATE EFFECT ON PTH RELEASE

PTH release is also influenced by plasma phosphate concentrations. Increased levels of plasma phosphate will lead to a net increase in PTH release, as well as PTH mRNA stability. In addition to this direct effect, high plasma phosphate will decrease serum calcium and 1,25(OH)2D production, causing an indirect increase in PTH release. Decreased levels of plasma phosphate will cause a decrease in PTH mRNA stability for an overall effect of decreased PTH activity.[1] In thyroparathyroidectomized animals, PTH is absent, and reabsorption of inorganic phosphate increases significantly and increases plasma inorganic phosphate levels. In primary hyperparathyroidism, PTH secretion is elevated, and plasma levels of inorganic phosphate are low. In this setting, steady-state urinary inorganic phosphate excretion is not markedly increased. This is because it depends largely on intestinal inorganic phosphate absorption. Lastly, dietary restriction of inorganic phosphate leads to close to 100% reabsorption of filtered inorganic phosphate and reduction of urinary phosphate to zero.

## MAGNESIUM EFFECT ON PTH RELEASE

Magnesium can act similarly to calcium on the CaSR to decrease PTH release in the chief cells when plasma magnesium levels are increased. When plasma magnesium concentrations are low, there will be a subsequent increase in PTH release. Interestingly, more severe hypomagnesemia will prevent the appropriate PTH release in the parathyroid gland in response to hypocalcemia, as well as prevent bone responsiveness to PTH for bone resorption. This mechanism is thought to involve increased activity of the $G_{q/11}$ and $G_i$ proteins coupled to the CaSR, leading to inhibition of PTH secretion and increased PTH degradation.[5]

## PTH ACTIONS

There are three types of PTH receptors (PTHR1, PTHR2, PTHR3), with PTHR1 responsible for pertinent physiological effects of the parathyroid hormone (see Figure 314.2). PTHR1

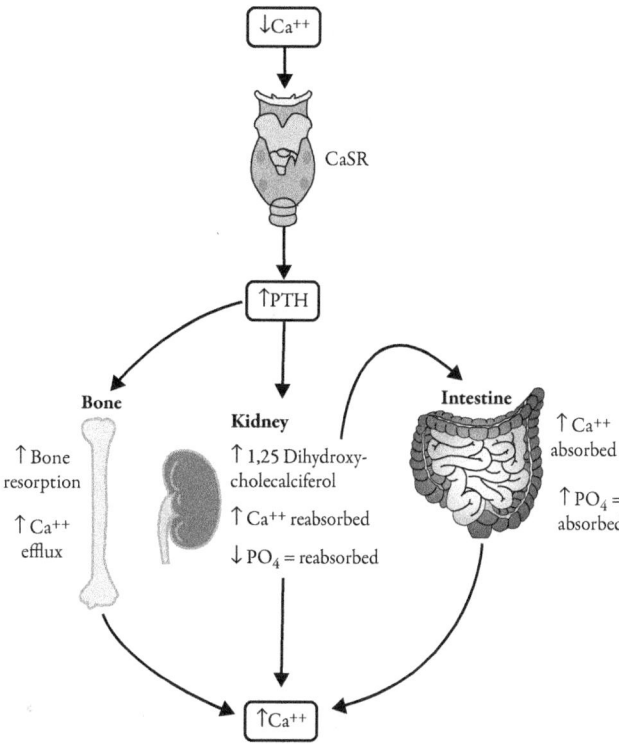

Figure 314.2. Summary of PTH effects at kidney, bone, and intestines.

is a stimulatory G protein-coupled receptor found in bone osteoblasts and the kidneys that utilizes multiple, second-messenger systems with cAMP, phospholipase C (PLC), and protein kinase C (PKC) to carry out its actions.[4]

## PTH ACTIONS IN KIDNEY

PTH directly stimulates active, transcellular calcium reabsorption in the distal tubules of the kidneys via increased insertion and opening of the apical calcium channels. Once calcium has entered the distal tubular cell from the lumen, it binds a vitamin D calcium-binding protein called calbindin D-28k that will carry it through the cytosol from the apical side to the basolateral side of the cell. Once at the basolateral membrane, calcium transport out of the cell occurs through $Ca^{2+}/Na^+$ exchanger and a $Ca^{2+}$ ATPase channel to bring calcium into the interstitium.[1] Decreased inorganic phosphate reabsorption in the kidneys occurs in response to PTH by increased internalization of Type IIa sodium-dependent phosphate transporters and their subsequent lysosomal degradation.[1] PTH also functions to induce activity of 1α-hydroxylase in the kidney at the proximal tubule to synthesize the metabolically active $1,25(OH)_2$ D from 25(OH)D and increase intestinal absorption of calcium and phosphate.

## PTH ACTIONS IN BONE

PTH in the bone stimulates release of calcium and phosphate from the bone matrix by first binding to PTHR1

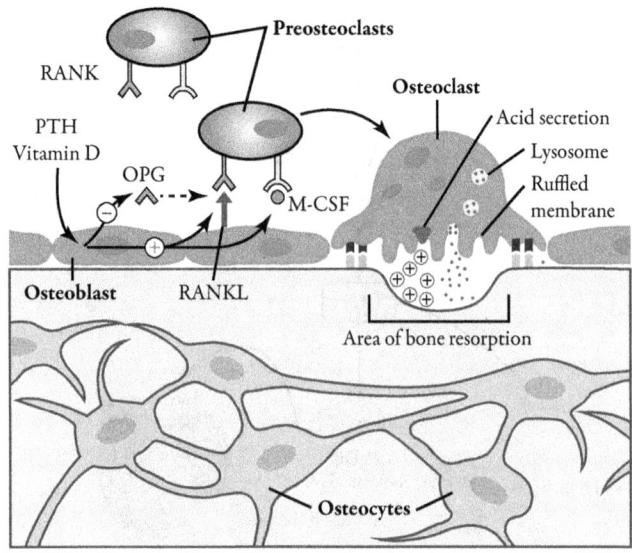

**Figure 314.3.** Illustration of PTH-mediated bone resorption.

on osteoblasts: this stimulates receptor activator of nuclear factor-κB ligand (RANKL) expression on the osteoblast outer surface and increased production of a growth factor, macrophage colony-stimulating factor (M-CSF), by the osteoblast (see Figure 314.3).[4] The RANKL on the osteoblasts will then bind to RANK on an osteoclast precursor that acts to initiate gene transcription required for maturation of osteoclasts with characteristic formation of a ruffled border. Osteoclasts bind to the bone surface with this ruffled border via β integrins, followed by fusion of acidic intracellular vesicles with the membrane. Hydrogen ions produced by carbonic anhydrase II can be carried across the membrane into the isolated extracellular microenvironment formed by use of H$^+$-ATPases. This acidification of the microenvironment makes dissolution of hydroxyapatite favorable and aids in lysosomal protease activation.[1] The products of this digestion (calcium, inorganic phosphate, and alkaline phosphatases) are endocytosed by the osteoclast to be released systemically into circulation. Osteoprotegrin (OPG) is a soluble decoy receptor that acts as a feedback regulator to bind and inhibit RANKL on osteoblasts. PTH inhibits OPG synthesis and secretion in order to decrease osteoblast inhibition and apoptosis.[4] Therefore, the overall goal of bone resorption is carried out by a combination of PTH-mediated increase of RANKL and a decrease of OPG.

## ANESTHETIC CONSIDERATIONS

### PREOPERATIVE

PTH directly effects calcium, which is critical in the mediation of muscle contraction, exocrine, endocrine, and neurocrine secretion, cell growth, and transport and secretion of fluids and electrolytes. Optimization of the patient's calcium levels prior to parathyroid surgery in the setting of hyperparathyroidism, along with monitoring post-parathyroidectomy for hypocalcemia, is crucial given the multitude of potential complications that can be seen. The major signs and symptoms of hypocalcemia include mental status changes, tetany, positive Chvostek and Trousseau signs, laryngospasm, hypotension, and dysrhythmias. Electrocardiographic evaluation may show prolongation of the QT interval or even heart block in severe cases. Treatment, often prompted by hypotension, involves intravenous infusion of 10% calcium chloride (1.36 mEq/mL) or calcium gluconate (0.45 mEq/mL).[6,7] When equivalent calcium doses are administered, both preparations are equally efficacious in restoring the calcium level to normal It should also be noted that hypocalcemia can interfere with the action of nondepolarizing neuromuscular agents.

### INTRAOPERATIVE

Train-of-four stimulation intraoperatively and serial calcium levels postoperatively with careful assessment of signs and symptoms consistent with hypocalcemia, including muscle weakness, will minimize morbidity and mortality. Extubation should be done with careful consideration of operative site to avoid trauma and subsequent hematoma formation compromising the airway in the setting of any related parathyroid surgery.[6,7]

### POSTOPERATIVE

Continue to monitor calcium levels and treat as needed.

## REFERENCES

1. Molina PE. Parathyroid gland and Ca2+ and PO4- regulation. In: Molina PE, ed. *Endocrine Physiology*. Vol 25. 4th ed. New York, NY: McGraw-Hill; 2013:1–27.
2. Fancy T, et al. Surgical anatomy of the thyroid and parathyroid glands. *Otolaryngol Clin North Am*. 2010;43(2):221–227.
3. Ritter CS, et al. Differential gene expression by oxyphil and chief cells of human parathyroid glands. *J Clin Endocrinol Metab*. 2012;97(8):E1499–E1505.
4. Melmed S, et al. Hormones and disorders of mineral metabolism. In: Bringhurst FR, Demay MB, Kronenberg HM, eds. *Williams Textbook of Endocrinology*. 13th ed. Philadelphia, PA: Elsevier; 2016:1253–1322.
5. Gardella TJ, et al. Parathyroid hormone and the parathyroid hormone receptor type 1 in the regulation of calcium and phosphate homeostasis and bone metabolism. In: Gardella TJ, et al., eds. *Endocrinology: Adult and Pediatric*. Vols. 1–2. 7th ed. Philadelphia, PA: Elsevier; 2016:969–990.e10.
6. Bajwa S, Sehgal V. Anesthetic management of primary hyperparathyroidism: A role rarely noticed and appreciated so far. *Indian J Endocrinol Metab*. 2013;17(2):235–239. doi:10.4103/2230-8210.109679
7. Miller RD. *Miller's Anesthesia*. 6th ed. Philadelphia, PA: Elsevier Churchill Livingstone; 2005.

# 315.

# ADRENAL CORTEX ANATOMY AND PHYSIOLOGY

*Brendan McCafferty and Nicholas Pesa*

## INTRODUCTION

The adrenal cortex of the human is the outer layer of the adrenal gland. It is devised into three distinct regions based on appearance, function, and molecules primarily secreted. These three layers are (1) the outer layer: zona glomerulosa; (2) the middle layer: zona fasciculata; (3) the inner layer: zona reticularis. All three of these layers produce distinct steroids deriving from cholesterol, and hence their unique histological appearance as well as function within the larger endocrine system and homeostasis (Figure 315.1).[1–5]

## ZONA GLOMERULOSA

The most superficial region of the cortex is the zona glomerulosa. This layer produces a group of hormones collectively referred to as mineralocorticoids. Aldosterone is the major mineralocorticoid produced. Aldosterone secretion is under tonic control by adrenocorticotropic hormone (ACTH), but is separately regulated by the renin-angiotensin system and by serum potassium. A decrease in blood volume will cause a subsequent decrease in renal perfusion pressure, which will lead to increases in renin secretion. Renin, an enzyme, catalyzes the conversion of

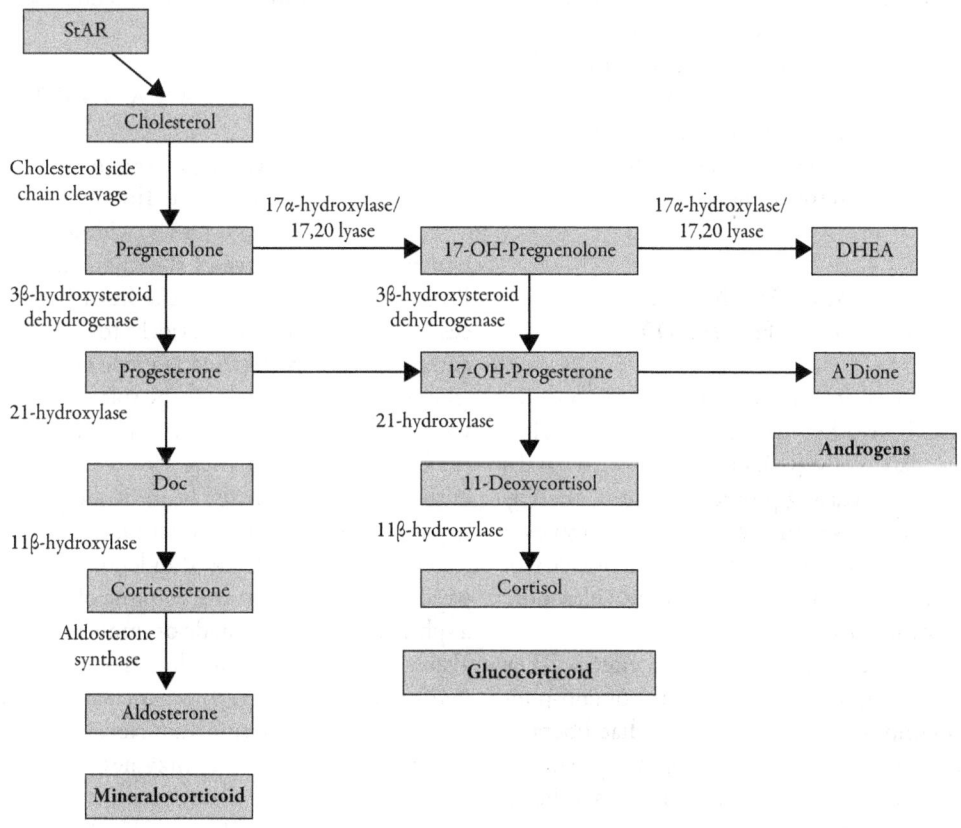

**Figure 315.1.** Overview of adrenal cortex and steps to produce mineralocorticoids, glucocorticoids, and androgens.
Reproduced with permission from Yeoh P. Anatomy and physiology of the adrenal gland. In: Llahana S, et al., eds. *Advanced Practice in Endocrinology Nursing.* Cham: Springer; 2019:645–655.

angiotensinogen to angiotensin I. Angiotensin I is converted to angiotensin II by angiotensin-converting enzyme (ACE). Angiotensin II acts on the zona glomerulosa to increase the conversion of corticosterone to aldosterone. Hyperkalemia also increases aldosterone secretion. Aldosterone's main physiological effects consist of an increase in renal Na+ reabsorption, increase in renal K+ secretion, and increase in renal H+ secretion.[2]

## ZONA FASCICULATA

The largest zone of the three zones, because of its high activity, is the cortisol-producing zone, the zona fasciculata, which lies in the middle of the adrenal cortex. The primary hormone produced by this zone is the glucocorticoid hormone, cortisol. Cells within the zona fasciculata have a foamy appearance because they are filled with small lipid droplets of stored cholesterol esters. These cells are very efficient at ingesting LDL from circulating blood, freeing the cholesterol from the LDL-lipoprotein, using the enzyme ACAT to esterify the cholesterol, and storing it as these aforementioned lipid droplets. The esterified cholesterol undergoes de-esterification by hormone-sensitive lipase (HSL) at the stimulation of ACTH.[5] It should be noted that the cells of the zona fasciculata can generate free cholesterol de novo, if needed, from acetate.

The free cholesterol undergoes a series of enzymatic reactions (5 in total) to form the ended product: cortisol. The rate-limiting step is actually the transfer of the free cholesterol from the cytoplasm through the outer mitochondrial membrane to the inner mitochondrial membrane and the free cholesterol's subsequent conversion to pregnenolone via the enzyme cholesterol desmolase.

## CORTISOL'S MECHANISMS OF ACTION ON THE BODY

Overall, glucocorticoids are essential for the response to stress, but they also have other mechanisms of action. They stimulate gluconeogenesis by (1) increasing protein catabolism in muscle and decreasing protein synthesis, thereby providing more amino acids to the liver for gluconeogenesis; (2) decreasing glucose utilization and insulin sensitivity of adipose tissue; (3) increasing lipolysis, which provides more glycerol to the liver for gluconeogenesis.[2]

Glucocorticoids have anti-inflammatory effects. They induce the synthesis of lipocortin, an inhibitor of phospholipase A2. Phospholipase A2 is an enzyme that liberates arachidonate from membrane phospholipids, providing a precursor for prostaglandin and leukotriene synthesis. Prostaglandins and leukotriene production is involved in the normal inflammatory response, so eliminating the precursor gives glucocorticoids anti-inflammatory properties. Glucocorticoids also inhibit the production of interleukin-2 and inhibit proliferation of T lymphocytes. Finally, they inhibit the release of histamine and serotonin from mast cells and platelets.

Glucocorticoids suppress the immune system. As stated earlier, glucocorticoids inhibit the production of IL-2 and T lymphocytes, both of which are critical for cellular immunity. This is why glucocorticoids are used to help prevent rejection of transplanted organs.[2]

Glucocorticoids provide maintenance of vascular responsiveness to catecholamines. Cortisol up-regulates $\alpha$-1 receptors on arterioles, increasing their sensitivity to the vasoconstrictor effect of norepinephrine. Thus, with cortisol excess, arterial pressure increases; with cortisol deficiency, arterial pressure decreases.[2]

## ZONA RETICULARIS

The deepest region of the adrenal cortex is the zona reticularis. This layer produces small amounts of sex hormones called androgens. These androgens supplement the androgens produced by the gonads. They are produced in response to ACTH and are converted in the tissues to testosterone and estrogens. In males, androstenedione is converted to testosterone via $5\alpha$-reductase.[2]

## PANCREAS ANATOMY

The pancreas is an elongated organ (approximately 15 cm) located behind the stomach. The right side of the pancreas is termed the "head" and is the widest part of the pancreas, which lies in the curve of the duodenum (the "pancreas"). Projecting inferiorly from the head is the uncinated process, which extends posteriorly toward the superior mesenteric artery. The tapered left side extends slightly upward (the "body") and ends near the spleen (the "tail"). Traveling within the entire pancreatic parenchyma from the tail to the head is the main pancreatic (Wirsung) duct. It connects with the bile duct in the head of the pancreas to form the hepatopancreatic duct, otherwise called the ampulla of Vater. This opens into the duodenum at the major duodenal papilla. Flow through the ampulla of Vater is controlled by a sphincter (of Oddi) made of smooth muscle. The pancreas also contains an accessory duct that communicates with the main pancreatic duct. The pancreas is made of two types of glands: the endocrine and exocrine gland. The exocrine gland secretes digestive enzymes. The endocrine gland, which consists of the islets of Langerhans, secrets hormones into the bloodstream (Figure 315.2).[4]

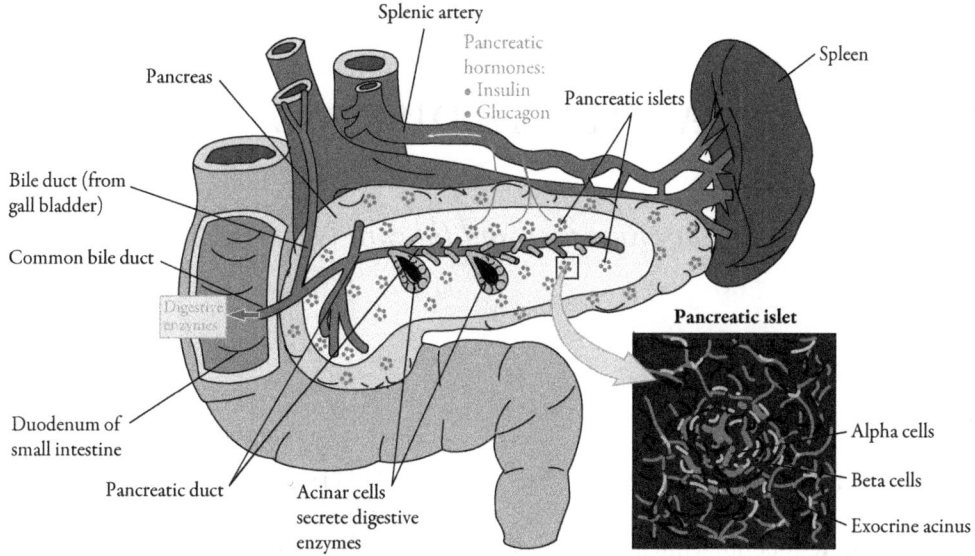

Labels on figure:
Splenic artery
Pancreatic hormones:
• Insulin
• Glucagon
Pancreas
Pancreatic islets
Spleen
Bile duct (from gall bladder)
Common bile duct
Digestive enzymes
Duodenum of small intestine
Pancreatic duct
Acinar cells secrete digestive enzymes

**Pancreatic islet**
Alpha cells
Beta cells
Exocrine acinus

**Figure 315.2.** Pancreas. The pancreatic exocrine function involves the acinar cells secreting digestive enzymes that are transported into the small intestine by the pancreatic duct. Its endocrine function involves the secretion of insulin (produced by beta cells) and glucagon (produced by alpha cells) within the pancreatic islets. These two hormones regulate the rate of glucose metabolism in the body. The micrograph reveals pancreatic islets. LM × 760.

Micrograph provided by the Regents of University of Michigan Medical School © 2012.

## REFERENCES

1. The endocrine pancreas: Anatomy and physiology. *Opentextbc.Ca*. March 6, 2013. opentextbc.ca/anatomyandphysiology/chapter/17-9-the-endocrine-pancreas/. Accessed May 15, 2020.
2. Costanzo LS. *Physiology*. Philadelphia, PA: Wolters Kluwer, 2019: 241–245.
3. The adrenal glands: Anatomy and physiology. *Openstax.Org*. 2012. openstax.org/books/anatomy-and-physiology/pages/17-6-the-adrenal-glands.
4. The pancreas. *John Hopkins Medicine*. 2019. www.hopkinsmedicine.org/health/conditions-and-diseases/the-pancreas. Accessed May 15, 2020.
5. Yeoh P. Anatomy and physiology of the adrenal gland. In: Llahana S, et al., eds. *Advanced Practice in Endocrinology Nursing*. Cham: Springer; 2019:645–655. https://doi.org/10.1007/978-3-319-99817-6_34

# 316.

# ADRENAL DISEASE

*Evgeney Romanov and Edward Noguera*

## INTRODUCTION

The adrenal glands are in the retroperitoneum in the medial aspect of the upper pole of each kidney. The fully matured adrenal gland is about 5 cm by 3 cm and is 1 cm think. The right gland is pyramidal and the left is oval shaped. Anatomically, the adrenals have a cortex and a medulla. The medulla secretes catecholamines and, functionally, is part of the sympathetic nervous system. The cortex has 3 different zones: glomerulosa, fasciculata, and reticularis. Each zone secretes different hormones.[1]

## ADRENAL PATHOLOGY

### CUSHING SYNDROME

See Table 316.1 for a summary of the mechanism and .

### CLINICAL FEATURES

Clinical features include truncal obesity (fat accumulation in the dorsocervical and supraclavicular fat pads), hypertension, fatigability, skin atrophy, and wide, purplish striae (abdomen is typical location), osteoporosis, proximal muscle weakness, skin hyperpigmentation (if ACTH excess), increased intravascular fluid volume and peripheral edema, psychiatric disturbances (depression, mania), increased likelihood of infections (due to impaired immunity), hyperglycemia, hyperlipidemia, hypokalemia, and metabolic alkalosis, which result from weak aldosterone-like effect of cortisol, leukocytosis (neutrophilia) from demargination of leukocytes.[2]

### DIAGNOSIS

1. Initial screening: An overnight (low-dose) dexamethasone suppression test is the initial screening test. Give the patient 1 mg of dexamethasone at 11 p.m. Measure the serum cortisol level at 8 a.m. If the serum cortisol is <5, Cushing syndrome can be excluded. If the serum cortisol is >5 (often >10), the patient has Cushing syndrome.

2. ACTH level: Once Cushing syndrome diagnosis is established, ACTH level should be measured. If it is low, the cause of high cortisol levels is likely an adrenal tumor or hyperplasia, not a pituitary disease or an ectopic ACTH-producing tumor.

3. High-dose dexamethasone suppression test:
   - In Cushing disease, the result is a decrease in cortisol levels (greater than 50% suppression occurs).
   - If cortisol suppression does not occur and plasma ACTH levels are high, an ectopic ACTH-producing tumor is likely the diagnosis.

4. Imaging tests (once hormonal studies have established the site of disease, e.g., pituitary, or adrenal): computed tomography (CT) scan or magnetic resonance imaging (MRI) help delineate the cause (tumor, location, size, and extension).

## ANESTHETIC CONSIDERATIONS

### Preoperative

Hypertension, hyperglycemia, and electrolyte imbalances should be well controlled. Fluid status, muscle weakness, and home dose diuretic responses should be assessed. Airway considerations include: inability or difficulties positioning patient for optimal airway management (i.e., truncal obesity, limited range of motion, limited space to maneuver standard blades, excessive neck pannus, severe osteopenia of cervical spine).[1,2]

### Intraoperative

Consider the size of the tumor and extension. For pituitary tumors, imaging and clinical symptoms should help establish what, if any, brain structures are compromised and if there is increased intracranial pressure. Document a neurological exam before induction of anesthesia. For adrenal tumors, imaging studies assess the compromise of adjacent structures. Appropriate plans for intravenous access, blood products, and massive fluid shifts are prompted if a large retroperitoneal tumor is in close proximity to inferior vena cava (IVC) or aorta. For patients with moderate to severe muscle weakness at baseline, titration and dosing of muscle relaxants is of paramount importance so residual weakness toward emergence of anesthesia is avoided. Refractory intraoperative hypotension due to a relative deficit of cortisol is possible. Consider dosing steroids intraoperatively. Special attention should be paid to patient positioning, padding of pressure points, and securement of limbs due to high prevalence of osteopenia and skin fragility.[1]

## Postoperative

For unilateral/bilateral adrenalectomy:

- Glucocorticoid replacement therapy at a dose equal to full replacement of adrenal output during periods of extreme stress. Hydrocortisone IV (50 mg q6h) can exert significant mineralocorticoid activity.
- Total dosage is reduced by 50% per day until a daily maintenance of steroids is achieved (20 to 30 mg/day of prednisone).
- Fludrocortisone can be added at a dosage of 0.05 to 0.1 mg/day postoperatively. Its dose should be reduced if congestive heart failure, hypokalemia, or hypertension occurs.

For solitary adrenalectomy: contralateral adrenal gland may compensate over time and glucocorticoid replacement therapy should be adjusted.

In case of unresectable tumor: continuous medical therapy with metyrapone is the treatment of choice.

## CONN SYNDROME

### CAUSE

Bilateral adrenal hyperplasia is the most common cause; mineralocorticoid-producing adrenal adenoma is the second most common cause.

### CLINICAL FEATURES

Clinical feature include hypertension, metabolic alkalosis, hypokalemia, and mild hypernatremia. There is no significant peripheral edema due to aldosterone escape mechanism (hypersecretion of sodium by kidneys in response to initial hypernatremia)

### DIAGNOSIS

- Elevated plasma aldosterone, low plasma renin
- Plasma aldosterone:renin ratio >20
- Adrenal suppression testing after oral saline load is used to confirm the diagnosis

*Table 316.1* MECHANISM AND PATHOLOGY OF CUSHING SYNDROME

| MECHANISM | PATHOLOGY |
| --- | --- |
| Overproduction of cortisol | Adrenal tumor, bilateral adrenal hyperplasia |
| Overproduction of ACTH | Paraneoplastic from lung tumors, kidney of pancreatic tumors |
| Exogenous glucocorticoid therapy | |

- Abdominal imaging (CT or MRI) and adrenal venous aldosterone sampling are used to differentiate adrenal tumor and bilateral adrenal hyperplasia.[1,2]

### ANESTHETIC CONSIDERATIONS

- Assessment of fluid status, hydration, and correction of hypovolemia or severe electrolyte abnormalities
- Hypertension and hypokalemia should be managed with spironolactone.
- Usual complications of chronic hypertension should be assessed.

## ADDISON DISEASE

### CAUSE

- Autoimmune adrenal destruction is the most common cause.
- Infections (tuberculosis, HIV, disseminated fungal)
- Hemorrhagic infarction
- Metastatic cancer
- Patients receiving chronic corticosteroid therapy may develop acute adrenal insufficiency during surgery due to hypothalamic-pituitary-adrenal axis suppression (tertiary adrenal insufficiency).
- Relative adrenal insufficiency is common in critically ill surgical patients with hypotension requiring vasopressors.

### CLINICAL FEATURES

- Fatigue, muscle weakness, anorexia, weight loss, nausea, vomiting, diarrhea. Only in primary adrenal insufficiency: diffuse hyperpigmentation due to increased ACTH level, hyponatremia and hyperkalemia due to mineralocorticoid deficiency. Vitiligo may be present in case of polyglandular autoimmune disease.
- Acute Addisonian crisis: abdominal pain, severe vomiting and diarrhea, hypotension, altered mental status, shock.

- Inadequate steroid replacement in patients receiving chronic corticosteroid therapy (rare) has features of refractory, distributive shock. Critically ill patients may not have classic symptoms and have a clinical picture of "sepsis without a source of infection."

### DIAGNOSIS

- ACTH, serum cortisol, and high-dose (250 μg) ACTH stimulation test
- Primary: low cortisol, high ACTH
- Secondary/tertiary: low cortisol, low ACTH

### ANESTHETIC CONSIDERATIONS

#### For Primary Adrenal Insufficiency

- In normal adult, adrenal glands produce 20 mg of cortisol and 0.1 mg of aldosterone/day with most of the hormone being secreted in the morning.
- To produce the stable concentration of hormone in plasma, the dosage is given twice daily with daily dosages being 50% higher.
- Prednisone: 5 mg in the morning, 2.5 mg in the evening. Hydrocortisone: 20 mg in the morning, 10 mg in the evening.
- Mineralocorticoid replacement is achieved with 0.05–0.1 of fludrocortisone per day.

#### For Secondary Adrenal Insufficiency

- Steroids are recommended. Mineralocorticoid replacement is not required.

### ACUTE ADRENAL INSUFFICIENCY

The clinical hallmark of acute adrenal insufficiency is persistent and profound shock that is refractory to fluids and commonly requires vasopressors. Typically, a patient has a history of adrenal disease or steroid use. Circulatory shock due to adrenal insufficiency usually requires invasive monitoring and titration of fluid resuscitation. Steroid replacement is indicated.[1,2] The response to steroids is very variable, and some patients respond within 24 hours after initiation of steroid replacement. Recommended doses are:

- Hydrocortisone, 100 mg IV bolus, followed by hydrocortisone 50mg IV q6h.
- If the patient stabilizes, steroid dose should be reduced starting day 2 and continued for at least 5 days to the minimum dose necessary to avoid hypotension.

### REFERENCES

1. Barash P, et al. *Clinical Anesthesia*. 8th ed. Lippincott Williams & Wilkins; 2017.
2. *Stoelting's Anesthesia and Coexisting Disease*. 7th ed. Elsevier; 2017.

# 317.

# BIOCHEMISTRY OF NORMAL BODY METABOLISM

*Felipe Vasconcelos Torres and Raquel Montagner Rossi*

## INTRODUCTION

Metabolism is defined by all the chemical reactions that take place in the human organism. Metabolic reactions can be divided into anabolic (synthetic) and catabolic (breakdown).

Anabolic reactions are essentially the synthesis of more complex substances using smaller, simpler molecules as building blocks.[1] They require energy, and are performed by the body when nutrients are readily available. Examples of anabolic reactions are gluconeogenesis and synthesis of glycogen, fatty acids, lipids, amino acids, proteins, and urea. Conversely, catabolic reactions involve the breakdown of complex substances into simpler ones. Examples of catabolic reactions are glycolysis, glycogenolysis, lipolysis, beta-oxidation of fatty acids, and degradation of amino acids and ketone bodies.

## THE ROLE OF THE LIVER IN BODY METABOLISM

The liver plays a central role in all metabolic processes in the body. Its functions include maintaining homeostasis, synthesis of molecules, energy storage and release, processing of nutrients and metabolization of toxic compounds. The following is a brief description of the metabolic functions of this remarkable organ.

## CARBOHYDRATE METABOLISM

The liver plays a major role in regulating blood glucose levels. In the fed state, a rise in glucose levels in the portal vein triggers glycogenesis, which is the synthesis of glycogen using serum glucose molecules. The opposite occurs during fasting, when low serum glucose levels trigger liver cells to break down glycogen (through glycogenolysis) or to create new glucose molecules from other intermediates (gluconeogenesis). The liver is also responsible for degrading fructose and galactose.

## LIPID METABOLISM

The liver performs oxidation of fatty acids for its own energy supply. Beta-oxidation of fatty acids to form acetyl-CoA can take place in all cells of the body, but it occurs most rapidly in hepatic cells.[2] During fasting, metabolism of fatty acids and glycerol from the breakdown of adipose tissue is significantly increased and exceeds the liver's energy needs. In this case, excessive acetyl-CoA is converted to ketone bodies, which are then released to the bloodstream to be used for energy by other organs. In addition, the liver also plays a central role in the metabolism of lipoproteins and the synthesis of cholesterol and phospholipids.

## PROTEIN METABOLISM

Liver cells are responsible for synthesizing almost all plasmatic proteins (with the exception of gamma globulins), including albumin and coagulation factors. They can also perform synthesis, deamination, and transamination of amino acids. Through the urea cycle, the liver helps maintain nitrogen balance in the body by converting ammonia—a toxic metabolic compound originating from the processing of amino acids by other tissues—to urea, a nontoxic substance that can be excreted by the kidneys. The glucose-alanine cycle is responsible for the transport of nitrogen—through alanine—from peripheral tissues to the liver, which, in turn, converts it to urea and releases glucose into the bloodstream.

## BODY METABOLISM IN FASTING AND IN POSTPRANDIAL STATES

The synthesis and breakdown of nutrients varies significantly in fasting compared to fed state. During the postprandial state, glucose and chylomicrons absorbed by the digestive system are sent to the bloodstream and are used by the body for fuel and for anabolic processes. Conversely, when there are no nutrients coming from diet, catabolic reactions occur and include glycogenolysis by the liver and

**FASTING** **POSTPRANDIAL**

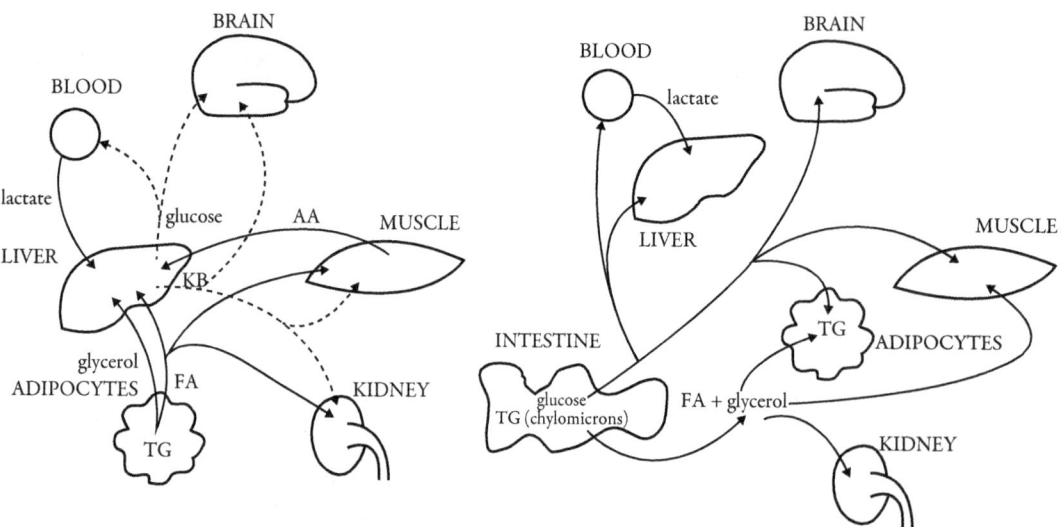

**Figure 317.1.** Integration of metabolism in fasting and postprandial states. Abbreviations: AA: amino acids; KB: ketone bodies; FA: fatty acids; TG: triglycerides.

muscle, release of fatty acids and glycerol from adipose tissue, and amino acids from muscle tissue. These catabolic reactions ensure the maintenance of appropriate cell metabolism (Figure 317.1).

## HOW DIFFERENT ORGANS MEET THEIR METABOLIC NEEDS

The metabolic machinery varies significantly from organ to organ, and therefore the role of glucose in energy metabolism for each cell is also organ dependent. Some organs are more strictly dependent on glucose for functioning, while others are more versatile and can use other substances, such as lactate and ketone bodies, for energy generation.

### BRAIN

Glucose is the only fuel for the brain, unless in a state of prolonged starvation. Brain tissue is not capable of storing glycogen or lipids, thereby requiring a continuous supply of glucose for functioning. During starvation (or in a ketogenic diet), the brain can have up to 50% of its energy derived from ketoacids (products of the metabolization of fatty acids in the liver), but the remaining 50% will still be dependent on glucose.

### STRIATED MUSCLE

Muscle tissue is very versatile. It can use fatty acids, glucose, and ketone bodies for energy. It is also able to store large amounts of glycogen and some lipids intracellularly. In resting muscle, up to 85% of energy is supplied by fat, while in active muscle this percentage decreases and the preferred fuel is glucose.

### CARDIAC MUSCLE

Myocytes are almost exclusively aerobic and have no glycogen storage. The heart can use glucose, fatty acids, lactate, acetoacetate, and ketone bodies as fuel.

### KIDNEYS

The kidneys have high energy requirements to support reabsorption of plasma solutes. They are responsible for the reabsorption of a vast amount of glucose as well; however, their main energy sources are fatty acids and ketone bodies.

### LIVER

Despite being involved in metabolic interchanges with many other organs, the α-ketoacids derived from the degradation of amino acids are the liver's own fuel.[3]

## RESPIRATORY QUOTIENT

Cellular respiration is the process that allows cells to generate the energy necessary to perform all their metabolic processes. In order to generate energy in the form of ATP, oxygen is consumed and carbon dioxide is produced. However, the ratio of $CO_2$ produced/$O_2$ consumed, also known as the respiratory quotient (RQ), varies with different nutrients that are processed. On a mixed diet, the RQ is approximately 0.8; in other words, for every 10 molecules of $O_2$ consumed, 8 molecules of $CO_2$ are produced. The RQ is 1 for carbohydrate, 0.8 for protein, and 0.7 for fat.[4]

## REFERENCES

1. Nelson DL, Cox MM. Part II: Bioenergetics and metabolism. In: Nelson DL, Cox MM, eds. *Lehninger Principles of Biochemistry*. 5th ed. page 487. W. H. Freeman; 2008:485–519.

2. Guyton AC, Hall JE. The liver as an organ. In: Hall JE, et al., eds. *Guyton and Hall Textbook of Medical Physiology*. 12th ed. Philadelphia, PA: Saunders Elsevier; 2011:839–840.

3. Berg J, Tymoczko J, Stryer L. Each organ has a unique metabolic profile. In: Berg JM, et al., eds. *Biochemistry*. 5th ed. New York, NY: W. H. Freeman; 2002:851–854.

4. Widmaier EP, Raff, Hershel, Strang KT. Respiration. In: Widmaier EP, et al., eds. *Vander's Human Physiology: The Mechanisms of Body Function*. 8th ed. New York, NY: McGraw Hill; 2001:442–484.

# 318.

# CARBOHYDRATES

*Felipe Vasconcelos Torres and Raquel Montagner Rossi*

## INTRODUCTION

Glucose plays a central role in energy metabolism. It is an energy-rich molecule, able to be stored as a polysaccharide, and also a versatile precursor for a number of biosynthetic pathways. When not used for synthesis of structural molecules, glucose will be mostly oxidized or stored. Storage of glucose in the human cells occurs in the liver and in skeletal muscle, and is done in the form of glycogen, a complex polysaccharide.

Oxidation of glucose can happen in two main pathways: the pentose phosphate pathway, in which glucose molecules are oxidized to pentoses (5 carbon sugars) that will be used as precursors for the synthesis of nucleotides and to regenerate the reducing agent NADPH; and the glycolytic pathway, which leads to energy generation for cells in the form of adenosine triphosphate (ATP). In this chapter, we will discuss the glycolytic pathway in further detail.

## THE GLYCOLYTIC PATHWAY

Glycolysis is a series of reactions that occur in the cytosol of the cell and lead to the splitting of the glucose molecule (a 6-carbon molecule) into 2 molecules of pyruvate (each with 3 carbon atoms). The first step of glycolysis is the phosphorylation of glucose to glucose-6-phosphate, which leads to entrapment of glucose inside the cell. This initial reaction is catalyzed by the enzymes glucokinase (found primarily in hepatocytes and pancreatic beta cells) and hexokinase (found in most tissues). After a series of reactions, two molecules of pyruvate are formed. This is also called the energy investment phase of glycolysis, because some ATP expenditure is required for the initial reactions to occur; however, during the second half of glycolysis, or energy-generation phase, ATP is also formed, leading to a small net gain of 2 ATP molecules at the end of the reaction chain. Keep in mind that glycolysis occurs in the cytosol and does not require oxygen.

It is important to note that glycolysis releases only a small fraction of the total available energy of the glucose molecule; the rest of the potential energy remains in the two molecules of pyruvate.[1] It is a resource, albeit inefficient, for energy generation by cells when oxygen supply is depleted (e.g., hypoxemia or strenuous exercise).

The glycolytic pathway can be further split into two pathways: aerobic and anaerobic. Different chemical

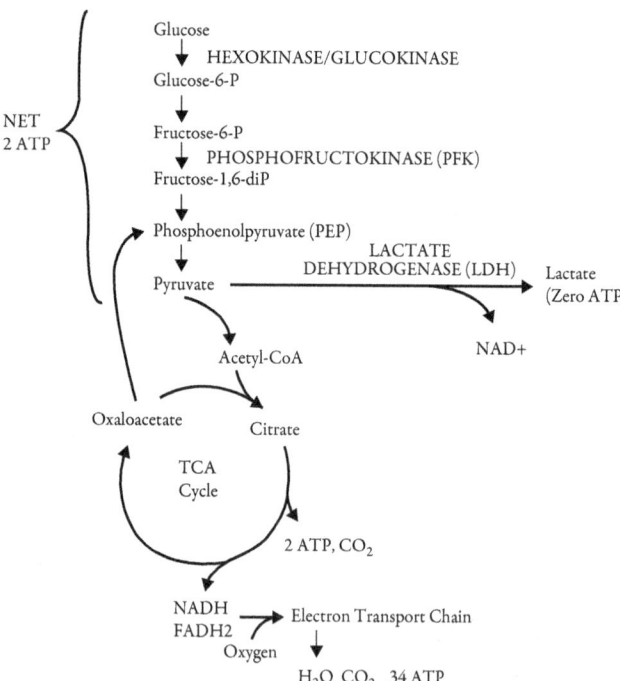

**Figure 318.1.** The glycolytic pathway.

processes are involved when oxygen is either present or absent (Figure 318.1).

## AEROBIC METABOLISM

The first steps of aerobic and anaerobic metabolism are essentially the same and end with the formation of pyruvate through glycolysis. Under aerobic conditions, where oxygen is available, tremendous amounts of energy can be produced by the cell. This is the main form of glucose metabolism in tissues with mitochondria.

Aerobic metabolism begins with the conversion of pyruvic acid molecules into acetyl coenzyme A (acetyl-CoA). Pyruvate molecules lose a carboxyl group and combine with coenzyme A, a derivative of pantothenic acid (vitamin $B_5$). Acetyl-CoA molecules then enter the TCA cycle (tricarboxylic acid cycle, or Krebs cycle), which occurs in the mitochondrial matrix. Through the TCA cycle, acetyl-CoA joins oxaloacetate, forming citrate. A series of redox reactions follow, with the formation of ATP and electron carriers (FADH and $NADH_2$) and the cycle continues with the regeneration of oxaloacetate.

Of note, products of the metabolism of fatty acids and amino acids are also able to enter the TCA cycle. However, oxaloacetate can be formed from glucose and some amino acids, but not from fatty acids. It can also be converted to pyruvate and re-enter the cycle.

The reduced electron carriers—FADH and $NADH_2$—will then pass their electrons on to the electron transport chain, a series of electron acceptors through which electrons travel until they reach cytochrome oxidase, which uses them to form water molecules. It is during the transport of these electrons, however, that energy is released and used by ATP synthase (or ATPase) to convert adenosine triphosphate (ADP) into huge amounts of ATP. This process is called oxidative phosphorylation.

## ANAEROBIC METABOLISM

When oxygen is unavailable or insufficient, or when there is an impairment of the oxidative pathway, oxidative phosphorylation cannot occur. However, as the initial steps of glucose breakdown do not require oxygen, a small amount of energy can still be produced by the cell through glycolysis.

When the two end products of the glycolytic reactions (pyruvate and hydrogen ions combined with NAD+ to form NADH and H+) begin to accumulate, they react with each other to form lactate, which diffuses out of the cell into the extracellular fluid and works as a "sinkhole," preventing negative feedback and, thus, allowing for glycolysis to continue for several minutes. When oxygen becomes available again, the lactic acid can then be rapidly converted back to pyruvic acid and used for energy. The enzyme responsible for converting pyruvate into lactate and back is called lactate dehydrogenase.

It is important to note that lactate production rises up only when oxygen usage is occurring at the maximum possible rate. In physiologic conditions it can happen due to increased demand (for example, when exercising vigorously), but could also be due to low availability of oxygen (for example: in anemia, carbon monoxide intoxication, and hypoxia/infarction).

## LACTATE FORMATION AND METABOLISM IN TISSUES

The direction of the reaction catalyzed by lactate dehydrogenase depends on both the intracellular concentrations of pyruvate and lactate, as well as the ratio of NADH/NAD+ in the cell. In the liver and heart, this ratio is lower than in exercising muscle, which allows them to oxidize lactate to pyruvate and use it for energy. Heart muscle is especially capable of oxidizing lactate, especially during heavy exercise when large amounts of lactate are released into the bloodstream.[2] Of note, red blood cells lack mitochondria and rely solely on anaerobic glycolysis for fueling, producing lactate even under aerobic conditions.

## REGULATION OF GLYCOLYSIS

Key enzymes that catalyze irreversible reactions are responsible for regulating the rate of glycolysis.[3] The most relevant enzymes are hexokinase, phosphofructokinase, and pyruvate kinase.

### PHOSPHOFRUCTOKINASE (PFK)

PFK catalyzes the conversion of fructose-6-phosphate to fructose-1,6-biphosphate and is the most important regulator of glycolysis. PFK is inhibited by high levels of ATP and citrate (high energy state). It is stimulated by AMP (a product of the conversion of ADP to ATP by the cell when in a low energy state).

### HEXOKINASE

Hexokinase catalyzes the first step of glycolysis and is inhibited by its product, glucose-6-phosphate (G6P). Of note, the liver has a different enzyme, glucokinase, which is not inhibited by G6P and has a much higher affinity for glucose than hexokinase, therefore allowing for its use for the synthesis of glycogen.

### PYRUVATE DEHYDROGENASE

This enzyme catalyzes the conversion of pyruvate to Acetyl-CoA. It is inhibited by ATP and NADH, and stimulated by ADP. The amounts of substrate (pyruvate) and product (acetyl-CoA) also regulate its action.

### REFERENCES

1. Nelson DL, Cox MM. Glycolysis, gluconeogenesis, and the pentose phosphate pathway. In: Nelson DL, Cox MM, eds. *Lehninger Principles of Biochemistry*. New York, NY: Worth; 2000: 528–539.
2. Guyton AC, Hall JE. Metabolism of carbohydrates, and formation of adenosine triphosphate. In: Hall JE, Guyton AC, eds. In: *Guyton and Hall Textbook of Medical Physiology*. Philadelphia, PA: Saunders Elsevier; 2011:809–817.
3. Berg JM, Tymoczko JL, Stryer L. The glycolytic pathway is tightly controlled. In: Berg JM, et al., eds. *Biochemistry*. 5th ed. New York, NY: W. H. Freeman; 2002:472–478.

# 319.

# RELATIONSHIP TO HORMONES

*Lucas Costa Santos and Raquel Montagner Rossi*

## INTRODUCTION

Bioenergetics is continuously adjusted in response to the various settings that the human body can be exposed to. Such changes are mediated by the nervous system and integrated between tissues primarily by the action of hormones.[1] Two peptide hormones—insulin and glucagon—play a major role in this process, aided by the action of the catecholamines epinephrine and norepinephrine as well as cortisol, among others. Variations in the levels of these hormones allow for the storage of energy during normal conditions and for its utilization in stressful situations.[2] This chapter aims to discuss the role of such hormones in controlling the utilization of energy in different situations.

## INSULIN AND THE FED STATE

In the setting of abundance of food and low demand for immediately available energy, the body is able to maintain an anabolic state. This means that the available nutrients can be stored in order to be used when necessary. Insulin, a peptide hormone produced by pancreatic β cells, plays a critical role in this process by favoring glycogenesis, synthesis of

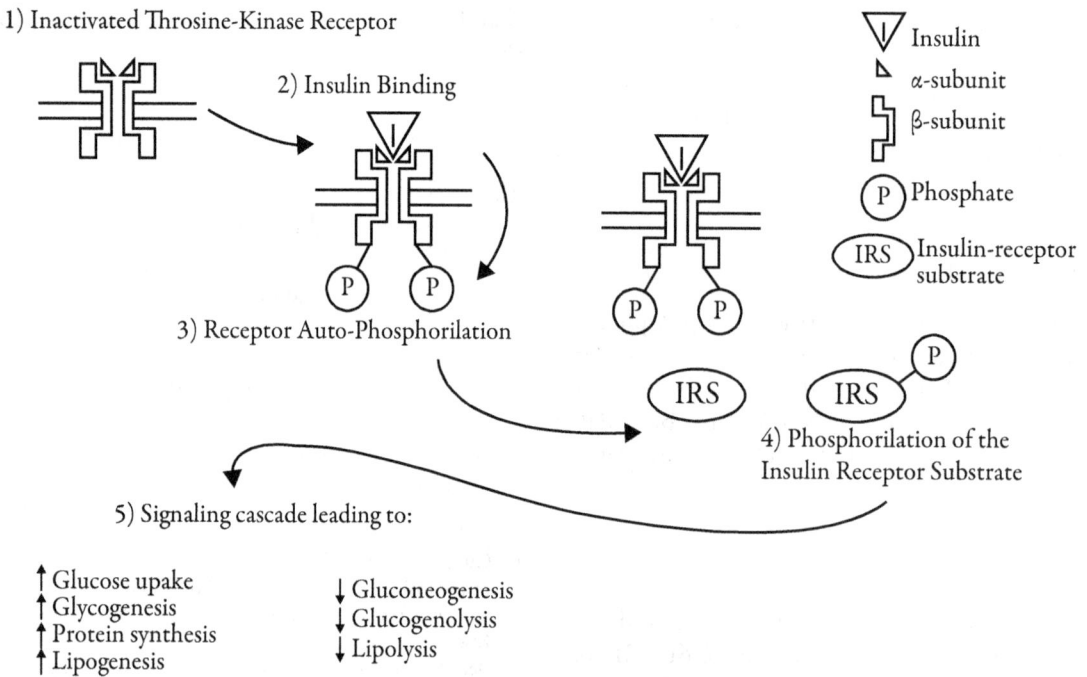

1) Inactivated Throsine-Kinase Receptor

2) Insulin Binding

3) Receptor Auto-Phosphorilation

Insulin
α-subunit
β-subunit
P  Phosphate
IRS  Insulin-receptor substrate

4) Phosphorilation of the Insulin Receptor Substrate

5) Signaling cascade leading to:

↑ Glucose upake          ↓ Gluconeogenesis
↑ Glycogenesis           ↓ Glucogenolysis
↑ Protein synthesis      ↓ Lipolysis
↑ Lipogenesis

**Figure 319.1.** Insulin signaling and metabolic effects.

proteins and triacylglycerols, as well as inhibiting the mobilization of these molecules.[1,2]

As shown in Figure 319.1, insulin acts by binding to the tyrosine-kinase receptor in the cell membrane of most tissues, especially in the liver, adipose tissue, and muscle, leading to its autophosphorylation and activation of a signaling cascade involving multiple insulin receptor substrates (IRSs). It promotes the uptake of glucose in the muscle and adipose tissue by increasing the availability of glucose GLUT-4 transporters in the cell membrane. At the same time, glycogen synthesis is stimulated in the muscle and liver, where gluconeogenesis and glycogenolysis are also inhibited by insulin.[2]

Concurrently, insulin facilitates the entry of amino acids in most tissues and promotes protein synthesis through the activation of translation factors. Similarly, adipose tissue responds by increasing the expression of lipoprotein lipases, which provides fatty acids that are incorporated into triacylglycerol molecules along with glycerol 3-phosphate provided by the increased glucose uptake, while hormone-sensitive lipases are inhibited in order to reduce lipid catabolism in this tissue.[2]

All this relates harmonically to the synthesis and regulation of insulin secretion, which involves the production of its inactive precursors preproinsulin and proinsulin. These are then cleaved in order to form the active form of this hormone, along with a connecting peptide (C-peptide) responsible for the proper folding of insulin. Both are then stored into cytosol granules and released by exocytosis. Insulin presents a short duration of action with a half-life of approximately 6 minutes due to the presence of insulin-degrading enzymes in the liver and kidneys, which allows for rapid changes in its circulating levels. Conversely, C-peptide has a broader half-life that corroborates its clinical significance in assessing the production and secretion of insulin.[1,2]

The secretion of anabolic hormones such as insulin is tightly coordinated with the production and release of their catabolic counterparts—glucagon and epinephrine—which we will discuss in the next chapter. Glucose is one of the main stimulators of insulin release by the pancreatic β cells, which act as glucose-sensing agents through the expression of GLUT-2 transporters and glucokinase. Upon entry and phosphorylation of glucose, adenosine triphosphate (ATP) is generated, leading to the secretion of insulin by closing membrane potassium channels.[1] Similarly, increased levels of amino acids and fatty acids lead to enhanced glucose-mediated insulin release. Finally, intestinal peptide hormones such as glucagon-like protein 1 (GLP-1) and gastric-inhibitory polypeptide (GIP) also increase the sensitivity of β cells to glucose, which accounts for the higher levels of insulin produced following oral administration of glucose compared to intravenous administration.[1,2]

Two other known hormones have important roles in the long-term regulation of metabolism—cortisol and growth hormone (GH)—while their effects are less evident in the short term. This is due to the fact that their actions are mainly mediated by gene transcription regulation, which takes some time to occur.[2–5]

## GROWTH HORMONE

Growth hormone (GH) is another anabolic peptide hormone which is secreted by the anterior pituitary. Sleep, stress, exercise, and low glucose levels—such as in a fasting state—trigger the release of GH into the bloodstream. Its anabolic effects include promoting protein synthesis and chondrocyte proliferation.[1] Through binding to cell membrane receptors, it triggers a complex intracellular signaling process mainly mediated by Janus kinase 2 (JAK2). One of the main results is the production of insulin-like growth factor 1 (IGF-1) by the liver. It acts on specific receptors on multiple tissues, similar to insulin receptors, and triggers a pathway that culminates in the activation of protein kinase B (Akt) and mitogen-activated protein kinase (MAPK). As a result, apoptosis is inhibited and proliferation is stimulated, accounting for the anabolic effects promoted by this hormone.[3,5]

Finally, despite its anabolic properties, it is also proposed that the counteracting effects of GH toward insulin are mediated through the inhibition of IRS phosphorylation by insulin receptors and by the degradation of IRS itself.[5] This leads to the promotion of gluconeogenesis and lipolysis, counterbalancing the hypoglycemic effects of insulin, and consequently elevating serum glucose levels.

In summary, we can see that the regulation of metabolism in various situations is mainly coordinated by hormones in a finely balanced interaction in their levels. While insulin and GH act on one side of this balance exerting anabolic effects during normal conditions, cortisol, glucagon, and catecholamines counteract during demanding situations in order to maintain metabolic homeostasis and energy supply to the body tissues.

## REFERENCES

1. Nelson DL, Cox MM. Bioenergetics and biochemical reaction types. In: Nelson DL, Cox MM, eds. *Lehninger Principles of Biochemistry.* 6th edition. New York, NY: W. H. Freeman; 2012:505–542.
2. Guyton AC, Hall JE. Energetics and metabolic rate. In: Hall JE, Guyton AC, eds. *Guyton and Hall Textbook of Medical Physiology,* 12th edition. Philadelphia, PA: Saunders Elsevier; 2011: 859–865.
3. Kim SH, Park MJ. Effects of growth hormone on glucose metabolism and insulin resistance in humans. *Ann Pediatr Endocrinol Metab.* 2017;22(3):145–152.
4. Seleznev IuM, Martynov AV. Permissive effect of glucocorticoids in catecholamine action in the heart: possible mechanism. *J Mol Cell Cardiol.* 1982;14(Suppl 3):49–58.
5. Laron Z. Insulin-like growth factor 1 (IGF-1): A growth hormone. *Mol Pathol.* 2001;54(5):311–316.

# 320.

# GLUCAGON AND CATECHOLAMINES

*Felipe Vasconcelos Torres and Lucas Costa Santos*

## INTRODUCTION

Hormones produced by the body play an important part in its metabolic response to different situations. Glucagon and epinephrine, in particular, play a central role in responding to stress. Along with cortisol and growth hormone, they oppose the effects of insulin and induce a counterregulatory response that improves the availability of energy to key tissues during crises.[1] This chapter describes the role of these hormones in the metabolic response to stress.

## GLUCAGON: A CATABOLIC HORMONE

Similar to insulin, glucagon is a peptide hormone produced by the pancreas—in this case by the α cells in the islets of Langerhans—that induces a catabolic response during stressful situations. Its synthesis is similar to the one described for insulin and involves the precursor molecule preproglucagon, which is cleaved to different end products in various tissues. For instance, while glucagon is the main product generated in the α cells, the intestinal L cells cleave preproglucagon into glucagon-like peptide-1 (GLP-1), one of the incretins mentioned in the previous chapter. In terms of duration of action, glucagon has a short half-life, comparable to insulin.[2,3]

As opposed to insulin, glucagon aims to maintain glucose levels during critical situations by promoting a catabolic response. Through binding to G-coupled receptors primarily on the surface of hepatocytes, this hormone activates adenylyl cyclase in the plasma membrane, leading to an enhanced conversion of adenosine triphosphate (ATP) into cyclic adenosine monophosphate (cAMP). The resulting reduced ATP/cAMP ratio activates protein kinase A (PKA) in the plasma and, thus, the phosphorylation of key enzymes,[2,3] as illustrated in Figure 320.1. Similarly to insulin, gene transcription is also altered by glucagon.

While having the liver as a primary target, glucagon promotes glycogenolysis and gluconeogenesis, which leads to a rapid rise in glucose levels. Moreover, the phosphorylation of acetyl-CoA carboxylase (ACC) in the adipose tissue allows for the breakdown of long-chain fatty acids through β-oxidation. The resulting free fatty acids are taken up by the liver and converted into ketone bodies, which are also used as energy sources.[2,3] Even though glucagon plays a role in lipolysis itself, it is in fact the catecholamines who are the main stimulators of hormone-sensitive lipases.[3,4] Finally, glucagon also increases the uptake of amino acids by the liver, which are released by muscle tissue, in order to provide yet another source for gluconeogenesis.[2,3]

## REGULATION OF GLUCAGON

The main stimulator of glucagon secretion is glucose. Low blood glucose levels trigger the release of glucagon by pancreatic α cells. Similarly to insulin, diet-derived amino acids also promote glucagon release. The rationale behind this is to prevent a potential hypoglycemic episode that could follow a protein-rich meal. Finally, secretion of epinephrine, mainly by the adrenal medulla, and norepinephrine released by the sympathetic nervous system also stimulate the release of glucagon by the pancreas. Conversely, the inhibition of glucagon secretion is mainly mediated by high blood glucose levels and by insulin itself.[1-3]

## CATECHOLAMINES: EPINEPHRINE AND NOREPINEPHRINE

Another important class of agents that act in a similar fashion as glucagon are the catecholamines, such as epinephrine and norepinephrine. These molecules are stored in the adrenal medulla, and are released in response to stress via sympathetic stimulation, with the goal of providing the body with enough energy sources during challenging situations, as well as increasing heart rate and vascular tone in order to redirect blood to key tissues and organs.[1,4]

Similarly, to glucagon, through binding to β-adrenergic receptors (which are G protein-coupled transmembrane

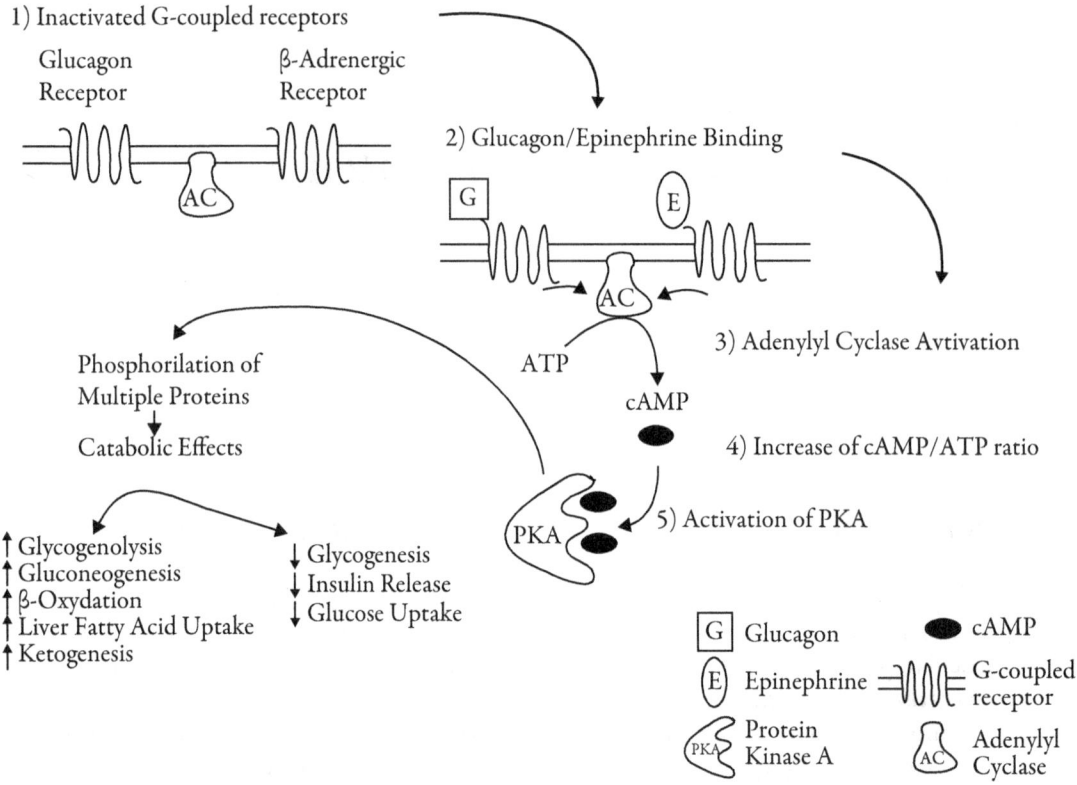

**Figure 320.1.** Cellular signaling and metabolic effects of glucagon and epinephrine.

receptors), catecholamines activate adenylyl cyclase. This results in elevated levels of cyclic AMP (cAMP) and the activation of protein kinase A (PKA), which, in turn, phosphorylates a variety of proteins. Consequently, catabolic effects are noted, such as upregulation of lipolysis and glycogenolysis, which provide the necessary energy sources. Also, catecholamines are able to override the effects of insulin in glucose uptake and to inhibit the secretion of insulin itself[2-4] (Figure 320.1).

## DEGRADATION OF CATECHOLAMINES

Catecholamines are degraded by two notable enzymes: monoamine oxidase (MAO) and catechol-O-methyltransferase (COMT). The resulting metabolites, vanillylmandelic acid (VMA) and homovanillic acid, are excreted in the urine and present a valuable clinical significance in the setting of increased catecholamine production and degradation. This is especially relevant in the presence of over-secreting adrenal tumors such as pheochromocytomas and neuroblastomas.[4]

## RELATIONSHIP TO CORTISOL

The metabolic effects of catecholamines are aided by the permissive effect of cortisol. Cortisol assists catecholamine action by two mechanisms: upregulation of adrenergic receptors on the cell surface, allowing for a higher availability for catecholamine binding; and binding of intracellular receptors that regulate gene expression. Through this last process, cortisol increases the synthesis of enzymes that are activated by the signaling processes triggered by catecholamines.[5]

It is notable that glucagon and catecholamines are the main promoters of catabolism in the setting of stressful conditions. As opposed to anabolic hormones, these exert their effects by enhancing glycogenolysis, gluconeogenesis, fatty acid breakdown, and ketogenesis. Their effects are mainly mediated by G protein-coupled receptors and the signaling cascades triggered by their interaction with such hormones. Finally, cortisol also plays a role in this process in a permissive fashion by altering gene expression and upregulating the exposure of target receptors on the cell membrane. All of this is critical in the metabolic response to stress in order to maintain energy availability and homeostasis.

## REFERENCES

1. Nelson DL, Cox MM. Bioenergetics and biochemical reaction types. In: Nelson DL, Cox MM, eds. *Lehninger Principles of Biochemistry.* New York, NY: Worth; 2000:528–539.
2. Guyton AC, Hall JE. Insulin, glucagon and diabetes mellitus. In: Hall JE, et al., eds. *Guyton and Hall Textbook of Medical Physiology.* Philadelphia, PA. Saunders Elsevier; 2011:939–950.
3. Harvey RA, Ferrier DR. Metabolic effects of insulin and glucagon. In: Harvey R, ed. *Lippincott's Illustrated Reviews: Biochemistry.* Philadelphia, PA: Wolters Kluwer Health; 2011:307–320.
4. Verly IRN, et al. Catecholamine excretion profiles identify clinical subgroups of neuroblastoma patients. *Eur J Cancer.* 2019;111:21–29.
5. Seleznev IuM, Martynov AV. Permissive effect of glucocorticoids in catecholamine action in the heart: Possible mechanism. *J Mol Cell Cardiol.* 1982;14(Suppl 3):49–58.

# 321.

# EFFECTS OF STRESS

*Allyson L. Spence and Elyse M. Cornett*

## INTRODUCTION

Stress, which may be defined as any condition, good or bad, that disrupts an individual's equilibrium, can alter the serum levels of various hormones, including catecholamines, glucocorticoids, prolactin, and growth hormone. Although stress is intended for protection, as it activates the "fight or flight" response, prolonged stress can lead to and/or worsen endocrine disorders. Furthermore, chronic stress can produce a reduction in neuroprotective hormones (e.g., dehydroepiandrosterone [DHEA]), reproductive hormones (e.g., gonadotropin-releasing hormone), and other metabolic hormones (e.g., triiodothyronine [T3]), thus leading to dysfunction in multiple body organ systems.[1]

## ACTIVATION OF THE SYMPATHETIC NERVOUS SYSTEM (SNS)

Stress activates the sympathetic nervous system to stimulate the release of catecholamines (e.g., epinephrine and norepinephrine), which causes sodium retention, increased cardiac output, bronchiolar dilation, and reduced intestinal motility.[1]

## HYPOTHALAMIC-PITUITARY-ADRENAL (HPA) AXIS

Overactivation of the HPA axis is a prominent response to both acute and chronic stress and can lead to increases in corticotrophin-releasing factor (CRF), adrenocorticotropic hormone (ACTH), and cortisol. This increased activity of the HPA axis is associated with increased fatigue, decreased cognitive abilities, and an increased risk of developing metabolic and psychiatric diseases (e.g., osteoporosis, depression, and hypothyroidism).[1]

## ETIOLOGY

Although many theories exist to explain the etiology of HPA axis dysfunction, most of these theories suggest that repetitive acute stressors and/or chronic stressors will lead to an overactivation of the HPA axis. As stressors continue in these individuals' lives, this over-responsiveness of the HPA axis may last for years before eventually transitioning into an underactive or nonresponsive state as the body adapts by reducing cortisol production. Although this is likely a protective response to prevent chronically high cortisol levels from leading to widespread bodily dysfunction (e.g., decreased immune response), the consequence can be just as dangerous, as patients may then suffer from hypercortisolism, which may then lead to an amplified immune response. This up-regulation of the immune system increases these individuals' susceptibilities to developing inflammatory diseases (e.g., autoimmune diseases).[1,2]

## DIAGNOSIS

### ACUTE STRESS DISORDER

Acute stress disorder can develop in individuals after experiencing and/or witnessing a traumatic event (e.g., acts of violence, motor vehicle crash, natural or man-made disasters, death of a loved one, diagnosis of a life-threatening illness). In order to be diagnosed with acute stress disorder, certain diagnostic criteria must be met. These criteria,

which are listed in the *Diagnostic and Statistical Manual of Mental Disorders* (DSM-5), include, but are not limited to, dissociative symptoms, re-experiencing the traumatic event, and marked symptoms of anxiety. Treatment options for patients experiencing an acute stress disorder include psychological first aid, cognitive behavioral therapy, and short-term pharmacological intervention.[3]

### HPA AXIS EVALUATION

Several diagnostic tools exist that can identify an HPA axis dysfunction. For example, clinicians may test the responsiveness of the adrenal gland to stress, which is typically done by collecting three morning saliva samples and testing them for cortisol levels to examine the cortisol awakening response. Although it is not as common, clinicians may also measure cortisol levels during an insulin-induced hypoglycemia, especially when ACTH deficiency is suspected.[2]

## ANESTHETIC CONSIDERATIONS

The perioperative period is associated with acute stress that can exacerbate symptoms of pain, anxiety, the surgical stress response, and the potential of anesthetic agents to produce neurotoxicity. Anesthesiologists should make conscious efforts to reduce this acute perioperative stress, and thus improve patient outcomes.[4]

### PREOPERATIVE

Clinicians can help reduce a patient's surgical stress and anxiety by educating patients on what they can expect during the perioperative period, encouraging them to engage in relaxation techniques (e.g., slow and deep breathing), and administering anxiolytics, such as benzodiazepines, prior to surgery.[4,5]

### INTRAOPERATIVE

Although general anesthesia is the most effective form of anesthesia to reduce the surgical stress response, this is not the best option for all surgical procedures. During procedures in which the patient is not under general anesthesia, clinicians can alleviate patient stress by preparing them during each step of the surgical procedure and/or readministering anxiolytics as necessary and as deemed medically appropriate. Additionally, thoracic epidurals may be superior to lumbar epidural anesthesia in suppressing the surgical stress response.[4,5]

### POSTOPERATIVE

Clinicians can alleviate postoperative patient stress by updating patients on their procedure, educating them on the next steps they should take, and/or administering pharmacological agents to alleviate any postoperative pain, as necessary and appropriate.[4,5]

## REFERENCES

1. Ranabir S, Reetu K. Stress and hormones. *Indian J Endocrinol Metab*. 2011;15(1):18–22.
2. Guilliams TG, Edwards L. Chronic stress and the HPA axis: Clinical assessment and therapeutic considerations. *Stand*. 2010;9(2):1–12.
3. Kavan MG et al. The physician's role in managing acute stress disorder. *Am Fam Physician*. 2012;86(7):643–649.
4. Borsook D, et al. Anesthesia and perioperative stress: Consequences on neural networks and postoperative behaviors. *Prog Neurobiol*. 2010;92(4):601–612.
5. Moraca RJ, et al. The role of epidural anesthesia and analgesia in surgical practice. *Ann Surg*. 2003;238(5):663–673.

# 322.

# PERIOPERATIVE MANAGEMENT OF INSULIN

*Jonathan I. Kim and Nathan Schulman*

## INTRODUCTION

Diabetes mellitus (DM) affects over 9% of people in the United States, necessitating increased surgical interventions secondary to cardiovascular and microvascular complications. The disease warrants careful assessment, as presentation involves a wide spectrum from asymptomatic to severe morbidity. Chronic dysfunction manifests as retinopathy, nephropathy, neuropathy, coronary disease, and hypertension, all of which form a complex interplay with acute surgical and anesthetic stressors.

Major goals of perioperative diabetes management center around avoidance of hypo/hyperglycemia, prevention of ketoacidosis/hyperosmolar states, as well as appropriate fluid and electrolyte balance (Figure 322.1). Within the bounds of extreme hypo/hyperglycemia, the ideal target for perioperative glucose is unclear, but correction of hyperglycemia improves mortality and hospital complications, while avoiding hypoglycemia similarly improves morbidity and mortality. Multiple trials and current guidelines recommend glycemic targets between 140 and 180 mg/dl.[1,2] For the anesthetist, the management of DM begins in the preoperative phase, extending through intraoperative and finally through postoperative management.

## ANESTHETIC CONSIDERATIONS

### PREOPERATIVE

Diabetic patients require a thorough history and physical examination for preoperative clearance. A distinction should be made between type 1 and type 2 DM given the higher incidence of ketoacidosis and subsequent requirement for basal insulin in type 1. Long-term sequelae of the disease, as mentioned in the Introduction of this chapter, should be reviewed. Assess baseline glycemic control, monitoring frequency, recent HgA1c, and average glucose, with particular note of extreme measurements and prior incidents of hypoglycemia or related hospitalizations. Hypoglycemia and its symptoms occur at levels below 70mg/dl. In alert patients with normal intake mechanisms, 15 g of carbohydrates can be given orally, while sedated patients can be given intravenous (IV) dextrose 25 g with repeated measurements every 5 to 10 minutes. Medication regimens including insulin, as well as dose timing, should be determined within the surgical context, including NPO (*nil per os*) initiation, timing and duration of the procedure, and type of anesthetic. Epidural and regional anesthesia minimally affect glucose and insulin activity versus general anesthesia.[3] As with all patients, but of particular importance in diabetics is the cardiopulmonary risk assessment with optimization

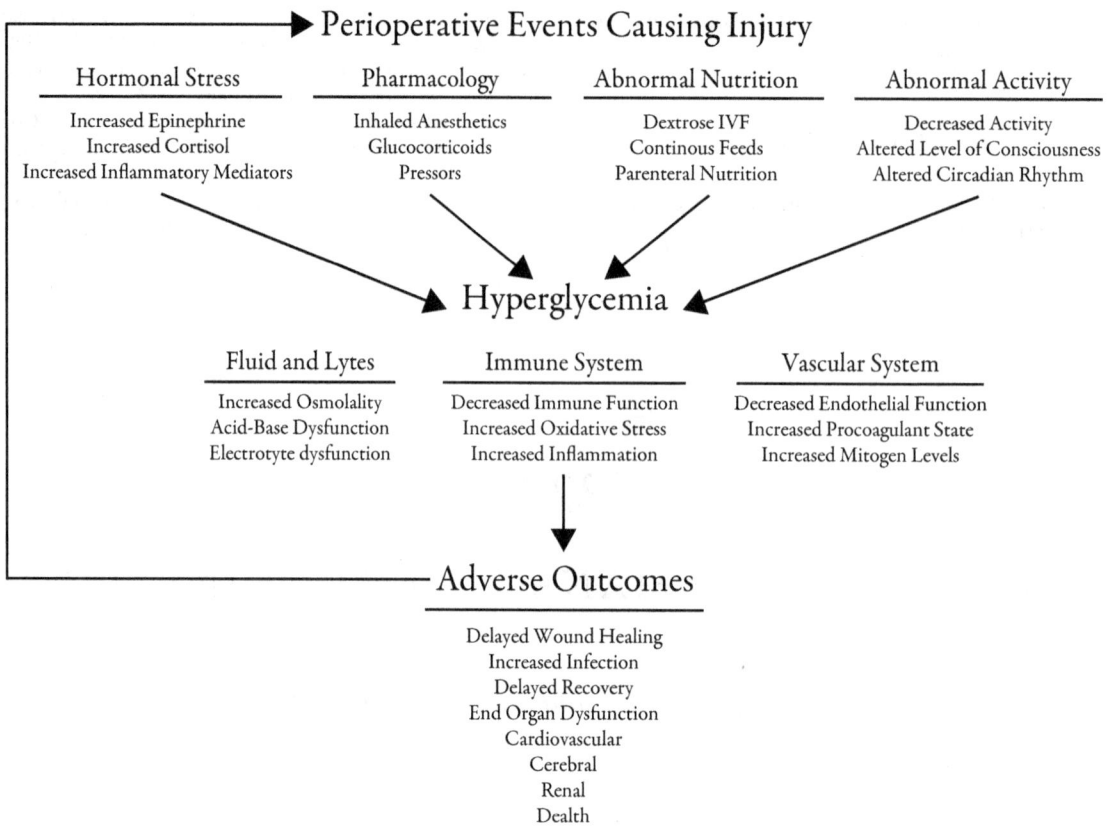

**Figure 322.1.** Perioperative Events Causing Injury
Reproduced with permission from Evans C, Lee J, Ruhlman M. Optimal glucose management in the perioperative period. *Surg Clin N Amer.* 2015;95(2):337–354.

of modifiable factors. Studies to include in a baseline screen include an electrocardiogram, serum creatinine, A1c if not recorded in the prior 4–6 weeks, and blood glucose.

## INTRAOPERATIVE

The intraoperative management of a diabetic patient can be divided by the dependence on home insulin or injectable medications, as well as length of procedure. Multiple approaches of target glucose maintenance exist, but currently there is no consensus of the optimal strategy. Protocols rely on expert opinion and are combined with hospital policy as well as personal experience. Accordingly, no model has been proven to reduce morbidity or mortality.[4]

Continuous insulin administration has similarly not demonstrated clear benefit and is often resource intensive. Unpredictable events as well as patient responses necessitate dynamic management with reliance on clinical judgement. Generally, diabetic patients should have surgery timed to prevent prolonged fasting.

Patients with diet-controlled DM rarely require any therapies perioperatively. In the event of hyperglycemia, short (regular) or rapid-acting insulin may be administered, with glucose checks every hour with intravenous use and every 2 hours with subcutaneous use.[5]

For patients with type 2 DM on oral agents, consensus guidelines recommend to continue their usual regimen until the morning of surgery. Many of the various classes of agents can cause perioperative complications. Metformin should be avoided in procedures involving intravenous contrast, renal hypoperfusion, increased lactate, and hypoxia when anticipated. DPP-4 and GLP-1 agents affect gastrointestinal motility, while thiazolidinediones may predispose to volume overload. Sulfonylureas may increase the incidence of hypoglycemia, while SGLT-2 inhibitors may worsen hypovolemia. In the event of hyperglycemia, similar to the diet-controlled patient, a supplemental short- or rapid-acting insulin may be titrated every 6 hours, with a transition to a basal/bolus regimen or resumption of oral agents with oral intake.

For insulin-dependent diabetics (both type 1 and 2) undergoing short procedures (estimated 2 hours or one meal skipped), it is recommended to omit short- and rapid-acting doses with maintenance of the basal dose. Patients with tighter baseline control or a history of hypoglycemia may require a reduction in basal dosing by 25%. Baseline metabolism requires half of normal insulin in the absence of oral intake, especially in type 1 patients with higher risk of ketoacidosis. With resumption of intake, home bolus doses can be administered as scheduled. Patients on continuous insulin-infusion devices can continue their usual rate if the device is properly secured. Blood glucose levels should be checked hourly, with higher frequency if measurements fall below 100 mg/dl. Fingerstick measurements may be less reliable in the critically ill, in the setting of vasopressors, or in hypotension, and laboratory methods are recommended in these cases. D5 at a rate of 75 to 125 cc/hour may be started if ongoing NPO status risks hypoglycemia.

For insulin-dependent diabetics (both type 1 and 2) undergoing long procedures, IV insulin is recommended over subcutaneous for multiple benefits. Studies comparing the routes found significant variability in glucose levels with subcutaneous delivery, likely from vasoconstriction and hypoperfusion. Additionally, infusions are easily titrated given a half-life of 5 to 10 minutes. Numerous algorithms combining insulin with potential glucose infusions have been published at different institutions. For lengthy procedures, especially with anticipated hemodynamic fluctuation, large fluid shifts, and vasopressors affecting subcutaneous delivery, intravenous administration is preferred. Titration will depend on patients' insulin resistance as well as procedure. For example, a coronary artery bypass graft can increase requirements by a factor of 10. Hourly serum glucose levels should be monitored in addition to electrolytes, including potassium and bicarbonate.

## POSTOPERATIVE

As with the preoperative and intraoperative phases, the postoperative phase attempts to minimize hypo/hyperglycemia.

Laboratory measurements direct care in the intraoperative phase, but hypoglycemic symptoms can be masked in the sedated patient and can therefore present after emergence as palpitations, anxiety, diaphoresis, paresthesias, and even a failure of emergence. During recovery, subcutaneous insulin may be used in the noncritically ill patients, with blood glucose checks every 2 hours at minimum, while a continuous insulin infusion is continued for the critically ill. Once patients are transitioned out of the post-anesthesia care unit (PACU) or intensive care unit (ICU) to the wards, administration of basal insulin should be started in addition to the sliding scale.[5]

## REFERENCES

1. Evans C, Lee J, Ruhlman M. Optimal glucose management in the perioperative period. *Surg Clin N Amer.* 2015;95(2):337–354.
2. Buchleitner A, et al. Perioperative glycaemic control for diabetic patients undergoing surgery. *Cochrane Data System Rev.* 2012;,.
3. Brandt M, et al. Effect of epidural analgesia on the glycoregulatory response to surgery. *Clin Endocrinol.* 1976;5(2):107–114.
4. Joshi G, et al. Society for ambulatory anesthesia consensus statement on perioperative blood glucose management in diabetic patients undergoing ambulatory surgery. *Anesth Analg.* 2010;111(6):1378–1387.
5. Duggan E, et al. Perioperative hyperglycemia management. *Anesthesiology.* 2017;126(3):547–560.

# 323.

# PROTEIN FUNCTION AS IMMUNOGLOBULINS AND HORMONES

*Dominika Lipowska James and Maryam Jowza*

## IMMUNE FUNCTION OF PROTEIN

One of the many important functions of proteins is immune protection. Immunoglobulins, also known as antibodies, are immunologically active plasma proteins involved in this process. Antibodies are specialized plasma proteins produced by B cells, which are inherent

to the proper function of humoral immunity. Simply put, their role is to identify and destroy pathogens, such as bacteria and viruses, that pose a threat to the organism. Immunoglobulins, as a class of molecules, have a unique ability to bind to a vast array of antigens, yet each antibody type is antigen specific.[1] This property is dependent on complex cellular mechanisms capable of altering B cell genetic makeup, and ultimately production of novel forms of immunoglobulins with altered antigen-binding sites. Each antibody is capable of recognizing specific antigens within the plasma or on the surface of the infected cells. Antibodies can then serve as cell-surface antigen receptors, leading to antigen recognition and initiation of cellular immunity.[1,2] Once exposed to a particular antigen, the human body is capable of fabricating antigen-specific antibodies ready for reactivation in an event of repeat exposure to the same pathogen. Pathogen deactivation may occur via:

- Antibody dependent cellular cytotoxicity: antibody provides a bridge between pathogen-infected cell and innate immune system cell
- Direct binding of antibodies to antigens, leading to neutralization of toxins and pathogens
  - Block infectivity of pathogens (bacteria, viruses, fungi, parasites) by interfering with pathogen-to-host-cell cellular attachment, or by triggering pathogen aggregation (IgM and IgA)
- Activation of the complement system (IgM and IgG antibodies) resulting in:
  - Pathogen lysis
  - Phagocytosis of pathogens opsonized with complement fragments
- Opsonization: attaching to and marking pathogen organisms for cytotoxic attack and phagocytosis by the innate immune system cells.

Structurally, immunoglobulins are heterodimeric proteins formed by joining of two identical heavy chains and two identical light chains in a shape of the letter Y (Figure 323.1). The two arms of this Y-shaped molecule, designated as Fab regions, are each composed of a heavy chain (dark blue), and a light chain (light blue), held together by dipeptide bonds. The most distant aspect of the Fab region is the antigen-binding portion of the molecule, and as such it is the only portion of the antibody where both chains are capable of structural alterations. This region is often referred to as the *hypervariable region*, as the modifications of this region allow the antibodies to develop specificity for new antigens. The Fc region is composed solely of two heavy chains (CH) with no variable domain. The Fc region is responsible for binding the antibody to its cellular receptors. At the junction of Fab and Fc regions, the two parallel fragments of the molecule are held together by disulfide bonds (DB).[1] There are five distinct antibody classes, which differ in structure and function: IgG, IgM, IgA, IgE, and IgD (Table 323.1).

IgM antibodies are in shape of a pentamer, capable of binding multiple antigens at the same time. Due to their pentameric structure, IgM antibodies are involved in early primary immune response, with their effect being widespread and antigen nonspecific. IgM antibodies use the process of opsonization to mark antigens for destruction through the process of complement activation. IgM antibodies function not only as the first line of immune defense, but also play a role in immunoregulation.[1] IgG antibodies are monomers, and are the second line of defense in response to infection. Their

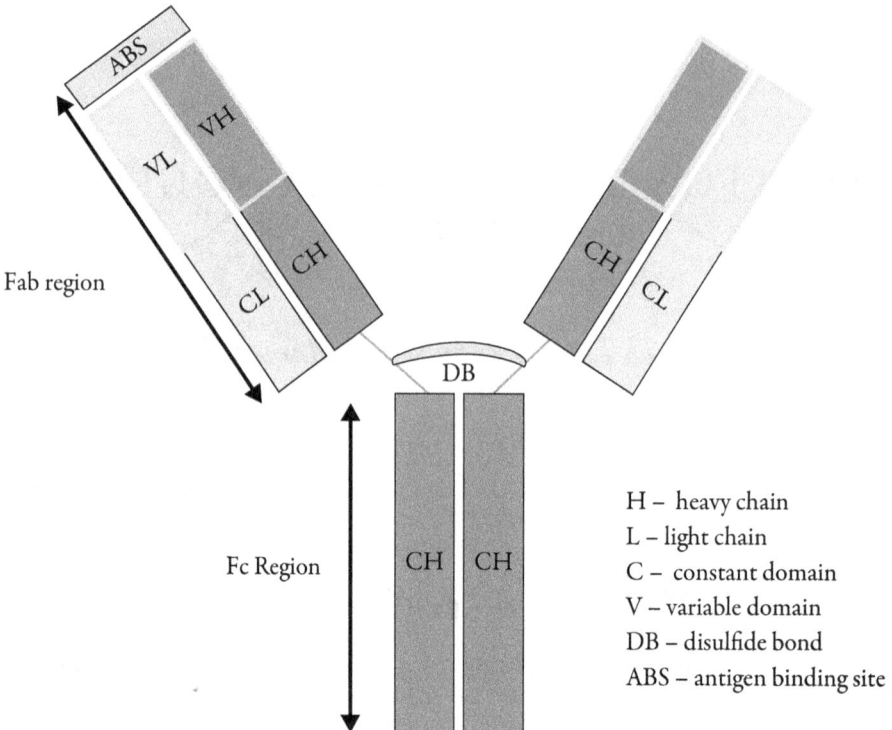

**Figure 323.1.** Structure of antibody.

H – heavy chain
L – light chain
C – constant domain
V – variable domain
DB – disulfide bond
ABS – antigen binding site

## Table 323.1 ANTIBODY CLASSIFICATION

| ANTIBODY CLASS | SHAPE | FUNCTION |
|---|---|---|
| IgM | Pentamer | Main antibody in early response Complement activation |
| IgG | Monomer | Main antibody in late response Complement activation Opsonization Cell-mediated cytotoxicity |
| IgA | Monomer Dimer | High in mucus membranes and in secretions |
| IgE | Monomer Heavily glycosylated | Type I hypersensitivity reactions, parasitic infections, autoimmune processes, venom protection |
| IgE | Monomer | Present on B-cell surfaces Homeostasis |

activity depends on opsonization, complement activation, and direct antigen deactivation.[2] Clinically, high-affinity IgG antibodies have been implicated in autoimmune diseases such as myasthenia gravis, lupus, and others. IgE antibodies have monomeric structure, are heavily glycosylated, and have been long recognized as the immunoglobulins involved in allergy response (asthma, atopic dermatitis) and type I hypersensitivity reaction. IgA antibodies, being present on mucosal surfaces, form the first line of defense against ingested or inhaled microorganisms. Clinically, IgA is associated with IgA nephropathy. Deficiency of antibodies leads to specific immune dysfunction syndromes based on the class of the immunoglobulin that is lacking.[2,3]

## HORMONAL FUNCTION OF PROTEIN

Human organ-system communication is a complex process that involves hormone molecules as messengers of the neuroendocrine system. In general, hormones can be divided into either steroidal or protein hormones. There are hundreds of recognized polypeptide hormones.

Polypeptide/protein hormones are often present in an inactive precursor form that requires proteolytic transformation for activation. Commonly, precursor hormones are proteolytically cleaved into more than one active hormone. Depending on size and configuration, peptide hormones can be further classified as amines, peptides, or protein hormones (Table 323.2).

Amine hormones are relatively simple molecules derived from a single amino acid, either tryptophan (hormone: melatonin) or tyrosine (hormone: thyroid hormones and catecholamines), via modification of their carboxyl groups.

## Table 323.2 HORMONE CLASSIFICATION

| HORMONE CLASS | HORMONE EXAMPLE | FUNCTION |
|---|---|---|
| Amine | EPI, NEPI, T3, T4, melatonin | Amino acid with carboxyl or amino group modifications |
| Peptide | Oxytocin, ADH, ACTH, prolactin, calcitonin, PTH, | Short chain of amino acids |
| Protein | GH Insulin Glucagon | Structurally complex 3-dimensional peptide chain |
| Glycoprotein | FSH, LH, TSH | Glycosylated protein |
| Steroid | Sex hormones Cortisol Aldosterone | Glycosylated protein Cholesterol based |

Unlike amine hormones, peptide and protein hormones are made of chains of amino acids. Some examples of peptide hormones include hormones produced by the pituitary gland, such as oxytocin, antidiuretic hormone, and prolactin. Protein hormones are significantly larger and more structurally complex. Examples of protein hormones include glucagon and insulin. Carboxylated protein hormones, such as lutenizing hormone, follicle-stimulating hormone, and thyroid-stimulating hormone, are called glycoprotein hormones. They are integral to proper growth, sexual development, and reproduction.[4,5]

Protein hormones, depending on the degree of their hydrophilicity, are transported in plasma, either in free state or bound to protein. Because they are hydrophilic, protein hormones are unable to cross cellular membranes, and exert their effect via transmembrane G-protein coupled receptors. Immune and neuroendocrine systems are intricately linked in their involvement of immune system function regulation.[4,5] Hormonal imbalances, such as hormone deficiency or excess, are each associated with a specific disease state (discussed in a different chapter).

## REFERENCES

1. Schroeder HW Jr, Cavacini L. Structure and function of immunoglobulins. *J Allergy Clin Immunol*. 2010 February;125(2 Suppl 2):S41–S52.
2. Thau L, Asuka E, Mahajan K. Physiology, opsonization. [Updated May 24, 2020]. In: *StatPearls* [Internet]. Treasure Island, FL: StatPearls; 2020 Jan–.https://www.ncbi.nlm.nih.gov/books/NBK534215/.
3. Kelley KW, et al. Protein hormones and immunity. *Brain Behav Immun*. 2007 May;21(4): 384–392.
4. Nussey S, Whitehead S. Endocrinology: An Integrated Approach. Oxford: BIOS Scientific Publishers; 2001. Chapter 1, Principles of endocrinology. Available from: https://www.ncbi.nlm.nih.gov/books/NBK20/
5. Anatomy & Physiology. OpenStax CNX. http://cnx.org/contents/14fb4ad7-39a1-4eee-ab6e-3ef2482e3e22@8.25

# 324.

# PROTEIN SYNTHESIS, STRUCTURE, AND FUNCTION

*Ryan Stuckey and Dominika Lipowska James*

## PROTEIN SYNTHESIS

The creation of a polypeptide chain occurs via series of complex and uniquely integrated steps referred to as *translation*. During this process, a messenger RNA (mRNA) molecule is utilized as a template. A transfer RNA (tRNA) molecule, carrying a specific amino acid, binds to the complementary mRNA segment on the ribosomal subunit. As the consecutive tRNA molecules enter the ribosomal complex binding to their designated mRNA sequences, transference of the amino acid leads to peptide chain elongation and ultimately release. This new polypeptide chain may then undergo a series of post-translational structural modifications, interacting with other polypeptide chains, leading to formation of a functional protein.[1,2]

Almost all plasma proteins are produced in the liver, with the exception of gamma globulins (antibodies), which are synthesized in the reticuloendothelial system. Clotting factor VIII is produced by vascular and glomerular endothelium, as well as by the sinusoidal cells in the liver.

## PROTEIN STRUCTURE

Twenty amino acids are utilized as the building blocks for protein synthesis. The structural components of amino acids are the central carbon connected to hydrogen molecule, a primary amino group (–NH$_2$), and a carboxylic acid (–COOH). The fourth linkage is a variable side chain called the R group. Each amino acid is connected by a peptide bond between the primary amine group of one amino acid and the carboxylic acid group of another amino acid. As additional amino acids are assembled, a three-dimensional structure is formed due to interactions between distant amino acids.[2]

There are four hierarchies of protein structure. The linear sequence of amino acids within the polypeptide chain is referred to as the primary structure. Amino acids located near each other form relationships and further distort the polypeptide chain into complexes referred to as either alpha helices or beta sheets, which comprise the secondary structure.

These localized regions then form relationships with adjacent regions to generate the polypeptide chain's tertiary structure (helix-loop-helix, beta barrel). Most proteins are composed of multiple polypeptide chains, referred to as subunits. A protein's quaternary structure is a description of how these subunits are associated with one another.[2]

## PROTEIN FUNCTION

Variation in the polypeptide amino acid sequence determines the subsequent polypeptide-folding pattern, leading to conformational protein changes, and the ultimate protein size and structure. Protein structure, in turn, governs its unique function within the body (Figure 324.1).

Proteins that are involved in catalysis of chemical reactions are called enzymes. Enzymatic proteins (transferases, lyases, hydrolases, isomerases, etc.) are able to facilitate various types of bodily reactions. Enzyme pseudocholinesterase (PCHE) is involved in the process of succinylcholine inactivation. The activity level of PCHE (influenced by quantity and functional quality of the enzyme) determines the number of succinylcholine molecules hydrolyzed per unit time. Function of the enzyme can be negatively affected by even a single amino acid substitution at or near the active site, leading to a substantial prolongation (4–8 hrs) of succinylcholine duration of action.[1-5]

Due to their complex, three-dimensional structure, proteins can also serve as transport molecules either by binding to, or structurally enclosing, its substrates, as can be exemplified by transport of cholesterol by lipoprotein. Lipoproteins are complex biomolecules designed to enclose and transport hydrophobic molecules (cholesterol) in hydrophilic medium (plasma). Other transport proteins include albumin and hemoglobin. Albumin plays a significant role in drug distribution, action, and clearance.

Hemoglobin (Hb) protein undergoes conformational change based on the substrate that it is exposed to. Hb is made up of four proteins (two alpha chains and two beta chains), with each protein attached to a heme unit. Each

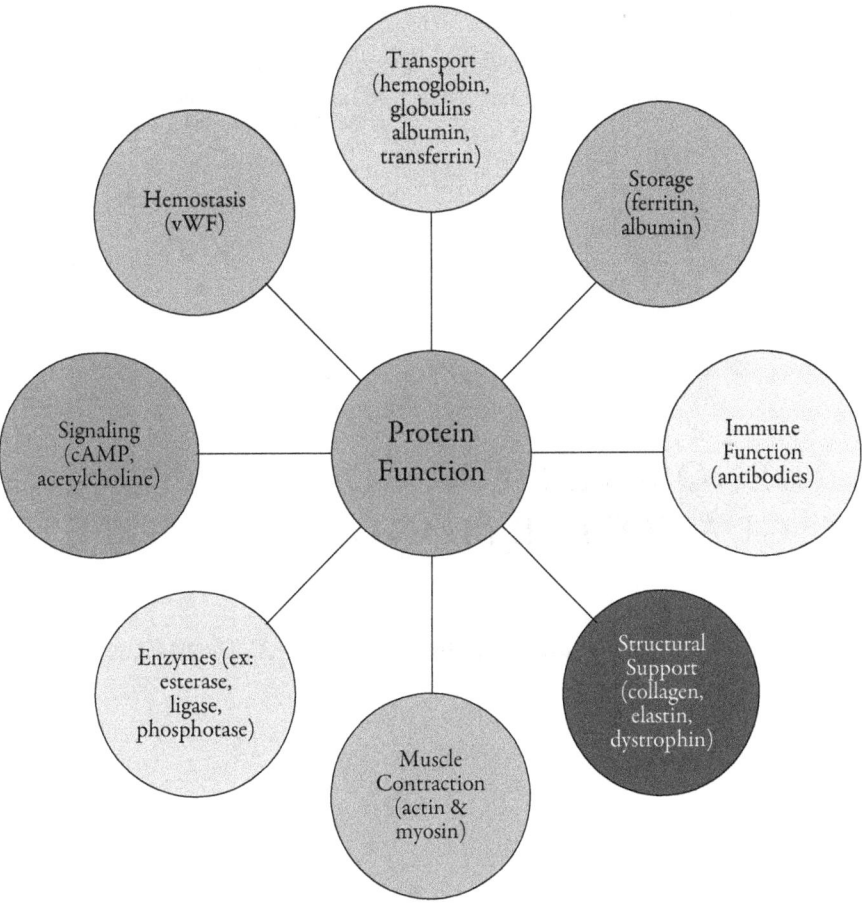

**Figure 324.1.** Proteins serve a variety of functions, enabled by their unique three-dimensional structure.

heme unit binds to one oxygen molecule. As each oxygen molecule becomes attached, the shape of Hg is augmented in a way that allows the remaining, unbound heme units to become more exposed to the available oxygen molecules in the plasma. This facilitates oxygen loading of the Hg molecule in oxygen-rich environments, as well as aids in the release of oxygen within oxygen-deprived tissues.[3]

Sickle cell disease is a medical condition where the change in the peptide amino acid order (substitution of valine for glycine at the 6th position in Hgb β chains) leads to alteration in Hgb structure and function. Deoxygenation of sickle hemoglobin (HbS) leads to an inadvertent binding of the adjacent HbS regions and inappropriate protein folding. This, in turn, results in distortion of the red blood cell (RBC) membrane (sickling) and RBS aggregation, culminating in small vessels occlusion, tissue ischemia, hemolytic anemia, and concomitant organ damage.[4]

Another condition reflecting the importance of protein as structural tissue elements is muscular dystrophy (MD). One of the primary function of proteins is their role as cellular building blocks and extracellular structural elements, providing support to cell membranes, intracellular organelles, and extracellular matrix, among many others. Dystrophin is a large protein that maintains the stability

and integrity of the cellular membrane. The dystrophin gene is highly susceptible to accrue mutations, most often deletions, leading to protein dysfunction and cellular death, resulting in a constellation of symptoms commonly referred to as MD,[5] a medical condition associated with progressive skeletal muscle denervation followed by replacement of muscle with adipose and connective tissue, resulting in weakness.

Proteins also serve as storage molecules. One of the most elegant examples of importance of the protein structure in relation to its function is exquisite three-dimensional folding of the ferritin protein into a symmetric spherical shell encapsulating the crystalline form of iron (Fe) in its center. Ferritin releases the Fe element in periods of iron scarcity. Excess of ferritin can lead to hemochromatosis, chronic hepatitis, and anemia.

## REFERENCES

1. Keegan MT. Prolongation of succinylcholine effect. *Faust's Anesthesiology Review* (4th ed., pp. 180–182). Philadelphia, PA: Elsevier; 2015.
2. Watson JD, Baker TA, Bell SP, Gann A, Levine M, Losic R. Weak and strong bonds determine macromolecular structure. *Molecular*

*Biology of the Gene* (6th ed., pp. 71–94). San Francisco, CA: Pearson/Benjamin Cummings; 2008.
3. Slinger P. Gas Exchange. *Stoelting's Pharmacology & Physiology in Anesthetic Practice* (5th ed., pp. 549–588). Philadelphia, PA: Wolters Kluwer Health; 2015.

4. Oprea AD. Hematologic disorders. *Stoelting's Anesthesia and Co-existing Disease* (6th ed., pp. 407–436). Philadelphia, PA: Elsevier; 2012.
5. Zhou J, Allen PD, Pessah IN, Naguib M. Neuromuscular disorders and malignant hyperthermia. *Miller's Anesthesia* (7th ed., Vol. 1, pp. 1171–1195). Philadelphia, PA: Churchill Livingstone/Elsevier; 2010.

# 325.

# CYCLIC ADENOSINE MONOPHOSPHATE (CAMP) AND CYCLIC GUANOSINE MONOPHOSPHATE (CGMP)

*Dominika Lipowska James and Ajay S. Unnithan*

## CYCLIC ADENOSINE MONOPHOSPHATE (CAMP)

Cyclic adenosine monophosphate (cAMP) is a small, hydrophilic molecule, specifically a cyclic nucleotide. It is synthesized from adenosine triphosphate (ATP) in a reaction catalyzed by an enzyme adenylyl cyclase (AC), which is located both within the cell membrane and in soluble form within the cytosol.[1] This reaction is triggered by an extracellular first messenger signal (i.e., a neurotransmitter, hormone, or growth factor) which interacts with a transmembrane receptor, called a G protein-coupled receptor (GPCR). Once this external signal acts on the GPCR, a component of the GPCR, called a G-protein, is activated and acts on AC to catalyze the reaction, which converts ATP to cAMP[1,2] (Figure 325.1).

Then cAMP diffuses throughout the cytosol of the cell and activates other proteins, including most prominently protein kinase A (PKA), as well as exchange protein activated by cAMP (EPAC). PKA phosphorylates other downstream enzymes involved in production of molecules responsible for carrying out multiple physiologic functions.[1,2] EPAC is a receptor group responsible for cellular functions such as gene expression, adhesion, exocytosis, and apoptosis. [3] PKA also phosphorylates a protein called phosphodiesterase (PDE) which acts to convert cAMP back to AMP, thereby terminating the action of the

cAMP. Through this negative feedback, cAMP serves to limit its own production.[1,2]

cAMP and its downstream effects have significant clinical relevance. It is involved in the coordinated response to circulating catecholamines, including beta-adrenergic stimulated lipolysis and glycogenolysis which helps to mobilize energy stores when needed.[1] In the heart, cAMP and its downstream effector PKA are involved with increasing myocardial contractile force, improving diastolic relaxation, while in the vascular system, activation of the cAMP signaling cascade leads to smooth muscle relaxation and vasodilation.[1] It has been shown that high levels of cAMP in the body may lead to suppression of the immune system, while being therapeutic in the setting of chronic obstructive pulmonary disease, asthma, and some autoimmune conditions.[1,2] In the kidneys, cAMP is involved in antidiuretic hormone–mediated retention of water, as well as parathyroid hormone–mediated calcium homeostasis.[1] The widespread downstream effects of the cAMP pathway provide for multiple targets for pharmacological agents aimed at treating many medical conditions. For example, many vasoactive agents like phenylephrine, norepinephrine, and epinephrine act via adrenergic receptors, which are GPCRs. Their actions on the cardiovascular system are a consequence of downstream effects of the signaling cascade initiated with the stimulation or inhibition of cAMP production. Specific PDE inhibitors work by inhibiting

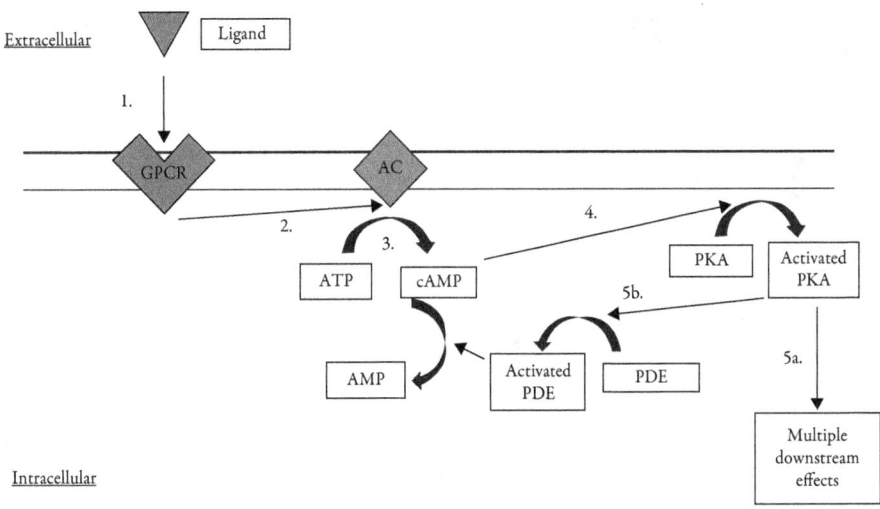

**Figure 325.1.** cAMP pathway. 1. An extracellular ligand (ex: neurotransmitter, hormone, etc.) acts on a transmembrane GPCR. 2. An activated G protein then acts on AC (in this figure presented in the transmembrane form, though it can also be in soluble form within the cell cytosol). 3. AC then acts to convert ATP to cAMP. 4. cAMP then activates PKA. 5a. Activated PKA goes on to phosphorylate multiple downstream proteins for a multitude of downstream physiologic effects. 5b. Activated PKA also activates PDE which deactivates cAMP back to AMP, thereby providing a negative feedback on cAMP production.

GPCR: G-protein coupled receptor; AC: adenylyl cyclase; ATP: adenosine triphosphate; cAMP: cyclic adenosine monophosphate; AMP: adenosine monophosphate; PKA: protein kinase A; PDE: phosphodiesterase.

PDE-induced deactivation of cAMP, thereby increasing cAMP levels. Milrinone is a PDE-III inhibitor which via increased cAMP levels leads to increased myocardial contractility and improved diastolic relaxation, both of which are of benefit in heart failure, while cilastazol, also a PDE-III inhibitor, leads to vasodilation of the vasculature and is used to treat claudication symptoms associated with peripheral vascular disease.[2]

## CYCLIC GUANOSINE MONOPHOSPHATE

Cyclic guanosine monophosphate (cGMP), similar to cAMP, is a hydrophilic, cyclic nucleotide formed from guanylyl cyclase (GC) via two main pathways. In one pathway, natriuretic peptides, atrial natriuretic peptide (ANP) and brain natriuretic peptide (BNP), act at the cell membrane via a membrane-bound GC to catalyze the formation of cGMP from guanosine triphosphate (GTP). In the second pathway, nitric oxide acts on a soluble form of GC in the cytosol to again catalyze the formation of cGMP[4] (Figure 325.2)

cGMP subsequently activates protein kinase G (PKG), which then carries out a number of downstream effects regulating numerous physiologic functions, similar to the action of PKA in the case of cAMP. cGMP catalyzes the formation of PDE, which converts cGMP back to GTP, providing a negative feedback on its own production.

PKG activation by cGMP leads to a variety of effects. In the vascular system, it leads to smooth muscle relaxation

and subsequently vasodilation. PKG can have both pro-angiogenic as well as anti-proliferative effects, depending on the particular GC form (soluble vs. membrane bound) utilized in the second messenger cascade.[4,5] In the neurological system, cGMP is involved in memory formation and retrieval, as well as in regulation of synaptic plasticity.[4] cGMP also plays a role in metabolism, in particular in regulation of insulin and glucagon release and function. Through its interactions in the hypothalamus, cGMP also has a role in the regulation of water intake.[4] It also has a role in the relaxation of gastrointestinal smooth muscle, thereby promoting intestinal motility.[4] cGMP also plays a role in regulation of coagulation by inhibiting platelet aggregation. Increasing the levels of cGMP via PDE-V inhibitors has been shown to improve renal function.[4]

Given its wide-ranging physiologic effects, cGMP, like cAMP has important clinical significance, especially in cardiovascular physiology, where the predominant downstream effect of cGMP activation is vasodilation. There are multiple pharmacologic agents which have been developed to target this molecular pathway for therapeutic effect. For example, in pulmonary arterial hypertension, inhaled nitric oxide is administered to induce pulmonary arterial vasodilation via nitric oxide–induced activation of cGMP. PDE-V inhibitors like sildenafil and tadalafil work to increase cGMP levels by inhibiting PDE deactivation of cGMP to GMP, thereby leading to vasodilation within the pulmonary vasculature. Milrinone also affects the systemic vasculature via its effects on cGMP. By inhibiting PDE-III, milirinone leads to increased cGMP levels, leading to vasodilation of systemic arteries and veins, which in

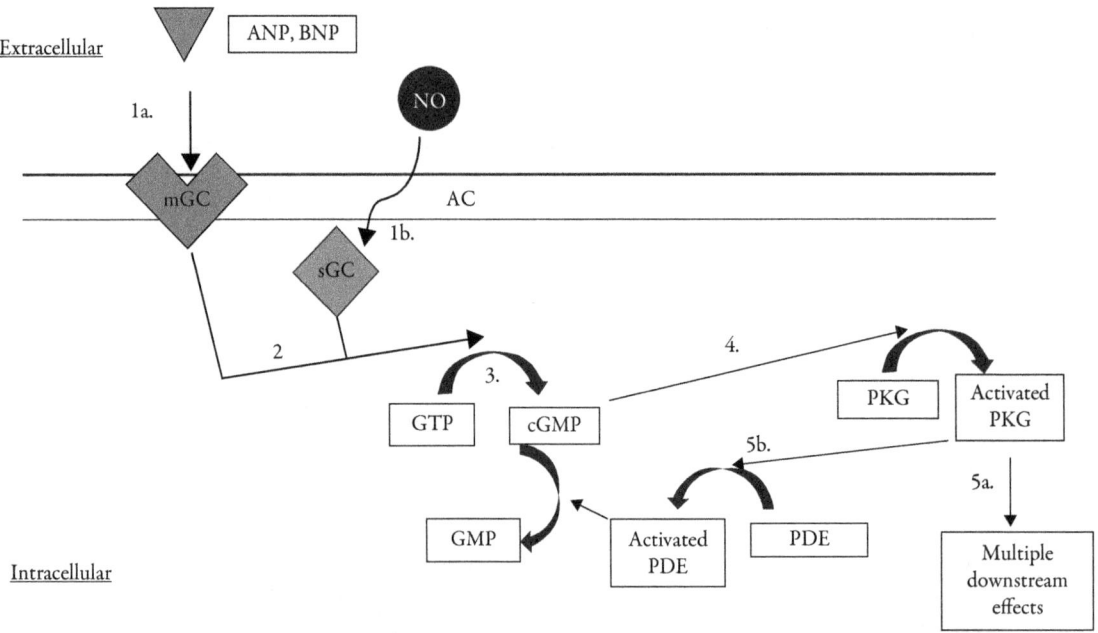

**Figure 325.2.** cGMP pathway. The pathway starts when 1a. ANP or BNP activates transmembrane GC or 1b. NO activates soluble GC within the cytosol. 2. Activated GC (either mGC or sGC) then acts to convert GTP to cGMP. 4. cGMP then activates PKG. 5a. Activated PKG goes on to phosphorylate multiple downstream proteins for a multitude of downstream physiologic effects. 5b. Activated PKG also activates PDE, which deactivates cGMP back to GMP, thereby providing a negative feedback on cGMP production.

ANP: atrial natiuretic peptide; BNP: brain natriuertic peptide; NO: nitric oxide; mGC: transmembrane guanylyl cyclase; sGC: soluble guanylyl cyclase; GTP: guanosine triphosphate; cGMP: cyclic guanosine monophosphate; GMP: guanosine monophosphate; PKG: protein kinase G; PDE: phosphodiesterase.

combination with its inotropic and lusitropic effects on the heart can be of benefit in heart failure.[5]

## CONCLUSION

cAMP and cGMP are critical second-messenger molecules which when stimulated produce numerous downstream cellular effects with wide-ranging physiologic consequences. They play a vital role in normal physiologic function, and the multitude of cascading pathways that are stimulated by their actions provide several pharmacologic targets for therapeutic interventions to manage pathological disturbances that occur in any number of clinical conditions.

## REFERENCES

1. Patra C, et al. Biochemistry, cAMP. [Updated August 16, 2020]. In: *StatPearls* [Internet]. Treasure Island, FL: StatPearls; 2020 Jan–.https://www.ncbi.nlm.nih.gov/books/NBK535431/.
2. Yan K, et al. The cyclic AMP signaling pathway: Exploring targets for successful drug discovery (Review). *Mol Med Rep*. 2016 May;13(5):3715–3723.
3. Almahariq M, et al. Cyclic AMP sensor EPAC proteins and energy homeostasis. *Trends Endocrinol. Metab*. 2014 Feb;25(2): 60–71.
4. Pasmanter N, et al. Biochemistry, cyclic GMP. [Updated November 13, 2019]. In: *StatPearls* [Internet]. Treasure Island, FL: StatPearls; 2020 Jan–.https://www.ncbi.nlm.nih.gov/books/NBK542234/
5. Kemp-Harper B, Schmidt HH. cGMP in the vasculature. *Handb Exp Pharmacol*. 2009;(191):447–467. doi:10.1007/978-3-540-68964-5_19.PMID:19089340.

# 326.

# LIPIDS

*Dominika Lipowska James and Shirin Ghanavatian*

## INTRODUCTION

Lipids are essential components of the human body, contributing to multiple biochemical processes such as energy storage, intracellular transport, and extracellular communication, and as structural building blocks of cellular membranes. Although cholesterol is often perceived as detrimental to human health, cholesterol in fact is a steroid molecule essential to the integrity of cell membranes and steroidogenesis. Cellular membranes are structured in a form of lipid bilayer made of cholesterol, phosphoglycerides, and sphingolipids, forming a diffusion barrier. The cellular lipid bilayer is spanned by integral membrane proteins of various functions, some creating ion channels for hydrophilic substrates, others being enzymes or participating in intracellular signaling pathways.

Cholesterol serves as a substrate for biosynthesis of most of the steroid hormones, from sex hormones (testosterone, estrogen, progesterone) to cortisol and aldosterone. Cholesterol also plays an important role in digestive processes by being a precursor of bile acids formation. Additionally, cholesterol is a precursor for vitamin D, which is essential in calcium and phosphorus metabolism.

Cholesterol is a lipophilic molecule and therefore requires hydrophilic lipoprotein particles to be transported in the plasma. Cholesterol is bound to either high-density lipoproteins (HDL) or low-density lipoproteins (LDL) for transport.

Plasma lipoproteins are divided into chylomicrons, very-low-density lipoproteins (VLDL), low-density lipoproteins (LDL), intermediate-density lipoproteins (IDL), and high-density lipoproteins (HDL).

Chylomicrons are secreted by intestinal epithelial cells and deliver cholesterol to the liver in the form of chylomicron remnants. VLDL is secreted by the liver and transports hepatic triglycerides (TGs) to the periphery. IDL particles are degradation products of VLDL and deliver TGs and cholesterol to the liver. LDL, which is also referred to as the "bad" cholesterol, delivers hepatic cholesterol to peripheral tissues and is internalized by target cells via receptor-mediated endocytosis. HDL, on the contrary, transports cholesterol from tissues to the liver. HDL is essential in apolipoproteins C and E formation, which play an important role in chylomicron and VLDL metabolism.

Triglycerides (TGs) are fatty acid esters of glycerol and the main constitute of body fat. Like cholesterol, hydrophobic TGs also use VLDLs for transport. TGs are often transported from liver to fatty tissues for storage as an energy source.

Notably, pulmonary surfactant is a lipoprotein-like mixture composed of phospholipids, triglycerides, cholesterol, and fatty acids. The lipid composition of surfactant opposes the high surface tension of the alveoli and prevents alveolar collapse and pulmonary edema. Surfactant deficiency leads to neonatal respiratory distress syndrome and impairment of gas exchange.[1,2]

## HYPERLIPIDEMIA/ HYPERCHOLESTEROLEMIA

Clinically, increased levels of plasma LDL and TGs, concomitant with low HDL levels, are associated with increased risk for development of cardiovascular disease (CVD). Polygenic hypercholesterolemia is the most common type of dislipidemia. Dyslipidemias are treated with modification of environmental factors in addition to medical therapy.

Prior studies have shown that increased levels of plasma total cholesterol, TGs, and particularly LDL particles are strongly associated with evolution of atherosclerosis and consequently CVD. In contrast, high levels of HDL cholesterol are considered protective, and low levels are considered a risk factor for development of CVD. Dyslipidemia is often considered a familial disease, particularly when the onset of occurs at a young age.[3,4]

## CLINICAL FEATURES

For most patients, hyperlipidemia is polygenic in nature; however, the manifestation of the disorder is considerably influenced by environmental factors such as obesity and high levels of dietary cholesterol. High LDL is of clinical importance, and elevated plasma LDL levels are referred to as *hypercholesterolemia*. Different hyperlipidemia conditions are listed in the following.

Polygenic hypercholesterolemia is the most common cause of hyperlipidemia and is considered a primary disorder causing an increase in plasma cholesterol when lifestyle factors are combined with susceptible genes. This condition is associated with the development of CVD.

Familial hypercholesterolemia is an autosomal dominant disorder due to absence or defect in the LDL receptor on the surface of cells, causing delayed removal of LDL from plasma. This condition affects 1 in 500 individuals and is the common genetic cause of premature CVD.

Familial hypertriglyceridemia is a common autosomal dominant disorder characterized by hepatic overproduction of VLDL particles. Moderate elevations of TGs usually occur during early adulthood. In the setting of contributors which elevate TGs, a severe hypertriglyceridemia and recurrent pancreatitis may develop. This condition is not associated with premature CVD development.

Familial combined hyperlipidemia is an autosomal dominant disorder clinically presenting similar to hypercholesterolemia and hypertriglyceridemia. It is characterized clinically by the absence of hyperlipoproteinemia, and its development occurs around puberty. Affected individuals have mild elevation in plasma lipid levels.

Familial dysbetalipoproteinemia is a genetic condition characterized by increased cholesterol and TGs level which manifests particularly in the presence of other genetic or environmental factors. Clinical evidence of hyperlipoproteinemia usually appears in early adulthood. The characteristic clinical findings are xanthoma striata and tuberoeruptive xanthomas. This disorder is associated with premature atherosclerosis and development of CVD.

## TREATMENT

Hyperlipidemia is usually a lifelong and progressive condition; therefore, early management is essential to prevent CVD.

Prevention and initial treatment modalities are focused on lifestyle modification, including weight loss, diet, smoking cessation, and exercise, with the possible addition of lipid-lowering medications if needed. Among these agents, statins are the most commonly utilized medications. Other less prescribed lipid-lowering agents are bile and resins, ezetimibe, fibrates, omega-3-fatty acids, and niacin.

## REFERENCES

1. Feingold KR, Grunfeld C. Introduction to lipids and lipoproteins. In: Feingold KR et al., eds. South Dartmouth, MA: Endotext; 2000.
2. Agassandian M, Mallampalli RK. Surfactant phospholipid metabolism. *Biochim Biophys Acta*. 2013;1831(3):612–625.
3. Ballantyne CM, et al. Hyperlipidemia: Diagnostic and therapeutic perspectives. *J Clin Endocrinol Metab*. 2000;85(6):2089–2112.
4. Cox RA, Garcia-Palmieri MR. Cholesterol, triglycerides, and associated lipoproteins. In: Walker HK, et al., editors. *Clinical Methods: The History, Physical, and Laboratory Examinations*. 3rd edition. Boston: Butterworths; 1990. Chapter 31.

# 327.

# SPECIFIC ORGAN METABOLISM

*Matthew J. Hallman and Dominika Lipowska James*

## INTRODUCTION

Metabolism is a broad topic that describes the complex biochemical reactions required to sustain life. Simply put, it is the process by which the body converts food into energy. At the level of each organ system, the biochemical energy produced, typically as adenosine triphosphate (ATP), is utilized to carry out its critical functions. Each organ system has unique aspects in terms of its metabolic requirements and what substrates it can use for metabolism.

The primary substrates for energy production are:

- Central nervous system (CNS): glucose (ketones during starvation)
- Skeletal muscle: glucose and fatty acids (ketones during starvation)
- Cardiac myocytes: fatty acids and glucose (ketones during starvation)
- Adipose tissue: fatty acids
- Red blood cells: glucose.

The liver serves as a center of multiple complex metabolic processes and is capable of converting glucose for storage into glycogen (in liver) or triglycerides (also occurs in peripheral tissues).[1,2] Conversely, the liver is also capable of extracting glucose from glycogen when energy is required. In times of glucose and fatty acid scarcity, the liver has the capacity to use protein as an energy source by converting it into ketone bodies.

## BRAIN METABOLISM

The primary substrate for energy production in the brain is glucose, except under states of starvation when ketone bodies (see section on Liver later in the chapter) may be utilized.[2,3] Unlike other parts of the body, the brain cannot change to anaerobic metabolism during periods of ischemia or hypoxia, and this is one of the factors that predispose it to anoxic injury more than any other organ. Cerebral metabolism plays a role in regulation of cerebral blood flow and many anesthetic agents, as well as decreased temperature, reduce *cerebral metabolic rate*. Metabolic products including hydrogen ions, adenosine, lactate, and ATP are thought to be involved in mediating this coupling of metabolism and flow.[2,3]

## HEART METABOLISM

Cardiac myocytes are more densely packed with mitochondria than their skeletal muscle counterparts and will preferentially utilize aerobic metabolism.[3] Under oxidative conditions, due to extremely high-energy requirements, fatty acids (FA) represent the main energy source for cardiac myocytes, with glucose also being utilized in normal states. Cardiac myocytes rely on the influx of the non-esterified FAs from the vascular reservoir. Under ideal conditions, cardiac myocytes consume 80%–90% of the maximum energy production of the electron transport chain via utilization of the following three cellular processes: tricarboxylic acid (TCA) cycle, oxidative phosphorylation, and transfer of ATP into storage molecule creatine, forming phoscreatine. Most of the energy used by myocardium serves the purpose of myocardiac contractility (70%), with the rest being utilized for the active transport of the calcium ions back within the smooth sarcoplasmic reticulum.[4] Ketone bodies are used when fatty acids and glucose are not available, and anaerobic metabolism can occur during periods of ischemia and hypoxia. The metabolic demands of the heart are dependent upon the work done by the heart (based on stroke volume, blood pressure, heart rate) and its efficiency. Heart failure is an example of reduced efficiency, and this disease state leads to an increase in cardiac oxygen consumption.[3]

## LIVER

The liver plays multiple important metabolic roles. These include maintaining levels of glucose, maintaining lipid homeostasis, and converting protein to energy in periods of

**Table 327.1** LIVER METABOLISM FUNCTION AND SIGNAL FOR RESPONSE

| LIVER METABOLIC FUNCTION | SIGNAL FOR RESPONSE |
| --- | --- |
| Glycogen formation | (+) Hyperglycemia, insulin<br>(–) Hypoglycemia, glucagon, catecholamines |
| Glycogenolysis | (+) Hypoglycemia, glucagon, catecholamines<br>(–) Hyperglycemia, insulin |
| Gluconeogensis | (+) Hypoglycemia, glucagon, catecholamines<br>*When glycogen stores depleted*<br>(–) Hyperglycemia, insulin |
| Lipogenesis | (+) Hyperglycemia, insulin<br>(–) Hypoglycemia, glucagon, catecholamines |
| Ketogenesis | (+) Hypoglycemia, glucagon<br>(–) Hyperglycemia, insulin |

starvation. For glucose control, the liver responds to insulin and high blood glucose levels by storing excess glucose as glycogen.[1,2] After glycogen stores are at capacity, the liver will convert excess glucose to fatty acids and triglycerides. The hepatocytes respond to glucagon, low blood glucose, or catecholamines by *glycogenolysis* (breaking down glycogen stores) to increase blood glucose levels. When glycogen stores are depleted, *gluconeogenesis* subsequently occurs. This process involves the creation of glucose from lactate, glycerol, and certain amino acids (alanine and glutamine)[2] (Table 327.1).

In states of starvation, after glycogen stores are depleted, the liver has the ability to produce other sources of energy outside of gluconeogenesis. The liver will metabolize aminoacids to ketone bodies that are used by other organs to generate energy. Through beta-oxidation, the liver will also metabolize triglycerides and fatty acids to actetyl coenzyme A and subsequently to ketone bodies. It is important to note that the liver cannot extract energy from ketone bodies for its own needs, but these ketone bodies are crucial for other essential organ systems in the fasting state.[2]

## MUSCLE

Skeletal muscles rely primarily on aerobic metabolism for energy production. Their primary oxidative substrates of choice are FAs, with glucose being utilized only during periods of high-intensity exercise or during the absorptive stage following a meal. Unlike cardiac myocytes, muscle tissue has a greater capability to sustain function with anaerobic metabolism when needed. In periods of high exercise, through the *lactic acid cycle*, muscles will convert glucose to lactic acid that is subsequently processed in the liver back to glucose (also known as the Cori cycle).[1,2]

## OTHER TISSUES

Adipose tissue utilizes FAs from its own stores of triglycerides for the source of energy and glucose in normal states. Human red blood cells and eye lenses are void of mitochondria; thus their ATP is derived via a process of lactic fermentation involving conversion of glucose into lactate.[1]

## REFERENCES

1. El Bacha T, Luz M, Da Poian A. Dynamic adaptation of nutrient utilization in humans. *Nature Education* 2010;3(9):8.
2. Pagel P, et al. Cardiac anatomy and physiology. *Clinical Anesthesia*. Philadelphia, PA: Lippincott Williams & Wilkins; 2013:239–262.
3. Dagal A, Lam, A. Anesthesia for neurosurgery. *Clinical Anesthesia*. Philadelphia, PA: Lippincott Williams & Wilkins; 2013:996–1029.
4. Pattel PM, et al. Cerebral physiology and the effects of anesthetic drugs. *Miller's Anesthesia*. Elsevier; 2014:387–422.
5. Sun LS, Schwarzenberger J, Dinavahi R. Cardiac physiology. *Miller's Anesthesia*. Elsevier; 2014:473–491.
6. Mushlin PS, Gelman S. Hepatic physiology and pathophysiology. *Miller's Anesthesia*. Elsevier; 2014:520–544.

# Part XXV

# NEUROMUSCULAR DISEASES AND DISORDERS

# 328.

# PREJUNCTIONAL COMPONENTS AND EVENTS

*Shaun Roche and Ruth E. Moncayo*

## INTRODUCTION

In 1942, Harold Griffith published a study documenting the effects of curare extract, a South American plant used for arrow poison, and its muscle relaxation abilities. Further development of neuromuscular blocking agents revolutionized the practice of anesthesiology by decreasing the dosage of anesthetic required to achieve immobility of the patient during surgery, resulting in their continued use in modern medicine. Basic understanding of the anatomy and physiology of the neuromuscular junction is required to appreciate the mechanism of action behind these neuromuscular blocking agents, their side effects, and anesthetic consideration in patients with neuromuscular disorders.

## PREJUNCTIONAL COMPONENTS

### MOTOR NEURONS, NEURONAL TRANSPORT SYSTEM

The neuromuscular junction (NMJ) is the nexus between a motor neuron and muscle cell.[1-3] The elements of the prejunctional part on the NMJ are represented by terminal nerve fibers of a large myelinated motor axon that originate in the ventral horn of the spinal cord of medulla, and further divides into 20 to 100 unmyelinated fibers, each of which innervates a single muscle fiber, forming the motor unit.[2,3] The area between the nerve ending and muscle cell is referred to as the synaptic or junctional cleft, and measures approximately 20 nm.[1,2] This junctional cleft is maintained by the basal lamina, and protein filaments which hold tight alignment between the nerve and muscle cell, promoting optimal conditions for communication across the synaptic cleft via acetylcholine (ACh).[2]

## PREJUNCTIONAL EVENTS

### ACETYLCHOLINE SYNTHESIS AND RELEASE, PREJUNCTIONAL COMPONENTS: SYNAPTIC VESICLES

Acetylcholine (ACh) is a neurotransmitter derived from the precursors choline and acetyl co-enzyme A.[1,2] Choline is regularly found in the extracellular fluid, and is mainly transported into the cytoplasm in direct proportion to sodium concentrations via a sodium-dependent choline transporter.[2] Acetyl co-enzyme A is produced within the mitochondria from pyruvate, derived from glucose during the process of glycolysis. Choline and acetyl co-enzyme A are synthesized into ACh by the enzyme choline acetyltransferase.[1,2] ACh is then subsequently stored within the cytoplasm until it is transported into vesicles for release across the synaptic cleft.[2]

The generation of an action potential promotes the release of ACh across the synaptic cleft.[2] As the action potential travels from the central nervous system down an axon, ion channels along the membrane of the axon open and close as the membrane reaches a threshold potential. The action potential promotes the opening of sodium channels, resulting in an influx of sodium ions into the axon, prompting depolarization of the membrane.[2] This depolarization promotes the opening of calcium channels, allowing an influx of calcium ions into the axon, and prompting the release of ACh stored within vesicles.[1,2] The site of neurotransmitter release is referred to as the active zone; the vesicles in these areas are clustered along thickened, electron-dense patches of membrane in the terminal portion of the nerve.[4] The process of docking, fusion, and release of ACh from synaptic vesicles is known as exocytosis.

Three proteins known as SNARE (soluble-N-ethylmaleimide-sensitive attachment protein receptors), which consist of synaptobrevin, syntaxin, and synaptosome-associated protein (SNAP-25), play a role in the exocytosis process.[2,3] During depolarization the binding of calcium, to calcium receptors within the SNARE proteins, promotes the formation of a ternary complex, forcing the vesicles into the nerve terminal membrane at the active zone, and stabilizing the vesicles in the docked state. After fusion and exostosis, the used vesicles and membrane components are recycled through an active process into the nerve terminal, where they are reused to form new vesicles (endocytosis), filled with ACh, and subsequently transported to the active sites for release.[4]

The outward flux of potassium via voltage-gated and calcium-activated potassium channels along the nerve terminal functions to restore membrane potential by limiting the entry of calcium into the nerve, and promoting repolarization.[2,3]

## PREJUNCTIONAL EVENTS

### MODULATION BY NICOTINIC AND MUSCARINIC PREJUNCTIONAL RECEPTORS

Nicotinic and muscarinic prejunctional receptors located on the motor nerve endings have been documented as having modulating effects on the release of ACh at the neuromuscular junction.[2] Studies have documented prejunctional nicotinic receptors promoting the availability of ACh via a positive feedback loop that increases levels of ACh during periods of muscle contraction.[2] Blockage of these prejunctional nicotinic receptors via nondepolarizing neuromuscular blockers decreases the speed at which ACh becomes available by inhibiting this positive feedback loop. This is believed to be the explanation behind the "fade" phenomenon seen with tetanic and train-of-four stimulation, after the administration of nondepolarizing neuromuscular blockers.[1,2] Two types of prejunctional muscarinic receptors, M1 and M2, have been documented. M1 has been described as potentiating the release of ACh, while M2 has been described as inhibiting the release of ACh, via modulation of calcium ion influx in the prejunctional membrane.[2] Blockage of M1 receptors would result in downregulation of the release of ACh, while blockage of M2 receptors would result in an increase in ACh release.

## REFERENCES

1. Butterworth J, et al. *Morgan and Mikhail's Clinical Anesthesiology.* 5th ed. New York, NY: McGraw-Hill Education; 2013:199–205, 224, 751.
2. Miller R. *Miller's Anesthesia.* 7th ed. Philadelphia, PA: Churchhill Livingstone; 2010:341–350, 356–358, 861–862, 885, 1032–1033, 1180–1181.
3. Khirwadkar R, Hunter JM. Neuromuscular physiology and pharmacology: An update. *Cont Educ Anesth Crit Care Pain.* 2012 Oct;12(5):237–244.
4. Themes U. Neuromuscular physiology and pharmacology [Online]. *Anesthesia Key.* 2020. https://aneskey.com/neuromuscular-physiology-and-pharmacology-2/.

# 329.

# POSTJUNCTIONAL COMPONENTS AND EVENTS

*Shaun Roche and Ruth E. Moncayo*

## INTRODUCTION

The development of neuromuscular blocking agents revolutionized modern-day surgery and anesthesiology, by allowing physicians to conduct surgical and invasive procedures under optimal conditions. Despite their widespread use, neuromuscular blocking agents still pose potential risks to patients, which makes an understanding of their mechanism of action paramount prior to their use. Understanding the anatomy of the neuromuscular junction and the events that occur to promote muscular contraction and relaxation allows physicians to prepare for potential intraoperative complications, physiological changes, and side effects associated with these medications.[1-3]

## POSTJUNCTIONAL COMPONENTS: MOTOR END PLATE AND ACETYLCHOLINE RECEPTOR

The motor end plate is a highly specialized region of the membrane of the muscle fiber. Its surface is deeply folded with multiple crests and secondary clefts, with nicotinic acetylcholine receptors (AChRs) densely packed within these folds. The release of acetylcholine (ACh) across the synaptic cleft by the motor axon ending binds to nicotinic cholinergic receptors along the motor end plate. This causes depolarization, and the cell becomes less negative compared with the extracellular surroundings. When a threshold of −50mV is achieved, compared to a resting potential of −80mV, voltage-gated sodium channels open, increasing the rate of depolarization and resulting in an end plate potential (EP) of 5–100 mV.[4] This in turn triggers the action potential that results in muscle contraction.

There are three known isoforms of the postjunctional nicotinic receptor, which are known as mature, immature or fetal, and alpha 7 receptors.[1,2] The receptor is composed of 5 protein subunits that are synthesized within the muscle cells, and these proteins are arranged in a cylindrical pattern, with a central pore allowing the flow of ions across the membrane of the muscle cell. The mature receptors have two alpha subunits, one beta, one delta, and one epsilon subunit. The immature or fetal receptors comprise two alpha subunits, one beta, one delta, and one gamma subunit[1,2] (the gamma subunit has replaced the epsilon). The alpha 7 receptors are composed of five alpha 7 subunits.[2]

## POSTJUNCTIONAL EVENTS: ACH BINDING TO ACH RECEPTORS, ION FLOW THROUGH ACH RECEPTOR

The alpha subunits serve as the binding site for ACh, and both alpha receptors must be bound simultaneously to promote the conformational change needed to open the ion channel, and the subsequent flow of sodium and calcium ions inside the muscle cell, and potassium out. The directional flow of these ions is based on their respective concentration gradients, and generate an end plate potential; this in turn triggers the muscle action potential that results in muscle contraction. Each neuromuscular junction (NMJ) is composed of approximately 5 million nicotinic receptors, but for each pulsation of ACh, approximately 500 000 of these ion channels open.[1,2] Despite this small fraction of channels opening, the resulting end plate

potential generated will depolarize the membrane. Closure of the ion channels occurs as ACh is hydrolyzed to acetate and choline by the enzyme acetylcholinesterase, located in the motor end plate membrane. Acetylcholinesterase is secreted by the muscle, and remains attached to the clefts of the motor plate by thin collagen threads linked to the basement membrane. This enzyme breaks down ACh within 1 second of being released, and allows for repolarization of the end plate.[1,2,4] In addition to postjunctional receptors in the motor endplate, AChRs can also be found outside the NMJ, and are referred to as extra-junctional receptors. Extra-junctional receptors can be found anywhere in the muscle membrane in very small numbers, though they are found in their greatest concentration around the end plate in the perijunctional zone. Denervation injuries and burns are associated with large increases in the number of extra-junctional receptors on the muscle membrane. These extra-junctional receptors have the structure of immature fetal receptors, which affects the physiology and pharmacology of the receptor, with increased sensitivity to depolarizing muscle relaxants, and decreased sensibility to nondepolarizing muscle relaxant.

## POSTJUNCTIONAL COMPONENTS: MUSCLE CELL

There are three muscle cell types in humans: skeletal, smooth, and cardiac. Myocytes are the cellular unit of muscles and contain thick filaments that are primary composed of myosin, and thin filaments which contain actin. As the muscle cells contract, these two layers slide across each other, following the sliding filament theory. Skeletal and cardiac muscles are known as striated because they contain repeating segments of contractile thin and thick filaments, known as sarcomeres. Smooth muscles are not arranged as repeating sarcomere units. The binding of ACh to the postjunctional nicotinic receptors prompts an action potential that penetrates into the muscle cell, resulting in the release of calcium from voltage-gated calcium channels in the sarcoplasmic reticulum of the muscle cell. Calcium binds to troponin (Tn) on the actin filament, promoting a conformational change in the Tn-Tm complex, which removes tropomyosin (Tm), uncovering a binding site, and allows for the interaction of the myosin head with actin. The myosin attached to actin is also bound to ADP + inorganic phosphate, which are released and prompt a power stroke that pulls that actin along with the myosin head. The binding of ATP to the myosin head detaches it from the actin binding side. ATP is converted to ADP + inorganic phosphate, and the energy produced from this reaction returns the myosin head to a cocked position. Smooth muscles do not contain Tn, and contraction is regulated by myosin regulatory light chain phosphorylation.[3] Calcium binds to calmodulin, and this complex activates the myosin light chain kinase, prompting phosphorylation of the myosin light chain, and allowing for the binding of actin and myosin.[2,3] Dephosphorylation of the myosin light chain kinase prompts relaxation.[3]

## UP- AND DOWN-REGULATION

*Up-regulation* is an increase in the number of ACh receptors on the postjunctional membrane in conditions involving decreased stimulation of the neuromuscular junction. This leads to hypersensitivity to ACh agonists and decreased sensitivity to antagonists. This phenomenon can lead to lethal potassium release after succinylcholine administration. Conditions that can lead to up-regulation include upper and lower motor neuron lesions, burns, severe infections, prolonged use of relaxants, muscle trauma, cerebral palsy, and chronic use of anticonvulsants. Chronic use of anticonvulsants does not lead to increase in potassium release after the use of succinylcholine.

*Down-regulation* develops in some conditions such as myasthenia gravis, organophosphate poisoning, and exercise conditioning. There is decreased sensitivity to ACh agonists and increased sensitivity to antagonists.

## REFERENCES

1. Butterworth J, et al. *Morgan and Mikhail's Clinical Anesthesiology.* 5th ed. New York, NY: McGraw-Hill Education; 2013:199–205, 215, 224, 748–755.
2. Miller R. *Miller's Anesthesia.* 7th ed. Philadelphia, PA: Churchhill Livingstone; 2010:341–358, 1032–1033.
3. Sweeney H, Hammers, D., 2018. Muscle contraction. *Cold Spring Harbor Perspect Biol.* 2018;10(2):p.a023200. https://cshperspectives.cshlp.org/content/10/2/a023200.full#abstract-1.
4. Ackroyd C, Gwinnutt C. Physiology of the Neuromuscular Junction. 2006. https://www.wfsahq.org/components/com_virtual_library/media/c12ca123e587cc180f2649a36d607dcc-a9ef1b2eee5101e31bd7308408a7dce5-20-Physiology-of-the-neuromuscular-junction.pdf.

# 330.

# PERIJUNCTIONAL CHANNELS

*Shaun Roche and Ruth E. Moncayo*

## INTRODUCTION

In 1942, Harold Griffith documented the effects of curare extract and its muscle relaxation abilities. Further development of neuromuscular blocking agents revolutionized modern-day surgery and anesthesiology, by allowing physicians to achieve optimal conditions for performing surgery. Prior to the administration of these neuromuscular blocking agents, a basic understanding of the composition and events associated with the neuromuscular junction is necessary to achieve adequate muscle relaxation in a safe way. This chapter will focus on the perijunctional channels associated with the neuromuscular junction.

## PERIJUNCTIONAL VOLTAGE-GATED CHANNELS

The neuromuscular junction is the area of associated between the terminal portion of the motor neuron and the muscle cell.[1,2] The generation of action potentials in the motor neuron promotes the opening of ion channels, which results in the release of acetylcholine across the synaptic cleft, where it binds to postjunctional nicotinic cholinergic receptors.[1,2] The binding of these receptors to acetylcholine results in the opening of ion channels, depolarization of the muscle cell membrane, and the generation of an action potential that promotes muscle contraction. The perijunctional zone refers to the area of the muscle immediately around the junctional area or motor end plate of the neuromuscular junction.[2] This zone contains a small density of acetylcholine receptors, and a large density of sodium channels.[1,2] The large concentration of sodium channels promotes an enhanced respond to the depolarization generated by the binding of acetylcholine to nicotinic acetylcholine receptors, and the perijunctional zone contains a greater density of these sodium channels compared to more distal parts of the muscle membrane.[2] These sodium channels allow for the wave of depolarization to travel along the muscle membranes and T-tubules, initiating contraction of muscle cells, through the release of calcium from the sarcoplasmic reticulum.[1]

These sodium channels have an upper and a lower gate, which limits the influx of sodium ions.[1] Both of these gates need to be open to allow for sodium ions to flow through the channel.[2] At rest the lower gate is open, but the upper gate remains closed, preventing this influx of sodium ions.[2] During depolarization, the voltage-dependent top gate opens, while the lower gate remains open, allowing for an influx of sodium ions.[1,2] The voltage-dependent gate will remain open until the termination of depolarization around the channel.[2] After the opening of the top gate, the time-dependent lower gate will close, stopping the flow of ions.[1,2] Once depolarization ceases, the voltage-dependent gate will close, and the time-dependent gate will reopen, returning the channel to a resting state.[1,2] The time-dependent gate cannot reopen until the voltage-gated gate closes.[2]

The depolarization caused by acetylcholine is very brief compared to depolarizing muscle relaxants, due to its rapid breakdown degradation by acetylcholinesterase.[2] The binding of depolarizing muscle relaxants to the alpha subunits of the acetylcholine receptor produces continuous stimulation of the receptor, depolarizing the end plate.[1,2] This prompts the opening of the outer gate, creating a continuous wave of depolarization to spread along the muscle cell. When the time-dependent lower gate closes, the voltage-dependent gate remains open. With the inability to open the lower gate, there is no influx of sodium ions through the channel, inhibiting perijunctional membrane depolarization, and preventing muscle contraction.[2] Additional ion channels downstream from those initially affected will remain in a resting state, unable to be depolarized by the inactive sodium channels.[1,2] As long as the depolarizing muscle relaxant remains bound to the receptor, the end plate will not undergo repolarization; this is known as a phase I block.[1]

Depolarizing muscle relaxants are not hydrolyzed rapidly by acetylcholinesterase, and elimination from the junction relies on plasma cholinesterase.[1] This process is known as accommodation, and if acetylcholine is released from the prejunctional aspect of the neuromuscular junction, it will not activate the inactivated sodium channels.[2] The process of accommodation does not occur in extraocular muscles, due to their expression of mature and fetal receptors.[2] Due

to this, the administration of succinylcholine can lead to prolonged contracture of these extraocular muscles.[2] The force of the contraction generated by these muscles can force the eye against the orbit, resulting in increased intraocular pressures.[2] So phase I is characterized by decreased contraction in response to a single twitch stimulus, decreased amplitude by sustained response to a continuous stimulus, train-of-four ration greater than 70%, absence of post-tetanic facilitation, and augmentation of neuromuscular blockade by anticholinesterase.

## CHANNEL BLOCKS, DESENSITIZATION BLOCKS, PHASE II BLOCKS

Different medications can alter the activity of the neuromuscular receptor without directly acting upon the acetylcholine binding site. Inhaled anesthetics, ketamine, cocaine, alcohols, and other medications can alter the ion channel, by altering the rate of channel opening and closure. If channel opening is slowed, the resulting decrease in ion flow would decrease the strength of depolarization. Conversely, prolonged channel opening could result in increased strength of depolarization. The impaired neuromuscular function associated with these medications is not overcome by the administration of cholinesterase inhibitors, and subsequent increase in perijunctional acetylcholine concentrations, due to receptor desensitization or channel blockade.[2]

A desensitization block occurs when a portion of receptors bound to an agonist does not undergo a confirmation change and opening of the ion channel associated with that agonist. There is evidence to suggest that desensitization is associated with the phosphorylation of a tyrosine unit within the receptor protein. However, the exact mechanism of desensitization is unknown.[2]

A channel block occurs when the flow of ions through a receptor is impaired, resulting in diminished or an absence of depolarization in the end plate. These blocks are separated into the closed-channel type, and open-channel type. The closed-channel block involves a drug within the channel that prevents the flow of ions, inhibiting depolarization. The open-channel block involves a drug that enters the ion channel but does not penetrate the channel, resulting in impaired ion flow through the channel. Medications such as cocaine, tricyclic antidepressants, naloxone, and more, have been associated with channel blocks. Both ion channel blocks result in the decreased flow of ions through the receptor, and subsequent prevention of depolarization, weakening or blocking neuromuscular transmission. Increasing the concentration of acetylcholine within the perijunctional zone will not overcome this type of block, because the site impacted is not the same as the acetylcholine binding site.[2]

Phase II blocks occur at junctional receptors that are exposed to high concentrations or prolonged administration of depolarizing neuromuscular agonists.[1,2] Initially the junction is depolarized by the depolarizing agonist, resulting in an efflux of potassium ions, and influx of sodium ions through the ion channels. The increased intracellular sodium concentration results in the increased activity of the sodium-potassium ATP pump, which transports sodium extracellularly in exchange for potassium, resulting in a gradual recovery of the membrane potential to normal. This recovery of membrane potential occurs despite continued binding of the agonist, and as long as the depolarizing medication is bound, the channel will remain open, allowing the continued exchange of ions.[2] Clinically, a phase II block resembles nondepolarizing muscle relaxant medications.[1] Reversal of a phase II block with acetylcholinesterase inhibitors is unpredictable.[2] Phase II is characterized by decreased contraction in response to a single twitch, tetanic fade, train-of-four ratio less than 30%, post-tetanic facilitation, and reversal of neuromuscular blockade with anticholinesterase.

## REFERENCES

1. Butterworth J, et al. *Morgan and Mikhail's Clinical Anesthesiology.* 5th ed. New York, NY: McGraw-Hill Education; 2013:200–205, 207–208.
2. Miller R. *Miller's Anesthesia.* 7th ed. Philadelphia, PA: Churchill Livingstone; 2010:344–346, 350–356.

# Part XXVI

# SPECIAL PROBLEMS IN ANESTHESIOLOGY

# 331.

# PHYSICIAN IMPAIRMENT AND DISABILITY

*Ramsey Saad and Joseph Salama Hanna*

## INTRODUCTION

Anesthesiology is a demanding specialty. The specialty involves making time-sensitive decisions and being able to react to the rapidly changing clinical situation efficiently and decisively. This chapter outlines some of the ethical and legal debates regarding physician impairment and ethical dilemmas regarding safe return to work while ensuring the protection of the public as well.

## PHYSICIAN IMPAIRMENT

According to the American Medical Association, *physician impairment* is defined as the inability to practice medicine with reasonable skill and safety to patients by reason of psychiatric or general-medical conditions.[1] One of the most common causes of this is substance abuse disorder (SUD), which can be a cause of disability among anesthesiologists as well as other physicians; however, other medical conditions could cause disability as well. Psychiatric disorders such as uncontrolled depression or anxiety, neurologic disorders such as dementia, or even changes that can occur with aging, such as decreased visual and hearing acuity, can all be causative or contributing factors to physician impairment.[2]

## DETECTION

The first step toward coming up with a management plan, as with any disease, is diagnosis. Certain conditions, such as visual and auditory impairment, can be detected by the physician him/herself. Other conditions, such as SUD, uncontrolled depression, and/or other psychiatric disorders and neurologic disorders, will need close observation from colleagues, family, and friends, and intervention in terms of bringing the concerns to the attention of the physician

and supervisors, with the goal of providing safe and effective treatment to the physician while maintaining his/her safety and that of the physician's patient population as a priority.

## COMMON SYMPTOMS OF SUD

Alcohol and prescription drug use are more common in physicians, as opposed to illicit drug use in the general population. Unique to anesthesiologists is the familiarity with intravenous (IV) drug dosages and familiarity with the technicality of IV access. The drug of choice for anesthesiologists is opioid, possibly for this reason.

Common signs of controlled substance abuse/diversion include:

- Initially, the anesthesiologist may appear more attentive at work, but with episodes of irritability and anger.
- Frequent volunteering for additional overnight calls
- Declining being relieved of clinical duties
- Frequent bathroom breaks
- Signing out excessive amounts of controlled substances for the assigned cases
- Uncontrolled pain postoperatively for patients
- The physician usually wearing long sleeves
- Weight loss and pallor are late signs.[3,4]

## APPROACH TO SUSPECTED OR CONFIRMED SUD

If the physician with active SUD has insight into the issue and enters treatment willingly, the approach would be multimodal, with monitoring and support from the physician's leadership, treating the physician in coordination with the Physician Health Program (PHP).

For those who do not seek assistance with this issue, honest feedback from a friend, family member, or colleague may be of use. Denial of SUD may be a characteristic of a severe form of SUD.

The goal of the intervention would be to present the facts objectively, voicing encouragement and motivation in a nonjudgmental fashion.

If a friend or colleague suspects SUD, and the physician is unwilling to seek attention regarding this, then leadership should be notified in order to address the next step. The goal of this would be patient safety, in addition to the physician's well-being. There should be a clear treatment and monitoring plan, and emphasis should be on immediate action.

Many physicians will be compliant with the plan. Given the sensitivity of the nature of the responsibilities of physicians and especially anesthesiologists, a more definitive approach should be taken in the event of physician refusal. The consequences of refusal should be made clear, such as disciplinary action and/or loss of medical license.[3]

## LEGAL CONCERNS

Legal counsel is highly recommended for both the physician seeking treatment for SUD and/or substance diversion, in addition to the institution for which the physician in question has medical privileges. The physician's state license may be at risk, in addition to the fact that the institution may face legal consequences in the event of failure to report, especially if adverse events occur involving the physician in question.

Consequences differ depending on state law; however, enrollment in PHPs are highly recommended, and frequently failure to comply with this may result in the case being referred to the corresponding State Medical Board.

Group therapy, though potentially beneficial, may pose a specific concern for physicians in terms of confidentiality.

## LONG TERM

Return to work is a topic of ethical and moral debate for the physician and the institution. On the one hand, after completing rehabilitation, the goal of return to work may encourage coming forward early and seeking help. The concern remains, though, in the event of relapse, potential harm to the physician and patients under his/her care; and in some instances the first sign of relapse, especially for opioid use, is death.[3,4]

## AMERICANS WITH DISABILITIES ACT

There is some protection offered to the physician by the Americans with Disabilities Act, more so with alcohol abuse. Regarding illegal substances, the physician must be enrolled in a treatment program to be provided some protection.[4]

Aging is not a disease. However, the physiologic changes that occur with aging must be taken into consideration, some of which, such as visual and auditory impairment, may be noticed by the physician. Other conditions, such as dementia or psychiatric disorders, may be more noticeable by colleagues and family members. The decision regarding return to work may be a joint one, between the treating physician, the anesthesiologist in question, and the medical institution.[2]

## REFERENCES

1. The Federation of State Physicians Health Programs. https://www.fsphp.org/ accessed on 12/23/2021.
2. Katz J. The impaired and/or disabled anesthesiologist. *Curr Opin Anesthesiol.* 2017;30:217–222.
3. Merlo L, et al. Substance use disorders in physicians: Epidemiology, clinical manifestations, identification, and engagement. Up-to-date last modified March 2019. Accessed on 12/23/2021. https://www.uptodate.com/contents/substance-use-disorders-in-physicians-epidemiology-clinical-manifestations-identification-and-engagement?search=substance%20abuse%20in%20physicians&source=search_result&selectedTitle=1~150&usage_type=default&display_rank=1
4. Bryson E, et al. Addiction and substance abuse in anesthesiology. *Anesthesiology.* 2008 Nov;109(5):905–917.

# 332.

# PHYSICIAN WELLNESS

*Joseph Salama Hanna and Ramsey Saad*

## BURNOUT

Burnout is a complex condition with a history in many disciplines. Based on his research, Freudenberger used "burnout" as shorthand for a psychological syndrome with three dimensions: emotional exhaustion, depersonalization, and reduced personal accomplishment. Maslach subsequently summarized the dimensions of burnout as "exhaustion," "cynicism," and "inefficacy," providing more identifiable definitions of each dimension that align well with her measurement tool. Those who score high in "exhaustion" feel overextended, their emotional and physical resources depleted. High scorers in "cynicism" (depersonalization) appear more callous or detached than would be expected for normal "coping." Those lacking confidence or feeling they have achieved little work success score high in the "inefficacy" (reduced personal accomplishment) dimension. Overall, sufferers from burnout are frequently exhausted, diminished in their ability to care, and feel as though their work makes little difference.[1]

## THE COMPONENTS OF WELLNESS

Hundreds of studies have confirmed the high prevalence of burnout, yet relatively few have examined or quantified the characteristics of physician wellness. Some studies have demonstrated that issues such as work-life balance, social and family support, adequate rest, and regular physical activity correlate with career satisfaction, improved sense of well-being, increased empathy, and decreased burnout. Physicians are particularly vulnerable to experiencing mental illness due to the nature of their work, which is often stressful and characterized by shift work, irregular work hours, and a high-pressure environment.[2] As opposed to physicians who neglect their health, physicians with healthy lifestyle habits have been perceived as more credible and motivating to their patients and the residents under their supervision. It has been shown that wellness behaviors in physicians are additive (the more behaviours adopted the better as their effects are additive); therefore, individuals should be encouraged to adopt a variety of approaches to best suit their individual needs.[3]

## KEYS TO BOOST PHYSICIAN WELL-BEING

- It is very important to find both meaning and purpose in work; healthcare providers have to work on creating a connection or alignment between work activities and what they personally find to be meaningful.[4]
- Healthy work environments are associated with job satisfaction, retention, and better patient outcomes.
- Alignment of healthcare professionals' values and expectations with those of the organization creates more engagement and rise in job satisfaction.
- Job control, flexibility, and autonomy
- Rewards can be either intrinsic or extrinsic. Intrinsic rewards occur when individuals perceive their work as meaningful, have job control, feel mastery over their work, and are mutually respected, while extrinsic rewards include appropriate financial compensation and explicit feedback on a job well done.
- Enhanced and supportive professional relationships with patients and colleagues provides a source of support that buffers against stress.
- Work-life conflicts can be reduced, and thus burnout reduced as well, when better balance is created between work schedules and personal life needs.

## REFERENCES

1. Stehman CR, et al. Burnout, drop out, suicide: Physician loss in emergency medicine: Part I. *West J Emerg Med*. 2019 May;20(3):485–494. doi: 10.5811/westjem.2019.4.40970
2. Mihailescu M, Neiterman E. A scoping review of the literature on the current mental health status of physicians and physicians-in-training in North America. *BMC Public Health*. 2019;19:1363. doi: 10.1186/s12889-019-7661-9
3. McClafferty H, Brown OW; Section on Integrative Medicine and Committee on Practice and Ambulatory Medicine. Physician health and wellness. *Pediatrics*. 2014 Oct;134(4):830–835.
4. Berg S. Magnificent 7: These are the keys to boosting physician well-being. *Am Med Assoc*. January 28, 2020. Magnificent 7: These are the keys to boosting physician well-being | American Medical Association (ama-assn.org)

# 333.

# PROFESSIONALISM AND LICENSURE

*Joseph Salama Hanna and Ramsey Saad*

## MEDICAL PROFESSIONALISM

Medical professionalism is a belief system in which group members ("professionals") declare ("profess") to each other and the public the shared competency standards and ethical values they promise to uphold in their work, and what the public and individual patients can and should expect from medical professionals. At the heart of these ongoing declarations is a three-part promise to acquire, maintain, and advance the following:

1. An ethical value system grounded in the conviction that the medical profession exists to serve patients' and the public's interests, and not merely the self-interests of practitioners;
2. The knowledge and technical skills necessary for good medical practice;
3. The interpersonal skills necessary to work together with patients, eliciting goals and values to direct the proper use of the profession's specialized knowledge and skills, sometimes referred to as the "art" of medicine.

Medical professionalism, therefore, pledges its members to a dynamic process of personal development, lifelong learning and professional formation, including participation in a social enterprise that continually seeks to express expertise and caring in its work.[1]

## CERTIFICATION AND LICENSURE

To obtain and maintain certification, a physician is expected to demonstrate the principles embodied in accepted statements of professional responsibility and ethical behavior (such as the Hippocratic Oath and the Declaration of Geneva); the precept of *primum non nocere* (first, do no harm); the application of moral principles, values, and ethical conduct to the practice of medicine; the skill, competence, and character expected of a physician; and compassion and benevolence for patients.[2]

## CERTIFICATION REQUIREMENTS

### ABA 2021 POLICY BOOK[3]

At the time of certification by the ABA, the candidate must:

A. Hold an unexpired license to practice medicine or osteopathy in at least one state or jurisdiction of the United States (U.S.) or province of Canada that is permanent, unconditional and unrestricted. Further, every U. S. and Canadian medical license the candidate holds must be free of restrictions. Candidates for initial certification and ABA diplomates have the affirmative obligation to advise us of any and all restrictions placed on any of their medical licenses, and to provide complete information concerning such restrictions within 60 days after their imposition or notice, whichever first occurs. Such information shall include, but not be limited to, the identity of the State Medical Board imposing the restriction as well as the restriction's duration, basis, and specific terms and conditions. Candidates and diplomates discovered not to have made disclosure may be subject to sanctions on their candidate or diplomate status. We must receive acceptable evidence of the candidate having satisfied the licensure requirement for certification by Nov. 15 of the Part 2 Examination administration year.

B. Have fulfilled all the requirements of the continuum of education in anesthesiology.

C. Have on file with the ABA a Certificate of Clinical Competence with an overall satisfactory rating covering the final six-month period of clinical anesthesia training in each anesthesiology residency program.

D. Have satisfied all Board examination requirements.

E. Have satisfactory professional standing (see Section 7.06).

F. Be capable of performing independently the entire scope of anesthesiology practice without accommodation or with reasonable accommodation (see Sections 1.02.A and 1.02.D).

*Table 333.1* MOCA 2.0 COMPONENTS[4]

| | |
|---|---|
| Medical License (Part 1) | Hold an active, unrestricted license to practice medicine in at least one jurisdiction of the United States (U.S.) or Canada. *Furthermore, all U.S. and Canadian medical licenses that a diplomate holds must be unrestricted.* |
| CME (Part 2) | 250 Category 1 CMEs of which 20 must be ABA-approved Patient Safety CMEs. Self-Assessment CMEs are no longer required. *If you previously completed Self-Assessment CMEs, you will get credit for them in MOCA 2.0.* |
| MOCA Minute (Part 3) | MOCA Minute° replaces the MOCA exam. Answer 30 questions per calendar quarter (120 per year by 11:59 p.m. EST on Dec. 31) and maintain a performance value of ≥.10, no matter how many certifications you are maintaining. *Diplomates certified in sleep medicine and hospice and palliative care medicine will need to take those recertification exams to maintain their subspecialty certifications.* |
| Quality Improvement (Part 4) | More options for activities with points awarded for each activity based on the time and effort associated with their completion. Diplomates must complete 25 points in Years 1–5 and 25 points in Years 6–10 for a total of 50 points per 10-year cycle. *If you are maintaining multiple certificates, these activities will be applied to all certificates.* |

Although admission into our examination system and success with the examinations are important steps in our certification process, they do not by themselves guarantee certification. The Board reserves the right to make the final determination of whether each candidate meets all of the requirements for certification, including A, E and F above, after successful completion of examinations for certification. ABA certificates in anesthesiology issued on or after Jan. 1, 2000, are valid for 10 years after the year the candidate passes the examination for certification. ABA certificates are subject to our rules and regulations, including our policy book, all of which may be amended from time to time without further notice.

A person certified by the ABA is designated a diplomate in publications of the American Board of Medical Specialties (ABMS) and the American Society of Anesthesiologists (ASA).

## MOCA 2.0 COMPONENTS

The following table (Table 333.1) illustrates the MOCA 2.0 components as published by ABA (American Board of Anesthesiology).[4]

## REFERENCES

1. ABMS Definition of Medical Professionalism (Long Form). Adopted by the ABMS Board of Directors, January 18, 2012. www.abms.org
2. Guidelines for Professionalism, Licensure, and Personal Conduct, The American Board of Family Medicine (ABFM), Version 2018-7. Adopted Effective April 30, 2018. Microsoft Word - Guidelines 2018-7 (theabfm.org)
3. ABA Policy Book (theaba.org)
4. http://www.theaba.org/MOCA/About-MOCA-2-0

# 334.

# ETHICS

*Joseph Salama Hanna and Ramsey Saad*

## ADVANCE DIRECTIVE

Advance directives are legal documents that allow a patient to spell out ahead of time what types of medical care the patient would want if he or she were ever unable to speak for him- or herself. These documents can also make things easier for the people who will need to make decisions for the patient should he or she become unable to make them.

Advance directives are especially important if patient is older than 65, has a serious life-threatening illness, such as advanced cancer, or end-stage heart or liver failure, and/or the person chosen by patient to be his or her health care proxy (decision-maker) is not a family member or legally married to the patient.

For the most useful kinds of advance directive, see Table 334.1.

## DNR SUSPENSION DURING SURGICAL INTERVENTION

Advance directives guide healthcare providers to listen to and respect patients' wishes regarding their right to die in circumstances when cardiopulmonary resuscitation is required, and hospitals accredited by the Joint Commission are required to have a do-not-resuscitate (DNR) policy in place. However, when surgery and anesthesia are necessary for the care of the patient with a DNR order, this advance directive can create ethical dilemmas specifically involving patient autonomy and the physician's responsibility to do no harm. Because of the potential conflicts between ethical care and the restrictions of DNR orders, it is critically important to discuss the medical and ethical issues surrounding this clinical scenario with the patient or surrogate prior to any surgical intervention. Practitioners are advised to first consider what is best for the patient and, when in doubt, to communicate with patients or surrogates and with colleagues to arrive at the most appropriate care plan. If irreconcilable conflicts arise, consultation with the institution's bioethics committee, if available, is beneficial to help reach a resolution. In a research study where the research team used a mixed-method, non-experimental qualitative study design to conduct audio-recorded interviews with 17 nonsurgical patients who had DNR orders, the patients in the study expected a discussion regarding any change in their DNR status before the day of surgery and thought they should have the option to maintain their DNR status.[12]

## HIPAA

The Health Insurance Portability and Accountability Act of 1996 (HIPAA) impacts all healthcare professionals. The administration simplification section of HIPAA includes specific regulations designed to protect the privacy of an individual's health records. These privacy regulations are not designed to impede upon essential healthcare practices, but do require that covered providers take reasonable steps to limit the use and disclosure of protected health information. Important aspects of the privacy regulations include the development of facility- or

*Table 334.1* **TYPES OF ADVANCE DIRECTIVE**

| | |
|---|---|
| Durable power of attorney | Allows the patient to choose someone to make medical decisions for him or her should the patient become unable to speak for him- or herself. |
| Living will | Document that tells healthcare providers what type of care the patient wants if he or she becomes unable to speak for him- or herself. |
| Do not resuscitate/Do not intubate order (DNR/DNI) | This is a form that must be signed by a doctor. It tells all healthcare providers that the patient has decided he or she does not want these treatments (breathing tube, CPR, feeding tube). |

practice-specific privacy policies, the development of a privacy manual, staff training on privacy policies and procedures, and the drafting and posting of a notice of privacy practices. In addition, authorization forms are mandated for instances of use and disclosure of public health information not related to treatment, payment, or healthcare operations.[3]

## REFERENCES

1. Sumrall WD et al. Do not resuscitate, anesthesia, and perioperative care: A not so clear order. *Ochsner J.* 2016 Summer;16(2):176–179.
2. Hiestand D, Beaman M. Perioperative do-not-resuscitate suspension: The patient's perspective. *AORN J.* 2019 Mar;109(3):326–334. doi: 10.1002/aorn.12612.
3. Lusis I, Hasselkus A. HIPAA privacy regulations. *Semin Speech Lang.* 2006 May;27(2):89–100.

# 335.

# INFORMED CONSENT

*Joseph Salama Hanna and Ramsey Saad*

## INFORMED DECISION-MAKING

Physicians have a legal and ethical responsibility to provide sufficient information to the patient so that he or she can make appropriate decisions. The physician is expected to carefully bring the patient into the medical decision-making process, addressing the patient's concerns, and creating reasonable expectations regarding outcomes. For consent to be valid, the patient must be competent. If a patient is deemed incompetent by a court of law, the duty of informed consent extends to the patient's proxy.[12]

In order to meet the requirements for effective, informed decision-making, a physician must disclose material facts, as well as appropriate additional disclosures (Table 335.1).

## COMMUNICATION

The physician should communicate in terms that patients and their families can understand. Elements of effective communication include focusing on the patient, using comprehensible language, offering educational material, and using interpreters when necessary.

## DOCUMENTATION

Patients may not accurately remember all the facts disclosed in teaching sessions.[3] Thus, the physician must document the content of informed consent sessions.

*Table 335.1* INFORMED CONSENTS COMPONENTS

| MATERIAL FACTS | ADDITIONAL DISCLOSURES |
| --- | --- |
| Diagnosis | Physicians must answer truthfully if asked about the number of similar procedures they have performed and their success rates. |
| Proposed treatment or procedure. | Advise patient of personnel and their respective roles, including residents, students, and equipment representatives. |
| Alternative treatment options, along with their risks and benefits | Inform patient of any additional procedures that may be predictably necessary for a successful outcome or that are recommended to prevent future health problems. |
| Risks and benefits of treatment | Disclosure of related financial conflict of interest |
| Risks of refusing treatment | |

## WITHDRAWAL OF CONSENT

Patients may withdraw consent at any time during a procedure, and the physician must then engage in a new informed consent discussion.[4]

## FAILURE TO OBTAIN CONSENT

Failure to provide the necessary, relevant information in a way that truly communicates with the patient may constitute ineffective, and therefore nonexistent, consent. There are two legal theories of recovery for failure to obtain informed consent: battery action and negligent nondisclosure.

## EMERGENCY SITUATIONS

In some cases, the need for consent may be outweighed by the need for urgent intervention, and the physician must proceed as expeditiously as the medical situation requires. If the patient cannot participate cogently, family members should be contacted if they are not present and if time allows. When available, living wills and durable powers of attorney should be consulted to determine who the surrogate decision-makers might be.

## REFERENCES

1. Marsha Ryan, Michael S. Sinha. Informed procedural consent. *UpToDate*. Last updated October 17, 2019. https://www.uptodate.com/contents/informed-procedural-consent
2. Berg JW, et al. *Informed Consent: Legal Theory and Clinical Practice*. 2nd ed. New York, NY: Oxford University Press; 2001.
3. Robinson G, Merav A. Informed consent: Recall by patients tested postoperatively. *Ann Thorac Surg*. 1976 Sep;22(3):209–212.
4. *Schreiber v. Physicians Insurance Company of Wisconsin*. 588 N.W.2d 26 (Wis. 1999).

# 336.

# MEDICAL ERRORS

*Joseph Salama Hanna and Ramsey Saad*

## CLASSIFICATION OF ERRORS

### ACTION-BASED ERRORS

Action-based errors include incidents such as accidental placement of a needle in the carotid artery during central venous cannulation, or endotracheal tube placement in the esophagus instead of the trachea.[1] These are relatively common but are usually identified and easily corrected (Table 336.1).

Prevention of action-based errors includes:

- Use of known safety precautions (e.g., use of ultrasound guidance for central line placement, use of end-tidal carbon dioxide [ETCO$_2$] for verification of endotracheal intubation)
- Use of standardized techniques
- Building redundancy into systems (e.g., two-person checks, use of both ultrasound guidance and transduction of a waveform from an 18-gauge needle or catheter that is inserted into a central vein prior to insertion of a larger 8.5 F introducer sheath)

### DECISION-BASED ERRORS

Decision-based errors happen mainly secondary to faulty knowledge or judgment; they are more insidious and

*Table 336.1* DEFINITIONS

| | |
|---|---|
| Patient safety | The avoidance, prevention, and amelioration of adverse outcomes or injuries stemming from the process of healthcare (US National Patient Safety Foundation, 1999). Freedom from accidental injury (Institute of Medicine, 2000)[2] |
| Adverse event | Unintended injury to patients caused by medical management (rather than the underlying condition of the patient) that results in measurable disability, prolonged hospitalization, or both (the Harvard Medical Practice Study, 1991, and the Utah and Colorado Medical Practice Study, 1999). Unintended injury or complication that results in disability, death, or prolonged hospital stay and is caused (including acts of omission and acts of commission) by healthcare management rather than the patient's disease (Quality in Australian Health Study, 1995) |
| Negligence | Failure to meet the standard of care reasonably expected of an average physician qualified to take care of the patient in question (Brennan et al., 1991)[3]. Care that fell below the standard expected of physicians in their community |
| Near miss | Any event that could have had an adverse patient consequence but did not, and was indistinguishable from a full-fledged adverse event in all but outcome (Barach and Small, 2000)[4] |
| Medical error | The failure of a planned action to be completed as intended (an error of execution) or the use of a wrong plan to achieve an aim (an error of planning) (Reason, 1990)[5]. An unintended act (either of omission or commission) or one that does not achieve its intended outcome (Leape, 1994)[6]. Deviations from the process of care, which may or may not cause harm to the patient (Reason, 2001)[7] |
| Medication error | The United States National Coordinating Council for Medication Error Reporting and Prevention defines a medication error as any preventable event that may cause or lead to inappropriate medication use or patient harm while the medication is in the control of the healthcare professional, patient, or consumer. Such events may be related to professional practice, healthcare products, procedures, and systems, including prescribing, order communication, product labeling, packaging, and nomenclature, compounding, dispensing, distribution, administration, education, monitoring, and use |
| Sentinel event | A sentinel event is a patient safety event that results in death, permanent harm, or severe temporary harm.[8] |

difficult to identify and correct than action-based errors.[9] Failure of critical thinking and cognitive biases may lead to inadequate risk assessment, incorrect diagnosis, and/or incorrect choices of treatment. Such errors may be compounded by persistence on an incorrect path. Since cognitive processes are similar in all humans, a situation that leads one individual to make an error will likely result in similar errors made by others.

Prevention of decision-based errors includes:

• Cognitive aids to decrease reliance on memory (e.g., mnemonics, algorithms, and computerized decision support)
• Simulation training for specific clinical scenarios
• Implementing evidence-based clinical practice guidelines.

## COMMUNICATION-BASED ERRORS

Communication failures occur commonly in the operating room setting and are the leading root cause of serious adverse events that result in patient harm.[10] Examples will be poor timing of the actual communication, missing or inaccurate content (incomplete report), wrong audience, and ineffective communication, resulting in failure to resolve the issue.

Prevention of communication-based errors includes:

• Employment of a preoperative briefing to ensure thorough communication among all members of the team before an intervention begins
• Use of structured communication
• Teamwork training to teach communication skills.

## REFERENCES

1. Joyce A. Wahr, Roberta Hines, Nancy A. Nussmeier. Safety in the operating room. *UpToDate*. Last updated August 31, 2021.
2. Grober ED, Bohnen JM. Defining medical error. *Can J Surg*. 2005;48(1):39–44.
3. Brennan TA, Leape LL, Laird NM, Hebert L, Localio AR, Lawthers AG, Newhouse JP, Weiler PC, Hiatt HH. Incidence of adverse events and negligence in hospitalized patients. *Results of the Harvard Medical Practice Study I. N Engl J Med*. 1991 Feb 7;324(6):370–376. doi:10.1056/NEJM199102073240604. PMID: 1987460.
4. Barach P, Small SD. Reporting and preventing medical mishaps: Lessons from non-medical near miss reporting systems. *BMJ*. 2000;320(7237):759–763. doi:10.1136/bmj.320.7237.759
5. Reason J. Human error. Cambridge: Cambridge University Press; 1990.

6. Leape LL. Error in medicine. *JAMA*. 1994 Dec 21;272(23):1851–1857.
7. Reason JT. Understanding adverse events: The human factor. In: Vincent C, ed. *Clinical risk management: enhancing patient safety.* London: BMJ Publishing Group; 2001:9–30.
8. https://www.jointcommission.org/en/resources/patient-safety-topics/sentinel-event/
9. Neuhaus C, et al. Applying the human factors analysis and classification system to critical incident reports in anaesthesiology. *Acta Anaesthesiol Scand*. 2018;62(10):1403–1411.
10. Arriaga AF, et al. A policy-based intervention for the reduction of communication breakdowns in inpatient surgical care: Results from a Harvard surgical safety collaborative. *Ann Surg*. 2011;253(5):849–854.

# 337.

# SHARED DECISION-MAKING

*Joseph Salama Hanna and Ramsey Saad*

## INTRODUCTION

Shared decision-making relies basically on both patient autonomy and informed consent. It recognizes the fact that patients have personal values that affect their interpretation of risks and benefits, and that these interpretations differ from those of the physician. Informed consent is at the core of shared decision-making,[1] i.e., without fully understanding the advantages and disadvantages of different treatment options, patients cannot fully engage in making informed and appropriate decisions.

## IMPORTANCE OF SHARED DECISION-MAKING

Shared decision-making helps providers and patients agree on a healthcare plan. When patients participate in decision-making and understand what they need to do, they are more likely to follow through.

In many situations, there is no single "right" healthcare decision because choices about treatment, medical tests, and health issues come with pros and cons. Shared decision-making is especially important in these types of situations:

- when there is more than one reasonable option;
- when no single option has a clear advantage.
- when the possible benefits and harms of each option affect patients differently.

## TIPS FOR SHARED DECISION-MAKING

The following six steps will help providers with shared decision-making.[2] They are adapted from the Informed Medical Decisions Foundation.

**Invite the patient to participate**: Inviting patients to participate lets them know that they have options and that their goals and concerns are a key part of the decision-making process.

**Present options**: Patients need to know the available options.

**Provide information on benefits and risks**: Provide balanced information based on the best available scientific evidence. Check back with patients to be sure they understand.

**Assist patients in evaluating options based on their goals and concerns**: To understand patients' preferences, ask them what is important to them and what they are concerned about.

**Facilitate deliberation and decision-making**: Let patients know they have time to think things over and ask them what else they need to know or do before they feel comfortable making a decision.

**Assist patients to follow through on the decision**: Lay out the next steps for patients, check for understanding, and discuss any possible challenges with carrying out the decision.

## REFERENCES

1. Whitney SN, et al. A typology of shared decision making, informed consent, and simple consent. *Ann Intern Med.* 2004;140(1): 54–59.
2. https://www.healthit.gov/sites/default/files/nlc_shared_decision_making_fact_sheet.pdf

# 338.

# DISCLOSURE OF ERRORS TO PATIENTS

*Joseph Salama Hanna and Ramsey Saad*

## INTRODUCTION

Silence and secrecy are increasingly considered ethically and legally unacceptable responses to medical injury, as can be seen in codes of professional ethics, healthcare organization accreditation standards, state apology laws, and "disclosure-and-offer" programs implemented by healthcare systems and liability insurers. The shift from prior practice, often a "deny-and-defend" approach, has not come with particularly effective, streamlined, or reassuring processes for providers who are called upon to make disclosures and apologies.[1,2] The Joint Commission standard states in RI. 1.2.2: "Patients and, when appropriate, their families are informed about the outcomes of care, including unanticipated outcomes."[3] We here review a recommended process for disclosing errors to patients that will take into consideration the duty of the physician to inform patient and family with the outcomes of care, while doing so in a carefully composed conversation maintaining moral and ethical obligations toward the patient and his or her family.

## RECOMMENDED PROCESS

- Informed consent: A well-executed informed consent session in advance of an interventional procedure will help to create realistic expectations for the patient, as it will alert that patient to the very real possibility that complications may arise.
- Initial discussion: At the initial contact with the patient and/or family when leaving the operating room, present the facts (as known at that time) of the surgical case and leave the remainder of the discussion until more is known.[4]
- Review policies: Before engaging in any additional communication regarding the event, review malpractice insurance contract provisions and contact the insurer.
- Involve risk management: Contact the hospital or health system counsel, as well as risk management, if the incident occurred in an institutional care setting.
- Participants and timing: Select key participants, as well as a suitable location and time. If a determination is made that the incident requires disclosure and/or an apology, a decision must be made about participants and their role in the dialogue. Those participants might include the surgeon, care-team members, and institutional representatives, as well as the patient and his/her invited guests.
- Statement and delivery: Carefully construct a statement and the parameters of the dialogue, and ensure calm, sympathetic, and sincere delivery. To avoid possible liability, based at least in part on the statements made, the apology in most jurisdictions should be limited to an expression of sympathy and compassion.[5]
- Documentation and follow-up: The dialogue should be objectively documented (in the patient's medical record if the discussion happens while the patient is in the hospital), and such documentations should

include the time, date, and location of the meeting; the individuals present; the disclosures made; the reactions of the patient and/or the patient's family; any promised follow-up; and next steps in treatment, if any.

## REFERENCES

1. Disclosure of errors in surgical procedures. *UpToDate.* Last updated January 13, 2020.

2. Sage WM, et al. How policy makers can smooth the way for communication-and- resolution programs. *Health Aff (Millwood).* 2014 Jan;33(1):11–19. doi: 10.1377/hlthaff.2013.0930.

3. Schroder JS. Disclosing medical errors: Practical, ethical and legal consideration, AHLA Seminar Materials, Hospitals and Health Systems Law Institute, Hollywood, Florida, February 12, 2004; AHLA-PAPERS P02120408: 1.

4. McMichael BJ, Van Horn RL. How to apologize effectively for medical errors. https://www.healio.com/primary-care/practice-man agement/news/online/%7B8ed41e3b-5695-40bd-aaf3-0831ed2bc b4d%7D/how-to-apologize-effectively-for-medical-errors

5. Zitter JM. Admissibility of evidence of medical defendant's apologetic statements or the like as evidence of negligence. *American Law Reports.* 2014;97:519 ʃ 3.

# 339.

# CORE COMPETENCIES

*Joseph Salama Hanna and Ramsey Saad*

## PRACTICE-BASED LEARNING AND IMPROVEMENT

The competency *practice-based learning and improvement* refers to the candidate's ability to investigate and evaluate patient care practices, appraise and assimilate scientific evidence, and improve the candidate's own practice of medicine, as well as the collaborative practice of medicine.

## PATIENT CARE AND PROCEDURAL SKILLS

The competency *patient care and procedural skills* refers to the candidate's use of clinical skills and ability to provide care and promote health in an appropriate manner that incorporates evidence-based medical practice, demonstrates good clinical judgment, and fosters patient-centered decision-making.

## SYSTEMS-BASED PRACTICE

The competency *systems-based practice* refers to the candidate's awareness of, and responsibility to, population health and systems of healthcare. The candidate should be able to use system resources responsibly in providing patient care (e.g., good resource stewardship, coordination of care).

## MEDICAL KNOWLEDGE

The competency *medical knowledge* refers to the candidate's demonstration of knowledge about established and evolving biomedical, clinical, and cognate sciences, as well as the application of these sciences in patient care.

## INTERPERSONAL AND COMMUNICATION SKILLS

The competency *interpersonal and communication skills* refers to the candidate's demonstration of skills that result in effective information exchange and partnering with patients, their families, and professional associates (e.g., fostering a therapeutic relationship that is ethically sound; using effective listening skills with nonverbal and verbal communication; being mindful of health literacy; and working effectively in a team, both as a team member and as a team leader).

## PROFESSIONALISM

The competency *professionalism* refers to the candidate's demonstration of a commitment to carrying out professional responsibilities; adhering to ethical principles; applying the skills and values to deliver compassionate, patient-centered care; demonstrating humanism; being sensitive to diverse patient populations and workforce; and practicing wellness and self-care.[1]

## REFERENCE

1. Standards for Initial Certification, American Board of Medical Specialties 2016. https://www.abms.org/board-certification/board-certification-standards/

# 340.

# APPROACH TO ANESTHESIOLOGY EXAMS

*F. Cole Dooley and Adrian Ching*

## INTRODUCTION

Residents in anesthesiology training programs take several exams to obtain board certification after their training. Yearly, residents take an in-training exam, typically in February. This exam consists of 200 multiple-choice questions given over approximately 4 hours and is meant to reflect progress through the knowledge expected of a graduate of an anesthesiology program. The American Board of Anesthesiology BASIC Examination is the first part of the staged exam process for board certification. It is typically offered in June and November, and it is taken after the first clinical anesthesiology year is completed. The content of this exam focuses on pharmacology, anatomy, physiology, and anesthesia equipment and monitoring. The ADVANCED Examination is taken after graduation from a residency training program and focuses largely on anesthesiology subspecialty knowledge and other advanced clinical issues. This exam is also administered in a multiple-choice question format.[1]

## LEARNING VS. STUDYING

When it comes to studying for exams, the most important aspect to remember is that these exams are meant to ensure that anesthesiology residents obtain the knowledge needed to practice as a consultant anesthesiologist. The most important preparation during training is to actively learn by reading voraciously and consistently. However, simply reading the material does not equate to learning; nor does it prove to be an effective means of preparing for a standardized exam. Reading must be an active process in which the learner summarizes, makes notes, and practices recalling information. An excellent means of practicing recalling information is to use available multiple-choice question banks.[2]

Studying for standardized exams can be difficult for several reasons, especially if simply reading material. In light of this, a few suggestions should be considered. First, the learner should focus their study using materials that are made available, specifically the content outlines from the American Board of Anesthesiology. It is often helpful to seek out short, concise summaries of many of the keywords. If knowledge appears to be lacking on a topic, a more in-depth text could be reviewed. Another important part of studying for a standardized exam is to complete practice questions that often come in the form of electronic question banks or a book of questions. Working through these questions allows the learner to assess their knowledge of a topic and to practice recall of the information, both in the context of how the questions will be asked on the exams. Most of these question sources also provide extensive answers to the questions that summarize the topic and discuss why other answers might have been wrong. These explanations often provide ideas as to how other aspects of the concept could be tested. Reading the explanations and studying carefully may be the most important lesson to be learned from question bank studying.

## APPROACHES TO ANSWERING QUESTIONS

When taking a multiple-choice test, one of the most frequent errors is misreading or misinterpreting the question. To avoid this, there are a number of strategies. First, read the question without looking at the answers, then ask what the question is asking; test takers may find it helpful to rephrase the question in their own words. A clear understanding of the question is imperative before proceeding to the answer section; the mind is generally the clearest immediately after reading the question. Once the question is understood, think of what is known about the subject and think of an answer. Look for an answer that matches that original thought. Marking off answers that appear clearly wrong can often lead to just two answers remaining.[3] For choosing between two answers, consider the following:

- Eliminate answers that are known to be wrong immediately.
- Quickly answer questions that are easy. This will allow more time for questions that are more difficult. Gut reactions are often correct.[3]
- *Always*, *never*, *must*, and *all* when appearing in an answer are generally wrong; *seldom*, *generally*, *probably*, and *usually* are generally correct.
- Look for grammatical clues based on tense and noun-verb agreement.
- Look for answers that belong to different categories. For example, if the question is a "what is the next best step in management" type, categorize the answers: are they all medications, interventions such as intubation,

or laboratory tests? An outlier could easily signal the right answer or allow it to be immediately eliminated. Choices that are very similar also may be able to be quickly eliminated.

- When answers are divided into categories, if a choice does not look like it fits with the others, it is probably wrong. If two answers are opposites, one of them is likely right. Make sure the answer chosen truly answers the question.
- Remember that all information in the question is valid. Do not make choices based on information that is included in the answer choices. Good test writers provide incorrect choices that may contain superfluous or distracting information. Remember that the correct answer answers the question.[3]
- Correct answers rarely present new information.[3]
- Questions are meant to be taken at face value; most would not write a question to be a trick. If a question appears to be a trick, it may be incorrectly read. Do not spend time focusing on scenarios where an answer may be true. Ensure that the answer selected actually answers the entire question. The correct answer rarely requires the test taker to make significant assumptions.[3]
- When making wild guesses, always choose the longest of the answers. Test writers need to make the correct answer unquestionably correct, so this often needs qualifiers and makes the answer choice longer. Wrong answers are distracters that generally do not need qualifiers and are shorter.[4]

## REFERENCES

1. American Board of Anesthesiology. Certification exams. 2020. https://theaba.org/certifications%20and%20exms.html.
2. Brown PC. *Make It Stick: The Science of Successful Learning*. Cambridge, MA: Belknap Press of Harvard Press; 2014:1–66.
3. Shain DD. *Study Skills and Test-Taking Strategies for Medical Students: Find and Use Your Personal Learning Style*. New York, NY: Springer; 1995:169–194.
4. Simplemost. *This Is the Best Way to Guess on Multiple Choice Tests, According to Research*. https://www.simplemost.com/best-way-guess-multiple-choice-test/. May 29, 2018.

# INDEX

*For the benefit of digital users, indexed terms that span two pages (e.g., 52–53) may, on occasion, appear on only one of those pages.*

Tables, figures, and boxes are indicated by *t*, *f*, and *b* following the page number

metabolism and, 779–80, 780*f*
non-clear liquids, 270
solids, 270
fatty acids (FA), 801
FBA (foreign body aspiration), 575
Fc region, immunoglobulin, 792
febrile non-hemolytic transfusion
   reactions (FNHTR), 739
febrile transfusion reactions, 750, 751*t*
feet, 17
femoral artery, 35
femoral nerve, 6
fenestrated capillaries, 644
fenoldopam, 209
fentanyl
   dopaminergic drugs and, 726
   effect on CFS production, 430
   electroencephalography and, 122
   pediatric anesthesiology, 225
   spinal adjuvants, 151–52
ferritin, 795
FESS (functional endoscopic sinus
   surgery), 582
FEV1 (forced expiratory volume in one
   second), 527, 528–29
fever and infection, 293
feverfew (*Tanacetum parthenium*), 170
FFP (fresh frozen plasma), 732*t*, 733,
   737, 738*t*
FI. *See* inspired gas concentration
fiberoptic devices, 323–24
fiberoptic intubation (FOI), 9–10
fibular nerve, 504*f*
Fick's law, 55, 552, 659
Fick's principle, 640*f*, 640–42, 653
filling phase, 619, 620*f*, 623, 624*t*
"finger-to-nose" test, 421
Fink, Bernard, 370
FIO₂ (fraction of inspired oxygen), 103
fire prevention and management, 135
first harmonic (fundamental frequency),
   119
Fisher's Exact test, 142
fish oil, 170
5-hydroxyindoleacetic acid (5-HIAA), 255
flow-inflating portable ventilation
   devices, 83
flowmeters
   limitations of, 51
   Ohmeda "link 25," 51*f*, 51
   overview, 49
   principles of, 50
   safety features of, 51
   structure of, 49–50, 50*f*
   Thorpe tube, 49–50
flow trigger, 103
flow velocity
   anesthetic considerations, 49
   determinants of, 48
   overview, 48
   as paths change, 48
   pressure, 41
   relationships that determine flow rate
      and resistance, 49*f*
   turbulent flow, 48–49
flow-volume loops, 534*f*, 535
fluid deficit calculations, 335–36
fluid-replacement strategies
   anesthetic considerations, 289–91
   general discussion, 289
   goal-directed volume management, 290
   liberal approach, 290
   restrictive approach, 290
fluid therapy
   ERAS protocol, 339–40
   intravenous fluid therapy, 334–37

fluid warmers, 125
fluoride toxicity, 174
fluoroscopy, 179
FN (false negative), 143
FNHTR (febrile non-hemolytic
   transfusion reactions), 739
focal ischemia, 425–26
FOI (fiberoptic intubation), 9–10
fondaparinux (ultra-low molecular weight
   heparin), 757, 758*t*
fontanelles, 24
foramen magnum, 22
forced expiratory volume in one second
   (FEV1), 527, 528–29
forced vital capacity (FVC), 527, 528–29
force of contraction, 632–33
forearms, 16–17
foreign body aspiration (FBA), 575
formoterol, 603–4
fossae, 22
FP (false positive), 143
fraction of inspired oxygen (FIO₂), 103
Frank-Starling curve, 631, 632*f*, 635
Frank-Starling law, 631–32, 633, 640
   anesthetic considerations, 631–32
   defined, 631
   general discussion, 631
Frank-Starling mechanism, 630
FRC (functional residual capacity),
   526–27, 542
fresh frozen plasma (FFP), 732*t*, 733,
   737, 738*t*
frontal lobe, 417, 418*f*, 481
full stomach, 270
functional endoscopic sinus surgery
   (FESS), 582
functional residual capacity (FRC),
   526–27, 542
fundamental frequency (first harmonic),
   119
FUSED CAR mnemonic, 563
FVC (forced vital capacity), 527, 528–29

GABA (gamma-aminobutyric acid)-ergic
   neurons, 470–71, 489
GABA A receptor. *See* gamma-
   aminobutyric acid A receptor
gabapentin, 400
   indications, 215
   intraoperative considerations, 244
   mechanism of action, 215
   metabolism of, 215
   perioperative management of, 275
   side effects, 215
gag reflex, 10
gain, ultrasound, 47
gamma-aminobutyric acid (GABA) A
   receptor, 191
   basal ganglia, 484–85
   benzodiazepines and, 197
   etomidate and, 195–96
   propofol and, 193
gamma-aminobutyric acid (GABA)-ergic
   neurons, 470–71, 489
ganglionic transmission
   acetylcholine, 460, 460*t*
   anesthetic considerations, 460, 461*t*
   general discussion, 459
   ligand gated sodium channels, 460
   norepinephrine, 460, 460*t*
   presynaptic VGCCs, 460
garlic (*Allium sativum*), 170
gas concentrations
   carbon dioxide analysis, 118
   oxygen analysis, 117

gases and vapors
   comparing, 175
   concentration effect, 55, 67*f*, 67–68
   diffusion of, 54
   effect on cardiovascular system, 174
   effect on central nervous system,
      173–74
   effect on hematologic system, 174–75
   effect on hepatic function, 174
   effect on neuromuscular function, 174
   effect on renal function, 174
   effect on respiration, 174
   overview, 173
   physical properties, 173
   second gas effect, 55*f*, 55
   solubility coefficients, 54
   toxicity, 175
   vapor pressure, 54
gas mixtures, 74
gastric aspiration, 374–75. *See also*
   aspiration
gastric content pH, 272
gastric fluid volume, 271–72
gastric-inhibitory polypeptide (GIP), 784
gastrointestinal (GI) system
   autonomic neuropathy, 461*t*
   drugs affecting LES tone, 712, 712*t*
   effect of intravenous opioid anesthetics
      on gastrointestinal motility, 184
   effect of nitrous oxide on, 71
   effect of NSAIDs on, 391
   effect of tricyclic antidepressants on,
      395
   enhanced recovery after colorectal
      surgery, 709–10
   esophagus, 711
   intestines, 711
   overview, 711
   perioperative management of chronic
      medications, 275
   PSNS effects on, 457*t*
   stomach, 711
GC (guanylyl cyclase), 797
G-coupled protein, vasoconstriction, 645
GCS (Glasgow coma scale), 280, 281
GDFT (goal-directed fluid therapy),
   339–40
gender
   defined, 449
   differences in pain and pain perception,
      449–50
general anesthesia
   acute postoperative and posttraumatic
      pain, 340–42
   airway devices, 322–24
   airway evaluation, 318–19
   airway management, 320–22
   analgesia, 313
   balanced anesthesia, 317
   colloid solutions, 337–39
   effect on cardiovascular system, 407
   endobronchial intubation, 327–28
   endotracheal tubes, 329–32
   ERAS protocol, 339–40
   excitement stage, 313
   general discussion, 313
   intravenous fluid therapy during,
      334–37
   medullary depression, 314
   neuroleptanesthesia, 317
   outpatient pediatric anesthesia,
      344–46
   sedation levels, 314–15, 315*t*
   stages of, 314*t*
   supraglottic secretion management,
      332–34

surgical airway, 324–26
surgical anesthesia, 313–14
total inhalation anesthesia, 316
total intravenous anesthesia, 315–16
genitalia, 18
gentamycin, 279–80
geriatric anesthesia, 264, 267*t*
Gerstmann syndrome, 481
GFCIs (ground fault circuit interrupters),
   93–94, 135–36
GFR (glomerular filtration rate), 157,
   246, 717
GH (growth hormone), 621, 785
GHRH (growth hormone-releasing
   hormone), 763, 764*f*
GIIb/IIIa receptors, 757, 757*t*
Gillespie, N. A., 313
ginger, 170
ginkgo biloba, 170
ginseng, 170
GIP (gastric-inhibitory polypeptide), 784
GI system. *See* gastrointestinal system
Glasgow coma scale (GCS), 280, 281
global ischemia, 425
glomerular filtration rate (GFR), 157,
   246, 717
glomerulus, 721
glossopharyngeal nerve (CN IX), 10, 507*f*
   carotid bodies, 510
   carotid sinus, 510
   general discussion, 508
   pharyngeal reflex, 509
   pharynx, 584
   upper respiratory tract, 588
glucagon, 691, 775*f*, 785–86, 786*f*
glucagon-like protein 1 (GLP-1), 784
glucocorticoids, 237, 735, 774. *See also*
   steroids
gluconeogenesis, 801–2
glucose, 779, 780
   aerobic metabolism, 782
   anaerobic metabolism, 782
   general discussion, 781
   glycolysis, 783
   glycolytic pathway, 781–82, 782*f*
glutamate, 484–85
glutamatergic neurons, 470–71
gluteal region, 17
Glycine max (soy isoflavones), 170
glycogenolysis, 801–2
glycolysis
   glucose, 781–82
   hexokinase, 783
   phosphofructokinase, 783
   pyruvate dehydrogenase, 783
glycopyrrolate, 513
GnRH (gonadotropin-releasing
   hormone), 763, 764*f*
goal-directed fluid therapy (GDFT),
   339–40
goal-directed volume management, 290
goblet cells, 601
Goldenhar syndrome (oculo-
   auriculovertebral dysplasia), 577
Golgi tendon reflex (inverse myotatic
   reflex), 439
gonadotropin-releasing hormone
   (GnRH), 763, 764*f*
G-protein, 796
G protein-coupled receptors (GPCRs),
   518, 796
Graham's law, 50
grapefruit, 170
gray matter, 437
great cerebral vein (of Galen), 492, 493*f*
great radicular artery, 438, 442, 444, 502

mathematics
  data mode, 142
  data types, 141, 141t
  diagnostic tests, 142–43
  mean, 142
  median, 142
  null hypothesis, 141–42
  statistical tests, 142
maxilla, 22
maxillary nerve (CN V2), 588
maximal expiratory pressure (MEP), 530
maximal inspiratory pressure (MIP), 530
maximum voluntary ventilation (MVV)
    test, 530
MCA (middle cerebral artery), 491, 492f
MCAS (mast cell activation syndrome),
    609–10, 611
McKay, R. E., 411
MCP (metacarpophalangeal) joints, 17
MD (muscular dystrophy), 795
MDMA, 188
MDR1 (multidrug resistance protein), 163
mean, data sets, 142
mean arterial pressure (MAP), 642, 650,
    651f
  baroreceptors, 655
  cerebral blood flow and, 423
  cerebral perfusion pressure, 249
  effect of general anesthesia on, 407
  intraocular pressure and, 245
mechanical ventilators, 102
  adaptive-support ventilation, 132–33
  assist-control ventilation, 132
  compliance curve, 130
  general discussion, 129
  inverse ratio ventilation, 132
  lung pressures, 129–30
  modes, 132–33
  positive-pressure ventilation, 130
  pressure-controlled ventilation, 132
  pressure-support ventilation, 132
  scalars, 130–31
  synchronized intermittent mandatory
    ventilation, 132
  volume-controlled ventilation, 132
mechanics
  blood pressure monitoring, 106–8
  carbon dioxide absorption, 84–86
  circle system, 78–80
  components of anesthesia circuit,
    75–77
  concentration effect, 67–68
  dead space, 73
  delivery of inhalation anesthetics,
    61, 62
  distribution of inhalation anesthetics,
    61–62
  Doppler ultrasound, 52
  echocardiography, 110–13
  elimination curves of anesthetic gas, 64
  flow, 48–49
  flowmeters, 49–51
  gases, 54–55
  gas mixtures, 74
  heart functions, 109–10
  heat, 74
  humidity, 74
  leaks, 74
  liquids, 54
  medical gas cylinders, 43–44, 45t
  monitoring methods, 95–97
  monitoring oxygen, 104–5
  neuromuscular function, 98–101
  nitrous oxides, 70–72
  non-circle systems, 81–82
  oxygen supply systems, 89–90

portable ventilation devices, 82–84
pressure measurement, 41–43
pressure regulators, 44
principles, 72–74
pulmonary ventilation, 101–4
rebreathing, 73
resistance gas flow, 72–73
safety features for anesthetic
    monitoring, 93–95
second gas effect, 68–69
toxicity of inhalation anesthetics,
    86–88
transducers, 43
ultrasound, 46
uptake curves of anesthetic gas, 63–64
uptake of inhalation anesthetics, 61, 62
vaporizers, 58–60
vapor pressure, 54, 56–57
waste anesthetic gas evacuation systems,
    91–92
mechanism of action
  carbamazepine, 215
  gabapentin, 215
  intravenous opioid anesthetics, 182
  local anesthetics, 216
  nonsteroidal anti-inflammatory drugs,
    390–91
  phenytoin, 214
mechanomyography (MMG), 100
median, data sets, 142
mediastinum, 593–94, 594f, 595f, 601
medical errors
  action-based errors, 820
  communication-based errors, 821
  decision-based errors, 820–21
  defined, 821t
  disclosure to patients, 823–24
medical gas cylinders, 43–44, 45t, 90t
medical knowledge core competency, 824
medication-assisted opioid withdrawal
  alpha-2 adrenergic agonists, 221, 222
  buprenorphine, 221–22
  general discussion, 221
  methadone, 221, 222
  naltrexone, 221, 222
medication assisted treatment (MAT)
  opioid SUD, 186–87
  substance use disorder, 185, 244
medulla, 486–87, 565–66, 720–21
medulla oblongata, 668
medullary arteries, 502
medullary depression, 314, 315t
megaloblastic anemia, 87
melatonin, 170
MELD (model of end stage liver disease)
    score, 160
memantine, 393
membrane potential, 445–46
meninges
  anatomy, 505
  clinical features of related conditions,
    505
MEP (maximal expiratory pressure), 530
meperidine
  effect on circulation, 183
  pediatric anesthesiology, 225
  renal dysfunction and, 381
mephentermine, 691
mepivacaine, 205
MEPs (motor evoked potentials), 122,
    122t, 442, 444, 445
mercury thermometers, 474
Merkel, G., 176
mesolimbic dopamine system, 185, 186f
messenger RNA (mRNA) molecules, 794
metabolic alkalosis, 563

metabolic derangements, 741
metabolic equivalents (METs), 229–30,
    276
metabolism
  anabolic reactions, 779–80
  barbiturates, 191
  brain and, 780
  carbohydrate metabolism, 779
  cardiac muscle and, 780
  catabolic reactions, 779–80, 780f
  effect of hypercarbia on, 559
  effect of hypocarbia on, 559
  effect of hypoxia on, 561
  fasting and, 779–80, 780f
  general discussion, 779
  kidneys and, 780
  lipid metabolism, 779
  liver and, 779, 780
  postprandial states, 779–80, 780f
  propofol, 193
  protein metabolism, 779
  respiratory quotient, 780–81
  striated muscle and, 780
metabolism of drugs, 147, 163–64
  benzodiazepines, 197
  carbamazepine, 215
  dexmedetomidine, 201
  etomidate, 196
  gabapentin, 215
  intravenous opioid anesthetics, 182–83
  ketamine, 199–200
  phenytoin, 214
metacarpophalangeal (MCP) joints, 17
metaproterenol, 603
metaraminol, 691
metarterioles, 661–63
metatarsophalangeal (MTP) joints, 17
metformin, 240, 790
methadone, 187, 221, 222, 244, 393
methemoglobinemia, 218, 553
methicillinresistant Staphylococcus aureus
    (MRSA), 278–79
methionine synthase, 87
methohexital, 192, 225
methoxamine, 691
methoxyflurane, 87, 161
methylene blue, 701–2
methylprednisolone, 606–7, 607t
metoprolol, 148
METs (metabolic equivalents), 229–30,
    276
mexiletine, 400–1
Meyer loop, 481
MH. See malignant hyperthermia
MI (myocardial infarction), 391
MIAVR (minimally invasive aortic valve
    replacement), 283
microcirculation
  anatomy, 661–62
  arterial inflow, 662
  function, 662
  general discussion, 661
  regulation, 662
  shock and, 663
  venous outflow, 662
microfilters, blood, 743–44
microlaryngeal endotracheal tubes, 330
microlaryngoscopy, 333
microshocks, 136, 136t, 136f
MICS. See minimally invasive cardiac
    surgery
midazolam, 482, 591
  metabolism of, 197
  as premedication, 235–36
  preoperative anesthetic considerations,
    198

midbrain, 486
middle cerebral artery (MCA), 491, 492f
middle ear, 71
middle fossa, 22
midline epidural, 26
MIDVAB (minimally invasive direct
    coronary artery bypass surgery),
    282–83
milk thistle (silymarin), 170
Miller blades, 323, 323t, 592
milrinone, 685–86, 796–97
MIMVS (minimally invasive mitral valve
    surgeries), 283
mineralocorticoids, 607t, 773–74
minimally invasive aortic valve
    replacement (MIAVR), 283
minimally invasive cardiac surgery
    (MICS)
  anesthetic considerations, 283–84
  aortic valve replacement, 283
  atrial fibrillation ablation, 283
  direct coronary artery bypass surgery,
    282–83
  general discussion, 282
  mitral valve surgeries, 283
minimal sedation, 314–15
minimum alveolar concentration (MAC)
  alcohol SUD, 186
  amphetamine SUD, 188
  barbiturate SUD, 188
  benzodiazepines, 188, 198
  cocaine use, 187–88
  defined, 176
  dexmedetomidine, 201
  electrolytes, 701
  factors that influence, 176–77, 177t
  MAC-awake value, 176
  MAC-BAR value, 176
  marijuana SUD, 187
  monitoring, 177
  monoamine oxidase inhibitors, 213
  opioid SUD, 187
  pediatric anesthesiology, 224t
  sevoflurane, 180
  volatile anesthetics, 176t
MIP (maximal inspiratory pressure), 530
mitral valve, 4
MMG (mechanomyography), 100
MOCA 2.0 components, 817, 817t
mode, data sets, 142
model of end stage liver disease (MELD)
    score, 160
moderate sedation, 314–15
moderator band, 630
molar substitution (MS) ratio, 338
molecular weight of gas, 547
monitoring methods
  basic, 95
  blood pressure, 104–5
  capnography, 95–96
  oxygen, 104–5
  pulse oximetry, 96–97
monoamine oxidase (MAO), 212, 454,
    458, 459, 513
monoamine oxidase inhibitors (MAOIs),
    240
  anesthetic considerations, 213
  clinical implications, 212–13
  general discussion, 212
  mechanism of, 212
  overview, 256
  perioperative management of, 275
monophasic defibrillators, 133–34
monosynaptic reflexes, 439, 439t
montelukast, 608–9
mood stabilizers, 275. See also depression

blood supply, 489
  components of, 489, 490*f*, 490*t*
  general discussion, 489
reticular formation (RF), 489, 520
retinal ischemia/infarction, 350
retinopathy of prematurity (ROP), 88
reverse-Trendelenburg position, 151
reversible antagonists, 167
Revised Cardiac Risk Index (RCRI), 229, 276, 285, 408
Reynolds number, 49
RF (reticular formation), 489, 520
rhabdomyolysis, 377
rheology, 423, 664
rhinitis (coryza), 581, 582, 610
rHuEPO (recombinant human erythropoietin), 749
right atrial pressure (RAP) curve, 624, 624*t*
right coronary artery (RCA), 675
rima glottidis, 586
rima vestibuli, 586
Ring-Adair-Elwyn (RAE) tubes, 330, 331*f*
Ringer's solution, 357
rise time, pulmonary ventilation, 104
Riva-Rocci, Scipione, 106
RLNs (recurrent laryngeal nerves), 10, 508–9, 594
rocuronium, 219–20
roots, spinal cord, 444
ROP (retinopathy of prematurity), 88
ropinirole, 724
ropivacaine, 205
rostral ventromedial medulla (RVM), 489–90, 519, 520–21
rotameters. *See* flowmeters
RQ (respiratory quotient), 780–81
RSI (rapid sequence induction), 321
RV (residual volume), 526

SABAS (short-acting β₂ agonists), 603
sacral hiatus, 15
sacral nerves
  anesthetic considerations, 504
  clinical considerations, 504
  general discussion, 503
  sacral plexus, 503–4
  spinal cord anatomy, 503
sacral plexus, 503–4
sacrum, 15, 26, 503
  sacral hiatus, 15
  sciatic nerve, 15
S-adenosylmethionine (SAMe), 170
SAFE trial, 338
safety features for anesthetic monitoring
  electrical systems in operating room, 94*t*
  intraoperative, 93–95, 93*t*
  preoperative, 93, 93*t*
Saklad, Meyer, 233
salivary glands
  afferent and efferent pathways, 465
  PSNS effects on, 457*t*
salmeterol, 603–4
salpingopharyngeus muscle, 583*t*
SAMe (S-adenosylmethionine), 170
SA node. *See* sinoatrial node
sarcomere length, 632–33
saturated vapor pressure (SVP), 56
saw palmetto, 170
SBP (systolic blood pressure), 650, 651*f*
scalars, ventilator, 131*f*
  flow-time scalar, 131
  volume-time scalar, 130
scalene muscles, 596
Schimmelbusch mask (open-drop anesthesia), 81

sciatic nerve, 6, 15, 503–4, 504*t*, 504*f*
SCM (sternocleidomastoid muscle), 3*f*, 3–4, 9, 593*f*, 596
scoliosis, 499
scopolamine patch, 409
SDB (sleep disordered breathing), 573
second gas effect, 55*f*, 55, 68–69, 163, 175
  alveolar gas concentration (FA), 68–69
  concentration effect and, 69, 70*f*
  nitrous oxide and, 71
SED (smoke evacuation devices), 179
segmental arteries, 501
segmental medullary arteries, 502
segmental spinal arteries, 501–2
seizures, 414
selective norepinephrine reuptake inhibitors (SNRIs)
  anesthetic considerations, 398
  mechanism of action, 397
  side effects, 397
selective serotonin reuptake inhibitors (SSRIs)
  adrenergic agonist interactions, 399
  anesthetic considerations, 398
  bleeding and, 399
  cytochrome P450 inhibition, 399
  drug-related complications, 240
  indications for, 397
  mechanism of action, 397
  perioperative management of, 275
  post-SSRI sexual dysfunction, 397
  serotonin syndrome, 398–99
  side effects, 397
self-inflating portable ventilation devices
  components of, 83*f*
  non-rebreathing valves, 83
  overview, 83
  oxygen reservoir, 83
  ventilation bag, 83
semi-closed circle system, 79
semi-open (non-rebreathing) system, 82
sensitive oxygen ratio system (S-ORC), 51*f*, 51
sensory dermatome map, 19*f*
sentinel events, 821*t*
sepsis, 293, 613, 702, 740
septum, 581
Sequential Organ Failure Assessment (SOFA), 702–3
serologic testing, 369
serotonin, 487
serotonin-norepinephrine reuptake inhibitors (SNRIs), 255–56, 275
serotonin syndrome, 256, 363–64, 363*t*, 398–99, 414
  anesthetic considerations, 363–64
  cocaine, 615
  etiology, 363
  symptoms, 363
  treatment, 363
serratus posterior muscle, 596
sevoflurane, 85
  boiling point, 57
  compared to other volatile anesthetics, 175
  effect on cardiovascular system, 174
  effect on CFS production, 430
  effect on renal function, 174
  neuromonitoring and, 124
  pediatric anesthesiology, 224
  pharmacologic properties of, 180, 180*t*
  reaction scheme for in presence of base, 87*f*
  saturated vapor pressure, 56
  toxicity risk, 87

vapor concentration, 56
  variable-bypass vaporizer, 58
sex
  defined, 449
  sex differences in pain and pain perception, 449
sex hormones, 621
SGA (supraglottic airway), 320–21
shared decision-making
  general discussion, 822
  importance of, 822
  tips for, 822–23
shivering, 302, 361
shock
  defined, 663
  pre- and post-capillary sphincter control, 663
  stages of, 663
short-acting beta-2 agonists (SABAS), 603
shoulders, 16
shunt measurement formula, 602
SIADH (syndrome of inappropriate antidiuretic hormone secretion), 765–66
sickle cell disease, 795
side stream capnography, 96
sigmoid sinus, 492, 493*f*
signal transduction, 517–18
sign test, 142
silymarin (milk thistle), 170
SIMV (synchronized intermittent mandatory ventilation), 103, 132
single-lumen endotracheal tubes, 327
single lung ventilation (SLV), 602
single twitch stimulation, 98–99
sinoatrial (SA) node, 620, 626*f*
  action potentials, 628
  as anatomical pacemaker of heart, 625
  conduction regulation, 681
  excitation-contraction coupling, 625
  general discussion, 680
  heart rate, 621
  myocardial contractility, 634
  stimulation from, 625–26
sinusoidal capillaries, 644
skeletal muscle contraction, 446–47
skull anatomy
  base of the skull, 22*f*
  embryology, 24
  fontanelles, 24
  general discussion, 20
  imaging studies, 7
  neurological anatomy, 24
  osseous anatomy, 20–22, 21*f*
  sutures, 24
  vascular anatomy of, 23
sleep disordered breathing (SDB), 573
slowed breathing exercises, 401
SLUDGE/BBB mnemonic device, 365, 366*b*
SLV (single lung ventilation), 602
small saphenous vein, 34
smart pumps, 138*t*
smoke evacuation devices (SED), 179
smoking
  anesthetic considerations, 572–73
  e-cigarettes, 572
  nicotine replacement therapy, 571–72
  perioperative smoking and, 571–73
SNARE (soluble-N-ethylmaleimide-sensitive attachment protein receptors) proteins, 805–6
SNP. *See* sodium nitroprusside
SNRIs (serotonin-norepinephrine reuptake inhibitors), 255–56, 275.
  *See also* selective norepinephrine reuptake inhibitors

SNS. *See* sympathetic nervous system
sNSAIDs (COX-2 selective NSAIDs), 390
soda lime, 84–85
sodium, 699–700
sodium bicarbonate
  alkalinization concentrations, 205
  bicarbonate buffer system, 204–5
  epidural adjuvants and, 152
  epidural anesthesia and, 205
  general discussion, 204
  pain management, 205
  peripheral nerve block and, 205
sodium-channel blockers, 400–1, 687–88, 688*t*
sodium cromoglycate (cromolyn), 609–10
sodium nitroprusside (SNP)
  anesthetic considerations, 207
  clinical applications, 207
  general discussion, 207
  pharmacodynamics, 207
  pharmacokinetics, 207
  side effects, 207
sodium-potassium pump, 445–46
SOFA (Sequential Organ Failure Assessment), 702–3
solubility coefficients, gases, 54
soluble-N-ethylmaleimide-sensitive attachment protein receptors (SNARE) proteins, 805–6
soma, 446
somatic afferents, 519, 520*f*
somatic pain, 519, 520*f*
somatosensory cortex, 514–15
somatosensory evoked potentials (SSEPs), 122, 122*t*, 442, 444, 445
somatostatin, 517
S-ORC (sensitive oxygen ratio system), 51*f*, 51
soy isoflavones (Glycine max), 170
SP (substance P), 402
spatial resolution, ultrasound, 47*f*, 47
spectrophotometry, 96
sphenoparietal sinus, 492
sphygmomanometers, 648
spinal accessory nerve, 593*f*
spinal accessory nerve (CN XI), 507*f*, 508
spinal adjuvants, 151–52
spinal anatomy, 25*f*
  anatomical landmarks, 27*f*
  anesthetic considerations, 26
  basic structure, 25
  cervical spine, 26
  coccyx, 26
  dural sac, 26
  epidural space, 26
  lumbar spine, 15, 26
  overview, 25
  sacrum, 26
  spinal ligaments, 27*f*
  subarachnoid space, 26
  subdural space, 26
  thoracic spine, 26
spinal anesthesia
  additives to, 308*t*
  backache, 302
  block height, 190
  cardiac complications, 302
  cardiovascular complications, 301
  cesarean sections, 307–8
  complications, 190
  contraindications for, 299
  duration of action, 190
  duration of blockade, 301
  gastrointestinal complications, 302
  general discussion, 151